Essential Oil Safety

Biography

Robert Tisserand

Robert is internationally recognized for his pioneering work in many aspects of aromatherapy. He started practicing as a therapist in 1969, founded a company to market aromatherapy products in 1974, and wrote the first book in English on the subject in 1977: *The Art of Aromatherapy*. Robert has written two further books including this one, co-founded several aromatherapy organizations, and has taught and lectured extensively. For 12 years, Robert was the principal of the Tisserand Institute in London, and during the same period he published and edited the International Journal of Aromatherapy. Today Robert lives in California and his activities include writing, online education, live events, and working as an independent industry expert. Robert is one of only two recipients of the Alliance of International Aromatherapists Lifetime Achievement Award. Follow his blog at www.roberttisserand.com/blog

Rodney Young

Originally trained as a chemist, Rodney obtained a BSc from the University of London in 1965 and a PhD in medicinal chemistry from the University of Essex in 1968. He worked for many years in the pharmaceutical industry as a research chemist, focusing on modulators of histamine, serotonin and inositol phosphates. Rodney has published widely in the field of scientific literature, and has taught at University College, London, Oxford Brookes University, Edinburgh Napier University, and the University of East London. He has a longstanding interest in the pharmacological and medicinal properties of plant natural products and in promoting evidence-based botanical medicine, and serves on the editorial boards of the Journal of Herbal Medicine and the Journal of Alternative and Complementary Medicine.

Content Strategist: *Claire Wilson/Kellie White*
Content Development Specialist: *Carole McMurray*
Project Manager: *Sukanthi Sukumar*
Designer: *Christian Bilbow*
Illustration Manager: *Jennifer Rose*
Illustrator: *Antbits Ltd*

Essential Oil Safety

A Guide for Health Care Professionals

SECOND EDITION

Robert Tisserand
Expert in Aromatherapy and Essential Oil Research
Ojai, CA, USA

Rodney Young PhD
Lecturer in Plant Chemistry and Pharmacology
University of East London, London, UK

Foreword by

Elizabeth M Williamson
Professor of Pharmacy and Director of Pharmacy Practice, University of Reading, UK;
Editor, Phytotherapy Research;
Chair, Herbal and Complementary Medicines Expert Advisory Group, British Pharmacopoeia Commission,
Medicines and Healthcare Regulatory Agency, Department of Health, UK

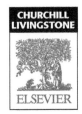

Edinburgh London New York Oxford Philadelphia St Louis Sydney Toronto 2014

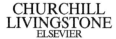

CHURCHILL
LIVINGSTONE
ELSEVIER

First edition 2002
Second edition 2014

ISBN 978-0-443-06241-4

British Library Cataloguing in Publication Data
A catalogue record for this book is available from the British Library

Library of Congress Cataloging in Publication Data
A catalog record for this book is available from the Library of Congress

Notices
Knowledge and best practice in this field are constantly changing. As new research and experience broaden our understanding, changes in research methods, professional practices, or medical treatment may become necessary.

Practitioners and researchers must always rely on their own experience and knowledge in evaluating and using any information, methods, compounds, or experiments described herein. In using such information or methods they should be mindful of their own safety and the safety of others, including parties for whom they have a professional responsibility.

With respect to any essential oils or products identified, readers are advised to check the most current information provided (i) on procedures featured or (ii) by the supplier or manufacturer of each essential oil or product to be administered, to verify the safest and most effective strategy for administration, including any contraindications. It is the responsibility of practitioners, relying on their own experience and knowledge of their patients, to make diagnoses, to determine the best treatment for each individual patient, and to take all appropriate safety precautions.

To the fullest extent of the law, neither the Publisher nor the authors, contributors, or editors, assume any liability for any injury and/or damage to persons or property as a matter of products liability, negligence or otherwise, or from any use or operation of any methods, products, instructions, or ideas contained in the material herein.

 ELSEVIER your source for books, journals and multimedia in the health sciences

www.elsevierhealth.com

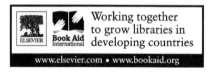 Working together to grow libraries in developing countries

www.elsevier.com • www.bookaid.org

The Publisher's policy is to use paper manufactured from sustainable forests

Printed in Great Britain
Last digit is the print number: 20 19 18 17 16 15

Contents

I warmly welcome the second edition of this book, expanded and updated, since the first edition has always been the first reference I go to for reliable information on the safety and composition of essential oils.

About 300 essential oils are commonly traded on the world market, which was estimated to be worth over $1000 million in 2013. They are very widely used in the cosmetics, pharmaceutical, food and household goods industries. About 20% of essential oils are consumed by the flavor industry for use in food products, about 20% by the pharmaceutical industry, and the rest by the fragrance industry, in cleaning products, hair and skin care, as well as in aromatherapy. So their safety is of huge importance to everyone, and although the information given in this book is highly relevant to aromatherapists, it is also an essential reference source for anyone dealing with essential oils, in any capacity.

There is no question that essential oils have pharmacological activity, and there is an extensive body of literature on this topic. In this book, the authors have critically appraised evidence from a variety of sources, both reliable and unreliable.

The effects of aromatherapy massage depend to a large extent on penetration through the skin, so general safety concerns are similar to those for essential oils even when ingested orally or inhaled. As befits a book about safety, toxicity in its many forms – including skin sensitization, genotoxicity, neurotoxicity and reproductive toxicity – is dealt with early in the book, very comprehensively, and in an impartial manner. It is as important to debunk myths about toxicity as it is to highlight it, because essential oils are used so widely and must be used with confidence.

Parts of the book are highly technical, which is necessary to make the points that must be made, and it is very well referenced. This ensures that the book also has the widest usage possible in the cosmetics and pharmaceutical industries, and that it is credible to the harshest of critics. It will help all healthcare practitioners, whether or not they eventually decide to recommend aromatherapy to their patients, and of course to aromatherapists, who will have confidence in their practice.

Elizabeth M Williamson

The authors gratefully acknowledge the considerable help of the following people in giving valuable information and advice.

For supplying or helping to source information on essential oil composition

Mohammad Abdollahi, Tehran University of Medical Sciences.

Julien Abisset, Greco, Grasse, France.

Jean-François Baudoux, Pranarom International, Ghislenghien, Belgium.

Olivier Behra, Antananarivo, Madagascar.

Tony Burfield http://www.users.globalnet.co.uk.

Chris Condon, Natural Extracts of Australia, Los Angeles, California, USA.

Charles Cornwell, Australian Botanical Products, Hallam, Victoria, Australia.

Ermias Dagne, Addis Ababa University, Addis Ababa, Ethiopia.

John Day, The Paperbark Company, Harvey, W.A., Australia.

Hussein Fakhry, A. Fakhry & Co., Cairo, Egypt.

Earle Graven, Grassroots Natural Products, Gouda, South Africa.

Jasbir Chana and Keith Harkiss, Phoenix Natural Products, Southall, Middlesex, UK.

Larry Jones, Spectrix, Santa Cruz, California, USA.

Daniel Joulain, Robertet, Paris, France.

Bill McGilvray, Plant Extracts International, Hopkins, Minnesota, USA.

Lucie Mainguy, Aliksir, Grondines, Quebec, Canada.

Butch Owen, Appalachian Valley Natural Products, Friendsville, Maryland, USA.

Rob Pappas, Essential Oil University Database.

Gilles Rondeau, Solarome, Mont Carmel, Quebec, Canada.

Gurpreet Singh, Guroo Farms, Rudrapur, India.

Olivier Sonnay, Olison, Switzerland.

Jessica Teubes (Jessica Lutge), Scatters, Randburg, South Africa.

Art Tucker, Dept. of Agriculture & Natural Resources, Delaware State University, Dover, DE, USA.

Elisabeth Vossen, Vossen & Co., Brussels, Belgium.

Naiyin Wang, Sinae Trading Company, Orpington, Kent, UK.

For other assistance

Anne Marie Api, RIFM, Hackensack, New Jersey, for information about melissa and lavender cotton oils.

Salaam Attar, Isabelle Aurel, Julia Glazer, Cathy Miller, Judith Miller, Elise Pearlstine and Stephanie Vinson for information about asthmatics reacting to essential oils.

Janetta Bensouilah, for comments on Chapter 5.

Jennie Harding, Rhiannon Harris and Danielle Sade, for help with the amount of oil used in massage.

Gabriele Lashly for German-English translation.

Bill McGilvray for safety information about blue cypress oil.

Deborah Rose for critiquing chapters for readability

Janina Sørensen, for Danish-English translation.

Art Tucker, for assistance with botanical nomenclature.

Joanna Wang, for Chinese-English translation.

The many books now available on the practice of aromatherapy usually touch on the possible adverse effects of certain essential oils, while naturally concentrating on their therapeutic properties. However, there is no text written with aromatherapy in mind which is concerned specifically and in detail with essential oil toxicology. This book is designed to fill that gap.

The fragrance and flavour industries already have their own guidelines for controlling essential oil safety. These, however, are not necessarily appropriate for aromatherapy.

At the time of writing there appear to be no regulations governing the sale or use of essential oils in aromatherapy that effectively protect the consumer. The increasing availability of undiluted essential oils, some of which undoubtedly present a potential hazard, is cause for concern. In the UK and the USA at least, it is currently possible to purchase, by mail order, the majority of the essential oils which we recommend should not be available to the general public.

We suspect that in many countries, there may be too few controls on the minority of essential oils which do present a hazard. We believe that the most responsible course of action for those, such as ourselves, who have information about known, or suspected toxicity, is to make it public. Both those who sell, and those who use essential oils, will then be in a better position to take informed decisions about which oils are safe to use, and in which circumstances.

We are not simply talking about banning or restricting certain essential oils. There is also a need to improve labelling, giving warnings where appropriate, and to make packaging safer, especially with regard to young children. There is a need for a greater awareness of the potential dangers among those who package, sell and use essential oils.

In recent years there have been many 'scare stories' in the media about the dangers of essential oils. Some of these have been quite accurate, but often the information given is misleading and based more on rumour than fact. We believe that it is vital for the aromatherapy community to address safety issues, and to take responsible action, in order to safeguard its future.

We are aware that a book such as this could have the effect of presenting essential oils as generally dangerous substances – this is certainly not our intention. On the contrary, there are several instances where we have shown that supposed dangers do not in fact exist. The majority of essential oils turn out to be non-hazardous as they are used in aromatherapy. The function of this book is to reassure, when appropriate, as well as to hoist some red flags.

The same intention to inform is behind our inclusion of physiology and biochemistry. We explain how different forms of toxicity arise and why the use of certain oils is sometimes inadvisable. We believe that this is much more useful than simply presenting summaries of 'safe' or 'dangerous' oils.

There are two approaches one can take when dealing with issues of safety. The first is to assume that the materials in question are hazardous until proven to be safe. This is the approach taken when dealing with pharmaceutical drugs. The second approach is to assume that substances are safe unless proven hazardous. This line is taken in the food and fragrance industries.

In general, we have taken the approach that essential oils are safe unless proven hazardous. It seems unnecessary to treat essential oils as pharmaceuticals, especially if they are only used externally. There are cases where we have flagged an essential oil as hazardous even though absolute proof may not be available. In practice one must steer a middle course, and use all the information available, both positive and negative.

In the context of these dilemmas we have attempted to give a balanced view. We acknowledge both that animal toxicity may be relevant to the human situation, and that experimental doses almost always greatly exceed those given therapeutically. We have given detailed information concerning the relevance or otherwise of specific animal tests to humans. Toxicologists increasingly acknowledge that giving excessive doses of a substance to a genetically in-bred mouse living in a laboratory may not have great relevance to the human situation.

Our hope is that this book constitutes a practical, positive basis for guidelines, both in the essential oil retail trade and the aromatherapy profession. While it is primarily written for the aromatherapy market, it will be of interest to all those who use essential oils, whether in fragrances, flavourings, toiletries or pharmaceuticals. Pharmacists, doctors, nurses and poisons units may find it a particularly useful summary.

This book replaces The Essential Oil Safety Data Manual by Robert Tisserand, first published in 1985. This text was largely an extrapolation of toxicological reports from the Research Institute for Fragrance Materials (RIFM). The RIFM data still form a very important part of the current volume which, however, contains more detail about a greater number of hazardous oils than its predecessor, and a great deal more toxicological and pharmacological information.

The aim of the book remains the same: to provide information for the benefit of all who are interested in the therapeutic use of essential oils, so that aromatherapy may be practised, and products may be developed, with the minimum of risk. This can only be accomplished if all those involved, in both the aromatherapy profession and the trade, are thoroughly familiar with the hazards which do exist, and which, in a few cases, are rather serious.

Robert Tisserand
Tony Balacs
Sussex, 1995

This revised edition took 12 years to complete, and is considerably longer than the previous edition. There are three reasons for the comprehensive revision. First, since the text was first published in 1995, there have been many notable developments in the area of essential oil safety. In addition to new data being published, many guidelines and restrictions have been revised or issued by various authorities, and we have introduced some of our own.

Second, significant changes and improvements have been made to the text, especially in the area of profiles, some of these in response to reader feedback. The structure of both the Essential Oil Profiles and the Constituent Profiles has been considerably elaborated, and new material has been added. This edition includes 400 Essential Oil Profiles, compared to 95 previously.

For each essential oil there is a full breakdown of constituents, and a clear categorization of hazards and risks, with recommended maximum doses and concentrations. All the compositional data for essential oils has been revised, expanded and referenced. There are 206 Constituent Profiles, and this section is 15 times that of the previous edition. Constituents are cross-referenced: each Constituent Profile lists the amount of that substance found in each of the 400 profiled essential oils.

Third, the structure of the book has been developed. There are now separate chapters on the nervous, urinary, cardiovascular, gastrointestinal, and respiratory systems. Some sections of text have moved from one chapter to another, and repetitive or outdated material has been deleted. We now have detailed safety advice on drug interactions, and overall there are more cautions. The new material is reflected in over 3,400 new references. A number of minor changes have also been made, such as the styling of references and the categorization of constituents.

The book's premise is that understanding safety is not primarily about knowing legal or institutional guidelines, but about understanding the biological action of essential oils and their constituents. There is a critique of current regulations, including some of the IFRA guidelines, and the EU 'allergens legislation'. There is considerable discussion of carcinogens, the human relevance of some of the animal data, the validity of treating an essential oil as if it was a single chemical (for example, discussing rose oil as if it contained nothing but methyleugenol) and the arbitrary nature of uncertainty factors. For carcinogens, we have given IFRA guidelines, EU guidelines and also our own guidelines for impacted essential oils.

Finally, when Tony Balacs and myself were in early stages of the revision, Tony decided that he could no longer commit the necessary time to the project and bowed out. An intensive search for a replacement co-author lead me to Rodney Young, who has honed considerably much of the pharmacology and chemistry, and has contributed massively to this extensive revision.

Robert Tisserand
Ojai, California
October 2012

Introduction

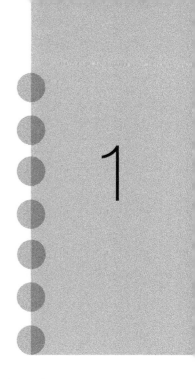

This book provides a framework of reference for those interested in the safe and effective use of essential oils in a cosmetic or therapeutic context. The information and guidelines contained herein are intended to help minimize any risk of harm associated with the use of these oils, while optimizing their beneficial effects. We have made rational assessments of risk by critically evaluating and extrapolating from available information relating to both the effects of essential oils and of their individual constituents, from in vivo and in vitro human and animal studies. We have read many excellent reports, as well as some seriously misguided ones.

A considerable amount of information about essential oils can be found in the printed literature, as well as on the internet. Much of the safety information available online is misleading, confusing, wrong or simply absent. Some websites promote potentially dangerous essential oils with no mention of possible dangers, though others make every effort to be safe. Misinformation is not difficult to find, even in the scientific literature. In one 'systematic review' of adverse reactions to essential oils, four of the reports cited pertain to fatty oils, not essential oils (Posadzki et al 2012). These are black seed, mustard, neem and tamanu. In the first two cases they are mistakenly referred to as essential oils even in the original research.

The quality of essential oils is an important issue for anyone using them therapeutically. Confidence in their safe use begins with ensuring that the oils have a known botanical origin and composition. In a case of purported tea tree oil allergy that was reported twice, analysis of the allergenic substance showed that it was not in fact tea tree oil (De Groot & Weyland 1992; Van der Valk et al 1994). With the advent of modern analytical techniques, the constituents of an essential oil can be determined with a high degree of accuracy. Despite these advances, many biological studies have been reported using essential oils whose composition has not been clearly stated or even determined. In several publications where essential oil constituents have been studied, low purity is a concern. This can lead to erroneous conclusions being made about the pure constituent. In other cases, the identity of constituents is ambiguous or unknown. This is especially true of compounds that exist as different isomers. Sometimes, mixtures of isomers have been used (e.g., α- + β-thujone), or the nomenclature employed has not been sufficiently specific to identify a single compound (e.g., farnesol, which exists as four different isomers). Such studies are of limited value as reproducibility cannot be guaranteed.

In some studies, observations were made only after administering extremely high doses. Consequently, an impression is created of greater risk than can be reasonably justified. In a carcinogenesis study of β-myrcene (which was only 90% pure), groups of rats and mice were given the equivalent of a human oral dose of 17.5 g, 35 g, or 70 g, every day for two years (National Toxicology Program 2010b). The authors justified the high doses on the basis that β-myrcene was not considered to be very toxic. Many animals died before the end of the study, the findings of which have no relevance to the use of essential oils containing β-myrcene.

Concerns about quality and purity apply to many studies of dermal adverse reactions, the results of which are often extrapolated and interpreted to an extent not justified by the poor standards of the research. The fact that the results of patch testing depend to a significant extent on the brand of patch used is a fundamental concern for the validity of this technique (Suneja and Belsito 2001; Mortz & Andersen 2010). There are also uncertainties about the vehicle used, the dispersion of test substance, and general reproducibility (Chiang & Maibach 2012). Patch testing may be useful for identifying the relative risk of different substances, but it cannot be used as a measure of allergy prevalence.

We are sceptical about the use of local lymph node testing in animals, and in vitro data showing constituent oxidation, as justifications for declaring a substance to be allergenic. Oxidation of certain constituents can and does take place, and it is a concern. However oxidation is a slow process, it does not always

http://dx.doi.org/10.1016/B978-0-443-06241-4.00001-1

increase the risk of skin reactivity, and in commercial products it is easily circumvented by the use of antioxidants, sometimes in combination with use-by or sell-by dates.

The term 'aromatherapy' was first coined by René-Maurice Gattefossé (1936). It can be defined as the use of essential oils, applied topically, orally, by inhalation or other means, to promote health, hygiene and psychological wellbeing. Aromatherapy is not a single discipline, but can include almost any application of essential oils to the human body. This would include natural perfumes (mixtures of essential oils, absolutes, etc.) and personal care products that contain them. The fact that essential oils have multiple end uses complicates the safety issue. While cosmetics are expected to encompass virtually zero risk, risk is acceptable in medicine because of potential benefits. There is also a 'middle ground', i.e., cosmeceuticals and hygiene products. For example, a small risk of skin reaction might be acceptable if the potential benefit is the prevention of MRSA (methicillin-resistant *Staphylococcus aureus*) infection. Proving safety is always a challenge, but especially when almost all the funding for research goes to single chemicals, and not to plant-derived products.

Aromatic plants have been used in traditional medicine for thousands of years in numerous forms, from the freshly harvested raw plant and its natural secretions to extracts and distillation products. Herbal preparations are administered by different routes according to the site of disease, most commonly orally, but also topically or by inhalation. A traditional and still popular oral preparation is the hot water infusion, or tea, and includes such plants as chamomile, lemon balm and lime. Topical application includes massage, which takes advantage of transdermal as well as pulmonary absorption, thereby giving oil constituents access to the systemic circulation, and thence to all parts of the body.

In parallel with popular aromatherapy, the application of essential oils is growing in food preservation, in farm animal health, and in agriculture, where many are classified as minimal-risk pesticides. In each case essential oils are replacing chemicals that are more toxic, or to which bacteria or pests have developed resistance. Antibiotic-resistant infectious disease is an area currently attracting significant research interest. Experimental evidence has shown a remarkable potential for essential oils, not only because they can kill resistant bacteria, but also because they can reverse resistance to conventional antibiotics.

The pharmaco-therapeutic potential of essential oils has been reviewed by Edris (2007) and by Bakkali et al (2008). In addition to infectious disease, potential applications include type 2 diabetes, cardiovascular disease, osteoporosis, and the prevention and treatment of cancer. Clinical successes include the treatment of liver cancer with *Curcuma aromatica* oil (Chen CY et al 2003), irritable bowel disease with peppermint oil (Grigoleit & Grigoleit 2005a), tinea pedis with tea tree oil (Satchell et al 2002a) and anxiety with lavender oil (Kasper et al 2010; Woelk & Schläfke 2010). Common uses of essential oils or their constituents in consumer health products include mouthwashes such as Listerine, liniments such as Tiger Balm, and products for the relief of respiratory symptoms, such as Vicks Vaporub.

We all consume essential oils when we eat food. Pecans, almonds, olives, figs, tomatoes, carrots, cabbages, mangoes, peaches, butter, coffee, cinnamon and peppermint naturally contain essential oils. Fresh aromatic plants typically contain 1–2% by weight of mainly fragrant monoterpenoid volatile compounds. When isolated by distillation as essential oils, the increased concentration of these constituents means that any biological properties are much more evident. Some of these properties may offer therapeutic benefits, but some may manifest as toxicity.

A toxic reaction is any adverse event that occurs following the contact of an external agent with the body. Toxicity in essential oils is an attribute we welcome when we want them to kill viruses, bacteria, fungi or lice, and human cells share some characteristics with these very small organisms. So it should not be totally surprising that some of the most useful antimicrobial essential oils, such as eucalyptus, garlic and savory, possess a degree of human toxicity. Toxicity can manifest in numerous ways. Depending upon the extent of damage and regenerative capacity, individual cells may die due to disruption of normal metabolic processes and inability to maintain cellular homeostasis, or whole organs may fail. Fortunately, most organs have substantial reserve capacity, and can recover.

Adverse reactions include abortion or abnormalities in pregnancy, neurotoxicity manifesting as seizures or retardation of infant development, a variety of skin reactions, bronchial hyperreactivity, hepatotoxicity and more. Interactions with chemotherapeutic or other prescribed drugs are a particular concern. In Chapter 4 and Appendix B we present the first summary of likely risk based on current information. A significant interaction between an essential oil and a drug will only become apparent when a certain dose (of essential oil) is administered. Regrettably, even in the academic literature, this factor is sometimes not properly considered.

Most accidents with essential oils involve young children, and are preventable. In the quantities in which they are most commonly sold (5–15 mL), essential oils can be highly toxic or lethal if drunk by a young child, and there have been a number of recorded fatal cases over the past 70 years. Perhaps the only reason that child fatalities have not increased with the current popularity of aromatherapy is because today most essential oils are sold in bottles with integral drop-dispensers. These make it more difficult for a toddler to drink large amounts. Most urgently, we would like to see 'open-topped' bottles (i.e., without drop-dispensers) of undiluted essential oil banned, and appropriate warnings printed on labels.

It is estimated that, in 1994, between 76,000 and 137,000 (a mean of 106,000) hospitalized patients in the USA had fatal adverse drug reactions (ADRs). Even taking the lower estimate of 76,000, fatal ADRs would rank sixth after heart disease (743,460), cancer (529,904), stroke (150,108), pulmonary disease (101,077), and accidents (90,523), and ahead of pneumonia (75,719) and diabetes (53,894). If we take the mean value of 106,000 fatalities from ADRs, this would mean that prescribed drugs had become the fourth leading cause of death in the USA, after heart disease, cancer and stroke. The overall incidence of fatal ADRs was 0.32% (0.23–0.41) and the overall incidence of non-fatal but serious ADRs was 6.7% (5.2–8.2) (Lazarou et al 1998). In the UK, over the years 1996–2000, the total percentage of reported ADRs ranged from 12% to 15% of all 'hospital episodes'. Fatal ADRs were estimated to be 0.35% of hospital admissions (Waller et al 2005). There has not been a single reported case of poisoning, fatal or non-fatal, from the oral administration of essential oils by a practitioner.

Comparing the safety of conventional medicine to medicinal aromatherapy, the ratio of 106,000 to zero is remarkable, although it must be said that the great majority of users do not ingest the oils. In reviewing the risks presented by essential oils, available evidence suggests that only a relatively small number are hazardous, and many of these, such as mustard and calamus, are not widely used in therapy. However, some commonly used oils do present particular hazards, such as lemongrass (teratogenicity), bergamot (phototoxicity) and ylang-ylang (skin sensitization). By limiting the doses and concentrations they are used in, we can prevent these hazards from presenting significant risk.

It seems to be widely believed that essential oils have not undergone any safety testing at all. It is not unusual to find statements such as 'The safety of essential oils for human consumption has not undergone the rigorous scientific testing typical of regulated drugs, especially in vulnerable populations such as children or pregnant women' (Woolf 1999). The assumption here that licensed drugs are extensively tested on children and pregnant women is extremely puzzling, but the idea that essential oils are not rigorously tested seems to be mostly due to ignorance. The information in this text is evidence of a considerable body of toxicology data, both on essential oils and their constituents.

We live in a world replete with toxic substances, yet 'hazard' should not be confused with 'risk'. The presence of a toxic substance (hazard) is only problematic if exposure is sufficiently great (risk). Context is often important too. Roasted coffee contains furan and benzo[a]pyrene, two known carcinogens, acrylamide, a probable carcinogen, in addition to glyoxal, methylglyoxal, diacetyl and hydrogen peroxide, all mutagens. Yet coffee is not considered carcinogenic. Almost all edible fruits contain acetaldehyde, a probable human carcinogen. But bananas and blueberries are not regarded as carcinogenic because the amounts of acetaldehyde are extremely small, and because there are large quantities of antioxidants, antimutagens and anticarcinogens also present in the fruits. It is a similar story with coffee.

Basil herb contains two rodent carcinogens – estragole and methyleugenol. Pesto is a particularly concentrated form of basil, yet the WHO has determined that the amounts of the two carcinogens in basil/pesto are so small that they present no risk to humans. Since that ruling, research has been published demonstrating that basil herb contains anticarcinogenic substances that counter the potential toxicity of the two carcinogens, and is itself anticarcinogenic (Jeurissen et al 2008; Alhusainy et al 2010). Some basil essential oils have been also shown to have anticarcinogenic effects (Aruna & Sivaramakrishnan 1996; Manosroi et al 2005).

Many essential oils, herb extracts and foods contain tiny amounts of single constituents that alone, and in substantial amounts, are toxic, but the parent natural substance is not toxic.

However, this scenario is rarely taken into consideration by the cosmetic regulatory bodies responsible for essential oils.

The most common type of dermal adverse reaction to an essential oil is allergic contact dermatitis, which has been reported for cinnamon bark, laurel leaf and tea tree, for example. There is some evidence that occupational exposure to essential oils is hazardous and can cause hand dermatitis. Adverse skin reactions are less emotive issues than poisoning, but they are much more common. The fact that essential oils are usually used in diluted form is not an absolute safeguard because allergic reactions are possible after repeated contact even with small amounts of allergen.

However, the flagging of essential oils or their constituents as allergens is reaching epidemic proportions. Most fragrant substances, under a sufficiently rigorous testing regime, will prove to have some degree of reactivity. If one reaction per 1,250 dermatitis patients patch tested (equivalent to perhaps 1 in 10,000 people using a product containing the same substance) is sufficient justification for labeling limonene as an 'allergen' (see Table 5.9) then all essential oils might qualify as allergens. However, regulating them beyond use is unreasonable, irrational and unnecessary. Safety and safety regulations are not always in harmony, in fact they often bear little resemblance. Therefore, the purpose of this text is to inform the reader about the safe use of essential oils, as distinct from simply informing the reader about legal requirements.

In this context, and in an attempt to balance the (in our opinion) dichotomy of sometimes over-regulated and sometimes under-regulated essential oils, many of the safety guidelines in this book are those of its authors. Inevitably, the translation of factual information into recommendations involves subjective judgment. We acknowledge that other interpretations are possible, particularly in the light of new information.

In recommending safe levels of exposure, we have drawn on both experimental animal data and cases of toxicity in humans. Our approach has been to critically review existing quantitative guidelines, to refine them where necessary, and to establish new guidelines where none already exist. To these ends, we have considered a wide range of published data relating to the toxicity of essential oils, and in some cases we have extrapolated from individual constituent data, even though this involves making certain assumptions. Where safe levels for dermal or oral use have been established previously we have tended to follow them, but we have not done so in every instance.

Where there are no established recommendations, we have assumed that oils are safe when diluted for dermal use except where experimental data show a potential risk, which we believe has not yet been appreciated. In some cases we have recommended that the oils should not be taken orally, but are safe to use topically. This is due to the higher dose levels of oral administration. In other cases we have indicated that specific essential oils should be avoided in certain vulnerable conditions, such as pregnancy, or that they should be used with special caution. For an easy reference list of contraindications, we draw the reader's attention to Appendix A.

Essential oil composition

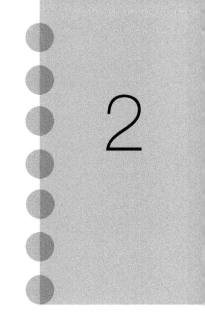

2

Essential oils

Plants are capable of synthesizing two kinds of oils: fixed oils and essential oils. Fixed oils consist of esters of glycerol and fatty acids (triglycerides or triacylglycerols), while essential oils are mixtures of volatile, organic compounds originating from a single botanical source, and contribute to the flavor and fragrance of a plant. Many of the single constituents found in essential oils are used by insects for communication, and are known as 'insect pheromones'. Though much more complex in plants, they fulfill a similar function—communication—generally as attractants to insects, occasionally as messages to other plants of the same genus. All these functions require volatility, and essential oils are also known as volatile oils. The word 'essential' is used to reflect the intrinsic nature or essence of the plant, and 'oil' is used to indicate a liquid that is insoluble in, and immiscible with, water. Oils are more soluble in lipophilic (non-polar, lipid-like) solvents such as chloroform or benzene.

Aromatic plants and infusions prepared from them have been employed in medicines and cosmetics for many thousands of years, but the use of distilled oils dates back only to the 10th century, when distillation as we know it today was developed (Forbes 1970). Solvent-extracted materials such as absolutes, resinoids and CO_2 extracts are much more recent inventions. Plants that produce essential oils belong to many different botanical species and are found throughout the globe. It is estimated that there are 350,000 plant species globally, and that 5% of these (17,500 species) are aromatic (Lawrence 1995g, pp. 187–188). Of these, more than 400 are commercially processed for their aromatic raw materials, about 50% being cultivated, and the rest being obtained either as by-products of a

The major essential oil-bearing plant families
Apiaceae (Umbelliferae)
Asteraceae (Compositae)
Cupressaceae
Lamiaceae (Labiatae)
Lauraceae
Myrtaceae
Pinaceae
Poaceae
Rutaceae
Zingiberaceae

primary industry or harvested in the wild. The principal ten essential oil-bearing plant families are listed in Box 2.1.

Being complex mixtures of chemical substances, every biological effect displayed by an essential oil is due to the actions of one or more of its constituents. In most cases the major contributor to a given toxic effect in an essential oil is identifiable. For example, we can state with confidence that the toxicity of wormwood oil is primarily due to its high content of thujone.

Isolation

The principal historical method for isolating essential oils was hydrodistillation, in which the plant material is boiled in water. A modern variation of this, in which steam is passed through the plant material, is now preferred for most essential oils. The use of water or steam subjects plant constituents to lower temperatures than would be needed for simple distillation, and is preferred because it carries a lower risk of decomposition. (Simple heating – 'dry distillation' – was used occasionally by early Persian distillers.) During steam distillation, volatile plant constituents are vaporized and then condensed on cooling to produce an immiscible mixture of an oil phase and an aqueous phase. The oil product is a complex mixture of mainly odoriferous, sometimes colored and frequently biologically active compounds—an essential oil. The aqueous layer is known as a hydrosol, aromatic water or hydrolat, and also contains odoriferous compounds but in much lower concentrations and in different ratios to the essential oil.

Most of the 2-phenylethanol in roses, for example, passes into the water phase during distillation since it is largely water-soluble, though a small amount is found in rose oil (rose otto). Rose is one of several essential oils produced by hydrodistillation—the roses are boiled, rather than being steamed. A very small number of essential oils are produced by dry distillation—no water is used (also known as destructive or empyreumatic distillation). This effectively burns the material, producing quite a different oil than if steam distillation or hydrodistillation had been used. Examples include cade and birch tar.

For a plant constituent to volatilize and undergo steam distillation, it must exert a significant vapor pressure at 100°C. Thus, liquids less volatile than water, as well as some solid compounds, may co-distil with water. Notable examples of such solids are furanocoumarin derivatives including psoralen and bergamottin. When these occur in essential oils in significant amounts, they are listed as 'non-volatile compounds' in the Essential Oil Profiles. Volatility is inversely proportional to molecular size, and while small molecules such as citronellol can be readily distilled, larger molecules mostly remain behind as a residue, such as a resin.

Ideally, the essential oil should be distilled from a single species, the whole of the essential oil should be recovered and none of its constituents should be removed intentionally during extraction, nor should any other substance be added. Not all essential oils, however, stand up to this definition, e.g., camphor oil which is fractionated, ylang-ylang oil (unless 'complete') and cornmint which is 'dementholized'. An essential oil, especially when distilled, is not necessarily identical in chemical composition with the oil that is present in the living plant. Quite often very high-boiling or low-boiling chemicals are simply 'lost' due to the nature of the distillation process, and due to economic and time constraints.

Although most constituents remain intact during distillation, a few undergo chemical changes. Chamazulene, for example, is not a natural product, but is formed by decomposition of its precursor, matricin, during steam distillation of blue chamomile oil. Garlic oil also contains substances that are formed from reactive precursors on distillation (Lawson et al 1992). Esters, such as linalyl acetate, may partially hydrolyze to alcohols during distillation. In other cases, undesirable 'artifacts' are formed during distillation, which are then removed during 'rectification' usually by fractional distillation, a process using a tall column that separates out single constituents or mixtures of compounds with similar boiling points. In some cases these constituents are removed because of their toxicity, such as the hydrocyanic acid in bitter almond oil, or the polynuclear hydrocarbons in cade oil. In the case of deterpenated oils, terpenes are removed in order to create an oil with unusual flavor and fragrance qualities.

Citrus oils may be extracted by cold pressing (expression). These cold-pressed oils are generally preferred for perfumery and aromatherapy, but distilled citrus oils are also made and are often used for flavor work, especially lime.[1] The phototoxic compounds found in citrus oils are relatively large, involatile molecules. Consequently they tend to be present in cold-pressed, but not in distilled citrus oils.

Essential oils can be obtained from many different parts of plants: flowers (rose), leaves (peppermint), fruits (lemon), seeds (fennel), grasses (lemongrass), roots (vetiver), rhizomes (ginger), woods (cedar), barks (cinnamon), gums (frankincense), tree blossoms (ylang-ylang), bulbs (garlic) and dried flower buds (clove). The oils are usually liquid, but a few are solid (e.g., orris) or semi-solid (e.g., guaiacwood), at room temperature. The majority of essential oils are colorless or pale yellow, although a few are deeply colored, such as blue chamomile, and European valerian, which is green.

Fresh aromatic plant material typically yields 1–2% by weight of essential oil on distillation, although a typical yield from roses is 0.015%, and rose otto is consequently highly priced. Fragrant oils can also be extracted with organic solvents, producing concretes, absolutes or resinoids, or with liquid carbon dioxide, producing CO_2 extracts. Some absolutes and resinoids are included in this text.[2]

Absolutes are produced from concretes. A concrete contains both fragrant molecules and plant waxes, and is made by washing the plant material with a non-polar solvent such as hexane. Concretes are used in their own right in perfumery, and are more or less solid. The concrete may then be washed with ethanol to dissolve out the fragrant molecules, separating them from the waxes. When the ethanol is evaporated off, this leaves what is known as an absolute. The much lower temperatures compared to distillation mean that delicate floral oils such as mimosa, that would not survive distillation, can be processed; and compounds that are water-soluble or of low volatility are more easily captured.

Composition

Essential oils typically contain dozens of constituents with related, but distinct, chemical structures. Each constituent has its characteristic odor and pattern of effects on the body. Most constituents are widely distributed throughout the plant kingdom. (+)-Limonene, linalool and the pinenes, for example, are found in a large number of essential oils, in fact very few contain none of these.

Although essential oils contain many different types of compound, one or two constituents often dominate their physiological action. Many of the properties of peppermint oil, for instance, can be attributed to its content of (−)-menthol (∼40%), and the action of eucalyptus is largely determined by its 1,8-cineole content (∼75%). Despite the fact that most constituents represent less than 1% of the whole oil, even these can have marked actions on the human body. For example, bergapten, one of the psoralens responsible for the phototoxicity of bergamot oil, is found at concentrations of about 0.3%.

In most cases, the percentage of a constituent varies within a certain range. For instance, the terpinen-4-ol content of tea tree oil is normally between 30% and 55%. Although terpinen-4-ol contents both above and below these ranges are possible, they are only rarely found in commercially produced tea tree oils. Some ranges are much narrower than the 25% seen here, while others are considerably broader. These variations may be due to factors that affect the plant's environment, such as geographical location, weather conditions, soil type and fertilizer used. They may also be due to factors such as the age of the plant and the time of day or year when it is harvested. Variations in yield, number of harvests or flowerings can result from growing the same plant in different locations. Differences in production techniques and manufacturing equipment will be apparent in the quality and composition of the resultant oil.

Seasonal variations, for example, can be seen in the 1,8-cineole content of Moroccan *Eucalyptus globulus* oil, which has a low of 62.4% in May and a high of 82.2% in July (Zrira & Benjilali 1996). Great variations in the menthone content of French *Mentha x piperita* oil can be seen, with lows of 6.1–8.1% in October and highs of 48.8–54.5% in June (Chalchat et al 1997). The α-thujone content of an Italian *Salvia officinalis* oil ranges from 29.7% in April to 48.8% in October (Piccaglia et al 1997). Elevation can also affect composition. In similar thyme plants grown in Turkey at elevations of 18 m and 1,200 m, oils extracted at full-flowering over three years

showed average *p*-cymol contents of 39.5% (lowland) and 28.3% (mountainous) (Özgüven & Tansi 1998).

Because they are processed differently to essential oils, resinoids and absolutes often contain constituents of low volatility that are rarely found in essential oils. These include benzenoid compounds such as benzyl acetate, benzyl salicylate, cinnamyl alcohol, methyl benzoate and coumarin. Benzyl cyanide, benzyl isothiocyanate, *cis*-3-hexenyl benzoate, indole and phytol occur exclusively in absolutes. On the other hand, compounds with high volatility, such as limonene, pinene and other monoterpenes, are only rarely present in absolutes, but are ubiquitous in essential oils.

A 'trace constituent' is one that is present in very small amounts. For instance, 1,8-cineole is found at about 0.002% in mandarin oil, some 40,000 times less than in eucalyptus oil. Mandarin oil has one major constituent, (+)-limonene, which along with other terpenes, accounts for some 95% of the oil. The remaining constituents, comprising at least 74 individual compounds, make up the other 5%. In the Essential Oil Profiles a trace constituent is flagged as 'tr', and generally occurs as the lower end of a range. For example, in the estragole chemotype of basil, the range of linalool is 'tr-8.6%'. Most trace constituents are not shown for reasons of space.

Chemotypes

These are plants of the same genus that are virtually identical in appearance, but which produce essential oils with different major constituents. Chemotypes (CTs) are named after the main constituent(s). Commercially produced thyme oils, for example, are extracted from the following seven chemotypes:

- carvacrol
- thymol
- thymol/carvacrol
- borneol
- geraniol
- linalool
- thujanol

The majority of thyme oils on the market are those rich in thymol and/or carvacrol, compounds with strong antibacterial properties, but which are also moderately irritant. The toxicity of some essential oils depends greatly on chemotype, notably basil, buchu, ho leaf and hyssop. Chemotypes are variants within a single botanical species, but in other cases, such as calamus or sage, a difference in botanical origin also entails significant compositional differences with important toxicological consequences. Clear labeling, with chemotype and botanical species, can therefore be of great importance in distinguishing between apparently similar essential oils.

Contamination

Contaminants are substances that are not natural constituents, artifacts of distillation, or adulterants (adulteration being intentional dilution or fabrication). They can include plasticizers and pesticides, or traces of solvent in solvent-extracted products. Because of their antimicrobial properties, essential oils are not generally subject to microbial contamination. Maudsley & Kerr (1999), for example, reported that eight essential oils were sterile and did not support the growth of seven bacterial species and *Candida albicans*.

Biocides

There are over 400 chemical biocides (pesticides or herbicides) that might be used on aromatic plants, and many of these do carry over during steam distillation (Briggs & McLaughlin 1974; Belanger 1989; Dikshith et al 1989). The products of solvent extraction (absolutes, resinoids and CO_2 extracts) are even more likely to retain any biocides, as are cold-pressed citrus oils. The transfer of the insecticide *chlorpyrifos* from roses to rose water, rose concrete and rose absolute, was 5.7%, 46.9% and 38.8%, respectively. Rose otto was not tested. Twelve days following application, no traces of *chlorpyrifos* were detectable in flowers or leaves (Kumar et al 2004).

Of 11 organochlorine pesticides screened in 148 cold-pressed lemon oils, 123 sweet orange oils, 121 mandarin oils and 147 bergamot oils produced in Italy in the years 1991–1996 (~20 samples per oil, per year) two pesticides (*tetradifon* and *difocol*) were detected, in addition to 4,4'-dichlorobenzophenone, a decomposition product of *difocol*. The detected range for a single pesticide was 0–5.95 ppm (Saitta et al 2000). A steady decline in the percentage of contaminated samples was seen over the six year period (Table 2.1). Dugo et al (1997) reviewed the organophosphorus and organochlorine pesticides in Italian citrus oils. They reported that since the 1960s, concentrations of pesticide ranging between 1.5 ppm and 450 ppm had been detected. Between 1983 and 1991, 12 organophosphorus pesticide residues were detected in 33 lemon oils, with total pesticide content ranging from 4.95–49.3 ppm. Of the 33 oils, 97.4% contained *methyl parathion*, 99.3% *ethyl parathion* and 98.4% *methidathion*. Di Bella et al (2004) found 0.26 mg/L and 0.20 mg/L of *difocol* in Calabrian bergamot oils from 1999 and 2000, respectively. *Tetradifon* was found at 0.06 mg/L for both years. Certified organic citrus oils are becoming widely available.

Propiconazole and *tebuconazole*, fungicides used to control rust in peppermint, were detected in the essential oil at 0.02–0.05 mg/kg and 0.01–0.04 mg/kg, respectively (Garland et al 1999). There is evidence of reproductive, hepatic and immunotoxicity for *propiconazole* (Wolf et al 2006; Goetz et al 2007; Martin et al 2007). Other investigations have found the insecticides *chlorpyrifos* and *carbofuran* in peppermint oil (Inman et al 1981, 1983), but failed to find the nematocide *oxamyl* in the same oil (Kiigemagi et al 1984). *Chlorpyrifos* exposure has been associated with low testosterone levels in US adult males, and with CNS (central nervous system) toxicity after neonatal exposure (Aldridge et al 2005; Meeker et al 2006). Overexposure to *carbofuran* has resulted in acute poisoning in both Nicaragua and Senegal, including some fatalities (McConnell & Hruska 1993; Gomes do Espirito Santo et al 2002).

Biocide use might feasibly alter essential oil composition. In three similar reports, the composition of sage oil and melissa oil was not significantly altered by the use of the pesticide *afalon WP50*, although only those chemicals expected to occur naturally in the oil were studied (Vaverkova et al 1995a, 1995b; Tekel et al 1997). However, in another study the use of *metribuzin* increased the linalool content of coriander seed oil (Zheljazkov & Zhalnov 1995).[3]

Sometimes the origin of xenobiotic substances found in essential oils is open to debate. One study found 2,4,6-trichloroanisole in Mexican lime, French orange leaf, Spanish rue and Bulgarian rue oils, but concluded that it was probably of microbial rather than pesticidal origin (Stoffelsma & De Roos 1973).

According to Hotchkiss (1994) most biocides are poorly absorbed through the skin, though *chlorpyrifos* and *carbofuran* are absorbed to a degree (Liu & Kim 2003; Meuling et al 2005). In vitro testing of human skin suggests that absorption depends on the solubility and molecular weight of the substance in question. *Methiocarb*, for instance, is relatively well absorbed, but *dimethoate* is not absorbed at all (Nielsen et al 2004). Dermal exposure to *methyl parathion* in rats resulted in acute toxic effects at 50 mg/kg, and only minimal toxicity at 6.25 or 12.5 mg/kg (Zhu et al 2001). These are very much higher doses than might be encountered from essential oil exposure.

It is feasible that an essential oil might enhance the dermal absorption of a biocide, and exposure through inhalation is also possible. The potential toxicity from biocides in essential oils is minimal, but still contributes to the total xenobiotic load, especially if biocides are also being ingested in foods, and zero exposure is surely preferable. Some of the reported allergic reactions to essential oils may be caused or enhanced by biocide residues, and not by the oils themselves (Wabner 1993).

Solvents

The use of benzene as a solvent for the extraction of concretes has declined considerably, but it is still in use. This well-documented carcinogen is listed under substances "known to be human carcinogens" by the NTP (National Toxicology Program 2005) and it is prohibited as a cosmetic ingredient in the European Union (EU) (Anon 2003a). The International Fragrance Association (IFRA) recommends that the level of benzene should be kept as low as practicable, and should not exceed 1 ppm in fragrance products (IFRA 2009). Traces of benzene may be present in absolutes processed from concretes extracted with it.

Cyclohexane is commonly used today as a replacement for benzene. Cyclohexane is made either by catalytic hydrogenation of benzene or by fractional distillation of petroleum, and may itself contain traces of benzene. Inhalation exposure of cyclohexane in rats indicates a NOAEL (no observed adverse effect level) of 500 ppm for both subchronic and reproductive toxicity

Table 2.1 Decline in percentage of citrus oils containing pesticides over a six year period

Year	1991	1992	1993	1994	1995	1996
Bergamot oil	50.0	52.6	31.6	35.0	40.0	26.3
Mandarin oil	94.7	90.0	80.0	77.3	75.0	50.0
Orange oil	94.7	77.8	78.3	68.4	68.2	54.5

Data from Saitta et al (2000).

(Kreckmann et al 2000; Malley et al 2000). Cyclohexane has not been evaluated for carcinogenicity, but it is not genotoxic. In a 2001 report by the Scientific Committee on Toxicity, Ecotoxicity and the Environment (CSTEE 2001) of the EU, it is suggested that human NOAELs of either 250 ppm or 1,200 ppm cyclohexane in air can be extrapolated from experimental data. *n*-Hexane, which is also used as a solvent, is neurotoxic (Tahti et al 1997). However, neither cyclohexane nor *n*-hexane present any risk of toxicity in the trace amounts present in absolutes. Other distillation/extraction solvents include polyethylene glycols, fluorocarbons and chlorofluorocarbons (Burfield, private communication, 2003).

As with biocides in essential oils, the likely risk of solvent toxicity from the use of absolutes is negligible, especially considering that the parts per million in an absolute are further diluted in an essential oil blend or aromatherapy product.

Phthalates

Phthalate esters, more commonly known as 'phthalates' (the 'ph' is silent), are a major group of plasticizing agents, and can occur either as (unintentional) contaminants or (intentional) adulterants in essential oils. They have long been used either simply to 'stretch' essential oils or to make unpourable resinoids more fluid. They are also ubiquitous contaminants in food and indoor air and are found, for example, in plastic food containers, plastic wrap, plastic toys, medical tubing and blood bags. Soft plastics, e.g., PVC, contain much higher concentrations of phthalates than hard plastics. In 1999, the EU banned the use of phthalates from some products, e.g., baby toys. In 2002, the FDA (Food and Drug Administration) advised that, if available, alternatives to phthalates should be used to keep plastics soft because certain devices could expose people to toxic doses. In the USA and Canada the chemicals have been removed from infant bottle nipples and other products intended to go in a baby's mouth, however the US Government has declined to ban the use of phthalates.

Although there has been some reduction in usage, total phthalate exposure may still be a problem. A study of 85 individuals in Germany found that 10 exceeded the tolerable daily intake value set by the EU for phthalates, and 26 exceeded the Environment Protection Agency's daily reference dose (Koch et al 2003). As a group, phthalates tend to be hepatotoxic, cause damage to the gastrointestinal tract, and demonstrate varying degrees of reproductive toxicity and carcinogenicity. They are also thought to be hormone disruptors (National Toxicology Program 1995; Duty et al 2003; Shea 2003; Seo KW et al 2004).

Not all phthalates are regarded as toxic. Diethyl phthalate (DEP), which is intentionally added to raw materials such as essential oils or resinoids, is apparently used because of its good safety profile. A comprehensive review of DEP by the Research Institute for Fragrance Materials (RIFM) concluded that, at the level of dermal exposure from its use in fragrance (0.73 mg/kg/day), there was no significant risk to humans with regard to skin reactions, carcinogenicity, reproductive toxicity or estrogenic activity (Api 2001a). The SCCNFP (Scientific Committee on Cosmetic Products and Non-Food Products, the EU regulatory body for cosmetics) concluded: 'the safety profile of diethyl phthalate supports its use in cosmetic products at current levels.

At present the SCCNFP does not recommend any specific warnings or restrictions under the currently proposed conditions of use' (SCCNFP 2001b, 2003c). However, this remains a controversial subject, and DEP is now widely avoided in the industry.

Phthalates other than DEP are found in essential oils. According to Naqvi & Mandal (1995) di-(2-ethylhexyl) phthalate (DEHP) has been a common adulterant of sandalwood oil. Of eight phthalates screened in Italian lemon, orange and mandarin oils in the years 1994–1996, one or both of two phthalates, diisobutyl phthalate (DIBP) and DEHP, were found in almost all samples, and dibutyl phthalate (DBP) was found in 8 of the total of 87 samples tested. Total phthalate concentrations up to 4 ppm were detected (Di Bella et al 1999). DBP, DIBP and DEHP were all detected in Calabrian bergamot oils from crop years 1999 and 2000, at concentrations ranging from 1.22–1.65 mg/L per phthalate. The phthalates are thought to derive from plastic materials used in the production process of citrus oils (Di Bella et al 2004).

Both DBP and DIBP are genotoxic in human mucosa and DBP is reproductively toxic in rats (Kleinsasser et al 2000, 2001; Zhang et al 2004). DEHP may cause reproductive and developmental toxicity, and is thought to be an endocrine disruptor (Gayathri et al 2004; Latini et al 2004). There is debate about whether it is a carcinogen in humans (Melnick 2001). Phthalate adulteration/contamination in essential oils is declining due to increasing legislation and awareness of phthalate toxicity. Diethyl maleate is not permitted as a cosmetic ingredient in the EU (Anon 2003a).

The intentional addition of phthalates to essential oils is of concern with regard to toxicity, especially since this involves much higher concentrations than phthalate contamination.

Adulteration

The purpose of adulteration is to increase profits by adding either odorous or non-odorous substances in order to dilute an essential oil or absolute. Odorous adulterants can include other essential oils, essential oil fractions or residues, synthetic aromachemicals similar to those found in the oil, or aromachemicals not found in the oil. Non-odorous adulterants, or 'extenders', include substances such as ethanol, mineral oil, isopropyl myristate, glycols, phthalates, and fixed oils such as rapeseed and cottonseed. Examples of adulteration are shown in Table 2.2.

The most costly essential oils and absolutes are highly subject to adulteration, for obvious reasons. These include jasmine and rose absolutes, sandalwood, neroli and rose essential oils. In other cases, the decision to adulterate depends on the relative market price of the oil and the proposed adulterant. Examples include may chang oil (synthetic citral), coriander seed oil (synthetic linalool) and tea tree oil (terpinen-4-ol, terpinenes). The cheapest essential oils, such as sweet orange and eucalyptus, are among the least likely to be adulterated.

'Passing off' is perhaps an extreme form of adulteration, since it means that none of the labeled material is present. For example, synthetic methyl salicylate may be passed off as wintergreen oil, or synthetic benzaldehyde as bitter almond oil. Mixtures of natural and synthetic ingredients are often passed

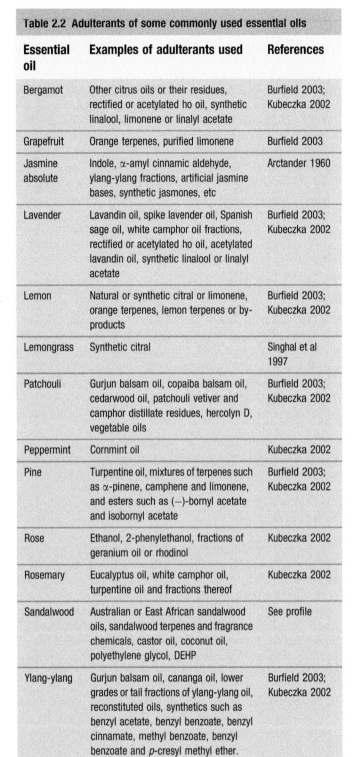

Table 2.2 Adulterants of some commonly used essential oils

Essential oil	Examples of adulterants used	References
Bergamot	Other citrus oils or their residues, rectified or acetylated ho oil, synthetic linalool, limonene or linalyl acetate	Burfield 2003; Kubeczka 2002
Grapefruit	Orange terpenes, purified limonene	Burfield 2003
Jasmine absolute	Indole, α-amyl cinnamic aldehyde, ylang-ylang fractions, artificial jasmine bases, synthetic jasmones, etc	Arctander 1960
Lavender	Lavandin oil, spike lavender oil, Spanish sage oil, white camphor oil fractions, rectified or acetylated ho oil, acetylated lavandin oil, synthetic linalool or linalyl acetate	Burfield 2003; Kubeczka 2002
Lemon	Natural or synthetic citral or limonene, orange terpenes, lemon terpenes or by-products	Burfield 2003; Kubeczka 2002
Lemongrass	Synthetic citral	Singhal et al 1997
Patchouli	Gurjun balsam oil, copaiba balsam oil, cedarwood oil, patchouli vetiver and camphor distillate residues, hercolyn D, vegetable oils	Burfield 2003; Kubeczka 2002
Peppermint	Cornmint oil	Kubeczka 2002
Pine	Turpentine oil, mixtures of terpenes such as α-pinene, camphene and limonene, and esters such as (−)-bornyl acetate and isobornyl acetate	Burfield 2003; Kubeczka 2002
Rose	Ethanol, 2-phenylethanol, fractions of geranium oil or rhodinol	Kubeczka 2002
Rosemary	Eucalyptus oil, white camphor oil, turpentine oil and fractions thereof	Kubeczka 2002
Sandalwood	Australian or East African sandalwood oils, sandalwood terpenes and fragrance chemicals, castor oil, coconut oil, polyethylene glycol, DEHP	See profile
Ylang-ylang	Gurjun balsam oil, cananga oil, lower grades or tail fractions of ylang-ylang oil, reconstituted oils, synthetics such as benzyl acetate, benzyl benzoate, benzyl cinnamate, methyl benzoate, benzyl benzoate and p-cresyl methyl ether.	Burfield 2003; Kubeczka 2002

off as melissa or verbena oils. In other cases, completely synthetic creations are either passed off as the natural oil, or added as adulterants. These 'reconstituted oils' are made by manually combining single constituents similar to those found in the natural oil, but typically leaving out most of the trace constituents. Reconstituted oils are sometimes declared as such, but may be sold as natural. Examples include ylang-ylang, neroli and rose.

Impurities in the synthetic chemicals used will also be present in amounts often ranging from 1–5%. For example, the presence of phenyl pentadienal, benzyl alcohol and eugenol in synthetic cinnamaldehyde forms the basis of its detection in cassia oil (Singhal et al 2001).

There are no tests that guarantee purity per se, but analysis by gas chromatography (GC) can be extremely useful (see Analytical techniques, below). The addition of a similar but cheaper essential oil, for example, will result in some compounds showing up on analysis that should not be there at all. The addition of a compound normally present in the oil will correspondingly reduce the percentages of all the other constituents, and some of these may then fall below normal minimum limits. The addition of a synthetic substance that is not in the natural oil will generally show up on a GC trace. One approach is to search for a single constituent that is present in the natural material, but is not commercially available, so it cannot be added. The concentration of this substance may be revealing, if indeed it is there at all.

Olfactory evaluation by a trained nose may be a useful adjunct to laboratory analysis, but it will not detect non-odorous adulterants. These, however, are usually detectable by testing physical parameters such as specific gravity, optical rotation, refractive index and solubility in alcohol, perhaps combined with GC testing.

Adulteration could feasibly increase toxicity, especially in the area of skin reactions. The co-presence of both contaminants and adulterants is also of concern.

Degradation

All organic materials are subject to chemical degradation. In the case of essential oils, this tends to occur on prolonged storage, under poor storage conditions, or when the oil is otherwise exposed to the air. When kept in dark, cool conditions in full, sealed containers the degradation is measured in months or years, but in unfavorable conditions, it can progress in a matter of days or weeks. The three principal factors responsible for essential oil degradation are:

- oxygen
- heat
- light.

Oxygen

Atmospheric oxygen can change the chemical composition of an essential oil by reacting with some of the constituents. Oxidation tends to occur more readily in essential oils rich in monoterpenes and other more volatile compounds. Most of the monoterpenes listed in Box 2.2 are alkenes, which are susceptible because carbon–carbon double bonds are reactive to oxygen. Unsaturated fats and oils become rancid for the same reason. However, not all oxidized monoterpenoid alkenes are high-risk allergens. In a multicenter study involving 1,511 consecutive dermatitis patients, only one (0.07%) tested positive to a 3% concentration of oxidized β-myrcene (Matura et al 2005).

One safety implication of chemical degradation is that we cannot be certain of the composition of a degraded oil unless it is retested, and we may therefore be using a mixture of uncertain composition in treatments. Oxidation can also affect the efficacy of an essential oil. Orafidiya (1993) found that oxidized lemongrass oil had lost much of its antibacterial activity when compared to fresh, unoxidized oil. In extensively oxidized samples, antibacterial activity was completely lost. Kishore et al (1996) reported that chenopodium oil lost its antifungal activity after 360 days, although storage conditions were not specified.

Another consequence of degradation is that it can render an essential oil more hazardous. Notably, terpene degradation in certain oils leads to compounds being formed that make the oils potential skin sensitizers, while fresh oils are safe to use. This especially applies to oils rich in α-pinene, δ-3-carene or (+)-limonene. Of five oxidation products of limonene identified by Karlberg et al (1992), (−)-carvone, and a mixture of (Z)- and (E)- isomers of (+)-limonene 1,2-oxide were potent skin sensitizers in guinea pigs, while (Z)- and (E)-carveol were not. Subsequent work identified two further oxidation products as allergens in guinea pigs, the (Z)- and (E)- isomers of limonene-2-hydroperoxide (Karlberg et al 1994a).

Cold (4–6°C) and dark storage of (+)-limonene in closed vessels prevents significant oxidation for 12 months. The addition of BHT (butylated hydroxytoluene, an antioxidant) to limonene retards oxidation to an extent depending on the purity of the materials and the ambient temperature, but in two of the tests oxidation was prevented in air-exposed limonene for 34 and 43 weeks, respectively. There was no direct correlation between the amount of BHT used and the time before oxidation could be detected, and after the BHT was consumed, oxidation proceeded at about the same rate as for limonene without BHT. The concentration of sensitizing oxidation products reached a peak after 10–20 weeks of air oxidation, and then declined due to polymerization of the oxidation products. After 48 weeks the identified oxidation products constituted 14% of the material (Karlberg et al 1994b).

The monoterpene content of lemon oil decreased from 97.1% to 30.7% in 12 months when the oil was stored at 25°C with the cap removed for three minutes every day. However, storage at 5°C, with the cap removed for three minutes once a month resulted in minimal degradation (Sawamura et al 2004).

Citrus oils are especially vulnerable, because they are high in (+)-limonene, and are not rich in antioxidant constituents. The most potent antioxidant constituent found in essential oils is eugenol, followed by thymol and carvacrol (Teissedre & Waterhouse 2000). In a study of different basil oils, there was a strong relationship between antioxidant activity and total phenolic content (Juliani & Simon 2002). Non-phenolic antioxidant constituents include benzyl alcohol, 1,8-cineole, menthol, menthyl acetate, methyl salicylate and thymoquinone (see Constituent profiles). Tea tree oils with a relatively high 1,8-cineole content may be less prone to oxidation, and therefore less prone to skin reactions, than those low in 1,8-cineole. If this was so it would be somewhat ironic, since the Australian tea tree industry has put great emphasis on low-cineole tea tree oils, in the mistaken belief that 1,8-cineole was a skin irritant.

Unsurprisingly, essential oils rich in antioxidant constituents invariably demonstrate antioxidant activity. The oil of *Achillea millefolium* subsp. *millefolium* showed significant antioxidant

activity, even though it only contained 24.6% of 1,8-cineole (Candan et al 2003). The antioxidant capacity of carvacrol-rich *Thymbra capitata* and 1,8-cineole-rich *Thymus mastichina* oils was compared to that of BHT in sunflower oil stored at 60°C. Both essential oils were much more potent, with *Thymus mastichina* showing 59% inhibition, compared with 20% for BHT (Miguel et al 2003b). Also see Table 9.3, especially those oils that are highly active against lipid peroxidation.

Heat

Heat will promote any endothermic (heat absorbing) chemical process because it helps reactants to overcome the activation energy barrier to react. The degrading effects of heat have not been widely researched, but the few published studies show great variation between different types of essential oil. Gopalakrishnan (1994) found that, in a cardamom CO_2 extract, concentrations of the more volatile constituents tended to decrease (presumably due to oxidation) and those of less volatile constituents to increase in the presence of heat (Table 2.3). In this study, clove oil and cardamom oil were kept at 28°C in airtight containers, and the initial analyses were compared with compositional data after 45 and 90 days. The cardamom oil showed significant degradation while the clove oil did not. Clove oil is low in monoterpenes and high in eugenol. CO_2 extracts of both plants, one of each kept at 0°C, the other at 28°C, were also compared after 45 and 90 days, and the samples kept at 28°C showed significantly more degradation than those kept at 0°C. The CO_2 extracts were more prone to degradation than the essential oils, though the reasons for this are not clear.

When samples of *Mentha piperita* and *Mentha viridis* oils were kept at 5°C and 27°C, there were no significant differences in degradation in either oil at different temperatures (Shalaby et al 1988). This may again be due to the fact that these oils are low in monoterpenes. Under good storage conditions, the composition of geranium oil did not alter markedly over a 24 month period (Kaul et al 1997). However, in a melissa oil stored in either glass or aluminum containers, and at either

Table 2.3 Percentages of the more volatile constituents of a cardamom CO_2 extract showing increased degradation at higher temperature

Constituent	0 days	90 days at 0°C	90 days at 28°C
α-Pinene	0.7	0.5	0.2
β-Pinene	4.3	2.0	0.3
Sabinene	2.8	1.4	0.1
(+)-Limonene	2.3	1.5	0.5
1,8-Cineole	27.0	21.8	14.7
Linalool	3.9	3.3	2.2
Terpinen-4-ol	2.0	2.1	2.0
α-Terpineol	5.9	5.5	4.4

Data from Gopalakrishnan (1994).

4°C or 27°C, considerable degradation occurred over 12 months in all four samples, with little difference between them. The concentrations of neral and geranial substantially increased while those of β-caryophyllene and citronellal decreased (Shalaby et al 1995). This report might point to a tendency for essential oils rich in citral or citronellal to readily degrade.

Light

Although well known to those in the essential oil industry, few papers have been published on the degrading effects of light. Light, especially UV (ultraviolet), is usually implicated in free radical reactions. In the case of oxidation, light will promote the formation of oxygen free radicals, which are highly reactive. An acidic emulsion of sweet orange oil was found to undergo significant changes in composition when exposed to UV light at 20°C for 50 minutes. These changes included decreases in neral, geranial and citronellal, and significant increases in carvone, isopulegol, carveol, linalool oxide and limonene oxide, as well as the appearance of at least 12 new constituents including piperitone, trans-β-terpineol, α-cyclocitral, photocitral A, menthone and isomenthone. This UV-initiated degradation is described as being clearly governed by photosensitized oxidation and intramolecular cyclyzation mechanisms (Ziegler et al 1991). Sweet fennel oil has been shown to oxidize more rapidly in light than in dark conditions (Misharina & Polshkov 2005).

Other factors

Resinification is another way in which essential oils degrade, and it is often preceded by oxidation. It is a process whereby discrete (usually small) molecules (monomers) joined together to form polymeric chains of two (dimers), three (trimers) or more monomers. A polymer is a long chain of molecules. The polymerization of ethene to give poly-ethene is one of the first known industrial examples. In so-called addition polymerizations, the reaction is started by a free radical, called an initiator. This may be an oxygen free radical. Several physical properties change with molecular size: viscosity increases, melting point increases, boiling point increases (i.e., volatility decreases), etc. This is due to intermolecular forces between chains. Resinification manifests as an obvious increase in viscosity, and can often be seen in old or improperly stored essential oils such as angelica seed, myrrh, taget and tarragon.

The presence of water in an essential oil causes spoilage. It can promote oxidation, lead to hydrolysis of molecules, and it causes essential oils to become opaque.

Prevention

Oxidation can be guarded against by proper storage and by the addition of antioxidants to susceptible essential oils or to preparations containing them. For all the reasons given above, it is important to store essential oils in dark bottles and away from direct sunlight and sources of heat. It is recommended that they are stored in a cool place, such as a refrigerator (but note that a few essential oils will become very viscous, and will be difficult to pour until warmed). The more air there is in a bottle of essential oil the more rapidly oxidation will take place. It would be preferable to store oils under an atmosphere of an inert gas, such as nitrogen, but this would be impractical for most practitioners.

Essential oils that readily degrade should be refrigerated and used within 12 months of end-user purchase or first opening. The addition of an antioxidant such as BHT to preparations made with oxidation-prone essential oils is recommended. To be fully effective, an antioxidant should be mixed with an essential oil shortly after extraction, and more may need to be added at the point of further decanting or processing. Naturally derived antioxidants include tocopherols, rosmarinic acid, ascorbyl palmitate and propyl gallate, though little is known about their relative efficacy in regard to essential oils. Mixing antioxidants often gives rise to a synergistic action.

An antioxidant could be regarded as an adulterant when added to an essential oil, though not if an adulterant is a substance added to increase profits. Whether added antioxidants would affect the status of an essential oil, for example organic certification, is a matter for debate. If benefits are weighed against risks, antioxidant addition to oxidation-prone essential oils could confer considerable benefit with negligible risk. Antioxidants are generally used at less than 0.1% concentration.

Combining essential oils may delay the onset of oxidation. A mixture of laurel leaf and coriander oils was shown to possess antioxidant activity, and it strongly inhibited the oxidation of sweet fennel oil constituents (Misharina & Polshkov 2005). Terpeneless (deterpenated) essential oils are available, particularly for citrus oils, with varying degrees of deterpenation. It would be safe to assume that these oils carry a reduced risk of toxifying degradation, although it should be remembered that most are not 100% terpene-free.

When an essential oil is incorporated into a formulation, the pH of the excipient may also affect stability. Perillyl alcohol was most stable at a pH of 5.9–6.0, when tested at four temperatures: 4, 25, 37 and 48°C. Significant degradation took place at pH values less than 4.0 (Gupta & Myrdal 2004).

Essential oil chemistry

Understanding the chemistry of essential oil constituents is a very useful basis for understanding essential oil toxicity. Before we explore the various ways in which essential oils might present hazards, we will need to have a basic familiarity with the chemical vocabulary.

Analytical techniques

Unraveling the chemistry of essential oils is a complex task. Many of the compounds that make up a given essential oil are only present in minute quantities and so are hard to detect. Some are very similar to each other and are difficult to distinguish with certainty, and some are simply hard to identify. The major constituents of the most common essential oils have been known for many years (Parry 1922), but it is only recently that some of the 'fine detail' has been revealed.

Modern methods routinely used for determining the composition of essential oils include GC, high performance liquid chromatography (HPLC), mass spectrometry (MS) and nuclear magnetic resonance (NMR) spectroscopy. Chromatographic techniques are used to separate essential oils into their individual constituents so that they can be identified by special techniques. GC is ideally suited to volatile compounds, and has revolutionized the detection of minor chemical constituents, especially when used in conjunction with MS and NMR spectroscopy. MS looks at the fragmentation patterns of compounds under ionizing conditions, and this information is used to deduce their structures. NMR elucidates the structures of molecules by examining the environment of specific atoms such as hydrogen, by looking at their characteristic nuclear spins. The sensitivity of analytical techniques for organic compounds has increased dramatically over recent years to the point where even trace constituents, including pollutants like pesticides, can be detected.

A GC trace of peppermint oil is shown in Figure 2.1. This identifies 1,8-cineole (10), menthone (24), isomenthone (25) and menthol (45) as a series of peaks collected at different times. The first peak to be collected, which is the most volatile compound in a particular essential oil, is designated peak number one, and so on, with subsequent compounds decreasing in volatility. When resolved, each peak usually represents a single chemical entity, and the area of a peak is proportional to the quantity of that compound in the essential oil. However, with some types of GC two or more compounds may appear as only one peak. This is why, for example, in the analyses of both Mexican and Persian lime oil, limonene and 1,8-cineole are shown as a single percentage (see Lime profile).

GC has, over decades, evolved from packed, to capillary, to multidimensional and, since the late 1990s, to two-dimensional, also known as GC × GC, in which the sample is subjected to analysis through two columns simultaneously. This allows for the separation of highly complex essential oils with closely eluting compounds, so what would show up as one peak on older GC equipment, may now be revealed as two or more identifiable peaks, sometimes as many as 10. This technique, which is still relatively new, means that all chiral compounds (for definition see Isomerism below) can be accurately separated and quantified. Because synthetic optical isomers are almost always prepared as mixtures, this represents an important development for the detection of adulterants, as it means that added synthetic compounds (such as citronellal or linalool) can be easily identified. (Multidimensional GC fulfills the same task, but with much less separation space, insufficient to show fine detail in many instances.)

The structure of organic compounds

In everyday speech, the word 'organic' is used to imply natural, untampered-with and wholesome. However, in chemistry, the same word is used to describe compounds that are composed mainly of the element carbon. Essential oils are made up of organic (i.e., carbon-based) compounds, as are the fixed or vegetable oils with which they are often mixed. Individual essential oil constituents contain atoms in addition to carbon, the most common being hydrogen and oxygen, and occasionally, nitrogen and sulfur. These elements are given symbols for ease of identification: C, H, O, N and S, respectively.

For those who wish to refer to other literature concerning essential oil toxicology or chemistry, it is useful to have an understanding of how molecules relate to one another in terms of similarities and differences in their chemistry. A quick way to do this is to compare their structural formulas.

An abbreviated structural formula of β-citronellol is shown in Figure 2.2A, indicating the different types of atoms represented by their letter symbols. For molecules of this size and larger, such formulas are difficult to recognize because their information content is complex, although for small molecules like water, H_2O, they are valuable.

In the structural formula shown in Figure 2.2B, lines have been included to show the types of bonds (single, double or triple) holding the atoms together. The wedge-shaped bond indicates that the methyl group, CH_3 projects toward the reader, and the dotted bond indicates that the hydrogen atom, H is

Figure 2.1 • Gas chromatographic trace of peppermint oil.

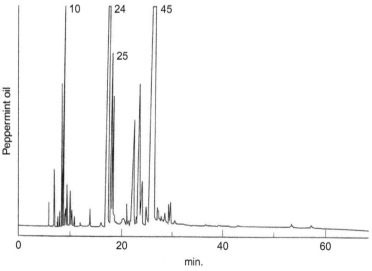

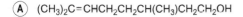

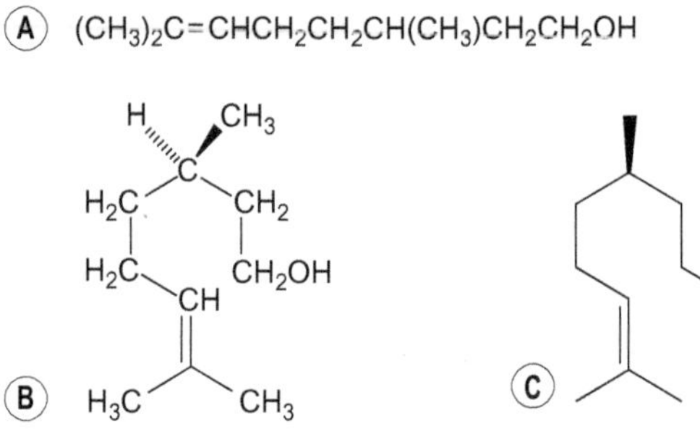

(A) $(CH_3)_2C=CHCH_2CH_2CH(CH_3)CH_2CH_2OH$

Figure 2.2 • Three different structural formulas of β-citronellol.

projected away from the reader. The information added by showing the bonds allows the structure of β-citronellol to be much more easily recognized.

We may simplify molecular structural diagrams by showing all the bonds, but omitting some or all of the carbon (C) and hydrogen (H) atom symbols. Any other atom type (such as oxygen or sulfur) is shown explicitly. This results in a simplified, or skeletal version of the structural formula (Figure 2.2C), which is particularly useful when representing very large molecules.

Although most molecules are three-dimensional rather than flat, they can usually be conveniently represented as two-dimensional projections. In many cases, these projections can be used to illustrate structural differences, such as that between the isomeric alcohols, geraniol and nerol (Figure 2.3).

Isomerism

Isomers are compounds with identical numbers and types of constituent atoms, but differ in the ways in which their atoms are arranged in the molecule.

Geraniol and nerol (Figure 2.3) are known as geometric isomers. They have different arrangements of atoms at each end of one of their carbon–carbon double bonds. Unlike carbon–carbon single bonds, double bonds are usually unable to rotate freely, and hence distinct isomers exist that are unable to interconvert. When atoms other than hydrogen are attached to the carbon atoms forming a double bond, and they lie on the same side of the double bond, the compound is referred to as a *cis*-isomer. When they lie on opposite sides of the bond, it is known as a *trans*-isomer.

Cis,trans-isomerism can also occur in cycloalkanes, where free rotation about a carbon–carbon single bond is restricted. In a compound lacking a hydrogen atom on one of its doubly bonded carbon atoms, assignment as either *cis-* or *trans-* is ambiguous. In such cases, assignments are made with respect to the largest atoms or groups. If the two largest groups lie on the same side of the double bond, a compound will be given the prefix *Z*. If they lie on opposite sides, it will be given the prefix *E*.

When a molecule contains a carbon atom to which four different atoms or groups are attached, that molecule is said to be chiral. Every chiral molecule has a mirror image, called an optical isomer, whose atoms and connections are identical, but whose arrangement in space is different. Like a left and a right hand, such pairs are similar, but not super-imposable. When in solution, optical isomers (or enantiomers) have the ability to rotate the plane of polarized light in opposite directions (clockwise and anticlockwise), and to the same extent. This rotation can be measured with accuracy, and helps distinguish such compounds. For example, (+)-carvone (or *d*-carvone) is dextrorotatory and rotates polarized light in a clockwise sense, while its enantiomer, (−)-carvone (or *l*-carvone) is levo-rotatory and rotates light in an anticlockwise sense (Figure 2.4). Although pairs of optical isomers are virtually identical in many of their properties, such as melting and boiling point, they can have quite different actions on biological systems due to the asymmetry of the macromolecules with which they interact.

(+)-Carvone is found in caraway oil and is responsible for its characteristic odor. The levo-rotatory isomer, (−)-carvone, smells minty and is the main constituent of spearmint oil. A mixture of equal amounts of the two isomers is known as (±)-, '*dl*' or 'racemic' carvone, and has been identified in gingergrass and lavandin oils. While isomeric chemicals often demonstrate similar biological properties, there are sometimes significant differences. For example, *cis*-anethole is more toxic than *trans*-anethole, and α-thujone is more toxic than β-thujone.

Another way of assigning stereochemistry to a chiral molecule is to use the *R-S* convention. Again, it is necessary to differentiate between the groups attached to the chiral carbon atom, and a priority system, based on the atomic numbers of atoms directly attached to the chiral atom and sometimes also their neighboring atoms, is used in a similar way to that described for the *E-Z* convention for alkenes. The structure is then drawn in a prescribed way, and the symbols (*R*) (rectus) or (*S*) (sinister) are assigned depending on the direction in which the groups

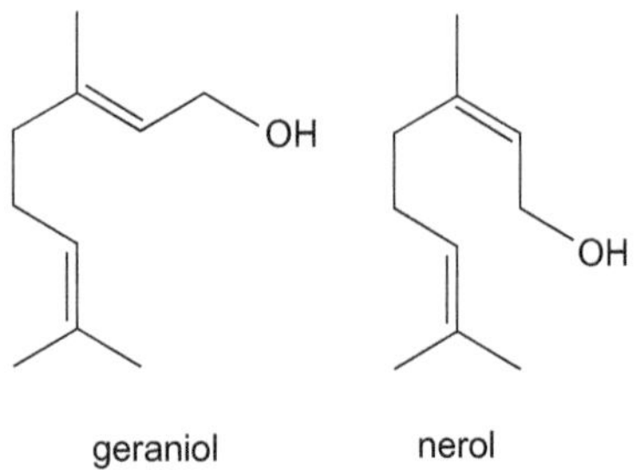

geraniol   nerol

Figure 2.3

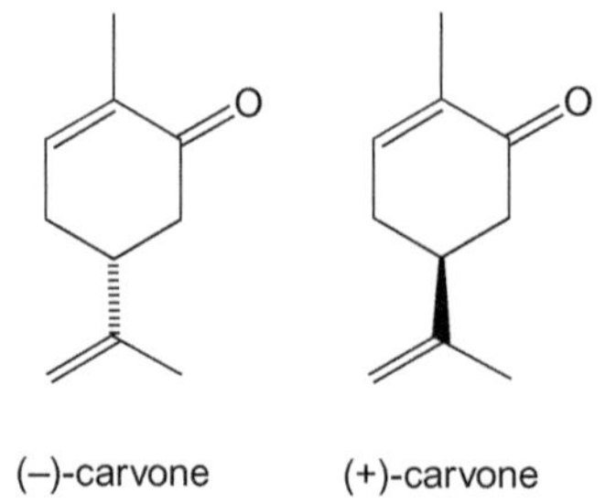

(−)-carvone   (+)-carvone

Figure 2.4

are viewed in order of decreasing priority, either clockwise or anticlockwise, respectively. The reader is referred to an organic chemistry textbook for further details.

For the sake of simplicity, specific isomers of many of the compounds listed in the boxes in this chapter are not mentioned explicitly.

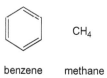

benzene   methane

Figure 2.5

Essential oil constituents

An essential oil constituent, like any organic compound, can be considered to consist of a relatively inert framework of atoms, mainly carbon and hydrogen (i.e., a hydrocarbon) to which one or more functional groups (see below) are attached.

By the term functional group, we mean an atom or a group of atoms that largely determine the characteristic chemical properties of any molecule containing it. In essential oils, most of the functional groups contain heteroatoms (atoms other than carbon) particularly oxygen, and include alcohols, phenols, aldehydes, ketones, esters and ethers. Functional groups replace hydrogen atoms in a hydrocarbon.

This does not mean that the hydrocarbon part of a molecule has no part to play in a compound's physical or chemical properties. On the contrary, it has an important influence on a compound's solubility and volatility, which are key factors in promoting access to odor and taste receptors. It might be better to consider functional groups as playing a specific role in intermolecular interactions, while the structural framework will play a relatively non-specific role.

Hydrocarbons are very soluble in lipids (i.e., they are lipophilic) but are very poorly soluble in water. Consider, for example, the differences between ethanol and cholesterol, both alcohols, but having very different hydrocarbon moieties. Ethanol is a volatile, water-soluble liquid that is readily absorbed into the bloodstream and transported around the body, while cholesterol is an involatile solid that is almost insoluble in water, but very soluble in lipids. It crosses cell membranes with difficulty, and is an important component of them.

Hydrocarbons

Hydrocarbons, which are composed entirely of carbon and hydrogen atoms, vary greatly in size and complexity. Those with open chains of carbon atoms are classified as aliphatic, and include alkanes, alkenes and alkynes. In alkanes, a simple example of which is methane, CH_4, all the atoms are joined together by single bonds. Alkenes have one or more carbon–carbon double bonds in their structure, while alkynes have one or more carbon–carbon triple bonds. Alkynes are not, however, normally found in essential oils. Frequently, alkanes and alkenes occur in ring or alicyclic structures, and include cyclohexane, C_6H_{12}, which contains a six-membered ring. The steroid hydrocarbon skeleton in cholesterol (mentioned above) is a much larger structure and is composed of four alicyclic rings. It is an example of a tetracyclic framework or moiety. Many essential oil constituents contain one or more rings, and are referred to as mono-, bi-, tri-, tetracyclic, etc.

Another class of hydrocarbons is known as aromatic. These compounds usually contain a benzene ring (C_6H_6), and include phenyl, benzyl, phenylethyl and phenylpropyl compounds, as well as polycyclic structures, such as naphthalene and benzo[a]pyrene. The name aromatic derives from the first benzene derivatives isolated from plants which were found to be pleasant smelling, e.g., wintergreen oil. Subsequently, however, less pleasant derivatives were discovered.

The structural formulas of methane and benzene are shown in Figure 2.5. Many essential oil constituents include a benzene ring in their structure, and these are known as 'benzenoid' constituents. Benzene is composed of six carbon atoms joined together into a ring, with one hydrogen atom attached to each. The benzene ring is often represented as a hexagon having alternate double and single bonds, although sometimes a circle is drawn inside the hexagon. In this book, we use the former convention.

The most commonly occurring compounds in essential oils are terpenoids and phenylpropanoids. Plant terpenoids are biosynthesized from isopentenyl diphosphate (IPD, Fig. 2.6) and its isomer, dimethylallyl diphosphate (DMAD). These so-called 'active isoprene units' both derive from the mevalonic acid and methylerythritol phosphate biosynthetic pathways. IPD then reacts with DMAD to give geranyl diphosphate. This C10 compound is the precursor of the monoterpenoids, so-named because they contain one pair of 5-carbon units. They comprise the simplest and most common class of terpenes found in essential oils. Two examples of monoterpenoids are (+)-limonene (Figure 2.7) and α-pinene.

The precursor of sesquiterpenes is farnesyl diphosphate. The basic sesquiterpene structure is composed of 15 carbon atoms (*sesqui* referring to one-and-a-half pairs of 5-carbon units). They are less abundant in essential oils than monoterpenes and because they have a larger molecular size, they are less volatile. Diterpenes, being still larger, are relatively rare in essential oils (phytol is an example). They are composed of 20 carbon atoms. Sesterterpenes (two-and-a-half pairs of 5-carbon units), triterpenes (three pairs of 5-carbon units) and tetraterpenes (four pairs of 5-carbon units) are also found in nature, but do not occur in essential oils (Table 2.4). (Triterpenes can be present in absolutes, such as mimosa.)

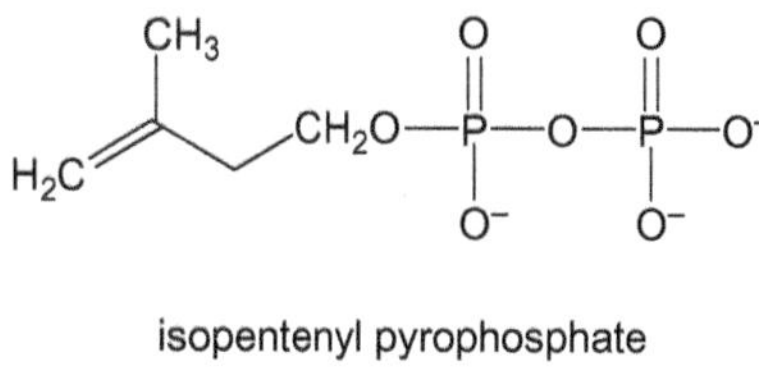

isopentenyl pyrophosphate

Figure 2.6

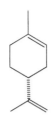

(+)-limonene

Figure 2.7

Table 2.4 Classes of terpenes		
Monoterpenes	2 × 5-carbon units	(C_{10})
Sesquiterpenes	3 × 5-carbon units	(C_{15})
Diterpenes	4 × 5-carbon units	(C_{20})
Sesterterpenes	5 × 5-carbon units	(C_{25})
Triterpenes	6 × 5-carbon units	(C_{30})
Tetraterpenes	8 × 5-carbon units	(C_{40})

Many terpenoid hydrocarbons are alkenes, and their names end in -ene (Box 2.2). They tend to possess low toxicity. The skin sensitizing effects of some terpene-rich oils is largely due to the formation of oxidation products on storage.

Phenylpropanoids, which are found in some essential oils, are synthesized via the shikimic acid biosynthetic pathway starting from phosphoenolpyruvate and erythrose 4-phosphate. They are characterized by having a chain of three carbon atoms attached to a benzene ring. Their main representatives in essential oils include the oxygenated hydrocarbons anethole, eugenol and safrole, which all possess a carbon–carbon double bond in the side chain (and are hence phenylpropenoid alkenes, or 'phenylpropenoids'). α-Asarone, β-asarone, estragole, methyleugenol and safrole are all phenylpropanoids that are rodent carcinogens (Box 2.3).

Box 2.2

Examples of terpenoid hydrocarbons

Monoterpenes	Sesquiterpenes
(−)-Camphene	(−)-Aromadendrene
δ-3-Carene	(−)-β-Bisabolene
p-Cymene	α-Cadinene
(+)-Limonene (Figure 2.7)	β-Caryophyllene
β-Myrcene	β-Cedrene
β-Ocimene	α-Copaene
α-Phellandrene	β-Elemene
α-Pinene	α-Farnesene
(+)-Sabinene	(+)-Germacrene D
α-Terpinene	β-Himachalene
Terpinolene	α-Humulene
α-Thujene	γ-Muurolene
	α-Zingiberene

Box 2.3

Examples of phenylpropanoids

(E)-Anethole
Parsley apiol
α-Asarone
Cinnamaldehyde
Chavicol
Cinnamic acid (see Figure 2.12)
Cinnamic alcohol
Elemicin
Estragole
Eugenol
Methyleugenol
Myristicin
Safrole

In some essential oils, such as pine, the hydrocarbons predominate and only limited amounts of oxygenated constituents are present. In others, such as clove, most of the constituents are oxygenated compounds. A few essential oils have sulfur-containing constituents, which do not come under either of the previous categories, and even fewer contain nitrogen.

Box 2.4 lists the various hydrocarbon moieties and functional groups that make up the structures of essential oil constituents. These are not limited to essential oils, but are found throughout

---

Box 2.4

Composition of compounds found in essential oils

Hydrocarbon moieties

Terpenoid (mono-, sesqui- and diterpenoids)
    Aliphatic (open-chain alkanes and alkenes)
    Alicyclic (cyclic alkanes and alkenes)
    Aromatic (benzene ring)
Phenylpropanoid
    Aromatic (benzene ring)

Functional groups

Alkenes
Alcohols
Phenols
Aldehydes
Ketones
Carboxylic acids
Carboxylic esters
Lactones
Ethers and oxides
Peroxides
Furans

Other compounds

Sulfur compounds
Nitrogen compounds
Inorganic compounds

nature. In certain instances, a compound may have more than one functional group. For example, eugenol is a phenol, an ether and an alkene, although it is commonly referred to as a phenol. Vanillin is a phenol, an ether and an aldehyde. Both contain benzene ring moieties.

Functional groups

We shall next review the main functional groups found in essential oil constituents, and give some examples. The symbols R and R′ represent generic hydrocarbon groups, and Ph represents a phenyl or benzene ring.

Hydrocarbon groups

Alkenes

In hydrocarbons, a carbon–carbon double bond has special chemical properties because of its electron density, and can be considered in a similar way to heteroatom-containing functional groups. Alkenes are common constituents of essential oils (Box 2.5). In constituents containing ring structures, the carbon–carbon double bond can form part of the ring (endocyclic alkenes) or can be part of a side chain (exocyclic alkenes, e.g., phenylpropenoids above).

Hydroxyl groups

Alcohols

Alcohols contain the hydroxyl functional group, and are perhaps the most varied group of terpene derivatives found in essential oils. The names of all alcohols end in -ol (Box 2.6). Monoterpene alcohols are not large in number, but occur in a great many number of essential oils. There are many sesquiterpene alcohols, but most of them are found in few essential oils. Alcohols are relatively non-toxic, are non-mutagenic, and possess low irritancy and allergenicity (Belsito et al 2008). Ethanol, best known as

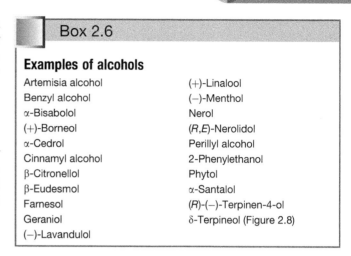

Box 2.6

Examples of alcohols

Artemisia alcohol	(+)-Linalool
Benzyl alcohol	(−)-Menthol
α-Bisabolol	Nerol
(+)-Borneol	(R,E)-Nerolidol
α-Cedrol	Perillyl alcohol
Cinnamyl alcohol	2-Phenylethanol
β-Citronellol	Phytol
β-Eudesmol	α-Santalol
Farnesol	(R)-(−)-Terpinen-4-ol
Geraniol	δ-Terpineol (Figure 2.8)
(−)-Lavandulol	

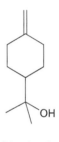

δ-terpineol

Figure 2.8

an ingredient of fermented alcoholic drinks, is not generally found as a natural component of any essential oil, partly because of its high volatility and water solubility, but it is found in rose otto, which is hydrodistilled.

Phenols

Like alcohols, phenols also have a hydroxyl group, and their names usually end in –ol (Box 2.7). However, in phenols, the -OH is attached to a benzene ring, which makes the -OH group very weakly acidic and fairly reactive. Consequently, phenols may be irritating to the skin and mucous membranes. The parent compound, phenol (or carbolic acid), is a disinfectant derived from coal tar and is not found in essential oils.

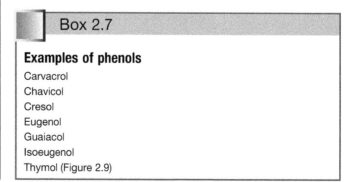

Box 2.5

Examples of alkene hydrocarbons

Endocyclic alkenes

δ-Cadinene	Apiole (dill and parsley)
α-Cedrene	(−)-Aromadendrene
Chamazulene	(−)-Camphene
α-Copaene	Eugenol
α-Gurjunene	Longifolene
α-Humulene	β-Pinene
α-Phellandrene	Safrole
α-Pinene	α-Santalene
α-Thujene	
	Acyclic alkenes
Exocyclic alkenes	α-Farnesene
(E)- and (Z)-anethole	β-Myrcene
	β-Ocimene

Box 2.7

Examples of phenols

Carvacrol
Chavicol
Cresol
Eugenol
Guaiacol
Isoeugenol
Thymol (Figure 2.9)

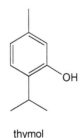

thymol

Figure 2.9

Carbonyl-containing groups

Aldehydes

These compounds contain the –CHO functional group, which is one of several examples of a carbonyl (C=O) -containing group. Aldehydes, which may be considered as partially oxidized primary alcohols, are widely distributed as natural essential oil constituents. Aldehydes have a slightly fruity odor when smelled on their own. They often cause skin irritation and allergic reactions. (A well-known aldehyde, not found in essential oils, is formaldehyde.) The names of aldehydes end in -al or -aldehyde (Box 2.8).

Box 2.8

Examples of aldehydes

Acetaldehyde	2-Dodecenal
Anisaldehyde	Geranial
Benzaldehyde	(1S)-(+)-Myrtenal
Cinnamaldehyde	Neral
Citral	(−)-Perillaldehyde (Figure 2.10)
β-Citronellal	Piperonal
Cuminaldehyde	Salicylaldehyde
2-Decenal	Vanillin
Dodecanal	

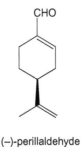

(−)-perillaldehyde

Figure 2.10

Ketones

Ketones are structurally similar to aldehydes and also possess a carbonyl group. Ketones can be produced by oxidation of secondary alcohols. They are relatively stable compounds and are not easily oxidized further. Bicyclic, monoterpenoid ketones have a tendency to be neurotoxic CNS stimulants. Ketones tend to be resistant to metabolism in the body and so are often excreted in the urine unchanged. (A well-known ketone, not found in essential oils, is the solvent, acetone). The names of ketones generally end in -one (Box 2.9).

Box 2.9

Examples of ketones

Artemisia ketone	Perilla ketone
(+)-Camphor	(+)-Pinocamphone
(−)-Carvone	Pinocarvone
(R)-(−)-Fenchone	(6S)-(+)-Piperitone
α-Ionone	(+)-cis-Pulegone
cis-α-Irone	(+)-β-Thujone (Figure 2.11)
cis-Jasmone	Thymoquinone
(−)-Menthone	ar-Turmerone
6-Methylhept-5-en-2-one	2-Undecanone
2-Nonanone	(1R,5R)-(+)-Verbenone

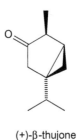

(+)-β-thujone

Figure 2.11

Carboxylic acids

Another category of carbonyl-containing functional groups is the carboxylic acid group, -COOH. Carboxylic acids are formed on oxidation of aldehydes, and are rarely found in essential oils because of their low volatility. They are weak acids and often have a pungent odor. Carboxylic acids are named after their hydrocarbon moiety, and have the suffixic acid (Box 2.10). Carboxylic acids are very reactive. They readily form esters with alcohols (or lactones when the alcohol group is within the same molecule) and amides with amines.

Box 2.10

Examples of carboxylic acids

Alantic acid
Anisic acid
Benzoic acid
(E)-Cinnamic acid (Figure 2.12)
(R)-(+)-Citronellic acid
Decanoic acid
α-(R)-Nepetalic acid
Phenylacetic acid
Valerenic acid

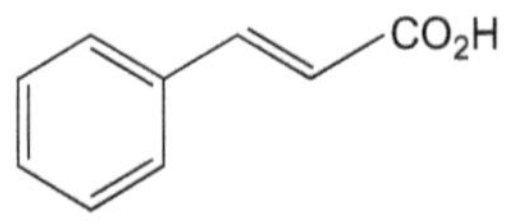

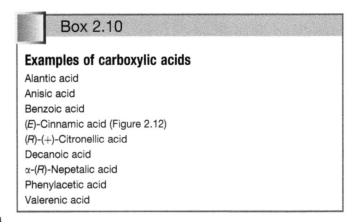

(E)-cinnamic acid

Figure 2.12

Carboxylic esters

These compounds often have an intensely sweet and fruity odor and can be produced from the corresponding terpene alcohol and a carboxylic acid. The highest levels are reached on maturity of the fruit/plant or on full bloom of the flower. In bergamot, as the fruit ripens, linalool is converted to linalyl acetate. In peppermint, (−)-menthol is converted to (−)-menthyl acetate (see Figure 2.13).

The names of esters generally contain the roots: -yl and –ate. The –yl derives from the parent alcohol, and the –ate from the parent carboxylic acid, e.g., linalyl acetate from linalool and acetic acid (Box 2.11).

Box 2.11

Examples of carboxylic esters

Benzyl acetate	(S)-(+)-Lavandulyl acetate
Benzyl benzoate	(−)-Linalyl acetate
Benzyl cinnamate	(−)-Menthyl acetate (Figure 2.13)
Benzyl salicylate	Methyl anthranilate
(−)-Bornyl acetate	Methyl benzoate
Butyl angelate	Methyl cinnamate
β-Citronellyl acetate	Methyl salicylate
β-Citronellyl formate	Neryl acetate
Dimethyl anthranilate	cis-Sabinyl acetate
Eugenyl acetate	α-Terpinyl acetate
Geranyl acetate	

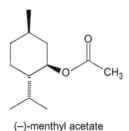

(−)-menthyl acetate

Figure 2.13

Lactones

Lactones are cyclic esters. Many simple examples occur in essential oils, as well as more complex molecules, which have low volatility. Sesquiterpene lactones are notorious for their tendency to be skin sensitizers (Warshaw & Zug 1996). Alantolactone, massoia lactone and dehydrocostus lactone are all potentially allergenic. The names of lactones are rather variable, although the suffixes -olide and -lactone are fairly common (Box 2.12).

Coumarin is a benzenoid lactone that is found in several essential oils, as well as in the form of derivatives. Consisting of two fused rings, it might be considered as a structural moiety as well as a functional group. Coumarin has a vanilla-like odor,

---

Box 2.12

Examples of lactones

Alantolactone
cis-Ambrettolide
Costunolide
Coumarin
Dehydrocostus lactone (Figure 2.14)
Massoia lactone
(Z,E)-Nepetalactone
(−)-Pentadecanolide

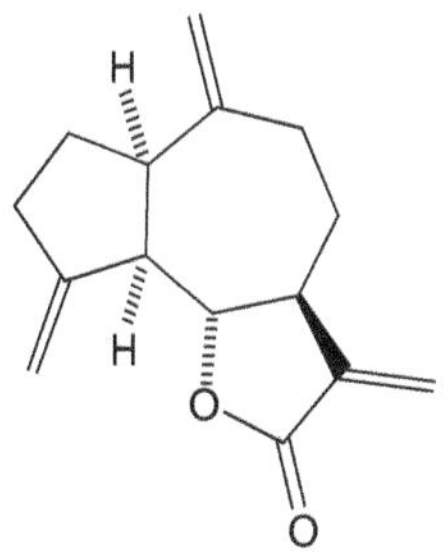

---

dehydrocostus lactone

Figure 2.14

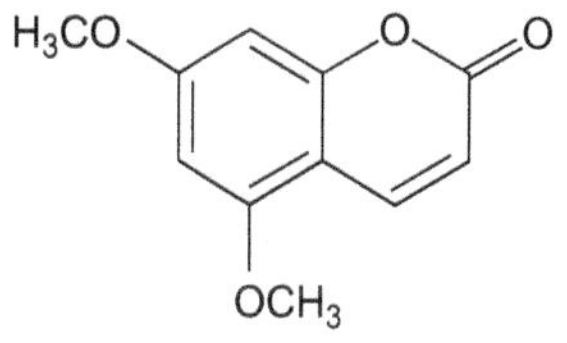

H₃CO ... OCH₃

citropten

Figure 2.15

and is responsible for the smell of new-mown hay. Citropten (Figure 2.15), the 5,7-dimethoxy derivative of coumarin, is phototoxic.

Oxygen-bridged groups

Ethers

Ethers are compounds in which an oxygen atom in the molecule is bonded to two carbon atoms. A number of ethers are illustrated in Figure 12.1, also see Box 2.13. Ethers also exist in cyclic forms, where an oxygen atom forms part of a ring. These ethers are also known as oxides. The most important oxide found in essential oils is cineole, which exists in two forms. The more abundant form is 1,8-cineole (see Figure 2.16). The other form, 1,4-cineole, occurs much more rarely in essential oils. Another type of cyclic ether is the epoxide. In this case, the oxygen atom forms part of a 3-membered ring with two carbon atoms. These are frequently formed during oxidative metabolism of alkenes, and are very reactive because the ring is highly strained. They may also form as degradation products, e.g., limonene 1,2-epoxide.

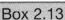

Box 2.13

Examples of ethers and oxides

Ethers	Oxides
(E)-Anethole	α-Bisabolol oxide A
Dill apiole	α-Bisabolone oxide A
β-Asarone	β-Caryophyllene oxide
p-Cresyl methyl ether	1,8-Cineole (Figure 2.16)
Elemicin	Geranyl oxide
Estragole	Linalool oxide A
Methyleugenol	(2R)-Nerol oxide
(Z)-O-Methyl isoeugenol	(−)-cis-Rose oxide
Phenylethyl methyl ether	Sclareol oxide
Myristicin	
Safrole	

Box 2.14

Examples of furans

α-Agarofuran
3-Butyl phthalide
(Z)-Butylidine phthalide
Dihydrobenzofuran
(Z)-Ligustilide
(6R)-(+)-Menthofuran (Figure 2.18)

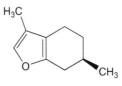

(6R)-(+)-menthofuran

Figure 2.18

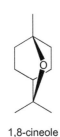

1,8-cineole

Figure 2.16

Furanocoumarins

Furan also forms part of the structure of furanocoumarins, of which there are several examples (Box 2.15). These compounds are typically phototoxic, and include bergapten (see Figure 2.19) found in many citrus fruit oils, and methoxsalen found in rue oil. Here, the furanocoumarin moiety might contribute as a functional group or, because of its size and rigidity, merely as a structural framework. In other words, it might participate in strong or weak intermolecular interactions.

Peroxides

In peroxides, two atoms of oxygen form a link between two carbon atoms. Peroxides are unusual, highly reactive chemicals that decompose easily at high temperatures (sometimes explosively) and on prolonged exposure to air or water. A typical example is the toxic ascaridole (Figure 2.17), found in wormseed oil. Few other peroxides exist in essential oils.

Box 2.15

Examples of furanocoumarins

Angelicin
Bergamottin
Bergapten (Figure 2.19)
Bergaptol
Byakangelicin
Imperatorin
Isopimpinellin
Methoxsalen
Oxypeucedanin
Psoralen

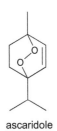

ascaridole

Figure 2.17

Furans

In furans, an oxygen atom is incorporated as part of a 5-membered ring. It is considered as an aromatic ring because it has chemical properties in common with benzene. Furan may also be regarded as a cyclic ether. Few essential oils contain furans, but menthofuran (see Figure 2.18) occurs in most mint oils. The names of some furans are given in Box 2.14.

bergapten

Figure 2.19

Other compounds

Sulfur compounds

These rather reactive and pungent molecules are found in only a few essential oils. They have relatively simple structures, and do not contain terpene or phenylpropanoid hydrocarbon moieties. The chemical names for sulfur-containing molecules usually include the letter sequences: sulf- or -thio- (Box 2.16) and include sulfides, disulfides, trisulfides, sulfoxides and isothiocyanates.

Box 2.16

Examples of sulfur compounds

Allyl isothiocyanate (Figure 2.20)
Allyl propyl disulfide
Benzyl isothiocyanate
Diallyl disulfide
Diallyl sulfide
Diallyl thiosulfinate (= allicin)
Dipropyl disulfide
Dimethyl disulfide
Methyl disulfide
Methyl allyl disulfide
Methyl allyl trisulfide
Phenylethyl isothiocyanate

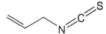

allyl isothiocyanate

Figure 2.20

Nitrogen compounds

Indole (Figure 2.21) is an alkaloid (alkali-like compound) that occurs in jasmine, and some other floral absolutes. It contains a benzene ring fused to a heterocyclic pyrrole ring (see Indole profile, Chapter 14).

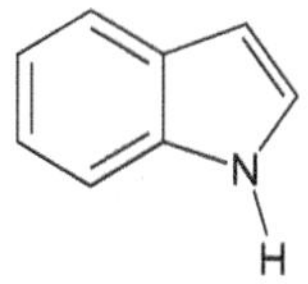

indole

Figure 2.21

Inorganic compounds

Hydrocyanic acid (hydrogen cyanide) is a highly toxic, inorganic acid that is found in bitter almond oil. It forms during distillation, but it is removed before the oil is used.

Summary

- A typical essential oil is a complex mixture of some 20–200 organic compounds, the great majority being present at levels of less than 1%. If sufficiently potent, these may still be important either therapeutically or toxicologically.
- Essential oils are moderately volatile and lipid-soluble, and have a very small degree of water solubility.
- Essential oils are either distilled or, in the case of citrus oils, cold-pressed. Other forms of aromatic extract include concretes, absolutes, resinoids and CO_2 extracts.
- There is a degree of variation in the concentrations of constituents in essential oils from the same species of plant. This is due to factors such as the plant's environment and growing conditions, harvesting and distillation techniques, or genetics.
- Plants of the same species that generate essential oils with quite different constituent profiles are called chemotypes. Chemotypes are genetically determined.
- Essential oils are not generally subject to microbial contamination.
- Contaminants such as phthalate esters and biocides may be found in essential oils, and traces of solvents such as cyclohexane may be present in absolutes.
- Essential oils are subject to adulteration, in which either odorous or non-odorous substances are added to increase volume and, therefore, profits.
- Contaminants and adulterants are generally detectable by laboratory analysis, such as GC, MS and NMR spectroscopy.
- Contamination or adulteration may increase toxicity.
- Some essential oils are very sensitive to the effects of light, heat, air and moisture. To avoid degradation, all essential oils should be stored away from direct sunlight in tightly stoppered dark glass bottles in a cool place such as a refrigerator.
- The addition of antioxidants to essential oils prone to oxidation (or preparations containing them) is recommended.
- Degradation can lead to increased hazards. The oxidation of some terpenes, for instance, makes them more likely to cause skin sensitization.
- Most toxic effects of essential oils are attributable to known constituents.
- Each essential oil constituent is composed of one or more functional groups attached to a hydrocarbon skeleton. It is the combined effects of these constituents that lend the oil characteristics such as odor, therapeutic properties and toxicity.
- The types of compound found in essential oils include hydrocarbons, alcohols, phenols, aldehydes, ketones, esters, ethers, peroxides, lactones, carboxylic acids, furans, furanocoumarins and sulfur compounds.
- Phenols are often irritants, aldehydes and sesquiterpene lactones may be skin sensitizers, some ethers are carcinogenic, and some bicyclic, monoterpenoid ketones are neurotoxic.

- Isomers are compounds that have identical numbers and types of constituent atoms, but differ in the ways in which their atoms are arranged in the molecule. Structural isomers differ in the way that their atoms are connected together, while geometric and optical isomers have the same connections between atoms, but different arrangements of atoms in space.

Notes

1. It is important, for reasons of clarity, to distinguish between the various types of oils and extracts, and not all of them are referred to as 'essential oils'. Unfortunately, however, there is no single word to describe the whole family of aromatic extracts, especially since for many people the word 'extract' connotes a material that is specifically not an essential oil.

2. CO_2 extracts are relatively new and little used, and consequently there is little or no toxicological data on them. However, they are used in aromatherapy, as are the even newer 'phytols'. Both CO_2 extracts and phytols (not to be confused with the constituent, phytol) more closely resemble the aromatic material as it occurs in the plant, than do essential oils, but they are both more costly.

3. β-Eudesmol, and various wood essential oils, mitigate the toxic effects of organophosphorus pesticides (Chiou et al 1995; Li et al 2006).

Toxicity

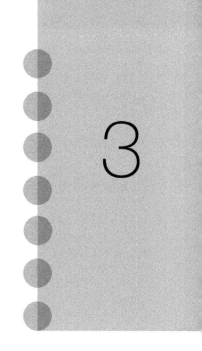

3

CHAPTER CONTENTS

This chapter addresses the identification, assessment and management of toxic risks associated with the use of essential oils.

Adverse effects

Toxicology is the study of harmful or adverse events which occur as a result of interactions between foreign substances (xenobiotics) and living systems. The Environmental Protection Agency (EPA) defines an adverse effect as 'any biochemical, physiological, anatomical, pathological, and/or behavioral change that results in functional impairment that may affect the performance of the whole organism or reduce the ability of the organism to respond to an additional challenge.' Not all xenobiotic effects are adverse, and the judgement of what constitutes an adverse effect is sometimes difficult.

Toxicity can manifest locally or systemically in a number of ways. It may involve the reversible or irreversible disruption of normal biochemical processes, which may result in impairment or loss of cell viability and regenerative capacity. In extreme cases, whole organs may fail and the organism may die. Localized acute toxicity usually affects organs responsible for absorption and elimination due to such factors as the presence of particular enzymes, local blood supply, and the organ's regenerative capacity. These include the skin, stomach, liver, intestines, lungs and kidneys. This kind of toxicity is named after the organ or tissue affected, e.g., nephrotoxicity for the kidneys and hepatotoxicity for the liver. Systemic toxicity may take the form of carcinogenicity, impaired immunity, changes in body weight, etc.

Toxicity also depends on the frequency of use and on the susceptibility of the individual. Individual sensitivity to potentially toxic substances can vary considerably, depending on such factors as age, sex, genetic profile, nutritional status and health status. These can be explained by differences in metabolic and eliminative capacity, drug interactions, and so on (Dybing et al 2002). Thus, infants, those taking prescription medication, pregnant women, the elderly, and people with life-threatening diseases may be at greater risk.

Toxic substances

Contact with potentially harmful substances is unavoidable. They are found in food, water, air, cleaning products, medications and toiletries, and are encountered both in the workplace and in the home. Among the 'poisons' found in commonly consumed foods are cyanogenetic glycosides (cyanide precursors) in apple seeds and almonds, teratogenic alkaloids in green potatoes, allyl isothiocyanate in cabbage and broccoli, and acetaldehyde, a carcinogen found in most fruits and many vegetables. The quantities of such toxic substances to which we are exposed do not normally represent a hazard because they are efficiently handled by the body's detoxification and other defense mechanisms. The process of risk assessment is described below.

In the case of medicines, a dose has to be found at which the therapeutic benefits outweigh any adverse effects. An approximate estimate of the window of drug safety can be gained from the therapeutic index (TI), as shown in Box 3.1. The larger the value of TI, the greater is the margin of safety. For commonly used drugs, TI varies from about 2 for digoxin to about 100 for diazepam. Notably, the TI for ethanol is about 10. The TI is regarded as a very rough measure of safety because it can vary between individuals, species, end-points and routes of administration. There is also the possibility of idiosyncratic toxic effects. A more useful estimate of drug safety is the standard margin of safety (Box 3.1), which compares the lowest dose required to produce a toxic effect with the highest dose required to produce a therapeutic effect. This estimate does not rely on the slopes of the dose–response curves being similar. A value of <1 would mean that a dose effective in 99% of a population would be toxic in more than 1% (Fleming 2003)

According to Paracelsus (1493–1541), all substances are potentially toxic, and their toxicity is related to the administered dose. However, it would be more accurate to say that the toxicity of a substance depends on its concentration at the site of damage and its inherent toxicity, i.e., its toxicokinetic (relating to its movement to its site of action) and toxicodynamic (relating to its actions on target sites) characteristics. These include:

- the dose and concentration applied
- the route of administration
- the mode of administration
- the bioavailability
- the mechanism of toxicity.

It should be borne in mind that a xenobiotic substance may be inherently toxic or it may be metabolized into a toxic substance in the body. For further details of toxicokinetics see Chapter 4.

Where information on the toxicity of essential oils in humans is available, we have used it preferentially throughout this book. Where such information is not available, we have attempted to extrapolate from more indirect data obtained from cell and animal studies. We have also considered the known actions of antitoxic constituents, as well as those of toxic ones.

Toxicity of mixtures

Toxicity testing is more frequently concerned with single pure substances than with mixtures, and sophisticated models have been developed to assess their safety. Essential oils, which are categorized by regulatory agencies as 'natural complex substances', present a particular challenge because they are not only mixtures, but different batches/sources/varieties contain different concentrations of toxic constituents. A standard approach to regulation, however, is to assume the highest level. This is not unreasonable, except that there is an assumption that the mixture will precisely reflect the toxicity of its constituents.

In many applications, two or more essential oils are frequently employed in combination. When those oils contain the same toxic constituent, or different constituents that exhibit the same type of toxicity, this should be taken into account when considering maximum safe doses. This could apply to skin irritants, allergens, phototoxins, neurotoxins, teratogens, carcinogens, hepatotoxins or drug interactors. In this book, we have assumed that such actions are additive. For example, lemongrass and lemon myrtle oils both contain citral, and both have limits of 0.7% for skin sensitization (and also teratogenicity) assuming 80% citral and a citral limit of 0.6%. But if both essential oils were used together, the limit would need to be 0.7% of the combined oils.

Interactions between compounds

The toxicity of a substance may be increased or decreased through interactions with other substances present in the body. In the case of an administered essential oil, interactions can occur between one or more of its constituents, as well as between a constituent and an orthodox drug or a food item.

Interactions between constituents in a mixture are notoriously difficult to predict. When two or more substances are co-administered, three outcomes are possible. The simplest is 'additivity', where the action and potency of the mixture are as predicted from the known actions and quantities of its constituents.[1] A second possibility is 'synergy' (sometimes referred to as synergism or potentiation). In this case, the mixture's

---

Box 3.1

Estimating the margin for drug safety

$$\text{Therapeutic index} = \frac{LD_{50}}{ED_{50}} \quad \text{or} \quad \frac{TD_{50}}{ED_{50}}$$

$$\text{Standard margin of safety} = \frac{LD_1}{ED_{99}} \quad \text{or} \quad \frac{TD_1}{ED_{99}}$$

Where LD_1 and LD_{50} are the doses causing deaths in 1% and 50% of a test population, or more generally, TD_1 and TD_{50} are the doses causing a toxic effect in 1% and 50% of a test population; ED_{50} and ED_{99} are the doses causing a therapeutic effect in 50% and 99% of the test population.

action is significantly greater than would be expected on the basis of additivity. In the context of pharmacology, this would be desirable because the therapeutic dose can be reduced. However, in terms of toxicology, an enhanced effect would be undesirable. The third possible outcome is 'antagonism', which is the opposite of synergy. On administering two substances simultaneously, the observed action is less than anticipated. While this may be unfavorable for a therapeutic effect, it would be beneficial for toxicity.

An apparently synergistic effect was seen when linalyl acetate, terpineol and ($\pm$)-camphor were tested individually or in pairs for in vitro activity against two human colon cancer cell lines. Neither camphor nor terpineol alone had any effect, linalyl acetate had a minimal effect, and linalyl acetate and terpineol together were moderately effective, causing 33% and 45% reduction in proliferation of the two cell lines. However, when all three compounds were used together, cell proliferation was reduced by 50% and 64% in the two cell lines. There was no toxic effect on normal intestinal cells (Itani et al 2008).

An antagonistic effect in essential oils is exemplified by the reduced toxicity of carvacrol in the presence of thymol (Karpouhtsis et al 1998). This apparently manifests in thyme oil high in thymol and/or carvacrol which contains a combined total of 30.9–79.9% thymol plus carvacrol (see Ch. 13, p. 266–267). The rat oral LD_{50} values of these constituents are 980 mg/kg and 810 mg/kg, respectively. (LD_{50} is defined under 'Acute oral toxicity' below.) If we assume an average LD_{50} for each of 895 mg/kg, then the LD_{50} of a thymol/carvacrol CT thyme oil would range from a possible 1,118–2,887 mg/kg. However, the rat oral LD_{50} of this type of thyme oil is 4,700 mg/kg, making it about half as toxic as would be predicted from the thymol and carvacrol content. Antagonism in skin sensitization is known as quenching. (+)-Limonene had a quenching effect on cinnamaldehyde sensitization in 3 of 11 human subjects, and eugenol had a similar quenching effect in 7 of the same 11 cinnamaldehyde-sensitive subjects. It is postulated that this may be due to competitive inhibition at the receptor level (Guin et al 1984). The same may be true of thymol and carvacrol, which are isomeric.

Like fruits and vegetables, essential oils contain complex mixtures of chemicals that may be harmful and/or protective. Plants are vulnerable to oxidative stress because they produce oxygen and reactive oxygen species during photosynthesis. As protection, plants biosynthesize an assortment of potent antioxidants. An antioxidant action is considered fundamental to many antitoxic effects, such as mitigating phototoxicity, allergenicity or mutagenicity. This can be seen, for example, in the antihepatotoxic actions of carvacrol, thymol and eugenol (Jiménez et al 1993; Kumaravelu et al 1995), the gastroprotective effect of 1,8-cineole (Santos & Rao 2001), the antinephrotoxic action of thymoquinone (Badary 1999) and the antimutagenic action of linalool (Berić et al 2007). Also see Table 9.3.

In other cases, an effect may be seen as either countering potential toxicity, or simply as therapeutic, e.g., the anticonvulsant effects of anise oil or cumin oil (Pourgholami et al 1999; Sayyah et al 2002b), the anti-asthmatic action of turmeric oil and may chang oil (Li et al 1998; Qian et al 1980) and the anticarcinogenic action of (+)-limonene and perillyl alcohol in skin cancer (Lluria-Prevatt et al 2002; Raphael & Kuttan 2003a, 2003b).

An observed effect may be enhanced or diminished by constituents in a mixture that do not express that effect directly themselves. For example, in essential oils that contain small amounts of carcinogens, the presence of large amounts of antioxidant, antimutagenic, anticarcinogenic constituents can render the oil non-carcinogenic (see Ch. 9, p. 183).

Although the toxicity of an essential oil cannot always be predicted from its chemical composition, the actions of major constituents tend to dominate. For example, the toxicity of methyl salicylate and wintergreen oil (~98% methyl salicylate) are essentially identical, the carcinogenicity of safrole is very similar to that of sassafras oil (62–90% safrole), and the potential for skin sensitization of cinnamaldehyde is very similar to that of cassia oil (73–90% cinnamaldehyde). In many other essential oils, toxic compounds occur only as minor constituents, and when there are antitoxic compounds present in much greater concentrations, toxicity is unlikely. When neither toxic nor antitoxic constituents predominate, assumptions as to outcome are more problematic.

Human toxicity

The number of incidents of an adverse reaction to an essential oil depends on:

- its inherent toxicity
- the number of people exposed to it
- the degree of exposure (oil concentration and time of exposure).

For example, the two most widely used essential oils in aromatherapy are lavender and tea tree, but there are more confirmed cases of both poisoning and adverse skin reactions for tea tree oil than there are for lavender oil. In this scenario, both the number of people exposed and the degree of exposure are similar, but tea tree oil is inherently more toxic. Similarly, cinnamon bark and spearmint oils are both widely used as flavoring agents in chewing gums, toothpastes and mouthwashes, but there are more reported oral adverse reactions for cinnamon than for spearmint.

Most cinnamon reactions are allergic, and such reactions are due to repeated exposure. Repeated exposure to toxic substances at subacute toxic doses may lead to a variety of chronic effects either due to accumulation of a substance in the body to a toxic level, or to a cumulative effect on tissues and/or organs. Here, we may be dealing with the same overt signs and symptoms of poisoning as for acute exposure, or different ones such as may result, for example, from chronic suppression of certain enzymes. This may be a consideration where products containing essential oils or their constituents are used on a regular basis.

Poisoning from accidental overdose is the most frequently reported type of toxicity in humans, followed by adverse skin reactions. (The latter may in fact be more prevalent, but only Sweden has a reporting system for these.)

Poisoning

Virtually all cases of serious poisoning from essential oils are a consequence of oral ingestion of the undiluted oil, in amounts much higher than therapeutic doses. Judging from the large quantities ingested, a few were probably suicides. (Death from essential oil overdose is slow, and can take from 15 minutes to 3 days.) Of the many non-fatal accidents, only two cases cite long-term ill effects, one involving wintergreen oil and one wormseed oil (Kröber 1936; Heng 1987). In fatal or near-fatal cases, a variety of signs and symptoms are possible, such as convulsions, vomiting, and rapid breathing, depending on the essential oil ingested (see Table 15.1).

Many cases of wintergreen oil poisoning have been recorded. In six cases of poisoning in adults, three people survived after ingesting 6 mL, 16 mL and 24 mL, and three died from ingestion of 15 mL, 30 mL and 80 mL (Stevenson 1937). None of these cases received any medical intervention. If we take an average of the non-fatal doses (15.3 mL), and an average of the fatal doses (41.7 mL), this gives a human median lethal dose of 0.2–0.6 mL/kg assuming the individuals were of average weight.[2]

Camphor and methyl salicylate, and the oils of clove, cinnamon and eucalyptus, are most frequently and consistently reported to cause toxicity. There are many instances of eucalyptus oil poisoning, and it is thought to be fatal to humans in oral doses between 30 mL and 60 mL (Gurr & Scroggie 1965).

In recent years, cases of tea tree oil ingestion have escalated in the USA, rising from 280 incidents and 11 adverse reactions in 2001, to 966 incidents and 30 adverse reactions in 2006. For comparison, adverse reactions to clove oil were 10 and 13 in the same two years (Table 3.1). With less frequency, ingestion of citronella, hyssop, pennyroyal, sage, sassafras, thuja or wormseed oil has all caused toxicity in humans. This may not be a comprehensive list, since most essential oils will probably cause serious problems if drunk in sufficient quantity. Availability can also influence statistics, as is suggested by the increase in tea tree cases.

The majority of cases of essential oil poisoning involve accidents with young children, often between 1 and 3 years of age. Approximately 75% of cases in the USA are in children up to 6 years old (Table 3.2). Parents (and consumers in general) need to be aware of the risks. Perhaps contrary to expectation, young children will

Table 3.1 Adverse reactions to essential oils in the USA

Essential oil	2001	2002	2003	2004	2005	2006
Clove	10	9	28	15	22	13
Cinnamon	22	13	24	34	29	18
Eucalyptus	8	9	6	12	5	3
Pennyroyal	1	0	4	1	5	0
Tea tree	11	9	28	30	35	30
Unknown oils	65	75	55	48	53	30

Information from: Bronstein et al 2007; Lai et al 2006; Litovitz et al 2001, 2002; Watson et al 2003, 2004, 2005. Information for specific oils not recorded before 2001.

Table 3.2 Essential oil incidents reported to the central toxicity database in the USA 1997–2006

Year	Total no. of exposures	Age			Outcome				
		<6	6-19	>19	None	Minor	Moderate	Major	Fatal
1997	3,990	2,720	508	651	1,021	1,224	67	4	0
1998	4,066	2,758	460	697	1,057	1,197	72	5	0
1999	4,099	2,772	435	779	958	1,166	78	9	1
2000	4,960	3,595	444	898	1,038	1,245	87	4	0
2001	6,456	4,842	509	1,088	1,547	1,422	93	7	0
2002	7,242	5,416	544	1,234	1,731	1,617	106	5	1
2003	7,310	5,561	568	1,162	1,810	1,498	117	3	0
2004	6,125	4,418	513	1,143	1,395	1,457	96	5	1
2005	7,282	5,422	567	1,239	1,699	1,462	110	6	0
2006	7,030	5,477	417	921	1,691	1,351	99	4	0

Information from: Bronstein et al 2007; Lai et al 2006; Litovitz et al 1998, 1999, 2000, 2001, 2002; Watson et al 2003, 2004, 2005.

drink an undiluted essential oil. One report tells of a 10-month-old infant who stood up in her crib, reached for a bottle of camphorated oil, removed the cap, and drank approximately 1 oz (about 30 mL) (Jacobziner & Raybin 1962a). In an Australian report of eucalyptus oil poisoning, 78 of 109 children of 5 years or less ingested solutions intended for vaporization, and the majority were ages 1–3 years (Day & Ozanne-Smith 1997).

Children are at risk because:

- their natural inquisitiveness leads them to examine materials by putting them in their mouths
- a liquid that is being examined by a child will probably be swallowed rather than sipped
- being smaller than adults, children are more susceptible to toxic substances
- metabolism in very young children is less effective than in adults.

Some unfortunate infants have died because a parent administered the essential oil by mistake, thinking it was, for example, castor oil. Some died because the essential oil was intentionally administered, either by a parent or doctor, who was not aware of the toxic consequences. But in most cases, a bottle of essential oil was within reach of the child and they were able to open it.

Essential oil poisoning in children is not a new problem. In 1953 Craig & Fraser (cited in Craig 1953) reported that of 502 cases of accidental poisoning in children (1931–1951, Aberdeen and Edinburgh), 74 were due to essential oils. Of 454 deaths from accidental poisoning in childhood that occurred in Britain during a similar period, 54 were caused by essential oils (Craig 1953). Statistics compiled for the USA show that in 1973 there were reports of 530 ingestions of camphor-containing products, 415 in children under the age of 5 years (Phelan 1976). The same year, doctors recommended that the sale of camphorated oil should be restricted (Bellman 1973). In all of these cases the products involved were over-the-counter (OTC) preparations, the majority being camphorated oil. Many OTC products contain camphor at 1–10% (Kauffman et al 1994). Camphorated oil contains similar quantities of camphor to several essential oils (20%), and the risk to young children from these oils is very similar.

There have also been serious toxic incidents in young children who have inhaled preparations containing essential oils that have been mistakenly instilled into the nasal cavity (see Ch. 6, p. 108).

Adverse skin reactions

There has never been a recorded fatality from the dermal absorption of an essential oil. Non-fatal systemic toxicity is possible, although this has occurred only very rarely. The true extent of adverse skin reactions to essential oils is not known, and estimates vary widely.

Photosensitivity

Among the essential oils known to increase light sensitivity, only the citrus oils are widely used. Oils of bergamot, lemon and lime are the most commonly reported causes of photosensitivity (see Ch. 5, p. 85). At the time of writing, the latest report we could find was for bergamot oil (Kaddu et al 2001). Fresh limes, often in use during sunny weather, are also a frequent cause.

Contact dermatitis

Most cases of contact dermatitis to essential oils are allergic as distinct from irritant, but in the context of this chapter, the difference is largely academic. Dermatologists have carried out thousands of patch tests using essential oils or, more commonly, constituents. This provides valuable information in terms of comparing the relative potencies of substances. However, only a small percentage of those reacting positively to a patch test actually have a skin problem that has been caused by an essential oil.

Only those essential oils used in patch testing can contribute to statistics, and the ones that are most commonly tested—sandalwood oil, jasmine absolute, narcissus absolute, tea tree oil, ylang-ylang oil—tend to be those used in previous patch tests. There are many reports of tea tree oil reactions (see below), but we could find none for narcissus absolute or sandalwood oil. There are a small number of cases each for ylang-ylang oil and jasmine absolute, as there are also for black seed oil and laurel leaf oil, though these last two are not routinely used in patch testing.

The essential oils used in patch testing also tend to be those for which allergenic constituents have not been identified. Testing does not usually include, for example, cinnamon bark oil, since its major constituent, cinnamaldehyde, is routinely used in patch testing. We found four cases of cinnamon oil allergy (presumably bark oil) over a 30 year period: one caused by skin contact with the undiluted oil (Sparks 1985), two from an ointment containing cinnamon oil (Calnan 1976), and one from a cinnamon oil mud bath (Garcéa-Abujeta et al 2005).

Skin allergies often follow an epidemiological pattern:

- a new cosmetic ingredient is introduced
- there are virtually no reports of adverse reactions
- its use becomes widespread
- over the course of several decades, reports of adverse reactions escalate
- use of the ingredient is restricted or otherwise reduced
- reports of adverse reactions decline.

Turpentine oil was a well-known contact allergen for a long time, mainly through occupational exposure, but when the mass paint industry replaced it with petroleum-based substitutes for paint thinning, reported cases of turpentine oil allergy decreased (Schnuch et al 2004a). Similarly, cold-pressed laurel berry oil (which contains some essential oil) was widely used as a conditioner for felt hats for about 100 years (1860–1960). By the 1940s it was recognized as a major cause of dermatitis, and the felt industry ceased using laurel oil in 1962. Since 1975, there have been no reports of laurel berry oil allergy.

Not every widely used essential oil causes skin problems. We found four case reports of confirmed dermatitis from citronella oil, but all of them were from contact with the undiluted oil and none of them is recent (Keil 1947; Lane 1922). Considering the extensive application of citronella oil in insect repellants for many decades, the apparent lack of skin reactions is notable. Similarly, in spite of the widespread use of lavender oil in the West since about 1990, we could only find only five confirmed instances of dermatitis from 1991–2000: two involved the undiluted oil being dripped onto pillows at night and causing facial dermatitis (Coulson & Khan 1999), two were cases with multiple sensitivities to essential oils (Schaller & Korting 1995;

Selvaag et al 1995), and one was an aromatherapist with hand dermatitis (Keane et al 2000).

Reported cases of tea tree oil allergy are more prevalent for this period. For the years 1991–2000, we found 29 cases, and in 21 of them the undiluted oil was used (Apted 1991; De Groot & Weyland 1993; Elliott 1993; Knight & Hausen 1994; Selvaag et al 1994, 1995; De Groot 1996; Bhushan & Beck 1997; Hackzell-Bradley et al 1997; D'Urben 1998; Rubel et al 1998; Khanna et al 2000; Varma et al 2000; Vilaplana & Romaguera 2000). One case was caused by airborne vapors, another by ingestion of the essential oil.

Even these few examples illustrate the increased risk of using undiluted essential oils on the skin. Single case reports are not a highly accurate reflection of incidence, since some cases are unrecorded. They do, however, give an approximation of the extent of a problem.

Adverse oral reactions

These may be caused by any product applied to the mouth or lips, such as mouthwash, toothpaste, toothpicks, lipstick, lip balm, etc. Adverse reactions include 'stomatitis', inflammation of the oral mucous membrane, and 'cheilitis', inflammation of the lips.

We found two case reports of cheilitis to spearmint oil in toothpaste (Poon & Freeman 2006; Skrebova et al 1998), but none for peppermint oil. For cinnamon, not always defined as cinnamon bark oil, Allen & Blozis (1988) reported 10 cases of cheilitis, most from chewing gum, Miller et al (1992) reported 14 cases of cinnamon stomatitis, and we identified a total of 39 further cases of oral adverse reactions (Cohen & Bhattacharyya 2000; Endo & Rees 2007; Tremblay & Avon 2008).

Other adverse reactions

Various other adverse reactions have been reported from clinical trials. In a wound healing pilot study, a 3% concentration of lemon myrtle oil caused increased pain and inflammation in some patients, and was discontinued (Kerr 2002). In a dandruff trial using 5% tea tree oil in a shampoo base, 1 of 63 patients reported mild scalp itching; however, 3 of 62 patients who used the shampoo base only reported the same symptom; one patient in each group reported mild scalp burning (Satchell et al 2002b). In a head lice repellent trial, a formulation with 3.7% citronella oil was administered daily for four months to the heads of 103 children. One child reported a slight itching and burning sensation (Mumcuoglu et al 2004).

In various trials involving the oral administration of peppermint oil or peppermint + caraway, there have been a small number of heartburn reactions, usually because patients chew capsules instead of swallowing them, and they are not meant to dissolve in the stomach (see Table 9.1).

Measuring toxicity

Animal toxicity

Although animal models can provide useful estimates for the toxicity of xenobiotics in humans, reliable predictions need to take account of any known toxicokinetic or toxicodynamic differences between the species. Many end-points have been used for the assessment of toxicity in animals, ranging from lethality to irritancy, not all of which are necessarily relevant to human exposure.

Acute toxicity refers to single or short-term repeated exposure (up to 24 hours) to a toxic substance. (It can be fatal, and, in humans, may result from either an intentional or accidental overdose, particularly in a young child.) For longer term exposure, terminology varies according to duration. Thus, if dosing is repeated for 14–28 days, it is known as subacute toxicity; if repeated over 90 days, it is termed subchronic toxicity; and if repeated for 12 months or longer is called chronic toxicity. Adverse effects from repeated-dose tests may include outward signs such as body weight reduction or growth inhibition, tissue abnormalities in organs or glands such as hypertrophy, hyperplasia or tumor formation, or cellular damage such as necrosis or DNA mutation.

The most commonly used animals for toxicity tests are rats and mice; hamsters or guinea pigs are used for some tests, and rabbits are normally used to assess dermal toxicity and eye irritation. Testing for adverse skin reactions, carcinogenicity and reproductive toxicity is discussed in the chapters covering those subjects, but alternatives to traditional animal testing for these are included below.

Toxicity tests approved by The Organisation for Economic Co-operation and Development (OECD) are listed in Box 3.2. This is a representative summary of currently used tests, but does not list every type of test referred to in this text.

Acute oral toxicity

First introduced in 1927, the conventional measure of acute toxicity is the LD_{50}: the dose that kills 50% of a group of animals, or median lethal dose. Different doses of the test substance are administered to matched groups of animals, usually rats or mice. LD_{50} values vary with species and route of administration. For instance, the acute oral LD_{50} value for wormseed oil in rats is 255 mg/kg, and 380 mg/kg in mice, and the acute dermal LD_{50} in rabbits is 415 mg/kg. Dermal LD_{50} values are generally similar to or higher than oral values, and the more invasive intraperitoneal (ip) LD_{50} is always lower than the oral value (Table 3.3).

Since the actual lethal dose of a substance varies with body size, the LD_{50} is expressed as milligrams of substance per kilogram of body weight. Therefore, the more toxic an essential oil is, the lower the value will be. The most toxic essential oil, boldo leaf, has an acute oral LD_{50} in rats of 130 mg/kg. The most toxic constituent (or in this case artifact) of any essential oil, hydrocyanic acid, has an estimated lethal dose in humans of 0.8 mg/kg.

Table 3.4 gives examples of human lethal doses assuming direct extrapolation from the animal data.

Table 3.5 illustrates the classifications that are generally accepted by toxicologists (Niesink et al 1996). Going by this standard, of the 200 or so essential oils that have been tested for acute oral toxicity, there are none that are either 'extremely toxic' or 'very toxic', the most toxic ones being 'moderately toxic'. The great majority of essential oils would fall into the 'slightly toxic' or 'non-toxic' categories. Table 3.3 lists some essential oils and constituents with LD_{50} values below 1 g/kg, but an average above this. Other essential oils, which have not

Box 3.2

The Organisation for Economic Co-operation and Development approved toxicity tests

Animal tests

Acute toxicity
    Oral
    Dermal
    Inhalation (>4 hours)
Subacute toxicity
    Oral (28 days)
    Dermal (21 or 28 days)
    Inhalation (14 or 28 days)
Subchronic toxicity (90 days)
    Oral
    Dermal
    Inhalation
Neurotoxicity (1–12 months or longer)
Uterotrophic bioassay (endocrine disruption)
Chronic toxicity (>12 months)
Carcinogenicity (18–24 months)
Genotoxicity
    Mammalian erythrocyte micronucleus (bone marrow or peripheral blood cells)
    Bone marrow chromosome aberration
    Rodent dominant lethal assay
    Mammalian liver unscheduled DNA synthesis (UDS)
    Mammalian spermatogonial chromosome aberration
    Mouse heritable translocation
    Mouse spot test
Reproductive and developmental toxicity
    Prenatal development
    One-generation reproduction toxicity
    Two-generation reproduction toxicity
    Reproduction/developmental toxicity screening
    Developmental neurotoxicity
Toxicokinetics (single or repeated dose)
Skin sensitization
    Guinea pig maximation test
    Local lymph node assay
Acute eye irritation/corrosion

Insect tests

Sex-linked recessive lethal test in *Drosophila melanogaster* (genotoxicity)

In vitro tests

Skin absorption
Skin corrosion
Phototoxicity
Genotoxicity

    Bacterial reverse mutation (Ames test)
    Saccharomyces cerevisiae miotic recombination
    Saccharomyces cerevisiae gene mutation
    Mammalian cell chromosome aberration
    Mammalian cell sister chromatid exchange
    Mammalian cell gene mutation
    Mammalian cell unscheduled DNA synthesis (UDS)

been tested for toxicity, might also fall into this group. These might include, for example, oils of mustard, horseradish, black seed, Western red cedar, lanyana and great mugwort, all of which contain substantial concentrations of moderately toxic constituents.

The LD_{50} is only a crude measure of toxicity as it uses an extreme end-point, and does not, for example, tell us anything about carcinogenesis or risks in pregnancy. In addition to the LD_{50}, much importance is now given to understanding the processes involved: what biochemical changes take place, how these happen and why. In recent years, alternatives to the LD_{50} have been developed – see Evolving legislation below.

Acute dermal toxicity

Acute dermal LD_{50} values are determined in a similar way to those for oral toxicity, except that the oil is applied to the skin instead of being given orally. (This is a measure of systemic toxicity, rather than toxicity to the skin itself.) Rabbits are routinely used, but rats or guinea pigs are also sometimes used. As with acute oral toxicity, there are problems in extrapolating the data to humans.

An acute dermal LD_{50} value of an essential oil is dependent as much on the percutaneous absorption of the constituents as on their toxicity. So long as human skin and rabbit skin absorb the oil at similar rates, the tests should provide useful information. However, there seems to be no evidence to this effect, and the absorption of chemicals is generally faster through laboratory animal skin (Hotchkiss 1994). In tests with six substances (Figure 3.1), including caffeine and cortisone, absorption rates were notably higher for rabbit than human skin (Bartek et al 1972). Although none of the substances tested were essential oils, they represent a wide range of chemical types and it is likely that many essential oil constituents will behave similarly. As with oral toxicity, metabolic differences between rodents and humans will also be important here.

Acute inhalation toxicity

In many situations involving the use of essential oils, a significant proportion of the constituents will evaporate and be inhaled. Since the respiratory tract is highly vascular and offers a large surface area for absorption, it is important to know the risk of any toxic effects from inhalation. Toxic effects can be assessed in animals by inhalation, but the findings are often qualitative because of uncertainties over the amounts of volatile substances inhaled.

Chronic toxicity

Testing entails repeated dosing for 12 months, or 24 months for carcinogens. The doses are lower than in acute toxicity, but there is a risk of cumulative effects. Blood levels can reach much higher values, and a xenobiotic substance may be taken up into tissues or bound to plasma proteins. It is also possible that it may lead to the development of tolerance as a result of enzyme induction or destruction.

Table 3.3 Toxicity ranking based on rodent LD$_{50}$ values, for orally administered substances

Essential oil	mg/kg value(s) obtained	Mean LD$_{50}$
Extremely toxic		
None		
Very toxic		
None		
Moderately toxic (oral)		
Boldo	130	130
Wormseed	255, 380	318
Wormwood (white)	370	370
Pennyroyal	400	400
Cedarwood (Himalayan)	500	500
Calamus (tetraploid form)	777	777
Thuja	830	830
Almond (bitter, unrectified)	960	960
Wormwood	960	960
Moderately toxic (dermal)		
Cassia	320[a]	320
Savory	340	320
Wormseed	415	415
Oregano	480	480
Cinnamon bark	690[a]	690
Rose absolute	800	800
Boldo	940	800

Constituents	mg/kg value(s) obtained	Mean LD$_{50}$
Extremely toxic		
Hydrocyanic acid	0.8	0.8
Very toxic		
None		
Moderately toxic (oral)		
Diallyl disulphide	130, 145, 260	178
α- and β-Thujone	190, 230	210
p-Cresol	207, 344	276
Allyl isothiocyanate	340	340
Coumarin	196, 202, 293, 680	343
α-Asarone	418	418
β-Pulegone	470	470

Continued

Table 3.3 Toxicity ranking based on rodent LD$_{50}$ values, for orally administered substances—Cont'd

Constituents	mg/kg value(s) obtained	Mean LD$_{50}$
Salicylaldehyde	520	520
β-Thujaplicin	775	775
Carvacrol	810	810
Constituents with LD$_{50}$ values close to 1 g/kg		
Methyl salicylate	700, 887, 1060, 1110, 1250	1001
p-Cresyl methyl ether	207, 1920	1064
2-Phenylethanol	600, 1150, 1790	1180
Methyleugenol	810, 1560	1185
Carvone	770, 1640	1205
Thymol	880, 980, 1800	1220
Moderately toxic (dermal)		
Citronellic acid	450	450
Cinnamaldehyde	590	450

[a]For ease of comparison this measurement has been changed from mL/kg to g/kg.

Table 3.4 Extrapolating rodent toxicity to humans

Toxicity	Essential oil	Rodent LD$_{50}$	Equivalent human lethal dose
Very toxic	None	–	–
Moderately toxic	Boldo oil	0.13 g/kg	9.1 g
Slightly toxic	Cornmint oil	1.25 g/kg	87.5 g
Non-toxic	Lemon oil	>5.0 g/kg	>350 g

The average human adult weighs about 70 kg, so a mean lethal dose of boldo oil would extrapolate to 0.13 g × 70 = 9.1 g. Many essential oils, such as lemon, have an LD$_{50}$ of 5 g/kg or more. For a 70 kg person, this is equivalent to a lethal dose of at least 350 g. This is over 1,000 times more than the maximum amount of 0.31 mL absorbed in an aromatherapy massage (30 mL of oil with 5% of essential oil, and 25% absorption).

Chronic toxicity is expressed in mg/kg/day, as parts per million (ppm) or % of the diet. In chronic toxicity there is usually a 'latency period', a period of time lapsing before any toxic effects appear. In addition to being dose-dependent, chronic toxicity is also dependent on frequency and total length of time of application. If the absorption rate of a substance exceeds the rate of biotransformation and excretion, then the 'body burden', the total amount in the body, will increase. For example, the continuous oral intake of high doses of (E)-anethole, induces

Table 3.5 Toxicity ratings used by toxicologists

Toxicity rating	Toxic dose
Extremely toxic	9 mg/kg or less
Very toxic	10–99 mg/kg
Moderately toxic	100–999 mg/kg
Slightly toxic	1–5 g/kg
Non-toxic	more than 5 g/kg

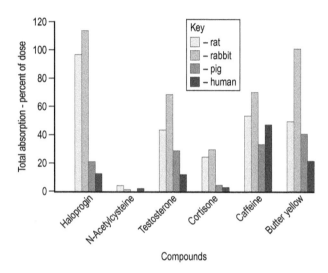

Figure 3.1 • Percutaneous absorption of several compounds in rats, rabbits, pigs and humans. (Reproduced with permission from Bartek M J, LaBudde J A, Maibach H I 1972 Skin permeability in vivo: comparison in rat, rabbit, pig and man. Journal of Investigative Dermatology 58:114-123. © Williams & Wilkins.)

hepatotoxicity in rats when the estimated daily hepatic production of anethole $1',2'$-epoxide, a reactive metabolite, exceeded 30 mg/kg body weight (Newberne et al 1999).

Cytotoxicity

Although cytotoxicity refers to toxicity to individual cells (cyto = cell), the actions of cytotoxic substances can compromise the functioning of whole organs and tissues. Estimates of cytotoxicity are made in vitro using cell cultures, so the test substance comes into direct contact with the cells. There are no complicating toxicokinetic mechanisms to consider, but dose extrapolation from cell to organism can be difficult. For example, information about toxicity to skin cells in vitro has limited value for predicting safe concentrations of substances for application to the skin, since cell cultures lack a protective epidermis. Nevertheless, cytotoxicity to skin cells generally correlates with skin irritation.

Mechanisms

Cell death may be promoted by electrophilic chemical species, free radicals (other than reduced forms of oxygen) or reactive oxygen species (ROS) (Niesink et al 1996). Cytotoxic ROS such as superoxide radicals and hydrogen peroxide are implicated in the etiology of many diseases, including cancer. They are produced in mitochondria during oxidative respiration, but their levels are normally moderated by cellular antioxidants. When these antioxidants become depleted, ROS levels rise and oxidative stress occurs (Ebadi 2001).

When a substance has an adverse effect on a bacterium, we describe it as an antibacterial rather than a cytotoxic effect, although the underlying mechanisms are similar to those that damage either cancer cells or normal cells. For example, the antibacterial activity of high concentrations of tea tree oil against *Staphylococcus aureus* paralleled cytotoxic activity to human skin cells, suggesting a similar mode of action probably involving the cell membrane and bacterial cell wall (Söderberg et al 1996). At lower concentrations, tea tree oil was lethal to methicillin-resistant *S. aureus* and yet not toxic to human fibroblasts (Loughlin et al 2008).

Eugenol, thymol and carvacrol are strongly antibacterial and antioxidant (Burt 2004; Lee KG & Shibamoto 2001; Teissedre & Waterhouse 2000), but methoxylated phenols can act both as antioxidants and pro-oxidants. Eugenol and similar compounds rapidly neutralize free radicals, but are themselves converted to phenoxyl radicals (ArO*). These radicals and their quinone methide products appear to be responsible for the compounds' cytotoxicity. The phenoxyl radical derived from eugenol is much more stable, and therefore less reactive, than ROS, thus affording an overall degree of protection (Fujisawa et al 2002).

Dosage

The actions of some oil constituents appear to depend on dosage. Eugenol was cytotoxic to human dental pulp fibroblasts in vitro (IC_{50} 0.9 mM), as were three other phenolic compounds, guaiacol (IC_{50} 9.8 mM), phenol (IC_{50} 4.5 mM) and thymol (IC_{50} 0.5 mM) (Chang et al 2000). At high doses, eugenol was also cytotoxic to guinea pig neutrophils by stimulating the release of superoxide radicals, reaching a plateau at 5 mM. Thymol was more potent, and *o*-cresol less potent than eugenol (Suzuki et al 1985). At a concentration higher than 3 mM, eugenol was cytotoxic to human oral mucous membrane cells, decreasing both cellular ATP and glutathione. However, at less than 1 mM, eugenol protected cells from the genetic attack of ROS, in part by inhibiting lipid peroxidation (Jeng et al 1994a). Essential oils of tea tree, manuka, eucalyptus, lavender and rosemary decreased the viability of human umbilical vein endothelial cells at 0.5% and above (Takarada et al 2004).

Lavender oil was cytotoxic to human dermal fibroblasts and endothelial cells in vitro at concentrations greater than 0.125% v/v. Linalool (35% of the oil sample) had similar toxicity to the essential oil, while linalyl acetate (51% of the oil sample) was more toxic. Membrane damage was suggested as the mechanism of toxicity of the three agents (Prashar et al 2004). Both eugenol and clove oil were cytotoxic to the same two cell types, clove oil at concentrations as low as 0.03%, indicating a potential for skin irritancy (Prashar et al 2006).

The cytotoxic concentrations for several essential oils are shown in Table 3.6. Even in wound healing, where there is no epidermal barrier, therapeutic concentrations that impart no apparent irritation or toxicity are one or two orders of

Table 3.6 Essential oil cytotoxicity to fibroblasts

Essential oil	Cytotoxic NOAEL (%, time)	Fibroblast cell type	Reference
Lavender	0.125%, 3 hours	Human dermal	Prashar et al 2004
Lemon myrtle	0.0005%[a], 4 hours 0.00005%[a], 24 hours	Human dermal	Hayes & Markovic 2002
Myrrh	0.01%[b], 3 hours 0.0036%[b], 24 hours	Human gingival	Tipton et al 2003
Tea tree	0.01%[c], 24 hours	Human gingival	Söderberg et al 1996
	<1.0%, 24 hours	Mouse embryo	Loughlin et al 2008

[a]Calculated as 5 and 0.5 mg/L
[b]EC_{50}
[c]Calculated as 100 mg/L

magnitude higher than in vitro cytotoxic concentrations, being used at 4–12% (Guba 1998/1999; Jandera et al 2000; Hartman & Coetzee 2002; Kerr 2002; Dryden et al 2004). However, lemon myrtle, the most cytotoxic of the four essential oils shown, did cause adverse effects in a wound healing pilot study when used at 3% (Kerr 2002).

Although cytotoxicity does correlate with irritancy, it is difficult to extrapolate any hard information from the above data to aromatherapy practice. Firstly, several mechanisms may be involved in cytotoxicity, both to normal and cancer cells; some may even be the same, such as depletion of glutathione. Secondly, we do not know enough about the mechanisms by which different essential oil constituents may cause cytotoxicity. In spite of these difficulties, specific types of cytotoxicity tests are in development, in order to replace certain animal tests.

Estimating risk

Extrapolating from animal data

Information on oral toxicity is useful for general safety assessment, and for estimating the risks involved in cases of accidental poisoning. However, problems are frequently encountered when extrapolating from rodents and other animal species. As already stated, xenobiotics frequently express toxicity differences between species due to differences in toxicokinetic and toxicodynamic characteristics (see Toxic substances above). Small animals have a large body surface area in relation to total body volume, and a higher metabolic rate, so relatively larger quantities of xenobiotics may be absorbed and metabolized. Although identifying the 'target organs' for toxicity is a stated aim of animal testing, those most commonly affected are the liver and kidneys, as elevated doses particularly impact the organs of excretion.

In some animal studies, the test substance is administered by gavage (stomach intubation) as dosage can be more accurately controlled than when the substance is mixed with feed.

However, this method can result in increased toxicity. For example, when cinnamaldehyde was given with corn oil by gavage to rats, doses of 940 mg/kg/day produced almost 100% mortality, while a similar dose in feed caused no deaths (Hébert et al 1994). Cases of gavage-related toxicity have also been reported for rodents receiving up to 2,137 mg/kg citral in corn oil for 14 days (Dieter et al 1993), up to 800 mg/kg benzyl alcohol in corn oil for 13 weeks (National Toxicology Program 1989a), up to 500 mg/kg benzyl acetate in corn oil for 2 years (National Toxicology Program 1986), and up to 1,000 mg/kg/day of methyleugenol in 0.5% methylcellulose over 2 years (National Toxicology Program 2000; Smith RL et al 2002).

Even when a substance is given in feed, the very high doses administered may overwhelm detoxifying mechanisms in ways that do not occur at lower doses, so linear extrapolation from high dose to low dose can lead to over-cautious regulation, especially for carcinogens. Small animals have much shorter lifespans than humans, and assuming that the effects on a rat over two years are equivalent to the effects on a human over 50 years is no more than an assumption. Interspecies differences pertinent to cancer are discussed on Ch. 12, p. 175.

For reasons such as these, the results obtained by animal testing cannot be easily extrapolated to humans, and this has created controversy for many years.

In a few instances, there is sufficient information to make comparisons between acute toxicity in humans and rodents. In the six cases of wintergreen oil poisoning in adults reported above (see Poisoning), a human median lethal dose of 0.2–0.6 mL/kg was estimated. This compares with an average LD_{50} of 1.0 g/kg for methyl salicylate in rodents (Table 3.3). If these figures are typical, wintergreen oil is some 1.5–4.5 times more toxic to humans on a bodyweight basis than it is to rodents, and data showing dietary methyl salicylate to be nontoxic to rats at 700–2100 mg/kg should not be extrapolated directly to humans (Packman et al 1961).

Fatalities in humans after ingesting 1,8-cineole-rich eucalyptus oil in doses between 30 mL and 60 mL (Gurr & Scroggie 1965) suggest that eucalyptus oil is more toxic to humans on a bodyweight basis than laboratory animals, since the acute oral LD_{50}

in rats for 1,8-cineole is 2.48 g/kg, and equivalent values in mice for *Eucalyptus camaldulensis* and *E. exserta* are 3.67 mL/kg and 3.75 mL/kg, respectively (Jenner et al 1964; Pho et al 1993).

In the case of pennyroyal oil, the animal data seem to correlate well with human toxicity. The rat acute oral LD_{50} for the oil is 400 mg/kg (Opdyke 1974), approximately equivalent to 1 oz of pennyroyal oil being fatal when ingested by an adult (Anon 1978).

These examples illustrate that circumspection is needed when applying animal data to the human use of essential oils, which in some cases may be up to six times more toxic to humans. Although cases of human poisoning permit a comparison of median lethal dose, they do not tell us what a safe dose is.

Alternatives to traditional animal testing

For safety reasons, and to comply with legal requirements, virtually every substance used in foods, medicines, cosmetics and toiletries, including most essential oils, has been tested for toxicity on animals. Due to the pressure of public opinion and lobbying by animal rights groups, the number of animal tests required for cosmetic ingredients is falling in many countries, and national prohibitions are in place in the UK, Germany, Austria and the Netherlands. The European Coalition to End Animal Experiments (ECEAE) has criticized acute toxicity testing on ethical grounds, and on the grounds of interspecies differences between rodents and humans (Langley 2005).

Evolving legislation

In 1970, up to 100 animals per species were required for an oral LD_{50} test. In 1981 new OECD guidelines reduced the number to 30, which was further reduced to 20 in 1987. The OECD currently has 30 member states, including the USA, Japan, Australia and most European countries, and regulates government agencies. In 2002, the OECD finally deleted the LD_{50} test as a requirement, replacing it with three possible alternatives: the fixed dose procedure (FDP), the acute toxic class method (ATC) and the up and down procedure (UDP). Each test has slightly different dosing procedures, and fulfills different regulatory requirements, but the general aim remains to estimate median lethality. Although these new tests all involve reductions in suffering and numbers of animals, they are still animal tests (Botham 2004b). The LD_{50} format is still used for acute dermal and inhalation toxicity.

Pharmaceutical drugs require more stringent testing than cosmetics or general use chemicals, in part because optimal dosage has to be very accurately determined. For all concerned, however, there is a great cost savings potential in moving from in vivo to in vitro testing. Animals have to be raised, fed, housed, cared for, and disposed of. The human labor involved is considerable, and carers often suffer emotionally. In 2008 18 pharmaceutical companies (including eight of the ten largest) petitioned to have acute toxicity studies in animals removed as a requirement for drug approval. It was proposed that the information gleaned is disproportionate to the 'substantial adverse effects experienced by some of the animals', and that sufficient information could be obtained from other animal tests, which have to be carried out anyway, but which do not have death as an end-point (Robinson et al 2008).

An update of the EU Cosmetics Directive includes a timetable for the replacement of animal testing in cosmetic products or ingredients. Over the originally planned 11 years of its implementation (2007–2018), this would necessitate the deaths of some 2–3 million animals, unless in vitro toxicity guidelines are adopted (Langley 2005). However, the timetable has proved unrealistic as it depends on acceptable alternatives being developed to specific deadlines. At the time of writing, there are no replacements for many toxicity end-points (Table 3.7). The EU has a separate initiative, REACH (Registration, Evaluation & Authorization of Chemicals) which requires new safety testing on thousands of cosmetic ingredients. Estimates of the numbers of rodents that would be killed in order to meet this requirement are in the tens of millions, and the direct conflict between REACH and the Cosmetics Directive in terms of animal testing remains unresolved.

Various types of cytotoxicity tests are currently being explored as possible alternatives for acute toxicity (Clothier et al 2008, Ukelis et al 2008). Similarly, efforts are being made to develop genotoxicity testing in such a way as to replace in vivo carcinogenicity testing. In silico methods (i.e., using computer modeling) are also being considered for genotoxins, carcinogens and skin allergens (see Patterns of toxicity below).[4]

In the USA, animal testing for certain types of finished products is mandatory, and there are notable conflicts between American and European legislation.[5] Global harmonization initiatives such as Globally Harmonized System (GHS) have been

Table 3.7 European Union timetable for the replacement of animal testing in cosmetics

Test	Original deadline	Update as of September 2012
Skin corrosion	2007	In place
Skin irritation	2007	In place
Skin penetration	2007	In place
Acute phototoxicity	2007	In place
Photogenotoxicity	2009	Possibly 2017
Eye irritation	2009	Possibly 2017
Acute toxicity	2009	Possibly 2017
Genotoxicity	2009	Possibly 2017
Skin sensitization	2013	2019 or later
Photoallergy	2013	No foreseeable deadline
Subacute & subchronic toxicity	2013	No foreseeable deadline
Carcinogenicity	2013	No foreseeable deadline
Chronic toxicity	2013	No foreseeable deadline
Reproductive toxicity	2013	No foreseeable deadline
Toxicokinetics	2013	No foreseeable deadline

launched in order to address such issues, and to attain greater regulatory commonality between countries. These initiatives also aim to harmonize test procedure guidelines, and to avoid unnecessary repetition of testing. However, regional differences may not be completely eroded for a long time.

Patterns of toxicity

A general indication of an essential oil's toxicity can sometimes be gained from the chemical structure of its constituents. However, making broad assumptions is unwise, especially since a chemical functional group can express quite different degrees and mechanisms of toxicity in different compounds. For example, sesquiterpene lactones are notorious skin sensitizers and furanocoumarins are generally phototoxic, but some are not; some aldehydes are skin sensitizers and some ethers are carcinogenic, but many are not. Phenols do tend to be irritants, and their irritancy may correlate with acid strength. Terpene hydrocarbons and alcohols tend to be relatively free from toxicity, as do esters, with two notable exceptions: methyl salicylate and sabinyl acetate. Many sulfur compounds are relatively toxic, and most neurotoxic constituents are bicyclic, monoterpenoid ketones. However, the hypothesis that all ketones, and therefore all ketone-rich essential oils, are neurotoxic, espoused by Franchomme & Pénöel (1990) and by Schnaubelt (1995), is not supported by the evidence.

Ford et al (2000) identified 49 structural moieties that predispose to toxic effects, whether topical, acute/systemic, or carcinogenic/mutagenic. Pilotti et al (1975) derived a good qualitative relationship between various functional groups and toxicity to mouse ascites tumor cell cultures. However, as is often the case, exceptions were found and the reader is advised to treat such observations with a degree of caution. While functional groups provide a useful basis for comparing essential oil constituents, they lack the specificity needed for reliably predicting actions on body tissues.

Mathematical models

Attempts to put toxicity prediction on a more quantitative footing have met with increasing success. Since the 1960s, mathematical models have been developed to account for a wide range of pharmacological data, which, when successful, can give valuable insights into the mechanisms of action. These so-called quantitative structure–activity relationships (QSAR) use physicochemical and structural parameters for each compound to describe electronic, spatial and hydrophobic factors, and relate them to measured biological end-points. In this way, toxicity predictions have been made for a series of acyclic terpenes on the basis of molecular spatial and electronic parameters (Lewis et al 1994).

Knowledge of the mechanism of action of toxic substances can be invaluable for predicting the toxicity of structurally related analogues. Allylbenzenes (with a 2,3-double bond) such as safrole, estragole and methyleugenol, are genotoxic, while propenylbenzenes (with a 1,2-double bond) such as isosafrole, (E)-anethole and methyl isoeugenol are non-genotoxic (Miller & Miller 1983). The allylbenzenes, unlike their propenyl analogues, undergo sequential 1-hydroxylation and sulfation,

leading to the formation of reactive carbonium ions which attack DNA. This mechanism is supported by semiempirical quantum mechanical calculations of the stability of the carbonium ions (Tsai et al 1994). However, two propenylbenzene analogues, α- and β-asarone, are hepatocarcinogenic in rodents. Hasheminejad & Caldwell (1994) have suggested that a novel activation route exists for alkenylbenzenes having a 2-methoxyl group in the aromatic ring.

On the basis of their skin penetration and metabolism, the allergenic effects of some essential oil constituents have been rationalized (Hostýnek & Magee 1997). Many other examples of QSAR as applied to toxicity have been published in the literature, but further discussion of these is beyond the scope of this book.

Although some quantitative models of carcinogenicity lack the predictive power required to set safe levels of exposure for new and untested chemicals in humans with confidence, the position is expected to improve over coming years as the database is expanded, and mechanisms of toxicity become elucidated.

Minimizing risk

Contact with potentially harmful chemicals is a hazard of modern life. Whether a particular scenario requires action depends upon the risks posed. One option is to withdraw a substance entirely, which may be appropriate when there is a significant probability of a serious threat to health. For a few essential oils, there is genuine concern about their use in aromatherapy, and in these cases we recommend complete avoidance (see Table 15.2)

A second option is to establish limits for safe exposure. This applies when there are concerns about damage to health based on indirect evidence, e.g., from animal testing, or evidence from humans of dose-related damage. In order to confidently set safe limits of exposure, we need to understand the nature of any risks, and to quantify them. For example, some essential oils are known to be neurotoxic from human accidents, and safe doses can be estimated for exposure to camphor and thujone. Several models exist for classifying maximum safe doses, and most of these use the NOAEL (no-observed-adverse-effect level) as a starting point (see Setting safe limits for exposure below).

A third option is specific label warnings, which are often appropriate where there are definable, vulnerable groups, such as children and pregnant women. In regard to adverse skin reactions, label warnings might be appropriate in some instances for people who are allergic to particular substances or for people with dermatitis or other skin conditions.

A fourth option is to provide a universal type of label warning, and/or to use restrictive closures to protect young children from accidentally harming themselves.

Risk assessment

The object of risk assessment is protection from serious or moderate health injury. Protection from non-serious health injury is also desirable, yet this needs to be moderated by considerations such as individual rights and freedoms, quality of life, and health benefits. Various frameworks have been proposed for the management of risk. A common approach is a four-step process:

- hazard identification
- dose–response analysis
- exposure quantification
- risk characterization.

Hazard identification aims to define the qualitative nature of a potential adverse event, and the strength of the evidence for that effect. For chemicals, this is done by drawing from toxicological and epidemiological data.

Dose–response analysis determines the relationship between dose and the probability or the incidence of effect. The complexity of this step derives mainly from the need to extrapolate results from experimental animals to humans, and/or from high to lower doses. In addition, the differences between individuals due to genetics or other factors mean that the hazard may be higher for particular groups. An alternative to dose–response estimation is to determine an animal NOAEL, with additional uncertainty factors (see Uncertainty factors below).

Exposure quantification aims to determine the amount of a substance (dose) that individuals and populations will be exposed to. As different locations, lifestyles and other factors are likely to influence this estimate, a range of possible values is generated. Particular care is taken to determine the exposure of susceptible populations.

In **risk characterization**, the results of the three previous steps are combined, and all the evidence 'weighted', to produce an estimate of risk. Because of the different susceptibilities and exposures, this risk will vary within a population. The decisions based on the application of risk assessment are sometimes based on a standard of protecting those most at risk. This problem raises the question of how small a segment of a population must be protected.

Risk assessment is an evolving area, and feedback is essential for improving the regulatory process. Realistic precautions should be taken, and they should be based upon factual information. In this book, we attempt to make realistic estimations of safe levels of exposure, as far as possible, based on and limited by the extent of known data. Bickers et al (2003a) give a detailed outline of the Research Institute for Fragrance Materials (RIFM)/International Fragrance Association (IFRA) approach to the safety assessment of fragrance materials, particularly in regard to chemical structure.

Setting safe limits for exposure

In recent years, a number of parameters have been suggested as estimates of the safety of commonly encountered substances. These include the reference dose (RfD), acceptable daily intake (ADI) and tolerable daily intake (TDI). These are all based on an observed animal NOAEL. The NOAEL is the highest daily dose that can be administered in a repeated-dose (usually 90 day) animal test without causing any observable toxic effects.[6] It is only a valid NOAEL if higher doses show progressive toxicity. However, dose levels are often spaced far apart, and an NOAEL is often not the true maximum dose that produces no adverse effect, but rather an arbitrary, relatively low dose that produces no adverse effect.

The ADI is an estimate of the safe level of daily intake of a substance over the lifetime of a human being. It has been applied by Joint Expert Committee on Food Additives (JECFA) and Joint Meetings on Pesticide Residues (JMPR) to chemicals such as food additives, veterinary drugs and pesticides that are relatively easy to control, and where safety problems have been identified (if there are no known safety problems, no ADI is set). For more toxic compounds, except carcinogens, estimates of tolerable, rather than acceptable intakes are used, such as the TDI. This is used for the intake of contaminants associated with foods. For contaminants that accumulate in the body, the provisional tolerable weekly intake (PTWI) is used by JECFA (Herrman & Younes 1999).

Uncertainty factors

As part of the extrapolation process from NOAEL to ADI, various 'uncertainty' or 'safety' factors are applied. For example, a safety factor of 10 is routinely used to allow for differences between animals and humans, and another factor of 10 to account for variation between individuals. This leads to an overall safety factor of 100, suggesting that only 1/100 of the dose found to be non-toxic in animals can be deemed safe in humans. Safety factors of 100 are invariably used in setting ADIs and TDIs.

NOAEL values for the cytotoxicity of lemon myrtle oil to human cell lines HepG2 (liver cancer) and F1–73 (normal skin cells) were calculated as 5 and 0.5 mg/L after 4 and 24 hours exposure, respectively. In attempting to extrapolate these values to the whole body, a factor of 5 was applied to account for differences in routes of administration, as well as a factor of 10 to account for variability in the human response. This resulted in RfD values of 0.1 and 0.01 mg/L corresponding to 4 and 24 hours exposure, respectively. The RfD values for citral, which comprised 92.3% v/v of the oil sample, were comparable to those of lemon myrtle oil, and are 5–50 times lower than the ADI for citral of 0.5 mg/kg set by JECFA (Hayes & Markovic 2002).

Composite uncertainty factors are now widely recognized as being too general and over-conservative. Moreover, there is no clear rationale either for choosing these values, or why they should apply to all chemicals equally. Neither is it sound to assume that all substances will be more toxic to humans than animals. When there is evidence that a substance is less toxic to humans than rodents, as is the case for some carcinogens, it is irrational to apply a safety factor that assumes the opposite scenario. Clearly, the use of arbitrary safety factors is far from satisfactory, and is likely to be of little practical value. As has been stated by others, this approach is 'without factual or scientific justification and, by implication, arbitrary and irrational...the system has fabricated quantitative illusions and deliberately foists the pretense of being scientific' (Gori 2001).

A first step in seeking to refine uncertainty factors has been suggested by subdividing the factor for human variability into two equal factors of 3.16 to cover toxicokinetic and toxicodynamic differences (Gundert-Remy & Sonich-Mullin 2002; Dorne 2004; Dorne & Renwick 2005). For further refinement, data specific to the toxic chemical in question will need to be used. This relies heavily on databases, which, for many substances, are still poorly developed. A 10-fold default factor should be the first

Table 3.8 ADI and TDI values compared to Tisserand & Young limits

Substance	Tisserand & Young daily oral limit (mg/kg)	ADI (mg/kg)	TDI (μg/kg)	Reference for ADI or TDI
(E)-Anethole	None	2		JECFA 1998
Benzaldehyde[a]	5	5		JECFA 2001a
Benzoic acid[a]	5	5		JECFA 2001a
Benzyl acetate[a]	5	5		JECFA 2001a
Benzyl alcohol[a]	5	5		JECFA 2001a
Benzyl benzoate[a]	5	5		JECFA 2001a
Carvone	25	1		Council of Europe 1992
1,8-Cineole	None	0.2		Council of Europe 2000
Cinnamaldehyde	None	1.25		Council of Europe 1992
Citral[a]	None	0.5		JECFA 1999a
Citronellol[a]	None	0.5		JECFA 1999a
Coumarin	0.6		100	EFSA 2004
Eugenol	None	2.5		JECFA 1982
Geranyl acetate[a]	None	0.5		JECFA 1999a
Linalool[a]	None	0.5		JECFA 1999a
Linalyl acetate[a]	None	0.5		JECFA 1999a
Menthofuran[b]	0.2		100	Council of Europe 1999
Menthol	None	0.2		JECFA 1999b
Methyl salicylate	5.0	0.5		JECFA 2001b
Octanal	None	0.1		JECFA 2002
Pulegone[b]	0.5		100	Council of Europe 1999
Thujone	0.1		10	Council of Europe 1999

[a]Group ADI
[b]Group TDI
ADI, acceptable daily intake; TDI, tolerable daily intake. TDI is used because these are considered more toxic compounds, so the intake is tolerable rather than acceptable. ADI and TDI values apply primarily to food additives, but are for total exposure from any source.

choice only in situations where available data is clearly inadequate (Dourson et al 1996).

New approaches

Since they are doses that often have virtually no biological effect, ADI and TDI values may be inappropriate for the therapeutic use of essential oils. Newer approaches such as the benchmark dose, however, may provide ways of making use of dose–response information. Our recommendation for thujone is based on a benchmark dose (Table 3.8). Another new tool for assessing toxic risk, the threshold of toxicological concern (TTC), has been used for evaluating the safety of cosmetic ingredients and impurities. TTC values are derived from chronic oral toxicity data for structurally related compounds where no chemical-specific toxicity data already exists (Kroes et al 2007). It involves a decision tree using questions that relate to whether the ingredient is suitable for assessment via the TTC approach, the presence or absence of structural alerts for genotoxicity and, depending on its structure, how the level of exposure relates to the relevant human exposure threshold.

The premise that structurally related compounds might exhibit similar toxic actions seems a reasonable starting point for estimating the toxicities of compounds where no data exists. However, without knowing the mechanisms of toxicity or the specificity of interactions that underlie them, the question remains as to how similar two compounds should be to justify such an approach. Enzymes and receptors can be very specific in their requirements for binding and subsequent actions, and frequently, subtle changes such as replacement of a single functional group can result in a large difference in biological action.

A combination of scientific uncertainty, a high degree of flexibility and reliance on individual experts makes it practically impossible to conduct a fully consistent and systematic assessment process. An in-depth study of a large number of risk assessments for selected substances has been published which highlights large and unsystematic differences between decisions made for different chemicals with similar adverse health effects (Hansson & Rudén 2006).

All these approaches are part of a process striving for a truly predictive model. It is justifiable to use the best information available at any time, and we have applied several essential oil constituent ADIs in this book. However, guidelines that virtually prohibit a substance on the grounds of ignorance cannot be justified.

Packaging and labeling

In a case report of clove oil poisoning, Hartnoll et al (1993) commented: 'Packaging and labeling of clove oil and other potentially toxic essential oils need to be urgently reviewed. If all these oils were sold in bottles that had child-resistant tops and were in restricted flow bottles, then even if a child managed to remove the top he/she would only be able to drink a very small amount. Also, the bottles need to be clearly labeled to indicate that the contents, if ingested, can be very toxic and urgent medical help should be sought if ingestion occurs.'

Since the mid-1990s, packaging and labeling of essential oils have both improved. Essential oils are now rarely found in bottles without flow restrictors, and appropriate warnings are much more prevalent on packaging. In the USA in the years 1997–2006, the number of cases of 'exposure' to essential oils reported to the American Association of Poison Control Centers has grown by 85%, but the number of serious cases of toxicity has not increased (see Table 3.2). In 1997 there were four serious cases out of 3,990 exposures (0.1%) and in 2006 there were four serious cases out of 7,377 exposures (0.05%). (An 'exposure' is defined as a call to a doctor or poison center, though most are without any adverse consequence.) So, while the number of exposures has increased, probably due to wider usage of essential oils, the percentage of these that are serious cases has decreased by 50%. This is likely due to more protective packaging. It is also worth noting that 95% of incidents were unintentional.

In the UK, there are no published statistics for reports to poison centers of essential oil exposure. A cross-sectional survey in the UK of parents with children aged 12–35 months suggests that consumer awareness of the risk essential oils pose to children is poor. From a number of household items surveyed, those least likely to be stored safely were essential oils (81%), oral contraceptives (80%), oven cleaner (78%) and bleach (74%); items least likely to be put away immediately after use were essential oils (77%), cough medicine (72%) and children's painkillers (69%). Parents perceiving essential oils as more harmful were more likely to store them safely (Patel et al 2008).

This low level of consumer awareness of risk is in contrast to the ubiquitous use of label warnings for essential oils in the UK, which suggests that child-resistant closures may be appropriate. They are clearly appropriate for the more toxic essential oils, and for both practical and safety reasons should perhaps be used for all essential oils. Safety guidelines for pure essential oils sold in a retail environment are given in Chapter 12.

Adverse event reporting

The reporting of an adverse event (AE) helps greatly to bridge the 'knowledge gap' between theoretical risk and real-world risk. A single case report may take the form of a letter or short report in an academic journal, and/or it may form a part of a reporting system, contributing to annual statistics. Published case reports help to pinpoint specific reactions to specific substances at specific or approximate doses, and may also help identify susceptible groups, or previously unknown drug interactions. AE reporting has, for example, identified interactions between topically applied methyl salicylate and warfarin, and the susceptibility of a subpopulation to menthol.

Essential oils are not classified as medications, and AEs are not reported under the usual 'pharmacovigilance' reporting system initiated by the WHO (World Health Organization) and used in most countries. In Europe they are classed as 'general use products'. Exposure to them is assessed alongside items such as herbal remedies, vitamins, food supplements and cosmetics.

In the USA there is a comprehensive summary of toxic reactions, which is published annually. Most essential oils associated with AEs are not identified by name, and only overall statistics concerning age and severity of reaction are included. The proportion of AEs that involved oral ingestion, inhalation or other route is not stated. In the UK, Australia, Canada and many other countries, the extent of reporting is not made public, and no statistics are published. Medical practitioners can contact their national database for information on a specific essential oil, but the usefulness of this system is limited since the information it contains is not openly shared. The Medical Products Agency in Sweden has a voluntary AE reporting system for cosmetics, though even here irritant or unusual reactions are apparently under-reported (Berne et al 2008). The FDA (Food and Drug Administration) is moving towards a reporting system for cosmetics, and it is being considered in the UK.

Current reporting systems for essential oil AEs are mostly inadequate. These shortcomings need to be urgently addressed, and aromatherapy associations can help by initiating their own system.

Summary

- Toxicology is the study of harmful interactions between xenobiotics and living systems. A xenobiotic may be inherently toxic, or it may be metabolized into a toxic substance.
- Toxicity is dependent on the dose, concentration, frequency of use, bioavailability and intrinsic toxicity of the substance, interactions with other xenobiotics, and the susceptibility of the individual. Environmental conditions, such as UV (ultraviolet) radiation, may also be important.
- Essential oils are complex mixtures that may contain both harmful and protective chemicals. Essential oil toxicity may be influenced by additivity, synergy or antagonism between constituents. Predicting the overall actions of such mixtures is often problematic.

- Qualitative predictions can sometimes be made about the toxicity of essential oil constituents from consideration of chemical structure, but this can be unreliable.
- Cases of poisoning often provide useful information about the general toxicity of specific essential oils in humans.
- Virtually all cases of serious poisoning from essential oils have arisen after oral ingestion. Aromatherapy massage is very unlikely to give rise to such poisoning.
- There have been many cases of accidental poisoning by essential oils in very young children. Parents and consumers in general need to be aware of this risk.
- The initial symptoms of essential oil poisoning often include mucosal irritation, epigastric pain, vomiting and diarrhea.
- Reports of poisoning and/or adverse skin reactions may increase with more widespread use of an essential oil. This has happened with tea tree oil, but not with lavender oil.
- Animal toxicology testing includes acute tests by oral, dermal, inhalation, subcutaneous and intraperitoneal routes. There are also repeated-dose and chronic tests, which take place over longer periods of time, and tests for reproductive toxicity, genotoxicity, carcinogenicity and adverse skin reactions.
- The LD_{50} is the median lethal dose, and varies with body size and species. There are no 'extremely toxic' or 'very toxic' essential oils, in the sense that none has an acute oral LD_{50} value lower than 100 mg/kg.
- Because of dosing, toxicokinetic and other interspecies differences, the results obtained by animal testing cannot be easily extrapolated to humans, and this has created controversy for many years.
- An uncertainty factor of 100 has been used historically in extrapolating toxicity data from cells and animals to humans. However, this practice has now been largely discredited on the grounds of being irrational and lacking scientific rigor.
- Estimates of cytotoxicity can be made fairly easily but extrapolation from cell to organism is difficult.
- The new European Chemicals Legislation (REACH) includes a timetable for the replacement of animal testing in cosmetic products or ingredients. However, some deadlines are unrealistic, as there is no replacement yet approved for acute toxicity, reproductive toxicity or carcinogenicity testing in rodents.
- The Global Harmonization Initiative may lead to increased regulatory commonality between countries.
- The NOAEL is the no-observable-adverse-effect level, or the highest daily dose that can be used without causing any observable toxic effects in an animal species.

- Essential oils should be adequately labeled, and should be sold in bottles with integral drop-dispensers.
- Child-resistant closures should be used for the more toxic essential oils. For both practical and safety reasons, they should perhaps be used for all essential oils.
- Adverse event reporting systems for essential oils are inadequate.

Notes

1. For two compounds, this might be expressed mathematically as: $E(d_a, d_b) = E(d_a) + E(d_b)$, where E represents a pharmacological or toxicological effect, and d_a and d_b are the doses of constituents a and b (Williamson 2000).

2. The variation in toxicity seen between these cases may be due to differences in factors such as body weight, metabolism, and individual health status. Four of the cases cited were between 21 and 28 years old, one was 55, and one was an adult, age unknown.

3. The LD_{100} is the dose required to kill 100% of the test animals (this is only rarely determined), while LD_0 is the theoretical highest single dose not causing any deaths. This last value is difficult to establish in practice, which is why the LD_{50} has become the standard reference for acute toxicity.

4. With the pressure of the REACH deadlines, the opportunity for private enterprise to have their brand of in vitro testing approved, and cheering from animal rights supporters, it should not be forgotten that, if the results of in vitro tests are honed to reflect those of animal tests, this may make them even less relevant to humans than animal testing.

5. One of the implications of the new European legislation is that certain categories of product (such as antiperspirants and sun care products) developed in the USA, which need to be tested on animals in order to meet the FDA's safety requirements, could not be imported into Europe. Conversely, products developed in Europe may not be accepted by the FDA.

6. The NOAEL for a carcinogen is extrapolated from two-year studies in rodents, which is virtually a lifetime for these animals. In the absence of any hard data, the maximum dose for a carcinogen may be estimated by taking the 90 day NOAEL for a substance and dividing by ten. Conversely, the maximum exposure limits for the carcinogens found in essential oils could be multiplied by a factor of ten for short-term exposure. However, although 90 days for a rat is equivalent to several years for a human, making such extrapolations is problematic.

Kinetics and dosing

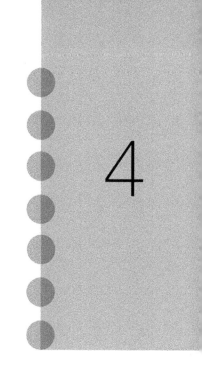

4

CHAPTER CONTENTS

The aim of the therapist in administering a physiologically active substance is to elicit the maximum therapeutic benefit while keeping any accompanying toxic or otherwise undesirable effects to a minimum. Depending upon the severity of the condition being treated, adverse effects can sometimes be tolerated, provided that a clear overall advantage can be demonstrated.

In order to work safely and effectively with essential oils, the therapist has a number of practical choices to make:

- the essential oil(s) to administer
- the route of administration
- the dose to administer
- the frequency of administration
- the medium or formulation in which to administer the essential oil
- additional factors such as timing of administration in relation to meals, baths or other activities.

In making a decision, the following factors may need to be taken into account:

- the desired therapeutic action(s)
- the intended site(s) of action

- the optimum concentration(s) of pharmacologically active constituent(s) desired at the target tissue or organ
- the maximum concentration(s) of toxic constituent(s) tolerated in any tissue or organ.

For many essential oil constituents, reliable quantitative information about the latter two points is not currently available. However, informed estimates can be made based on the limited amount of existing data on the toxicity and fate of essential oils and different classes of pure compounds after they have been administered by different routes. Since each constituent in a mixture is processed by the body in different ways, the metabolic fate of an essential oil must be understood in terms of its individual constituents. This argument should also apply to compounds that exist as mixtures of isomers, unless proof of identical properties has been demonstrated.

To add another level of complexity, the actions of constituents studied in isolation often differ from their actions when given as part of a mixture. Many examples have been quoted in the literature of the benefits of administering compounds as mixtures, often obtained from plant sources, including reduced toxicity. For example, the unexpected lack of genotoxicity and carcinogenicity in essential oils or extracts containing safrole (Ishidate et al 1984; Bhide et al 1991a; Choudhary & Kale 2002), and the reduced acute toxicity in essential oils containing thymol (Karpouhtsis et al 1998). Such benefits may occur as a result of interactions between constituents, phenomena that were discussed in Chapter 3.

To establish a rational basis for determining the optimum dose and frequency for administering essential oils by any route, it is necessary to take account of factors that affect the concentrations of individual constituents in the bloodstream and in various other tissues at different times. We shall therefore begin by reviewing the different ways in which chemical substances move into and within the body by examining their absorption, distribution, metabolism and excretion, together known as pharmacokinetics.

Absorption

Bioavailability

Bioavailability is one of the main parameters to consider when choosing a route for administering an essential oil. The bioavailability of a substance is defined as the proportion of an administered dose that reaches the systemic circulation unchanged. It depends on the following factors:

- the substance administered
- the mode and route of administration
- the recipient.

The substance administered

The passage of molecules inwards through the skin, unlike sweating which is an active, energy-requiring process, occurs mainly by passive diffusion (Grandjean 1990). We know that the rate of passive diffusion of a substance through the skin, as with any cell membrane, depends on its concentration gradient (i.e., the difference between its concentrations on either side), and is given by Fick's first law.[1] It is also influenced by solubility in aqueous and lipid media (i.e., hydrophilicity and lipophilicity, respectively) and its molecular size. These aspects are discussed below.

The mode and route of administration

Bioavailability depends on the route of administration, dosage form, frequency of dosing and the length of time over which administration occurs. If a substance is introduced by intravenous injection, its bioavailability, by definition, will be 100%. If given by any other route, this value will be less than 100%. It is important to know whether, and under what conditions, essential oil constituents enter the blood circulation, and how they are distributed within the body, because these factors will have important implications from a toxicological point of view.

The bioavailability of some essential oil constituents administered by different routes has been reviewed (Kohlert et al 2000). In most studies, these compounds are reported to be quickly absorbed after oral, dermal and inhalational administration, though it is concluded that there is a general lack of good quality pharmacokinetic data in humans. Table 4.1 gives the peak serum concentrations of some constituents administered by different routes. Although the first three compounds in this table seem to have an extremely low bioavailability from dermal application, the study that most closely approximates to an aromatherapy massage is the one by Jäger et al (1992a), which involved an abdominal massage with 2% lavender oil in peanut oil for 10 minutes (also see Figure 4.2). This may be because the essential oil was being inhaled as well as being dermally absorbed.

The recipient

Bioavailability is subject to biological variation. No two individuals will handle the same substance in the same way, and even the same individual will handle the same substance in different ways at different times, because of factors such as health status, nutritional status, age, integrity of skin, and metabolism (see Pharmacogenetics below). For example, in atopic dermatitis, the skin is likely to be broken so its function as a barrier to exogenous substances is compromised (see Percutaneous absorption below). This has obvious implications not only for the choice and dose of an oil for its therapeutic effects, but also for minimizing its toxicity.

The routes most commonly used for administering essential oils include dermal, inhaled, oral, rectal and vaginal.

Dermal administration

In aromatherapy massage, essential oils are usually applied to the skin diluted in a vegetable oil vehicle. Recipients may benefit in three ways: from absorbing essential oil constituents through the skin, from absorbing constituents via inhalation, and from the massage itself. Commercial aromatherapy products also elicit their actions after skin application and/or inhalation.

It is important to know how quickly, and to what extent components of essential oils and vegetable oils penetrate human skin and find their way into the circulation. It is also pertinent to

Table 4.1 Peak serum concentrations of essential oil constituents following different routes of administration in humans

Preparation administered	Constituent detected	Peak serum concentration (ng/mL)	Route of administration	Time to peak (minutes)	Reference
Pinimenthol ointment	Camphor[a]	1	Dermal	–	Schuster et al 1986
Suntan preparation	Bergapten	1	Dermal	–	Moysan et al 1993
Pinimenthol ointment	α-Pinene[a]	10	Dermal	–	Schuster et al 1986
Bergamot oil	Bergapten	235	Dermal	360	Wang & Tso 2002
2% Lavender oil	Linalyl acetate[a]	100	Dermal/inhalation	20	Jäger et al 1992a
2% Lavender oil	Linalool[a]	120	Dermal/inhalation	20	Jäger et al 1992a
Thymol (1.08 mg)[b]	Thymol	93.1	Oral	120	Kohlert et al 2002
GeloMyrtol (300 mg)[c]	1,8-Cineole	238	Oral	–	Zimmermann et al 1995
Peppermint oil (180 mg)	(−)-Menthol	1,492	Oral	100	Mascher et al 2001

[a]Isomer not specified
[b]Administered in the form of a Bronchipret TP tablet
[c]1,8-Cineole is the main active ingredient

understand the factors that aid or hinder dermal penetration. Surprisingly, these questions have received little attention in the literature, apart from some toxicological studies.[2]

For many years, biologists believed that the skin formed an impervious barrier to the outside world. We now know that this is not the case and that many substances are dermally absorbed to some degree.[3] Volatile chemicals have been detected in human breath following dermal exposure (Thrall et al 2000). Nevertheless, the skin is still an important protective barrier, limiting the rate at which potentially harmful substances enter the body, as well as preventing the loss of body fluids. Apart from its outer, horny layer the skin has other means of protection, including sweating, detoxifying enzymes and certain immune mechanisms (Hotchkiss 1994).

Several studies have shown that human skin is less permeable than that of most experimental animals such as rodents (Bartek et al 1972; Garnett et al 1994; Beckley-Kartey et al 1997), although there are exceptions (Yourick & Bronaugh 1997). In the latter study, coumarin passed more easily through human skin than rat skin. Therefore, caution is needed in extrapolating animal data to humans, and in this text we have ignored most existing animal data.

The structure of the skin

The skin is the largest organ in the human body. It is essentially a water-resistant barrier about 3 mm thick, consisting of an outer epidermis (F) and a deeper dermis (G) (Figure 4.1). The outer layer of the epidermis, the stratum corneum (B), is the main physical barrier to free access by external chemicals, and incorporates dead epidermal cells embedded in a lipid matrix. The main lipids are ceramides (41%), cholesterol (27%), cholesterol esters (10%), fatty acids (9%) and cholesterol sulfate (2%)

(Tanojo et al 1998). This matrix, where lipids form a highly convoluted mass, is primarily responsible for the very low permeability of the stratum corneum to water (Potts & Francoeur 1991). Below the stratum corneum lies the remainder of the epidermis (the 'viable' epidermis) consisting of living cells arising in the deep epidermis, which become flatter as they rise to the surface and replace exfoliated dead cells. Below the epidermis is the dermoepidermal junction, and then the much thicker dermis, containing nerves, sweat glands, sebaceous glands, hair follicles, blood vessels and lymph vessels. Beneath the dermis lies subcutaneous tissue, primarily fat (H).

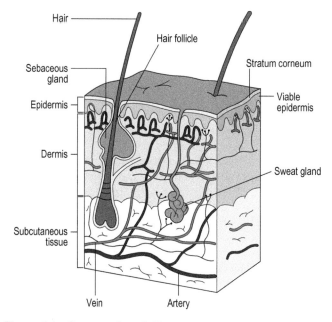

Figure 4.1 • Cross-section of skin.

The absorption characteristics of skin differ between individuals and between different areas of the body. The apparent permeability coefficients (P_{app}) of 13 of the most abundant constituents of Damask rose oil were estimated following application of the oil to human abdominal, breast and upper arm skin in vitro. Significant differences were observed for the permeation of some constituents. For example, eugenol was found to permeate breast and abdominal skin with similar efficacy, but failed to penetrate upper arm skin, while β-pinene was found to permeate upper arm skin significantly better than abdominal skin. It was argued that these differences were related to chemical structure, but overall, no application site was considered preferable to the others (Schmitt et al 2010).

There are a few structural differences between black and white skins. These include a higher total lipid content but a lower amount of ceramides in black skin, and fewer cell layers (although equal thickness) in white stratum corneum (Berardesca & Maibach 1996). However, there is no convincing evidence of important differences in percutaneous absorption between different colored skins.

Percutaneous absorption

Since the cells of the stratum corneum are not living, they are incapable of registering a physiological response to toxic chemicals. Therefore, before an essential oil constituent can cause a toxic response in the skin, or indeed anywhere else in the body, it must first cross the stratum corneum. Two pathways are theoretically available for this: the intercellular route (between the skin cells) and the transcellular route (through them) (Michaels et al 1975). The intercellular regions are full of lipids structured in multi-lamellar arrays, through which more than one route of molecular diffusion can be envisaged, and there are data to support this view (Albery & Hadgraft 1979; Bunge et al 1999).

A third possible route of entry, through the hair follicles, bypasses the stratum corneum altogether (Scheuplein & Blank 1971; Meidan et al 2005). Lipophilic substances might diffuse preferentially through hair follicles and sebaceous ducts using sebum, a lipophilic secretion, as a transport medium. This might explain why, for example, the flux of coumarin across human scalp skin is higher than for human abdominal skin (Ritschel et al 1989). Terpinen-4-ol has been found in the hair follicles of cattle udder skin after application of 5% tea tree oil in a variety of vehicles. Its concentration in sebum was 0.16–0.43%, depending on the vehicle used (Biju et al 2005).

There is good evidence that many essential oil constituents travel from the skin surface to the stratum corneum, then to the dermis and the blood circulation. In a study using isolated human skin, methyl salicylate penetrated both the stratum corneum and the dermis, and was also detected in subcutaneous tissues.[4] This was due to direct tissue penetration, and not redistribution by the systemic blood supply (Cross et al 1998).

Once a constituent has been absorbed, the epidermis may act as a reservoir, retaining a proportion for up to 72 hours before it crosses the dermoepidermal junction, enters the dermis, and then the blood capillaries (Chidgey & Caldwell 1986; Beckley-Kartey et al 1997; Hotchkiss 1998). The majority is absorbed within 24 hours. In an ex vivo dermal absorption study with tea tree oil, 2.75% of the applied dose, mainly terpinen-4-ol, crossed the epidermis, and 0.3% was retained in it after 24 hours (Cross et al 2008).

Following dermal application of a cosmetic tanning lotion containing bergamot oil to the forearm skin of 11 healthy volunteers, bergapten was detected in the dermis after 220 minutes (Makki et al 1991). In a similar study, bergapten was found in the dermis, and also in plasma after repeated applications (Moysan et al 1993). In a further study, bergamot oil, emulsified jojoba oil containing bergapten, and cleansing foam with bergamot oil were each applied to the forearms of volunteers. The skin was left uncovered. Bergapten was detected in the stratum corneum after 120 minutes, and in the volunteers' blood after 240 minutes (Wang & Tso 2002). Since bergapten is not volatile, there is no possibility of inhalatory absorption; it could only have reached the bloodstream via the skin.

An analgesic ointment containing methyl salicylate was applied topically to the thighs of 12 human volunteers twice daily for four days. Blood concentrations of 0.31–0.91 mg/L of methyl salicylate were detected within 1 hour of application, rising to a maximum of 2–6 mg/L after the seventh application. Urinary recovery of methyl salicylate and metabolites during the first 24 hours averaged 175.2 mg (Morra et al 1996). In a study of camphor, menthol and methyl salicylate applied undiluted to human volunteers by skin patch for eight hours, peak blood levels were 16.8, 19.0 and 26.8 ng/mL, respectively, for four patches, and 29.5, 31.9 and 41.0 ng/mL, respectively, for eight patches. Systemic exposure was said to be low, in spite of the long period of time and large number of patches (Martin et al 2004).

There is one report that closely approximates to what happens in an aromatherapy massage. Peak plasma concentrations of two lavender oil constituents were detected 20 minutes after the oil had been applied by massage; after 90 minutes, concentrations had fallen close to zero (Figure 4.2). In this study, 1.5 g of 2% lavender oil in peanut oil was massaged over the abdomen for 10 minutes, and blood samples were drawn

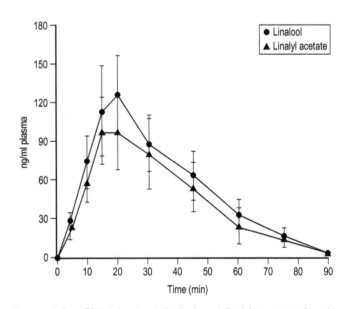

Figure 4.2 • Blood levels of linalool and linalyl acetate after the application of lavender oil by massage. (Reproduced with permission from Jäger et al 1992a Percutaneous absorption of lavender oil from a massage oil. Journal of the Society of Cosmetic Chemists 43:49-54. © The Society of Cosmetic Chemists.)

from the arm (left cubital vein) 0, 5, 10, 20, 30, 45, 60, 75, and 90 minutes after finishing the massage. The two constituents measured were linalool (24.8% of the oil) and linalyl acetate (29.6% of the oil). Linalool peaked at 120 ng/mL plasma after 20 minutes (Jäger et al 1992a).

This study did not control for inhalation and pulmonary absorption. However, in an earlier report by Schuster et al (1986) subjects inhaled 'clean' air, and plasma concentrations of α-pinene, β-pinene, camphor, δ-3-carene and (+)-limonene were determined over a period of three hours. In 12 human volunteers, 2 g of Pinimenthol ointment (containing eucalyptus oil, pine needle oil, menthol, camphor) was applied over a 400 cm^2 area of skin, and plasma levels peaked at between 1 ng/mL (camphor) and 10 ng/mL (α-pinene) after 10 minutes.

Permeability and absorption kinetics of essential oil constituents are influenced by the composition of the essential oil, the vehicle, the skin, and certain environmental factors.

After application to uncovered excised human skin, varying amounts of essential oil constituents have been absorbed (Table 4.2). A proportion of the volatile compounds evaporate, but occlusion reduces loss and increases skin permeation. The maximum percentages of any essential oil constituent absorbed dermally over 24 and 72 hours were 33% and 50%, respectively, for coumarin (Beckley-Kartey et al 1997). However, coumarin is rarely found in essential oils, and the 24 hour maximum of 5.9% for benzyl alcohol is more typical. If we assume that a

further 50% (of the 5.9%) is absorbed over the next 48 hours, this would extrapolate to about 8.8%. In Table 4.3 we have rounded this up to 10%, and this is the maximum we have assumed for almost all essential oil constituents in setting safety limits for dermal application. Using this parameter, the maximum quantity absorbed from dermal application in 24 hours (0.15 mL) is therefore less than that of oral dosage (0.22–0.66 mL, as shown in Table 4.7). The high levels of skin absorption for methyl salicylate reported by Moody et al (2007) may, in part, be due to the use of acetone as a vehicle. Acetone disrupts the barrier function of skin in mice mainly by removing corneocytes and extracting nonpolar lipids (Rissmann et al 2009; Kamo et al 2011).

No datum is currently available for the percentage skin penetration of α-thujone or methyleugenol, but values can be estimated from their permeability coefficients, which are directly related.[5] The in vitro skin permeability coefficient (P_s) of a substance can be measured by applying it in a suitable vehicle to human epidermis in a thermostatic diffusion cell. P_s values for (−)-camphor, (−)-carvone, 1,8-cineole, (−)-linalool, (−)-menthol, α-thujone, (−)-menthone and (E)-anethole ranged from 1.51×10^{-3} cm/h to 0.14×10^{-3} cm/h (Gabbanini et al 2009). α-Thujone has a similar P_s value to (−)-linalool (0.62×10^{-3} cm/h and 0.82×10^{-3} cm/h, respectively) using reconstructed human epidermis of unstated origin (Gabbanini et al 2009). Methyleugenol has a similar reported apparent

Table 4.2 The percentage absorption of essential oil constituents over a 24 hour period through uncovered, excised human skin

Constituent	% Absorbed	Skin sample	Vehicle	Concentration applied	Reference
γ-Terpinene	0	Female breast and abdomen	Aqueous solution[a,b]	5% Tea tree oil	Nielsen & Nielsen 2006
α-Terpineol	0	Female abdomen	Ethanol	20% Tea tree oil	Cross et al 2008
Methyl isoeugenol	0.9	Lower abdomen	Ethanol/water 70/30 v/v	10 mM	Jimbo et al 1983
Isoeugenol	0.9	Lower abdomen	Ethanol/water 70/30 v/v	10 mM	Jimbo et al 1983
Terpinen-4-ol	1.5	Female abdomen	Ethanol	20% Tea tree oil	Cross et al 2008
Linalool	2.8 / 3.6	Not stated / Not stated	Diethyl phthalate / Ethanol/water 70/30 v/v	4% w/v / 4% w/v	Lapczynski et al 2008g
Geraniol	3.5 / 7.3	Not stated / Not stated	Diethyl phthalate/ethanol 3:1	2% / 5%	Gilpin et al 2010
Citronellol	3.8 / 4.7	Not stated / Not stated	Diethyl phthalate/ethanol 3:1	2% / 5%	Gilpin et al 2010
Benzyl alcohol	5.9	Lower abdomen	Ethanol/water 70/30 v/v	10 mM	Jimbo et al 1983
Methyl salicylate	11 / 17 / 32	Female breast and leg	Acetone	200 mM / 20 mM / 2 mM	Moody et al 2007
Coumarin[c]	33	Female breast	Ethanol	0.02%	Beckley-Kartey et al 1997

[a]1% Tween, 0.9% NaCl, 98.1% water
[b]% absorption after 48 hours
[c]52% coumarin was absorbed over 72 hours. None of the other studies measured absorption for this long

Table 4.3 Maximum dermal absorption of essential oil constituents

Concentration of essential oil in excipient	Maximum quantity of essential oil constituents likely to be percutaneously absorbed (in mL) per quantity of product applied, assuming 10% absorption					
	5 mL	10 mL	15 mL	20 mL	25 mL	30 mL
1%	0.005	0.01	0.015	0.02	0.025	0.03
2%	0.01	0.02	0.03	0.04	0.05	0.06
3%	0.015	0.03	0.045	0.06	0.075	0.09
4%	0.02	0.04	0.06	0.08	0.1	0.12
5%	0.025	0.05	0.075	0.1	0.125	0.15

permeability coefficient (P_{app}) to linalool and geraniol, i.e., 5.23×10^{-5}, 3.87×10^{-5} and 3.22×10^{-5} cm/s, respectively, for human abdominal skin, and 6.29×10^{-5}, 4.12×10^{-5} and 4.11×10^{-5} cm/s for human breast skin (Schmitt et al 2010). Therefore, it is reasonable to assume that the dermal absorption of methyleugenol and α-thujone is within the range of 2–5%.

Molecular size and solubility

The stratum corneum has both hydrophilic and lipophilic regions. Highly water-soluble molecules, such as glucose, have difficulty passing through lipid-rich regions, while highly lipid-soluble substances, such as cholesterol, have a low probability of crossing the aqueous regions. In general, lipophilic substances cross the dermal barrier more readily and more extensively than hydrophilic ones (Wester & Maibach 2000). However, some water solubility is important too, to facilitate the passage of a substance from the dermis into the bloodstream.[6] We would therefore expect substances that pass most readily from the surface of the skin into the bloodstream to have a favorable balance between water and lipid solubility (Hansch and Fujita 1964, Wepierre et al 1968).[7]

Attempts to derive mathematical models for the dermal penetration and absorption of topically applied substances are still being refined (Williams & Riviere 1995).

A convenient measure of the relative solubilities of a substance in lipid and aqueous media is its partition coefficient (P), usually expressed in its logarithmic form, $\log_{10} P$.[8] For the dermal absorption of essential oil constituents, an optimum log P value of 2–4 (for the n-octanol/water system) has been proposed (Cal 2006b), and in an in vitro study of human skin penetration, terpinen-4-ol penetrated the epidermis and dermis more rapidly than 1,8-cineole, α-pinene and β-pinene (Cal et al 2006). However, no clear relationship with log P is apparent here. Log P (octanol/water) values for a range of essential oil constituents are given in Table 4.4.

The uptake into, and the elimination of (±)-β-citronellol, (±)-linalool and linalyl acetate from human skin were studied in vitro. All compounds easily penetrated all layers of the skin, and (±)-linalool promoted its own uptake. No clear relationship between absorption or elimination and log P values was seen, and the most lipophilic compound, linalyl acetate, was the least well absorbed (Cal & Sznitowska 2003). However, in a study

Table 4.4 $\log_{10} P$ (octanol/water) values for some essential oil constituents

Constituent	$\log_{10} P$	Reference
Benzyl alcohol	1.1	Gluck et al 1996
Vanillin	1.2	Niknahad et al 2003
Guaiacol	1.3	Tisserand & Young[a]
Coumarin	1.4	Tisserand & Young[a]
Benzaldehyde	1.5	Pybus & Sell 1999, p190
(E)-Cinnamaldehyde	1.9	Niknahad et al 2003
Benzyl acetate	2.0	Tisserand & Young[a]
Bergapten	2.0	Saïd et al 1997
Methyl salicylate	2.3	Tisserand & Young[a]
Eugenol	2.4	Tisserand & Young[a]
Isoeugenol	2.6	Tisserand & Young[a]
α-Terpineol	2.8	Cross et al 2008
1,8-Cineole	2.8	Cal 2006c
Methyleugenol	2.9	Tisserand & Young[a]
Terpinen-4-ol	3.0	Cal 2006c
Citral	3.0	Tisserand & Young[a]
Methyl isoeugenol	3.1	Tisserand & Young[a]
Estragole	3.1	Tisserand & Young[a]
Thymol	3.2	Tisserand & Young[a]
(E)-anethole	3.3	Tisserand & Young[a]
(+)- and (−)-Linalool	3.4	Lapczynski et al 2008e, 2008f
Carvacrol	3.4	Tisserand and Young[a]
(+)- and (−)-Citronellol	3.6	Lapczynski et al 2008b, 2008c
Linalyl acetate	4.1	Cal 2006c
γ-Terpinene	4.4	Cross et al 2008
α- and β-Pinene	4.4	Cal 2006c
(+)-Limonene	4.5	Cross et al 2008
α-Santalol	5.0	Bhatia et al 2008d
α-Terpinene	5.5	Cross et al 2008
Nerolidol	5.7	Lapczynski et al 2008h
Farnesol	5.8	Lapczynski et al 2008d
δ-Cadinene	6.5	Cross et al 2008

Constituents with log P values within the range of 2–4 are thought to penetrate skin more readily than those with log P values either higher or lower (Cal 2006b). Lower values indicate greater water solubility, and higher values indicate greater lipid solubility
[a]This book, calculated for the octanol/water system using the CLogP algorithm in ChemDraw Ultra 6.0

comparing a wide range of compounds, including some essential oil constituents, a highly significant linear relationship between percutaneous absorption across excised human skin in vitro and octanol/water log P values, and an inverse relationship with molecular mass, was found (Cronin et al 1999).

Permeability enhancement

Many essential oil constituents appear to enhance their own dermal uptake and that of other substances. Some, such as methyl salicylate, may do this in part by acting as rubefacients,[9] increasing local capillary blood flow (Cross et al 1999). Others temporarily alter the transport properties of the stratum corneum, through interacting with the intercellular lipids (Williams & Barry 1991). They can either be applied as a skin pre-treatment, or may be formulated with the vehicle. For example, carveol, α-terpineol and terpinen-4-ol significantly boosted permeation of water and ethanol in isolated human epidermis after 4 hours (Magnusson et al 1997). Similarly, (+)-limonene enhanced the permeation of citronellol and eugenol, and both α-pinene and β-myrcene enhanced phenylethanol permeation (Schmitt et al 2009). When 1–2 mL of undiluted terpenes were applied to a small area of uncovered human skin for 12 hours, 8.9% of the applied dose of (+)-limonene, 26.2% of 1,8-cineole and 39.6% of nerolidol were detected in the stratum corneum. These compounds appear to enhance their own accumulation by disrupting the integrity of intercellular lipid bilayers (Cornwell et al 1996).

In simple terms, essential oils mix with skin lipids, reduce their barrier function by making them slightly more hydrophilic, and thereby ease their own passage through to the dermis. Some terpenes enhance the skin's transport properties so efficiently that they have been used to increase the percutaneous absorption of various medications.

This could be a problem with topical drugs. 5-Fluorouracil (5-FU) is a prescription pharmaceutical used in a cream base at 5% as a treatment for sun-damaged skin cells. In a study using excised human skin, pre-treatment with four essential oils enhanced the dermal absorption of 5-FU, from 2.8-fold for anise oil, to 34-fold for eucalyptus oil (Williams & Barry 1989). The transdermal absorption of other drugs, not normally applied to the skin, is enhanced by essential oils and constituents, for example aspirin ((+)-limonene, in vivo, human), indomethacin (cardamom oil, in vivo, rabbit), and nicrorandil (carvone, in vivo, human) (McAdam et al 1996; Huang et al 1999; Krishnaiah et al 2006).

For medications, controlled dosage is important for safe and effective treatment, and any enhancement from coincidental aromatherapy could have adverse effects. Therefore essential oils should not be applied to skin to which any medication is applied, or on which drug patches are being used (e.g., hormone or nicotine patches). In various animal studies, both eucalyptus oil and camphor enhanced nicotine absorption (Nuwayser et al 1988).

A recent study attempted to rationalize the permeability-enhancing ability of a group of 49 terpenes (Kang et al 2007). The permeability coefficient of haloperidol through excised human skin appeared to be related to lipophilicity, molecular weight, boiling point, terpene type and the presence or absence of certain functional groups. However, the applicability of this relationship to other drug types is not known.

The delivery vehicle and concentration

When administered in a vehicle, the tendency of a substance to leave that vehicle and diffuse through the skin is related to the difference in lipophilicity between substance and vehicle. Being predominantly lipophilic, essential oil constituents tend to move from aqueous to lipid environments. Thus, when applied to the skin diluted in a vegetable oil, its constituents will diffuse into the skin more slowly than when they are dispersed in a semi-aqueous medium (Florence & Attwood 1998). This has been shown for benzyl alcohol, isoeugenol and methoxsalen using human epidermis (Gazith et al 1978; Jimbo et al 1983). When (±)-linalool or terpinen-4-ol were applied to human skin in vitro at 5% in three different vehicles, the absorption rates of the terpenes into the stratum corneum decreased from hydrogel to grapeseed oil to a mineral oil-in-water emulsion (Cal 2006a).

Compounds with molecular masses greater than 500 usually have more difficulty passing through skin than smaller ones (Cronin et al 1999). These include triacylglycerols (fatty acid esters), which are found in vegetable oils. Being highly lipophilic, triacylglycerols are likely to penetrate the stratum corneum which contains fatty acids, but may not penetrate any further. Free fatty acids, however, combine lipophilicity with molecular masses well below 500, and can therefore be absorbed through skin.

The transdermal absorption of fatty acids may be further promoted by some essential oil constituents. A preparation containing various concentrations of 1,8-cineole, ethanol and borage oil containing ~25% γ-linolenic acid (GLA) enhanced the in vitro permeation of GLA through full-thickness pig skin (Ho et al 2004). Conversely, the permeation of several drugs through mouse skin was greatly enhanced by the addition of unsaturated fatty acids in propylene glycol, the most effective being oleic acid. Saturated fatty acids were mainly less effective (Oh et al 2001; Gwak & Chun 2002). Using full-thickness human skin, the permeation of tamoxifen was enhanced either by the addition of borage oil or GLA. These effects were explained by the formation of solvation complexes with greater penetrant properties (Karia et al 2004; Heard et al 2005). Permeation enhancement has also been reported using oleic, palmitoleic and linoleic acids in combination with benzyl alcohol (Nanayakkara et al 2005).

Although an oil is not an ideal vehicle for promoting the absorption of lipophilic substances (Bowman & Rand 1980), the rate of passage across the skin will increase with concentration according to Fick's first law.[1] For this reason, we would expect the constituents of undiluted essential oils may diffuse into the skin more rapidly than when they are diluted in a vehicle. For example, when linalyl acetate was applied undiluted to human skin in vitro, absorption into the stratum corneum, viable epidermis and dermis were all noted, but when diluted at 0.75% in hydrogel, grapeseed oil or emulsion, no absorption was seen (Cal & Sznitowska 2003; Cal 2006b).

In some applications, a slow absorption rate of essential oil constituents may be desirable from a safety point of view (and also a therapeutic one, if the aim is to keep oils at the site of application for as long as possible, e.g., in case of certain skin conditions).

In regard to safety, the application of undiluted essential oils to the skin is controversial. It is proscribed by most aromatherapy schools and practitioner associations. Trade organizations such as the UK's Aromatherapy Trade Council require their members to include a safety statement on bottles of essential oils to the effect that the oil should not be used undiluted on the skin. On the other hand, the 'raindrop technique' involves the application of undiluted essential oils, specifically: oregano (2–4 drops), thyme (3–5 drops), basil (6–10 drops), cypress (6–10 drops), wintergreen (6–10 drops), marjoram (6–10 drops) and peppermint (6–10 drops), making a total of 35–59 drops (Essential Science Publishing 2004).[10]

There are reasons for avoiding this practice, especially in vulnerable groups such as infants, children or the elderly. First, the risk of skin reactions increases with essential oil concentration (see Ch. 5, p. 72) and the widespread use of raindrop technique could lead to an escalation of skin allergy to essential oils. Undiluted thyme and oregano oils, for example, pose a risk of skin irritation. Second, when essential oils are applied undiluted to the skin, percutaneous absorption may lead to relatively high constituent concentrations in the bloodstream, which increases the risk of systemic toxicity. Wintergreen oil, for example, is moderately-to-severely toxic, and many basil oils are potentially carcinogenic, with recommended dermal use levels of below 2% (see Chapter 13, Basil profiles). Finally, the risk of drug interactions is increased. Topically applied methyl salicylate can increase the anticoagulant effect of warfarin, causing side effects such as internal hemorrhage (Le Bourhis & Soenen 1973), and wintergreen oil contains 98% methyl salicylate.

There may be scenarios in which undiluted essential oils can be safely and profitably applied to the skin, possibly in the medical treatment of localized infections, and where benefits outweigh risks this may make sense. However, most practitioners should avoid using essential oils in this way, and encouraging untrained people to apply concentrated essential oils to themselves or others is unwise and unsafe. Table 4.5 gives recommended maximum concentrations for general massage purposes, and these also apply to any application to large areas of skin. For local application, concentrations greater than 5% may be appropriate. For wound healing (cuts, burns, sores and ulcers), concentrations between 4% and 12% can be both safe and effective (Guba 1998/1999; Jandera et al 2000; Hartman & Coetzee 2002; Kerr, 2002; Dryden et al 2004).

Hydration, temperature and pressure

Hydration of the stratum corneum, such as occurs during a bath or shower, facilitates essential oil absorption (Bowman & Rand 1980). For example, the dermal penetration of terpenes increased when essential oils were put in hot bath water, although inhalation was not controlled for (Römmelt et al 1974). By measuring the amount of salicylate excreted in urine, an early, very detailed study concluded that methyl salicylate permeation through the skin of the hand is greatly enhanced by prolonged prior immersion in hot water. It was also found that massage of the hand increased dermal absorption by 34–158%, depending on the experimental parameters (Brown & Scott 1934). This may be due to the stimulating effect of massage on blood flow, though in a study using excised human skin, pressure alone

increased the transcutaneous absorption of caffeine by up to 1.8 times (Treffel et al 1993).

A rise in temperature of $10\,^{\circ}C$ in the oil or oil suspension in which volunteers' hands are immersed increases the rate of percutaneous absorption several-fold, presumably because of enhanced capillary circulation in the area (Hotchkiss et al 1992). The use of an aqueous medium does not mean an increase in skin reactivity. In a small study of hand dermatitis patients allergic to hydroxycitronellal, there were no reactions when the fingers were immersed in water containing 0.025% of the substance (Heydorn et al 2003c).

Volatility and occlusion

When applied to warm, unoccluded (uncovered) skin, in general, the smaller constituents are more volatile than the larger ones. The more volatile essential oil constituents partially evaporate, reducing the amounts available for absorption. This may partly explain why only a small proportion (2.61%) of benzyl alcohol (liquid, boiling point (bp) = $108\,^{\circ}C$) is absorbed even though it readily partitions through the skin (Jimbo et al 1983), while a much higher proportion (33.0%) of coumarin (solid, bp = $301\,^{\circ}C$) is absorbed (Beckley-Kartey et al 1997). Both substances were applied, diluted in ethanol, to unoccluded, excised human abdominal skin (benzyl alcohol) or breast skin (coumarin) and assessed after 24 hours.

If the skin is occluded with a non-permeable material after application of an undiluted essential oil, absorption into the bloodstream is greatly increased (Wester & Maibach 1983; Bronaugh et al 1990). Using epidermal tissue from six donors and 70/30 v/v ethanol/water as a vehicle, the total amount of linalool absorbed after 24 hours was 3.57% for unoccluded skin, and 14.1% for occluded skin (Lapczynski et al 2008g). Occlusion changes the temperature and hydration of the skin, as well as minimizing evaporation, and these physical factors affect absorption (Wester & Maibach 1983).

Trauma

When the skin is damaged or diseased, the rate of absorption of applied substances can be significantly faster. For example, the severity of atopic and seborrheic dermatitis in children correlates with the percutaneous absorption of hydrocortisone (Turpeinen 1988). Similarly, increasing human skin barrier damage correlates with increased dermal penetration of salicylic acid (Benfeldt et al 1999). A larger concentration of bergapten was found in the skin of psoriatic patients than in volunteers with healthy skin following application of a topical gel (Colombo et al 2003).

In inflammatory skin diseases, such as psoriasis and atopic dermatitis, there is decreased barrier function, allowing easier dermal penetration (Madison 2003). Barrier disruption produces a cytokine response and an increase in epidermal Langerhans cell density, which may promote inflammation (Ghadially 1998). In atopic dermatitis, there is a significant decrease in the production of certain skin lipids, which in part explains the barrier disruption (Schafer & Kragballe 1991). The increased absorption results in a greater risk of skin reactions, creating a negative cycle (Wester & Noonan 1980).

Surprisingly, even non-diseased areas of skin can show barrier dysfunction, whether on parts of the body not affected by skin disease, or in people whose condition has only recently resolved (Berardesca et al 1990). Factors that can negatively affect skin barrier function include psychological stress and chronic alcoholism (Garg et al 2001; Brand & Jendrzejewski 2008). In any type of skin disease, essential oils should always be applied with caution.

Age

Neonatal skin is much thinner than adult skin (Lund et al 1999). The skin of pre-term infants is approximately 2.5 times more permeable than adult skin, and before 30 weeks gestation it is 100–1,000 times more permeable (Fischer 1985; Barker et al 1987). Before 30 weeks gestation, the epidermis is thin, has only a few cell layers, and a poorly formed stratum corneum, but by 34 weeks it has largely matured, and by 37 weeks drug absorption and trans-epidermal water loss (TEWL) has considerably reduced (Harpin & Rutter 1983; Evans & Rutter 1986). Epidermal barrier properties undergo a number of significant changes during the first 4 weeks of life, including a decrease in surface pH and an increase in surface hydration (Visscher et al 2000). These progressive adaptation processes continue until 12 weeks (Hoeger & Enzmann 2002). Therefore children up to three months are at increased risk of skin damage from topically applied agents.

In the elderly, a number of radical changes take place in the skin (Roskos & Maibach 1992). The corneocytes become less adherent to one another, there is a flattening of the dermoepidermal interface, and the number of melanocytes and Langerhans cells decreases (Fenske & Lober 1986). There is an overall thinning of the epidermis, and TEWL increases significantly, the result being greater permeability, which is further accentuated in photo-aged skin (Lavker et al 1986; Wilhelm et al 1991). This process is due to a reduction in stratum corneum lipids and a profound abnormality in cholesterol synthesis (Elias & Ghadially 2002). Barrier recovery from dermal injury is approximately three times slower in people over 80 than in those of 20–30 years of age (Ghadially et al 1995). In elderly people, the risk of sensitization may decrease due to a reduction in the number of Langerhans cells, although the reduction in barrier function may more than compensate for this. In a comparison of 41 healthy volunteers with a mean age of 24 years and 82 volunteers with a mean age of 75 years, 37% of the older group reacted to at least one of 22 allergens on patch testing, compared with 15% of the younger group (Mangelsdorf et al 1996).

Other factors

Studies of human skin at different times of day suggest that permeability is higher in the evening and at night than in the morning (Yosipovitch et al 1998). Deeply pigmented skin has superior barrier integrity and function compared to less pigmented skin (Reed et al 1995).

Dermal dosing

For both practitioner and recipient safety, it is important to limit the amounts of essential oil used in aromatherapy. It is equally necessary to limit dermal dosing for essential oils that contain, for example, carcinogenic, neurotoxic, or phototoxic constituents. Maximum dermal use levels for these oils are given in the profiles.

The total quantity of essential oil absorbed into the body from an aromatherapy massage varies according to:

- the total quantity of oil(s) applied
- the dilution of the essential oil in the vehicle
- the vehicle in which the essential oil(s) is/are dispersed
- the total area of skin to which the oil is applied
- the health and integrity of the skin
- the age of the recipient
- the temperature and moisture content of the skin
- the extent to which the skin is covered after the massage
- how soon the skin is washed following the massage
- the essential oil(s) used.

Using the first five variables, it is possible to make an approximate estimate of the range of quantities that will be absorbed. The percentage dilution used for massage over a large area of skin is commonly between 2% and 3%, but with a minimum of 1% and maximum of 5%. The usual vehicle is a vegetable oil such as sweet almond oil, and the total quantity of essential oil applied ranges between a minimum of 5 mL and a maximum of 30 mL for a full-body massage (Harding, Harris, Sade, private communications, 2005). The maximum number of full-body applications in 24 hours is one. The smallest quantity of total essential oil likely to be applied in practice is therefore 0.05 mL, and the largest quantity is 1.5 mL. Table 4.6 is a key to calculating various dilutions of essential oil. Using Imperial units, a simple approach is as follows:

0.1% = 1 drop of essential oil per ounce of excipient
1% = 10 drops of essential oil per ounce of excipient
2% = 20 drops of essential oil per ounce of excipient, etc.

Since 1 mL of essential oil is equivalent to 20–40 drops, depending on the type of dropper used (Svoboda et al 2001), 0.15 mL is equivalent to 3–6 drops of essential oil.

Infants and children

Great caution is necessary for infants. Since neonatal skin does not mature until three months of age, it is more sensitive and more permeable to essential oils. A newborn is also less equipped to deal with any adverse effects than an adult

Table 4.5 Age-related recommended and maximum concentrations of essential oils for massage

Age	Essential oil concentration	
	Recommended (%)	Maximum (%)
Premature infant	0	0
Up to 3 months	0.1	0.2
3–24 months	0.25	0.5
2–6 years	1.0	2.0
6–15 years	1.5	3.0
15+ years	2.5	5.0

These concentrations are not research-based, and should be taken as helpful suggestions rather than absolute rules. The particular oils used and the health status of the individual are also important factors.

Table 4.6 Calculating essential oil concentrations

Desired % of essential oil	Number of drops of essential oil needed for 8 different volumes							
	5 mL	10 mL	15 mL	20 mL	25 mL	30 mL	50 mL	100 mL
0.03	0.05	0.1	0.14	0.2	0.23	0.27	0.5	1
0.05	0.1	0.15	0.2	0.3	0.4	0.5	0.75	1.5
0.07	0.1	0.2	0.3	0.4	0.5	0.6	1	2
0.1	0.15	0.3	0.5	0.6	0.75	0.9	1.5	3
0.2	0.3	0.6	0.9	1.2	1.5	1.8	3	6
0.3	0.5	0.9	1.4	1.8	2.25	2.7	4.5	9
0.4	0.6	1.2	1.8	2.4	3	3.6	6	12
0.5	0.75	1.5	2.25	3	3.75	4.5	7.5	15
0.6	0.9	1.8	2.7	3.6	4.5	5.4	9	18
0.7	1	2	3	4.2	5.25	6.3	10.5	21
0.8	1.2	2.4	3.6	4.8	6	7.2	12	24
0.9	1.35	2.7	4	5.4	6.75	8	13.5	27
1.0	1.5	3	4.5	6	7.5	9	15	30
1.1	1.7	3.3	5	6.6	8.25	9.9	16.5	33
1.2	1.8	3.6	5.4	7.2	9	10.8	18	36
1.3	2	4	6	8	9.75	11.7	19.5	39
1.4	2	4.2	6.3	8.4	10.5	12.6	21	42
1.5	2.25	4.5	6.75	9	11.25	13.5	22.5	45
1.6	2.4	4.8	7.2	9.6	12	14.4	24	48
1.7	2.5	5	7.7	10	12.75	15	25.5	51
1.8	2.7	5.4	8	10.8	13.5	16	27	54
1.9	2.9	5.7	8.6	11.4	14.25	17	28.5	57
2.0	3	6	9	12	15	18	30	60
2.5	3.75	7.5	11.25	15	18.75	22.5	37.5	75
3.0	4.5	9	13.5	18	22.5	27	45	90
3.5	5.25	10.5	15.75	21	26.25	31.5	52.5	105
4.0	6	12	18	24	30	36	60	120
4.5	6.75	13.5	20.25	27	33.75	40.5	67.5	135
5.0	7.5	15	22.5	30	37.5	45	75	150

The numbers in the table refer to drops of essential oil. Although we have given precise figures, fractions of drops may be rounded up or down to the nearest whole drop. These figures assume that 30 drops of essential oil = 1 mL. For instance, a 0.4% dilution of bergamot oil will be obtained by mixing three drops of bergamot oil in 25 mL of vehicle, or 6 drops in 50 mL. These figures are averages, as the number of drops per mL can vary from 20 to 40, according to the type of dropper used (Svoboda et al 2001).

because of a lower metabolic capacity, i.e., enzymes present in lower concentrations.[11] These cautions apply even more to premature babies, and here it would be prudent to avoid all use of essential oils.

When massaging or applying essential oils to children, the total dose applied will be less than for adults because of their smaller body size. Recommended and maximum % concentrations of essential oils for children are given in Table 4.5.

We recommend that infants are not given baths containing essential oils unless the oils have been previously dispersed in a water-soluble medium. This is to guard against skin irritation from undispersed oils, and could be applied in fact to any age group.

Inhalation

Inhaled substances pass down the trachea into the bronchi, and from there into finer and finer bronchioles, ending at the microscopic, sac-like alveoli of the lungs, where gaseous exchange with the blood mainly takes place. The alveoli are extremely efficient at transporting small molecules, such as essential oil constituents, into the blood. This efficiency increases with the rate of blood flow through the lungs, the rate and depth of breathing, and with the fat-solubility of the molecules (Breuninger et al 1970; Römmelt et al 1987).

The olfactory epithelium, though small, also acts as an absorptive membrane and a high proportion of the molecules that come into contact with the nasal mucosa are absorbed into the general circulation (Gilman et al 1980). Essential oil constituents absorbed via inhalation may enter the bloodstream and reach the central nervous system (CNS) with relative ease. Easy access to the CNS may have safety implications, especially if potentially neurotoxic compounds are being inhaled. There might be particular risks for people with CNS pathologies, such as epilepsy.

When eight male volunteers were exposed to air concentrations of 10, 225 or 450 mg/m^3 of 97% pure (+)-limonene during light physical exercise, mean respective capillary blood concentrations were 1.5, 11.0 and 21.0 µmol/L after one hour, and 1.5, 12.5 and 23 µmol/L after two hours. Up to 70% of the higher two doses was absorbed into the blood. The authors suggested that it might take three days for the highest dose to be eliminated entirely. The doses of (+)-limonene used were equivalent to evaporating 1–40 g in a 100 m^3 room (2 m × 5 m × 10 m). The subjects experienced no irritation or CNS-related symptoms, or any significant changes in lung function variables (Falk-Filipsson et al 1993).

In two similarly constructed studies, the human pulmonary uptake was ~60% for inhaled α-pinene, and ~70% for δ-3-carene at the two higher doses. Total uptake increased linearly with increasing exposure, and the total blood clearance was high. In both reports there were no changes in lung function at the higher levels, but some airway irritation was observed (Falk et al 1990, 1991a). When two male and two female volunteers inhaled air passed over 4 mL of 1,8-cineole for 20 minutes, peak plasma concentrations of 459–1,135 ng/mL were attained after 14–19 minutes, with average absorption half-lives of 3.4 minutes for males, and 10 minutes for females (Jäger et al 1996). No irritation was reported.

In experiments with mice, after one hour of continuous inhalation, the plasma concentrations of various constituents (coumarin, α-terpineol, linalool, linalyl acetate) were in the range of 2–10 ng/mL (Jirovetz et al 1991, 1992). Similarly, one hour after 0.5 mL of rosemary oil was evaporated in sealed cages, the air concentration of 1,8-cineole (39% of the oil) was 13.7–15.6 nL/mL. After 60 minutes of inhalation, the mean plasma concentration of 1,8-cineole (in five mice) increased linearly from 4.5 to 15.5 nL/g blood, depending on the amount of rosemary oil evaporated (0.1–0.6 mL/cage) (Kovar et al 1987).

Inhalation is an important route of exposure because of the role of odor in aromatherapy, but from a safety standpoint it presents a very low level of risk to most people. Even in a relatively small closed room, and assuming 100% evaporation, the concentration of any essential oil or constituent is unlikely to reach a dangerous level, either from aromatherapy massage or from essential oil vaporization. The only likely risk would be from prolonged exposure (perhaps 30 minutes or more) to relatively high levels of essential oil vapor, such as could occur when directly sniffing from a bottle of undiluted oil, or moderate exposure (perhaps 10 minutes or more) to high concentrations of neurotoxic constituents such as pinocamphone or thujone. However, there is currently insufficient information to define what constitutes an inhalational risk.

Inhalation dosing

Inhalation is a useful route for administering essential oils (as vapors) when a local action on any part of the respiratory tract is required. For example, thyme oil or blue chamomile oil can be inhaled for their antibacterial or anti-inflammatory actions, respectively. However, dosing by this route is difficult to estimate and control because of inherent uncertainties including the proportions of evaporated constituents entering the nose, duration of inhalation, methods used to evaporate an oil, etc. In any case, it is unlikely that sufficient essential oil vapor will be inhaled under normal conditions to represent a toxic hazard. On the other hand, toxicity is more likely to result from accidental instillation of oils.

The Swedish occupational exposure limit to inhaled terpenes such as δ-3-carene, α-pinene and β-pinene is 150 mg/m^3 (Eriksson et al 1997). The reported sensory irritation threshold for inhaled limonene in humans is above 80 ppm, while the NOAEL was estimated to be 100 ppm in mice (Larsen et al 2000).

Oral administration

Advantages of the oral route include that it is convenient for the patient, allows for greater precision in dosing, and the bioavailability of oil constituents is often high. For example, after ingestion of GeloMyrtol forte capsules, a treatment for bronchitis and sinusitis, the bioavailability of 1,8-cineole, the main ingredient, was 95.6% (Zimmermann et al 1995).

Most oral preparations can be formulated so that they have little or no taste and gastrointestinal irritation is often minimal or non-existent. Much larger amounts can be administered than by other routes, so great care must be exercised if prescribing in this way. Those medical practitioners who favor the oral route are frequently treating infectious diseases that require heavy dosing. However, any hazards are also magnified proportionately.

One disadvantage of oral dosing with essential oils is that some of the constituents might irritate the gastrointestinal mucosa, which is generally more sensitive to insult than skin. Since irritation is concentration-dependent, it is important that the essential oil is efficiently dispersed or dissolved in an appropriate vehicle before being swallowed. Preferred methods would be to administer essential oils either in capsules, dissolved in a lipophilic medium such as a vegetable oil, or in aqueous alcohol. As well as preventing gastric irritation, dispersal aids efficient and steady absorption. Note that high viscosity (such as that of vegetable oils) has been shown to slow absorption from the gastrointestinal tract (Gerarde 1960).

Oral administration always carries the potential for inducing nausea and vomiting, and the presence of food has unpredictable effects on absorption into the bloodstream. Digestive enzymes can break down some types of essential oil constituents, for example esters may be hydrolyzed in the stomach. After absorption from almost all regions of the gastrointestinal (GI) tract, most substances pass directly to the liver, where a significant proportion is deactivated in first-pass metabolism but some, paradoxically, are made more toxic.

Virtually all recorded cases of serious poisoning with essential oils have occurred after the ingestion of large amounts of essential oil (see Chapter 3), although these amounts are generally much higher than therapeutic doses.

Oral dosing

In various studies, the quantities of essential oils that have been taken orally by adults over a 24 hour period range from 0.05–1.3 mL (Table 4.7). The typical oral dosage range (0.22–0.66 mL) is approximately ten times greater than the amount typically absorbed from massage (0.03–0.06 mL). We have assumed that 100% of any oil administered orally is absorbed. Although this is unlikely in every instance, it is appropriate for a worst-case scenario.

If oral dosage is 10 times greater than for massage, this constitutes a reasonable basis for making a clear distinction between the two in terms of safety. Absorption into the bloodstream after dermal application is slower than after oral dosing, and the mucous membranes of the GI tract are likely to be more readily penetrated (due to blood capillaries close to the surface) and more easily irritated than skin, therefore requiring greater caution. With oral administration there is a greater risk of overdose, of gastric irritation, and of interactions with medications. Therefore only practitioners who are qualified to diagnose, trained to weigh risks against benefits, and have a knowledge of essential oil pharmacology should prescribe essential oils for oral administration.

Frequency of dosing

The frequency of oral dosing for any therapeutic substance is determined by factors such as optimum plasma concentration, duration of treatment and patient compliance. Most importantly, the elimination half-life tells us how often we need to dose to maintain a certain blood concentration. For conditions where this is important, e.g., in treating infections, essential oils are often given three times per day (Belaiche 1979). As can be seen from Table 4.8, there is considerable variation in the elimination half-lives of constituents. Although three daily doses might be appropriate for some oils, the same regimen for thymol-rich oils, for instance, may lead to adverse effects due to accumulation of thymol.

Since there is little information concerning the safety of oral dosing over a period of several days or weeks, individual cases should be carefully monitored by the supervising primary care practitioner.

Infants and children

The dosage of a drug is normally reduced for children in proportion to body weight, so that approximately the same amount of drug per kg of body weight is administered. So, for a 30 kg

Table 4.7 Daily oral doses of essential oil-based medicines

Medication	Daily dose	Condition	Reference
Anise oil	300 mg	Dyspepsia	Blumenthal et al 1998
1,8-Cineole	200 mg × 3	Sinusitis	Kehrl et al 2004
Cinnamon bark oil	50–200 mg	Loss of appetite, dyspepsia	Blumenthal et al 1998
Eucalyptus oil	300–600 mg	Respiratory catarrh	Blumenthal et al 2000
Fennel oil	0.1–0.6 mL	Dyspepsia	Blumenthal et al 1998
GeloMyrtol forte[a]	300 mg × 4	Acute bronchitis	Matthys et al 2000
Geranium oil	0.45 mL	Stress and hypertension	Nozaki 2001
Gouttes aux essences[b]	90–120 mg × 3	Acute bronchitis	Ferley et al 1989
Juniperberry oil	20–100 mg	Dyspepsia	Blumenthal et al 1998
Oregano oil	200 mg × 3	Intestinal parasites	Force et al 2000
Peppermint oil + Caraway oil	90 mg × 2 50 mg × 2	Dyspepsia	May et al 2000
Peppermint oil	0.2–0.4 mL × 3	Irritable bowel syndrome	Reynolds 1993
Peppermint oil	450 mg × 2	Irritable bowel syndrome	Cappello et al 2007

Daily totals range from 50 mg (cinnamon bark oil) to 1,200 mg (GeloMyrtol forte), or 0.05–1.3 mL.
The majority of daily doses range from 200–600 mg (0.22–0.66 mL)
[a]Main active ingredient by volume is 1,8-cineole, and also contains (+)-limonene and α-pinene
[b]Contains peppermint, cinnamon, clove, lavender and thyme oils.

(66 lb) child, a normal oral dose of essential oil would be 0.1–0.4 mL (~3–12 drops) in 24 hours (i.e., 30/70 of the adult dose of 0.25 mL to 1 mL). This would be given in three daily doses of ~1–4 drops per dose. We do not recommend oral dosing in children weighing less than 20 kg (44 lb).

Alternatively, if a child's weight is not known, Young's or Dilling's formulas could be applied to give an approximate dose based on age alone.[12]

Rectal administration

Suppositories are sometimes used as alternatives when oral dosing results in significant breakdown of essential oils in the gastrointestinal tract or by first-pass metabolism in the liver, and

Table 4.8 Elimination half-lives of some essential oil constituents

Constituent	Route	Animal (sex, if known)	Half-life (hours)	Reference
β-Asarone	Oral	Rat	0.9	Wu and Fang 2004
δ-3-Carene	Inhalation	Human (M)	4.5	Filipsson 1996
1,8-Cineole	Inhalation	Human (F)	2.95	Jäger et al 1996
1,8-Cineole	Inhalation	Human (M)	0.5	Jäger et al 1996
Cinnamaldehyde	Intravenous	Rat (M & F)	1.7	Yuan et al 1992
Coumarin	Dermal	Human (M)	1.7	Ford et al 2001
(+)-Limonene	Inhalation	Human (M)	1.25	Falk-Filipsson et al 1993
(+)-Limonene	Oral	Rat	5.6	Chen et al 1998
(−)-Menthol*	Oral	Human (M & F)	0.9	Gelal et al 1999
Methyleugenol	Oral	Human (M & F)	1.5	Schecter et al 2004
Methyl salicylate	Bath	Human	2.4–4.0	Pratzel et al 1990
α-Pinene[†]	Inhalation	Human (M)	4.8	Filipsson 1996
β-Pinene[†]	Inhalation	Human (M)	5.3	Filipsson 1996
Thymol	Oral	Human (M)	10.2	Kohlert et al 2002

[†]Isomer not specified
*Half-life for menthol glucuronide

where high systemic concentrations are desired. Another advantage is that it is the most efficient way to administer a remedy locally to the lower colon. Being lined with a mucous membrane, the rectum is highly sensitive to irritation, especially if the essential oil is unevenly dispersed. Rectal administration of 1,8-cineole, menthol or thymol resulted in respectively high, moderate and zero elimination via the lungs in rats (Grisk & Fisher 1969).

Formulations can be based on lipophilic or hydrophilic vehicles. The same principles that apply to partitioning of substances across the skin also apply to mucous membranes. Thus, cocoa butter, a lipophilic vehicle, is especially useful for delivering hydrophilic substances. The same cautions about concentration and dispersal apply as for oral administration, as mucous membrane irritation is likely with some oils.

Vaginal administration

Pessaries are formulated in a similar way to suppositories, but are placed into the vagina for local absorption. They provide a convenient route for administering essential oils for the treatment of vulval and vaginal infection or irritation. Alternatively, essential oils can be applied in aqueous douches. The main

safety considerations are similar to those for oral and rectal administration. The mucous membrane lining the vagina is highly sensitive to irritation, and care is needed to ensure that the essential oil is administered in appropriate amounts and is evenly dispersed. Some form of emulsification will therefore be required for douches.

There are very few reports of vaginal or vulval reactions to essential oils. There is one alleging a connection between vulvovaginitis and both tea tree oil and the lavender absolute content of a lavender gel (confusingly, the lavender absolute is also referred to as 'lavender oil absolute' and 'lavender oil'). However, clinical relevance is questionable, especially for lavender absolute, which patch tested positive at 10%, but not at 2% (Varma et al 2000).

When 92 women with vulval complaints were patch tested, 35 had positive allergic reactions, 15 of which were considered relevant to their clinical condition, most of these being allergies to topical pharmaceutical products. There were four reactions to the fragrance mix (see Chapter 5), one to 2% oxidized (+)-limonene, and one to 2% isoeugenol, but none of these were clinically relevant (Nardelli et al 2004).

In terms of safety, a distinction should be made between fragranced products such as intimate wipes, washes, fragrances, etc., intended for frequent application to the female genitalia, and the therapeutic application of essential oil-based preparations to treat vulvovaginitis. Essential oils such as tea tree and geranium may eliminate the infective cause, and directly reduce inflammation (Blackwell 1991; Maruyama et al 2008). For intimate use products, a safety factor of 20 has been suggested in extrapolating from skin to mucosal exposure (Farage et al 2003). For therapeutic products, essential oil concentrations of 1–5% have been proposed, but clinical data are sparse, and it would appear that adverse reactions are rare.

Distribution

The distribution of substances within the body is largely determined by their solubility in the various aqueous and fatty body compartments. In a similar way to that whereby substances reach the bloodstream from their sites of administration, tissue distribution also depends on the relative lipid and water solubility of the substance in question. However, passage from blood into the tissues varies between different tissues. Lipophilic substances are readily taken up into the liver, while water-soluble compounds tend to remain primarily in the blood or move to other aqueous compartments. Diffusion into the brain requires a substance to be appreciably lipophilic because tight junctions between adjacent endothelial cells lining its blood vessels (the so-called blood–brain barrier) force it to pass by the intracellular route. Essential oil constituents are able to penetrate the blood–brain barrier, and have been observed to interact with various receptor sites in the brain, such as those for GABA and glutamate (Aoshima & Hamamoto 1999; Elisabetsky et al 1999).

Once absorbed into the bloodstream, the extent to which a substance is taken up by different body tissues depends partly on the amount of blood they receive. Tissues that receive a high proportion of the cardiac output include the brain, kidneys, lungs and exercising skeletal muscle. When at rest, however, skeletal muscle has a relatively low throughput of blood. Usually, the tissues and organs most affected by toxic substances are those exposed to high blood concentrations.

The liver, which carries out a large number of biotransformations, is subject to site-specific toxicity since innocuous substances may be converted into toxic ones that exert local effects. While the blood–brain barrier offers some protection to the adult brain, these barriers are less effective in the peripheral nervous system and in the immature brain, and are therefore more susceptible to toxic compounds. The lungs are also exposed to a high throughput of inhaled air, which may carry toxic gases, vapors and fine particles.

Accumulation in tissues

Being predominantly lipophilic, mono- and sesquiterpenes would be expected to spend a short time in the bloodstream before being redistributed first to muscle, and then over a longer period of time to fat. However, repeated high doses can lead to toxicity due to accumulation. This may explain why a woman who ingested 20 drops of thuja oil twice a day for five days, had a seizure and fell after the tenth dose (Millet et al 1981).

Uptake into body fat is an important factor in the distribution of lipophilic compounds, as fat can act as a reservoir, slowly removing compounds from, and releasing them back into the blood circulation. This will be more important in obese individuals. While localized in fat, most substances are unable to exert any pharmacological or toxicological actions.

Essential oil constituents probably remain in fatty tissues for several hours or days.[13] For example, rats and mice eliminated all of an oral dose of citral (up to 1 g/kg) within 72 hours and 120 hours, respectively, and after dermal application of benzyl acetate to rats, virtually all the absorbed dose was excreted within 24 hours (Phillips et al 1976; Chidgey et al 1987). Citral is significantly more lipophilic than benzyl acetate, as suggested by their calculated log P (octanol/water) values of 3.0 and 2.0, respectively.[8]

Fat tissue is poorly served with blood vessels, so equilibration of a substance with blood is slow. If body fat were to be significantly reduced, for example in malnutrition, toxic effects could result from a short-term release of accumulated substances.

In experimental animals, thymol, carvacrol, eugenol and guaiacol (log P (octanol/water) = 3.2, 3.4, 2.4 and 1.3, respectively)[8] redistributed rapidly to the blood and kidneys following oral administration (Schröder & Vollmer 1932). Most of an intravenous dose of (E)-anethole (log P = 3.3) given to mice was accumulated by the liver, lungs and brain (Le Bourhis 1968). In rats, citral (log P = 3.0) was rapidly and completely absorbed from the GI tract and then redistributed equally to all the tissues (Phillips et al 1976). Following an intragastric dose of 500 mg/kg linalool (log P = 3.4) in rats, 96% was excreted within 72 hours (Parke et al 1974b). The data in Table 4.9 show that relatively small amounts of constituents are excreted following inhalation. Slower excretion probably indicates a longer time in body tissues, compared to oral administration.

Binding to plasma proteins

The blood contains a number of soluble proteins that can bind to, and form reversible complexes with, many circulating small molecules. The protein most commonly implicated is albumin, which is present in very high concentration in the blood in healthy subjects. Because of its high concentration, its effect on the concentration of free small molecules can be large. The proportion of a drug that exists at any time in its bound state depends on the affinity of albumin for that substance. If a small amount of a substance with a high affinity for albumin enters the bloodstream, it will effectively be mopped up, leaving very little free in the circulation. In this way, plasma proteins function in a similar way to adipose tissue.

Although a wide range of drugs and hormones are known to bind to plasma proteins to varying degrees, little is known about essential oil constituents. While most have properties that might favor binding to plasma proteins (Florence & Attwood 1998), many reports indicate that they are rapidly cleared from the body. This suggests that protein binding, and therefore accumulation in the bloodstream, is relatively unimportant for essential oil constituents (Kohlert et al 2000).

In rats, β-elemene was absorbed and eliminated rapidly and distributed widely in the body after ip or iv administration despite being 97% bound to plasma proteins, suggesting rapid rates of uptake and release from proteins (Wang & Su 2000). After oral dosing, 98.5% of bergapten and 77.5% of methoxsalen became reversibly bound to serum proteins, principally albumin (Artuc et al 1979) and following intravenous and oral administration, the plasma protein binding of (+)-limonene was 55.3% (Chen et al 1998). Binding to human serum albumin has also been demonstrated for borneol, safranal and thymoquinone (Kanakis et al 2007; Hu & Chen 2009; Lupidi et al 2010).[14]

C-(1R)-(+)-β-pulegone metabolites are thought to bind to α_{2u}-globulin in male rats (Chen LJ et al 2003). This plasma protein is specific to male rats, and causes 'protein droplet' nephropathy. (+)-Limonene 1,2-oxide, a metabolite of (+)-limonene, also binds reversibly to α_{2u}-globulin (Lehman-McKeeman et al 1989).

While bound to plasma protein (or stored in fatty tissue) a compound will be unable to express any pharmacological or toxicological activity. In addition, bound compounds will be unavailable for possible biotransformation and excretion (see later sections), and so their lifetime in the body will be prolonged. Compounds that bind to the same plasma proteins can also influence each other's actions by competing for binding sites. Because essential oil constituents will probably bind to some extent to plasma proteins, there is a theoretical possibility that they could interact with some drugs (Figure 4.3).

As with orthodox drugs, there may be a case for reducing the dosage of essential oils given orally to patients with kidney or liver disease since their plasma albumin levels may be depressed, and there is likely to be a greater proportion of free molecules in the blood (Bowman & Rand 1982). However, since most essential oil constituents studied have fairly short half-lives (Table 4.8) and their blood levels following a typical aromatherapy massage will be relatively low, protein binding is not likely to have any significant consequences for their actions or those of co-administered drugs.

Table 4.9 Excretion of some essential oil constituents in mammals

Species	Constituent	Route	Urine	Feces	Exhaled air	Reference
Cat	(Z,E)-Nepetalactone	Oral	86–94%	1–2%	1–12%	Waller et al 1969
Rat	Isoeugenol	Oral	>85%	10%	<0.1%	Badger et al 2002
Rat	Cinnamaldehyde	Oral	80–85%	3–7%	NS	Sapienza et al 1993
Rat	Cinnamic acid	Oral	87.8%	0.8%	NS	Nutley et al 1994
Rat	Indole	Oral	80%	10%	2%	Scheline 1991
Rat/mouse	Allyl isothiocyanate	Oral	75%	1–5%	13–15%	Ioannou et al 1984
Rat	Citral	Oral	61%	17%	20%	Phillips et al 1976
Mouse	Piperonal	Oral	89%	3.2%	1.1%	Kamienski & Casida 1970
Rat	Linalool[a]	Oral	58%	15%	23%	Parke et al 1974b
Rat	(+)-Limonene	Oral	60%	5%	2%	Igimi et al 1974
Rabbit	(+)-Limonene	Oral	72%	7%	NS	Kodama et al 1974
Rabbit	Eugenol	Oral	>70%	NS	NS	Schröder & Vollmer 1932
Human	Eugenol	Oral	95%	NS	NS	Fischer et al 1990
Rat	Safrole	Oral	92%	None	NS	Benedetti et al 1977
Human	Safrole	Oral	88%	NS	NS	Benedetti et al 1977
Rat	Vanillin	Oral	41–47%	NS	NS	Scheline 1991
Rabbit	Vanillin	Oral	69%	NS	NS	Scheline 1991
Human	Vanillin	Oral	73%	NS	NS	Scheline 1991
Human	Estragole	Oral	31–54%	0%	12.9%	Sangster et al 1987
Human	Anethole	Oral	63.5–67%	NS	19.8%	Sangster et al 1987
Human	β-Pinene[a]	iv	NS	NS	3%	Römmelt et al 1974
Human	Camphene[a]	iv	NS	NS	3.6%	Römmelt et al 1974
Human	α-Pinene[a]	Inhalation	NS	NS	8%	Falk et al 1990
Human	δ-3-Carene	Inhalation	0.001%	NS	3%	Falk et al 1991a

The values given above represent the percentage of radiolabel excreted, frequently as metabolites, following administration of a radiolabeled constituent.

NS = not studied

[a]Isomer not specified

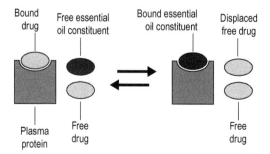

Figure 4.3 • Schematic diagram of interaction between an essential oil constituent and a drug at a plasma protein.

Metabolism

Metabolism is a process whereby a substance is chemically changed into one or more different substances in the body, each having its own physicochemical properties and biological actions. Metabolism has two main consequences. Firstly, a metabolite is usually more hydrophilic than its parent compound, and it will therefore be eliminated more rapidly via the kidneys (see Excretion below). Secondly, a metabolite usually has different pharmacological and/or toxicological properties compared to its parent compound. Once in the body, all organic compounds are susceptible to metabolism, although they may be metabolized by different routes and at different rates. The liver is the most important metabolizing organ though the skin, nervous tissue, kidneys, lungs, intestinal mucosa, blood plasma, the adrenals and placenta also have this ability.

In a similar way to other kinetic processes discussed in this chapter, it is important to appreciate that essential oils are mixtures, each constituent of which has its own metabolic fate. It is therefore inappropriate to speak of the metabolism of an essential oil. Typically, a compound will go through several stages of transformation, and each constituent may be subsequently eliminated from the body by one or more routes. Since biotransformation can also occur along several metabolic pathways at the same time, numerous metabolites may be created from a single compound. It is also worth noting that essential oil constituents that are predominantly lipophilic will have different tissue binding characteristics from their polar biotransformation products.[14] Metabolites, being less lipophilic than their precursors, are less likely to represent a toxic threat because they will be cleared from the body faster, and are less likely to linger in fatty tissues and on blood proteins.

The body is capable of carrying out many different kinds of biotransformation reactions on both exogenous and endogenous substances. These reactions are divided into so-called phase I and phase II reactions. Often, these reactions occur in sequence, but sometimes, one or both steps may be omitted. Figure 4.4 illustrates the possible routes and outcomes for a substance that has entered the body.

Phase I reactions

These are mainly concerned with introducing or unmasking polar and reactive functional groups, such as hydroxyl, amino and thiol groups. The most common phase I reactions are hydrolysis, oxidation and reduction, and they occur primarily in the liver.

Hydrolysis

Hydrolysis is a process whereby a compound is broken down into simpler compounds, and is accompanied by the chemical incorporation of water. Almost all tissues contain enzymes that catalyze hydrolysis, but the highest concentrations are found in the liver. Enzymes that hydrolyze esters are called esterases, and many of these enzymes are relatively non-specific and will accept a wide range of substrates. The esters commonly found in essential oils, such as linalyl acetate and geranyl propionate, are almost certainly metabolized in this way. The products of

ester hydrolysis are the parent carboxylic acids and alcohols. For example, methyl cinnamate is hydrolyzed to cinnamic acid and methanol, and methyl salicylate is hydrolyzed to salicylic acid and methanol.

Oxidation

Oxidation reactions are used very widely in the body to prepare molecules for conjugation. They usually involve the addition of an oxygen atom to a carbon, nitrogen or sulfur atom, or the removal of a hydrogen atom. An important reaction is the hydroxylation of benzene rings to give the corresponding phenols. Sometimes, bonds are cleaved under oxidizing conditions, for example, when alkyl groups are removed from ethers to give alcohols or phenols. (E)-Anethole is metabolized in this way to give the phenol analogue. The liver is the most important organ of oxidation, although the lung, kidney, skin, placenta and small intestine are also important.

The most important group of oxidative enzymes are the mixed function cytochromes P_{450} (CYP) of which there are more than 50 types in man. They can oxidize an extremely wide range of foreign molecules, including many pharmaceutical drugs, and are known to metabolize essential oil constituents.[15] (+)-Limonene, for example, is oxidized by CYP2B enzymes (Miyazawa et al 2001a). CYP enzymes often detoxify molecules, rendering them inactive, but they can also activate some molecules to highly reactive metabolites capable of seriously damaging the liver or other organs. Menthofuran, for example, is oxidized by CYP enzymes to reactive and hepatotoxic metabolites that irreversibly bind to cellular proteins in the liver (Madyastha & Raj 1990; Thomassen et al 1991).

Reduction

This reaction is far less important than oxidation and hydrolysis as a route for detoxification and elimination. Reduction essentially concerns the addition of hydrogen atoms to, or the removal of oxygen atoms from a substrate. In other words, it is the opposite of oxidation. Oral cuminaldehyde, for example, is primarily oxidized, though some reduction also occurs (Scheline 1991 p. 90). α-Ionone metabolism involves both oxidation and reduction (Ide & Toki 1970). Many microorganisms present in the gut possess reductive enzymes, but it is unlikely that these will play a significant part in the metabolism of essential oil constituents.

Phase II reactions

Phase II reactions are also known as conjugation reactions. They are those in which substances are combined with polar endogenous molecules in order to substantially reduce their lipid solubility and prepare them for excretion. Most drugs and essential oil constituents undergo reactions of this type (Bowman & Rand 1982). Included within this section are glucuronidation, sulfation, and glutathione conjugation.

Glucuronidation

Glucuronidation is the most common phase II reaction occurring in humans and many animals, and is nearly always a route

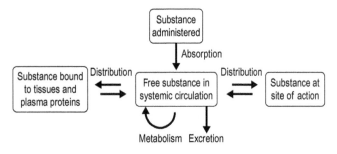

Figure 4.4 • Absorption, distribution, metabolism and excretion.

for detoxifying foreign substances. Glucuronides are formed by molecules that contain hydroxyl groups (alcohols and phenols), carboxylic acid groups and amino groups in the presence of a glucuronyl transferase enzyme.[16] Many essential oil constituents fall into one of the former two categories, and are eliminated from the body at least partly as glucuronides. Citronellal, for example, is largely conjugated with glucuronic acid, and a proportion is excreted as a dicarboxylic acid (Scheline 1991 p. 87). These conjugates are excreted in the urine if the molecular weight of the parent compound is 300 Da or less, as they are for most essential oil constituents. Glucuronides of higher molecular weights are likely to enter the gastrointestinal tract (for example, if excreted in the bile), where they may be hydrolyzed back to the parent compound.

Sulfation

Sulfate conjugation is almost as important as glucuronidation as a metabolic reaction. This reaction is catalyzed by sulfotransferase enzymes, which are present in the liver and other organs. Sulfate conjugates are extremely polar, and are therefore excreted readily via the kidneys. These enzymes are quickly saturated in the presence of large amounts of substrate. In the case of safrole, estragole and methyleugenol, this reaction is regarded as a toxification reaction, because in each case one of the metabolites, 1'-sulfooxysafrole, 1'-sulfooxyestragole and 1'-sulfooxymethyleugenol, is believed to be either the proximate or ultimate carcinogen.

Glutathione conjugation

Glutathione is a tripeptide that has a very reactive thiol functional group. It reacts with a wide range of foreign substances, catalyzed by glutathione transferase enzymes, to form glutathione conjugates, which are often converted to simpler conjugates such as N-acetylcysteine derivatives before being eliminated. Glutathione performs a protective role by reacting with, and mopping up reactive toxic molecules (e.g., free radicals) before they can damage DNA or proteins. It is thus a very important pathway for detoxifying a wide range of toxic substances taken into the body from the environment, especially since DNA damage can lead to the development of cancers. The liver is the main organ for carrying out glutathione conjugation reactions in the body.

A very small number of essential oil constituents are known to deplete hepatic glutathione (see Ch. 9, p. 127), and this could increase vulnerability to mutagens, as well as leading to hepatotoxicity. However, a large number of constituents induce glutathione S-transferase, thereby offering protection from mutagenesis (Box 4.1). (To induce an enzyme means to increase its rate of synthesis.) When this effect has been recorded, we have listed it in the relevant essential oil or constituent profile under Carcinogenic/anticarcinogenic potential.

Dermal metabolism

The skin contains many important enzymes that can transform exogenous chemicals into different compounds. Most are found in the suprabasal layers of the epidermis, though UDP-glucuronosyltransferase is found in the stratum corneum

---

Box 4.1

Essential oils and constituents that induce glutathione S-transferase

Constituent

Anethofuran (Zheng et al 1992d)

Benzyl isothiocyanate (Wattenberg 1983)

(+)-Carvone (Zheng et al 1992d)

β-Caryophyllene (Zheng et al 1992c)

β-Caryophyllene oxide (Zheng et al 1992c)

Citral (Nakamura et al 2003)

Diallyl disulfide (Munday & Munday 2001; Sheen et al 2001; Wu et al 2001; Fukao et al 2004)

Diallyl sulfide (Munday & Munday 2001; Sheen et al 2001)

Diallyl trisulfide (Munday & Munday 2001; Fukao et al 2004)

Eugenol (Yokota et al 1988; Zheng et al 1992c; Vidhya & Devaraj 1999)

Geraniol (Zheng et al 1993a, 1993b)

α-Humulene (Zheng et al 1992c)

(+)-Limonene (Zheng et al 1992d, 1993a, 1993b)

Methyl allyl trisulfide (Wattenberg et al 1985)

Myristicin (Ahmad et al 1997; Zheng et al 1992b)

Essential oil[a]

Ambrette (residues) (Lam & Zheng 1991)

Angelica root (Lam & Zheng 1991)

Basil (holy) (Aruna & Sivaramakrishnan 1996)

Basil (linalool CT) (Lam & Zheng 1991)

Basil (pungent) (Singh A et al 1999, 2000)

Bergamot terpenes (Lam & Zheng 1991)

Caraway (Lam & Zheng 1991)

Cardamon (Banerjee et al 1994)

Celery seed (Lam & Zheng 1991; Banerjee et al 1994)

Chamomile (type unspecified) (Lam & Zheng 1991)

Coriander seed (Banerjee et al 1994)

Cumin (Aruna & Sivaramakrishnan 1996)

Dill weed (Lam & Zheng 1991)

Eucalyptus terpenes (Lam & Zheng 1991)

Fennel (sweet) (Lam & Zheng 1991)

Galangal rhizome (type unspecified) (Lam & Zheng 1991)

Garlic (Wu et al 2001, 2002)

Ginger (Lam & Zheng 1991; Banerjee et al 1994)

Grapefruit (Wattenberg et al 1985)

Hop (Lam & Zheng 1991)

Lemon (expressed) (Wattenberg et al 1985)

Lemongrass (type unspecified) (Lam & Zheng 1991)

Lime terpenes (Lam & Zheng 1991)

Nutmeg (type unspecified) (Banerjee et al 1994)

Orange (type unspecified) (Wattenberg et al 1985)

Oregano (Lam & Zheng 1991)

Parsley leaf (Lam & Zheng 1991)

Peppermint tail fractions (Lam & Zheng 1991)

Sandalwood (E. Indian) (Banerjee et al 1993)

Spearmint (Lam & Zheng 1991)

Tangerine (Wattenberg et al 1985)

Thyme (type unspecified) (Lam & Zheng 1991)

Tomar seed (Banerjee et al 1994)

[a]The potency of essential oils for enzyme induction will vary with composition

---

(Oesch et al 2007). Dermal enzymes can catalyze phase I reactions, including oxidation, reduction and hydrolysis, as well as phase II conjugation reactions, though with varying efficiency. Esterase enzyme activity is particularly high, 99% of benzyl acetate being hydrolyzed to benzyl alcohol in human skin (Hotchkiss 1998). Dermal glycine conjugation seems to be

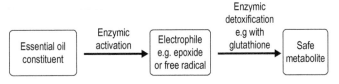

Figure 4.5 • Electrophile detoxification.

much less efficient than in the liver. In cultured human skin cells, only 2% of benzoic acid was converted to hippuric acid, compared to 98% in cultured liver cells (Nasseri-Sina et al 1997). Coumarin is unchanged during human transcutaneous absorption, suggesting an absence of certain CYP isoforms (Beckley-Kartey et al 1997).

Cinnamaldehyde is progressively metabolized to cinnamic acid and cinnamyl alcohol in human skin (Weibel & Hansen 1989a, 1989b), and both alcohol dehydrogenase and aldehyde dehydrogenase are involved. It is thought that unmetabolized cinnamaldehyde may bind to host proteins eliciting an immune reaction, and this may explain why such reactions depend on concentration (Cheung et al 2003). CYP1A1 and CYP3A5 seem to be mainly responsible for the metabolism of geraniol in human skin, partially transforming it into geranial (Hagvall et al 2008).

Most of the CYP isoforms found in the liver are also found in human skin (Baron et al 2001; Ahmad & Mukhtar 2004). However, their activity in the skin is generally low compared with the liver, and it is possible that a high dermal concentration of essential oil may overwhelm detoxification capacity. In a study of 15 CYP1-4 genes, all were expressed, though CYP2C8 was not. Unlike in the liver, those most highly expressed were CYP2S1 and CYP4B1 (Du et al 2006b). There are major interspecies differences in dermal CYP expression (Rolsted et al 2008), which may have important implications in extrapolating data from animal studies, such as dermal LD_{50} values, to humans. As in the liver, some dermal enzymes may activate chemicals, making them more toxic (see Toxification below).

Isomer differences

Sometimes, isomers of the same compound are metabolized differently, and this can have implications for toxicity. For example, (1S)-(−)-β-pulegone is less toxic than (1R)-(+)-β-pulegone, and this has been linked to the lower levels of p-cresol and piperitone metabolites formed (Madyastha & Gaikwad 1998). When incubated with rat or human liver microsomes (R)-(−)-carvone was converted to 4R,6S-(−)-carveol, while (S)-(+)-carvone was converted to 4S, 6S-(+)-carveol (Jäger et al 2000). After being given separately to human subjects at doses of 300 mg topically, rapid uptake was followed by stereoselective metabolism of the (R)-(−)-enantiomer, while no metabolism of the (S)-(+)-enantiomer could be detected (Jäger et al 2001).

Pharmacogenetics

This is about how a person's genetic make-up affects their response to medicines. Most importantly, genetic variations between individuals determine which metabolizing enzymes (generally CYP isoforms) their body will produce and which

ones not. These variations, called polymorphisms, are generally related to racial type (Johnson et al 2005). For example, codeine has no analgesic effect unless it is metabolized to morphine, but almost 10% of people of European ancestry do not produce the enzyme necessary (CYP2D6) for this transformation. Sex differences have also been found. There is evidence for females having higher CYP2A6, CYP2B6 and CYP3A4 activity, and lower CYP1A2 and CYP2E1 activity. However, the wide cross-variability between ethnicity and sex makes definitive statements difficult (Andersson et al 2008).

Differences in the way humans metabolize essential oil constituents have not been widely studied, but do not appear to be uncommon. Pharmacogenetic variations have been recorded for coumarin (see Ch. 9, p. 129) and methyleugenol (see Ch. 12, p. 175) and these have important toxicological consequences. Menthol cannot be metabolized by people with glucose-6-phosphate dehydrogenase (G6PD) deficiency (Olowe & Ransome-Kuti 1980; Hardisty & Weatherall 1982). This mostly affects African Americans, and people who reside in Africa, the Middle East and Southeast Asia.

It has been postulated that genetic factors may determine an individual's susceptibility to allergic contact dermatitis (Khan et al 2006). This has not yet been demonstrated for any essential oil constituent, but it has for sensitization to phenylenediamine, an ingredient of some hair dyes and color cosmetics (Nacak et al 2006).

Although the study of pharmacogenetics is about 50 years old, a detailed understanding of its implications is only now emerging, and it is currently the subject of intense research (Goldstein & Tate 2005). However, there is no accessible test, as yet, to determine an individual's metabolic profile.[17]

Implications for toxicity

Whether essential oil constituents are toxic or not, metabolism facilitates their excretion from the body via the kidneys. In addition, a toxic substance may be converted into a metabolite with little or no toxicity (detoxification or inactivation), or a non-toxic substance may be converted into a toxic substance (toxification or activation). Detoxification is more common for essential oil constituents, but toxification also occurs, notably in potentially carcinogenic propenylbenzene derivatives such as safrole, estragole and methyleugenol.

It should be remembered that metabolic enzyme activity varies between individuals, and changes with age. It is low in neonates, where metabolic capacity is still developing, and in the elderly, where liver and kidney function is declining. Thus, caution is indicated in cases where reduced enzyme activity could pose a risk, and smaller amounts of essential oils should be administered to these age groups.

Toxification

As we have seen, many substances that are introduced into the body, or which find their way there accidentally, undergo biotransformation. If they are pharmacologically active, this process usually results in loss or reduction of their activity, but not always. Some substances are activated into toxic metabolites (Madyastha & Moorthy 1989). A well-known example is that of acetaminophen (paracetamol), a commonly used analgesic that can cause fatal hepatotoxicity and nephrotoxicity when taken in overdoses (Nelson & Gordon 1983). A small proportion of the drug is oxidized by hepatic CYP enzymes to an electrophile (N-acetyl-p-benzoquinone imine, NAPQI) which reacts irreversibly with local cellular proteins and kills cells in which metabolism has occurred (Timbrell 2000). At lower doses, glutathione removes NAPQI by reacting with it, but at high doses glutathione is overwhelmed and becomes depleted. The metabolism of substances to electrophiles, which must then be detoxified, is illustrated in Figure 4.5.

A similar process of bioactivation is responsible for the hepatotoxicity of (+)-pulegone and estragole. (+)-Pulegone is metabolized in the liver to menthofuran via a highly reactive metabolite which can bind irreversibly with liver proteins, thereby destroying the liver (Thomassen et al 1990). Fatal poisoning with (+)-pulegone may be associated with very low plasma (+)-pulegone and menthofuran levels of 18 ng/mL and 1 ng/mL, respectively (Moorthy et al 1989b; Anderson et al 1996).

Enzymes in the skin may also activate chemicals, making them more toxic. These include CYP enzymes, which convert a small number of essential oil constituents (safrole, estragole and perhaps others) into potentially carcinogenic compounds (see Ch. 12, p. 167). However, it is not known how efficient dermal CYP is in this regard. The more efficient it is, the greater the risk will be from estragole-rich essential oils such as basil when they are applied to the skin.[18]

Excretion

The main organs of excretion are the kidneys, liver, lungs and skin. For many substances, the most important of these is the kidney, which functions as a filter for the blood. All substances, including essential oil constituents present in the bloodstream, pass through the kidneys, and most are filtered and leave the blood. Large molecules such as proteins are not small enough to be filtered, and if a compound binds significantly to plasma proteins, it will not be filtered, and excretion will be slowed. This will increase the lifetime of that substance in the body. Once filtered, substances may regain access to the bloodstream by passive diffusion. However, this will only occur if they have sufficient lipophilicity. After metabolism, many compounds will have become appreciably less lipophilic.

Because essential oil constituents are somewhat volatile and exert low vapor pressures, small quantities diffuse from the bloodstream across membranes, to be excreted via the lungs on exhaling. Metabolites, which tend to be more soluble in the blood, are less likely to be excreted in this way. Very small amounts of essential oil constituents may be released into various body secretions, including sweat, saliva and milk. In the latter case, it is important for any nursing mother who is receiving essential oils to be aware that oil constituents are likely to be ingested by the baby.

As can be seen in Table 4.9, following oral administration, essential oil constituents are primarily excreted in the urine, with exhaled air and feces as secondary routes of elimination. However, urinary excretion seems to be a very minor route for inhaled constituents. Most are metabolized, while a few are excreted unchanged. Relatively few studies have been carried out to determine the fate of essential oils after dermal or intravenous administration. Those that have, suggest that constituents are rapidly eliminated from the body.

Efficiency of elimination

High clearance and short elimination times mean that accumulation in tissues is improbable from normal doses, whatever the route of administration. For example, at 72 hours less than 0.25% of isoeugenol remained in the tissues following either oral or iv administration of 156 mg/kg to rats (Badger et al 2002). Rats and mice eliminate virtually all of a single oral dose of citral (up to 1 g/kg) within 72 hours and 120 hours, respectively (Phillips et al 1976). After dermal application of benzyl acetate to rats, virtually all the absorbed dose is excreted within 24 hours (Chidgey et al 1987). In both rats and mice given 250 mg/kg of anethole, >95% of the dose was recovered, the majority in the 0–24 hour urine (Bounds & Caldwell 1996).

The biphasic or triphasic elimination profile of most essential oil constituents suggests that they are efficiently distributed from the blood into other tissues (Kohlert et al 2000). After intravenous injection of a mixture of terpenes, the initial phase (absorption into the tissues) lasted 3–4 minutes, and the secondary phase (elimination) 60–65 minutes (Kleinschmidt et al 1985). Transdermal or inhalational absorption of α-pinene was followed by an initial phase with a half-life of five minutes, and a secondary phase with a half-life of 26 to 38 minutes. Following inhalation, a third and longer phase was determined with an elimination half-life of 695 minutes (Falk et al 1990). Coumarin is rapidly and extensively absorbed from the skin of both humans and rats, and is readily distributed and excreted. Peak plasma concentrations were achieved at, or before, one hour after application of 0.2 mg/cm^2 to the skin, and mean plasma half-lives were 1.7 hours and 5 hours, respectively (Ford et al 2001). The elimination half-lives of some essential oil constituents are shown in Table 4.8.

Drug interactions

When the pharmacological or toxicological consequences of administering two or more drugs concurrently cannot be directly attributed to their individual actions, a drug interaction is said to occur. This can be especially problematic for drugs with narrow therapeutic indexes (i.e., when the therapeutic dose is close to the toxic dose), or when blood plasma levels must be maintained within a specified range (see Chapter 3).

It is difficult to predict the probability of essential oil interactions with drugs, as a wide array of mechanisms could be involved. For example, there could be competition for binding sites in tissues or on plasma proteins; there could be competition for specific cell surface or intracellular receptor sites; there could be a change in gut flora composition or in gut motility; metabolic enzymes may be induced or inhibited. Detailed information is scarce in most cases, but interactions with enzymes may be common.

A list of incompatibilities between pharmaceutical drugs and essential oils is shown in Table 4.10.

Table 4.10 Drug interactions

A. Possible incompatibilities from all routes of administration

Essential oils	Drug	Reason for incompatibility	References
Birch (sweet), wintergreen	Warfarin (anticoagulant)	Methyl salicylate inhibits platelet aggregation, and exacerbates blood thinning	Le Bourhis & Soenen 1973; Chow et al 1989; Yip et al 1990
Camphor (brown)[a], sassafras[a,b]	CYP1A2 substrates[c]	Safrole inhibits CYP1A2, which could potentiate drug action	Ueng et al 2005
Lemongrass, may chang, myrtle (honey), myrtle (lemon), tea tree (lemon-scented)[b]	CYP2B6 substrates[c]	Constituents of these oils inhibit CYP2B6, which could potentiate drug action	Seo KA et al 2008
Balsam poplar, chamomile (blue, all CTs (chemotypes)), mugwort (great), sage (wild mountain), tansy (blue), yarrow (chamazulene CT)[b]	CYP2D6 substrates[c]	Constituents of these oils inhibit CYP2D6, which could potentiate drug action	Ganzera et al 2006
Betel[a], camphor (brown)[a], camphor (yellow)[a], sassafras[a,b]	CYP2E1 substrates[c]	Safrole inhibits CYP2E1, which could potentiate drug action	Ueng et al 2005

B. Possible incompatibilities if the essential oils are taken in oral doses

Essential oils	Drugs	Reason for incompatibility	References
Betel[a], camphor (yellow)[a], chamomile (blue, α-bisabolol oxide A CT), chamomile (blue, α-bisabolol / (E)-β-farnesene CT), mugwort (great), tansy (blue), yarrow (chamazulene CT)[b]	CYP1A2 substrates[c]	Constituents of these oils inhibit CYP1A2, which could potentiate drug action	Ueng et al 2005; Ganzera et al 2006
Basil (lemon), bergamot (wild), citronella, finger root, geranium, jamrosa, lemon balm (Australian), lemon leaf, melissa, palmarosa, thyme (geraniol CT), thyme (lemon), verbena (lemon)[b]	CYP2B6 substrates[c]	Constituents of these oils inhibit CYP2B6, which could potentiate drug action	Seo KA et al 2008
Chamomile (blue, α-bisabolol / (E)-β-farnesene CT)[b]	CYP2C9 substrates[c]	Constituents of these oils inhibit CYP2C9, which could potentiate drug action	Ganzera et al 2006
Chaste tree, cypress (blue), jasmine sambac absolute, sandalwood (W Australian)[b]	CYP2D6 substrates[c]	Constituents of these oils inhibit CYP2D6, which could potentiate drug action	Ganzera et al 2006
Ho leaf (camphor CT)[b]	CYP2E1 substrates[c]	Safrole inhibits CYP2E1, which could potentiate drug action	Ueng et al 2005
Chamomile (blue, α-bisabolol / (E)-β-farnesene CT), mugwort (great), sassafras[a], tansy (blue), yarrow (chamazulene CT)[b]	CYP3A4 substrates[c]	Constituents of these oils inhibit CYP3A4, which could potentiate drug action	Dresser et al 2002; Ganzera et al 2006
Ajowan, anise, anise (star), araucaria, atractylis, basil (estragole CT)[a], basil (holy), basil (Madagascan)[a], basil (pungent), bay (W. Indian), betel[a], birch (sweet), cassia, chervil[a], cinnamon bark, cinnamon leaf, clove bud, clove leaf, clove stem, cornmint, fennel (bitter), fennel (sweet), garlic, lavandin, leek, marigold (Mexican)[a], Marjoram wild (carvacrol CT), Myrtle (aniseed), onion, oregano, oregano	Aspirin (antiplatelet) Heparin (anticoagulant) Warfarin (anticoagulant)	Constituents of these oils inhibit platelet aggregation, and could exacerbate the blood-thinning action of these drugs	Rasheed et al 1984; Fenwick & Hanley 1985; Chiariello et al 1986; Murayama & Kumaroo 1986; Barrie et al 1987; Takenaga et al 1987; Janssens et al 1990; Chen et al 1996; Wang et al 2000; Enomoto et al 2001; Ballabeni et al 2004; Yoshioka & Tamada 2005; Hsu et al 2006; Huang et al 2007a; Lee 2006; Tognolini et al 2006; Tsai et al 2007

Continued

Table 4.10 Drug interactions—Cont'd

B. Possible incompatibilities if the essential oils are taken in oral doses—Cont'd

Essential oils	Drugs	Reason for incompatibility	References
(Mexican), patchouli, pimento berry[a], pimento leaf, pine (ponderosa), ravensara bark[a], savory, tarragon[a], tejpat, thyme (borneol CT), thyme (limonene CT), thyme (spike), thyme (thymol and/or carvacrol CTs), wintergreen			
Birch tar[a], buchu (pulegone CT)[a], calamint (lesser)[a], pennyroyal[a]	Acetaminophen (paracetamol) (non-opioid analgesic)	Constituents of these oils could exacerbate glutathione depletion	Gordon et al 1982; Swales & Caldwell 1992; Choi et al 2001
Buchu (pulegone CT)[a], calamint (lesser)[a], pennyroyal[a]	Phenobarbitone (phenobarbital) (sedative hypnotic)	Phenobarbitone induces enzymes that could exacerbate pulegone hepatotoxicity	Moorthy et al 1989a
Basil (holy), basil (pungent), bay (W. Indian), betel[a], cinnamon leaf, clove bud, clove leaf, clove stem, parsleyseed, parsnip, pimento berry[a], pimento leaf, sweet vernalgrass, tejpat	MAOIs including isocarboxazid, moclobemide, phenelzine, selegiline, tranylcypromine	Constituents of these oils inhibit MAO enzymes, which could affect blood pressure and cause tremors, confusion, etc.	Truitt et al 1963; Huong et al 2000; Tao et al 2005
	Pethidine (meperidine, demerol) (opioid analgesic)	Possible potentiation of serotonin causing agitation, delirium, headache, convulsions, and/or hyperthermia	Reynolds 1993
	SSRIs including citalopram, escitalopram, fluoxetine, paroxetine, sertraline	Potentiation of CNS serotonin levels which could cause serotonin syndrome	Izumi et al 2006
	Indirect sympathomimetic drugs including ephedrine, amphetamine	Possible hypertension, tachycardia and arrhythmias	Sjöqvist 1965
Anise, anise (star), basil (lemon), black seed, cassia, cinnamon bark, dill, fennel (bitter), fennel (sweet), fenugreek, geranium, lemon leaf, lemongrass, marjoram (wild, carvacrol CT) may chang, melissa, myrtle, myrtle (aniseed), myrtle (honey), myrtle (lemon), oregano, savory, tea tree (lemon-scented), thyme (spike), turmeric, verbena (lemon)	Antidiabetic drugs including glibenclamide, tolbutamide, metformin	Constituents of these oils influence blood sugar levels and may cause hyperglycemia or hypoglycemia	Al-Hader et al 1993, 1994; Essway et al 1995; Mølck et al 1998; Sepici et al 2004; Babu et al 2007; Chung et al 2010; Ping et al 2010; Hamden et al 2011; Modak & Mukhopadhaya 2011; Boukhris et al 2012; Lekshmi et al 2012
Anise	Diuretic drugs including bendroflumethiazide (bendrofluazide), furosemide (frusemide), spironolactone	This oil contains constituents that have antidiuretic actions	Kreydiyyeh et al 2003

[a]Since this oil should not be taken in oral doses, there is no drug interaction warning in the corresponding essential oil profile
[b]These oils are proposed as being the most potent overall inhibitors of CYP isozymes involved in the metabolism of commonly prescribed drugs. Inhibitory rankings have been calculated by dividing the abundance (%) of known CYP-inhibiting constituents by their IC_{50} or K_i values (μM), and, in the case of multiple inhibitory constituents, calculating their sum
[c]See Appendix B

Modulation of liver enzymes

Some essential oil constituents increase the production of certain metabolic enzymes. This action is referred to as enzyme induction. Induction of a particular enzyme may increase the rate at which a medication is metabolized, and thereby decrease its blood levels and therapeutic actions. Inhibitors of drug metabolizing enzymes would have the opposite effect, causing blood levels to rise, and possibly increasing any side effects. Cytochrome P_{450} enzymes, along with UDP-glucuronosyltransferases, are the ones primarily responsible for drug metabolism.

Cytochrome P_{450}

The CYP enzymes are found in microsomes, primarily in the liver, but also in other areas of the body, notably the small intestine. Almost all the research is conducted in rat liver microsomes. It is thought that these enzymes originally evolved in order to metabolize plant chemicals such as toxic alkaloids and terpenoid compounds, so it is not surprising that many essential oils and constituents affect their activity.

The CYP enzymes are classified into numbered families. About 17 are found in humans, and 1, 2 and 3 are the families that mainly degrade xenobiotics such as essential oil constituents and drugs. Subfamilies are identified by a letter: CYP1A, CYP1B, etc. Finally, individual genes are identified by a number, for example CYP2B1. Each individual variant is called an 'isoform' or 'isozyme', and there are about 50 in humans. In order to understand possible drug interactions, it is necessary to identify which CYP isoform is being targeted, and more recent research generally does so.

Induction

We have already seen that pulegone can be converted to more toxic compounds, and this is catalyzed by CYP1A2, CYP2E1 and CYP2C19 (Khojasteh-Bakht et al 1999). Drugs that induce one or more of these enzymes (e.g., phenobarbitone) will therefore increase pulegone's hepatotoxicity (Moorthy et al 1989a). Since such drugs are widely prescribed, the use of pulegone-rich essential oils can be especially hazardous, but this type of toxification interaction is rare among essential oil constituents. In many cases, enzyme induction results in decreased rather than increased toxicity because conjugation enables toxic chemicals to be excreted more easily. It can also cause blood levels of drugs to fall, which might expose patients to serious health problems. However, very high doses of essential oils are usually required to cause significant induction.

Early research reported the induction of CYP enzymes as a group. Borneol, cedrene, 1,8-cineole, geraniol, (+)-limonene, myristicin, safrole and terpineol had been reported to induce CYP by the mid-1980s (Parke & Rahman 1969, 1970; Hashimoto et al 1972; Chadha & Madyastha 1984; Ioannides et al 1985; Madyastha & Chadha 1986).[19] CYP induction may go through phases. After three days of oral dosing in rats at 600 mg/kg/day, linalool increased hepatic CYP by 50%, but its activity decreased to control values after 3 further days of dosing (Chadha & Madyastha 1984). In other linalool research, CYP was depressed on day seven, but showed a 50% increase after 30 days of dosing at 500 mg/kg/day (Parke et al 1974a).

Eugenol increased the activities of the enzymes EROD and PROD when administered to rats by gavage at 1,000 mg/kg/day for 10 days, while 250 and 500 mg/kg/day had no significant effect. EROD and PROD are used as selective markers for CYP1A1 and CYP2B1, respectively. Similarly dosed at 125 or 250 mg/kg/day, (E)-anethole did increase EROD activity, but not significantly (Rompelberg et al 1993). In rats, gavage doses of linalool increased the activity of cytochrome $b5$ (Parke et al 1974a), which is part of the respiratory enzyme chain, but only at 500 mg/kg/day for 30 days.

Essential oil inhalation can also cause enzyme modulation. When rats were exposed to bedding sprayed with an ether solution containing 3% cedarwood oil for 48 hours, CYP was induced, and hexobarbital-induced sleeping times were reduced to 27.9% of controls (Wade et al 1968). In rats, inhalation of cedrene (isomer unspecified) vapor, for either 2 or 6 days at a concentration resulting in a dose of 60 mg/kg/day, showed a 30% increase in CYP content. The total daily dose of cedrene absorbed during the period of inhalation was sufficient to cause similar effects to those from either oral or ip administration (Hashimoto et al 1972). Little useful information can be extrapolated from these intensive exposures.

In humans, inhalation of an aerosol containing 1 mL of 1,8-cineole for 10 minutes per day for 10 days reduced plasma levels of aminopyrine in four of five volunteers. Similar reductions were observed for three other drugs when inhaled by rats (Jori et al 1970). When administered to rats as an aerosol inhalation over 4 days, 1,8-cineole significantly reduced pentobarbitone-induced sleeping times, and induced liver microsomal CYP. However, guaiacol, menthol, α-pinene, β-pinene and *Pinus pumilio* oil had no effect (Jori et al 1969).

Even though inhaled essential oil vapors can interfere with drug metabolism, it would appear that this only occurs after prolonged inhalation. There is no evidence that CYP inhibition occurs following external essential oil administration as used in aromatherapy, and this seems unlikely.

The CYP-inducing activities of a number of essential oils and constituents in rat liver microsomes are shown in Table 4.11A. In every case substantial doses were administered, either by the oral or ip routes. It is highly unlikely that humans would be exposed to equivalent quantities of oils under normal conditions, and we therefore believe that essential oils offer no significant risk of affecting blood levels of drugs in humans through CYP induction when used topically or orally.

Inhibition

Several oils and constituents have been found to inhibit CYP enzymes. Pentobarbitone-induced sleeping times in mice were prolonged by anise oil, nutmeg oil, (E)-anethole, (+)-carvone and (−)-carvone, when injected ip either simultaneously or 30 minutes prior to the drug. Injection of the natural compounds 24 hours prior to the drug had no effect. The authors commented that the effects were not of sufficient magnitude or duration to be of concern (Marcus & Lichtenstein 1982). Single doses of β-myrcene were given to male rats one hour before pentobarbitone administration. At 250 and 400 mg/kg body weight (bw), there was no effect, but at 1,000 mg/kg bw there was a significant increase in sleeping time, thought to be due to

Table 4.11 Essenial oils and constituents that affect cytochrome P450 isozyme

A. Cytochrome P_{450} inducers

Isozyme	Essential oil or constituent	Activity increase (dose)	Preparation	Reference
CYP1A1	Rosemary oil	3.8 × (5 g/kg in diet for 2 weeks)	Male rat liver microsomes	Debersac et al 2001
	Methoxsalen	ca 3.3 × (2.5 g/kg in diet for 6 weeks)	Female rat liver microsomes	Diawara et al 1999
	Bergapten	ca 2.4 × (2.5 g/kg in diet for 6 weeks)		
	β-Myrcene	1.5 × (1 g/kg by gavage for 24 hours)	Female rat liver microsomes	De-Oliveira et al 1997a
	1,8-Cineole	significant increase (800 mg/kg/day po for 3 days)	Male rat liver microsomes	Kim NH et al 2004
CYP1A1/2	Myristicin	ca 17 × (96 mg/kg ip)	Male rat liver microsomes	Jeong & Yun 1995
	Eugenol	2.5 × (1 g/kg/day by gavage for 10 days)	Male rat liver microsomes	Rompelberg et al 1993
CYP1A2	Rosemary oil	1.7 × (5 g/kg in diet for 2 weeks)	Male rat liver microsomes	Debersac et al 2001
	Diallyl sulfide	2–5 × (0.2% in diet for 13 days)	Male rat liver microsomes	Haber et al 1995
	Diallyl disulfide[a]			
CYP2B1	Hinoki wood oil	17 × (300 mg/kg/day ip for 5 days)	Male rat liver microsomes	Hiroi et al 1995
	Hibawood oil	11 × (300 mg/kg/day ip for 5 days)		
	Hinoki leaf oil	4.6 × (300 mg/kg/day ip for 5 days)		
	1,8-Cineole	15 × (300 mg/kg/day ip for 5 days)		
	Cadinene[b]	15 × (300 mg/kg/day ip for 5 days)		
	α-Pinene[b]	12 × (300 mg/kg/day ip for 5 days)		
	Borneol[b]	7.3 × (300 mg/kg/day ip for 5 days)		
	Limonene[b]	significant increase (5% w/w in diet for 2 weeks)	Female rat liver microsomes	Maltzman et al 1991
	β-Myrcene	13–23 × (1 g/kg by gavage for 24 hours)	Female rat liver microsomes	De-Oliveira et al 1997b
CYP2B1/2	Rosemary oil	24 × (5 g/kg in diet for 2 weeks)	Male rat liver microsomes	Debersac et al 2001
	Farnesol[c]	5.3 × (females); 6.4 × (males) (1 g/kg/day by gavage for 4 weeks)	Rat liver microsomes	Horn et al 2005
	Myristicin	ca 24 × (96 mg/kg ip)	Male rat liver microsomes	Jeong & Yun 1995
	α-Ionone[d]	significant increase (300 mg/kg po)	Male rat liver microsomes	Jeong HG et al 2002
	β-Ionone[e]	significant increase (300 mg/kg po)		
	1,8-Cineole	significant increase (400 mg/kg/day po for 3 days)	Male rat liver microsomes	Kim NH et al 2004
	Diallyl sulfide	5–15 × (0.2% in diet for 13 days)	Male rat liver microsomes	Haber et al 1995
	Diallyl disulfide[a]	7–36 × (0.2% in diet for 13 days)		
	Eugenol	3.4 × (1 g/kg/day by gavage for 10 days)	Male rat liver microsomes	Rompelberg et al 1993
CYP2B2	Limonene[b]	significant increase (5% w/w in diet for 2 weeks)	Female rat liver microsomes	Maltzman et al 1991
CYP2E1	Myristicin	2.5 × (96 mg/kg ip)	Male rat liver microsomes	Jeong & Yun 1995
CYP3A1/2	Farnesol[c]	4.4 × (1 g/kg/day by gavage for 4 weeks)	Female rat liver microsomes	Horn et al 2005
	1,8-Cineole	significant increase (800 mg/kg/day po for 3 days)	Male rat liver microsomes	Kim NH et al 2004
CYP3A2	Hinoki wood oil	2.1 × (300 mg/kg/day ip for 5 days)	Male rat liver microsomes	Hiroi et al 1995
	Hibawood oil	1.9 × (300 mg/kg/day ip for 5 days)		
	Cadinene[b]	2.4 × (300 mg/kg/day ip for 5 days)		
	1,8-Cineole	1.9 × (300 mg/kg/day ip for 5 days)		
CYP4A1	Citral	2.0 × (1.5 g/kg/day by gavage for 5 days)	Male rat liver microsomes	Roffey et al 1990
CYP4A1-3	Farnesol[c]	1.6 × (females); 5.4 × (males) (1 g/kg/day by gavage for 4 weeks)	Rat liver microsomes	Horn et al 2005

Continued

Table 4.11 Essenial oils and constituents that affect cytochrome P450 isozyme—Cont'd

A. Cytochrome P$_{450}$ inducers—Cont'd

Isozyme	Essential oil or constituent	Activity increase (dose)	Preparation	Reference
CYP4A2	α-Pinene[b]	1.6 × (300 mg/kg ip once a day for 5 days)	Male rat liver microsomes	Hiroi et al 1995
CYP19	Farnesol[c]	3.2 × (1 g/kg/day by gavage for 4 weeks)	Male rat liver microsomes	Horn et al 2005

B. Cytochrome P$_{450}$ inhibitors

Isozyme	Essential oil or constituent	IC$_{50}$	K$_i$	Preparation	Reference
CYP1A1	Bergamottin	0.010 μM[f], 0.057 μM[g]		male rat liver microsomes	Baumgart et al 2005
	Isopimpinellin	0.015 μM[f], 1.36 μM[g]			
	Angelicin	0.31 μM[f], 11.7 μM[g]			
	Methoxsalen	1.07 μM[f], 2.44 μM[g]			
CYP1A2	Chamomile (blue) oil	1.59 μg/mL		human recombinant microsomes	Ganzera et al 2006
	(E)-Spiroether	0.47 μM			
	(Z)-Spiroether	2.01 μM			
	Chamazulene	4.41 μM			
	Safrole	5.7 μM		bacterial membranes	Ueng et al 2005
CYP1B1	Perillyl alcohol[b]	1.5 μM		MCF-7 cells	Chan et al 2006
CYP2A6	Bergamot oil		0.81 μg/mL	rabbit liver microsomes	Williamson 2010
	Lime oil		1.4 μg/mL		
	(6R)-(+)-Menthofuran		2.5 μM	human liver microsomes	Khojasteh-Bakht et al 1998
	Methoxsalen		1.9 μM	human liver microsomes	Koenigs et al 1997
	Safrole	12.0 μM		bacterial membranes	Ueng et al 2005
CYP2B1	Methoxsalen		2.9 μM	male rat liver microsomes	Koenigs and Trager 1998
	(−)-α-Pinene	0.087 μM		female rat liver microsomes	De-Oliveira et al 1997a
	(+)-α-Pinene	0.089 μM			
	β-Myrcene	0.14 μM			
	(+)-Limonene	0.19 μM			
	α-Terpinene	0.76 μM			
	Citral	1.19 μM			
	Citronellal	1.56 μM			
	(±)-Camphor	7.89 μM			
	β-Ionone	0.03 μM		female rat liver microsomes	De-Oliveira et al 1999
	1,8-Cineole	4.7 μM			
	(−)-Menthol	10.6 μM			
	α-Terpineol	14.8 μM			
CYP2B6	Citral		6.8 μM	human liver microsomes	Seo et al 2008
	Geraniol[b]		10.3 μM		
	Borneol[b]		9.5, 22 μM	human liver microsomes	Kim et al 2008
	Isoborneol[b]		5.9, 26 μM		
CYP2C9	Chamomile (blue) oil	14.3 μg/mL		human recombinant microsomes	Ganzera et al 2006
	α-Bisabolol[b]	46.1 μM			
	Chamazulene	59.3 μM			
	Farnesene[b]	73.1 μM			

Continued

Table 4.11 Essenial oils and constituents that affect cytochrome P450 isozyme—Cont'd

B. Cytochrome P_{450} inhibitors—Cont'd

Isozyme	Essential oil or constituent	IC_{50}	K_i	Preparation	Reference
CYP2D6	Chamomile (blue) oil	8.49 µg/mL		human recombinant microsomes	Ganzera et al 2006
	Chamazulene	1.06 µM			
	α-Bisabolol[b]	2.18 µM			
	Farnesene[b]	4.80 µM			
	(E)-Spiroether	34.8 µM			
	(Z)-Spiroether	57.6 µM			
	Safrole	110 µM		bacterial membranes	Ueng et al 2005
CYP2E1	Tangerine oil		4.3 µg/mL	rabbit liver microsomes	Williamson 2010
	Bergamot oil		6.4 µg/mL		
	Mandarin oil		7 µg/mL		
	Petitgrain oil		7.6 µg/mL		
	Lemon oil		8 µg/mL		
	Orange oil		8 µg/mL		
	Grapefruit oil		9 µg/mL		
	Lime oil		10 µg/mL		
	Neroli oil		10 µg/mL		
	Garlic oil	significant reduction (500 mg/kg po for 1-3 days)		male rat liver microsomes	Kwak et al 1995
	Diallyl sulfide	significant reductions (0.2% in diet for 13 days)		male rat liver microsomes	Haber et al 1995
	Diallyl disulfide[a]				
	Safrole	1.7 µM		bacterial membranes	Ueng et al 2005
CYP3A	Oxypeucedanin[b]	1.8 µM		human liver microsomes	Guo et al 2000
	Isopimpinellin	1.9 µM			
	Methoxsalen	2.9 µM			
	Bergapten	3.1 µM			
	Psoralen	5.1 µM			
	Bergamottin	22 µM			
CYP3A4	Chamomile (blue) oil	4.97 µg/mL		human recombinant microsomes	Ganzera et al 2006
	(Z)-Spiroether	6.13 µM			
	(E)-Spiroether	7.14 µM			
	Chamazulene	7.58 µM			
	α-Bisabolol[b]	15.8 µM			
	Farnesene[b]	38.1 µM			
	Peppermint oil		35.9 µg/mL	human liver microsomes	Dresser et al 2002
	(−)-Menthol		87.0 µM		
	(−)-Menthyl acetate		124 µM		
	DHB[h]	1.2 µM		human liver microsomes	Messer et al 2012
	Bergamottin	4.5 µM			
	Bergaptol	77.5 µM			
	Bergapten	19 µM, 36 µM		human liver microsomes	Ho et al 2001
	Methoxsalen	35 µM, 39 µM			
	Psoralen	116 µM, 257 µM			
	Safrole	43.5 µM		bacterial membranes	Ueng et al 2005

[a]80% pure

[b]Isomer not specified

[c]A mixture of (Z,Z)-farnesol (11.09%), (Z,E)-farnesol (25.08%), (E,Z)-farnesol (24.59%) and (E,E)-farnesol (38.77%)

[d]90% pure

[e]95% pure

[f]In the presence of light

[g]In the absence of light

[h]6',7'-Dihydroxybergamottin (not found in essential oils)

an increase in pentobarbitone bioavailability (Freitas et al 1993). However, this is an extremely high dose.

Peppermint oil was a moderately potent reversible inhibitor of CYP3A4 activity in vitro in human liver microsomes. Possibly through this mechanism, it increased the bioavailability of felodipine (a calcium antagonist used to control hypertension) in 12 healthy volunteers when given orally at 600 mg (Dresser et al 2002). However, it is not clear from this small study whether there is potential for a clinically relevant interaction. In rats, 100 mg/kg of peppermint oil tripled the bioavailability of cyclosporine, an immune-suppressant drug (Wacher et al 2002). The implication of this finding for humans is uncertain, but this is a high dose of essential oil.

Grapefruit juice inhibits the metabolism of many medications (Fuhr 1998). The constituent primarily responsible is 6,7-dihydroxybergamottin (DHB), a furanocoumarin (FC) not present in grapefruit oil, which inhibits CYP3A4 (Paine et al 2005). However, citrus oils contain other FCs that inhibit CYP3A4, namely, bergamottin, bergapten and bergaptol. Based on the IC_{50} values (Table 4.11B) and the concentrations of these FCs in expressed citrus oils, the CYP3A4 inhibitory potencies of grapefruit and all other citrus oils is extremely low, and not likely to cause drug interactions.

Evaluating risk

A summary of essential oils and constituents that induce or inhibit CYP isozymes is shown in Table 4.11. Some constituents induce one CYP isoform, yet inhibit another, and some both induce and inhibit the same isoform. Unsurprisingly, CYP modulation varies with dose, but it can also vary with sex. Tested in rats, 1 g/kg/day of oral farnesol for 28 days induced CYP2B1/2, CYP2C11/12 and CYP3A1/2 in females, but not in males, while CYP19 was induced only in males (Horn et al 2005).

Orthodox drugs are metabolized by a range of CYP isozymes (most commonly, CYP3A4), therefore, inhibition of these enzymes will increase their concentrations and half-lives in the bloodstream. Examples of some commonly prescribed drugs are presented in Appendix B showing the CYP isozymes mainly responsible for their metabolism. In theory, therefore, caution should be exercised when the oils and constituents listed in Table 4.11B are taken in combination with drugs where these drug parameters are critical. In order to compare the relative CYP-inhibitory potencies of essential oils, we divided the abundance (%) of known CYP-inhibiting constituents by their IC_{50} or K_i values (µM), and in the case of multiple inhibitory constituents, calculated their sum. Although IC_{50} and K_i values are related, they are not necessarily equivalent, due to differences in experimental conditions. However, we believe that these calculations offer a useful guide to the most potent oils, and these are listed in Table 4.10 (the first section under 'Possible incompatibilities'). As previously stated, we see no material risk in the use of essential oils that induce CYP enzymes.

Monoamine oxidase

Monoamine oxidase (MAO) is an enzyme that breaks down certain neurotransmitters, including serotonin, dopamine, epinephrine and norepinephrine. Myristicin, a constituent of nutmeg oil, appears to inhibit rodent brain MAO, as does nutmeg oil, albeit in higher doses than myristicin (Truitt et al 1963). Myristicin is less potent as a MAO inhibitor than standard drugs such as tranylcypromine and iproniazid, and this might be explained by its lack of a basic nitrogen atom. Eugenol, which is structurally similar to myristicin, dose-dependently inhibited human MAO-A with a K_i value of 26 µM, and inhibited human MAO-B to a much lesser extent (Tao et al 2005). Coumarin inhibited mouse brain MAO, with an IC_{50} value of 41.4 µM (Huong et al 2000).

We recommend that oral doses of essential oils rich in myristicin, eugenol or coumarin are not taken in conjunction with MAO inhibiting antidepressants, due to possible blood pressure changes, tremors, confusion, etc. (Table 4.10). It is also inadvisable to take these oils alongside sympathomimetic drugs such as ephedrine, as potentially dangerous cardiovascular changes may occur (Sjöqvist 1965). Selective serotonin reuptake inhibiting (SSRI) antidepressants should not be taken with MAO inhibitors, as this can lead to a serious drug reaction called serotonin syndrome (Izumi et al 2006). Combining pethidine with MAO inhibitors can cause serious side effects (Reynolds 1993). [The MAO inhibiting action of essential oils such as nutmeg and clove is probably related to their antidepressant action (Tao et al 2005).] Caution is also advised when these oils are ingested in conjunction with certain foods. Those containing tyramine, which include cheese, may precipitate a hypertensive crisis (Blackwell & Mabbitt 1965), while tryptophan-containing foods may lead to elevated serotonin levels.

Other enzymes

1,8-Cineole, given to rats either sc (500 or 1,000 mg/kg/day for 4 days) or by aerosol for 5–8 days (amount absorbed not known), produced a marked increase in the activity of glucuronyltransferase (GTA), which only returned to normal after up to 20 days. GTA is a key enzyme in both drug metabolism and endogenous detoxification. Nutmeg oil, thuja oil, turpentine oil, camphor, menthol and thymol (all 500 mg/kg/day sc for 4 days) had no effect (Hohenwallner & Klima 1971). Eugenol dose-dependently increased the levels of hepatic UDP-glucuronyltransferase when given in the diet at 1%, 3% or 5% for 23 days (Yokota et al 1988).

Modulation of drug transport

Another potential site for interactions between essential oils and drugs is P-glycoprotein (P-gp). P-gp is an ATP-dependent transport protein found in plasma membranes, including those of intestinal epithelial cells, which actively transports many drugs into the intestinal lumen. Using LLC-GA5-COL150 cells transfected with human MDR1 cDNA encoding P-gp, the intracellular accumulation of [³H]digoxin was found to be inhibited by a number of essential oil constituents including (R)-$(+)$-citronellal, α-terpinene, terpinolene, (S)-$(−)$-β-citronellol and $(−)$-β-pinene, with IC_{50} values ranging from 167 to 608 µM (Yoshida et al 2005, 2006). The importance of this mechanism in the context of essential oils altering the blood concentrations of different drugs is not clear, but the magnitude of these particular IC_{50} values suggests that it might be marginal.

Blood clotting

Several clinical cases raise the question of a possible potentiating effect of topically applied salicylates on the action of the anticoagulant, warfarin, and the kind of symptoms this can cause. An 85-year-old woman was admitted to hospital with acute cardiovascular problems, and was prescribed heparin, followed by warfarin. Some weeks after leaving hospital she returned, suffering from gross vaginal bleeding and subcutaneous hemorrhaging on various parts of her body. Her blood hemoglobin had fallen from 117 g/L to 80 g/L. The previous week she had liberally applied a preparation containing menthol and methyl salicylate to her arthritic joints (Le Bourhis & Soenen 1973).

Two further cases of interaction between warfarin and topically applied methyl salicylate are reported by Chan (1998). In both cases, medicated balms were used containing 15% and 50% methyl salicylate. In a fourth case, a 68-year-old man taking warfarin liberally applied topical trolamine salicylate to his neck and shoulders on several recent occasions because of pain (Le Bourhis & Soenen 1973).

Another salicylate, acetylsalicylic acid (aspirin) can increase the risk of hemorrhage in patients taking warfarin. Animal models have demonstrated that high salicylate levels decrease hepatic synthesis of vitamin K-dependant coagulation factors (Le Bourhis & Soenen 1973). The possibility that methyl salicylate may complicate the use of anticoagulant drugs other than warfarin, aspirin and heparin, has not been established.

Summary

- Because toxicity is dose-related, extremely small amounts of 'toxic' substances can be ingested without causing any harm.
- The amount of essential oil absorbed from a full-body massage ranges between 0.01 mL and 0.15 mL. For oral doses, the quantity taken within a 24-hour period typically ranges from 0.1–1.3 mL.
- For safety reasons, practitioners should generally avoid using undiluted essential oils on the skin.
- When massaging children of 15 years or under, the concentration of essential oil used should be reduced according to the age of the child. Essential oils should not be used on premature infants.
- To guard against skin irritation, infants should not be given baths with essential oils unless these have been previously dispersed in a water-soluble medium. This guideline could be applied to any age group.
- In most scenarios, we can only discuss the metabolic fate of an essential oil by describing that of its constituents.
- Because of their small molecular size and their favorable lipid/aqueous solubility, most essential oil constituents are able to cross the stratum corneum, travel to the dermis, and from there enter the blood supply.

- The intercellular lipid matrix of the stratum corneum, and the equally lipid-rich hair follicles provide possible transdermal routes for essential oil constituents.
- Dermal absorption of essential oil constituents is enhanced by warmth, massage, hydrating the skin before oil application, and covering the skin following massage.
- Essential oil constituents are absorbed into the skin more rapidly from semi-aqueous media such as gels or emulsions than they are when mixed with vegetable oils.
- In any type of skin disease, essential oils should be applied with caution, as there is an increased the risk of skin reactions.
- Oral dosing is convenient, allows for precision in dosing, and for relatively high doses to be administered. The risks of oral dosing include accidental overdose, drug interactions and gastric irritation.
- The quantities of essential oils used in pessaries, douches and suppositories vary, and could result in appreciable levels of constituents reaching the bloodstream. Rectal and vaginal dosing also carry the risk of local mucous membrane irritation.
- Essential oil constituents may reach the blood supply through inhalation, primarily via the lungs, but also via the mucosa of the upper respiratory tract. Molecules absorbed via the nasal mucosa probably have easy access to the CNS.
- There may be a risk of neurotoxicity from the inhalation of high concentrations of neurotoxic constituents such as pinocamphone or thujone, but there is currently insufficient information to define what constitutes an inhalational risk.
- Essential oil constituents are fairly rapidly absorbed, distributed, metabolized and excreted by all routes of administration. Significant long-term accumulation in any tissues is improbable at doses normally used.
- Through metabolic action essential oil constituents are detoxified or, in rare cases, made more toxic.
- The most important types of reaction which essential oil constituents undergo in the liver are oxidation, hydrolysis, glucuronide conjugation and glutathione conjugation.
- Isomers of compounds are often metabolized differently, and this can have implications for toxicity.
- Once in the body, most essential oil constituents are excreted via the urinary tract after being metabolized, although some are also excreted in the feces and in the expired air. Small amounts may also be excreted through the skin.
- Both ethnicity and gender affect the mix of metabolizing enzymes in an individual, and the presence or absence of a particular enzyme will affect how certain xenobiotics are metabolized. Pharmacogenetics is the study of how people's genetic make-up affects their response to medicines.
- Essential oil constituents may increase or decrease the activity of enzymes that metabolize drugs, the most important being the cytochrome P_{450} (CYP) family. This might lead to an increase or decrease in the blood levels of a drug, both being undesirable. Side effects may also be increased.
- There are a number of known and suspected drug interactions involving essential oils, including wintergreen

oil with warfarin (known), and peppermint oil with felodipine (suspected).

- Essential oils should not be applied to skin on which any medications or drug patches are being used, as the oils may dramatically increase the bioavailability of the drug.
- Certain groups of patients—those with chronic disease, the old, the very young, and those with kidney and liver disease—are less able to handle any foreign substances entering the body. They should be closely monitored for strong or unusual reactions.

Notes

1. Fick's first law can be stated as: $J = -D(d_c/d_x)$ where J is the rate of diffusion, D is the diffusion coefficient, and d_c/d_x is the concentration gradient across the skin.

2. Human skin absorption can be studied using fresh, healthy skin taken from patients undergoing surgery, usually mastectomy or cosmetic breast surgery. A section of skin, including the dermis, is removed and kept at 32 °C (normal skin temperature) in a special chamber. The underside of the skin is continually bathed in a solution that mimics the flow of blood. This keeps the skin alive and metabolically active for at least 24 hours by providing nutrients and oxygen and carrying away waste products. After applying a chemical to the surface of this skin, the rate and degree of absorption can be measured.

3. Some chemicals can have disastrous effects when transcutaneously absorbed. For example, in the 1970s hexachlorophene was used as an antiseptic in baby soaps and talcs, and caused brain damage and even death in some babies after it penetrated their skin. There is good evidence that many toxic substances can be absorbed through the skin to lethal effect, including arsenic, cyanide, phenol and plant alkaloids. This can be profoundly influenced by the vehicle used for administration.

4. Franz (1975) found a qualitative correlation between data from in vitro studies using human skin and human in vivo absorption. Quantitatively, however, the correlation was less than perfect, although the in vitro method adequately distinguished compounds of low permeability from those of high permeability and ranked them in approximately the same order found in vivo.

5. At steady state, the amount (Q) of a substance that passes through the skin is related to its skin permeability coefficient (P_s) by the equation: $Q = P_s (C_D - C_R) t$, where C_D and C_R are the concentrations of the substance in the donor and receptor chambers of the diffusion cell, and t is the time of permeation (Gabbanini et al 2009).

6. Although essential oil constituents are predominantly lipophilic, some, notably those with oxygen-containing functional groups, are also soluble to a limited extent in water. Water solubility is thought to be necessary for the odor of essential oils to be detected by the olfactory receptors.

7. In a study of psoralen analogues, Saïd et al (1997) found that 8-methoxypsoralen (8-MOP) and 5-methoxypsoralen (5-MOP) crossed whole human skin and epidermis more easily than 4,5,8-trimethylpsoralen (TMP), and suggested that the latter compound was essentially retained in the keratin of the stratum corneum. TMP is much more lipophilic than the other psoralens.

8. The partition coefficient (P) of a substance is defined as the ratio of its solubility in a lipid solvent, such as olive oil or *n*-octanol, to that in water. High values reflect a preference for lipid, while low values indicate a preference for aqueous media (i.e., lipophilic and hydrophilic behaviour, respectively). $Log_{10}P$ rather than P values, are normally used for making comparisons between compounds, and it should be noted that log P values differ somewhat between solvent systems. Traditionally, log P values were measured experimentally, but computer programs are now available to calculate them to within about 0.5 log units. Our own values quoted in this book were calculated using the CLogP algorithm provided in ChemDraw Ultra 6.0 (CambridgeSoft), and refer to the octanol/water system. They have all been truncated to one decimal place.

9. A rubefacient is literally a substance that causes reddening of the skin when applied locally. This occurs due to dilatation of the blood capillaries. Other substances that act in this way include the pungent constituents, zingiberene (in *Zingiber officinale*) and piperine and capsaicin (in *Capsicum minimum*).

10. Raindrop technique is a controversial practice, developed by Gary Young in the USA. The seven undiluted oils are dripped onto the back in sequence in order to 'correct defects in the curvature of the spine' by killing the viruses and/or bacteria that are said to be the cause of scoliosis, etc. How essential oils can be expected to remedy structural spinal deformities is not explained. Any reddening of the skin is said to indicate 'that positive benefits are being imparted' (Essential Science Publishing 2004).

11. Although many studies reveal that developing infants have difficulty in metabolizing xenobiotics, and are more vulnerable than adults to the toxic effects of environmental chemicals, infants may be less vulnerable and more resilient to a few drugs and chemicals (Brent 2004).

12. Young's formula gives the proportion of the adult dose as: age of child/(age of child + 12). For example, the dose for a 6-year-old child would be 6/(6 + 12) = 1/3 of the adult dose. Using Dilling's formula, the proportion of the adult dose is given as: age of child/20. So, the dose for a 6-year-old child would be 6/20 = 3/10 of the adult dose.

13. Unlike essential oil constituents, highly lipophilic compounds such as steroids may remain in body fat for weeks or even months before being completely eliminated. Fatty tissue effectively 'drags' highly fat-soluble compounds out of other tissues (Bowman & Rand 1982).

14. Although the metabolism of substances in animals often reflects that in humans, there are instances when it does

not. For example, phenylethyl alcohol, a component of rose oil, is toxic when given orally to rats, but in humans it is metabolized to phenylacetic acid, a naturally occurring, non-toxic compound (Ford 1991).

15. If two substances oxidized by the same CYP isoform reach the enzyme at the same time, there will be some degree of competition, and the rates of metabolism may be reduced for both substances.

16. Cats are severely deficient in glucuronyl transferase, and so are not well equipped to metabolize essential oil constituents. Cats, therefore, may be particularly susceptible to essential oil toxicity.

17. In some scenarios, different patients will require a different dose of the same drug to elicit a similar response. If hereditary traits are taken into account before starting drug treatment, the type of drug and its dosage can often be tailored to the needs of the individual patient (Roots et al 2004). Medications that turn out to be hepatotoxic to a small subset of the population are not uncommon. Idiosyncratic drug reactions made up

20% of cases of severe liver injury requiring hospitalization in a US study involving 307 patients, and in the years 1998–2003, two pharmaceuticals were withdrawn by the FDA because of problems due to hepatotoxicity (Lee 2003).

18. In 1775, an English doctor named Percivall Pott noticed an increase in scrotal cancer in chimney sweeps, and postulated skin contact with soot as a causal factor. Recent studies have established that the polycyclic aromatic hydrocarbons found in soot are converted by the CYP enzymes in the skin into reactive compounds that can damage cellular DNA in a way that can lead to cancer (Hotchkiss 1994).

19. Ioannides et al (1985) observed that compounds containing intact allyl and methylenedioxyphenyl groups (safrole, isosafrole and myristicin) were potent inducers of CYP, while compounds containing an intact allyl group only (estragole and methyleugenol) were not.

The skin

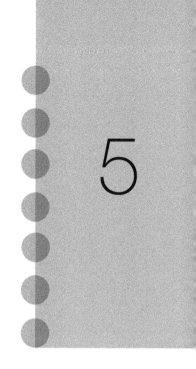

5

CHAPTER CONTENTS

Adverse skin reactions

Adverse skin reactions are of prime importance, since essential oils are commonly applied to the skin. Compared to most other types of toxicity, skin reactions are difficult to predict. There is disagreement about the level of risk, and about the relevance of toxicity data for single, synthetic constituents to whole essential oils. In this chapter we discuss these issues in relation to current legislation. We describe the various types of skin reaction, listing the essential oils most likely to cause them, along with maximum dermal use levels. We discuss the implications of fragrance allergy data, and the pros and cons of patch testing.

Fragrance is the second most common cause of skin allergy, after nickel. However 'fragrance' is not a single substance; it is a term that encompasses thousands of chemicals and hundreds of essential oils. There is a tendency to cite screening data from dermatology clinics as if it represented risk to the general population, but this is a misrepresentation of the data. Moreover, risk needs to be balanced with benefit. If every substance that has caused at least one known allergic reaction was forbidden in personal care products, there would be no personal care products, and if every essential oil was used at a level that presented zero risk, there would be no benefits at all.

Types of reaction

Inflammation caused by contact of any substance with the skin is known as contact dermatitis, and this is sub-divided into irritant contact dermatitis (ICD), allergic contact dermatitis (ACD), pigmented contact dermatitis (PCD) and photocontact dermatitis, or photosensitization (Figure 5.1). Each of these is discussed later in the chapter. 'Sensitization', a word often used in this text, is the first stage in the process of acquiring ACD. Similarly 'irritation' may lead to ICD.

Irritation from essential oils is often regarded as less of a problem than sensitization, and there are fewer clinical data. Although the two types of reaction are generally considered distinct, irritation can be a factor in promoting sensitization, since the reduced barrier function facilitates access to the cells that could mount an immune reaction, and some consider all contact allergens also to be irritants.

Some essential oil constituents are haptens. A hapten is a small reactive molecule which, when coupled with a protein, can initiate the formation of antibodies. Irritation by a hapten can cause an immediate inflammatory reaction and may also cause prime cells in the skin (Langerhans cells) to react to contact with the same substance in the future. Whether or not ACD develops following the initial irritation may depend on the skin concentration of the hapten and its duration of contact with the skin (Saint-Mezard et al 2003a; Bonneville et al 2007).

Determining factors

The severity of a skin reaction varies with factors such as the anatomical site of exposure, the total area of skin exposed, the frequency and duration of exposure, the substance applied, its total quantity and concentration, the vehicle used, whether or not occlusion is used, the presence of inflammation or diseased skin, and the degree of percutaneous penetration (Boukhman & Maibach 2001; Basketter et al 2002a).

Environmental conditions should not be forgotten. The presence of ultraviolet (UV) light is the determining factor in photosensitization, and ambient temperature and humidity can influence general sensitivity. With both the fragrance mix (FM; see The fragrance mix below for definition) and turpentine oil, cool and dry conditions correlated with an increase of mild adverse reactions, compared to warmer and more humid weather (Uter et al 2008).

There are three primary factors that determine skin reactivity, and all of the above involve aspects of one or more of the following:

- dose metrics (quantity and concentration of substance)
- degree of percutaneous absorption of substance
- degree of reactivity between substance and immune system.

Dose metrics is the easiest of the three to control, because it does not depend on the individual. Unfortunately, the same dose of a substance may induce a reaction in one person and not in another. A further complication is that the same substance may vary in its effect, depending on what other substances are present, since this can affect percutaneous absorption. Although there is some knowledge about the pharmacokinetics of oils, gels, etc., in relation to the skin, little is known about essential oil constituents in this regard.

The high degree of variability in individual reactions to the same substance is due to differences in percutaneous absorption, and differences in reactivity due to either genetics and/or frequency of exposure. Genetic variation impacts many relevant factors such as antioxidant status, skin barrier function, cytokine expression and the concentration of regulatory T cells that modulate immune responses (Schnuch et al 2010). Although it is not yet possible to accurately predict or control susceptibility, the following section highlights some known vulnerable groups.

Susceptible individuals

In Tables 14.1–14.5 the average percentage of individuals reacting to a fragrance material varies according to the group being tested, with susceptibility increasing from healthy volunteers (not shown in the tables), to dermatitis patients, to patients suspected of cosmetic or fragrance allergy, to known fragrance-sensitive patients, and finally to patients known to be sensitive to the material being tested. Cosmetic-sensitive patients are a subset of dermatitis patients in general. For example, of 281,100 dermatitis patients, 13,216 had contact dermatitis, and of these 713 were related to cosmetic ingredients (Adams et al 1985). Similarly, of 18,747 dermatitis patients, 1,781 had contact dermatitis and 75 were allergic to cosmetic products (De Groot 1987). It can be assumed that these differences are determined by the variables discussed above. In assessing risk, the degree of susceptibility of one group of individuals should not be applied to another.

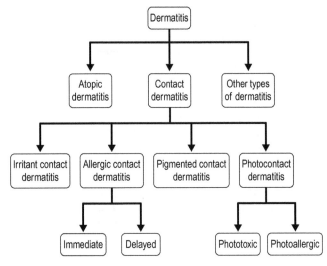

Figure 5.1 • Classifications of dermatitis.

Health status

Adverse skin reactions are determined by the health of the individual in a number of ways. In order to produce adverse effects, most irritants or allergens must cross the stratum corneum to reach the viable epidermis. If an essential oil is applied to damaged, diseased or inflamed skin the condition may be worsened, since larger amounts than normal may be absorbed and adverse reactions are more likely to occur.

Psychological stress can have an adverse effect on skin health. Several mechanisms have been proposed:

- it can reduce skin barrier integrity through the increased production of glucocorticoids (Denda et al 2000)
- it can enhance skin sensitization, possibly because the immune system is primed to mount an optimal response. In mice, acute stress just prior to sensitization greatly magnified the reaction of Langerhans cells and T cells to a hapten; this was mediated by norepinephrine (Saint-Mezard et al 2003b)
- it increases the release of a neuropeptide called 'substance P' from nerve endings in the skin, and this triggers the release of inflammatory cytokines from mast cells (Kawana et al 2006).

Interestingly, cutaneous allergic reactions were suppressed at both induction and elicitation phases in mice, by inhalation of the synthetic odorant 'citralva' (Hosoi & Tsuchiya 2000). It has been suggested that inhalation of anxiolytic odorants prevents the release of substance P and the consequent inflammatory cascade (Hosoi et al 2003). In mice, valerian oil inhalation reduced stress-induced plasma corticosterone levels (Hosoi et al 2001), presumably because it is anxiolytic.

Chronic illness and old age are often associated with reduced antioxidant status (see Ch. 12, p. 170) and this may increase skin reactivity. Endogenous antioxidants such as glutathione help prevent the formation of allergen-protein adducts, an important step in skin sensitization, and also help protect the skin against UVA-induced phototoxicity (Lutz et al 2001; Meewes et al 2001). Both scenarios involve reactions with free radicals, as does photocarcinogenesis. When oxidative stress overwhelms the skin's antioxidant capacity, this leads to degenerative processes, which may include DNA damage (Briganti & Picardo 2003).

Age

In a survey of 57,779 adult dermatitis patients, the prevalence of fragrance allergy increased with advancing age, probably due to increasing cumulative exposure to fragrances (Uter et al 2001). In Europe, the frequency of fragrance allergy among dermatitis patients is low in the first two decades of life (2.5–3.4%). It gradually increases in females after the age of 20 to peak in the 60s at 14.4% of those tested, with a decline to 11.6% in the 80s. The prevalence in males rises more slowly and peaks at 13.7% in the 70s, declining to 10.8% in the 80s (Buckley et al 2003). The number of Langerhans cells is significantly reduced in aged skin, which may explain why it is less reactive to allergens (Kligman 1979; Fenske & Lober 1986).[1]

Children up to three months old are theoretically at greater risk of skin sensitization due to the immaturity of their skin and its barrier function. However, contact allergies are in fact rare in young children, possibly due to a lack of exposure to allergens. Nickel and topical medications are among the most common causes of infant ACD (Carder 2005). In a survey of 304 unselected infants, no reproducible positive reactions to the FM were found at either 12 or 18 months (Jøhnke et al 2004). This does not mean that infant contact with fragrance materials or essential oils is devoid of risk; in fact intensive exposure may predispose a child to skin allergy problems later in life. In a Turkish survey of children with contact dermatitis, there was one reaction to the FM in 84 children aged 2–8 (1.2%) and four reactions in 89 children aged 9–16 (4.5%) (Onder & Adisen 2008).

Gender

According to Scheinman (1996) women are 3–4 times more likely to be affected by fragrance sensitivity than men. In one report the male/female distribution was 26.5/74.4% for the fragrance mix (ratio 2.8:1), and 17.6/82.4% for its constituents (ratio 4.7:1), in another the female/male ratio for the fragrance mix was 2.3:1 (Lunder & Kansky 2000; Temesvári et al 2002). A Swedish report of hand eczema found that ICD was much more common in women than men (Meding 1990).

The higher susceptibility of women may be due to a greater use of fragranced products, or because women are inherently more susceptible to skin allergies. Modjtahedi et al (2004) concluded that females are more at risk of ACD because of different exposure patterns, and not because of differences in intrinsic skin characteristics. However, women have more vigorous cellular immune reactions than men, and testosterone has been shown to suppress immune function (Darnall & Suarez 2009). Cytokine production decreased in men but increased in women, following a psychosocial stress test. Differences in response were also evident between women at different stages of the menstrual cycle (Kirschbaum et al 1999). These findings suggest that hormonal parameters do affect susceptibility, but because of differences in immune reactivity, not skin permeability.

Genetics and race

Individual susceptibility is in part dependent on genetic factors. For example, carriers of defective genes for certain isoenzymes of glutathione S-transferase or N-acetyltransferase are more susceptible to skin allergy (Lutz et al 2001; Nacak et al 2006). This may be because reduced antioxidant status leads to greater reactivity to allergens.

Atopic dermatitis is a highly heritable condition, with 81 reported genetic markers in people of Asian or Caucasian racial origin. Some of these genes are associated with skin barrier dysfunction, and more than half are associated with the immune response (Barnes KC 2010). There are conflicting data as to whether atopic dermatitis is a risk factor for ACD, though it is thought to be a risk specifically for type I allergic reactions. Those who consider it a risk factor include Larsen et al (1996b), Manzini et al (1998) and Mortz et al (2001). Those finding no association include Giordano-Labadie et al (1999), Mortz et al (2002) and Schafer T et al (2001). One study found atopic dermatitis to be a risk factor for hand dermatitis in massage therapists (Crawford et al 2004). The prevalence of atopic dermatitis varies considerably with age, race and location. In a pediatric practice in San Diego, California, incidence was 2% for Hispanics, 2.8% for non-Hispanic whites, 3.2% for people of mixed race, 3.7% for blacks, 5.6% for non-Filipino Asians and 8.5% for Filipinos (Baker RB 1999). In adults, prevalence varies from 0.2% in Scotland (>40 years) to 3.1% in the Netherlands (Herd et al 1996; Verboom et al 2002).[2]

It is now recognized that a subset of the population is susceptible to multiple contact allergies, defined as positive patch tests to three or more allergens. It is estimated that 5% of contact dermatitis patients are 'polysensitized'. These patients are more easily sensitized, 80% are women, and increased risk is associated with atopic dermatitis, leg ulcers and old age (Carlsen 2009). Polysensitization is thought to be due to genetic factors (Schnuch et al 2007b). The increased susceptibility to patch testing is evident at both induction and elicitation stages, and has been linked to genetic markers for TNF-α and IL-16 (Carlsen et al 2008; Schnuch et al 2008). Both of these cytokines are involved in the inflammatory response to an allergen, and corresponding genetic over-expression could therefore increase susceptibility to contact dermatitis (Reich et al 2003; Westphal et al 2003). It is not known whether polysensitization represents a distinct phenotype.

In a review encompassing 8,610 white and 1,014 black dermatitis patients, it was concluded that there were no differences in the overall response rate to a variety of allergens. Although some differences were seen in reactions to specific allergens, these are probably due to differences in exposure determined by ethnicity (Deleo et al 2002). There were no significant racial differences in adverse reactions to eugenol, cinnamaldehyde or cinnamic alcohol in 887 white and 114 black dermatology patients (Dickel et al 2001). Further to the particular sensitivities discussed in the section covering Pigmented contact dermatitis below, a report from Korea highlights a relatively high reactivity to sandalwood oil and cinnamic alcohol, both tested at 2%, in 422 dermatitis patients (80% female) with suspected fragrance allergy. A total of 35 fragrance chemicals and seven essential oils or absolutes were tested (An et al 2005).

Variables of application

The variables affecting percutaneous absorption are described in Chapter 4, and can be listed as:

* the substance applied (lipid and water solubility, molecular size, etc.)
* the circumstances of application (area of body, presence of occlusion, etc.)
* skin permeability (age, skin health, etc.).

In this section, further aspects are discussed that impact whether or not an adverse reaction will occur.

Dose metrics

Skin reactivity to an allergen is highly concentration-dependent and this is clearly seen in Table 5.1. As the concentration of cinnamaldehyde is reduced, the number of people reacting decreases from 100% to zero. Concentration dependency is also seen in mixtures of fragrance materials, and in essential oils (Santucci et al 1987; Selvaag et al 1995; Frosch et al 2005b). Although there are inconsistencies, the data in Tables 13.1–13.4 and 14.2–14.6 indicate that overall, the percentage of allergic reactions increases in relation to the concentration of the test substance used for test subjects with similar classifications of

Table 5.1 Cinnamaldehyde patch tests in dermatitis patients known to be sensitive to 2% cinnamaldehyde

Concentration used	Percentage who reacted	Number of reactors
2.0%	100%	18/18
1.0%	83%	15/18
0.5%	61%	11/18
0.1%	27%	5/18
0.05%	17%	3/18
0.02%	6%	1/18
0.01%	0%	0/18

(Data from Johansen et al 1996a)

skin disease. (Note that concentrations used in patch testing are measured by weight, not by volume.)

However, the critical exposure determinant for evaluating skin sensitization risk is 'dermal loading', or dose per unit area of skin exposed, and not simply the total dose applied or the total area of application (Robinson et al 2000). Concentration and vehicle have been used in the theoretical risk assessment of cinnamaldehyde-containing products (Gerberick et al 2001a). Since all allergens show dose–response and threshold characteristics, it should be possible to use them safely, so long as they are incorporated at concentrations well tolerated by most individuals.

Frequency of exposure

Repeated exposure to the same substance over time is widely considered to increase the risk of adverse reaction. This probably explains why infants show no reactivity to the fragrance mix. However, frequent exposure to a *low-risk* fragrance allergen may not lead to a high incidence of ACD.

Fenn (1989) analyzed 400 fragranced products, and listed the most used fragrance constituents (by volume %) and the percentage of products containing them in the USA and the Netherlands. These include, for example, linalool (90% USA, 91% Netherlands), 2-phenylethanol (82%, 79%), and linalyl acetate (78%, 67%). It is notable that these three constituents have very low reported incidences of sensitization. In a paper reporting on patch tests in eleven European dermatology clinics, with all 48 of the materials listed by Fenn (1989), only 10 tested positive and only one of these (citronellol) is in the top ten ranking for either country. Each material was tested on 100 or more dermatitis patients, and clinical relevance of the positive reactions was not established in a single case (Frosch et al 1995a). Therefore, frequency of exposure does not necessarily increase risk, even though it can be a factor in ACD.

The substance applied

Clearly, some essential oils are more likely to cause adverse reactions than others, and the presence and concentration of a relatively potent allergen is a major factor in ACD. The presence of adulterants or contaminants may also be a factor. The oxidation of essential oil constituents can increase risk (see Ch. 2, p. 10–11) because the oxides and peroxides formed are more reactive. This is seen with (+)-limonene, δ-3-carene and α-pinene and is due to the formation of oxidation products, some of which are more sensitizing than the parent compound (see Chapter 14, Constituent Profiles). However, the fact that an essential oil constituent is capable of being oxidized does not automatically mean that the use of an essential oil containing it presents a significant allergenic risk.

Once oxidation has begun it is difficult to halt, but the onset of oxidation can be prevented for a period of weeks, months or years by storage under nitrogen, by keeping a product cool, by screening it from UV rays, and by the addition of antioxidants such as (synthetic) butylated hydroxytoluene (BHT) or (natural) α-tocopherol. The efficacy of other natural antioxidants with regard to essential oil oxidation has not been much studied, but these include other tocopherols, rosmarinic acid, propyl gallate and ascorbyl palmitate. Combinations may be more effective than single chemicals. We recommend that effective antioxidant systems are used in preparations containing essential oils prone to oxidation.

In general, aged products are more likely to cause sensitization reactions. However, cinnamaldehyde may be markedly less allergenic in aged preparations, where it has oxidized to cinnamic acid, and in mixtures in which it can react with alcohols and/or amines to form non-allergenic compounds.

Quenching

In 1976, RIFM published a brief report indicating that human sensitization to citral, cinnamaldehyde and phenylacetaldehyde could be reduced by the presence of other constituents. Citral sensitization was 'quenched' by α-pinene or (+)-limonene, phenylacetaldehyde sensitization by 2-phenylethanol, and cinnamaldehyde sensitization by either (+)-limonene or eugenol (Opdyke 1976 p. 197–198). A further RIFM study found that sensitization from 86% pure nootkatone was counteracted when mixed with (+)-limonene 1:4 (IFRA 2009).

Seven subsequent and more rigorous studies have demonstrated similar quenching effects, three in guinea pigs and four in humans. Citral induced sensitization reactions in guinea pigs at concentrations above 0.5%, and this effect was reduced by the co-presence of an equal quantity of (+)-limonene. It was concluded that the quenching effect operates at two levels, induction and elicitation, and it was suggested that (+)-limonene may interact with node macrophages and Langerhans cells to block delayed hypersensitivity (Hanau et al 1983). A similar quenching effect of (+)-limonene on citral was seen in human volunteers (Api & Isola 2000). (+)-Limonene had a quenching effect on cinnamaldehyde sensitization in 3 of 11 human subjects, and eugenol had a similar effect in 7 of the same 11 cinnamaldehyde-sensitive subjects. It is postulated that this may be due to competitive inhibition at the receptor level (Guin et al 1984).

In 10 people who developed urticaria after cinnamaldehyde had been applied to the skin, six had a greatly diminished reaction when it was applied combined with eugenol (Allenby et al 1984). Eugenol caused a reduction in non-immune immediate contact urticaria induced by cinnamaldehyde, benzoic acid or sorbic acid, even when it was applied 60 minutes prior to application of cinnamaldehyde, and the effect was not eliminated by washing (Safford et al 1990).

In contrast to these reports, Basketter & Allenby (1991) found no evidence of cinnamaldehyde quenching by eugenol in human subjects with a history of cinnamaldehyde allergy. (This study was criticized by Nilsson et al 2004 for using only one concentration of allergen and quenching agent, making detection of any inhibitory effect difficult.) Basketter (2000) reviewed quenching, concluding that it was unproven, although his critique did not include reference to Allenby et al (1984) or to Guin et al (1984).

Subsequent work by researchers in Sweden has provided what may be the first conclusive evidence for quenching. A significant inhibitory effect on (R)-(−)-carvone sensitization in guinea pigs was seen when induction was carried out along with a structural analogue, either (R)-methylcarvone or (2R,5R)-dihydrocarvone (Karlberg et al 2001). In a further study, linalool quenched (R)-(−)-carvone sensitization, showing that structural similarity between sensitizer and quenching agent is not important. The quenching effect was not due to anti-inflammatory activity (Nilsson et al 2004). In both reports, the inhibitory effect lasted 48 days on re-challenge.

Quenching may be responsible for some unexpected results in essential oil testing. For example, citral was significantly sensitizing in maximation tests at concentrations ranging from 2–8% (Opdyke 1979a p. 259–266). However, when similarly tested, essential oils of lemongrass and may chang, both rich in citral, were not sensitizing when tested at 4% and 8%, respectively (Opdyke 1976 p. 455, p. 457, Opdyke & Letizia 1982 p. 731–732). Lemongrass oil tested at 5% (equivalent to 4% citral) was not sensitizing in two further maximation tests, nor were there any reactions to 4% citral + 1% (+)-limonene in a human repeat insult patch test with 118 volunteers (Api 2000; Api & Isola 2000). Both lemongrass and may chang oil contain (+)-limonene as well as citral.

The International Fragrance Association (IFRA) rejected limonene-citral quenching on the basis that no evidence of the phenomenon could be seen in local lymph node assay (LLNA) testing or in some guinea pig assays (Lalko & Api 2008). The argument that animal data are more relevant to human risk than are human data is a curious one.

Since quenching is a form of antagonism, it makes sense that such a phenomenon would exist. Synergy and antagonism are commonly seen in the interaction of mixtures with the human body, and there is good evidence of synergy in relation to fragrance materials and ACD (Lepoittevin & Mutterer 1998; Matura et al 2003). Several dermatologists, for example De Groot et al (1993) have reported cases who do not test positive to the FM, but who do test positive to one of its constituents. This type of false-negative reaction may be due to quenching. Temesvári et al (2002) found that, of 104 FM-negative patients, 18 (11.9%) subsequently tested positive to one or more of six of the eight constituents. Clearly, mixtures of fragrance materials can lead to both synergistic and antagonistic phenomena.

Quenching does not totally eliminate adverse reactions, but significantly reduces their severity. Antagonism in mixtures may be due to competition between different molecules for the active site of an enzyme in the skin that converts

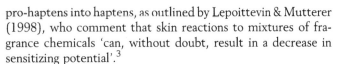

pro-haptens into haptens, as outlined by Lepoittevin & Mutterer (1998), who comment that skin reactions to mixtures of fragrance chemicals 'can, without doubt, result in a decrease in sensitizing potential'.[3]

Other types of substance can also be quenching agents. In many cases a major step in antigen formation involves reaction with oxygen radicals (Bezard et al 1997). Antioxidants can reduce the potency of haptens that form full antigens in this way. For example, either ascorbic acid or α-tocopherol reduced the sensitization response when applied to the skin before limonene-2-hydroperoxide, a product of limonene oxidation (Gafvert et al 2002). Antioxidants, such as lutein or ascorbic acid, offer protection by inhibiting histamine release, thereby reducing the severity of an allergic reaction (Mio et al 1999; Lee et al 2004). Since topically applied lavender oil prevents induced anaphylaxis and histamine release in mice and rats (Kim & Cho 1999), the potential therefore exists to use mixtures of antioxidant essential oils to prevent oxidative skin damage (Wei & Shibamoto 2007b). Also see Table 12.4.

The above arguments have considerable ramifications for aromatherapists, dermatologists and regulators. It may be convenient for regulators to assume that a given concentration of, say, citral, always presents the same level of risk, no matter what other substances may be present and no matter whether it is a synthetic material or an essential oil constituent. However, such an approach is unsatisfactory because it does not reflect reality. In order to assess the probable allergenicity of an essential oil, the oil should be assessed, rather than assumptions being made on the basis of one or two of its constituents.

Patch testing

Dermatologists use patch testing to determine the chemical cause of contact dermatitis in a patient. Patients are either screened with what are considered to be the most likely allergens, or the ingredients of a suspect product are tested. From screening tests, there are data covering thousands of patients, but only a small number of essential oils or constituents, i.e., the ones commonly tested. In order to proactively identify high-risk substances many more have been tested using animal models, and various in vitro and in silico models are in development to replace these. For a person with contact dermatitis, the only alternative to patch testing is total or selective avoidance of products applied to the skin.

Patch testing is usually carried out by dermatologists or other health care workers trained in the procedure. Materials being tested are applied to healthy skin on the inside of the forearm or more commonly the upper back. Occlusive patches made specifically for the purpose are used, such as Finn Chamber 8 mm 'blanks' to which a prepared concentration of essential oil in petrolatum can be added (but these are only sold to doctors). Patches are left in place for 48 hours, and the area of skin being tested should not be washed or exposed to sunlight or other sources of UV light. An initial assessment is made one hour after removal, and a second assessment is made 48 hours later. Any irritation response will be apparent at this point. Many dermatologists recommend that, when testing for sensitization, a final assessment should be made seven days after application.

Table 5.2 Grading of adverse skin reactions to patch tests

Code	Strength of reaction	Signs
+?	Doubtful	Mild redness only
+	Weakly positive	Red and slightly thickened skin
++	Strongly positive	Red, swollen skin with individual small water blisters
+++	Extremely positive	Intense redness and swelling with coalesced large blisters or spreading reaction
IR	Irritant	Red skin improves once patch is removed

Do not use undiluted essential oils for patch testing. Mix the test oil at 5% w/w with petrolatum (petroleum jelly). Bandages are not recommended for patch testing, but if used, they should be latex-free and all edges should be adhesive. Plastic, waterproof bandages may be a good choice. Any reaction seen is scored according to the International Contact Dermatitis Research Group system, as illustrated in Table 5.2. It is sometimes difficult to determine whether a reaction is irritant or allergic, and whether a very slight reddening should be classed as a reaction at all. Doubtful reactions are classed as '?', 'IR/?' or '+?'. Dubious allergic reactions can be as high as 25% of those recorded (Frosch et al 2005b).

If there is a positive result, any of the following may be present: redness, itching, swelling and papules (small, solid blisters). An irritant reaction is most prominent immediately after the patch is removed and fades over the next day. An allergic reaction usually takes a few days to develop, so may be more prominent sometime after the patch is removed. A substance that causes an allergic reaction should be avoided completely if possible. Repeated exposure may increase the severity of the reaction.

Two methods used in research are the maximation test and the human repeated insult patch test (HRIPT). A maximation test is typically conducted on 25 healthy volunteers by utilizing five alternate day 48-hour occluded induction applications of test material. Following a 10–14 day rest period, 48-hour challenge applications are made to naïve sites, either with or without pre-treatment with sodium lauryl sulfate (a skin irritant), until a maximal response is obtained (Lalko & Api 2006). This method has been widely used by RIFM in its sensitization testing of fragrance materials. The HRIPT usually involves 100 subjects and a total of nine 24-hour occluded applications of test material over three weeks, followed by a two week rest period. A single 24-hour challenge is then made to a naïve site with the same material (Lalko & Api 2006).

Some consider patch testing for research purposes (as opposed to identifying the source of ACD in an individual) to be unethical.

Interpreting patch test data

Flaws in research design are apparent in reports of fragrance allergy, among the most fundamental being a lack of clear and consistent criteria both for the diagnosis of ACD, and the absence of grading of the response to a test material. Many studies do not record reactions to the vehicle alone, as a control. Some studies have small numbers of participants and in many, unclear provenance and/or purity of the materials being tested is an issue (merely stating the name of the supplier does not clearly identify a substance. Single chemicals are available in various grades of purity, and essential oils can vary greatly with chemotype and origin). Almost none of the reports in which essential oils or absolutes are patch tested give a detailed compositional breakdown. Problems such as these considerably reduce the significance of the research, and yet such papers are widely cited as definitive, simply because they are published in peer-reviewed journals.

Most patch tests are conducted using petrolatum as a diluent, even though petrolatum is, albeit rarely, a clinically relevant cause of allergy (Kundu et al 2004; Rios Scherrer 2006; Tam & Elston 2006). In one study of skin reactions to fragrance materials, one person out of 167 (0.6%) had an allergic reaction to 100% petrolatum, and two (1.2%) had an irritant reaction to it (Larsen et al 1996b). In an analysis of data from 79,365 patients patch tested with petrolatum, 0.3% had unconfirmed positive reactions (Schnuch et al 2006). **This suggests that reaction rates of 0.3% or less to fragrance materials have no significance.** (The 0.3% figure does include doubtful reactions, but so do many of the reports of adverse reactions to fragrant substances.)

False-negative reactions may occur in maximation tests due to the small size of the test group (25 volunteers) and yet the rate of positive findings is sometimes so great as to suggest distortion with false positives (Marzulli & Maibach 1980). Albert Kligman, who designed the test, cautioned: 'It must be thoroughly understood that the maximation procedure does not directly assess safety in use (except when negative). It does not predict the incidence of sensitization in a population of users' (Kligman 1966). Approximately 50% of reactions to the fragrance mix are thought to be false positives (see Fragrance mix, below).

Patch testing is commonly carried out using a battery of potential allergens, not all of them fragrance materials. 'Excited skin syndrome' (ESS), or 'angry back' is characterized by multiple reactions to allergens (Bruynzeel & Maibach 1986). Patients with ESS may have a disposition to develop sensitivities to unrelated allergens, and the close proximity of the patches may be an exacerbating factor (Brasch et al 2006, Duarte et al 2002b). In one analysis, ESS developed in 39 of 630 dermatitis patients or 6.2% (Duarte et al 2002a). An 'angry back' reaction to patch testing may or may not suggest polysensitization (described above, under Genetics and race).

Another reason for false-positive reactions is the misidentification of irritants as allergens (Kligman 1998). A further problem is discordance between patch test systems, of which there are several. In using two different patch test systems, TRUE Test missed 50% of the clinically relevant FM reactions that were detected using Finn Chambers (Suneja & Belsito 2001). Although the Finn Chambers system appears to be more accurate in detecting clinically relevant fragrance allergy, TRUE Test is the only commercial system approved in the USA. When both TRUE Test and Trolab were used to test the FM simultaneously in 5,006 dermatitis patients, 218 (4.4%) reacted to TRUE Test,

464 (9.3%) reacted to Trolab, and 187 (3.7%) reacted to both (Mortz & Andersen 2010). There is clearly a significant problem when the results of patch testing are so dependent on which brand of patch is used.

'Clinical relevance' refers to whether a positive reaction to a patch test is relevant to the patient's presenting condition. In one study of 702 patients, clinical relevance was not established in almost one third of cases with positive patch tests (Frosch et al 1995b). In a meta-analysis of ACD data that adjusted for clinical relevance, the prevalence of FM allergy in dermatitis patients was 3.4%, 3–4 times less than typical estimates (Krob et al 2004). Storrs (2007) found that, 'many persons…have positive patch test reactions, but few of these individuals have clinical allergies to fragrances.' Similarly, Hostýnek & Maibach (2003b, 2004b, 2004c) found that a clear cause–effect relationship has only infrequently or rarely been established for citronellol, geraniol and linalool, in spite of these being cited as frequent causes of ACD.

To summarize, a substantial percentage of patch tests using fragrant materials on dermatitis patients generate either false positives or are clinically irrelevant, and there are design flaws in much of the research. As regards the general population, because of threshold considerations, only a very small percentage of those who test positive to a fragrance material will develop related clinical manifestations (Kimber et al 1999). The patch testing data from the FM and its constituents do not readily extrapolate to actual use, because the severe conditions of patch testing are much more likely to result in allergic reactions. There are multiple reasons for this.

The incidence of patch test reactions to low molecular weight chemicals depends, not simply on the size of the patch used, nor on the total dose or concentration of substance applied, but on the dermal loading (the dose per area of exposed skin) expressed as $\mu g/cm^2$ (Friedmann 1990; Friedmann et al 1983a, 1983b; White et al 1986). Hostýnek & Maibach (2004a) suggest that 1% of an ingredient in a perfume spray results in a dermal loading of 26 $\mu g/cm^2$ of that ingredient (Gerberick et al 2001a). However, a patch test using 1% of the same ingredient has a dermal loading 11, 21, 38 or 68 times greater, depending on which of four patch test systems is being used: Finn Chamber 8 mm, Professional Products 1.9 cm × 1.9 cm, Webril 2 cm × 2 cm or Hill Top Chambers 19 mm, respectively (Robinson et al 2000). Therefore a patch test with 1% tea tree oil presents a higher risk than a product containing 1% tea tree oil. The concentrating effect of occlusion (see Ch. 4, p. 46), combined with the relatively long duration of exposure, adds considerably to the severity of patch testing.

The threshold concentration for eliciting a positive reaction varies inversely with the severity of the induction regime. So, the higher the percentage of substance used to initially induce the allergic response, the lower the percentage of the same substance that will elicit an allergic reaction. Therefore normal exposure to weak allergens, such as some fragrance materials, may induce 'sub-clinical' allergic states (a low-level induction state), in which no skin reaction occurs under normal conditions of use. However, the more severe conditions of patch testing may elicit a positive reaction. Consequently, dermatologists sometimes induce positive reactions that would not occur under everyday use conditions (Hostýnek & Maibach 2004a).

For example, two dermatology patients became sensitized to sesquiterpene lactone mix when it was used on them in patch testing (Kanerva et al 2001b). In patients with multiple contact allergies, the risk of acquiring additional allergies increases with repeated patch testing (Carlsen 2009).

All of the above explains why patch testing with essential oils and fragrance materials suggests a much higher level of ACD incidence than is apparent from consumer complaints, or from the experience of most aromatherapists. It also means that realistic safe levels of fragrance materials are greater than a no effect concentration established in a series of patch tests would indicate. True prevalence or incidence rates from the use of naturally or synthetically fragranced products, whether in the general population or in dermatitis patients, cannot be determined from patch test data (Naldi 2002).

Patch testing is an indispensable tool for identifying the cause of a pre-existing skin allergy, and dermatologists consider the severe testing conditions appropriate for detecting susceptibilities that might otherwise have gone undetected. Unfortunately they may also be inducing or eliciting reactions that might not otherwise have occurred. Some consider that the risk of inducing sensitization is appropriate in diagnostic testing, but not when screening healthy volunteers (Basketter et al 1997; Uter et al 2004). There is debate about the circumstances in which patch testing should be used in clinical aromatherapy.

Irritation

Irritation causes reversible skin damage, and is less severe than corrosion. Corrosive chemicals, which include acids and alkalis, usually act on the surface of the skin, disrupting its function as a barrier. Strong alkalis, for example, may dissolve the stratum corneum, allowing water to be lost from the tissues and harmful substances to penetrate into deeper layers of the skin. In this scenario, direct damage to the skin is usually of greater importance than the inflammatory response. Some essential oils, such as horseradish and mustard, can produce severe skin irritation, but corrosion has only been noted for p-cresol, a major constituent of birch tar oil.

Irritants act on the first exposure, the reaction is rapid and the severity is highly dependent on dilution. For example, patch tests were performed on 28 dermatitis patients who were not allergic to turpentine oil with various concentrations of freshly distilled, unoxidized δ-3-carene, (+)-limonene, α-pinene or β-pinene, all major constituents of turpentine oil. Concentrations of 70–80% were irritating in most patients, at 50% weak reactions were obtained 'in some cases' but no reactions were seen at 25–30% (Pirilä et al 1964).

Although ICD, or 'primary irritation', is not an allergic reaction, it is now seen as a more complex event than was previously thought. There is strong evidence that IL-1α plays a key role, with the assistance of TNF-α, leading to the release of inflammatory cytokines and chemokines from skin cells. In most cases, this cascade of events is triggered by disruption of the epidermal barrier, and there are multiple ways in which keratinocytes signal barrier disruption to other cell types (Fluhr et al 2008).

Inflammation is said to be a fundamental characteristic of ICD. However, there is one type of ICD, known as 'sensory irritation' in which there is subjective irritation (itching, stinging, burning or tingling) with no clinical signs of inflammation (Fluhr et al 2008). People with sensitive skin may have either sensory irritation, or 'normal' irritation.

Sensitive skin

In a large minority of people there is an increased susceptibility to irritants, or even to cosmetic ingredients not normally thought of as irritants. Sensitive (hyper-irritable) skin has only been recognized by dermatologists since the late 1980s when, in a group of 74 females, a correlation was seen between subjective stinging and erythema on patch testing with sorbic or benzoic acid (Lammintausta et al 1988). It was realized that skin with a normal appearance could be functionally abnormal, and that a stinging sensation might not be accompanied by any visible reaction (Maibach et al 1989).

Sensitive skin may be genetically determined, independent of atopy; blacks in general have less irritable skin than whites of Northern European extraction. In fact people classed as skin phototype I or II (Table 5.3) are sensitive not only to UVB, but also to chemicals in general. This may be related to the number of cell layers in the stratum corneum, and/or to barrier function (Frosch 1992 p. 45–46).

Sensitive skin tends to be drier, redder, and less supple than the norm. In the West, approximately 40% of the population considers that they have sensitive skin (Berardesca et al 2006). There is currently no recognized test for it, and there are almost certainly several sub-types, with different mechanistic triggers. We do know that barrier function is a critical factor in skin discomfort, and it is highly dependent on the integrity of the stratum corneum lipids (Farage et al 2006). This, in turn, is susceptible to increases in psychological stress (Garg et al 2001). Psychological stress, however, can be a factor in any type of ICD.

Table 5.3 Skin phototypes

Skin phototype	Typical features	Tanning ability
I	Pale white skin, blue/hazel eyes, blond/red hair	Always burns, does not tan
II	Fair skin, blue eyes	Burns easily, tans poorly
III	Darker white skin	Tans after initial burn
IV	Light brown skin	Burns minimally, tans easily
V	Brown skin	Rarely burns, tans darkly easily
VI	Dark brown or black skin	Never burns, always tans darkly

Sensitive skin is sometimes defined as a non-immunologically mediated skin inflammation, which is the result of intolerance to stimuli that are normally well tolerated. In these cases it may be prudent to cease use of all cosmetics, then reintroduce them one at a time at intervals of 1–2 weeks, in order to identify irritant products (Pons-Guiraud 2004). In addition to cosmetics, weather and psychological stress are important self-reported factors in sensitive skin (Farage 2008).

Identifying irritants

The classifications for irritants given in Box 5.1 and Table 5.4 are our own, and are based only on human testing. Massoia and wild mountain sage oils are provisionally classified based on their content of massoia lactone. It is possible that chemicals formed during oxidation were responsible for the irritation seen in Siberian fir needle and dwarf pine oils. The irritation responses caused by lemon myrtle and lemon verbena oils are probably due to citral, and other citral-rich oils may also possess some irritancy. The same may be true of essential oils rich in cinnamaldehyde or thymol.

Industrial safety guidelines (CPL: Classification, Packaging and Labeling) list several essential oils as 'R38 – irritating to the skin', but this is in relation to handling the undiluted material in bulk, and in most cases the listing seems to be based on animal testing. For example, the following undiluted essential oils have been moderately or markedly irritating to rabbit, guinea pig, mouse or pig skin: clove leaf (Opdyke 1978 p. 695), summer savory (Opdyke 1976 p. 859–860), taget (Opdyke & Letizia 1982 p. 829–830), parsley leaf (Opdyke & Letizia 1983 p. 871–872), oregano (Opdyke 1974 p. 945–946) and may chang (Opdyke & Letizia 1982 p. 731–732). Yet these essential oils, all listed as R38 – irritating to the skin, were non-irritant when tested in dilution on human skin. Other essential oils with the R38 classification include melissa, tea tree and turpentine.[4]

Some of the skin irritation data in the RIFM monographs are based on tests using rabbits; a substance is applied undiluted and the skin is then covered. This tells us little about the risk of irritation when the same substance is applied in dilution to uncovered human skin. Some essential oils that are irritating to rabbit skin seem to have no such effect on human skin, for example sandalwood (Opdyke 1974 p. 989–990). Consequently, little weight has been given to the rabbit data in this book. Several alternative in vitro methods have been developed for identifying skin irritants, some of which use reconstituted human skin models (Botham 2004a).

Box 5.1	
Skin irritant constituents	
High risk	**Moderate risk**
Allyl isothiocyanate	Benzoic acid
Benzyl isothiocyanate	Carvacrol
Masssoia lactone	p-Cresol
	Thymol

Table 5.4 Grading of skin irritancy for essential oils and absolutes

Substance	Maximum for skin[a]
High risk: dermal maximum of 0–0.1%	
Horseradish oil	No safe level
Mustard oil	No safe level
Massoia oil[b]	0.01%
Moderate risk: dermal maximum of 0.2–1.0%	
Immortelle absolute	0.5%
Sage oil (wild mountain)[b]	0.7%
Garlic oil	No set limit
Low risk: dermal maximum of 1.1–20%	
Oregano oil[c]	1.1%
Marjoram oil wild (carvacrol CT)[c]	1.2%
Oregano oil (Mexican)[c]	1.2%
Savory oil (winter)[c]	1.2%
Thyme oil (carvacrol / thymol CT)[c]	1.3%
Ajowan oil[c]	1.4%
Savory oil (summer)[c]	1.4%
Thyme oil (spike)[c]	1.4%
Thyme oil (limonene CT)[c]	2.1%
Thyme oil (borneol CT)[c]	3.3%
Fir needle oil (Siberian)	No set limit
Pine oil (dwarf)	No set limit

Note: Fig leaf absolute and parsleyseed oil are irritants, but are restricted for other types of toxicity.
[a]See Adjusting safe doses and concentrations (see Ch.13, p. 189)
[b]For massoia lactone content
[c]For thymol and/or carvacrol content

Sensitization

The most common skin reaction to fragrance materials is sensitization, or ACD, which shows on light-colored skin as a bright red rash, and on darker colored skin as a darker area. This is the visible sign of tissue damage caused by substances such as histamine released in the dermis due to an immune response. There are four classes of allergic reaction that can manifest on the skin, although only types I and IV can be induced by essential oils or other fragrant materials:

Type I: immediate hypersensitivity
Type II: cytotoxic hypersensitivity
Type III: immune complex hypersensitivity
Type IV: delayed hypersensitivity.

Temesvári et al (2002) found that, of 294 positive patch tests with fragrance materials, 90.2% were type IV, 6.1% were type I, and 3.7% involved both types of reaction. In addition to types I and IV, there is a complication related to ACD, known as PCD (see below).

Immediate hypersensitivity

Immediate hypersensitivity (type I) is also known as immediate contact urticaria or contact urticaria syndrome, and the reaction occurs very rapidly. Common causes include insect bites and ingested peanuts. It is mediated by IgE antibodies, which bind to the surface of mast cells. Within minutes of skin contact by an antigen, the mast cells release histamine and other factors, causing an inflammatory reaction. Both immunologic and non-immunologic type I reactions were proposed by Maibach & Johnson (1975). According to De Groot & Frosch (1998), cases of immediate contact urticaria to fragrance materials are most commonly non-allergic, even though caused by the liberation of histamine. However, the non-allergic mechanism is not completely understood, and may involve other factors such as prostaglandins. Cinnamaldehyde, and other essential oil constituents, can cause urticarial reactions (Safford et al 1990).

Anaphylaxis is an extreme form of immediate hypersensitivity. It is a life-threatening reaction involving massive histamine release, which can lead to breathing difficulties and low blood pressure. The only recorded instance of anaphylaxis due to skin contact from an essential oil or constituent was to cinnamaldehyde, when a woman was being tested with constituents of the fragrance mix (see Box 5.3) (Diba & Statham 2003). There is also one recorded case of anaphylactic shock from fragrance inhalation (see Ch. 6, p. 106).

Delayed hypersensitivity

In type IV reactions, little or no effect is evident on first exposure (induction, or sensitization) to a substance. On subsequent exposure to the same material (elicitation, or challenge phase), an inflammatory reaction occurs, just as rapidly as in a type I reaction. Induction takes 10–15 days to become established, and may precede elicitation by several years. The severity of the elicitation response can seem out of proportion to the concentration of substance present, and in rare cases very unpleasant reactions are evoked by minute quantities. Hives may occur, in which wheals are formed on the skin. These normally last 15–30 minutes.

The offending allergen may be a drug, a household or industrial chemical, a cosmetic ingredient, a plant, or an essential oil constituent. In addition to fragrances, common causes of ACD include nickel, formaldehyde, cosmetic preservatives, clothing dyes and, in North America, poison ivy. An atypical type IV reaction that only manifests in the presence of UV light is known as photoallergy, and this is discussed in the section on Photosensitivity below.

The mechanisms involved in type IV hypersensitivity are quite well understood. Most allergenic chemicals are haptens: chemically reactive molecules too small to be recognized by the immune system, until they bind to skin proteins in the dermis. Cinnamaldehyde-protein adducts, for example, have been detected in human skin (Elahi et al 2004). Paraphrasing Saint-Mezard et al (2004), the two stages involve the following steps:

Induction

* haptens come into contact with the skin, and penetrate the dermal barrier
* in the epidermis, the haptens bind to peptides at the surface of Langerhans cells
* langerhans cells bearing hapten–peptide complexes migrate from the epidermis to local lymph nodes
* in the lymph nodes, CD8+ T cells are 'primed' by the Langerhans cells to recognize the haptenated peptide as an antigen
* the CD8+ T cells migrate from the lymph nodes into the bloodstream.

Elicitation

* a second skin contact with the same haptens occurs
* the haptens are taken up by skin cells that already express haptenated peptide complexes
* specific T cells are activated in the epidermis and dermis
* an inflammatory process is triggered, involving the release of cytokines, chemokines and histamine, and apoptosis of keratinocytes
* leukocytes migrate from the blood to the skin, causing skin lesions
* immune cells are recruited leading to amplification of the response.

The priming of T lymphocytes in the lymph nodes is central to this process, and sufficient quantities of both hapten and Langerhans cells must be available for the allergenic response to be fully enacted (Kimber et al 2008). Finally, CD4+ T cells 'call off' the inflammatory reaction, and the skin lesions disappear, unless there is repeated exposure to the same haptens. The mechanistic basis of ACD is illustrated in Figure 5.2, and has been reviewed by several research groups (Basketter et al 1995, Belsito 1997, Fyhrquist-Vanni et al 2007). Fragrance allergens, such as isoeugenol and cinnamaldehyde, significantly alter the expression of Langerhans cell-surface proteins, while sodium lauryl sulfate, an irritant, does not. This shows a clear distinction between sensitization and irritation (Verrier et al 1999).

Essential oil constituents may be metabolized in the dermis to reactive metabolites, from pro-haptens to haptens. For example, isoeugenol is oxidized to a highly reactive paraquinone methide in mouse skin (Bertrand et al 1997). A proportion of cinnamyl alcohol (a pro-hapten) is converted by enzymes in human skin, to cinnamaldehyde (a hapten). Interestingly, cinnamaldehyde is in turn 'detoxified' in the skin to cinnamyl alcohol and cinnamic acid, and the extent of this detoxification is dependent on the amount of available enzymes (Smith et al 2000; Cheung et al 2003). This would explain why increasing concentrations of an allergen result in increasing incidence of sensitization.[5]

We know that thresholds exist for both induction and elicitation of allergic responses, although these are not absolute

Figure 5.2 • Induction and elicitation. (Reproduced with permission from Saint-Mezard P, Rosières A, Krasteva M et al 2004 Allergic contact dermatitis. European Journal of Dermatology 14:284-295.)

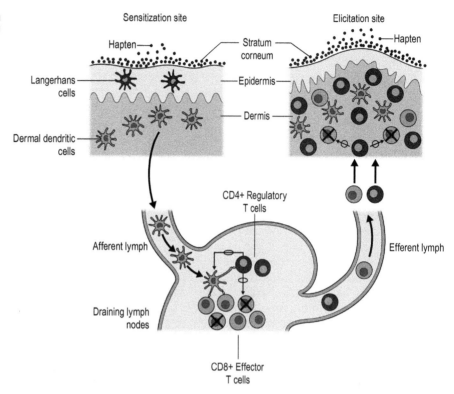

values (Kimber et al 1999; Andersen et al 2001). Variation between individuals at the induction stage may be due to differences in susceptibility to acquired sensitization (Kimber et al 2008). Thresholds in skin contact sensitization are both quantitative, for example, in the degree of protein haptenation, and qualitative, in terms of the type of immune response that is engaged. The existence of thresholds is evidenced by the observation that only a proportion of those exposed to a substance become sensitized and, of this group, only a proportion develop ACD (Kimber et al 1999).

In cross-sensitization, an individual reacts to a substance that is chemically and structurally similar to the one that caused the original sensitization (Basketter et al 1995).

Allergic contact dermatitis

Allergic contact dermatitis is the usual clinical consequence of delayed hypersensitivity. In addition to being elicited through direct skin contact, ACD may be elicited through airborne contact or ingestion. Airborne contact dermatitis has been reviewed by Dooms-Goossens & Deleu (1991), De Groot (1996) and Schaller & Korting (1995). It is more frequently caused by fine particles than by volatile molecules, but in any case is very rare: less than 0.2% of dermatitis patients (Komericki et al 2004). Although individuals who react to dermal testing do not always react when the same substance is given orally, foods such as citrus fruits and spices can play a role in 'systemic' contact dermatitis (Forsbeck & Skog 1977; Salam & Fowler 2001).

Skin reactions are generally limited to the area of skin to which the allergen is applied, but more widespread reactions occasionally occur (Bruynzeel et al 1984; Seidenari et al 1990a; Dharmagunawardena et al 2002). An individual with skin contact allergy to a fragrance material may have more frequent and more severe eye and airway symptoms to the same airborne substance (Elberling et al 2004).

Pigmented contact dermatitis

The term 'PCD' was coined by a Danish dermatologist, who described an epidemic of melanosis in Copenhagen (Osmundsen 1970). Although the cause was eventually found to be a whitener in a laundry detergent, PCD can also be precipitated by rubber products, azo dyes, cosmetics and fragrances. A distinguishing characteristic of PCD is a triggering of skin hyperpigmentation without the stimulus of UV light. Unlike photosensitivity, it occurs only in a very small percentage of individuals. Reactions are non-eczematous, are usually on the face, are more commonly seen in women than men, and are generally limited to darker-skinned individuals. It is thought that, in these cases, melanin passes into the upper dermis when the dermoepidermal junction is severely disturbed by inflammatory processes in the skin (Trattner et al 1999).

In a report from Spain, a 27-year-old Caucasian female developed dark brown hyperpigmentation on her face. Patch tests were positive for geraniol and lemon oil, and were not UV-dependent (Serrano et al 1989). In a review of 29 cases of PCD in Israel, four had positive and relevant reactions to the fragrance mix (Trattner et al 1999). In tests using guinea pigs with moderately colored skin, 100% jasmine 'oil' and 20% ylang-ylang oil caused hyperpigmentation that followed contact allergy, while 100% benzyl salicylate was a much less potent inducer of PCD. It was noted that it could take up to 30 days to reach a plateau of pigmentation, in comparison with about seven days for UVB irradiation. As part of the test procedure, the animals were injected with Freund's complete adjuvant, an inflammatory substance. This test was said to resemble the hyperpigmentation often seen in Asian skin (Imokawa & Kawai 1987).

In Japan, in the 1960s and 1970s, there were reports of women developing areas of brown hyperpigmentation, invariably on the face. It was determined through systematic patch testing that the major causative agents were coal tar dyes and fragrances. Materials frequently implicated included jasmine absolute, the essential oils of ylang-ylang, cananga, geranium, patchouli and sandalwood, and the constituents benzyl alcohol, benzyl salicylate, geraniol and β-santalol. Major Japanese cosmetic companies stopped using various sensitizers in their products in 1977, and since 1978 the incidence of this condition is said to have decreased significantly.

The term 'pigmented *cosmetic* dermatitis' was coined by Nakayama et al (1984) to describe the cases seen in Japan. Biopsies suggested that the hyperpigmentation was due to melanin being released from cells in the basal layer of the epidermis when they were attacked by lymphocytes (Nakayama 1998). According to De Groot & Frosch (1998), the condition is virtually unknown in Western countries and is limited to central and eastern Asian races. However, pigmented cosmetic dermatitis is now seen either as a variant of PCD or as the same condition (Trattner et al 1999; Shenoi & Rao 2007).

Subsequent patch testing in Japan does not support the view that Japanese people are any more susceptible than Caucasians to ACD from the essential oils and constituents listed above, with the possible exception of sandalwood oil and benzyl salicylate (Itoh 1982; Sugai 1994; Sugiura et al 2000). However, there is an increased susceptibility to PCD, which is no doubt genetic. Hyperpigmentation is the most common cosmetic skin complaint in people of Asian ethnicity, who have a greater predisposition to congenital and acquired pigmentary skin disorders than other racial groups (Kurita et al 2009, Yu et al 2007).

Identifying allergens

Very widespread consumer exposure to an allergen can lead to a contact allergy epidemic, as has occurred with preservatives such as formaldehyde and methyldibromo glutaronitrile (Thyssen et al 2007). Such epidemics are controlled by restricting the amount of allergen permitted in consumer products, though such measures are often not taken until allergies have become widespread. Most regulatory agencies are now alert to the need to identify potential epidemics before they occur. Patch testing is of course the mainstay of identifying causative substances.

In the 1970s cinnamaldehyde was implicated as among the most serious potential allergens, and so too were lactones, such as those found in costus and elecampane oils. More recently attention has been focused on isoeugenol and oakmoss absolute, and the number of reactions to cinnamaldehyde has declined (Nguyen et al 2008). Temesvári et al (2002) report 14.8% of

dermatitis patients testing positive to isoeugenol, 13.1% to oakmoss absolute and 20.6% to cinnamyl alcohol.

Table 5.5 is a guide to the risk of skin sensitization, and is based on essential oil and/or constituent data. IFRA guidelines are given, as are our recommendations. Garlic oil is rarely used on the skin, and there are few clinical data, but sensitization is most commonly linked to diallyl disulfide, including one case of systemic contact dermatitis (Delaney & Donnelly 1996; Fernandez-Vozmediano et al 2000; Pereira et al 2002). The essential oils that only develop an allergic potential after oxidation has set in are listed in Box 5.2.

Skin sensitivity reactions are idiosyncratic, and identification of the causative allergen(s) and their subsequent withdrawal generally leads to a resolution of the problem.

The fragrance mix

A standard mixture of eight components in a base of petrolatum, known as the fragrance mix (FM), has been routinely used to screen for ACD in susceptible individuals since the late 1970s (Box 5.3). The components were originally used at 2% w/w each (totaling 16%) but, since this proved too irritating, the concentration was reduced to 1% each (Larsen 1977; Wilkinson JD et al 1989). Two FM ingredients, α-amyl cinnamic aldehyde (incorrectly reported as α-amyl cinnamic alcohol in some papers) and hydroxycitronellal are not found in essential oils. The emulsifier sorbitan sesquioleate is also present in the FM, at 5%. Since many fragrance-sensitive individuals react to Peru balsam (the raw material, not the essential oil), this is frequently tested in addition to the FM.

The average percentage of dermatitis patients reacting to the FM from ten sets of figures was 9.56%, with a low of 4.1% and a high of 15.0%.[6] De Groot & Frosch (1998) estimated a range of 6–11%, and a multicenter study gave a figure of 10.5% for Central Europe (Schnuch et al 1997). White races are more susceptible than Asians to the FM, and to isoeugenol and oakmoss. Benzyl salicylate allergy is more common in Asia than in Europe or the USA (Larsen et al 1996a).

The percentage of the general population reacting to the FM is naturally lower than the 10% or so of dermatitis patients. FM allergy prevalence rates of 0.5%, 1.1%, 1.8%, 1.8% and 1.8% (mean 1.4%) have been found in five European studies that collectively patch tested 81,609 people (Seidenari et al 1990b; Nielsen & Menné 1992; Mortz et al 2002; Schnuch et al 2002a; Dotterud & Smith-Sivertsen 2007). This suggests that there is a sevenfold difference in the relative risk of fragrance allergy between dermatitis patients and the general population ($10 \div 1.4 = 7.14$). However, extrapolating FM data to the real-world risk presented by actual fragrances or essential oil use, is more complex than this, and can only ever be a rough approximation (see Interpreting patch test data above).

It is estimated that the FM identifies only 60–80% of people with fragrance allergy (Larsen et al 1998; Trattner & David 2003). An improvement has been reported by including additional substances in the mixture such as benzyl salicylate and benzyl alcohol (Larsen et al 1998). Citral has also been cited as one of the most common non-FM allergens (Frosch et al 2002a; Heydorn et al 2003b). Of the essential oils and absolutes tested, ylang-ylang oil has provided a relatively high percentage

Table 5.5 Grading of skin sensitization

Substance	Maximum for skin[b]	Reference
High risk: (dermal maximum of 0–0.1%)		
Elecampane oil	No safe level	IFRA
Fig leaf absolute	No safe level	IFRA
Costus oil	No safe level	IFRA
Massoia oil	0.01%	Tisserand & Young (no safe level IFRA)
Saffron oil/absolute	0.02%	IFRA (for safranal content)
Lavandin absolute	0.03%	Tisserand & Young
Cassia oil	0.05%	IFRA (for cinnamaldehyde content)
Cinnamon bark oil	0.07%	IFRA (for cinnamaldehyde content)
Oakmoss absolute	0.1%	IFRA
Treemoss absolute	0.1%	IFRA
Lavender absolute	0.1%	Tisserand & Young
Moderate risk: (dermal maximum of 0.2–1.0%)		
Tea leaf absolute	0.2%	IFRA
Verbena absolute (lemon)	0.2%	IFRA
Clary sage absolute	0.25%	Tisserand & Young
Ginger lily absolute	0.3%	Tisserand & Young
Peru balsam oil	0.4%	IFRA
Clove bud oil	0.5%	IFRA (for eugenol content[a])
Cinnamon leaf oil	0.6%	IFRA (for eugenol content[a])
Clove leaf oil	0.6%	IFRA (for eugenol content[a])
Clove stem oil	0.6%	IFRA (for eugenol content[a])
Opopanax oil	0.6%	IFRA
Styrax oil	0.6%	IFRA
Tejpat	0.6%	IFRA (for eugenol content[a])
Jasmine absolute	0.7%	IFRA
Myrtle oil (lemon)	0.7%	IFRA (for citral content[a])
Lemongrass oils	0.7%	IFRA (for citral content[a])
Sage oil (wild mountain)	0.7%	Tisserand & Young (for massoia lactone)
Basil oil (pungent)	0.8%	IFRA (for eugenol content[a])
May chang oil	0.8%	IFRA (for citral content[a])
Narcissus absolute	0.8%	Tisserand & Young
Tea tree oil (lemon-scented)	0.8%	IFRA (for citral content[a])
Ylang-ylang oil/absolute	0.8%	IFRA[a]
Cananga oil	0.8%	IFRA[a]

Continued

Table 5.5 Grading of skin sensitization—Cont'd

Substance	Maximum for skin	Reference
Bay (WI)	0.9%	IFRA (for eugenol content[a])
Lemon leaf oil	0.9%	IFRA (for citral content[a])
Melissa oil	0.9%	Tisserand & Young (for citral, IFRA 0.63%)
Myrtle oil (honey)	0.9%	IFRA (for citral content[a])
Verbena oil (lemon)	0.9%	Tisserand & Young (for citral, no safe level IFRA)
Basil oil (holy)	1.0%	IFRA (for eugenol content[a])
Ginger lily absolute	1.0%	Tisserand & Young (for isoeugenol content)
Low risk: dermal maximum of 1.1–20%		
Lemon leaf oil	1.1%	IFRA (for citral content[a])
Basil oil (lemon)	1.4%	IFRA (for citral content[a])
Basil absolute (linalool CT)	1.5%	IFRA (for eugenol content[a])
Spearmint oil	1.7%	IFRA (for carvone content[a])
Sandalwood oil (East Indian)	2.0%	Tisserand & Young
Benzoin resinoid	2.0%	Tisserand & Young
Tolu balsam resinoid	2.0%	Tisserand & Young
Balsamite oil	2.3%	IFRA (for carvone content[a])
Bakul absolute	2.9%	IFRA (for cinnamyl alcohol content[a])
Basil oil (linalool CT)	3.3%	IFRA (for eugenol content[a])
Lemon balm oil (Australian)	3.4%	IFRA (for citral content[a])
Thyme oil (lemon)	3.7%	IFRA (for citral content[a])
Jasmine absolute sambac	4.0%	IFRA
Bergamot (wild)	5.7%	IFRA (for geraniol content[a])
Jamrosa oil	6.2%	IFRA (for geraniol content[a])
Palmarosa oil	6.5%	IFRA (for geraniol content[a])
Tea tree oil	15.0%	Tisserand & Young
Geranium oil	17.5%	IFRA (for geraniol content[a])
Citronella oil	18.2%	IFRA (for geraniol content[a])
Catnip oil	No set level	Tisserand & Young
Perilla oil	No set level	Tisserand & Young

[a]Based on IFRA category 4: body oils, lotions. Asafoetida oil, black seed oil, garlic oil and onion oil might fall into this category also
[b]See Adjusting safe doses and concentrations (see Ch.13, p. 189)
IFRA, International Fragrance Association 2009

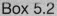

Box 5.2

Essential oils with possible increased risk of sensitization if oxidized

Angelica oils	Larch
Anise	Lemon balm (Australian)
Caraway	Lemon leaf
Celery oils	Longoza
Cistus	Mastic
Citrus fruit oils	Myrtle (aniseed)
Curry leaf	Pepper (black)
Cypress	Pepper (Sichuan)
Dill oils	Pepper (white)
Elemi	Pine oils
Fennel oils	Pteronia
Ferula	Ramy bark
Fir oils	Sage (blue mountain)
Fleabane	Spruce oils
Frankincense oils (most)	Star anise
Galbanum	Sumach (Venetian)
Gingergrass	Tana
Grindelia	Tea tree
Hemp	Tick bush
Juniper oils	Turpentine
Kanuka	Verbena (white)

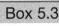

Box 5.3

Composition of the fragrance mix

1% Cinnamyl alcohol
1% Cinnamaldehyde
1% α-Amyl cinnamic aldehyde
1% Hydroxycitronellal
1% Eugenol
1% Isoeugenol
1% Geraniol
1% Oakmoss absolute
5% Sorbitan sesquioleate (an emulsifier)
87% Petrolatum

of responses, as has lemongrass. Table 5.6 compares reactions to the FM and to several essential oils. New fragrance materials not found in essential oils are also being identified as allergens. Hydroxyisohexyl 3-cyclohexene carboxaldehyde, a widely used aromachemical also known as Lyral, causes allergic reactions in 2–3% of dermatitis patients tested (Johansen et al 2003b), and it is now included in the patch test 'standard series' in Germany (Geier et al 2002). α-Hexylcinnamic aldehyde has also been cited as a potential allergen (Larsen et al 1998).

However, whether such testing truly identifies people with fragrance allergy is open to question. False-positive reactions to the FM are frequently cited, and the combination of its components may lead to a synergistic action (Santucci et al 1987). Johansen et al (1998a) found that a combination of two fragrance allergens in individuals allergic to both substances had a synergistic effect; the 1:1 mixtures elicited responses as if the doses were three to four times higher than those actually used. In four separate European studies, the probability that a patient with a positive reaction to the FM will have a reaction to any of its individual components was 50–56%, suggesting that one of every two FM reactions is a false positive (Frosch et al 1995b; Naldi 2002; Schnuch et al 2002b; Heydorn 2003b).

The emulsifier sorbitan sesquioleate (SSO), which is used at 5% in the FM, is itself an allergen (Tosti et al 1990) and it can increase reactions to the FM by 13.2%. In one small study, the addition of SSO increased allergic reactions to individual constituents by these amounts: eugenol 20%, isoeugenol 35%, oakmoss 39%, geraniol 66%, cinnamaldehyde 500% (Frosch et al 1995b). Orton & Shaw (2001) reported 12 clinically relevant cases of SSO allergy, which had caused false-positive FM results. Enders et al (1991) considered that SSO was not allergenic, but that it could cause false-positive results when mixed with the FM.

There have been reports of allergies to the FM increasing over the years 1979–1992 (Johansen & Menné 1995), 1992–1996 (Marks et al 1998) and 1985–1998 (Johansen et al 2000). These and other results suggest increasing reactions to fragrance materials (Becker et al 1994; Katsarou et al 1999). However, subsequent data point to a reversal of this trend. In a multicenter project (1996–2002), reactions to the FM increased from 10.2% in 1996 to 13.1% in 1999, and then showed a steady decline to 7.8% in 2002 (Schnuch et al 2004a). This may be due to a reduction of consumer exposure to FM ingredients in fragranced products in recent years.

Individual FM constituents have their own trends. Allergic reactions to cinnamaldehyde are decreasing over time, possibly because it is being used less in personal care products (Johansen & Menné 1995; Marks et al 1995, 1998; Buckley et al 2000; Nguyen et al 2008). Reactions to oakmoss absolute are high and have shown no signs of decreasing, either from 1979–1992 or from 1996–2002 (Johansen & Menné 1995; Schnuch et al 2004a). In a retrospective analysis of 3,636 patients, the incidence of reactions to patch testing with 1% isoeugenol showed a year-on-year increase in the UK. This may be due to an increased use of compounds chemically similar to isoeugenol (White et al 2007). There was no change in the frequency of reactions to geraniol in the UK from 1980 to 1996, in spite of a general upward trend for the period (Buckley et al 2000).

If we look at skin assays that address reactions to actual fragrances on the general population, the data show very much lower responses. From a total of 11,632 patch tests (on 10,400 subjects) with consumer products containing either eugenol as such, or clove leaf oil, there was only one instance of induced hypersensitivity at 0.05% eugenol, and one of pre-existing sensitization at 0.09% (Rothenstein et al 1983). Similarly, data from a total of 16,530 patch tests indicates that, as present in consumer products and fragrance blends, cinnamyl alcohol has no detectable potential to induce hypersensitivity (Steltenkamp et al 1980b), nor does citral, after 12,758 patch tests were conducted with products containing it (Steltenkamp et al 1980a). Cinnamaldehyde, when tested alone at concentrations up to 0.008%, or in consumer products at up to 0.6%, elicited no pre-existing hypersensitivity reactions in any of the 4,117 patch tests that constituted the survey (Danneman et al 1983).

Table 5.6 Comparison of fragrance mix allergy to some essential oils

Fragrance material	Concentration used in testing	Percentage of patients showing an allergic response		
		Lowest[a]	Highest[a]	Average[a]
Fragrance mix	8%	9.3%	17.9%	11.4%
Ylang-ylang I oil	2%	1.6%	6.2%	2.6%
Ylang-ylang II oil	2%	1.3%	6.2%	2.5%
Lemongrass oil	2%	0.3%	2.9%	1.6%
Narcissus absolute	2%	0.7%	3.4%	1.3%
Jasmine absolute	5%	0%	2.7%	1.2%
Sandalwood oil	10%	0.5%	2.1%	0.9%
Patchouli oil	10%	0.3%	1.3%	0.8%
Spearmint oil	2%	0%	1.9%	0.8%
Dwarf pine needle oil	2%	0.3%	1.9%	0.7%
Cedarwood oil[b]	10%	n/g	n/g	0.6%
Peppermint oil	2%	n/g	n/g	0.6%

Results of patch testing in 1,606 consecutive dermatitis patients in six European centers (Frosch et al 2002b)

n/g, not given

[a]The lowest and highest figures from the different centers are shown, in addition to the average positive response

[b]Type of oil unspecified

In a Swedish study over 4.5 years (January 1994 through to June 1998) there was no significant difference in either frequency of complaints about products with and without fragrance, or in a paired comparison of 17 products marketed both with and without fragrance. The fragranced leave-on products contained up to 770 ppm, and the fragranced wash-off products up to 84 ppm of between 0 and 7 of the FM ingredients (Barany & Loden 2000). While this finding might not be very meaningful in many countries, in Sweden it is significant, as there is a simple and much-used system for such complaints. This suggests that a level of 0.07% would be safe for FM ingredients in leave-on products.

Enders et al (1989) found that only 69 of 142 (42.6%) patients who tested positive to the 8% FM in 1982/83, still tested positive to it in 1987. In 18 patients with previously positive patch tests, only 20 out of 26 tests (77%) were still positive on repeat testing (Soni & Sherertz 1997). This raises the possibility of eventual habituation to allergens in some people. It seems unlikely that the large difference seen by Enders et al could be totally explained by false positives in the earlier tests that did not show up on later testing.

Aromatherapy and allergic contact dermatitis

Essential oils and aromatherapy have been reported as causing ACD. For example, a 39-year-old woman who had used aromatherapy products for two to three years, developed an erythematous eruption on her face and chest that rapidly resolved when she stopped using the products (Weiss & James 1997). Dermatitis in a 53-year-old was caused by sensitization to airborne vapors of lavender, jasmine and rosewood (Schaller & Korting 1995).

Commercial aromatherapy products may be more likely to cause ACD than a visit to an aromatherapist, since fragrance allergy is particularly associated with deodorant use, and with the irritant potential of the surfactants used in foaming products (Johansen et al 1998b). Many cosmetic preservatives are also well-known potential allergens. Reactions to a lotion containing 5% tea tree oil were reduced when the lotion base was reformulated (Veien et al 2004). Products are often used on more sensitive areas of skin, such as the face and axillae, and are generally used with more frequency, than are essential oils in aromatherapy practice. However, essential oils may be used at higher concentrations in aromatherapy practice, and practitioners may be less able than manufacturers to control the problems associated with essential oil oxidation.

If 1.8% of the general population is FM sensitive, and if the FM represents 70% of all fragrance allergies, then 2.57% of the population will be sensitive to fragrance. However, for all the reasons outlined above, this does not represent actual risk from fragrance use. Allowing for the 50% of false positives in FM testing reduces this to 1.3%, and even this is an arbitrary number that does not represent real-world risk, merely reactivity to patch testing. In addition, 'fragrance' includes many synthetic materials not found in essential oils. In a group of 102 Peru balsam-sensitive individuals, twice as many reacted to fragrance constituents as did to essential oils such as ylang-ylang and lemongrass (Hausen 2001). This suggests a higher risk of allergy from synthetic fragrance than from essential oils.

Ylang-ylang, lemongrass and tea tree, three of the most allergenic of the commonly used essential oils, may be used as case examples. Ylang-ylang oil at 2% elicited positive reactions in 2.0%, 2.5% and 2.6% of dermatitis patients (Rudzki et al 1976; Frosch et al 2002b). Lemongrass oil, tested at 2%, elicited allergic responses in 1.6% (25 of 1,606) of dermatitis patients (Frosch et al 2002b). In a multicenter study in Germany and Austria, 5% tea tree oil tested positive in 1.1% (36 of 3,375) of dermatitis patients (Pirker et al 2003). A differential of 7 can be used to extrapolate to the general population (explained in the previous section), plus a factor of 11 to allow for dermal loading and the intensive conditions of patch testing. Therefore the real risk of an allergic reaction from using these essential oils at 2–5% could be estimated as 0.01–0.03% of the general population.

Most other essential oils commonly used in aromatherapy will pose a lower level of risk than this, and most aromatherapy preparations will contain lower concentrations of these particular essential oils than those used in these tests. Therefore the skin allergy risk from aromatherapy in general, if such a risk can be quantified, may be less than 0.01% (1 in 10,000) of the general population, about 100 times less than the number who show as FM sensitive on patch testing.

The clinical use of essential oils in the treatment of, for example, wounds, burns or leg ulcers is a different scenario to personal care products or massage oils. Higher concentrations of essential oil may be required, yet benefit may outweigh risk. Patch testing prior to essential oil use may be useful.

Occupational risk

It is well known that certain occupations, such as nursing and hairdressing, entail an increased risk of irritant or allergic hand dermatitis. We identified 11 reports of occupational ACD in aromatherapists.

On developing dermatitis, some aromatherapists test positive to multiple essential oils. Some of these might be due to ESS or to sensitivity to a constituent found in all of the oils. One aromatherapist showed marked sensitivity to benzoin and 13 essential oils, and moderate sensitivity to a further five (Selvaag et al 1995). In a further two cases, one had moderate or marked sensitivities to 20 essential oils, and the other to 15. Most of the essential oils used by these last two aromatherapists contained α-pinene, which on subsequent patch testing was positive in both cases (Dharmagunawardena et al 2002). Three aromatherapists presenting with contact dermatitis all had multiple relevant contact allergies (Taraska & Pratt 1997). In one of two cases reported by Boonchai et al (2007), there was sensitivity to 8 of 10 single or blended essential oils tested. Further reports of occupational ACD in aromatherapists include Bilsland & Strong 1990; Cockayne & Gawkrodger 1997; Sánchez-Pérez & García-Díez 1999; Keane et al 2000; Bleasel et al 2002; Maddocks-Jennings 2004; Trattner et al 2008.

The risk of skin sensitization to an aromatherapist using essential oils in massage is almost certainly higher than to recipients of the treatment, since the practitioner will be exposed to skin contact for many more hours per week. In addition,

repeated friction may be a factor in hand dermatitis of massage therapists. In a report of 57,779 dermatitis patients in 52 occupations, masseurs or physiotherapists had a relatively high prevalence of moderate or marked FM contact dermatitis, at 5.9% (Uter et al 2001). Regular use of hand cream has been shown to counteract the increased roughness and dryness caused by frequent hand washing (Kampf & Ennen 2006).

In a study of hand dermatitis in massage therapists, the use of "aromatherapy products in oils, creams or lotions" increased risk by 3.27 times. Atopic dermatitis was an even greater risk factor, with an odds ratio of 8.06. These data came from a survey in which 356 massage therapists (57% of those asked) in Philadelphia completed a questionnaire. Of these, 47% reported using aromatherapy oils or creams, and 39% aromatherapy candles or burners. The 12-month prevalence of hand dermatitis in the respondents was 15% by self-reported criteria, and 23% by a symptom-based method. Another factor was frequent hand washing; the use of detergents is known to exacerbate fragrance-related ACD (Crawford et al 2004).

The results of this survey may have been biased by those who had experienced symptoms being more likely to take part. It should also be noted that some of the 'aromatherapy' massage oils, creams and candles referred to in this report could contain synthetic fragrances, so the survey may not be a true reflection of the risk of essential oils.

There is a probable occupational risk of ACD from essential oils, especially hand dermatitis. Ways to reduce this risk include:

* using lower concentrations of essential oils for massage
* avoidance of high-risk and moderate-risk essential oils
* avoidance of oxidized essential oils
* avoidance of detergents for hand washing
* use of hand cream after hand washing
* wearing thin plastic disposable gloves (not latex, as it can cause severe allergy)
* ensuring adequate ventilation.

Adequate ventilation is an important safety measure generally, and airborne contact with the skin could theoretically increase the risk of dermatitis. If a practitioner should develop dermatitis, consultation with a dermatologist may lead to identification of the allergen(s) responsible, which should then be avoided. Wearing plastic gloves for a period of time may be useful in this scenario. Individuals with a history of atopic dermatitis should be wary of a career involving regular skin contact with essential oils. The sensitivities to multiple essential oils in some of the reports cited above suggest the possibility of polysensitization (see Genetics and race above).

Photosensitization

Photosensitization, is a reaction to a substance applied to the skin that occurs only in the presence of UV light in the UVA range, and it may be either phototoxic or photoallergic. Phototoxicity may lead to photocarcinogenesis. However, in the absence of UV light, photoallergic and phototoxic chemicals are not damaging to DNA, and some demonstrate anticarcinogenic activity. Similar reactions may occur following ingestion of photosensitizing chemicals, though these are likely all phototoxic, and not photoallergic (White 1995).

The clinical outcome of photosensitization is known as 'photocontact dermatitis'.

Photoallergy

This is an uncommon type of skin reaction to UV light; an allergic reaction without pigmentation. (Although confusingly, photoallergy can cause a pigmentation reaction similar to phototoxicity.) It is an acquired reactivity dependent either on an immediate antibody reaction or a delayed cell-mediated one (Epstein JH 1999). Photoallergens have been shown to bind to proteins in the skin under the influence of UV light (Pendlington & Barratt 1990). The most common photoallergens are chemicals used as sunscreens. Three fragrance materials not found in essential oils, musk ambrette, 6-methylcoumarin and 7-methoxycoumarin, are photoallergens, and are banned by IFRA for fragrance use.

Some consider that there are no photoallergic essential oils (Kaidbey & Kligman 1981; Scheinman 1996). However, a case of photoallergy to sandalwood oil was reported by Starke (1967) and there is one report of photoallergy to lavender oil concerning a 45-year-old female in Spain (Goiriz et al 2007). Two instances of photoallergy to diallyl disulfide have been reported, so garlic oil must also be considered a potential cause (Alvarez et al 2003; Scheman & Gupta 2001).

The test for photoallergy is known as the photopatch test. Twin patches of test substance are applied, one of which is exposed to UV light, and photoallergy is diagnosed if there is a reaction only in that patch. UVA is normally used, though UVB may also be used. Positive reactions to sandalwood oil were seen in 3 of 138 patients (2.2%) who were photopatch tested in the USA by Fotiades et al (1995), and 2 of 1,050 probable photodermatitis patients (0.19%) in Italy (Pigatto et al 1996). In Japan, there were no reactions in a total of 838 dermatology patients tested with 2% santalol, nor in 106 tested with 5%, nor in 327 tested with 10% (Bhatia et al 2008b).

Other substances that have been used for photopatch testing include the FM, eugenol, alantolactone, Peru balsam and oakmoss absolute (Gould et al 1995). In 1,050 patients with probable dermatitis, bergamot oil and alantolactone each elicited responses in two individuals, and the FM elicited 23 (Pigatto et al 1996). Both eugenol and costus root oil have produced photoallergic reactions in dermatitis patients, and oakmoss absolute and cinnamaldehyde can be photoallergic in patients with sunlight sensitivity (Addo et al 1982). However, it should be remembered that this is a very rare type of reaction. When the FM was photopatch tested on 111 people with suspected photocontact dermatitis, there were no positive reactions (Katsarou et al 1999).

Phototoxicity

Like many flat, polycyclic molecules, furanocoumarins (FCs) form complexes with DNA by intercalating between adjacent base pairs. On irradiation with UVA light, these complexes become activated and form covalent bonds first with one, and then a second adjacent pyrimidine base, resulting in cross-linking. This leads to the generation of inflammatory mediators causing a subsequent erythema response which can manifest as inflamed and painful skin as in sunburn, and in severe cases, extreme blistering. These clinical effects are delayed, peaking 36–72 hours after UVA exposure. A post-inflammatory hyperpigmentation follows the acute reaction, and may last for weeks or months (Gould et al 1995). Higher concentrations of FCs, and/or longer exposure to UV light, increase the severity of the reaction.

FCs are found primarily in citrus fruit oils, and in relatively small amounts, generally less than 3%. However, even if an essential oil is diluted to 1%, so that 0.03% or less of FCs are present, phototoxic effects may still occur. Extensive burns can also result from oral ingestion of FCs in combination with UV exposure (Nettelblad et al 1996). Some of the FCs found in essential oils are listed in Table 5.7. FC molecules are composed of a furan ring attached to a bicyclic coumarin structure. When the furan ring is attached to the coumarin 6,7-bond, it forms a linear FC, or psoralen (Figure 5.3). When the furan ring is attached to the coumarin 7,8-bond, it forms what is known as an angular FC, or an angelicin (Figure 5.3). Psoralen and angelicin are also the names of single compounds.

FCs demonstrate different degrees of phototoxicity (Table 5.7), in fact four (bergamottin, bergaptol, isobergapten and isopimpinellin) are non-phototoxic (Kavli et al 1983; Ivie & Beier 1996; Bode et al 2005; Messer et al 2012). Psoralen is the most potent, followed by methoxsalen, then bergapten, then oxypeucedanin (Joshi & Pathak 1983; Naganuma et al 1985; Bode & Hansel 2005). The risk of phototoxicity depends on the type and amount of phototoxic substance present. Box 5.4 shows the concentration at which each phototoxic essential oil is considered safe to use on the skin, based on IFRA guidelines. Any higher percentage is considered to entail risk.

The FCs are relatively non-volatile molecules and are generally found in expressed (cold-pressed) citrus fruit oils, but not in distilled citrus fruit oils. It is possible to remove (or, more correctly, considerably reduce) the bergapten in bergamot oil. The resulting oil is known as 'bergaptenless' bergamot, or bergamot FCF (furanocoumarin-free). This oil is regarded as having an inferior fragrance to the oil in its natural state (Dubertret et al 1990a). At the time of writing, other FC-free citrus oils are becoming available. FCs are removed by fractional distillation.

Clinical data

About a century ago it was noticed that dermally applied bergamot oil could produce reddening of the surrounding skin after exposure to an ultraviolet lamp, with subsequent blistering 24–72 hours later, followed by abnormally dark pigmentation (Kavli & Volden 1984). The patches of darkened skin can remain for many years. The condition was first described in 1916 and has been called berloque dermatitis, bergapten dermatitis and phytophotodermatitis (Young et al 1990).

Studies in the 1950s and 1960s revealed that a reaction took place between FCs and the skin, in the presence of UV light (Musajo et al 1953, 1954, 1966; Pathak & Fitzpatrick 1959). In 1970, problems with a tanning lotion containing bergamot oil were reported in France (Meyer 1970). In 1972, Urbach

Table 5.7 Light-related risks of some furanocoumarins and lactones

Constituent	Degree of phototoxicity	Photomutagenic	Photocarcinogenic	Type[a]
Psoralen	Strong	Yes	Yes	LF
Methoxsalen	Strong	Yes	Yes	LF
Bergapten	Strong	Yes	Yes	LF
Angelicin (isopsoralen)	Moderate	Yes	Weak	AF
Imperatorin	Moderate	Yes	Not known	LF
Citropten	Moderate	Yes	Not known	Lac
Oxypeucedanin	Moderate	Not known	Not known	LF
Isoimperatorin	Weak	Not known	Not known	LF
Bergamottin	Negligible	Negligible	Not known	LF
Isobergapten	Negligible	Not known	Not known	AF
Isopimpinellin	Zero	No	Unlikely	LF
Bergaptol	Zero	No	Unlikely	LF
7-Methoxy-5-geranoxycoumarin	Not known	Not known	Not known	Lac

These are listed in approximate descending order of phototoxic potency
[a]LF, linear furanocoumarin (psoralen); AF, angular furanocoumarin (angelicin); Lac, lactone

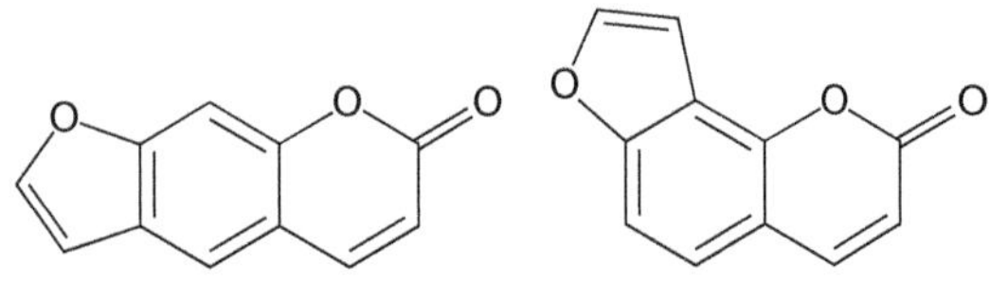

psoralen   angelicin

Figure 5.3

& Forbes found that severe phototoxic effects were experienced when humans were treated with expressed bergamot oil and simulated sunlight (unpublished report, cited in Opdyke 1973 p. 1031–1033). Other studies have confirmed the phototoxicity of dermally applied bergamot oil in humans (Zaynoun et al 1977a, 1977b) and in hairless mice (Gloxhuber 1970).

There are few detailed cases. A woman was treated for minor burns after a 20-minute session on a sunbed, taken immediately after a sauna with lemon oil. A few drops of the oil had been placed in a pot in the sauna room, and the burns were to one arm and leg (Anon 1992a). In a second, more serious case, a female adult sustained severe, full-thickness burns following a 20-minute sunbed session, which was taken 15 minutes after the self-application of undiluted bergamot oil. Blistered burns slowly developed during the following 48 hours, at which time she was admitted to hospital where she remained for seven days (name withheld, private communication, 1993).

There are similar reports of distressing skin lesions and burns that occur after applying bergamot oil to the skin and exposing it to UV light (Nettelblad et al 1996; Clark & Wilkinson 1998; Cocks & Wilson 1998; Kaddu et al 2001). We could find no reports of lime oil phototoxicity, but 11 cases due to skin

Box 5.4

IFRA recommended maximum use levels to avoid phototoxic reactions

High risk: maximum dermal use level

Fig leaf absolute: none
Verbena oil: none[a]

These should not be used on the skin, or in products intended for retail at any concentration

Low to moderate risk: maximum dermal use level[c]

Taget oil: 0.01%
Taget absolute: 0.01%
Rue oil: 0.15%
Mandarin leaf oil: 0.17%
Bergamot oil: 0.4%
Cumin oil: 0.4%
Lime oil (expressed): 0.7%
Angelica root oil: 0.8%
Orange oil (bitter, expressed): 1.25%
Lemon oil (expressed): 2.0%
Laurel leaf absolute[b]: 2.0%
Grapefruit oil (expressed): 4.0%

Treated skin should not be exposed to sunlight or UV lamps for 12–18 hours, if used at levels higher than those indicated. Consumer products should not contain these essential oils at levels higher than those indicated.[ab]

[a]We do not agree with this restriction. See Verbena (lemon) oil profile
[b]From Bouhlal et al (1988b)
[c]See Adjusting safe doses and concentrations (see Ch. 13, p. 189).

contact with fresh limes were reported in 1941, and up to 2001 there have been ten further reports (Sams 1941; Wagner et al 2002a). Skin contact with fresh lemons can cause the same reaction (Khokhar et al 2004). The rind of fresh Persian limes and Mexican limes was found to contain 128.7 μg/g and 20.9 μg/g of bergapten, respectively, in addition to other FCs (Nigg et al 1993).

None of the clinical studies addresses the issue of safety thresholds.

Susceptible individuals

In a study of 63 volunteers, differences in eye color, age, sex and ability to tan did not significantly affect phototoxic responses to bergamot oil. Skin color was a significant factor, but there was no statistical difference between those with skin described as fair, sallow and light brown (Table 5.3). The average concentration of bergamot oil required to produce a phototoxic response in these individuals was 2.4%, compared to an average of 15% in those with dark brown or black skin. A suntan gave light skin some extra protection (Zaynoun et al 1977a, 1977b). Although people with darker skin have some increased tolerability to FC phototoxicity, they are as susceptible as Caucasians to skin conditions caused by sunlight (Kerr & Lim 2007).

People with oculocutaneous albinism have reduced skin pigmentation, and are at an increased risk of photosensitivity and skin cancer (Suzuki & Tomita 2008).

Phototoxic essential oils

Most phototoxic essential oils are found in the plants of two botanical families, Rutaceae and Apiaceae (Table 5.8), possibly due to evolutionary divergence. The only other families of aromatic plants associated with phototoxicity are the Asteraceae

(taget) and the Moraceae (fig). FCs can also be found in roots, including angelica, taget, celery, parsnip and carrot (Ivie et al 1982; Downum 1992; Gral et al 1993; Nivsarkar et al 1996; Bang Pedersen & Pla Arles 1998).[7] (But note that FCs are destroyed by cooking.)

Some essential oils from Apiaceae plants that might be expected to be phototoxic are not. Angelica seeds, dill leaves and parsley leaves, for instance, are all known to contain FCs (Ojala et al 1999; Müller et al 2004), but none of the equivalent essential oils is phototoxic (see Essential oil profiles, Chapter 13). Parsley leaf oil in fact typically contains 0.002% bergapten (www.ifraorg.org/view_document.aspx?docId=22594 accessed November 12th 2012), which is not sufficient to cause a phototoxic reaction. Low-level phototoxic effects have been found for caraway seed oil, but these are not considered significant (Opdyke 1973 p. 1051).

FC molecules are larger than most essential oil constituents, and in their pure form they are non-volatile solids. However, FCs can pass over during distillation, since small amounts are found in the distilled oils of angelica root, lime, mandarin leaf, parsley leaf, rue and taget (Lawrence 1989 p. 43; McHale & Sheridan 1989; IFRA 2009; SCCP 2005a), most of which are phototoxic.[8] There is evidence that rue is phototoxic, and bergapten and methoxsalen have been found both in the leaves and the corresponding steam-distilled oil (Yaacob et al 1989; Schempp et al 1999). It is likely that any FCs in plant material would carry over into absolutes and CO_2 extracts, since these processes extract heavier molecules than steam distillation. Phototoxicity has been confirmed in rue absolute (Bouhlal et al 1988b).

A number of citrus oils are not phototoxic (Box 5.5). Neither satsuma oil nor yuzu oil has been tested for phototoxicity. However, since bergapten is found in all phototoxic citrus oils at 100 to 3,000 ppm, the absence of bergapten in satsuma oil and yuzu oil down to a detection limit of 0.1 ppm is good evidence that these oils are not phototoxic. No information could be found on the phototoxicity of the citrus fruit oils from combava or clementine.

Both celery and lovage leaves contain FCs, as do parsnip seeds and roots. Khella oil is reported to contain the FCs marmesine and 8-hydroxybergapten (Franchomme & Pénöel 1990).

Table 5.8 Botanical grouping in relation to phototoxicity

Rutaceae	Apiaceae
Known to be phototoxic	
Bergamot oil	Angelica root oil
Fig leaf absolute	Cumin oil
Grapefruit oil	
Lemon oil (expressed)	
Lime oil (expressed)	
Mandarin leaf oil	
Orange oil (bitter, expressed)	
Rue oil	
Possibly phototoxic	
Clementine oil	Angelica root absolute
Combava fruit oil	Angelica root CO_2 extract
Skimmia oil	Celery leaf oil
	Celery seed absolute
	Cumin seed absolute
	Cumin seed CO_2 extract
	Khella oil
	Lovage leaf oil
	Parsnip oil

Box 5.5

Non-phototoxic citrus fruit and leaf oils

Bergamot oil (FCF)
Lemon oil (distilled)
Lemon leaf oil
Lime oil (distilled)
Mandarin oil
Orange oil (sweet)
Orange leaf oil
Satsuma oil (expressed)*
Tangelo oil
Tangerine oil
Yuzu oil (expressed or distilled)*

*Assumed from negligible bergapten content.

Bergapten has twice been reported as being present in skimmia oil (Lawrence 1989 p. 37), while a third report failed to detect any (Mathela et al 1992). These possibly phototoxic essential oils (none has been tested) are listed in Table 5.8, along with some absolutes and CO_2 extracts of Apiaceae plants that are known or suspected to contain FCs.

FCs may not be the only phototoxic constituents in essential oils. Both taget herb and root contain α-terthienyl, a thiophene, which is strongly phototoxic (Kagan et al 1980; Rampone et al 1986). Although no reports could be found showing α-terthienyl as a component of the essential oil, the oil's phototoxicity is apparently due to this thiophene content (Meynadier 1983, cited in Burfield 2004). Mandarin leaf oil has not been tested for phototoxicity, but it contains up to 60% dimethyl anthranilate, a phototoxic ester (Opdyke 1979a p. 273).

Managing risk

There is generally no phototoxic risk if the oils are used in a product that is either not applied to the body or is washed off the skin, such as shampoo, bath preparation or soap. However, essential oils can adhere to the skin if used in a sauna or steam inhalation. There is no risk if the skin to which the oils are applied is covered in such a way as to prevent UV rays from reaching them. Lightweight clothing fabrics only have a sun protection factor of 5–15, whereas heavy, substantial clothing blocks out most UV (Dayton 1993). The use of sunscreens in a potentially phototoxic preparation will reduce the risk of phototoxicity to some degree. There is no risk if non-phototoxic citrus oils are used, such as distilled or furanocoumarin-free oils.

If several phototoxic oils are used together, the risk is assumed to increase proportionally. For instance, bergamot and cumin oils both have maximum dermal use levels of 0.4%. If both are used in a product in equal proportions, the maximum safe percentage will be 0.2% for each, not 0.4% for each. When using deterpenated (folded) citrus fruit oils, we recommend checking with the supplier for phototoxicity risk. Deterpenated citrus oils are generally produced from distilled oils, which possess zero or very low phototoxicity, but the process of deterpenation may increase the total percentage of phototoxic constituents.

FCs are found in some common foodstuffs, notably parsnips, celery and grapefruit juice, and high dietary consumption of these will increase the total FC load. The safety factor between possible dietary intake and phototoxic threshold has been estimated as 2–10 (Schlatter et al 1991). Therefore food intake can increase risk.

The sensitivity of the skin to a phototoxic chemical increases during the first hour after application, remains at a peak for the next hour, and then decreases over the following eight hours (Table 5.9). This is certainly true for bergamot oil (Zaynoun et al 1977a, 1977b) and the same time course will probably hold for other phototoxic oils. The steady increase and then gradual decrease mirrors the time taken for the FCs to reach the dermis, and then to pass beyond it. Dubertret et al (1990b) confirmed that human skin photosensitivity is maximal two hours after application of an alcohol-based fragrance containing bergamot oil. As can be seen in Table 5.9, a 0.5% concentration of bergamot oil produced no phototoxic reactions in human volunteers, 1% was safe after eight hours, and 2.5% was safe after 10 hours.

We recommend that skin treated with phototoxic oils at levels higher than those maximum use levels, should not be exposed to UV light for 12–18 hours. A 15% or 20% concentration of bergamot oil can still produce a phototoxic reaction 12 hours after application and undiluted oils can produce reactions for 18 hours or longer. A 0.5% concentration of methoxsalen (roughly equivalent to undiluted bergamot oil in terms of phototoxic potential) continued to produce phototoxic reactions for 36 hours, but ceased after 48 hours (Zaynoun et al 1977a, 1977b).

Photocarcinogenesis

The main causative factor in most human skin cancers is solar ultraviolet light. Chronic exposure to UVB causes changes to skin cells that can eventually lead to full malignancy. The three major skin cancers are associated with mutations in different genes: p53 (squamous cell carcinoma), PATCHED gene (basal cell carcinoma) and p16 (melanoma) (Cleaver & Crowley 2002). Certain chemicals, such as coal tar and some FC molecules, are photocarcinogenic.

Table 5.9 The response of five volunteers to varying concentrations of bergamot oil and subsequent UV irradiation of the skin

Concentration in ethanol	Number of positive responses at different time intervals (hours)								
	0	0.5	1	2	4	6	8	10	12
0.5%	0/5	0/5	0/5	0/5	0/5	0/5	0/5	0/5	0/5
1.0%	0/5	1/5	2/5	3/5	2/5	1/5	0/5	0/5	0/5
2.5%	0/5	3/5	4/5	3/5	2/5	1/5	1/5	0/5	0/5
5.0%	0/5	3/5	5/5	5/5	2/5	2/5	2/5	0/5	0/5
Total	0/20	7/20	11/20	11/20	6/20	4/20	3/20	0/20	0/20

(Reproduced by permission from Zaynoun S T, Johnson B E, Frain-Bell W 1977 A study of bergamot and its importance as a phototoxic agent. Contact Dermatitis 3: 225–239, © 1977 Munsgaard International Publishers Ltd., Copenhagen, Denmark.)

Photocarcinogenesis is the initiation of cancer by UV light, or by a chemical in the presence of UV light. As with most cancers, the carcinogenic process is preceded by genotoxicity (see Ch. 12, p. 166). Most FCs are believed to form stable adducts with pyrimidine bases in DNA (Ortel et al 1991), and DNA-photoadducts have been seen with bergapten and methoxsalen, both in vitro and in vivo (Pathak et al 1986; Amici & Gasparro 1995). However, photocarcinogenesis does not always follow phototoxicity. This may be because cell death precludes the development of DNA damaged cells, and/or because ROS-mediated toxicity from some FCs is easily repaired.

Photogenotoxicity

Of the phototoxic compounds found in essential oils only three, bergapten, methoxsalen and psoralen, are known to be strongly photogenotoxic and photocarcinogenic. However, virtually all of the phototoxic oils contain bergapten and/or psoralen. Methoxsalen is only found in rue oil.

In the presence of UV light, FCs can become inserted in between DNA bases, forming easily repaired adducts (monoadducts). Psoralens can, in addition, form inter-strand cross-links in DNA (biadducts), but angelicins do not form cross-links (Grossweiner 1984; DFG 2006). Biadducts have been seen with bergapten, psoralen, methoxsalen and imperatorin, but not angelicin (Bissonnette et al 2008). It has been suggested that psoralens are therefore more likely to be genotoxic, but the evidence does not support this view. Angelicins can also be photogenotoxic and photocarcinogenic, as has been seen with angelicin and citropten (Ashwood-Smith et al 1983; Mullen et al 1984; Alcalay et al 1990). Bergaptol, bergamottin and isopimpinellin are not photogenotoxic (Schimmer & Kühne 1990; Morlière et al 1991; Aubin et al 1994; Ivie & Beier 1996; Bode et al 2005; Messer et al 2012).

Antigenotoxicity

Photosensitivity and phototumorigenicity in the skin are both associated with the production of oxygen radicals, especially singlet oxygen radicals, a process known as 'photo-oxidative stress' (Gocke 2001; Llano et al 2003; Bode & Hansel 2005). The role played by ROS is central to the growth inhibition of skin cells and 'accelerated aging' seen in photoaged skin (Dalle Carbonare & Pathak 1992; Ma et al 2002).

French or English lavender oil, and to a lesser extent Japanese lavender oil, linalool and linalyl acetate, demonstrated a singlet oxygen radical quenching action in the skin of mice exposed to UVA, dose-dependently suppressing ROS generation (Sakurai et al 2005). Myrrh oil is a singlet oxygen quencher that protects against peroxidation of skin lipids prone to photo-oxidation (Auffray 2007). Similarly, cinnamaldehyde protects human skin cells in vitro from oxidative stress induced by singlet oxygen, and has been proposed as a preventative of photocarcinogenesis (Wondrak et al 2008).

Essential oils of *Origanum compactum*, *Artemisia herba alba* and Madagascan *Cinnamomum camphora* protect against nuclear DNA damage in the yeast *Saccharomyces cerevisiae* induced by methoxsalen plus UVA (Bakkali et al 2006). The genotoxic mechanism may involve interference with the normal processing of mutagenic lesions either by promoting oxidative stress, or initiation of apoptosis and necrosis (Bakkali et al 2005, 2006). Because perillyl alcohol inhibits UVB-induced tumorigenesis in mice, it is being considered as a potential chemopreventive agent in skin cancer (Barthelman et al 1998, Stratton et al 2000). Similarly, α-santalol, applied to mouse skin at 5%, significantly inhibited UVB-induced tumor development (Bommareddy et al 2007, Dwivedi et al 2006).

Kaul et al (2007) have reviewed the use of both oral and topical antioxidants to combat photoaging. Topically applied BHT (an antioxidant) had no effect on methoxsalen phototumorigenesis (Black et al 1989). However, some dietary protection against phototoxicity is offered by carotenoids, flavonoids and tocopherols (Giles et al 1985; Lee et al 2004; Sies & Stahl 2004).

Susceptibility to both FC phototoxicity and photocarcinogenesis, may, therefore, be reduced by diet and by other essential oils.

PUVA therapy

There is a great deal of clinical information from the therapeutic use of methoxsalen in PUVA (psoralen + UVA) therapy, which was first used in the 1940s (Pathak & Fitzpatrick 1992). PUVA therapy entails the oral administration of high doses of methoxsalen (0.5–0.7 mg/kg), plus UVA irradiation 2–4 times a week for an average of 12 weeks. It is often used in the treatment of vitiligo, severe cases of psoriasis, and certain other skin conditions (De Wolff & Thomas 1986; Momtaz & Fitzpatrick 1998). It helps control the abnormal proliferation of skin cells, and there is in vitro evidence that PUVA therapy may be helpful in treating melanoma (Carneiro Leite et al 2004).

However, PUVA therapy can also lead to methoxsalen-DNA adducts in normal skin cells (Besaratinia & Pfeifer 2004), and people with Caucasian skin who undergo long periods of therapy are at risk of squamous cell or basal cell carcinoma (Bruynzeel et al 1991, McKenna et al 1996, Seidl et al 2001, Stern & Lange 1988). There are also reports indicating an increased risk of melanoma, a more virulent type of skin cancer, though not until 15 years after PUVA therapy (Stern et al 1997, 2001).

In a 5+ year follow-up, Murase et al (2005) reviewed 4,294 long-term PUVA patients in Japan, Korea, Thailand, Egypt and Tunisia, and concluded that people with ethnically darker skin (Asian or Arabian-African) are not at risk from non-melanoma skin cancers. However, in documenting 1,380 long-term PUVA patients of different skin phototypes, Stern et al (2001) noted that while there was a decreased incidence in skin phototypes IV, V or VI, there was still some occurrence of non-melanoma cancers in these groups after a 20+ year follow-up. The same researchers found that malignant melanoma did not occur in long-term PUVA patients with skin phototypes IV, V or VI, though it did in patients with lighter skin. Complete protection from PUVA-related melanoma was also seen in a type of mouse with hyperpigmented skin, in spite of the presence of melanoma-inducible oncogenes (Kato et al 2007).

In PUVA therapy, the total dose of UVA given varies, and is a major factor in the incidence or otherwise of skin cancers. In a meta-analysis of nine reports, and adjusting for baseline squamous cell carcinoma (SCC) incidence, high-dose PUVA therapy was associated with an increase in SCC, while low-dose

PUVA therapy was not (Stern & Lunder 1998). High-dose was defined as more than 200 treatments, or 2,000 J/cm^2, and low-dose as less than 100 treatments, or fewer than 1,000 J/cm^2. For comparison, measurements of daylight UVA in Glasgow varied from 4 J/cm^2 in December to 69 J/cm^2 in June (Moseley et al 1983).

The data from PUVA therapy suggest that there is an increased risk of skin cancer from high *oral* doses of methoxsalen, plus high-dose UVA irradiation of compromised skin. However, the risk from *dermal* FCs is lower. In a 14-year follow-up of 158 psoriasis patients who received methoxypsoralen baths instead of oral dosing, there was no correlation between treatment and skin cancer incidence (Hannuksela-Svahn et al 1999). In PUVA bath therapy, plasma levels of methoxsalen varied from <5 to 34 ng/mL, according to the severity of the disease (Gómez et al 1995). The uptake of methoxsalen into psoriatic plaques is more than double that for normal stratum corneum, but is still only 0.25% of the applied dose and only 2.5% of an oral dose, a significant reduction in the possible toxic hazard (Anigbogu et al 1996).

The skin cancer risk from oral bergapten may be lower than that of methoxypsoralen in humans. No increase in skin cancer incidence was reported during a 14-year observation of 413 light-skinned psoriasis patients who had received PUVA therapy with bergapten (McNeely & Goa 1998).

Collectively, the data from PUVA therapy suggest that oral methoxsalen + high-dose UVA radiation in people with skin disease increases the long-term risk of non-melanoma skin cancer. The risk of melanoma is increased for skin phototypes I, II and III only. No association with any skin cancer has been demonstrated from low-dose PUVA therapy, from topically applied methoxsalen, or from oral bergapten + UVA. It is important to note that long-term PUVA therapy is more hazardous than chronic sunlight exposure (Stern & Laird 1994; Stern 1998) and therefore cannot be used to directly estimate risk associated with sunlight.

Mouse data

Studies in hairless mice show that oral doses of methoxsalen + UVA similar to those used in humans lead to skin cancers, but not to other types of cancer, that topically applied bergapten or methoxsalen plus UVA give rise to a similar incidence of skin cancer, and that bergamot oil containing bergapten is similarly photocarcinogenic (Dunnick et al 1991; Young et al 1983, 1990; Zajdela & Bisagni 1981). When bergapten was applied to hairless mouse skin in concentrations of 5, 15 and 50 ppm, even the lowest dose resulted in tumors, some benign and some malignant, in the presence of UV light (Young et al 1990); 15 ppm of bergapten is equivalent to a 0.4% dilution of a typical commercial bergamot oil.

The bergapten/UV light procedure was carried out every weekday for 75 weeks, in many cases more than half the lifespan of the mice. The authors point out that mice are thought to be less capable of DNA repair than humans, and that mouse data cannot be used to predict absolute human risk (Young et al 1990). More recent findings support this view in relation to the repair of UV-induced DNA damage (Hanawalt 2001; Van Zeeland et al 2005). Bergapten is the only phototumorigenic constituent in bergamot oil, and even low concentration sunscreens completely inhibit bergapten-enhanced phototumorigenesis.

Risk/benefit considerations

It has been claimed that bergapten can help prevent sunlight-related skin cancer, since tanned skin is more protective against sunlight damage (Young et al 1990). An initial study on pigs showed that bergamot oil, plus a sunscreen, provided good protection against epidermal cell damage from UV light (Sambuco et al 1987). In further human studies, a tan gained with bergapten resulted in less DNA damage than one gained without it (Young et al 1988, 1991). The levels of bergapten used, 15–45 ppm, are similar to those causing photocarcinogenesis in mice, cited above. 'Ultimately, the question of the addition of bergamot oil (containing 5-MOP) to sunscreens must be addressed in terms of risk–benefit analysis. We present evidence that the judicious use of 5-MOP-containing sunscreens may confer benefit against solar DNA damage in people who seek a tan' (Young et al 1991).

There is clearly a theoretical risk from oral FCs, though it should be stressed that in some studies there was no incidence of skin cancer, and in most the incidence was very low. Dubertret et al (1990a) comment that reported phototoxic side effects from perfumes are very rare, and that there are no reports of increased incidence of epithelial tumors on skin sites that are habitually perfumed. The human PUVA data with bergapten suggest a lower level of risk to humans than mice, and in vitro DNA-repair assays support this view. Mouse data therefore cannot be directly extrapolated to humans in risk assessment. Curiously, both bergapten and bergamot oil exhibit selective, photo-induced cytotoxicity to A375 (human malignant melanoma) cells in vitro (Menichini et al 2010).

Safety thresholds

The IFRA maximum for furanocoumarins is 15 ppm. It has been proposed that manufacturers of cosmetic products in EC countries be required to limit the maximum content of 'furocoumarin-like substances' to 1 ppm (SCCNFP 2003b). This limit appears to be an arbitrary figure, and the proposal is based on the assumption that all FCs are photomutagenic. However, since bergaptol, bergamottin and isopimpinellin are neither phototoxic nor photomutagenic, all FCs should not be treated as posing equal risk. The SCCNFP opinion is apparently based on the unsound assumption than rodent or in vitro data can be used to assess human safety thresholds (Hanawalt 2001; Van Zeeland et al 2005; Kejlová et al 2007).

We know that methoxsalen, under certain conditions, can be photocarcinogenic in humans, and that bergamot oil is photocarcinogenic in hairless mice. However, there is not enough information to identify safety thresholds for dermally applied FC-containing essential oils in humans.

Managing adverse skin reactions

Once an allergic reaction begins it cannot be halted, but any essential oil remaining on the surface of the skin should be removed by washing the skin with soap, preferably unperfumed. More detailed guidelines for first aid procedures are given in Box 15.1. Most allergic skin reactions do not last more than 30 minutes, but they can be very unpleasant.

A long-term approach to dealing with intolerance to cosmetics and perfumes in general is complete avoidance of all cosmetic and cleaning products for a period of time (Scheman 2000). The avoidance period varies in individual cases from several weeks to 12 months, after which time cosmetics may be gradually reintroduced (Wolf et al 2001).

Practitioners should check with new clients/patients to find out whether they have ever experienced skin reactions to essential oils, perfumes or fragranced products, and whether they have a personal or family history of atopic dermatitis. If they have, extra care may need to be taken in the selection of essential oils and the concentrations used. Even if safety guidelines are carefully followed, practitioners may encounter idiosyncratic skin reactions at some time. If this occurs, a visit to a dermatologist might help identify the essential oils or constituents responsible.

We recommended that practitioners do not conduct *routine* pre-emptive patch testing in order to check the safety of an essential oil preparation before using it on a client/patient, although it may be a wise choice if there is reason to believe that an adverse skin reaction is likely. See Patch testing above, for a full description.

Regulation

Since the early 1970s the fragrance industry has controlled product safety through a set of voluntary guidelines: the IFRA Code of Practice. This requires, for example, that certain materials are not used at all, and others are used at specific maximum concentrations. However, compliance was poor initially, and there were signs of increasing fragrance allergy in the 1980s and 1990s. Many of the IFRA guidelines have now been adopted by the EU and enshrined into law, as an attempt to reduce adverse reactions. As a response to those who felt that the IFRA guidelines were not sufficiently far-reaching, further measures have been taken.

In Europe, this has resulted in Directive 2003/15/EC Amending The Cosmetics Directive 76/768/EEC (The 7th Amendment), which lists 26 fragrance materials as skin allergens (SCCNFP 1999). Of these, 16 occur in essential oils (Table 5.10). The 7th Amendment requires that any cosmetic product sold in an EU member state and containing a listed material must declare it on the ingredients list if it occurs at more than 100 ppm (0.01%) in a wash-off product or 10 ppm (0.001%) in a leave-on product. From Table 5.10 it can be seen that some of these materials occur in very few essential oils or absolutes.

The EU Cosmetics Directive 7th Amendment

The 7th Amendment can be criticized in its criteria for selection, one draft of which includes this statement: 'Positive patch test data from more than one patient in more than one independent center should be present.' Surely two reactions to a substance should not be sufficient to qualify it as a high-risk

Table 5.10 Essential oil constituents listed as allergens in the EU

Constituent	No. of essential oils or absolutes containing more than 1.0%
Limonene	211
Linalool	180
Geraniol	49
Eugenol	27
Citral	20
Benzyl benzoate	18
Citronellol	15
Farnesol	15
Coumarin	10
Benzyl alcohol	8
Benzyl salicylate	5
Cinnamaldehyde	5
Isoeugenol	5
Cinnamyl alcohol	4
Benzyl cinnamate	2
Anisyl alcohol	1

allergen? But the criteria for selection of fragrant allergens have never been made clear by the SCCP. No consideration seems to have been given to the notion that a great many fragrance materials are probably very low-risk contact allergens. For example, small numbers of dermatitis patients have reacted to β-caryophyllene, cyclohexyl acetate, α-damascone, 3,7-dimethyl-7-methoxy-octan-2-ol, ethylene dodecanedioate, hedione, nerol, α-irone, methyleugenol, methylisoeugenol, 3-phenyl-1-propanol, piperonal, α-terpineol and thymol (Frosch et al 2002a, 2002b; Larsen et al 2002). And this from only three reports in which researchers tested these materials. Therefore, the existence of a handful of reports of adverse reactions does not indicate a high level of risk.

Relative risk

The EU labeling requirement for allergens has since been taken to mean much more than that, yet the listing of a substance as an 'allergen', though now widely cited, has been poorly considered. No allowance was made for the fact that some fragrance materials are considerably more potent allergens than others (Table 5.11). It is especially surprising to see cinnamaldehyde and linalool treated by the EU as if they presented an equal degree of risk. The data in Tables 14.1A and 14.5A show that, while an average of 2.5% (518/20,606) of dermatitis patients reacted to 1–5% cinnamaldehyde, only 0.05% (13/25,164) reacted to 5–20% linalool, 50 times less. If we look at both compounds tested at 5%, 29.2% of patients reacted to cinnamaldehyde while not one of 1,399 patients reacted to linalool. It is

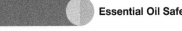

Table 5.11 Relative risk of purported EU allergens

Substance tested	Concentration used	Number of +, ++ or +++ reactions		Total no. of reactions	Total % reactions
		Schnuch et al 2007a	Heisterberg et al 2011		
Tree moss absolute	1%	45/1,658	50/1,503	95/3,161	3.0%
Oakmoss absolute	1%	46/2,063	31/1,503	81/3,566	2.27%
Cinnamaldehyde	1%	21/2,063	20/1,503	41/3,566	1.15%
Isoeugenol	1%	26/2,063	14/1,502	40/3,565	1.12%
Farnesol	5%	38/4,238	5/1,502	43/5,740	0.75%
Cinnamyl alcohol	1%	13/2,063	10/1,501	23/3,564	0.64%
Citral	2%	13/2,021	4/1,502	17/3,523	0.48%
Eugenol	1%	11/2,065	4/1,502	15/3,567	0.42%
Coumarin	5%	8/2,020	3/1,503	11/3,523	0.31%
Citronellol	1%	9/2,003	1/1,503	10/3,506	0.29%
Geraniol	1%	10/2,063	0/1,502	10/3,565	0.28%
Benzyl alcohol	1%	7/2,166	2/1,508	9/3,674	0.24%
Linalool	10%	7/2,401	1/1,397	8/3,798	0.21%
Benzyl cinnamate	5%	6/2,042	1/1,503	7/3,545	0.20%
Benzyl salicylate	1%	2/2,041	3/1,503	5/3,544	0.14%
Limonene	2%	3/2,396	0/1,399	3/3,795	0.08%
Anisyl alcohol	1%	1/2,004	1/1,503	2/3,507	0.06%
Benzyl benzoate	1%	1/2,003	0/1,503	1/3,506	0.03%

disturbing to realize that linalool was listed as an allergen on the basis of only five positive reactions spread over a five-year period. Although the EU retrospectively justified this decision on the basis that oxidized linalool is allergenic, the first oxidation data were published in 2002, three years after the legislation was drafted.

In contrast, a report by an ECETOC (European Center for Ecotoxicology and Toxicology) taskforce, lays the groundwork for the classification of chemicals as allergens in Europe. It proposes four categories and notification levels: extreme (0.003%), strong (0.1%), moderate (1%) and weak (3%). The task force closely examined various ways to ascertain the relative potency of sensitizers (Kimber et al 2003). Several essential oil constituents were included as examples, and all of them were provisionally categorized as either moderate (cinnamaldehyde, isoeugenol) or weak (citral, eugenol, linalool) sensitizers. So, while the 7th Amendment requires notification of linalool if over 0.001%, the ECETOC taskforce proposes a threshold of 3%.

The relative risk of the purported EU allergens has been investigated by Schnuch et al (2007a) and by Heisterberg et al (2011); Table 5.11 summarizes their findings (the substances not found in essential oils are not included here). Earlier we explained why a reaction rate of 0.3% or less from patch testing could be considered negligible. Bearing in mind that data from patch tests does not represent real-world risk, do these numbers suggest safety thresholds, and if so where? We believe it is self-evident that the first four substances in Table 5.11 should be restricted, and equally, that the last four (or six, or seven) should not be restricted. To quote Schnuch et al (2007a): 'In this group, true allergenicity is in doubt, considering the possibility of false-positive reactions, and of doubtful or irritant reactions.'[9] The authors conclude that fragrance companies that totally avoid the 26 'allergens' may be putting consumers at risk, by using alternative fragrance materials that are less well studied from a toxicological standpoint.

Others have noted that the citral skin sensitization data in particular are confounded by probable confusion with irritation, and the research on anisyl alcohol is hardly sufficient to draw any conclusions at all. A comparison of skin reaction data for various constituents in dermatitis patients, not including those known to be cosmetic- or fragrance-sensitive, is shown in Table 5.12A. This is yet another viewpoint for relative risk, and yet such constituent data cannot necessarily be extrapolated to essential oils containing those constituents. 'Concordance' between reactions to certain constituents and essential oils containing them was evaluated by Uter et al (2010). They found that concordance was good for lemongrass oil and citral, and for clove oil and eugenol, but it was non-existent for lemon

Table 5.12 Comparison of skin reaction data for various essential oil constituents in dermatitis patients

A. Comparison of patch test data from dermatitis patients to show relative risk for some of the purported EU allergens

Constituent	Percentage who reacted	Number of reactors	Concentration used	Chronological range of data	References
Cinnamaldehyde	1.96%	374/19,047	1%	1987–2011	Santucci et al 1987; Nethercott et al 1991; Frosch et al 1995a, 1995b; Marks et al 1995, 1998; Belsito et al 2006; Schnuch et al 2007a; Heisterberg et al 2011
Isoeugenol	1.37%	125/9,100	1%	1987–2011	Santucci et al 1987; Frosch et al 1995a, 1995b; Tanaka S et al 2004; Schnuch et al 2007a; Heisterberg et al 2011
Farnesol	0.73%	94/12,800	5%	2000–2011	Sugiura et al 2000; Frosch et al 2004, 2005a; Schnuch et al 2004b, 2007a; Heisterberg et al 2011
Citral	0.67%	47/7,049	2%	2000–2011	De Groot et al 2000; Frosch et al 2005a; Schnuch et al 2007a; Heisterberg et al 2011
Eugenol	0.56%	39/6,948	1%	1987–2011	Santucci et al 1987; Frosch et al 1995a, 1995b; Schnuch et al 2007a; Heisterberg et al 2011
Cinnamyl alcohol	0.54%	37/6,838	1%	1987–2011	Santucci et al 1987; Frosch et al 1995a, 1995b; Schnuch et al 2007a
Geraniol	0.33%	23/6,939	1%	1987–2011	Santucci et al 1987; Frosch et al 1995a, 1995b; Schnuch et al 2007a; Heisterberg et al 2011
Citronellol	0.30%	25/8,426	1% or 5%	1995–2011	Frosch et al 1995a, 2002a, 2005a; Heydorn et al 2002, 2003b; Schnuch et al 2007a; Lapczynsky et al 2008b; Heisterberg et al 2011
Benzyl salicylate	0.28%	17/6,127	1%, 2% or 5%	1995–2011	Frosch et al 1995a; De Groot et al 2000; Heydorn et al 2003b; Schnuch et al 2007a; Heisterberg et al 2011
(+)-Limonene	0.23%	15/6,601	2% or 3%	1987–2011	Santucci et al 1987; Frosch et al 2002b; Schnuch et al 2007a; Heisterberg et al 2011
Benzyl cinnamate	0.23%	10/4,292	5%	2001–2011	Wöhrl et al 2001; Schnuch et al 2007a; Heisterberg et al 2011
Linalool	0.16%	9/5,623	10% or 20%	2000–2011	De Groot et al 2000; Schnuch et al 2007a; Heisterberg et al 2011
Benzyl benzoate	0.11%	6/5,024	1%, 2% or 5%	1982–2011	Mitchell et al 1982; Ferguson & Sharma 1984; Heydorn et al 2003b; Schnuch et al 2007a; Heisterberg et al 2011

B. Comparison of patch test data from dermatitis patients to show relative risk for some essential oils and absolutes tested at 1% or 2%

Essential oil or absolute	Percentage who reacted	Tisserand & Young dermal maximum	No. of reactors	Concentration used	Chronological range of data[a]	References
Oakmoss absolute	2.03%	0.1%	159/7,831	1%	1976–2011	Santucci et al 1987; Frosch et al 1995b; Schnuch et al 2007a; Heisterberg et al 2011
Ylang-ylang oil	1.32%	0.8%	107/8,102	2%	2002–2006	Frosch et al 2002b; Pratt et al 2004; Belsito et al 2006
Lemongrass oil	0.98%	0.7%	50/5,106	2%	2001–2010	Wöhrl et al 2001; Frosch et al 2002b; Paulsen & Andersen 2005; Uter et al 2010
Narcissus absolute	0.92%	0.8%	40/4,369	2%	2002–2010	Frosch et al 2002b; Paulsen & Andersen 2005; Uter et al 2010

Continued

Table 5.12 Comparison of skin reaction data for various essential oil constituents in dermatitis patients—Cont'd

B. Comparison of patch test data from dermatitis patients to show relative risk for some essential oils and absolutes tested at 1% or 2%

Essential oil or absolute	Percentage who reacted	Tisserand & Young dermal maximum	No. of reactors	Concentration used	Chronological range of data	References
Jasmine absolute	0.7%	0.7%	54/7,703	2%	1987–2006	Santucci et al 1987; Pratt et al 2004; Belsito et al 2006
Peppermint oil	0.45%	4.4% (for hepatotoxicity)	12/3,124	2%	1987–2005	Santucci et al 1987; Frosch et al 2002b; Paulsen & Andersen 2005
Sandalwood oil	0.38%	2.0%	11/3,342	2%	1987–2007	Santucci et al 1987; Frosch et al 2002b; Paulsen & Andersen 2005

[a]No pre-1987 data is included in this table

oil or orange oil and limonene. For example, although eight of 1,585 dermatitis patients reacted to lemon oil, none of the eight reacted to limonene.

Table 5.12B is a comparison of relative risk for essential oils that we have extrapolated from clinical data. While such data are subject to variability, we believe that the large numbers involved greatly compensate for this.

Further critique

The EU allergens legislation can be criticized for its general lack of rigor. For example, it does not account for the fact that significant allergenicity in limonene and linalool is only postulated after oxidation has set in. There are three considerations here. Firstly, considerable oxidation needs to take place before peroxides and hydroperoxides are formed, and it has not been demonstrated that this occurs in commercial products (Hostýnek & Maibach 2008). Secondly, the addition of appropriate antioxidants to these materials considerably reduces the rate of oxidation (Karlberg et al 1994b). Finally, material risk from oxidized limonene or linalool in essential oils has not been demonstrated. Hostýnek and Maibach (2008) conclude that: 'Regardless of the possibility that autoxidation may enhance the allergenic potential of this substance [linalool] it is not yet documented as a major fragrance allergen.'

The possible contribution to allergenicity of impurities in synthetic aromachemicals (which are used in virtually all of the research) has been pointedly ignored by the SCCP. Most of the data on coumarin allergy are unreliable since they do not indicate a clear purity of the material used (Floch et al 2002). Vocanson et al (2006, 2007) have since demonstrated that 99.9% pure coumarin is not allergenic, and that reactivity in coumarin of lower purity is due to the impurities it contains. Therefore, there is no longer any rationale for classing naturally occurring coumarin as an allergen.

The coumarin used in dematological tests is 95–99% pure, but no information is given about the 1–5% of impurities present. If the allergenicity of a synthetic compound is due to impurities, then the same compound, as it occurs in nature, cannot be assumed to be allergenic. This finding sheds new

light on the earlier opinion of the SCCNFP, that there is no '...difference in allergenicity between a fragrance ingredient synthetically produced or extracted from a natural product' (SCCNFP 2003e). The purities of commercially available citral (95–96%), citronellol (95–99%) and farnesol (90–96%) are of particular concern. It is worth noting that the FDA requires the toxicity assessment of any impurity occurring in a pharmaceutical drug at 0.1% or more (Kruhlak et al 2007).

Enantiomeric differences between natural and synthetic compounds have also not been taken into account. This is important, since there are often considerable enantiomeric differences between naturally occurring and synthetic compounds, and ACD is enantiospecific (Benezra 1990; Benezra et al 1985; Ford et al 1988b; Warshaw & Zug 1996).

The 7th Amendment is based on the premise that the percentage of reactions to the FM indicates the percentage of people who actually react to fragrances. However, the FM data are suspect on several grounds already discussed, and extrapolation from these to actual fragrance use has no scientific basis. The fact that the great majority of the FM data only examine risk to dermatitis patients is given no weighting. A mixture of eight more or less high-risk fragrance materials in an 8% dilution cannot accurately reflect the risk from mixtures derived from a palette of up to 2,500 substances. And, quenching is given no credence.

If the aim of this legislation was to identify the most potent allergens in fragrances, then this was a laudable one. Unfortunately, many materials are included which are clearly not potent allergens. The resulting misinformation has created regulatory chaos and confusion in the affected industries.

The IFRA Quantitative Risk Assessment

More recently, IFRA has radically changed its approach to safety guidelines, and now bases these on a highly complex 'quantitative risk assessment', or QRA. This takes into account a large number of variables including human data, animal data, product type and other factors (Api & Vey 2008; Api et al 2008). There are concerns: that the science has too many gaps; that the resulting guidelines are too complex; that the IFRA/RIFM/REXPAN lobby is funded by corporations with vested interests; and that the QRA approach, though being heavily 'sold' as the way forward for the fragrance industry, has been rushed through without being vetted by independent scientists, and without proper consultation with affected industries.

The IFRA QRA is based on the following:

- skin allergenicity is dependent on dose per unit of skin area ($\mu g/cm^2$). IFRA also expresses this as an EC3 value, the estimated concentration of a substance necessary to cause a threefold increase in lymph node cell proliferation. A 'moderate' skin sensitizer, for example, would fall within the range of 100–1,000 $\mu g/cm^2$, which corresponds to 1–10% w/w
- a NESIL (no expected sensitization induction level), expressed as a percentage, can be extrapolated from HRIPT data and/or from LLNA data
- EC3 values, derived from LLNA data, can be extrapolated to humans using a sensitization assessment factor (SAF)
- the SAF is similar to the uncertainty factors used in extrapolating NOAEL data to human risk. The intention is to 'scale down' in anticipation of (1) inter-individual variability, (2) vehicle/product matrix effects, and (3) 'use considerations' (basically, product type)
- the inter-individual SAF used by IFRA is always 10. The matrix SAF is either 1 or 3, depending on product type, and the use SAF is 1, 3, 10 or 20.

On Ch. 5, p. 78 we explained the crucial role played by T lymphocytes in lymph nodes in the process of skin sensitization. In the LLNA, the test substance is topically applied to the ears of female mice, daily for three days. After two rest days, [^{3}H] methyl thymidine is injected into the tail vein. Five hours later the mice are killed, and suspensions of lymph node cells are prepared. The incorporation of thymidine is measured, and expressed as ^{3}H disintegrations per minute (dpm) per lymph node. Higher dpm values are said to correlate with greater skin sensitizing potential (Gerberick et al 2007).

Both IFRA and others acknowledge that the LLNA can sometimes give rise to false positives because of irritation. The LLNA does not account for possible differences between mouse and human in skin absorption or dermal metabolism of a substance. Crucially, the data given to support the correlation of LLNA-derived EC3 values to human sensitivity are not robust, even though they show a reasonable qualitative relationship. For example, isoeugenol has an HRIPT-derived value of 69, and an LLNA-derived value of 450 (Gerberick et al 2001b). If there was a good correlation, we could expect to see a correlation equation with statistics. There is also a lack of clear division between different classifications in some cases, e.g., cinnamic aldehyde (moderate) and citral (weak) have similar NOELs. And, there is only one compound in the non-sensitizers classification where NOEL can be compared to LLNA data.

IFRA has a long history of publishing guidelines, while holding back some of the data they are based on. With the QRA, the HRIPT-derived EC3 values are given but not the raw data, and it is not clear how the NESIL values have been arrived at. The uncertainty factors used by IFRA (Felter et al 2003) may seem cautious, but they are arbitrary and unscientific. The 'Use SAF' is partly based on a classification system that assumes specific relative skin sensitivities for different areas of the body. For example: 'The plantar foot arch was about 12-fold less permeable than the skin of the back, while the scalp and axillae were about 2-fold higher, and the forehead was about 3-fold higher.' However, the comparative data on this are extremely thin, and insufficient to support the complex regulatory framework built on them.

In a review of skin sensitization and dose–response assessment, Van Loveren et al (2008) make the point that the LLNA has not been validated, and also that (Q)SAR data are insufficient, though both may be useful in a weight-of-evidence exercise. They stress the importance of elicitation data derived from sensitized dermatology patients. Since the relevance to human risk, even of single constituents, has not been fully validated, making the further assumption that constituent data can be routinely applied to essential oils, stretches the model beyond believability.

The challenges of this approach were encapsulated by Juryj Hostýnek (1998): 'Furthermore, absorption of an individual fragrance component will depend on its concentration in the formula, on the presence of solvents and other constituents acting as adjuvants or penetration enhancers, on component volatility, and the interdependence of these, and other factors. If one is to estimate the absorption of an individual component per unit area of skin and, ultimately, of the potential for its total absorption, a further process of assumptions and simplifications becomes necessary in order to arrive at a model of actual exposure. Such an analysis of multiple parameters…. appears extremely arduous.'

Table 5.13 show our response to the IFRA QRA that had been published at the time of writing. Our opinion is based on the clinical data found in the appropriate essential oil or constituent profile, some of which is summarized in Tables 5.11 and 5.12.

The SCCP has rejected IFRA's QRA approach (SCCP 2008). Among the reasons given are these:

- the weight-of-evidence guidelines have no general validity and scientific support is missing
- no scientific data is given to support the levels identified by the model as safe for the consumer other than the calculations in the model itself. No validation has been done nor has a strategy been provided
- risk assessment is made for 33 product categories. The many product categories imply a precision of the model unsupported scientifically
- as for established fragrance allergens causing allergy in the consumer, clinical and epidemiological data must be used as the critical decision point in risk assessment
- aggregated exposures are not considered in the dermal sensitization QRA, but should be given priority. Occupational exposures are neither considered
- the proposed model seems not to take account of that significant proportion of the population who suffers from skin disease (e.g., dermatitis).

There is also criticism of the HRIPT, on the basis that it is not yet validated, and that it is generally considered unethical.

Discussion

Many of the EC regulations seem unjustified, since all allergens are treated as presenting equal risk, and some conclusions are

Table 5.13 Comment on IFRA Guidelines for constituents and essential oils to avoid skin allergenicity

Oil constituent	IFRA Category 4[a]	Our comment	Recommendation
Isoeugenol	0.02%	Too restrictive	0.2%
Cinnamaldehyde	0.05%	Reasonable	0.05%
Perillaldehyde	0.1%	Insufficient data	No limit
Benzaldehyde	0.27%	No need for a limit	No limit
Cinnamyl alcohol	0.4%	Reasonable	0.4%
Eugenol	0.5%	Reasonable	0.5%
Citral	0.6%	Reasonable	0.6%
Anisyl alcohol	0.7%	No need for a limit	No limit
(+)-Carvone	1.2%	Insufficient data	No limit
(−)-Carvone	1.2%	Reasonable	1.2%
Farnesol	1.2%	Insufficient data	No limit
Coumarin	1.6%	No need for a limit	No limit
Benzyl cinnamate	2.1%	No need for a limit	No limit
Benzyl alcohol	2.7%	No need for a limit	No limit
Geraniol	5.3%	Reasonable	5.3%
Benzyl salicylate	8.0%	No need for a limit	No limit
Citronellol	13.3%	No need for a limit	No limit
Benzyl benzoate	26.7%	No need for a limit	No limit

Essential oil	IFRA Category 4[a]	Comment	Recommendation
Massoia oil	No safe level	Too restrictive	0.01%
Verbena oil (lemon)	No safe level	Too restrictive	0.9%
Oakmoss absolute	0.1%	Reasonable	0.1%
Treemoss absolute	0.1%	Reasonable	0.1%
Tea leaf absolute	0.2%	Reasonable	0.2%
Peru balsam oil	0.4%	Reasonable	0.4%
Jasmine absolute (grandiflorum)	0.7%	Reasonable	0.7%
Cananga oil	0.8%	Reasonable	0.8%
Ylang-ylang oils	0.8%	Reasonable	0.8%
Melissa oil	0.63%	Insufficient data	0.8%
Jasmine absolute (sambac)	4.0%	Reasonable	4.0%

[a]IFRA maximum concentrations for body creams, oils and lotions

based on flawed assumptions. At the same time, the EC is critical of the IFRA guidelines for not being sufficiently stringent, and for including some invalid assumptions. The basic approach to risk assessment is outlined on Ch. 3, p. 34, and typically includes (Q)SAR analysis, exposure assessment, pre-clinical testing, and clinical testing (Kimber et al 2002). However, as Tony Burfield has been at pains to point out, clinical testing is virtually non-existent for phototoxic essential oils, and taget oil, for example, is restricted in spite of the lack of a single relevant case of phototoxicity being reported. Risk assessment is supposed to consider theoretical and in vitro data *in combination with* clinical data, not instead of it.

Surely no one would argue with the notion of minimizing risk, but defining this in regulatory terms is clearly not easy. The EC approach seems to be based on a zero risk aim, protecting 100% of the population. However, the only way to achieve this would be to prohibit the use of all fragrances, cosmetics and household products. People with dermatitis deserve as much protection and consideration as anyone else, and yet zero risk to all people is neither realistic nor practical. IFRA's QRA is elaborate, and probably covers all the right bases. It certainly goes a long way toward accounting for relative risk. However its foundations are weak and too many assumptions have been made. It could be said that the EU over-emphasizes dermatological data, and the QRA under-emphasizes it.

Summary

- Compared to most other types of toxicity, adverse skin reactions are difficult to predict. Patch testing is useful for identifying the cause of an existing allergy.
- The three principal categories of adverse skin reaction relevant to essential oils are irritation, sensitization and photosensitization.
- The factors that affect adverse skin reactions all involve one or more of the following: dose metrics (quantity and concentration of substance); degree of percutaneous absorption of substance; degree of reactivity between substance and immune system.
- The most common skin reaction to fragrance materials is sensitization, which causes ACD. It is generally a delayed hypersensitivity reaction that manifests as a rash.
- Skin sensitization is idiosyncratic. Identification of the causative allergen(s) and their subsequent withdrawal generally leads to a resolution of the problem.
- Skin reactivity to an allergen is partly dependent on factors such as genetic profile and psychological stress, both of which can influence antioxidant status. Models that predict dermal loading and percutaneous absorption do not control for such factors.
- In sensitization, little or no effect is evident on first exposure to a substance, but an inflammatory reaction occurs on subsequent exposure to the same material, or to a similar substance with which there is cross-sensitization.
- The mechanisms involved in sensitization are quite well understood, and generally involve the binding of haptens to dermal proteins. The allergen is then large enough to be recognized by antigens on Langerhans cells, which interact with T-helper cells, leading to the release of histamine from mast cells.
- It is well established that thresholds exist for both induction and elicitation of allergic responses. Induction describes the acquisition of skin sensitization in a previously naïve individual. Elicitation describes a clearly discernible cutaneous reaction in a previously sensitized subject.
- Children up to three months old are at greater risk of skin sensitization due to the immaturity of their skin, and women are 3–4 times more likely to be affected by fragrance sensitivity than men.
- There are some differences in skin reactivity that are determined by age, sex, race or skin color. In general, allergenicity does not differ much with race.
- People with a history of atopic dermatitis may be at greater risk of skin sensitization.
- There is an occupational risk of skin sensitization to aromatherapists and other practitioners using essential oils in massage. There are ways in which this risk can be reduced, such as the avoidance of high-risk oils, and monitoring of the concentrations of specific materials.
- Oxidized essential oils are more likely to cause adverse skin reactions. It is recommended that effective antioxidants be used in preparations containing oxidation-prone essential oils.
- Practitioners should check with new patients to find out whether they have ever experienced skin reactions to essential oils, perfumes or perfumed substances, and whether they have a history of atopic dermatitis.
- The existence of quenching in skin sensitization has been questioned, but there are some good data supporting the hypothesis.
- The EU has listed 26 fragrance chemicals as skin allergens, 16 of which occur in essential oils. Our interpretation of the clinical literature is that only some of these should be classed as allergens. Some only become allergenic upon oxidation, and this is preventable with antioxidants.
- The 'FM' is used to estimate fragrance allergy prevalence, estimated to be 1.8% of the general population. However, data from patch testing cannot simply be extrapolated to estimate risk from essential oil use, which may be less than 0.01% of the general population, or one in 10,000 people.
- Phototoxicity is a skin reaction that occurs in the presence of a phototoxic chemical and ultraviolet light in the UVA range, leading to the formation of ROS, and to chronic sun damage on the skin.
- The most common phototoxic agents found in essential oils are the furanocoumarins, such as bergapten, which can be phototoxic even at very low concentrations. There are maximum safe percentages for phototoxic essential oils.
- If deterpenated citrus oils are used, the maximum percentage should be reduced in proportion to concentration to avoid phototoxicity. Deterpenated oils are classed according to their degree of concentration, e.g., $3\times$, $5\times$, $10\times$, etc.
- Skin that has been exposed to phototoxic oils at levels higher than the maximum should not be exposed to UV light (sunlight, sunbeds) for at least 12 hours.
- Skin color is a factor in determining susceptibility to phototoxicity.
- Sunscreens afford some protection from phototoxicity.
- A diet high in furanocoumarin-containing foods (celery, parsnips, grapefruit juice, etc.) may increase phototoxic risk, while a diet rich in carotenoids, flavonoids and tocopherols may reduce it.

- Some phototoxic furanocoumarins are potentially photocarcinogenic. Safety thresholds have not been established.

Notes

1. Other researchers estimate that ACD (though not specifically a fragrance mix allergy) generally reaches the incidence seen in adults by age 10 (Kütting et al 2004). A Portuguese study of 562 schoolchildren found the highest prevalence of ACD in the 5–6 year age group, with prevalence in the 7–8, 9–10 and 11–12 age groups all being significantly lower (Barros et al 1991).

2. From 1999 data, the incidence of ACD in Germany was estimated to be between and 0.017% and 0.7% per annum (Schnuch et al 2002a). From major population studies conducted in the US and in EU countries, the incidence of ACD in the general population was estimated at 1% in 1999 (http://www.theucbinstituteofallergy.com/_up/tuioa_com/images/europeanallergywp-summary_tcm114-11424.pdf). For a chronic condition like ACD, prevalence in the general population will be higher than (annual) incidence. The prevalence of ACD to cosmetics in Belgium has been estimated at 1–3% (Kohl et al 2002).

3. Cutaneous allergic reactions can be suppressed at both induction and elicitation phases by inhalation of anxiolytic odorants (Hosoi & Tsuchiya 2000). It is thought that stress causes mast cell activation through an increase in substance P (a neuropeptide) and that odorant inhalation may prevent this occurring (Hosoi et al 2003). In mice, valerian oil inhalation reduced stress-induced plasma corticosterone levels (Hosoi et al 2001).

4. A scale (the Draize scale), based on the production of erythema, edema and eschar, has been used to quantify levels of irritancy. Health Canada has suggested a mean Draize score of 5.1–8.0 for severe to extreme irritation, with scores of 3.1–5.0 and 1.6–3.0 assigned to moderate and mild irritation, respectively (www.hc-sc.gc.ca/hecs-sesc/ghs/sa/pcp_table2.html). A scale proposed by the FDA comprises eight grades of irritation, from 0 (no evidence of irritation) to 7 (strong reaction spreading beyond test site) (www.fda.gov/cder/guidance/2887fnl.htm#APPENDIX%20A).

5. Quantitative structure–activity relationships (QSAR) have been applied predictively to contact allergens (Basketter 1998; Patlewicz et al 2001, 2004). A theoretical basis has been proposed for the differential sensitizing ability for different benzoquinones, including thymoquinone (Cremer et al 1987). Possible reasons for the differences in sensitizing potential of eugenol, isoeugenol and methyleugenol are explored by Itoh (1982). Aldehydes can form Schiff bases with primary amines, and Schiff bases have a higher affinity for cell-surface proteins. Theoretically, because this moiety remains longer in the stratum corneum, it is more likely to contribute to sensitization (Scheinman 1996). The skin sensitization of cinnamaldehyde is probably initiated by protein Schiff base formation (Weibel & Hansen 1989a; Patlewicz et al 2001). QSAR and fragrance sensitization was reviewed by Hostýnek et al (1998).

6. Reactions to the FM in 'cosmetic-sensitive' dermatitis patients are naturally higher, and range from 19.2–47.3% (Malten et al 1984; Adams & Maibach 1985; Broeckx et al 1987; De Groot et al 1985; De Groot 1987; Larsen et al 1996a). In one report, 80% of adverse reactions to cosmetics were due to ACD mainly involving the face, eye and upper arm. Fragrant substances were common causative agents (Eiermann 1982). Johansen et al (1997) reported a significant correlation between cosmetic-sensitive dermatitis patients and a positive patch test to the FM.

7. Many researchers believe that the phototoxicity of some secondary plant metabolites has arisen independently several times in evolution as a defense mechanism against infestation by bacteria, fungi, parasites and insects. Some of the toxic effects associated with phototoxic compounds, such as oxidative stress and adduct formation, make them extremely potent antiviral agents (Hudson 1989).

8. Verbena oil is not very powerfully phototoxic. Out of six samples tested, three were phototoxic when applied undiluted; one of these was not phototoxic at 12.5%, and another was not phototoxic at 50% (Opdyke & Letizia 1982 p. 137S-138S).

9. A similar ranking order has been proposed by Germany's Informationsverbund Dermatologischer Kliniken (Information Network of Departments of Dermatology) or IVDK. They have listed cinnamaldehyde, isoeugenol, oakmoss and treemoss as potent allergens, cinnamyl alcohol as a less potent allergen, citral, eugenol and farnesol as "rarely found as allergens", and the rest as "risk of being an allergen is too small to consider".

The respiratory system

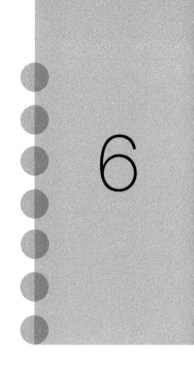

Due to their large surface area, rich blood supply, and the thin membrane separating air and blood, the lungs are very efficient organs for the absorption of gases and volatile substances from the air. The mucous membranes of the nasal cavity and pharynx make a contribution to gas exchange, but much less so. Conversely, exhalation may contribute to the excretion of blood-borne volatile compounds that have reached the bloodstream by any route. The lungs are therefore exposed to airborne toxic vapors as well as xenobiotic chemicals carried in the bloodstream. In addition to carcinogens and other toxins entering the body, the respiratory system is susceptible to irritation and allergic reactions. The significance of the lungs as ports of entry to the body is reflected in the presence of important local detoxifying enzymes.

Many factors affect air quality. The major contributors to the indoor aerial environment are bio-odorants (including human body odor, molds, and animal-derived materials), tobacco smoke, volatile household materials (found in cleaning agents, new carpet and paint) and fragranced products such as deodorants, perfumes and air fresheners (Cone & Shusterman 1991). Outdoor sensitivities can be triggered by vehicle exhaust, pesticides, dust storms and plants (Bener et al 1996; Baldwin et al 1997, 1999). Smoke from fires can also cause problems, whether indoors or outdoors.

Essential oils may be inhaled incidentally because they are present in the ambient air from plant emissions, personal care products, household products, etc., or because they are intentionally vaporized (in candles, essential oil vaporizers, aromatic baths or steam inhalations). Reasons for intentional use include relaxation, masking unpleasant odors, and reducing airborne molds, bacteria or viruses. In order to alleviate symptoms of respiratory disease, essential oils may be used in environmental or steam inhalation, or applied to the chest in the form of a 'rubbing ointment'.

Many essential oils and essential oil constituents have significant antimicrobial activities, and hence offer potential benefits in respiratory infections. For example, the vapors of cinnamon, thyme, and oregano essential oils, and their constituents, cinnamaldehyde, thymol, and carvacrol, were effective against Gram-negative bacteria (*Escherichia coli*, *Yersinia enterocolitica*, *Pseudomonas aeruginosa*, and *Salmonella choleraesuis*), Gram-positive bacteria (*Listeria monocytogenes*, *Staphylococcus aureus*, *Bacillus cereus*, and *Enterococcus faecalis*), molds (*Penicillium islandicum* and *Aspergillus flavus*), and a yeast (*Candida albicans*) (López et al 2007).

Inhaled essential oils might also be harmful, and fundamental safety questions that should be addressed include:

- can essential oils contribute to poor air quality?
- can essential oils cause respiratory disease?
- can essential oils exacerbate the symptoms of pre-existing respiratory disease?
- what are the NOAELs for inhaled essential oil vapors?
- under what circumstances is risk increased or reduced?

Inhalation toxicity is an emerging field of study, and even for recognized respiratory diseases, causal relationships with inhaled substances have not been fully elucidated. In addition, there is enormous scope for new compounds to be formed in the atmosphere, especially indoors. This combination of incomplete understanding and chemical complexity make it difficult to draw clear conclusions and establish safety guidelines. Adding to this complexity, there is sometimes uncertainty about whether a patient has asthma, chronic obstructive pulmonary disease (COPD), multiple chemical sensitivity (MCS), or some other respiratory complaint.

Most of the data in this chapter concern inhalation, but other routes of administration may also be pertinent to the respiratory system (see Pulmonary toxicity). Neurological effects from inhalation are covered in Chapter 10.

Volatile organic compounds

A volatile organic compound (VOC) is defined by the US Environmental Protection Agency (EPA) as 'any compound of carbon, excluding carbon monoxide, carbon dioxide, carbonic acid, metallic carbides or carbonates, and ammonium carbonate, which participates in atmospheric photochemical reactions' (www.epa.gov/iaq/voc2.html accessed April 28th 2012). There are hundreds of identified VOCs, including toxic substances such as chloroform, formaldehyde, acetaldehyde, benzene, toluene, xylene and styrene,[1] as well as some essential oil constituents. VOCs form photochemical oxidants, including ozone, that have adverse effects on health, materials, crops and forests. Common sources of VOCs in the home include hair sprays and air fresheners, which may contain volatile propellants in addition to a high proportion of low molecular weight fragrance chemicals.

Much has been published concerning the adverse respiratory and neurological effects of VOCs in general. The regular use of air fresheners and aerosols in the home has been strongly correlated with an increased incidence of diarrhea in infants and headache in new mothers. Total VOC concentration was estimated from measurements of toluene (Farrow et al 2003). If exposure is high enough, VOCs can cause **sensory irritation**. VOCs that have been associated with reduced respiratory function and/or asthma include formaldehyde, benzene, ethylbenzene and 1,4-dichlorobenzene (Rumchev et al 2002, 2004; Elliott et al 2006). Although few essential oil constituents have been implicated, long-term exposure to moderate concentrations of mixtures containing terpenes entails possible health risks, and the term 'air freshener' may often be a misnomer (Anderson & Anderson 1997a).

Adverse effects of airborne substances

The two principal adverse effects of ambient essential oils and other inhaled substances are **bronchial hyper-reactivity** (BHR), and **sensory irritation** (SI), which includes both eye and airway irritation. Sensory irritation is non-allergic, although it can exacerbate allergic conditions; BHR can be allergic or non-allergic in origin, and may be associated with respiratory disease such as asthma, allergic rhinitis, or COPD.

A controversial, asthma-like syndrome, known as sensory hyper-reactivity (SHR) is not an allergic reaction and has no known etiology, but may be associated with inhalation of fragrant substances. SHR can be viewed as both an adverse reaction and a respiratory disorder—we have included it under **Respiratory disease**.

Sensory irritation

When an odorous substance is sufficiently pungent, trigeminal or vagal afferent C fibers in the nose, mouth and eyes are activated (see Transient receptor potential channels below). This sensory system, called the common chemical sense (CCS), may have evolved as a warning system for potentially hazardous chemicals. It is distinct from olfaction (i.e., the sense of smell), and also reacts to chemicals with no detectable odor, such as tear gases and capsaicin (an alkaloid from Cayenne pepper fruit). It evokes sensations such as irritation, tickling, burning, warming, cooling, and stinging in the nasal and oral cavities and in the cornea, via pain receptors and the trigeminal nerve. Eye irritation may be a good assay for CCS sensitivity, as smell does not interfere with it (Millqvist 2006). Effects may be exacerbated by low humidity.

When 66 healthy males were exposed for 2.75 hr to a mixture of 22 VOCs, including α-pinene, at 0 and 25 mg/m^3, a significant majority associated the VOC exposure with increasing headache, degrading air quality, and general discomfort (Otto et al 1990). There is evidence that younger people and allergic rhinitis sufferers are more sensitive than others to VOC sensory irritation (Shusterman et al 2003). A survey of 643 young adults found self-reported illness from inhaling air that carried chemicals from paint, new carpet, perfume (all sources of VOCs), vehicle exhaust or pesticides. A total of 66% reported feeling unwell from one or more of these sources, and 15% to four or more. From a possible list of 11 symptoms, the most commonly reported were daytime sleepiness, daytime fatigue, difficulty concentrating, headache, irritability, and joint or muscle pain (Bell et al 1993). This picture is similar to that of MCS (see Sensory hyper-reactivity).

Sensory irritation may be over-reported, since subjective impressions may be biased by expectation, and researchers have found separating odor perception from true irritation to be a challenge. When two groups of people inhaled methyl salicylate, perceived nose, throat and eye irritation was 5–10 times more intense in the group told it was an industrial solvent, than in those informed it was a natural extract (Dalton 2003). However, objective evidence of nasal mucous membrane irritation (measured as increased neutrophil influx) in humans was found after inhalation of 25 mg/m^3 of mixed VOCs for 4 hours (Koren et al 1992).

Table 6.1 RD$_{50}$ concentrations of some VOCs in male mice[a]

Substance	RD$_{50}$ (ppm)	Calculated irritation threshold (0.03 × RD$_{50}$)
Chlorine[b]	3.5	0.1 ppm
Formaldehyde[b]	4	0.1 ppm
1-Octen-3-ol[c]	35	1 ppm
3-Octanol[c]	256	7 ppm
Benzaldehyde	363	11 ppm
(+)-α-Pinene	1,053	31 ppm
(+)-Limonene	1,076	32 ppm
(+)-β-Pinene	1,279	38 ppm
(+)-δ-3-Carene	1,345	40 ppm
Menthol	1,653	50 ppm
3-Octanone[c]	3,360	101 ppm
(−)-β-Pinene	4,663	158 ppm
(−)-α-Pinene	Inactive	No limit

RD$_{50}$ is the concentration that depresses the respiratory rate by 50%

[a]All values from tests in OF1 species, except for formaldehyde and (+)-limonene, which were BALB/CA species

[b]Chlorine and formaldehyde, not essential oil constituents, are shown for comparison

[c]Minor constituent (up to 5%) of a small number of essential oils

Benzaldehyde data are from Steinhagen & Barrow (1984) and menthol from Luan et al 2006. All other data are from Nielsen et al (2007a), and include data cited therein.

The essential oil constituents most commonly cited as sensory irritants are listed in Table 6.1. When inhaled by mice, δ-3-carene caused a dose-dependent decrease in breathing rate due to SI, but there was no deterioration of lung tissue (Kasanen et al 1999). When δ-3-carene was inhaled by humans, there was an increase in pulmonary irritation when the concentration increased from 225 ppm to 450 ppm (Falk et al 1991a). Sulfur compounds are also irritants. Inhalation of mustard oil, for example, greatly irritates the eyes and the upper airway mucous membranes (Von Skramlik 1959).

The respiratory tract is intimately connected with the ears and eyes by a mucous membrane, and thus exogenous irritants may affect tissues at one or more of these different anatomical sites. Eye irritation can be provoked by perfume in patients with a history of BHR to chemical triggers (Millqvist et al 1999; Elberling et al 2005), and eye reactions were confirmed in 8 of 21 such susceptible patients in a double-blind study (Elberling et al 2006).

Not all essential oil constituents are sensory irritants. Coumarin, 2-phenylethanol, octanoic acid and vanillin were virtually undetectable by nasal pungency in anosmics or via nasal localization in normosmics at room temperature (Cometto-Muñiz 2005a). These compounds are regarded as being 'nontrigeminal', and are therefore unlikely to pose any risk of SI. The exposure of rats or hamsters to finished fragrance in the ambient air at up to 50 mg/m^3 for 4 hours/day, 5 days/week for 13 weeks resulted in no toxicologically significant effects. The fragrances included, as major components, coumarin, 2-phenylethanol and benzyl acetate (Fukayama et al 1999).

Terpene oxidation

The irritant and sensitizing actions of many, often aged, essential oils have been ascribed to oxidation products of various constituents, especially unsaturated compounds (see Chapter 2). This could be due to oxygen (O_2) as well as ozone (O_3) and other oxidants. Experiments in mice suggest that respiratory irritation can be caused by oxidation products of α-pinene and of (+)-limonene, two common constituents of indoor air (Wolkoff et al 1999; Clausen et al 2001). Ozone is a powerful oxidizing agent. It reacts readily with alkenes to form unstable ozonides, which go on to form aldehydes, ketones or carboxylic acids that are more reactive and irritating than their alkene precursors. Short-lived oxidizing radicals such as hydroxyl may also be formed, especially during daylight hours, and these also react with alkenes (Calogirou et al 1999).

Ground-level ozone increases during very hot, sunny weather, especially in cities, since it is photochemically formed in the presence of nitrogen dioxide (from vehicle exhaust) and man-made VOCs.[2] High ozone levels have been epidemiologically correlated with respiratory hospital admission in young children and the elderly, and with asthma morbidity in children (Gielen et al 1997, Yang et al 2003). An increase in outdoor ozone will lead to indoor ozone increases.

In mice, ozone irritancy was marked by shallow breathing followed by a decrease in the respiratory rate. The NOEL of ozone was estimated to be about 1 ppm during 30 minutes exposure. No major effect occurred in resting humans at about 0.4 ppm (Nielsen et al 1999). At 0.5 ppm, ozone did not augment the irritancy of 50 ppm (+)-limonene in mice, suggesting that the NOAEL of ozone is approximately 0.5 ppm (Wilkins et al 2003).

Respiratory parameters were measured in mice for 60 minutes during inhalation exposure to a mixture of 3.4 ppm ozone, and 47 ppm (+)-α-pinene, 51 ppm (+)-limonene, or 465 ppm isoprene. Due to reaction, the ozone concentration at the point of exposure fell to <0.35 ppm. Upper airway irritation was a prominent effect, as was the development of airflow limitation that persisted for at least 45 minutes after exposure. The effects were reversible within six hours, suggesting that terpene oxidation products may have adverse effects of moderate duration on the airways (Rohr et al 2002). In 10 healthy humans, blink frequency increased by 17% following exposure to the vapors of a 10-minute-old mixture of 92 ppb (+)-limonene and 101 ppb ozone. This increase was accompanied by weak eye irritation, presumed to be caused by oxidation products of limonene (Nøjgaard et al 2005). (+)-Limonene itself is not a strong eye irritant.

Of concern in the context of essential oils is the potential of ozone to react with airborne unsaturated terpenes well below their NOEL concentrations to form irritant compounds and sub-micron particles (Wainman et al 2000; Wolkoff et al 2000). This has been demonstrated for α-pinene, β-pinene, camphene, p-cymene and (+)-limonene (Lamorena et al 2007). Increases in the indoor concentrations of sub-micron particles of up to tenfold over controls were observed for (+)-limonene in the presence of ambient ozone (Weschler & Shields 1999). The extent to which ultrafine particles contribute to airway irritation is, however, uncertain. When mice were exposed to a mixture of 0.05 ppm ozone and 35 ppm (+)-limonene for 30 minutes, the respiratory rate decreased by more than 30%; 75% of the SI here was explained by formaldehyde and residual (+)-limonene (Wolkoff et al 2008).

The relevance of these animal data to human exposure to essential oils in the presence of ozone is questionable. The concentration of 0.05 ppm ozone used in the Wolkoff et al (2008) study is in accordance with the classification of 'good air quality' as defined by the Pima County Department of Environmental Quality/US EPA (http://www.airinfonow.com/html/ed_ozone.html accessed April 28th 2012). The 0.8 ppm concentration of ozone used in the Sunil et al (2007) study, however, is greater than the range described as 'very unhealthy' in the same guidelines. At this concentration, ozone alone might be expected to cause significant respiratory distress including difficulty in breathing, cough, phlegm, and reduce peak expiratory flow rate in children with mild asthma, and possibly lower airway inflammation.

Apart from its presence in the atmosphere, ozone is formed in vivo as part of the inflammatory response, being released by neutrophils and other white cells. Although terpene oxidation products may be irritating to bronchial tissues, they represent much less of an irritant threat than ozone. It therefore appears reasonable that inhaled alkenes such as (+)-limonene might afford protection against the damaging effects of endogenous ozone, and may have a beneficial scavenging role in asthma. Inhaled (+)-limonene significantly prevented bronchial obstruction in rats constantly exposed to 125 ppm of (+)-limonene for 7 days by means of an electric scented oil warmer. This was therefore a close approximation to the circumstances of essential oil vaporization (Keinan et al 2005).

In rats, age differences have been observed in responses to (+)-limonene oxidation products. When female rats were exposed to a mixture of 6 ppm (+)-limonene and 0.8 ppm ozone for 3 hours, 2 month-old animals showed endothelial cell hypertrophy, perivascular and pleural edema and thickening of alveolar septal walls. In 18-month-old animals, only patchy accumulation of fluid within septal walls in alveolar sacs and subtle pleural edema were noted (Sunil et al 2007). This shows that the pulmonary inflammatory response is significantly attenuated in older, compared to younger rats.

We caution against the use of monoterpene-rich essential oils in high-ozone environments (Tamas et al 2006). It would be sensible to minimize indoor concentrations of ozone in aromatherapy treatment rooms by removing sources such as photocopying machines, laser printers and ozone-generating air cleaners.[3] As noted above, ozone is itself a respiratory irritant, and low levels are often present in offices. Both high humidity and increased ventilation reduce the irritancy of mixtures of limonene and ozone (Weschler & Shields 2000; Wilkins et al 2003).

Thresholds

Sensory irritation has been found to slow respiration, and the airborne concentration of a chemical required to depress the respiratory rate in animals by 50% (RD_{50}) is accepted as a standard measure of sensory irritation by the American Society for Testing and Materials (ASTM E981-04).[4] Mouse log RD_{50} values correlate well with log (LOAEL) values in humans, suggesting that RD_{50} is a useful predictor of safe public exposure levels (Kuwabara et al 2007). RD_{50} values for various VOCs in mice are shown in Table 6.1.[5] In humans, RD_{50} concentrations of these substances are expected to produce intolerable irritation, and it has been suggested that $0.03 \times RD_{50}$ might be a close approximation to the tolerable threshold value in humans (Schaper et al 1993).

The reported airborne sensory irritation threshold for inhaled (+)-limonene in humans is above 80 ppm, while the NOAEL was estimated to be 100 ppm in mice (Larsen ST et al 2000). These data are consistent with the calculated $RD_{50} \times 0.03$ of 32 ppm for (+)-limonene (see Table 6.1). The American Industrial Hygiene Association has set a limit of 30 ppm for (+)-limonene (0.003%, or 167 mg/m^3) for workers continually exposed to it. The Swedish occupational exposure limit for inhaled terpenes is 150 mg/m^3 (Eriksson et al 1997). This is approximately equivalent to the vapors of 7 drops of essential oil per cubic meter (150 mg (+)-limonene = 0.238 mL (density is 0.842 g/mL). If there are 30 drops per mL (Table 4.6) this makes 7.14 drops).

(+)-Limonene is not a strong eye irritant. The threshold for eye irritation assessed in 12 healthy individuals was 1,250 mg/m^3 (224 ppm). δ-3-Carene had a similar threshold, and α-pinene and α-terpineol were less irritating (Molhave et al 2000).

Four parameters have received much attention as measures of the detectable actions of airborne VOCs. These are the odor threshold (measured in normosmic subjects), nasal pungency threshold (measured in anosmic subjects), eye irritation threshold and nasal localization (left versus right) (measured in both normosmic and anosmic subjects). All four parameters were determined for δ-3-carene, p-cymene, linalool, 1,8-cineole, geraniol and cumene vapors. The three trigeminally mediated thresholds were about three orders of magnitude higher than the corresponding odor thresholds, which ranged between 0.1 and 1.7 ppm. Trigeminal chemosensitivity was comparable between the nose and the eyes, and between normosmics and anosmics. Only 1,8-cineole and δ-3-carene consistently caused eye irritation, at 235 and 1,636 ppm, respectively (Cometto-Muñiz et al 1998a, 1998b).

Good quantitative correlations have been reported between both the human nasal pungency and eye irritation thresholds of various nonreactive VOCs, including esters, aldehydes, ketones, alcohols, carboxylic acids, aromatic hydrocarbons and pyridine, and various calculated physicochemical parameters. These equations have been interpreted as implying that potency is determined by the ease of transport of the VOCs from air into the receptive tissues (Abraham et al 1996, 1998, 2001). An equation for odor thresholds has been derived by including an extra parameter to describe molecular length (Abraham et al 2001).[6]

An essentially similar approach has been taken by Hau et al (1999), who related the nasal pungency of VOCs to measured partition coefficients between octanol and water, and between air and water. A common irritation receptor site was proposed for all VOCs. More recent statistical models for predicting the sensory irritation (logRD$_{50}$) of reactive and nonreactive VOCs using various calculated constitutional, topological, electronic, and other descriptors have been proposed by Luan et al (2006).

Bronchial hyper-reactivity

In people with BHR, also known as bronchial hyper-responsiveness, there is an exaggerated tendency for the smooth muscle of the tracheobronchial tree to contract in response to a given stimulus, compared to normal individuals. (For testing, either methacholine or histamine is commonly used to provoke a response.) The most prominent manifestation of this contraction is a decrease in airway caliber that can be readily measured with a spirometer. BHR is a diagnostic feature of asthma, and is also a concern in other respiratory diseases. In sensitive individuals, BHR may be elicited by dust mites, pollen or other triggers. It is more prevalent in atopic individuals, and in the young and the elderly.

A correlation was found between BHR and the concentration of (+)-limonene in the home in a Swedish epidemiological study including 47 people with asthmatic symptoms and 41 without. Of those with symptoms, 72% were women. Spirometric testing showed correlations between variability of peak expiratory flow and concentrations of α-pinene and δ-3-carene. Terpene concentration correlated with nocturnal breathlessness or tightness of the chest. The maximum concentration of terpenes was very low, $1.0 \, mg/m^3$, with an average of 64% (+)-limonene, 21% α-pinene and 15% δ-3-carene (Norbäck et al 1995). High average concentrations of CO_2 were also noted, presumably due to poor ventilation. None of the correlations reached a level of significance needed to support causation. Respiratory symptoms were more common in dwellings with dust mites, or dampness and microbial growth.

Also in Sweden, sawmill workers exposed to aerosol wood, including α-pinene, β-pinene and δ-3-carene, experienced slightly reduced lung function measured by spirometry (FVC, FEV_1 and MMF, see Table 6.2) although this did not deteriorate upon further acute exposure (Hedenstierna et al 1983).

These reports suggest that some airborne terpenes could induce low-to-moderate BHR, though there is no evidence of allergy. Låstbom et al (1998, 2000, 2003) found that prior skin sensitization to δ-3-carene increased BHR to inhaled δ-3-carene in isolated guinea pig lungs, suggesting an allergic mechanism. However, we could find no other evidence for such an effect, and a review of the literature by Nielsen et al (2007b) found little support for the allergy-promoting effects of indoor VOCs. Neither eugenol nor isoeugenol sensitized the respiratory tract in a mouse immunoglobulin E (IgE) test, even though both compounds elicited positive responses in skin sensitization tests (Hilton et al 1996). IgE is associated with atopy, allergic asthma and allergic rhinitis. However, although it may play a role in eczema, it is not associated with contact dermatitis and type IV skin allergy. In a study of BHR to perfume and fragranced products, no significant association was found with atopy, suggesting that the BHR was not IgE-mediated (Elberling et al 2005). In 11 patients with contact allergy to isoeugenol, there were no adverse respiratory effects from inhaling $1 \, mg/m^3$ of isoeugenol for 60 minutes (Schnuch et al 2011).

Transient receptor potential channels

An important mechanism in both normal sensory irritation and hyper-reactivity is the interaction of inhaled substances with transient receptor potential (TRP) ion channels located in the airways (Table 6.3). These channels are divided into several subfamilies, including the TRPV (vanilloid), the TRPA (ankyrin) and the TRPM (melastatin) groups. The TRPV subfamily includes channels that are critically involved in nociception and thermo-sensing (Vennekens et al 2008).

TRPV1 and TRPA1 especially, are activated by pungent compounds in spices (Iwasaki et al 2008), and such activation may contribute to MCS, asthma, chronic cough, and other conditions exacerbated by airway reactivity. TRPA1 is activated by chlorine, reactive oxygen species (ROS), and noxious constituents of smoke and smog, initiating irritation and airway reflex responses (Bessac & Jordt 2008). Ovalbumin is used to induce experimental allergic airway hyper-reactivity in mice. However, in TRPA1-deficient mice, there was an almost complete lack of BHR, inflammatory cytokine activity and other signs characteristic of asthma following ovalbumin injection (Caceres et al 2009).

TRPV1 is predominantly expressed in the cell membranes of afferent sensory neurons. On stimulation, they release neuropeptides that trigger effects such as airway inflammation, bronchoconstriction and cough (Adcock 2009; Takemura et al 2008). Evidence in experimental animals and patients with airway disease indicates a marked hypersensitivity to cough induced by TRPV1 agonists (Materazzi et al 2009). Patients with allergic rhinitis have an increased itch response to TRPV1 stimulation (Alenmyr et al 2009). Therefore, TRPV1 receptor antagonists have been proposed as therapeutic candidates (Takemura et al 2008).

(−)-Menthol is a TRPV1 receptor antagonist (Mandadi et al 2009) and so may be therapeutic for cough. Inhaled at 30 µg/L, (−)-menthol reduced evoked cough in guinea pigs by 56% (Laude et al 1994). An inhaled mixture of 75% (−)-menthol and 25% 1,8-cineole significantly reduced cough evoked by citric acid compared to pine oil or plain air in healthy individuals (Morice et al 1994).

Table 6.2 Some pulmonary function parameters measurable with a spirometer

FVC	Forced vital capacity	The total amount of air that can be forcibly exhaled after full inspiration
FEV_1	Forced expiratory volume in one second	The amount of air forcibly exhaled in one second
FEV_3	Forced expiratory volume in three seconds	The amount of air forcibly exhaled in three seconds
MEFR	Maximum expiratory flow rate	Maximum forced flow rate during full expiration
MMF	Maximum mid-expiratory flow	The mean forced expiratory flow during the middle half of the FVC
FEF	Forced expiratory flow	Same as MMF
$FEF_{25\%}$	Forced expiratory flow 25%	The mean forced expiratory flow during the first 25% of the FVC
VC	Vital capacity	The maximum volume of air that can be exhaled after a maximal inspiration

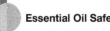

Table 6.3 Examples of substances that interact with transient receptor potential channels

A. TRPV1 agonists (provoke cough, irritant, may cause pain)

Substance	Reference
Capsaicin	Masamoto et al 2009
Citric acid	Canning et al 2006
Cigarette smoke constituents	Andrè et al 2008
Smog constituents	Bessac & Jordt 2008
Allyl isothiocyanate	Ohta et al 2007
Citral	Stotz et al 2008

B. TRPV1 antagonists (inhibit cough, may reduce pain)

Substance	Reference
(−)-Menthol	Mandadi et al 2009

C. TRPA1 agonists (perceived as pungent, may irritate)

Substance	Reference
Allyl isothiocyanate	Iwasaki et al 2008
Carvacrol	Lee et al 2008
Cinnamaldehyde	Iwasaki et al 2008
Citral	Stotz et al 2008
Diallyl disulfide	Koizumi et al 2009
Diallyl trisulfide	Koizumi et al 2009
Perillaldehyde	Bassoli et al 2009
Thymol	Lee et al 2008

D. TRPM8 agonists (produce cold sensation)

Substance	Reference
(−)-Menthol	Masamoto et al 2009
1,8-Cineole	Masamoto et al 2009

Respiratory disease

In light of all of the above, an important question is whether any essential oils are safe to use by inhalation for respiratory disease, especially since BHR is an issue in many such diseases. The use of pine oil in preparations for acute respiratory infections is particularly relevant, since it is almost entirely composed of (+)-limonene, δ-3-carene and α-pinene.

It is possible that exposure to an airborne substance slightly above its safety threshold level might be more damaging over time than relatively short-term inhalation (<1 hour) with greater airborne concentrations, such as seen below. This has been demonstrated with bergamot oil inhalation, which reduced heart rate and blood pressure in 100 healthy subjects when inhaled in the ambient air for one hour, but increased these beyond baseline when inhaled for longer periods of time (Chuang et al 2012).

Acute respiratory tract infections

The most common upper respiratory tract infection is the common cold. Others include sinusitis, pharyngitis, tonsillitis and croup. Acute infections of the lower respiratory tract include acute bronchitis and pneumonia. Some of the symptoms of acute respiratory tract infections are the same as those elicited by VOCs, such as dryness, irritation, tickling, burning and stinging (in the eyes, and the nasal and oral cavities) and headache.

Pinimenthol ointment is an over the counter (OTC) antibacterial expectorant product used for the treatment of upper respiratory infections. Its active ingredients are 20% eucalyptus oil, 17.78% pine needle oil (containing α-pinene, β-pinene, δ-3-carene and (+)-limonene as major constituents) and 2.72% menthol by weight. In a post-marketing observational study, data were collected from 3,060 patients who had used the ointment. The tolerability was rated as excellent or good by 96.7% of physicians and 95.7% of patients. A total of 22 patients (0.7%) reported adverse reactions, which included:

- hypersensitivity skin reactions – 10 (0.33%)
- cough – 6 (0.2%)
- obstructive respiratory tract symptoms – 5 (0.16%)
- hypersensitivity reactions of mucous membranes – 4 (0.13%).

It was concluded that Pinimenthol ointment is well tolerated by both adolescents and adults (Kamin & Kieser 2007). In animal studies, inhaled Pinimenthol vapor reduced bronchospasm by 50% (Schäfer & Schäfer 1981).

In a smaller study, 24 non-smoking adults with common colds were randomly assigned to inhale air with either steam or a mix of 9% eucalyptus oil, 35% camphor and 56% menthol w/w for 1 hour. The mean concentration of aromatic compounds in the inspired air was 56 µg/L, and consisted of 38% camphor, 33% 1,8-cineole, 15% menthol and 14% α-pinene. In the aromatic inhalation group, only 6 out of 22 measured spirometric parameters significantly improved when measured after 20 minutes, and 14 had improved when measured at 60 minutes. These included FVC, FEV_1, FEV_3 $FEF_{25\%}$ and MEFR (see Table 6.2) (Cohen & Dressler 1982).

Vicks VapoRub, Olbas products and Pinimenthol are all widely used OTC medicines with very few reports of adverse reactions when they are used as instructed. However, infants may react adversely. A case of severe respiratory distress was reported in an 18-month-old girl with a supposed upper respiratory infection after Vicks VapoRub was applied under her nose. In subsequent laboratory studies, Vicks VapoRub was found to stimulate mucin secretion and mucociliary transport velocity in vitro in the lipopolysaccharide-inflamed ferret airway in a similar way to that caused by exposure to irritants (Abanses et al 2009). The product's label cautions against using it on children under 2 years of age. Also see Infants and nasal instillation, below.

Chronic obstructive pulmonary disease

COPD describes a group of progressive lung diseases including chronic bronchitis and emphysema. COPD is characterized by difficulty in breathing, due to narrowing of the airways. It is unclear whether the role and mechanisms of hyper-reactivity in COPD are similar to those in patients with asthma, or whether the underlying pathophysiologic abnormalities are different for both diseases (Grootendorst & Rabe 2004).

The application of 7.5 g Vicks VapoRub ointment [a decongestant, cough suppressant and analgesic remedy containing camphor (4.8%), menthol (2.6%) and eucalyptus oil (1.2%)] enhanced lung mucociliary clearance in 12 long-term smokers with chronic bronchitis in a controlled, single-blinded trial. Progressive improvements were recorded at 30 and 60 minutes, but there was no further effect over the following five hours, despite further application of the inunction (Hasani et al 2003).

In a study published in Russian, 96 patients with chronic bronchitis breathed air containing 0.1 mg/m^3 of essential oil vapors for 40 minutes per day. There was a significant increase in mean Tiffeneau index (the ratio between FEV_1 and VC) and a decrease in total serum IgE.[7] Neither the essential oils used nor the duration of therapy is mentioned in the summary (Eremenko et al 1987).

Allergic rhinitis

Seasonal allergic rhinitis, triggered by pollen from trees, grasses, etc., or by fungal spores is the most common allergic disease. Perennial (or persistent) rhinitis may be allergic, where precipitating factors include animal hair, house dust mites or certain chemicals, or it may be non-allergic, where smoke, foods or medications may be responsible. Patients often report a combination of symptoms such as itching, sneezing, rhinorrhea, nasal obstruction, eye redness and tear flow (Remberg et al 2004). A substantial subset of individuals with allergic rhinitis (and 100% of those with non-allergic rhinitis) are hyper-reactive to non-allergic triggers (Shusterman & Murphy 2007).

In an open label pilot study, a nasal spray was used by 12 people with allergic rhinitis and/or asthma, 7 of whom also had allergic conjunctivitis. The spray consisted of 0.4% v/v southernwood (*Artemisia abrotanum*) essential oil and 2.5 μg/mL of various flavonoids from the same plant source (principally centaureidin, castacin and quercetin dimethyl ethers), in 80/20 v/v water/ethanol. The essential oil contained approximately 50% davanone and 40% cineole, but no thujone. The spray was used up to six times daily, either in response to or in anticipation of symptoms, which were subjectively scored by patients. Pronounced symptom relief for 'up to several hours' was experienced in allergic rhinitis, allergic conjunctivitis and bronchial obstruction, and efficacy was judged as being equivalent to that of previously used antihistamines or decongestants. All 12 patients reported a mild-to-moderate stinging sensation lasting a few seconds after using the spray (Remberg et al 2004).

Asthma

Asthma is a chronic disease characterized by acute episodes of reversible airflow obstruction leading to wheezing, coughing and difficulty in breathing. These episodes can be triggered by viral infection, exercise, stress, irritants or allergens. Essential oils are mixtures of volatile compounds, some of which conform to the US EPA definition of VOCs (see above), and represent a possible risk as potential irritants or allergens. Occupational asthma is caused by exposure to inhaled substances, and essential oils could theoretically be causative.

Causative agents

A broad range of chemicals is associated with occupational asthma, particularly those that contain nitrogen, oxygen or sulfur, as part of acid anhydride, isocyanate, amine, imine, and carbonyl groups. Increased risk has also been associated with certain functional groups, including carbonyl and amino, when they occur twice within the same molecule (Jarvis et al 2005). However, this latter description does not apply to any of the compounds listed in our Essential Oil Profiles, Chapter 13. A website that maintains a record of substances considered to have caused occupational asthma lists almost 300, but no essential oils, and only three essential oil constituents (carene, (+)-limonene and styrene) are listed (http://www.nems.nih.gov/Sustainability/Documents/NIH%20Asthma%20Report.pdf, accessed November 24th 2012). There have been two reports of occupational asthma that were reasonably attributed to chronic inhalation of turpentine vapors, although it is likely that in one case, colophony was partly responsible (Hendy et al 1985; Dudek et al 2009). Turpentine vapors contain δ-3-carene and (+)-limonene. (Note that occupational exposure means almost constant exposure during working hours.)

Irritant asthma is also known as reactive airways dysfunction syndrome (RADS). It begins within 24 hours of a single exposure to a high concentration of irritant fumes, and there are no recorded cases of such induction by essential oils or essential oil constituents (Alberts & Do Pico 1996). In irritant asthma, there is damage to the tissues that line the airways, with loss of surface cells and resultant chronic inflammation and airway dysfunction (Currie & Ayers 2004; Demeter et al 2001). A variant of RADS known as irritant induced asthma (IIA) is only evoked after repeated, often moderate exposure for several weeks or months. Controversy exists as to whether moderate irritant exposures can cause asthma, and there may be little difference between IIA and SHR.

The majority of asthma cases are allergic, not irritant. Asthma attacks were induced in a 40-year-old woman, with no previous history of respiratory disease, due to an allergic response to menthol (Dos Santos et al 2001). In spite of this, the anti-inflammatory and bronchodilatory action of menthol strongly suggests a therapeutic effect in asthma in most people (Wright et al 1997; Juergens et al 1998c). In a pilot study, four weeks of menthol inhalation reduced airway excitability in asthma patients (Tamaoki et al 1995).

The allergic response in asthma is due to pro-inflammatory mediators, such as leukotrienes, cytokines, TNF-α and histamine, some of which are derived from arachidonic acid metabolism. There is evidence of essential oils having possible anti-allergic effects. Since chamazulene inhibits the formation of inflammatory prostaglandins and leukotriene B4, essential oils containing it may be therapeutic in allergic asthma or rhinitis (Safayhi et al 1994). Similarly, cedarwood deodar oil has anti-inflammatory effects attributed to the inhibition of leukotriene synthesis and mast cell stabilizing activity (thus preventing histamine release) (Shinde et al 1999a). Ajowan oil, lavender oil, bergapten and eugenol have all shown antihistaminic effects (Kim et al 1997; Kimura & Okuda 1997; Kim & Cho 1999; Boskabady & Shaikhi 2000) and eugenol, α-humulene and β-caryophyllene inhibit TNF-α production (Kim et al 1997;

Passos et al 2006). In a randomized controlled trial (RCT) in asthma patients, 200 mg/day of oral 1,8-cineole reduced airway inflammation, allowing a reduction in oral steroid dosage (Juergens et al 2003). This effect is probably related to the inhibition by 1,8-cineole of both cytokines and arachidonic acid pathways (Juergens et al 1998a, 1998b).

There is one report of anaphylactic shock when a female medical assistant with no history of asthma or reactions to fragrance was assaulted by a patient, who pumped three sprays of an unknown perfume in her face (Lessenger 2001).

In conclusion, there is no evidence that essential oils can *cause* either irritant or allergic asthma, but there is evidence suggestive of therapeutic effects.

Trigger factors

Although changes in air quality can adversely affect the severity of asthma symptoms, identifying causative agents is difficult since there are many possibilities, including particulate matter, spores and VOCs. Among the most clearly established are tobacco smoke, vehicle exhaust, mold and formaldehyde, which is a VOC. An increase in the prevalence of asthma has been correlated with VOC emission from newly painted surfaces in the home (Wieslander et al 1997). When 680 Swedish asthma and/or rhinitis patients were questioned, 79% reported that their symptoms were elicited by either birch twigs or strong-smelling flowers such as hyacinth and lilac (Eriksson et al 1987).

Several reports describe the symptoms of asthma being exacerbated by perfume (Shim & Williams 1986; Bener et al 1996; Baldwin et al 1999; Baur et al 1999). In an RCT of 29 asthmatic adults, exacerbations occurred in 36%, 17% and 8% of patients with severe, moderate and mild asthma, respectively, following inhalation from commercial perfume strips found in magazines (Kumar et al 1995). In a second RCT, subjective symptom reports and objective measures were used to assess the exacerbation of symptoms in moderate asthmatics, mild asthmatics and non-asthmatics. Subjects inhaled a fragranced aerosol product. Moderate asthmatics reported more nasal congestion than non-asthmatics, but there were no exposure-related changes in ocular redness or nasal mucosal swelling in any of the groups. It is suggested that reports of asthmatic symptom exacerbation may in part be due to perception triggered by other sensory cues (Opiekun et al 2003).

No literature describing the exacerbation of asthma symptoms by essential oils could be found, but seven people responded to an online request for information. The consensus from these individuals is that it is not uncommon for any strong fragrance, whether synthetic or natural, to induce an asthma attack, but all seven claimed to be more susceptible to commercial fragrances than essential oils.[8] The severity of an attack is strongly linked to the ambient concentration of essential oil or fragrance, and if this is low enough no crisis will be provoked. Of the seven individuals, one was particularly susceptible to lavender oil and one to geranium oil (Salaam Attar, Isabelle Aurel, Julia Glazer, Cathy Miller, Judith Miller, Elise Pearlstine, Stephanie Vinson, private communications, 2006).

Brochospasm

Bronchospasm is a problem in many respiratory conditions, and there is ex vivo evidence of bronchodilatory effects for essential oils of ajowan, anise, angelica root, basil, clove, sweet fennel and rose (Reiter & Brandt 1985; Boskabady & Shaikhi 2000; Boskabady & Ramazani-Assari 2001; Boskabady et al 2004, 2006); similarly, for the constituents carvacrol and 1,8-cineole (Boskabady & Jandaghi 2003, Coelho-de-Souza et al 2005). Although inhaled isothiocyanates and other sulfur compounds are pungent and irritant (Table 6.3), when given orally they have anti-asthmatic effects in mice, inhibiting bronchospasm (Dorsch et al 1984, 1987, 1988). In treating asthma, oral administration may therefore be more effective and less risky than methods involving inhalation for certain essential oils.

However, there is evidence that rubbing ointments may be useful. In a review of 165 adolescents with asthma, 127 (77%) used the bronchodilating inhaler albuterol as the first treatment for their last asthma attack, and 18 (11%) used rubbing ointments. Both groups were similar in asthma severity, mean age, gender and ethnicity. Subjects in the rubbing ointment group said they were less likely than those in the albuterol group to have made an emergency department (ED) visit over the past 12 months or over their lifetime. After controlling for asthma severity, the use of rubbing ointment was therefore associated with lower asthma morbidity as measured by ED visits (Reznik et al 2004).

Multiple chemical sensitivity

MCS is a controversial diagnosis and, while there are many theories, no established physiological basis has been identified for MCS (Lacour et al 2005). The symptoms are diverse and ephemeral, and no controlled testing has been found that reliably reproduces them (Staudenmayer 2001). This is in spite of large numbers of people self-reporting illness, although the *symptom* of feeling ill from chemical odors may be more common than the *syndrome* of MCS (Miller CS 1996).

MCS (re-named by the WHO in 1996 as 'idiopathic environmental intolerance') is a widespread problem that crosses all demographic groups (Caress et al 2002; Kreutzer et al 1999). A telephone survey of 1,054 randomly selected USA residents found 11.2% reporting an unusual hypersensitivity to common chemical products, including perfume, and 2.5% who had been medically diagnosed as having MCS (Caress & Steinemann 2004). In a similar survey of 4,046 Californian residents, 15.9% reported hypersensitivity to common chemicals, and 6.3% disclosed an MCS diagnosis. Of the 461 (11.4%) respondents who reported an asthma diagnosis, 19.0% had also been diagnosed with MCS, and 4.6% reported feeling 'very sick' when exposed to cologne, aftershave or perfume (Kreutzer et al 1999). Consistently, more women than men consider themselves odor-intolerant (Bell et al 1993; Kreutzer et al 1999; Ross et al 1999; Caress et al 2002; Johansson et al 2005; Bailer et al 2008).

It is widely accepted that chemical exposure can cause adverse effects and even disease. MCS symptoms are initially induced by acute or chronic exposure to a chemical substance, and in this sense MCS is identical to IIA. However, people with MCS become sensitive to very low concentrations, and progressively exhibit a multitude of symptoms in response to an increasing number of chemicals (Miller CS 1996). The substance inducing susceptibility is commonly an organic solvent, a pesticide, or cigarette smoke, and only very rarely a fragrance (Ross et al 1999).

However, perfume is a common trigger. Among a group of individuals with MCS, the most common triggers were cleaning products (88.4%), tobacco smoke (82.6%), perfume (81.2%), pesticides (81.2%) and vehicle exhaust (72.5%) (Caress et al 2002). Other commonly reported triggers include air fresheners, fresh paint, new carpet and formaldehyde (Gibson & Vogel 2009). Objective assessment may not validate self-reported susceptibility. In a double-blind study, 20 MCS patients were exposed to either plain air or to airborne concentrations of the substances to which they were susceptible. Both exposures were masked with one of three essential oils, and lasted for periods varying from 15 minutes to several hours. The patients could not distinguish actual exposure from sham exposure, nor did their reported physical symptoms, for up to 72 hours, correlate with actual exposure (Staudenmayer et al 1993).

MCS is thought by some to be psychosomatic, and either related to excessive concerns about environmental toxins, or to stress, either one leading to an increased association between odors and disease (Bailer et al 2008). It would not be surprising if psychological stress could increase sensitivity to inhaled substances. In mice, stress intensifies skin reactions to topically applied substances (Saint-Mezard 2003a, 2003b). Even low doses markedly amplify gene expression related to neurogenic inflammation (Nakano 2007). An olfactory-limbic 'neural sensitization' mechanism has been proposed for MCS, in which there is a progressive amplification of responsivity with repeated exposure, even to very low concentrations (Bell et al 1997).

Meggs (1993) has proposed that MCS is a disorder of the regulation of neurogenic inflammation. (As a clinician, he had seen inflammatory lesions in the nasal mucous membranes of people with MCS.) Neurogenic inflammation is a general term describing the local release from afferent neurons of inflammatory mediators, such as substance P. Preclinical studies have associated neurogenic inflammation with airway symptoms, possibly due to epithelial damage (Barnes PJ 1992).

In a Japanese study, people with self-reported MCS had significantly higher plasma levels of substance P, vasoactive intestinal peptide and nerve growth factor (NGF) than did healthy controls. After 15 minutes of inhaling 3.13–3.42 mg/m^3 of VOCs from fresh paint (while sitting in a freshly painted room) plasma levels of the same substances were even further elevated in the MCS group, as was histamine, but not in the control group. For example, mean NGF levels after VOC inhalation were 156 in the control group, and 1,696 in the MCS group (Kimata 2004). Interestingly, odorant inhalation suppressed stress-induced cutaneous allergic reactions in female volunteers, by preventing an increase in plasma levels of substance P (Hosoi et al 2003).

The relationship between odor perception and symptomatic reaction is complex, and the perception of a fragrance is partly determined by context and expectation. The inhaled irritancy of three odorants was rated as significantly more intense by subjects when given a verbal negative bias by researchers (Dalton 1999). People with MCS may perceive odors differently, even though their olfactory acuity may be no greater than normal. Significantly more women with MCS rated common household smells as unpleasant than either men with MCS or women without MCS (Ojima et al 2002).

A range of factors has been proposed to explain MCS, including immunological, neuropsychological, sociological and toxicological, none of which work adequately in isolation. In spite of the frustrations in understanding the mechanisms involved, MCS is increasingly recognized as a disease entity (Winder 2002). In a survey of 691 Danish GPs, the cause of MCS was perceived as multi-factorial by 64.3%, as somatic/biologic by 27.6%, and psychological by 7.2% (Skovbjerg et al 2009).

Sensory hyper-reactivity

SHR has been proposed as a subdivision of MCS, specifically applying when cough and other airway symptoms are present (Millqvist et al 2005). SHR is characterized by upper and lower airway symptoms induced by inhaled substances such as those listed above. Common symptoms include rhinitis, hoarseness, coughing, phlegm, dyspnea and eye irritation, with some individuals also experiencing fatigue and headache. This picture could suggest allergic rhinitis and/or asthma, but in SHR there is little or no response to antihistamines or inhaled corticosteroids, no bronchial obstruction after provocation, and no sign of IgE-mediated allergy (Millqvist 2006). However, there is a correlation with an increase in NGF immediately following capsaicin exposure, which is consistent with the concept of increased neuronal sensitization (Millqvist et al 2005).

In two similar single-blind RCTs, patients with hyper-reactive respiratory symptoms were exposed to either perfumed or unperfumed air. It was concluded that eye irritation, cough and shortness of breath could be provoked by perfume in these patients (Millqvist & Löwhagen 1996; Millqvist et al 1999).

Neither MCS nor SHR sufferers in general have an unusually acute sense of smell, and research in Sweden has focused on the possible involvement of increased trigeminal sensitivity. A series of small-scale trials lends support to this idea, with greater susceptibility in self-diagnosed SHR sufferers to inhaled capsaicin, which is non-odorous, but induces cough through a trigeminal mechanism (Millqvist et al 1998; Millqvist 2000; Ternesten-Hasséus et al 2006). In 17 patients with a minimum of 12 months history of SHR, 15 tested positive to capsaicin inhalation, while 16 self-reported perfume and 14 reported fragrant flowers as triggers (Ternesten-Hasséus et al 2007). Since women more commonly report odor intolerance, it is noteworthy that they have a greater capsaicin cough sensitivity than men (Yamasaki et al 2007).

Neither capsaicin sensitivity nor self-perceived odor intolerance necessarily indicate MCS or SHR. In one report, only 16 of 103 people with self-reported SHR showed an increased sensitivity to capsaicin (Johansson et al 2006). In a random sample of 401 Swedish teenagers, 11 tested positive to capsaicin, and 3 of these (0.9% of the total) were also classed as hyper-reactive to 'chemicals and scents' by questionnaire (Andersson et al 2008). There are probably overlaps between allergic rhinitis, IIA and SHR (Baldwin et al 1999).

Olfactory hypersensitivity

Migraine is the only disease associated with a pronounced increase in olfactory sensitivity. Even between episodes, migraine sufferers show greater olfactory hypersensitivity to vanillin than controls (Snyder & Drummond 1997). They also display abnormal cerebral activation patterns in response to olfactory stimulation (Demarquay et al 2008).

Of 807 people with migraine, 41.2% experienced osmophobia (an aversion to smells) during an attack, compared with none of 198 people with tension headaches (Zanchin et al 2007). 'Perfume or odor' was reported as a migraine trigger in 45.5% of 673 patients: 22.7% occasionally, 10.2% frequently, and 12.6% very frequently (Kelman 2004). In an earlier study, 11 of 50 migraineurs (22%) reported that either pleasant or unpleasant odors could precipitate an attack (Blau & Solomon 1985). This suggests that great care is required in treating migraine sufferers with essential oils.

There may be a hormonal factor in migraine. Before puberty and following menopause, migraine incidence is the same for both sexes, but in women of reproductive age it is approximately three times greater than in men (Raña-Martínez 2008). In many women, migraines coincide with menstruation (Crawford et al 2009). The relationship between hormones and olfaction, however, is complex. On average, women have a more acute sense of smell than men, though the difference is not great. Fluctuations of olfactory acuity with menstrual cycle have been observed, but the data are inconsistent, and may vary between odorants. Correlations between olfactory acuity and pregnancy are similarly inconclusive (Doty & Cameron 2009). The shared association of nausea and vomiting in both migraine and pregnancy may be due to a common genetic/hormonal mechanism (Heinrichs 2002; Wang et al 2008).

It has been experimentally demonstrated that marked increases in olfactory acuity are possible after repeated exposures to odorants in people with average baseline sensitivity to those compounds. An average increased sensitivity of five orders of magnitude was observed, but only in females of reproductive age (not men, nor older or younger females). This suggests that the olfactory-induction process may be associated with female reproductive behaviors such as pair bonding and kin recognition (Dalton et al 2002). The same phenomenon was observed by Diamond et al (2005), who reported that the increased sensitivity only occurred when the women consciously focused on what they were smelling, and only when odorants were used at no more than just-perceivable levels. This 'focused attention' is reminiscent of the correlation between 'modern health worries' and MCS observed by Bailer et al (2008).

Pulmonary toxicity

Perilla oil contains perilla ketone, and unusual chemotypes may contain the related substituted furans, egomaketone and isoegomaketone. These are all potent agents that, when consumed, can cause fluid build-up in the lungs of animals. This lung-specific toxicity is of most concern to farmers whose cattle or sheep may graze on the perilla plant. Pulmonary toxicity has also been induced by perilla ketone, both in cattle and in laboratory rodents, when given by ip or iv injection (Wilson et al 1977). There are no reports of perilla oil causing any problems in humans, and it is extensively used in food flavorings in Japan (Wilson 1979). However, we believe that perilla oil should be used with caution due to its potential for pulmonary toxicity.

There is one report of an association between niaouli oil inhalation and acute respiratory infection (lipid pneumonia, a potentially serious condition) in a 4 month-old infant (Decocq et al 1996). The authors caution against essential oil inhalation by infants, a caution with which we concur.

The respiratory system may be a conduit for toxicity that manifests in other parts of the body. For example, male mice were allowed to breathe airborne volatile constituents emitted by commercial cologne and air freshener products for up to one hour, once or twice a day for two days. Some animals exhibited tremors, stupor, coma, convulsions, twitching, limb paralysis or difficulty in breathing. It was suggested that this test might have a predictive role for common sensitivities to products containing essential oils in humans (Anderson & Anderson 1997b). These mostly neurotoxic effects were presumably induced by significant airborne concentrations.

In animals, chronic inhalation of terpinyl acetate caused changes in the CNS, blood and liver. The minimum active concentration was $10 \, mg/m^3$ or 1.25 ppm (Rumiantsev et al 1993). Citral was not fetotoxic in rats when administered to females at up to 68 ppm as an aerosol/vapor mixture for 6 hours per day for 10 days, but it was maternally toxic at this level. The NOAEL for maternal toxicity was 34 ppm ($212 \, mg/m^3$) (Gaworski et al 1992).

Infants and nasal instillation

Studies have shown that non-convulsant CNS effects are likely following inhalation of 1,8-cineole (Kovar et al 1987; Stimpfl et al 1995). Instillation, or introducing drops into the nose, can result in serious consequences, as significant quantities can be absorbed through a combination of oral ingestion, inhalation and local absorption. Nasal instillation of Olbas Oil (which contains approximately 45% 1,8-cineole and 20% menthol) caused severe respiratory distress in a 4-month-old boy, who immediately collapsed, breathing rapidly, turning blue, wheezing and coughing. He recovered fully within a week (Wyllie et al 1994). An almost identical case involving a 6-month-old child, mistakenly given Olbas Oil instead of saline drops, was reported by Crandon & Thompson (2006).

There are other reports of non-fatal, but serious toxicity in children who have had solutions containing (−)-menthol (4 cases), or 1,8-cineole (9 cases) nasally instilled (Melis et al 1989). Their ages ranged from 1 month to 3 years 9 months. The effects of poisoning included irritated mucous membranes, rapid heart rate, labored breathing, nausea, vomiting, vertigo, muscular weakness, drowsiness and coma. The most serious symptoms, including coma, were seen in a child of under two months, who had 1 mL of an unspecified menthol solution instilled into his nose. Some of the others suffered no more than mucous membrane irritation.

In most cases the drops were given accidentally, instead of another, safer preparation. No details were given regarding the amounts of (−)-menthol or 1,8-cineole administered, so it is difficult to extrapolate to essential oils. Clearly, peppermint and eucalyptus oil would be implicated, and these are among the oils commonly used as decongestants. Other essential oils, administered in this way, could cause similar problems, and we recommend that peppermint, cornmint, and any oil with 40% or more 1,8-cineole should not be applied to the face of infants or children, or otherwise inhaled by them.

The action of (−)-menthol and 1,8-cineole on the airways of young children can be partly explained by the fact that both substances are TRPM8 agonists (Table 6.3), producing a sensation of cold, though (−)-menthol is more potent (Masamoto et al 2009). Either cold air or (−)-menthol slowed respiration in guinea pigs, due to stimulation of cold receptors (Orani et al 1991). (−)-Menthol inhalation slows respiration in newborn dogs for the same reason (Sant'Ambrogio et al 1992), and in premature infants respiration is either slowed or temporarily ceases (Javorka et al 1980).

Summary

- Some essential oils contain compounds which are a potential cause of eye and airway irritation.
- The essential oil constituents most commonly cited as irritants are the monoterpenes α-pinene, β-pinene, δ-3-carene and (+)-limonene.
- In spite of the fact that these four compounds can cause BHR, the clinical data suggest that these compounds, and essential oils containing them, may be therapeutic when used to treat respiratory disease.
- It is possible that long-term, ambient inhalation of essential oils is more insidious than short-term inhalation, and duration of exposure is at least as important as concentration.
- Levels of environmental fragrance should be maintained at minimal concentrations.
- There are increased risks to young children and the elderly, and in the presence of high levels of ambient ozone. Those most at risk may also include aromatherapists.
- Concentrations of ozone in aromatherapy treatment rooms should be minimized by removing sources such as photocopying machines, laser printers and ozone-generating air cleaners.
- Adequate ventilation, and adequate humidity levels in dry environments, help to minimize airway irritation.
- Essential oils are not a significant *cause* of respiratory disease, but inhaled fragrant molecules can *trigger* attacks in people with asthma or MCS.
- Anyone with diagnosed asthma or COPD, or anyone reporting airway hyper-reactivity to fragrances, paint fumes or turpentine should be wary of direct inhalation of any essential oil vapor.
- We recommend a maximum of 1% of essential oil for aromatherapy massage in those with diagnosed asthma, or anyone reporting airway hyper-reactivity to fragrances, paint fumes or turpentine and in atopic children.

- Since odors can trigger migraine, great care is required in treating migraine sufferers with essential oils.
- Perilla is the only essential oil suspected of causing pulmonary toxicity.
- Essential oils with a high content of menthol or 1,8-cineole should not be applied to the faces of infants or children.

Notes

1. One of these compounds, styrene, can occur in cassia oil at up to 0.1%.
2. The stratospheric ozone layer extends upward from about 6 to 30 miles, and shields the Earth's surface from solar ultraviolet radiation. However, ground-level (tropospheric) ozone is a pollutant that is a potential hazard to human, animal and plant health. It is a major component of urban smog (www.epa.gov/ozone accessed June 27th 2012).
3. See www.epa.gov/iaq/pubs/ozonegen.html for EPA comments on the benefits and risks of ozone-generating air cleaners.
4. Inhaled gases can cause respiratory depression by irritating (stimulating) nerves in the nasal cavity. Respiratory depression, in turn, decreases the rate of delivery of those gases to the stimulated nerves, potentially leading to a complex feedback response. The ordinary differential equation model describes the dosimetry of these reactive gases in the respiratory tract, with particular focus on the physiology of the upper respiratory tract, and on the neurological control of respiration rate due to signalling from the irritant-responsive nerves in the nasal cavity. The ventilation equation is altered to account for an apparent change in dynamics between the initial ventilation decrease and the recovery to steady state as seen in formaldehyde exposure data. Further, the model is evaluated and improved through optimization of particular parameters to describe formaldehyde-induced respiratory response data and through sensitivity analysis. The model predicts the formaldehyde data well, and hence it is thought to be a reasonable description of the physiological system of sensory irritation. The model is also expected to translate well to other irritants (Yokley et al 2008).
5. The differences between α-pinene enantiomers and between β-pinene enantiomers may be due to differences in binding to a sensory irritant receptor (Nielsen et al 2005).
6. When homologous series of acetate esters, alcohols, aldehydes and carboxylic acids were studied, eye irritation could not be detected beyond certain chain lengths. Decyl acetate, 1-undecanol, dodecanal, and heptanoic acid were the shortest homologs that failed to produce eye irritation. These cut-off points have been rationalized in terms of molecular size, where increasing chain length supposedly renders them unable to interact effectively with human chemesthetic receptors (Cometto-Muñiz & Cain 1991; Cometto-Muñiz et al 2005b, 2007).
7. Values of 100 x FEV_1/VC below 75% are considered to indicate abnormal pulmonary ventilation.

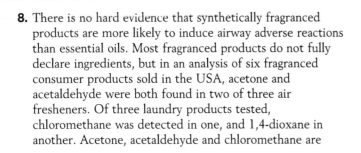

8. There is no hard evidence that synthetically fragranced products are more likely to induce airway adverse reactions than essential oils. Most fragranced products do not fully declare ingredients, but in an analysis of six fragranced consumer products sold in the USA, acetone and acetaldehyde were both found in two of three air fresheners. Of three laundry products tested, chloromethane was detected in one, and 1,4-dioxane in another. Acetone, acetaldehyde and chloromethane are respiratory irritants; acetaldehyde and 1,4-dioxane are carcinogens, and chloromethane is a refrigerant, no longer used because of its high toxicity. Quantities were not determined (Steinemann 2009). In a similar report, the constituents most commonly found in the microenvironments of tested consumer products such as perfumes, soaps and deodorants were, in descending order, toluene, methylene chloride, ethanol and 1,1,1-trichloroethane (Wallace et al 1991).

The cardiovascular system

7

The cardiovascular system comprises the heart, the blood, and the vessels through which blood flows. The heart is a pump whose function is to ensure that the body tissues receive adequate blood to supply their need for oxygen, glucose, fats, amino acids and other nutrients. In addition, the rate of blood flow out of the tissues must be sufficient to remove waste products and toxins, and to prevent fluid accumulation.

The heart

There are very few known effects of essential oils on the heart, except when taken in overdose. Cardiovascular consequences of human poisoning from various essential oils include irregular heartbeat (tansy), rapid heartbeat (wintergreen), cardiovascular collapse (eucalyptus) and congestive heart failure (wormwood) (Eimas 1938; Gurr & Scroggie 1965; Grieve 1978; Weisbord et al 1997). Damage to the heart has been seen after fatal doses of wintergreen and wormseed oils (Eimas 1938; Opdyke 1976 p. 713–715).

Heart activity is dependent upon the movement of calcium ions into myocardial cells, and substances that inhibit this influx, the so-called calcium channel blockers, have a depressant effect on the heart. They act on slow calcium channels to reduce contractility and electrical conduction in the heart. They also act on vascular smooth muscle to reduce vascular tone (see Calcium channel blockade below). Bisabolol, carvacrol, β-caryophyllene oxide, eugenol, (+)-carvone, (−)-menthol, thymol and possibly (E)-anethole, block calcium channels in cardiovascular cell membranes (Schafer et al 1986; Teuscher et al 1989; Sidell et al 1990; Sensch et al 2000; Damiani et al 2004; Magyar et al 2004). The same effect has been observed with peppermint oil (Hills & Aaronson 1991). In addition, β-caryophyllene oxide strongly inhibited potassium ion fluxes, while eugenol exerted a smaller effect (Sensch et al 2000).

Thujone had a depressant action on the isolated rabbit heart, affecting both systole and diastole. A preliminary fall in pressure was followed by a rise, and these were explained in terms of a direct action on heart muscle, and an action on the vasomotor center, respectively (Florey and Student, 1968).

Heart rate and rhythm

A depressant effect on dog heart has been observed following the iv administration of 1–2 mL per kg doses of a "saturated solution" of sage oil in 33° alcohol (equivalent to 18.9% v/v ethanol) (Caujolle & Franck 1945a). Geraniol, thymol and (−)-carvone all had a depressant action on frog heart function, when a 10% aqueous emulsion was injected into the femoral lymphatic sac, e.g., geraniol has an effect at 180 mg/kg or higher, but not at 90 mg/kg (Lysenko 1962). These findings imply that only high doses of these constituents affect the heart. Camphor produced a rise in heart rate in isolated rabbit heart, via a direct effect on heart muscle (Christensen and Lynch 1937). In humans, the predominant effect on the heart appears to be depressant. However, one report suggests that camphor can sensitize the heart to epinephrine (adrenaline) (Saratikov et al 1957).

The only known negative effects from essential oils in moderate doses apply to menthol and peppermint. Mentholated cigarettes and peppermint confectionery have been linked to cardiac fibrillation in patients prone to the condition while being maintained on quinidine, a stabilizer of heart rhythm (Thomas JG 1962). This might be explained by an interaction between menthol and quinidine, but no precedent for this could be found. Bradycardia (slowing of heartbeat) has been reported in an individual addicted to menthol cigarettes (Luke 1962). Menthol-rich oils (cornmint and peppermint) should probably be avoided altogether in cases of cardiac fibrillation.

Blood pressure

Pressure in the blood circulatory system varies according to the phases of the cardiac cycle, and the proximity of the different vessels to the heart. It is regulated principally by the rate and force of contraction of the heart, by the caliber of the resistance vessels, mainly the arterioles, and by the volume of blood in the system. Blood pressure (BP) is at its highest in the aorta and other main arteries when the ventricles contract (in systole) and is at its lowest when the ventricles are relaxed (in diastole), as well as in the veins and venules throughout the cardiac cycle.

There is an ongoing debate about the relationship between BP and cardiovascular disease. It is now thought that the risk of cardiovascular disease begins when systolic and diastolic pressures are 115 and 75 mmHg, respectively, and that this doubles with each increment of 20 and 10 mmHg, respectively. It has also been suggested that individuals with systolic and diastolic readings of 120–139 and/or 80–89 mmHg, respectively, should

be classified as prehypertensive, and may need to adopt health-promoting lifestyle changes (Chobanian et al 2003).

Any excessively elevated or prolonged increase in BP (hypertension) is undesirable because it increases the work of the heart and can lead to irreversible changes to organs including the blood vessels, heart, kidneys and brain. The most common form of hypertension (in 90–95% of cases) is known as 'primary' or 'essential' hypertension, where no single causal factor can be identified. Rather, a number of predisposing or risk factors are likely to be present, including smoking, excessive drinking of alcohol, a stressful life, poor diet and lack of exercise. Some people have a genetic predisposition to hypertension (Coy 2005; Imumorin et al 2005).

Temporary fluctuations in BP are normal and harmless in a healthy individual. They may be due to a variety of factors such as psychosocial demands or changes in physical activity. It should be stressed that psychological factors can play a role in raising or lowering BP (Whyte 1983; Linden & Moseley 2006). Substance use can also lead to the elevation of BP, salt and caffeine being two examples. In a hypertensive individual, though small fluctuations may not be harmful, regular, moderate increases can be damaging.

Animal and ex vivo studies

The essential oils most commonly cited in aromatherapy texts as being contraindicated in hypertension are hyssop, thyme, rosemary and sage (Table 7.1). Similar advice is repeated in other books and on many websites, but very little supporting evidence could be found in the scientific literature. The original source for this information appears to be Valnet (1990), first published in French in 1964. In this text, the four essential oils are claimed to be hypertensive, and in each case two references are given. One is Caujolle & Franck (1944b), but this is a mistake since this paper concerns lavender, lavandin and spike lavender oils only. The other reference is a thesis by R. Cazal, published in 1944. We were not able to locate a copy of this. Data on these and other essential oils are outlined below.

Table 7.1 Essential oils reputed to raise blood pressure in aromatherapy texts

Essential oil	Valnet 1964	Tisserand 1977	Franchomme & Pénöel 1990	Battaglia 1997	Davis 1999	Pitman 2004
Black pepper	–	–	–	–	√	–
Camphor	–	√	–	–	–	–
Eucalyptus	–	–	–	–	–	√
Hyssop	√	√	–	√	√	√
Peppermint	–	–	√	–	√	–
Rosemary	√	√	–	√	√	√
Sage	√	–	–	√	√	√
Thyme	√	–	–	√	–	√

Valnet 1964 p. 220, 260, 272, 288; Tisserand 1977 p. 201–204; Franchomme & Pénöel 1990 p. 374; Battaglia 1997 p. 295; Davis P 1999 p. 153; Pitman 2004 p. 343.

Convulsants

There is a complex relationship between convulsants and BP (Freeman 2006). Intracranial hypertension can lower the seizure threshold, and for example in eclampsia, both hypertension and seizures are seen. In a report of nine distressed neonates whose BP was continuously recorded, three had generalized seizures, during which mean aortic pressure increased dramatically (Lou & Friis-Hansen 1979). However, a sudden drop in BP can also precipitate seizures (Agrawal & Durity 2006).

When injected iv in convulsant doses, both wormwood oil and hyssop oil produce a sudden drop, then rise in BP, the convulsions coinciding with BP elevation. After apparently extensive testing in cats, Coombs & Pike (1931) concluded that 'oil of absinthe' (wormwood oil) produced a hypotension that initiated the seizures, and that the muscular contraction of the seizures caused the spike in hypertension. BP dropped below baseline after a seizure, and did not rise until the next seizure took place. In some instances, doses below the convulsive threshold caused a fall in BP that was so precipitous it was fatal.

The type of wormwood oil used in this study is not stated, but the commercially available oil was the β-thujone CT (Parry 1922 p. 288; Guenther 1949–1952 vol 5 p. 494; Arctander 1960 p. 661–663). The wormwood oil was diluted to 5% v/v in 95% ethanol, and the minimum convulsive dose was 0.08 mL/kg bw of the solution, so 0.004 mL/kg (3.6 mg/kg) for the oil. Clonic convulsions were produced, with tonic limb extension appearing at just under a lethal dose (Pike et al 1929). Similarly, injecting dogs iv with 1–2 mL of a 'saturated solution' of hyssop oil in 33° alcohol resulted in an initial fall in BP, followed by a rise, accompanied by clonic convulsions, both lasting 3–4 minutes (Caujolle & Franck 1945b).

The convulsant constituents of wormwood oil and hyssop oil are the thujones and pinocamphones, respectively. In cats, camphor caused an initial fall in BP lasting 2–10 minutes, followed by a rise of 8–30 mmHg above normal and lasting for up to 30 minutes, when given intravenously at only 5 mg/kg (Christensen & Lynch 1937). Considering that this was a sub-convulsant dose, the longer hypertensive phase is interesting. However, whether camphor is hypotensive or hypertensive has been debated for more than a century. Topically applied camphor is likely to cause local vasodilation (Futami 1984).

Sage oil, which can cause convulsions, contains varying amounts of camphor and 1,8-cineole though camphor usually predominates. When ~1 g/kg of alcohol saturated with sage oil was given iv to dogs there was no increase in BP, and in some cases a slight fall was observed (Caujolle & Franck 1945a). An intravenously administered aqueous-alcoholic extract of sage caused a moderate but prolonged hypotensive effect in cats (Todorov et al 1984).

In early 20th century reports, benzyl alcohol apparently caused hypotension and convulsions in experimental animals (MMWR 1982). In low birth weight infants exposed to benzyl alcohol, toxic symptoms included respiratory distress and hypotension (Benda et al 1986; Sreenan et al 2001). Many infants also had central neural depression or seizures (Anon 1982).

Calcium channel blockade

One proven way of lowering BP is to reduce the flow of calcium ions into heart and vascular muscle using calcium channel blockers. Apart from relaxing the heart, these drugs also reduce the tone of the arteries and arterioles, thereby decreasing the resistance to blood being pumped by the heart. Peppermint oil and its major constituent (–)-menthol both have calcium channel blocking actions. This explains why (–)-menthol dilates systemic blood vessels after iv administration, and why peppermint oil reduces smooth muscle spasm in the gut (Rakieten & Rakieten 1957; Grigoleit & Grigoleit 2005b; Hawthorn et al 1988; Hills & Aaronson 1991).

A hypotensive action has been reported for thyme oil in a Russian paper (Kulieva 1980). This is consistent with the calcium channel blocking actions of its major constituents thymol and carvacrol (Magyar et al 2004), and the hypotensive action of carvacrol (Aydin et al 2007) and of topically applied thymol (Futami 1984). We could find no information on peppermint oil and BP, but topically applied menthol reduces blood pressure for a short time through an effect on local tissues (Futami 1984; Ragan et al 2004), and the calcium channel blocking effect of both peppermint oil and menthol (cited above, under The heart) makes a hypertensive action unlikely.

In mice, cinnamon bark oil caused variable changes in BP after ip dosing at 100 mg/kg (Powers et al 1961). Cinnamaldehyde was hypotensive when administered to anesthetized dogs at 5–10 mg/kg iv. In guinea pigs, a lower dose of 1 mg/kg iv caused a small fall in BP. The authors inferred that this action was mainly due to peripheral vasodilation mediated by calcium channel blockade, similar to that caused by papaverine (Harada & Yano 1975). In a recent study, a range of 1 μM to 1 mM of cinnamaldehyde dose-dependently relaxed prostaglandin $F_{2\alpha}$, norepinephrine and KCl-stimulated rat aorta. It was suggested that a combination of endothelium-dependent and -independent effects were responsible. One of the latter mechanisms is thought to involve the blocking of calcium channels (Yanaga et al 2006).

Undefined mechanisms

Other essential oil constituents with hypotensive actions caused by direct vasodilation include, in order of decreasing potency, linalool, citronellol, nerol, geraniol, α-terpineol and 1,8-cineole. These compounds caused a 25% fall in systolic pressure, in doses from 9.2–26.3 mg/kg, when administered iv to dogs in an emulsion (Northover & Verghese 1962). Intravenous 1,8-cineole was dose-dependently hypotensive in normotensive rats at 0.3–10 mg/kg, and decreased heart rate at the highest dose (Lahlou et al 2002a). Soares MC et al (2005) reported that 1,8-cineole probably has a calcium channel blocking action. Spike lavender oil (28.0–34.9% 1,8-cineole) injected iv in dogs resulted in a slight reduction in BP, followed by a rapid return to normal (Caujolle & Franck 1944b). The essential oil of *Hyptis fruticosa* was hypotensive in normotensive rats at 5–40 mg/kg iv, and caused concentration-dependent relaxation of phenylephrine-stimulated isolated rat superior mesenteric artery at 1–1000 μg/mL (Santos et al 2007). Although this oil is not commercially available, it is interesting to note that it contains 16.8% 1,8-cineole, as well as 12.3% bicyclogermacrene and 11.3% α-pinene (Menezes et al 2007). The action of eucalyptus oil will undoubtedly reflect that of 1,8-cineole.

Single iv injections of eugenol (1–10 mg/kg) elicited immediate and dose-dependent hypotension in rats (Lahlou et al 2004), and similar results were found for eugenol-rich *Ocimum gratissimum* leaf oil when given to hypertensive rats (Interaminense et al 2005). Intravenous administration of either 1–20 mg/kg of *Alpinia zerumbet* leaf oil (~40% terpinen-4-ol) or 1–10 mg/kg of terpinen-4-ol, elicited dose-dependent decreases in mean aortic pressure in rats (Lahlou et al 2002b). The hypotension induced by 1,8-cineole, eugenol or tepinen-4-ol appears to be due to direct vascular relaxation, rather than by affecting sympathetic tone. Northover & Verghese (1962) reached the same conclusion.

Both geranium and lavender oils lowered BP in dogs when administered iv in a 'saturated alcoholic solution' at 1–2 g/kg (Clerc et al 1934). Similarly, an aqueous suspension of carrot seed oil, injected iv into dogs, produced dose-dependent falls in BP (Bhargava et al 1967). Taget oil was hypotensive in dogs, reducing BP by up to 50% for 45 minutes after an iv dose of 50 mg/kg (Chandhoke & Ghatak 1969). Essential oils of angelica (type unspecified), calamus, zedoary and tomar seed each caused a transient fall in BP and heart rate when injected iv into dogs at 0.01–0.05 mL/kg (Chopra et al 1954). Intravenous doses of 0.2–1.6 mg/kg black seed oil dose-dependently decreased arterial BP in rats (El Tahir et al 1993). This action is in part due to the main constituent, thymoquinone, which counteracted induced increases in systolic BP in rats when given orally at 0.5 or 1 mg/kg/day (Khattab & Nagi 2007). In cats, β-eudesmol at 10 mg/kg iv precipitated a hypotensive response of 50–69% that lasted for 5–6 hours, but at a dose of 5 mg/kg iv, there was no effect (Arora et al 1967).

(+)-Limonene, which constitutes 16.4–24.4% of black pepper oil and 44.2% of white camphor oil, lowered monocrotaline-induced pulmonary hypertension in rats, when given orally at 400 mg/animal/day for up to 21 days (Touvay et al 1995). The farnesyltransferase inhibitory activity of limonene was suggested as being linked to this action.

Human oral studies

In a clinical study, 14 of 15 hypertensive patients who ingested 0.45 mL/day of geranium oil for two months showed significant improvement in their condition. They also showed a reduction in cortisol levels (Nozaki 2001). Two small-scale controlled trials showed preliminary clinical evidence for garlic oil having a hypotensive action. When taken in capsules at 18 mg/day for four weeks by normotensive volunteers, the oil reduced mean (presumably systolic) pressure from 94 mmHg to 88 mmHg, compared with a 2.3 mmHg mean reduction in the placebo group in a two period, cross-over trial with 10 volunteers per group. However, this 'garlic oil' was cold-pressed from fresh garlic (Barrie et al 1987). A second randomized-controlled trial in 27 normotensive trained male runners noted a mean drop of 4.5 mmHg in systolic pressure following daily ingestion of 2.3 mg steam-distilled garlic oil in capsules for 16 weeks (Zhang et al 2001).

Inhalation effects

Temporary hypertension has been recorded following the inhalation of certain of essential oils. Grapefruit, fennel, black pepper or tarragon oil caused a slight increase of systolic BP in humans after being inhaled for either three or seven minutes (Haze et al 2002). It is feasible that these effects may have been due to psychological factors. Human inhalation of ylang-ylang oil caused a significant reduction in BP, which was thought to be psychologically mediated (Hongratanaworakit & Buchbauer 2004). After 10 minutes of inhaling cedrol, both systolic and diastolic pressures were reduced in healthy male and female Japanese volunteers due to a reduction in sympathetic and an increase in parasympathetic activity (Dayawansa et al 2003). Conversely, inhalation of grapefruit oil for 10 minutes raised BP in rats, due to the enhancement of sympathetic and the suppression of parasympathetic activity (Shen et al 2005, Tanida et al 2005). This appears to indicate a physiological effect.

Inhalation of lavender oil by rats resulted in a fall in mean arterial BP, which is consistent with iv data cited above. The effect was thought to be autonomically mediated, and was eliminated following induced anosmia (Tanida et al 2006). However, 30 minutes of lavender oil inhalation by 30 healthy young men had no effect on BP, though other effects were seen (Shiina et al 2008). In the summary of an article published in Korean, once daily inhalation of a mixture of lavender, bergamot and ylang-ylang oils for four weeks was said to lower BP in patients with essential hypertension (Hwang 2006).

Both psychological and pharmacological processes were determined to be responsible for increases in BP in humans following 30 minutes inhalation of (+)-limonene (systolic), (–)-limonene (systolic), (+)-carvone (diastolic), or (–)-carvone (systolic and diastolic) (Heuberger et al 2001). For example, fragrance-induced subjective ratings of increased alertness correlated significantly with increases in BP. However, these same compounds, when not administered by inhalation, may be hypotensive.

In a human study that prevented inhalation, 1 mL of 20% sandalwood oil or α-santalol in peanut oil was applied to the abdominal skin of volunteers, resulting in a small but significant reduction in both systolic and diastolic pressures compared to control subjects. This was presumably due to a physiological effect resulting from transdermal absorption (Hongratanaworakit et al 2004).

Discussion

Increases in BP have been recorded in both animals and humans on essential oil administration, but it is not known whether any of the data indicate a risk to people with hypertension. In all of the cited studies, animals and humans with normal BP were tested. Most of the early (1940s) research was carried out by injecting dogs intravenously with moderately large doses of essential oils diluted in ethanol. In some of these, the precise quantity of essential oil used is not known, since only the amount of the total solution is given. Both increases and decreases in BP were recorded. Dermal administration of essential oil constituents can cause reductions in BP due to local effects. Conversely, most inhalation studies have reported BP increases.

Intravenous administration leads to a direct action on the vascular system, which is primarily due to calcium channel antagonism (Lahlou et al 2005). In inhalation studies, the effects are autonomically mediated, and in humans, psychological factors may come into play. In both rats and humans, elevations of BP were seen in conditions that reflect those of intentional and fairly intensive essential oil inhalation. Since soft tissue massage reduces BP, the only potential risks seem to be either from overdoses of certain convulsant essential oils, and from intensive (as distinct from incidental) inhalation.

Oral garlic oil is possibly the most likely to reliably reduce high BP, but there is no evidence that this would exacerbate an already established hypotension. The action of garlic oil is clearly not due to psychological factors nor, presumably, are the effects seen for other essential oils in animal studies. However, in those involving human inhalation, psychological factors are likely to play a part, and the effects are autonomically mediated. In contrast, iv administration leads to a direct action on the vascular system, which is primarily due to calcium channel antagonism (Lahlou et al 2005). A formulation containing fenugreek oil inhibited angiotensin-converting enzyme (ACE) in plasma and kidney when fed to male alloxan-diabetic rats. ACE inhibitors are now commonly used in the treatment of hypertension (Hamden et al 2011).

The mode of administration can play a significant role in the resulting effect. For example, hypertension and convulsions can both be caused by acute methyl salicylate poisoning. However, topically applied methyl salicylate lowers BP through local effects (Futami 1984; Ichiyama et al 2002; Dawson et al 2004). We have already seen that in rats, (+)-limonene lowered BP on iv injection, but raised it on inhalation. Since different effects on BP seem to be possible from different methods of administration, those from inhalation or dermal absorption should not be assumed to reflect those of iv administration.

There is no research that shows whether the use of single or blended essential oils can lead to a significant increase in BP during an aromatherapy massage, but this seems unlikely since soft tissue massage itself tends to reduce both systolic and diastolic pressure (Holland & Pokorny 2001, McNamara et al 2003; Aourell et al 2005).

Conclusion

Eucalyptus, camphor, pine, thyme and peppermint oils should be scratched from cautionary lists. Hyssop and sage oils are only a risk in convulsant oral doses, and lower doses are very likely to be hypotensive. Therefore, they should not be contraindicated in hypertension. It is likely that rosemary oil follows the same pattern. Inhalation data suggest that essential oils presenting a risk include grapefruit, lemon, caraway, black pepper, fennel, tarragon and other oils high in carvone or limonene. However, in the human studies the increases were only slight.

There is no clear evidence that essential oils have adverse effects on the control of BP in humans. Some essential oils may present a risk to some classes of hypertensive patient, in certain dose/route combinations, and there may be a theoretical argument for exercising caution in certain cases of hypertension and hypotension. However, until we know more about where the risks lie, there is no case for contraindication of any essential oils.

Blood

Blood is regarded as a circulating tissue. It consists of erythrocytes (red cells), leukocytes (white cells) and thrombocytes (platelets) suspended in plasma, an aqueous medium containing proteins and ions. Key functions of blood are to transport oxygen, nutrients (including glucose) and hormones to different tissues, and to transport carbon dioxide, metabolic waste products and toxins away from tissues to the organs of excretion. Blood also conducts heat around the body.

Blood disorders arise as a result of abnormal concentrations of enzymes, hemoglobin or other proteins in plasma, or from abnormalities in the structure of blood cells. These factors can lead to impaired transport to and from the tissues with such consequences as weakness, as well as susceptibility to infections and decreased surveillance to pre-cancerous cells. As far as essential oil constituents are concerned, effects on coagulation, involving platelets, are the most common.

Defects in heme synthesis (which takes place in the liver and bone) are discussed in Chapter 9, under Porphyrin production.

Thrombocytes

Thrombocytes (platelets) play an important role in hemostasis, by plugging and repairing damaged blood vessels, thus preventing blood loss. They also participate in a cascade of events that leads to blood clotting by triggering the release of a series of coagulation factors. In the first step, platelets are activated by various substances, including collagen from damaged tissue, as well as ADP (adenosine diphosphate) and thromboxane A2, secreted by activated platelets. Activation causes platelets to become adhesive, which facilitates their attachment to damaged tissues and to each other to form clumps. The penultimate step in coagulation is the formation of fibrin from fibrinogen. Fibrin filaments enmesh platelets and red and white blood cells to form a plug, which contracts to form a clot. Because this is a multi-step process, separate in vitro tests are often carried out for inhibition of platelet aggregation by collagen, ADP, arachidonic acid, or other substrates.

Although the blood clotting mechanism is essential for controlling blood loss, it can also lead to ischemic diseases such as strokes and heart attacks, due to thrombosis and consequent obstruction of blood flow. In order to maintain an optimal supply of blood to tissues, various mechanisms exist to prevent excessive and counterproductive clotting.

Blood coagulation can be affected by a number of exogenous substances, including essential oils, and can be a particular cause of concern when administered in overdose. In a fatal case of pennyroyal oil toxicity, there was bleeding from injection sites as well as the vagina (Sullivan et al 1979). In other cases, blood-thinning activity may result from relatively low doses. In a small-scale trial with 20 healthy volunteers, a daily oral dose of 18 mg cold-pressed garlic oil for four weeks reduced mean platelet aggregation by 16.4% compared to placebo (Barrie et al 1987). Both garlic and onion oils possess antiplatelet activity, onion oil being more potent than garlic (Fenwick & Hanley 1985). Since onion and leek oils share over 60% of their constituents, it seems likely that leek oil will possess a similar action. Three constituents of garlic oil, diallyl sulfide, diallyl disulfide and diallyl trisulfide, showed dose-dependent inhibition of ADP-induced aggregation of isolated human platelets in vitro at 5–10 μM. At these concentrations, they also exhibited a protective effect against glucose-induced oxidation in erythrocyte membranes and platelets (Chan et al 2002). Another constituent, methyl allyl trisulfide, also inhibits platelet aggregation (Boullin 1981; Fenwick & Hanley 1985).

In a report on the in vitro antiplatelet activity of 23 essential oils, the most potent against a range of stimulants were *Ocotea quixos* (a non-commercial oil containing 27.8% cinnamaldehyde and 21.6% methyl cinnamate), *Artemisia dracunculus* (70% estragole) and *Foeniculum vulgare* (75.8% (*E*)-anethole). *Origanum vulgare* (54.4% carvacrol and 14.3% thymol), and *Thymus vulgaris* (8.0% carvacrol and 6.8% thymol) oils were the most potent inhibitors of arachidonic acid-induced platelet aggregation with IC$_{50}$ values of 1.9 and 4.7 μg/mL, comparable with that of aspirin. Among all 23 essential oils, antiplatelet and clot dissolving activity correlated with their content of phenylpropanoid or phenolic constituents. Essential oils with a negligible action included clary sage, cypress, lemongrass, rosemary, Dalmatian sage Scots pine and turmeric (Tognolini et al 2006).

Inhibition of platelet aggregation has been confirmed for cinnamaldehyde, (*E*)-anethole, estragole, eugenol, carvacrol and thymol. Cinnamaldehyde inhibited the aggregation of human platelets in vitro, and anticoagulant activity was seen in mice after a combination of oral and ip dosing (Huang J et al 2007a). Confirmation of platelet aggregation has also been demonstrated for (*E*)-anethole and estragole, which inhibited aggregation of rabbit platelets induced by ADP, collagen or arachidonic acid as potently as aspirin (Yoshioka & Tamada 2005). Both thymol and carvacrol inhibited arachidonic acid-induced platelet aggregation, with potencies over 30 times greater than that of aspirin. Thymoquinone, *p*-cymene, (–)-menthol and (–)-menthone were virtually inactive (Enomoto et al 2001).

The essential oil of *Foeniculum vulgare* and (*E*)-anethole both demonstrated significant antithrombotic activity in vivo in mice at oral doses of 30 mg/kg/day for five days. This may be due antiplatelet and clot-destabilizing properties, in addition to a vasorelaxant action (Tognolini et al 2007).

Dose-dependent antiplatelet activity, due to an antiprostaglandin action, was demonstrated by eugenol and isoeugenol, which were both as potent as indomethacin. Myristicin, elemicin and safrole were 100 to 1,000 times less potent, and linalool, α-pinene, β-pinene, camphene, α-terpineol and terpinen-4-ol were inactive (Rasheed et al 1984; Janssens et al 1990). Eugenol similarly inhibited platelet aggregation induced by arachidonic acid, collagen, epinephrine (adrenaline) or ADP (Chen SJ et al 1996). Inhibition of platelet aggregation has been reported for verbenone and for *ar*-turmerone, but borneol, 1,8-cineole and sabinene had no effect (Lee HS 2006; Chiariello et al 1986). Both bergapten and imperatorin (the latter found at very low levels in expressed lemon and lime oils) demonstrated strong antiplatelet aggregation activity in vitro (Chen IS et al 1996).

There was a synergistic effect between the constituents of lavandin grosso oil, in inhibiting platelet aggregation induced by arachidonic acid, U46619, collagen and ADP, with IC$_{50}$

values of 51, 84, 191 and 640 μg/mL, respectively. The major constituents of the oil tested were linalyl acetate (36.2%), linalool (33.4%), camphor (7.6%) and 1,8-cineole (5.8%), which individually possessed only very weak antiplatelet activity in the presence of the four agonists, compared to that of the whole oil (Ballabeni et al 2004). Patchouli oil displays antiplatelet activity, as does α-bulnesene, one of its major constituents (Hsu et al 2006; Tsai et al 2007). β-Eudesmol is also significantly active, reducing arachidonic acid-induced platelet aggregation by 88% at 240 μM (Wang et al 2000).

Cornmint oil, menthol and menthone were found to be only weak inhibitors of collagen and ADP-induced platelet aggregation with IC$_{50}$ values in the millimolar range (Murayama & Kumaroo 1986).

Acceleration of blood coagulation has been reported for allyl isothiocyanate in rats, when given at 20 mg/kg/day iv for 7 days. Blood coagulation time was decreased by 43%, which was thought to be due to an increase in plasma phospholipids; this effect was largely reversed by co-administration of thyroxine (Idris & Ahmad 1975). However, the essential oil of *Wasabia japonica* roots, which contains a number of isothiocyanates including allyl isothiocyanate (79%), inhibited arachidonic acid-induced rabbit platelet aggregation in vitro with an IC$_{50}$ value of 112.1 μg/mL. Allyl isothiocyanate had an IC$_{50}$ in the same test of 1.7×10^{-3} M (Kumagai et al 1994).

Topically applied methyl salicylate can inhibit platelet aggregation systemically (Tanen et al 2008). The anticoagulant drug interaction issues with methyl salicylate are covered on Ch. 14, p. 598. Methyl salicylate-rich essential oils should be avoided by oral and non-oral routes.

We have contraindicated oral dosing of essential oils where there is clinical evidence of coagulation inhibition (Box 7.1A). We have cautioned oral dosing for essential oils with significant in vitro data either for the essential oil, or for constituents occurring at >25%: lavandin oil, leek oil, patchouli oil, and essential oils containing (*E*)-anethole, carvacrol, cinnamaldehyde, estragole, β-eudesmol, eugenol or thymol (Box 7.1B).

Erythrocytes

Erythrocytes (red blood cells) are responsible for carrying oxygen to, and carbon dioxide from, tissues. To perform efficiently, these cells must contain an optimum amount of hemoglobin, which requires an adequate level of iron in the body. A deficiency of iron and/or hemoglobin is a cause of anemia, a condition characterized by symptoms such as fatigue, shortness of breath on exertion and poor concentration due to poor oxygenation of body tissues.

Casearia sylvestris essential oil, and two of its constituents, β-caryophyllene (18.1%) and α-humulene (4.7%) caused significant hemolysis in human erythrocytes in vitro with maximal concentrations not causing hemolysis (MCnH) values of 156.2, 96.3 and 98.9 μg/mL, respectively. Human erythrocytes were among the most sensitive of seven species tested (Da Silva et al 2008). *Casearia sylvestris* oil is not commercially produced. Thymoquinone, a major constituent of black seed oil, triggered phospholipid scrambling and shrinkage of human erythrocytes in vitro at 3 μM and above, after 48 hours

Box 7.1

Essential oils that affect blood coagulation

A. Essential oils that are known to, or are very likely to, inhibit blood coagulation

Birch (sweet)
Garlic
Onion
Wintergreen

B. Essential oils that may inhibit platelet aggregation based on in vitro data either for the oil or a major constituent

Ajowan
Anise
Anise (star)
Araucaria
Atractylis
Basil (estragole CT)
Basil (holy)
Basil (Madagascan)
Basil (pungent)
Bay (W. Indian)
Bee balm (lemon)
Cassia
Chervil

Cinnamon bark
Cinnamon leaf
Clove bud
Clove leaf
Clove stem
Fennel (bitter)
Fennel (sweet)
Lavandin
Leek
Marigold (Mexican)
Marjoram wild (carvacrol CT)
Myrtle (aniseed)
Oregano
Oregano (Mexican)
Patchouli
Pimento berry
Pimento leaf
Ravensara bark
Savory
Tarragon
Tejpat
Thyme (borneol CT)
Thyme (limonene CT)
Thyme (thymol and/or carvacrol CTs)
Thyme (spike)

Oral administration of the above listed essential oils is either contraindicated (list A) or cautioned (list B) in these circumstances:

- If taking anticoagulant drugs such as aspirin, heparin and warfarin
- Breastfeeding mothers[a]
- Hemophilia
- Peptic ulcer
- Internal bleeding
- Severe hepatic or renal impairment
- Hypertensive or diabetic retinopathy
- Thrombocytopenia (decreased platelet count)
- Vasculitis
- Up to one week before or after major surgery or childbirth

[a]This is precautionary, and is a controversial contraindication even within conventional medicine, for 'novel' anticoagulant drugs. If they are known to pass into breast milk, then contraindication is very likely.

These erythrotoxic effects are part of a more general cytotoxic effect that may also impact cancer cells. We believe that there is currently insufficient information for specific contraindications.

In contrast, some essential oil constituents have been shown to exert a protective effect on erythrocytes. For example, eugenol dose-dependently inhibited the hemolysis of erythrocytes induced by liver S9 fraction-treated carbon tetrachloride, presumably by protecting them from oxidative stress (Kumaravelu et al 1996).

Glucose

Glucose is the body's main source of energy, and therefore blood glucose concentrations must be tightly controlled. Numerous hormones contribute to this goal including glucagon which increases blood concentrations, and insulin which decreases blood levels. If blood glucose levels fall below the normal range (hypoglycemia) a person may feel lethargic and experience impaired mental functioning, or even brain damage in extreme cases. Chronic high blood levels (hyperglycemia) may implicate diabetes, which can be accompanied by such problems as eye, kidney, heart and/or nerve damage.

Several essential oils and constituents have been shown to exert hypoglycemic effects in animal models. A melissa oil with an unusually high citral content (65.4% geranial and 24.7% neral), when fed to male mice at 0.015 mg/day for six weeks, caused a 65% reduction in blood glucose, a significant increase in serum insulin levels, and an improvement in glucose tolerance, compared to a control group. The authors explained this by enhanced glucose uptake and metabolism in the liver and adipose tissue, and inhibition of hepatic gluconeogenesis (Chung et al 2010). Similarly, gavage doses of 10, 15 or 20 mg/kg/day citral for 28 days, dose-dependently lowered plasma insulin levels and increased glucose tolerance in obese rats (Modak & Mukhopadhaya 2011). When a laboratory-distilled Tunisian geranium oil was given to alloxan-induced diabetic male rats at 75 and 150 mg/kg/day po for 30 days, blood glucose was reduced by an amount comparable with that elicited by glibenclamide (600 µg/kg), while hepatic glycogen concentration increased (Boukhris et al 2012).

Dietary fenugreek oil (for composition see Fenugreek Profile, Chapter 13) fed to male alloxan-diabetic rats at 5%, significantly inhibited α-amylase and maltase activity in the pancreas and plasma. It also improved glucose tolerance and helped to protect pancreatic β-cells (Hamden et al 2011). Turmeric oil dose-dependently inhibited glucosidase enzymes more effectively than the antidiabetic drug acarbose. Its main constituent, ar-turmerone (45.0–58.0%), showed potent α-glucosidase ($IC_{50}=0.28$ µg) and α-amylase ($IC_{50}=24.5$ µg) inhibitory activity (Lekshmi et al 2012).

Myrtle oil reduced blood glucose by 51% in alloxan-diabetic rabbits four hours after an oral dose of 50 mg/kg, but had no effect on serum insulin concentrations (Sepici et al 2004). In rabbits, 50 mg/kg ip of black seed essential oil reduced blood glucose in fasting normal and alloxan-diabetic animals (Al-Hader et al 1993). Here again, the mechanism of action did not appear to be insulin-mediated. Significant reductions in blood glucose levels in both normal and alloxan-diabetic rats

exposure, though loss of membrane integrity was not significant until 20 µM. These changes are precursors to hemolysis (Qadri et al 2009). Citral exhibited in vitro hemolytic activity in erythrocytes (species not stated) at $3.0–5.9 \times 10^{-4}$ M. A non-specific free radical-peroxide mechanism has been suggested (Segal & Milo-Goldzweig 1985).

The essential oil of freshly distilled *Tagetes minuta* leaves caused significant decreases in erythrocyte and hemoglobin levels when administered orally for 14 days to rats at 125 µL/kg bw. There were also increases in mean corpuscular volume, mean corpuscular hemoglobin and neutrophils (Odeyemi et al 2008).

were reported one hour following subcutaneous injections of dill (type unspecified), sweet fennel, Dalmatian sage and white wormwood oils at 27, 21.5, 39 and 18.75 mg/kg, respectively (Essway et al 1995). In contrast, Eidi et al (2005) found no significant change in serum glucose levels in streptozotocin-diabetic rats for up to five hours after ip administration of 0.042, 0.125, 0.2 or 0.4 mL/kg of Dalmatian sage oil.

Gavage doses of 25, 50 or 100 mg/kg/day of cinnamon bark oil for 35 days decreased plasma glucose concentrations in KK-A^y diabetic mice (Ping et al 2010). Cinnamaldehyde, at oral doses of 5, 10 or 20 mg/kg/day for 45 days, dose-dependently decreased plasma glucose concentrations in streptozotocin-diabetic male rats, and 20 mg/kg markedly increased plasma insulin levels (Babu et al 2007). Wild *Satureja khuzestanica* oil (93.9% carvacrol) significantly reduced plasma glucose concentrations in diabetic rats when given orally at 100 mg/kg/day for 21 days. It was thought that inhibition of liver phosphoenol-pyruvate carboxykinase may contribute to this action (Shahsavari et al 2009). Other carvacrol-rich essential oils will probably have similar effects. Plasma glucose concentrations were significantly reduced in rats after gavage dosing with (1*R*)-(+)-β-pulegone at 160 mg/kg/day for 28 days. The authors suggested that this might be due to inactivation of glucose-6-phosphatase (Mølck et al 1998). Apart from (+)-pulegone, it is interesting to note that most of the essential oils exerting hypoglycemic activity here contain constituents that possess a carbonyl group, commonly as aldehydes or ketones. Some phenols also seem to be active. Nevertheless, it must be stated that these compounds do not necessarily share a common mechanism of action.

Hyperglycemic effects have also been seen. In normal rabbits, 25 mg/kg im rosemary oil produced 20–55% increases in plasma glucose levels above those of control animals after 60–120 minutes, and a 30% decrease in serum insulin levels (Al-Hader et al 1994). Anise oil significantly enhanced the absorption of glucose in rat jejunum. This action correlated with an increase in Na$^+$/K$^+$ ATPase activity (Kreydiyyeh et al 2003). Because anise oil and sweet fennel oil both affect glucose metabolism, we have included other (*E*)-anethole-rich essential oils in Box 7.2. We have not included essential oils that we recommend should not be taken in oral doses.

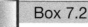

Box 7.2

Essential oils that should be used with caution orally in diabetic subjects whose blood glucose levels are being controlled by orthodox drugs

Anise	Lemon leaf
Anise (star)	Lemongrass
Basil (lemon)	May chang
Black seed	Melissa
Cassia	Myrtle
Cinnamon bark	Myrtle (aniseed)
Dill	Myrtle (honey)
Fennel (bitter)	Myrtle (lemon)
Fennel (Sweet)	Tea tree (lemon-scented)
Fenugreek	Turmeric
Geranium	Verbena (lemon)

Oral ingestion of the essential oils listed in Box 7.2 is cautioned in diabetic subjects whose blood glucose levels are being controlled by orthodox drugs.

Summary

- There is no hard evidence that any essential oil, by any route, exacerbates either hypertension or hypotension as used in aromatherapy.
- Patients taking anticoagulant drugs, and other at risk individuals, should avoid oral administration of essential oils that inhibit platelet aggregation.
- Emerging research indicates that some essential oils may be cytotoxic to erythrocytes, but there is currently insufficient information for specific contraindications.
- Experimental evidence suggests that some essential oils can increase or decrease blood glucose concentrations. Oral ingestion of these is cautioned in anyone taking medication to control blood sugar levels.

The urinary system

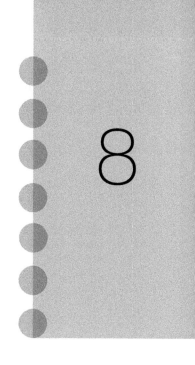

8

The kidneys, which form part of the urinary system, are the body's main organs of excretion. They remove waste products associated with normal body metabolism, as well as drugs and other foreign molecules and their metabolites from the bloodstream. Another key function of the kidneys is to maintain homeostasis by regulating the body's water, electrolyte and pH levels. The functional unit of the kidney is the nephron, a microscopic arrangement of tubules for exchange of substances between the blood and the urine.

The composition of the urine is regulated by three processes: glomerular filtration of blood plasma, passive reabsorption of substances from the filtrate back into the blood, and active secretion from the blood to the tubular fluid. Many water-soluble substances are subjected only to glomerular filtration before being excreted in the urine, and some hydrophilic drugs and drug metabolites are eliminated in this way. The more hydrophilic essential oil constituents, such as terpenoid alcohols, aldehydes and ketones are excreted in this way, at least in part.

Lipophilic substances, including many drugs, diffuse back through the tubule walls into the bloodstream to varying degrees, and so the liver has a key role to play in rendering these substances more water-soluble to ensure their eventual elimination. Many essential oil constituents are sufficiently lipophilic to come into this category, particularly the hydrocarbons.

Nephrotoxicity

The kidneys are susceptible to toxicity from xenobiotics because they receive a high proportion of the cardiac output. Moreover, cells of the nephron are particularly vulnerable, being exposed to substances both in the blood and in the urine. The cells in the proximal tubules have the greatest concentration of CYP enzymes in the nephron, and are therefore vulnerable to toxins derived from bioactivation in the same way as the liver.

Overdose or prolonged ingestion of over-the-counter non-steroidal anti-inflammatory drugs such as paracetamol (acetaminophen), acetylsalicylic acid (aspirin) and phenacetin can lead to necrosis of renal tissue, which is a common cause of life-threatening renal insufficiency. In West Germany in 1983 an average of 13% of patients who registered for hemodialysis had overdosed on analgesics (Niesink et al 1996). Acetylsalicylic acid is chemically related to methyl salicylate, a constituent of several essential oils, which can also cause renal problems if taken in excessive amounts. In a fatal poisoning incident, a 17-month-old child was given 4 mL of methyl salicylate in error. On autopsy, the kidneys were swollen and highly congested, with some degeneration of the tubules (Hughes RF 1932).

However, there are very few known adverse effects for essential oils in relation to the urinary system. In most cases, essential oil constituents are efficiently metabolized and excreted in humans except in cases of overdose and/or renal disease.

Acute dosing

Renal problems caused by essential oils in humans are rare and have all been associated with oral overdose. One teaspoon of wintergreen oil proved fatal in a child aged 22 months, with autopsy showing abnormalities in the heart, liver and kidneys (Eimas 1938; Kloss & Boeckman 1967). Kidney damage was seen on autopsy in children of 2 and 12 years, who died after being given 16 drops and 30 drops, respectively, of wormseed oil (Wolf IJ 1935). Wormseed oil is toxic even at low doses because of its depressant action on the heart, and toxic signs include significant renal damage (Van Lookeren Campagne 1939; Opdyke 1976 p. 713–715).

In one of the few fatal cases of pennyroyal oil poisoning, the ingestion of an unknown quantity by a woman resulted in rapid destruction of the kidney tubules, with death following massive urea leakage into the blood (Vallance 1955). A 31-year-old man was hospitalized with renal failure after ingesting 10 mL of wormwood oil. He fully recovered after 17 days (Weisbord et al 1997). Severe damage to kidney tissue has also been observed in several cases of poisoning from high-dose parsley apiole ingestion (Lowenstein & Ballew 1958; Amerio et al 1968; Colalillo 1974).

In each of these cases, the substances causing nephrotoxicity were not only taken in high doses, but they are all known to be toxic. Wormwood and wormseed oils should not be administered by any route, and pennyroyal, parsleyseed and wintergreen oils should not be taken by mouth, and have dermal use limits. In one rare instance, methyl salicylate toxicity was implicated as a cause of kidney damage after high-dose dermal administration and application of a heat pad (Heng 1987).

Very high doses of some essential oils have been nephrotoxic in experimental animals. A single oral dose of rue oil at 400 mg/kg was fatal in guinea pigs due to liver, adrenal and kidney damage (Leung & Foster 2003). Severe liver and kidney damage have been seen in LD_{50} tests with essential oils of calamus and sassafras (Von Skramlik 1959; Abbot et al 1961).

As with essential oils, some of their constituents are nephrotoxic to rodents after acute dosing. Sublethal oral doses of benzyl cyanide were nephrotoxic in rats, causing increased excretion of protein, amino acids and glucose (Guest et al 1982). p-Cresol is nephrotoxic in high doses by any route, and can cause uremia (Wu ML et al 1998a; Lesaffer et al 2001; De Smet et al 2003). Benzyl cyanide is only found in four absolutes (ginger lily, karo karoundé, orange flower and nasturtium), and p-cresol is only found in oils of birch tar and cade oils.

Subacute and subchronic dosing

There were histological changes in the kidneys of rats dosed by gavage with 73.5 mg/kg of cinnamaldehyde for 90 days, along with proteinuria, creatinuria, and increased activities of renal, serum and urinary enzymes. Animals were not affected by lower doses (Gowder & Devaraj 2008).

Very high doses (4 mL/kg) of methyl salicylate, applied to the skin of rabbits, five days a week for up to 96 days, caused early deaths and kidney damage. Lower (but still high) doses, 0.5, 1.0, or 2.0 mL/kg, caused a higher than normal incidence

of 'spontaneous' nephritis (Webb & Hansen 1963). Since all doses were toxic, no NOAEL was established. Some other esters show signs of moderate nephrotoxicity on subchronic oral dosing at high levels. When rats were given isobornyl acetate at 15, 90 or 270 mg/kg/day for 90 days, there were signs of nephrotoxicity at the two higher dose levels (Gaunt et al 1971). Rats were given octyl acetate, 5 days per week for 90 days, at 100, 500 or 1,000 mg/kg. After 45 days of dosing, effects seen in the high-dose group included increased kidney weight and, in males only, evidence of hydrocarbon nephropathy (Daughtrey et al 1989a). The NOAEL of 100 mg/kg is equivalent to a human adult dose of 14 g of *Boswellia papyrifera* oil.

Alcohols can also produce renal effects in rodents at elevated doses. In a 90-day study, rats were given dietary *cis*-3-hexenol at 310, 1,250 and 5,000 ppm. No effects were seen at the lower two doses, but at the high dose, the relative kidney weight was increased in male rats (Opdyke 1974 p. 909–910). When male and female rats were administered 0, 25, 100 or 400 mg/kg of 3-octanol for 90 days by gavage, some kidney damage was seen in males at the two higher doses (Lindecrona et al 2003). Both *cis*-3-hexenol and 3-octanol are only very minor constituents of essential oils. When 400 mg/kg of terpinen-4-ol was administered orally to rats for 28 days there were no changes in function or morphology of the kidneys and therefore no nephrotoxicity (Schilcher & Leuschner 1997). This is equivalent to a human adult dose of about 65 g.

When angelica root oil was given orally to rats for 56 days at 0.5, 1.0, 2.0 or 3.0 g/kg, there was weight loss and decreased activity at the higher two doses, and deaths were associated with severe liver and kidney damage (Von Skramlik 1959). These are massive doses for any substance, and it seems surprising that any rats would have even survived on them for so long.

Juniper oil has been mentioned frequently in connection with kidney damage. It has been claimed that, when given orally, 'juniper' can irritate the kidneys, and that it is contraindicated in kidney disease. However, while other preparations made from juniper may be problematic in kidney disease, no evidence could be found to support this claim for the essential oil (see Juniper profile, Chapter 13). One investigation of the purported nephrotoxicity of juniper oil found none. Up to 1 g/kg was administered orally to rats for 28 days and no changes in kidney function or morphology were seen (Schilcher & Leuschner 1997).

Chronic dosing

When the rodent carcinogen safrole was given in the diet to male and female rats at 390 ppm or 1,170 ppm for 24 months, congestion and significant cellular changes were observed in the kidneys at the higher level (Abbot et al 1961).

Species-specific effects

In adult male rats, both oral 1,8-cineole and (+)-limonene produced renal accumulation of a soluble protein, α_2u-globulin with associated microscopic abnormalities (Kanerva & Alden 1987; Kristiansen & Madsen 1995; Lehmann-McKeeman et al 1989; Saito et al 1991). This 'protein droplet' nephrotoxicity can lead to the formation of kidney tumors, but it is specific to male rats, and does not occur in humans (Kanerva et al 1987; Webb et al 1989, 1990; Hard et al 1993). Specific binding to α_2u-globulin of male (but not female) rats has also been observed for pulegone and its metabolites menthone or menthofuran when given orally at doses of 80, 80, or 60 mg/kg, respectively, in corn oil. However, this binding did not result in accumulation of the protein (Ferguson et al 2007). Renal tubule necrosis was seen in rats of both sexes given gavage doses of β-myrcene ranging from 250–4,000 mg/kg/day for 14 weeks (National Toxicology Program 2010b). This is likely a function of the massive doses used.

Other compounds are nephrotoxic on low-level dosing. Oral methoxsalen was dose-dependently nephrotoxic in rats given 37.5 or 75 mg/kg/day for two years (National Toxicology Program 1989b). However, methoxsalen is only a trace constituent, and even achieving the lower dose would require the impossible ingestion of 8 kg of rue oil (0.032% methoxsalen) by a 70 kg human. Allyl isothiocyanate was toxic to rat kidney at 40 mg/kg given by gavage for up to six weeks, but no toxicity was seen at 10 mg/kg (Lewerenz et al 1988). Given to male and female rats and mice at 50 mg/kg for 14 days, it caused thickening of the bladder wall in male mice (National Toxicology Program 1982). The three isothiocyanates found in commercially available essential oils (allyl, benzyl and phenylethyl) are particularly irritating to the urinary system in rats (Bechtel et al 1998). Allyl isothiocyanate is a constituent of mustard and horseradish oils, which are too toxic and irritant to use in essential oil therapy. When consumed in food, the extreme pungency of mustard and horseradish should normally restrict intake to relatively low levels.

Antinephrotoxicity

Protective effects have been observed for some essential oils and constituents, and these are summarized here.

Juniper oil has shown a renoprotective action, completely reversing the decrease in inulin clearance caused by tacrolimus (a drug used to prevent the rejection of transplanted tissue) in rats (Butani et al 2003). Thymoquinone protects the kidneys from the damaging effects of two anticancer drugs in rodents. Given orally to rats at 5 mg/kg/day for 5 days, it significantly reduced renal damage induced by ifosfamide (Badary 1999). Low-dose single injections of either thymoquinone or isoeugenol similarly ameliorated cisplatin nephrotoxicity in rats (Badary et al 1997; Rao et al 1999a). One week of daily oral dosing with 50 or 100 mg/kg of garlic oil attenuated the effect of iron nitrilotriacetate (a potent nephrotoxic agent) in rats (Iqbal & Athar 1998). Blue chamomile oil reduced plasma urea to normal concentrations in rabbits with induced glomeronephritis (Grochulski & Borkowski 1972).

Diuresis

When freshly distilled anise oil was added to the drinking water of rats at 0.05% (approximately 30 mg/kg), it exerted a significant antidiuretic effect but did not affect water intake. The oil increased the activity of renal Na^+/K^+ ATPase, an enzyme which increases the tubular reabsorption of sodium and therefore water

retention, at concentrations as low as 0.025 nL/L, peaking at 250 nL/L (Kreydiyyeh et al 2003). Administration of 350 mg/kg of the essential oil of a 'white-headed' Roman chamomile to rats by sc and ip injection resulted in decreases in water elimination from 93.04% (controls) to 46.85% (sc) and 28.10% (ip) of the water administered. The major constituents of this oil were butyl angelate and isoamyl angelate (Rossi et al 1988).

Nothing can be meaningfully extrapolated from the massive dose of chamomile oil used here. However, the antidiuretic action of anise oil signals the need for caution when taken orally by people with edematous disorders or renal insufficiency, as well as in those taking diuretic medication.

Conclusions

Essential oil constituents that are nephrotoxic in rodents at low or moderate oral dose levels include benzyl cyanide, p-cresol and allyl isothiocyanate (Box 8.1). Of other constituents given subchronically to rodents, the NOAELs for isobornyl acetate (15 mg/kg) and 3-octanol (25 mg/kg) are close to the upper oral dose range for an essential oil. Since 3-octanol is not found at more than 2.6% in any essential oil, no caution is needed for normal use. However, the NOAEL of isobornyl acetate is equivalent to a human adult dose of 3.2 g of hemlock spruce oil, which therefore warrants a specific caution when administered orally.

Nephrotoxicity is a feature of salicylate poisoning. Older people are particularly vulnerable because both hepatic metabolism and renal clearance of salicylates reduce with age, and chronic nephrotoxicity can occur with marginally high salicylate concentrations (Durnas & Cusack 1992). For these and other reasons, there are oral and dermal maximums for wintergreen and sweet birch oils.

People with renal disease are more vulnerable to nephrotoxicity, and so oral administration and dosage of any essential oil should be carefully considered. Since patients with renal failure have an increased risk of bleeding complications, oral administration of anticoagulant essential oils should be avoided (Box 8.1).

Summary

- Some essential oils cause kidney damage when taken in overdose.
- Extrapolation from the constituent data in rodents suggests that oils of horseradish, mustard (allyl isothiocyanate) and

---

Box 8.1

Materials that have a demonstrated potential for nephrotoxicity at therapeutic doses

Allyl isothiocyanate – the major constituent of horseradish and mustard oils

Parsley apiole – a major constituent of parsleyseed oil

Benzyl cyanide – found in several absolutes at low concentrations

p-Cresol – a major constituent of birch tar oil, a minor constituent of cade oil

Wormseed oil

birch tar (cresols) can cause damage to healthy human kidneys in therapeutic doses.

- Male rats are particularly susceptible to nephrotoxicity from certain compounds. These include (+)-limonene, 1,8-cineole, *cis*-3-hexenol, 3-octanol, octyl acetate and allyl, benzyl and phenylethyl isothiocyanate.

- Caution is advised when anise oil is taken orally by people with edematous disorders, renal insufficiency, or when taking diuretic medication.

- In spite of statements to the contrary, we could find no evidence that juniper oil is nephrotoxic.

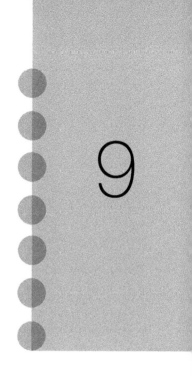

The digestive system

The digestive system comprises the entire gastrointestinal (GI) tract from the mouth to the anus, as well as associated organs including the liver, gallbladder and pancreas. Its purpose is to mechanically and chemically break foods down into small molecules that can be absorbed into the bloodstream or lymph, mainly via the small intestine. Chemical breakdown is affected by digestive enzymes secreted by the tract and accessory organs, as well as hydrochloric acid secreted by the stomach. The GI tract is protected from the corrosive actions of these enzymes and acid by a mucous membrane composed of epithelial cells which secrete mucus and fluid.

The oral (ingested) route is a common and often convenient route for administering medicines where systemic distribution is required, but substances taken by this route will be subject to first-pass metabolism in the liver. Alternatively, substances may be applied to different parts of the GI tract (without being ingested) for their local effects. Thus, oral hygiene products such as toothpastes and mouthwashes are applied to the oral cavity, while suppositories may be applied rectally for local or systemic actions. Substances absorbed systemically in the lower part of the rectum are not subjected to first-pass metabolism.

Each of these routes is utilized for delivering essential oils and their individual constituents for therapeutic purposes. However, being thinner and more fragile than skin, and lacking a protective keratinized cell layer, the mucous membrane is more sensitive to insult and is more permeable. Therefore, undiluted essential oils should not be taken orally, nor applied to the mouth or rectum.

The gastrointestinal tract

The principal risk of administering essential oils or their constituents to any part of the GI tract is irritation and inflammation of the mucous membrane. This has occasionally been reported following overdose, for example with wormseed oil (Opdyke 1976 p. 713–715), but does not always occur, such as in a case of tea tree oil overdose (Del Beccaro 1995). The concentration of essential oil is an important determining factor, as are the total dose and frequency of exposure. Repeated exposure, therefore, increases the risk of irritation.

There have been very occasional reports of oral sensitivity to peppermint oil and menthol, with burning, ulceration and/or inflammation either on contact or after excessive, prolonged use (Morton et al 1995; Rogers & Pahor 1995; Fleming & Forsyth 1998). Considering the widespread use of peppermint oil, such reactions are rare. In contrast, we found reports of 63 oral adverse reactions to cinnamon bark oil as an ingredient of toothpastes, chewing gums or food flavorings. Symptoms invariably included either erosion of mucosal tissues or allergic reaction, sometimes extending to the lips (Allen & Blozis 1988; Miller et al 1992; Cohen & Bhattacharyya 2000; Endo & Rees 2007; Tremblay & Avon 2008).

In tests performed on one of us (RT) and two other volunteers, 0.02 mL of various undiluted essential oils was applied to a small area on the inside of the mouth, which was kept open to prevent dilution of the oil with saliva. Subjective observations were made for up to 3 minutes, and any irritation became apparent 15–30 seconds after application. Essential oils rich in cinnamaldehyde, eugenol, carvacrol or thymol generally produced the most severe reactions. Other constituents that are probable mucous membrane irritants include allyl isothiocyanate, ethyl acetate and p-cresol (see Constituent profiles, Chapter 14). High concentrations of perillyl alcohol may also irritate the alimentary mucosa (Hudes et al 2000).

Adverse effects other than irritation are possible from essential oil ingestion, at least with very high doses. In clinical trials using perillyl alcohol in the treatment of various cancers, doses ranging from 2,400–8,400 mg/m^2 per day[1] (equivalent to approximately 62–218 mg/kg) produced strong GI side effects that increased with dose. These included nausea, vomiting, satiety and eructation, and may have been exacerbated by the large amount of soybean oil that the perillyl alcohol was mixed with (Ripple et al 1998, 2000; Liu et al 2003; Murren et al 2002; Bailey et al 2002, 2004, 2008).

Medicines containing essential oils may be formulated in different ways depending on the desired pharmacokinetic characteristics, for example, enterically coated capsules for dyspepsia and irritable bowel syndrome. These dissolve preferentially in the relative alkalinity of the small intestine (pH about 8) but not in the acidic stomach environment. Table 9.1 shows recorded adverse effects from clinical trials. In these, the incidence of side effects is regarded as low, and equal to or better than that of more conventional medications.

Dose-related effects

Mucous membrane irritation is concentration-dependent. For example, although mustard oil is a severe irritant (Leung & Foster 2003), at 0.125%, it was only slightly irritating to the human oral mucous membrane (Simons et al 2003). As mentioned in Chapter 2, phenolic compounds have a particular tendency to be irritants. Applied for 5 minutes to the tongues of dogs, undiluted eugenol caused erythema and occasionally ulcers (Lilly et al 1972); applied to rat labial mucosa and observed for up to 6 hours, it caused swelling, cell necrosis and vesicle formation (Kozam & Mantell 1978); applied to mouse mucous membrane, it progressively destroyed epithelial cells, causing an acute inflammatory response (Fujisawa et al 2001).

When rats were given 150 mg eugenol po (~450 mg/kg), there was gastric epithelial damage, with punctate hemorrhages in the pyloric and glandular regions (Hartiala et al 1966). However, given orally at 10–100 mg/kg, it reduced the number of ulcers and the severity of lesions induced by ethanol and platelet activating factor (Capasso et al 2000), and doses of 5–50 μg/kg reduced tongue edema in mice (Dip et al 2004). Evidently, lower concentrations of eugenol have the opposite effect to higher ones on mucous membranes. Markowitz et al (1992) reported that low concentrations of eugenol exerted anti-inflammatory and local anesthetic effects on dental pulp, but high concentrations were cytotoxic, and could cause extensive tissue damage.

Although thymol, another phenol, is said to irritate the gastric mucosa (Reynolds 1993), oral *Lippia sidoides* leaf oil, consisting of 66.7% thymol, dose-dependently inhibited alcohol-induced gastric lesions when given at 1, 5 or 10 mg/kg.

Table 9.1 GI reactions in clinical trials using oral doses of essential oils and constituents

Substance	Single dose × doses per day	Number of reactions	Adverse reactions	Reference
Oregano oil	200 mg × 3	0/14	None	Force et al 2000
Peppermint oil	450 mg × 2	1/28	Heartburn[a]	Cappello et al 2007
	187 or 374 mg × 3	0/21	None	Kline et al 2001
	187 mg × 3–4	1/52	Heartburn	Liu et al 1997
Peppermint oil + caraway oil	90 mg / 50 mg } × 2	2/47	Heartburn, nausea[a]	May et al 2000
	90 mg / 50 mg } × 2	8/60	1[a] + 7 Unstated	Madische et al 1999
1,8-Cineole	200 mg × 3	1/76	Heartburn[a]	Kehrl et al 2004
Perillyl alcohol	4,340–14,260 mg/day in divided doses	Not recorded, but a majority	Nausea, vomiting, satiety, eructation	Ripple et al 1998, 2000; Murren et al 2002; Bailey et al 2002, 2004, 2008; Liu et al 2003

[a]Adverse reactions assessed by the researchers as being unrelated to the essential oil medication. In the other cases, causation by the test medication could not be ruled out. Since peppermint oil relaxes the lower esophageal sphincter, chewing enterically coated capsules, instead of swallowing them whole, can cause heartburn. This has happened in some trials.

This effect reduced slightly as the dose was further increased to 50 and 100 mg/kg (Monteiro et al 2007). *Origanum onites* oil (64.3% carvacrol, an isomer of thymol) protected rats against colonic damage induced by trinitrobenzene sulfonic acid (TNBS), used at 0.1 or 1.0 mg/kg intrarectally in olive oil. Ulceration, mucus cell depletion and inflammation were all significantly reduced (Dundar et al 2008). These phenomena may be related to the concentration-dependent, pro-oxidant/antioxidant action of phenols.

In tests of gastric toxicity in rats, essential oils of *Ocimum basilicum* (22% eugenol), *Ocimum gratissimum* (30% thymol) and *Cymbopogon citratus* (66% citral), diluted in corn oil, were administered by gavage in doses of 50, 500, 1,000, 1,500, 2,000, 3,000 or 3,500 mg/kg/day for 14 days. NOAELs for functional damage to the stomach were 1,500, 1,000, and 1,000 mg/kg, respectively. Higher doses caused erosion of the stomach mucosa and disappearance of the surface epithelium (Fandohan et al 2008).

Essential oils with non-phenolic major constituents may also be protective. Cardamon oil (26.5–44.6% 1,8-cineole) inhibited ethanol-induced gastric irritation and ulcerative lesions in rats at 40 mg/kg, although 12.5 mg/kg had no effect (Jamal et al 2006). This gastroprotective action may be related to antioxidant activity of 1,8-cineole (Santos & Rao 2001). Pre-treatment with 1,8-cineole by rectal instillation at 200 or 400 mg/kg, in an emulsion with Tween 80, attenuated TNBS-induced colonic damage in rats, and caused repletion of glutathione (Santos et al 2004).

Gastroprotective and, where known, gastrotoxic doses of essential oils and constituents are shown in Table 9.2.

Excipients

In order to prevent GI irritation, orally dosed essential oils need to be dispersed in a vehicle, such as a gel or fixed oil. In a study to assess the efficacy of peppermint oil in reducing gastric spasm during endoscopy, a 1.6% concentration of peppermint oil emulsified in water (using a surfactant) was sprayed directly onto the pyloric ring in 50 patients; there were no side effects (Hiki et al 2003). Colpermin capsules contain 187 mg of peppermint oil in a thixotropic gel to ensure adequate dispersal in the bowel (Liu et al 1997), while Mintoil capsules contain 225 mg of peppermint oil and 45 mg of a starch that absorbs oils (Cappello et al 2007). In a study of 14 patients with enteric parasites, tablets containing 200 mg of emulsified oregano oil were used. The emulsification process was said to increase the surface area of the essential oil by six orders of magnitude (Force et al 2000).

The liver

The liver is the largest internal organ of the body. It is a remarkable structure in many respects, not least in its ability to carry out so many life-supporting functions. It makes enzymes and plasma proteins, it recycles red blood cells and stores their iron, it is the main heat producer of the body, it is involved in vitamin manufacture, it metabolizes almost every ingested nutrient, and it detoxifies drugs and other xenobiotics. Because blood is

Table 9.2 Gastrotoxic and gastroprotective doses of orally dosed essential oils and constituents in experimental animals

Substance	Gastrotoxic dose (mg/kg)	Gastroprotective dose (mg/kg)	Reference
Essential oil			
Cardamon oil	–	50	Jamal et al 2006
Lavandin oil grosso	–	100	Barocelli et al 2004
Lemongrass oil WI	1,500	–	Fandohan et al 2008
Lippia sidoides oil	–	10–100	Monteiro et al 2007
Vassoura oil	–	50–500	Klopell et al 2007
Constituent			
(*E*)-Anethole	–	30–300	Freire et al 2005
β-Caryophyllene	–	1–150	Tambe et al 1996
1,8-Cineole	–	50–200	Santos & Rao 2001
(−)-α-Bisabolol	–	8–80	Torrado et al 1995
	–	100–200	Moura Rocha et al 2010
Eugenol	~450	10–100	Capasso et al 2000
Linalool[a]	–	33	Barocelli et al 2004
Linalyl acetate[a]	–	36	Barocelli et al 2004
Nerolidol[a]	–	50–500	Klopell et al 2007
Thymoquinone	5–20		El-Abhar et al 2003

[a]Isomer not specified

delivered to the liver directly from most of the digestive tract, its exposure to potentially toxic chemicals is high.

Hepatotoxicity

Some xenobiotic compounds cause direct injury to liver cells, while others are metabolized by CYP enzymes to toxic substances, notably highly reactive molecules called electrophiles.[2] If a xenobiotic is absorbed in quantities sufficient to overwhelm detoxifying enzymes, the liver itself becomes subject to injury.

This may be an acute event, or it may progress over time. Electrophiles may cause necrosis (cell death), in some cases with depletion of hepatic glutathione. The main types of liver injury caused by xenobiotics are: hepatocellular necrosis, steatosis (fatty degeneration), cholestasis (obstruction of bile flow), granulomas (small nodules) and vascular lesions. Essential oils may not be implicated in these last two. Oxidative stress, steatosis and CYP enzyme induction are closely associated with hepatic cancer. Because the liver bioactivates carcinogens, it is the primary target for cancers from DNA-reactive molecules.

Essential oil constituents have been reported to increase porphyrin production, disrupt protein synthesis, interfere with metabolic enzymes, or cause various microscopic or macroscopic structural changes. A few constituents are only hepatotoxic to a subset of the population (Pharmacogenetic toxicity, below). Sufficiently high doses can be lethal. In cases of fatal toxicity from parsley apiole ingestion, considerable liver damage is generally found post mortem (Lowenstein & Ballew 1958; Amerio et al 1968; Colalillo 1974). Similarly, autopsy results indicate that fatal doses of camphor can damage the liver (Smith & Margolis 1954; Siegel & Wason 1986). Although the liver has a substantial capacity to regenerate following injury, this capacity is not unlimited, and is reduced in some individuals due to age, disease or lifestyle factors.

Liver function tests

Liver impairment typically presents as general malaise, either with or without jaundice, and is most commonly assessed by means of 'liver function tests'. When hepatic cells are damaged, they release increased quantities of certain enzymes into the blood (Box 9.1). Liver function tests measure the levels of these, and of bilirubin. Liver damage may be categorized as hepatocellular (mainly ALT elevation) or cholestatic (mainly ALP elevation), though mixed types of liver injury are common (Bénichou 1990).

An essential oil of *Salvia officinalis* containing 17.4% α-thujone, 3.9% β-thujone and 3.3% camphor was not toxic to rat hepatocytes at 200 nL (of essential oil dissolved in DMSO) per mL of cell suspension or less. However at 2,000 nL/mL a significant increase in LDH and decrease in glutathione occurred, indicating cell damage (Lima et al 2004).

Deteriorating liver function was a feature in a case of near-fatal poisoning in a 2-year-old boy who ingested 5–10 mL clove oil (Hartnoll et al 1993). Similarly, a 15-month-old boy developed acute liver failure after ingesting 10–20 mL clove oil (Janes et al 2005). Administered orally at 600 mg/kg, eugenol, the major constituent of clove oil, caused liver damage in mice

whose livers had been experimentally depleted of glutathione (Mizutani et al 1991). However, oral administration of 1,000 mg/kg eugenol to rats with normal livers did not deplete glutathione, in fact the activity of glutathione S-transferases (see Glutathione depletion, below) was induced after two weeks of treatment (Vidhya & Devaraj 1999). There is clearly a risk of hepatotoxicity from elevated doses of eugenol, but it is not known whether this is associated with glutathione depletion. Eugenol, however, is hepatoprotective in low (therapeutic) doses (see Hepatoprotection, below). The dose-dependent action of eugenol in relation to the liver is similar to its effect, and that of other phenols, in relation to the GI tract and mucous membrane irritation (discussed above).

Oxidative stress

Safrole caused reversible lipid peroxidation and oxidative DNA damage in rat liver, as evidenced by dose-dependent increases in serum ALT and AST activities, on ip dosing at 250–1,000 mg/kg (Liu et al 1999). Intraperitoneal injection of 500 mg/kg of benzaldehyde or benzyl alcohol in rats caused a significant increase in the rate of reactive oxygen species formation in hepatic mitochondrial fractions (Mattia et al 1993). Benzaldehyde was subsequently found to inactivate glutathione peroxidase with a K_i value of 15 mM (Tabatabaie & Floyd 1996).

Visible lesions

Parenchymatous degeneration is the mildest form of liver degeneration. The hepatocytes become swollen, and uptake of water may cause the formation of apparently empty cytoplasmic areas (Niesink et al 1996 p. 687). Dietary methyl salicylate, fed to dogs at 150 or 350 mg/kg for 2 years, caused the formation of abnormally large liver cells, with both macroscopic and microscopic signs of hepatotoxicity. However, these adverse effects were not apparent from doses of 500 mg/kg for 9 days, 250 mg/kg for 52 days or 50 mg/kg for 2 years (Webb & Hansen 1963). Gavage doses of 200 mg/kg/day (−)-menthol in soybean oil for 28 days resulted in vacuoles appearing in the hepatocytes of 4 out of 20 rats. Lower doses were not tested, and the finding has not been replicated (Thorup et al 1983b). This is 13 times the recommended maximum oral adult dose for peppermint oil of 1.2 mL (1,080 mg) (Table 4.7). In studies on isolated rat hepatocytes, 0.1–4.0 mM (−)-menthol had a slight inhibiting effect on the release of ALT, AST and LDH, and was therefore protective at this concentration range (Manabe et al 1987).

Microscopic liver lesions in rats appeared after oral administration of safrole or estragole at 650 mg/kg/day for 4 days (Taylor et al 1964). A single ip injection of 300 mg/kg estragole in mice was hepatotoxic to adult females, but not to adult males or to suckling offspring of either sex (Vasil'ev et al 2005). Dose-dependent hepatotoxicity (paler and smaller livers) was observed in pregnant female mice following savin oil administration at 15, 45 and 135 mg/kg/day sc during 10 gestational days (Pages et al 1989b). Savin oil has been reported to cause liver lesions in guinea pigs suggestive of a degenerative hepatitis (Patoir et al 1938a, 1938b).

Box 9.1

Liver function test enzymes

ALP – alkaline phosphatase
ALT – alanine transaminase
AST – aspartate aminotransferase
LDH – lactate dehydrogenase

Fatty degeneration

Fatty degeneration is also known as steatosis. The accumulation of fat (triglyceride) globules within liver cells results in deterioration of tissue and diminished functioning. A seriously fatty liver becomes enlarged, and can contain as much as 50% fat instead of about 5%. Safrole caused liver enlargement in rats after administration at 150 mg/kg/day for 32 weeks (Gray et al 1972). When fed to rats at 1,000 ppm or 10,000 ppm for up to 370 days, safrole caused hepatic fatty degeneration and there was an increased incidence of neoplasms at both dietary levels (Homburger et al 1962). The exposure of rat hepatocytes to micromolar quantities of α-asarone in vitro caused morphological and ultrastructural changes, fat accumulation and inhibition of protein synthesis (López et al 1993).

Porphyrin production

Some individuals are not able to properly biosynthesize heme, a building block of hemoproteins including hemoglobin and myoglobin, a protein found in certain muscles. Molecules called porphyrins are used in heme biosynthesis, and heme synthesis defects are also known as 'porphyrias'. Heme synthesis defects are a rare underlying cause of some types of anemia. (+)-Camphor, α-pinene and α-(−)-thujone (a sample containing 3% β-(+)-thujone) increased the production of porphyrin in primary chick embryo liver cell cultures at 100 μM and above (Bonkovsky et al 1992). These were the only substances tested. This suggests caution in patients with underlying defects in hepatic heme synthesis, such as acute hepatic porphyrias. Ingestion of a mouthwash caused a clinical crisis in an 18-year-old female with hereditary hepatic porphyria. The mouthwash contained 1,8-cineole, menthol, thymol and methyl salicylate, but only 1,8-cineole was active in in vitro testing. The patient admitted drinking 'substantial quantities' of the mouthwash over a period of several months (Bickers et al 1975).

Little is known about the bioavailability of these constituents when applied topically, although peak blood levels of camphor were reported to reach a maximum of 0.2 μM after being applied undiluted to human skin (Martin et al 2004). It is therefore unlikely that topical application of essential oils will present any risk. Because camphor, pinene and cineole are ubiquitous in essential oils, and because other unknown constituents might also be active, we caution the use of all essential oils orally in people with heme synthesis defects.

Glutathione depletion

Many of the chemical reactions that take place in the liver generate reactive molecules such as electrophiles and free radicals. For the protection of its own cells, the liver contains a substance called reduced glutathione (GSH), a tripeptide incorporating a thiol group, which neutralizes these reactive molecules before they can damage DNA or protein. The reaction between GSH and an electrophile is catalyzed by a glutathione S-transferase enzyme to form an S-substituted glutathione conjugate. Glutathione is synthesized in two steps from its component amino acids, catalyzed by the enzymes γ-glutamylcysteine synthetase and glutathione synthetase.

Glutathione depletion occurs in the presence of large amounts of a reactive substance. In this scenario, reactive molecules are free to attack and seriously damage liver and blood cells, before the glutathione is replaced. Severe damage can be fatal, and is due to cell death around the central vein, leading to liver failure and/or hemolytic anemia.[3]

An oral overdose of an essential oil could be absorbed in sufficient quantities to deplete hepatic glutathione, although only a few oils are known to present such a risk. When either pennyroyal oil or (1R)-(+)-β-pulegone was administered ip to mice, doses of 300 mg/kg decreased hepatic glutathione to ~75% of control levels in three hours, and 400 mg/kg caused extensive hepatic necrosis (Gordon et al 1982). Glutathione depletion by pulegone or pennyroyal oil at lower doses has not been investigated.

Ingestion of almost 30 g pennyroyal oil by a woman was survived with few consequences other than vomiting, following treatment with N-acetylcysteine, which promotes glutathione replenishment (McCormick & Manoguerra 1988). A 22-month-old girl survived after ingesting <20 mL of pennyroyal oil. She was given gastric lavage, followed by activated charcoal, sorbitol and N-acetylcysteine. Ten hours after ingestion, her liver function tests were normal (Mullen et al 1994). Sullivan et al (1979) reported the ingestion of 30 mL of pennyroyal oil by an 18-year-old girl resulting in massive hepatic necrosis. Liver function tests became abnormal 24 hours after ingestion; she lapsed into coma and died on the sixth day in hospital from brain stem dysfunction due to liver damage. The only intervention was the administration of plasma and platelets.

Cassia bark oil depletes glutathione in experimental animals (Choi et al 2001), as do (E)-cinnamaldehyde and salicylaldehyde (see Constituent profiles, Chapter 14), two of its constituents. Cinnamaldehyde was administered ip to rats at 0.5 mL/kg (Boyland & Chasseaud 1970). Salicylaldehyde is more toxic to hepatocytes, but cinnamaldehyde depletes glutathione more extensively (Niknahad et al 2003). As an α,β-unsaturated carbonyl compound, (E)-cinnamaldehyde reacts with cellular nucleophiles such as glutathione, and there is good evidence that alkenal-mediated oxidative stress contributes to cytotoxic/genotoxic cell damage (Janzowski et al 2003). In addition, α,β-unsaturated carbonyl compounds, including (E)-cinnamaldehyde, irreversibly inhibit human glutathione S-transferase P1-1 (Van Iersel et al 1997). However, since at 25 or 50 mg/kg ip in rats, cinnamaldehyde reduced the activity of glutathione S-transferase, but did not deplete glutathione, its hepatotoxic action only manifests at very high doses.

Salicylaldehyde is not found in significant concentrations in any commercially available essential oils. p-Cresol rapidly depletes hepatic intracellular glutathione in rat liver ex vivo (Thompson et al 1994, 1996). Since birch tar oil contains p-cresol as a major constituent, it probably has a potential for glutathione depletion.

High doses of (E)-anethole and (E)-anethole 1',2'-epoxide (AE), a reactive metabolite, deplete glutathione (Marshall & Caldwell 1992, 1993). The toxicity of (E)-anethole is due to AE, different amounts of which are produced in different species. The quantities of (E)-anethole-rich essential oils used in aromatherapy pose no risk (see (E)-Anethole profile, Chapter 14).

Administration of 125 mg/kg ip of coumarin to male Sprague-Dawley rats depleted hepatic glutathione after 2 hours and caused hepatic centrilobular necrosis after 24 hours. A marked reduction of GSH levels was also observed in vitro. The coumarin metabolite, coumarin 3,4-epoxide is responsible for this toxicity (Lake et al 1984, 1999). Since the epoxide is the major metabolite in rats but only a minor one in humans, and is detoxified much more efficiently in humans (see Coumarin below), glutathione depletion is not an issue in humans.

It would be prudent to avoid oral administration of certain essential oils in people taking drugs such as acetaminophen (paracetamol), which rapidly consumes hepatic glutathione. Box 9.2 lists essential oils high in $(1R)$-$(+)$-β-pulegone and p-cresol.

Hepatocellular toxicity

$(6R)$-$(+)$-Menthofuran, a minor constituent of peppermint and cornmint oils, is a major metabolite of $(1R)$-$(+)$-β-pulegone. It is hepatotoxic because it destroys CYP enzymes, as does pulegone (see Constituent profiles, Chapter 14). Unlike pulegone, menthofuran does not deplete glutathione (Thomassen et al 1990). Menthofuran is oxidized by CYP enzymes to form reactive and hepatotoxic metabolites capable of irreversibly binding to cellular proteins, quickly destroying the liver (Madyastha & Raj 1990; Thomassen et al 1991). The reactive intermediate, 8-pulegone aldehyde (an α,β-unsaturated aldehyde) may be the ultimate toxicant from $(1R)$-$(+)$-β-pulegone or $(6R)$-$(+)$-menthofuran. Its rate of formation is 5–10 times faster from $(6R)$-$(+)$-menthofuran than from $(1R)$-$(+)$-β-pulegone in mouse, rat and human microsomes (McClanahan et al 1989; Madyastha & Raj 1990; Nelson et al 1992a; Thomassen et al 1992).

Hepatoprotection

A number of essential oils and constituents have demonstrated experimental hepatoprotective effects, restoring enzyme and/or bilirubin levels to normal values (Table 9.3). For example, thymoquinone (found in black seed oil) protected mice against

Table 9.3 Hepatoprotective effects of essential oils and constituents

Substance	Animal	Dose	Inducing agent	Reference
Essential oil				
Fennel (sweet) oil	Rat	0.4 mL/kg[a]	CCl_4	Özbek et al 2003
Garlic oil	Mouse	200 mg/kg ip	Acetaminophen	Kalantari & Salehi 2001
Thyme oil[b]	Rat	125 mg/kg ip	CCl_4	Jiménez et al 1993
Constituent				
Bergapten	Mouse	25 or 50 mg/kg po	Acetaminophen	Liu et al 2012
Carvacrol	Rat	73 mg/kg ip	I/R	Canbek et al 2008
	Rat	125 mg/kg ip	CCl_4	Jiménez et al 1993
Diallyl disulfide	Rat	100 µmols/kg po	CCl_4	Fukao et al 2004
Eugenol	Rat	10.7 mg/kg ip	CCl_4	Kumaravelu et al 1995
	Rat	100 mg/kg po	Iron	Reddy & Lokesh 1996
Thymol	Rat	125 mg/kg ip	CCl_4	Jiménez et al 1993
	Mouse	300 mg/kg po	CCl_4	Alam et al 1999
Thymoquinone	Mouse	12.5 mg/kg ip	CCl_4	Mansour et al 2001
	Mouse	100 mg/kg po	CCl_4	Nagi et al 1999

CCl_4, carbon tetrachloride; I/R, ischemia-reperfusion
[a] Mode of administration not stated
[b] *Thymus zygis* (74% thymol)

induced liver damage at doses of 100 mg/kg po and 12.5 mg/kg ip, though not at 25 or 50 mg/kg ip (Nagi et al 1999; Mansour et al 2001). When administered orally to mice at 1, 2 or 4 mg/kg/day for 5 days, thymoquinone dose-dependently induced hepatic glutathione S-transferase and quinone reductase (Nagi & Almakki 2009). Essential oils that induce glutathione S-transferase are also likely to be hepatoprotective (Box 4.1). As part of an experimental protocol to assess chemopreventive activity, male rats were dosed with 200 mg/kg/day po of black seed oil for 14 weeks. Gross and microscopic examination of the liver revealed no histopathological changes (Salim & Fukushima 2003). This dose is equivalent to 54–110 mg/kg thymoquinone.

Eugenol reduced the release of ALT at 0.1–4.0 mM, and of LDH at 0.001–4.0 mM in isolated rat hepatocytes (Manabe et al 1987). Similarly, daily oral administration of 100 mg/kg eugenol in 1 mL groundnut oil to rats for 10 days reduced

---

Box 9.2

Constituents and corresponding essential oils that have a demonstrated potential for hepatotoxicity

$(1R)$-$(+)$-β-pulegone

Pennyroyal (European): 67.6–86.7%
Pennyroyal (N. American): 61.3–82.3%
Calamint (lesser): 17.6–76.1%
Buchu (pulegone CT): 31.6–73.2%
Pennyroyal (Turkish): 66.7%

p-Cresol

Birch tar: major constituent

We advise caution in oral dosing of these oils in people with liver disease, such as cirrhosis and hepatitis, people with alcoholism, and in anyone concurrently taking acetaminophen (paracetamol).

elevated serum levels of ALT, AST and LDH, induced by iron (Reddy & Lokesh 1996).

In studies on isolated rat hepatocytes, the release of AST was dose-dependently increased by 0.2–4.0 mM thymol (Manabe et al 1987). However, in vivo, 125 mg/kg ip thymol (in an emulsion with Tween 80) showed considerable protection against carbon tetrachloride-induced hepatotoxicity in rats (measured as a reduction in ALT release), combined with a marked radical scavenging activity (Jiménez et al 1993). Similar protection was seen in mice, a single oral dose of 300 mg/kg thymol acting as a free radical scavenger of lipid peroxidation (Alam et al 1999).

Pharmacogenetic toxicity

Coumarin

Coumarin is found in a small number of essential oils and absolutes. It may present an increased risk to a small percentage of individuals. In clinical trials in Ireland using coumarin as an anticancer agent, 0.37% of the patients developed abnormal liver function that was considered treatment-related. The majority of the 2,173 patients took 100 mg/day of coumarin for 1 month, followed by 50 mg/day for 2 years (the other patients were taking between 25 and 2,000 mg/day). Eight patients showed abnormal liver function (as assessed by serum bilirubin, ALP, ALT and AST levels), which began 1–6 months after the commencement of therapy, and returned to normal on stopping the coumarin (Cox et al 1989).

In a crossover clinical trial in the USA, 138 women with lymphedema of the arm (after treatment for breast cancer) took 400 mg of coumarin or placebo daily for 6 months, followed by a 6 month crossover period. There were no abnormal liver function indices during a placebo period, but during coumarin therapy, nine women (6.5%) had elevated AST, and one also developed jaundice (Loprinzi et al 1999). In a third clinical trial in Germany, 114 Caucasian patients being treated for chronic venous insufficiency took 90 mg/day of coumarin for 16 weeks. Four patients (3.5%) had elevated AST and/or ALT that was considered either possibly or probably coumarin-related, and began at about four weeks. A past history of hepatitis was a significant risk factor (Schmeck-Lindenau et al 2003). In a similar German trial, there were no adverse events in 115 patients (Vanscheidt et al 2002).

These findings suggest that oral coumarin, taken for 4 weeks or longer at 90 mg/day or higher, causes hepatotoxicity in 0.4–6.5% of a largely Caucasian population of individuals with a history of various health problems.

Three primary metabolites have been identified for coumarin in humans and rodents: coumarin 3,4-epoxide (CE), the major metabolite in rats and mice, but a minor product in humans; 7-hydroxycoumarin, the major metabolite in humans, but a minor product in rats and mice; and 3-hydroxycoumarin, a minor metabolite in rats, mice and humans (Rietjens et al 2008). CE is an unstable compound that has been considered to be hepatotoxic (Born et al 2002). It spontaneously rearranges in aqueous solution to o-hydroxyphenylacetaldehyde (o-HPA), now thought to be the main hepatotoxic intermediate, or it can be conjugated with glutathione. o-HPA can be detoxified by conversion to o-hydroxyphenylacetic acid (o-HPAA), a process

that occurs more than 50× faster in humans than in rats (Vassallo et al 2004).

In studies of Jordanian volunteers, the relative importance of coumarin 7-hydroxylation and 3-hydroxylation was highly variable. One individual out of 103 was found to be deficient in CYP2A6, the enzyme responsible for 7-hydroxylation, due to a single amino acid substitution. In this case, approximately 50% of an oral dose of 2 mg coumarin was excreted as 2-hydroxyphenylacetic acid, the end-product of coumarin 3-hydroxylation (Hadidi et al 1997, 1998).

Subsequently, several population-based studies have identified CYP2A6 pharmacogenetic variations in Chinese, Iranian, Japanese, Malaysian, Thai and Vietnamese populations (Emamghoreishi et al 2008; Mahavorasirikul et al 2009; Peamkrasatam et al 2006; Veiga et al 2009; Xu et al 2002; Yusof & Gan 2009). It is clear that considerable inter-individual variability exists in the metabolism of coumarin to 7-hydroxycoumarin. Any reduction in CYP2A6 activity means that the epoxidation and 3-hydroxylation pathways take on a greater significance (Farinola & Piller 2007). However, clinical evidence suggests that coumarin hepatotoxicity is not linked to CYP2A6 polymorphism (Burian et al 2003), and even when 7-hydroxylation is deficient, the risk posed by o-HPA will still be significantly lower in humans than rats when exposed to similar doses on a body weight basis (Rietjens et al 2008).

In 2004, the European Food Safety Authority (EFSA) set a tolerable daily intake (TDI) of 0.1 mg/kg for coumarin. This is based on the hepatotoxic NOAEL of 10 mg/kg/day in a two-year dog study, and an uncertainty factor of 100 (www.efsa.europa.eu/en/efsajournal/pub/104.htm accessed April 28th 2012). According to the EFSA, humans are unlikely to produce toxicologically relevant concentrations of o-HPA following low level exposures when CYP2A6-mediated 7-hydroxylation greatly exceeds CE formation. Felter et al (2006) have suggested a reference dose (acceptable daily exposure level for a lifetime) of 0.64 mg/kg/day, based on 16 mg/kg/day NOAEL in female rats, with a total uncertainty factor of 25. They point out that this is likely a conservative value, and is protective for all health endpoints, including cancer.

Menthol

Essential oils containing large amounts of (−)-menthol are likely to cause liver problems in people deficient in the enzyme glucose-6-phosphate dehydrogenase (G6PD), which is usually involved in detoxifying menthol. Menthol provokes severe neonatal jaundice in babies with a deficiency in G6PD.[4] When they were given a menthol-containing dressing for their umbilical stumps, menthol accumulated in their bodies (Olowe & Ransome-Kuti 1980). This is an enzyme deficiency inherited by 400 million people worldwide, though most are asymptomatic throughout their life. It primarily affects people in Africa, the Middle East, South-East Asia and Brazil (Cappellini & Fiorelli 2008). G6PD deficiency is also gender linked; 12% of male African Americans are G6PD deficient, but only 3% of females (Hardisty & Weatherall 1982).

Menthol should clearly be avoided, at least in oral doses, by anyone with a deficiency of this enzyme. Such people will characteristically have had abnormal blood reactions to at least one of the following drugs, or will have been advised to avoid them:

- antimalarials
- sulfonamides (antibacterial)
- chloramphenicol (antibacterial)
- streptomycin (antibacterial)
- aspirin (analgesic, antiplatelet).

Choleretics

A key function of bile, which is produced in the liver, is to emulsify fats in order to aid their digestion and absorption. Some essential oils and their constituents are choleretic (meaning they promote the secretion of bile), notably peppermint oil, menthol and geranyl acetate (Trabace et al 1994). Although choleretics are useful in the treatment of gallstones and other disorders of the digestive tract, they are contraindicated in cases where the flow of bile has been severely obstructed (cholestasis) (Fujii et al 1994). Cholestasis leads to bile salts, fats and bilirubin accumulating in the blood.

Summary

- For oral or rectal administration, essential oils should be prepared in an appropriate medium and dose in order to avoid GI tract irritation.
- GI side effects from high-dose perillyl alcohol for cancer treatment include nausea, vomiting, satiety and eructation. In clinical trials with other constituents or essential oils, at doses about 14 × lower, adverse effect incidence is low, and equal to or better than that of more conventional medications.
- Hepatotoxicity from essential oil constituents is generally due to the formation of highly reactive metabolites. These may trigger cell death, in some instances with glutathione depletion, and sufficiently high doses can be lethal.
- Liver impairment typically presents as general malaise, either with or without jaundice, and is most commonly assessed by means of 'liver function tests' in which the activity of certain liver enzymes is measured.

- We advise caution for oral dosing of essential oils containing large amounts of $(1R)$-$(+)$-β-pulegone or p-cresol in anyone with alcoholism, liver disease, or who is concurrently taking paracetamol (acetaminophen), since this could result in depletion of glutathione, an important detoxifying enzyme co-factor.
- Salicylaldehyde is hepatotoxic, but is not found in any essential oils in quantities sufficient to cause problems.
- Eugenol, (E)-anethole and methyl salicylate are hepatotoxic, but only in doses much higher than those used for therapeutic purposes. Thymol and $(-)$-menthol may also fall into this category of substances. Eugenol and thymol are hepatoprotective in moderate doses.
- People deficient in the enzyme G6PD should avoid oral doses of essential oils containing large amounts of $(-)$-menthol (cornmint and peppermint).

Notes

1. Drug dosage is occasionally measured as milligrams per square meter of body surface.
2. Electrophiles, which are deficient in electrons, have an affinity for molecules with electron-rich centers. Unfortunately, most biological molecules, including proteins and DNA, provide suitable electron-rich centers and are quickly attacked by any electrophile that comes into contact with them.
3. A commonly used pharmaceutical drug that can cause liver damage in this way is acetaminophen (paracetamol). This drug is metabolized in the liver to a highly reactive electrophile which is neutralized by reacting with local glutathione (see Toxification section in Chapter 4). If sufficient electrophile is formed, the liver's glutathione stores will become exhausted, and cellular damage will ensue as liver proteins are attacked. This is why a paracetamol overdose is likely to be fatal.
4. Jaundice-like symptoms have also been seen after oral administration of estragole and isosafrole (Taylor et al 1964), both of which are hepatotoxic in a number of species (Caujolle & Meunier 1958).

The nervous system

The nervous system comprises the central nervous system (CNS) and the peripheral nervous system (PNS). Nervous tissue, especially in the CNS, is particularly vulnerable to toxic substances because it has a very limited capacity to regenerate, and if nerves are damaged they may not recover. Although the CNS receives a significant proportion of the cardiac output, it is protected from many blood-borne xenobiotics by the blood–brain barrier,[1] which permits access to only the more lipophilic substances. However, most essential oil constituents are moderately lipophilic and some will be neurotoxic, at least in high doses.

Neurotoxicity

A neurotoxic substance causes temporary (reversible) or permanent (irreversible) disruption by interfering with the structure and/or function of neural pathways, circuits and systems. Reversible behavioral changes may include cognitive function deficits, effects on mood or sleep (CNS), and muscular effects such as weakness, numbness and alterations in motor coordination (CNS and PNS). Developmental neurotoxicity (by definition caused during pregnancy or lactation) may disrupt behavioral, learning, or other developmental patterns (see Ch. 11, p. 158).

Cumulative, or even short-term exposure to a neurotoxin may lead to irreversible damage and chronic abnormalities. Known neurotoxins include industrial solvents such as toluene and trichloroethylene, metals such as mercury and lead, and organophosphates, often used in pesticides and nerve gases. Reversible neurotoxicity has been recorded for the minor essential oil constituent p-cresol.[2] Styrene, which can occur at up to 0.1% in cassia oil, is generally regarded as neurotoxic (Gagnaire et al 2006). Hydrocyanic acid, found in unrectified bitter almond oil, is a potent neurotoxin (Reynolds 1993).

Wormseed oil is powerfully neurotoxic, and oral ingestion has caused visible edema of the brain and meninges. In most cases of wormseed oil poisoning, considerable CNS damage is seen at autopsy, particularly in the brain (Van Lookeren Campagne 1939; Opdyke 1976 p. 713–715). Because of its high toxicity, this oil should be avoided altogether by any route of administration. Wintergreen oil is a less potent neurotoxin. In overdose, it causes death through cardiopulmonary arrest and respiratory failure. In a review of fatal salicylate poisoning cases, 18% had nervous system abnormalities on autopsy (McGuigan 1987).

Structural changes

Structural alterations to the CNS have been seen in repeated dose animal tests using some essential oil constituents. Given orally to rats for 28 days, (−)-menthone produced cerebellar lesions at 400 and 800 mg/kg/day, but not at 200 mg/kg/day (Madsen et al 1986). Also in 28-day studies, dietary (1R)-(+)-β-pulegone and peppermint oil were reported to produce microscopic lesions in the white matter of the rat brain and the cerebellum, respectively (Thorup et al 1983a; Olsen & Thorup 1984; Spindler & Madsen 1992), although other studies have failed to reproduce these lesions using peppermint oil (Mengs & Stotzem 1989; Mølck et al 1998). When male rats were exposed to 300 ppm turpentine vapor for 6 hours daily, 5 days per week for 8 weeks, α-pinene accumulated in brain tissue (Savolainen & Pfäffli 1978). The structural effects seen in these studies are reversible, but long-term exposure at such levels may lead to irreversible damage.

Phytol

Refsum's disease is a rare recessive familial disorder characterized by peripheral neuropathy, cerebellar ataxia, retinitis pigmentosa, as well as bone and skin changes (Berkow & Fletcher 1992). Its neurological component involves malformations of myelin sheaths around nerve cells, and is caused by an accumulation of phytanic acid in the plasma and tissues due to a deficiency of phytanic acid hydroxylase, an enzyme which metabolizes phytanic acid (Steinberg et al 1966). Phytanic acid is a metabolite of phytol, a constituent of jasmine absolute (and also many foods).

Phytol is only found at significant levels in jasmine absolute, and this is not taken orally. Even externally it is not normally used at more than 1%. A whole body massage using 30 mL of oil with jasmine absolute at 1% would entail a maximum of 0.006 mL of phytol being applied to the skin, not all of which is absorbed. Therefore very much less phytol would be absorbed than the dietary 0.5% found to cause no adverse effect in rats over 15 months (Steinberg et al 1966). However, some caution may be appropriate in people with Refsum's disease.

Functional effects

Some essential oil constituents have functional CNS effects that are pharmacological in origin, but may be detrimental to safety, even to the point of being dangerous. These include sedatives and psychotropics, many of which act by modulating γ-aminobutyric acid (GABA), N-methyl D-aspartate (NMDA), opioid or cannabinoid receptors. These are discussed below.

CNS stimulation or depression resulting from essential oil use is generally reversible at moderate doses, with only minor disruption of function. There is one report of dizziness, incoordination, confusion and fatigue in mice exposed to the vapors of commercial fragrances for one hour (Anderson & Anderson 1998). Sensory irritation (see Ch. 6, p. 100) is also a form of neurotoxicity, since it involves an alteration in neurological function.

It is interesting to note that in isolated cell or animal models, some essential oils and constituents protect nervous tissue from damage, often through antioxidant mechanisms.[3]

CNS stimulant activity

Both CNS stimulation and CNS depression are manifestations of functional neurotoxicity, since they can alter normal modes/states of cognition, alertness and coordination. CNS stimulants include many ketones, which reduce sleep duration and can also cause seizures (see Table 10.3). Not all CNS stimulants are convulsants, but this is the most important safety issue related to CNS stimulation by essential oils.

Convulsants

Convulsions are a functional manifestation of neurotoxicity and are an aspect of CNS stimulation. The terms *convulsion* and *seizure* are both used to describe involuntary changes in behavior, which may involve movement, function, sensation or awareness. They can range in severity from sudden, violent muscle contractions, often accompanied by loss of consciousness, to sensations of fear, visual disturbances or 'lost contact with the outside world' lasting for a few seconds.

Seizures are caused by abnormal electrical activity in the brain leading to loss of synchronization of neuronal activity. Symptoms depend on where in the brain the disturbance occurs. *Focal* or *partial* seizures originate from a localized area, while *generalized* seizures originate from more than one area. Partial seizures may develop to become generalized and involve loss of consciousness. Generalized seizures are classified according to their effect on the body and include the following:

- an *absence* (petit mal) seizure is characterized by a sudden, temporary change in behavior such as a loss of conscious activity or rapid blinking, and may not be noticed by others. These seizures typically occur in people under 20 years of age and last only a few seconds, followed by a full and rapid recovery
- a *clonic* seizure is characterized by rapidly alternating contraction and relaxation of muscles
- a *tonic* seizure is characterized by sustained muscle contraction or tension
- a *tonic-clonic* (grand mal) seizure includes characteristics of both tonic and clonic seizures. During the tonic phase, a sufferer may cry out, become incontinent, lose consciousness and fall to the ground. Muscle contraction may be extreme, and respiration may cease. The clonic phase involves generalized rhythmic jerking.

When chronic and recurrent, unprovoked seizures are classified as epileptic and may require medical intervention. Seizures may be precipitated by a number of mechanisms. These include a diminution of GABAergic transmission (as occurs with thujone and pinocamphone) and a drastic reduction in blood supply to the brain (as may happen in some LD_{50} tests).

The immature nervous system is more susceptible to toxic substances because the blood–brain barrier is less effective than that of the adult brain (Saunders et al 2000). There is also a greater susceptibility to seizures because the developing brain exhibits features that enhance neuronal excitability (Jensen 1999, Veliskova et al 1994). Changes that take place in the brain at a relatively young age reduce this excitability and the consequent susceptibility to seizures (Sperber et al 1999). Because of sex-determined differences in brain development, male children have a higher incidence of unprovoked seizures than do females (Veliskova et al 2004).

The ketones pinocamphone, (±)-camphor and α- and β-thujone can all cause convulsions (see below) at non-lethal doses in mice, while (1R)-(+)-β-pulegone has been implicated in convulsions at non-lethal doses in humans, when ingested as a constituent of pennyroyal oil (see Pulegone, below). Overdoses of methyl salicylate have also induced seizures. Essential oils containing significant amounts of these compounds therefore present a dose-dependent risk, though this may be modified by the co-presence of anticonvulsant constituents. Table 10.1 shows the maximum safe dermal and oral exposure for each of these constituents. The rationale for these amounts is explained by the appropriate constituent profile, and is also based on the data in Table 4.6. Table 10.2 lists the essential oils requiring dose limitation to avoid neurotoxicity.

Pinocamphone

Pinocamphone is convulsant and lethal to rats above 0.05 mL/kg ip (Millet et al 1981). The only essential oil that contains more than 5% is the pinocamphone CT of hyssop. Both pinocamphone and isopinocamphone act as GABA$_A$ receptor antagonists, a characteristic of some convulsants (Höld et al 2002).

Hyssop oil

'Hyssop oil' normally refers to the pinocamphone CT. The convulsant effects of hyssop oil were first researched in the 19th century. Doses of 2.5 mg/kg were injected ip into dogs, producing almost immediate seizures (Cadéac & Meunier 1891). In subsequent tests, injecting hyssop oil at 1–2 mL revealed a biphasic response. During the first phase, blood pressure fell, breathing became rapid, and random clonic movements appeared. The second phase was characterized by hypertension, rapid heartbeat and numerous clonic contractions (Caujolle & Franck 1945b). In rats, convulsions appeared for hyssop oil at single doses of 130 mg/kg ip, and the mean non-toxic dose was 80 mg/kg (Millet et al 1979). When administered to rats at 20 mg/kg ip for 15 days, cortical effects began to appear after 3–4 days, becoming stronger and more frequent thereafter (Millet et al 1980). Diazepam protected mice against the convulsant effects of hyssop oil (Höld et al 2002). The convulsant action of hyssop oil is assumed to be due to its content of pinocamphone (31.2–42.7%) and isopinocamphone (30.9–39.2%).

The amounts of hyssop oil used in these animal tests were generally high, but there are three reported cases of low-dose hyssop oil ingestion by humans resulting in convulsions. The first case was of a 6-year-old whose mother frequently gave him 2–3 drops of hyssop oil for his asthma. During one severe attack, he was given 'half a coffee spoon' (perhaps ~1 mL) shortly after which he suffered a convulsion. He fully recovered after three days in hospital (Arditti et al 1978). In the second case, an 18-year-old girl ingested 30 drops of hyssop oil to treat a cold. One hour later she lost consciousness for 10 minutes, during which she suffered generalized contractions and bit her tongue (Arditti et al 1978). In the third case a 26-year-old woman took 10 drops of hyssop oil on each of two consecutive days, and had a seizure on the second day (Millet et al 1981).

There is clearly a risk of seizures from ingested hyssop oil, although it should be noted that there is a linalool chemotype with ~50% of linalool, and only 0.5–1.0% of pinocamphone. The risk of seizures from the linalool CT is probably negligible, especially since linalool is an anticonvulsant (see Unilateral action below).

Thujone

A mixture of α- and β-thujone was convulsant and neurotoxic when administered ip to rats (Millet et al 1980). Subcutaneous thujone was convulsant but not lethal in mice at 590 mg/kg (Wenzel & Ross 1957) and in rats at 36 mg/kg (Sampson & Fernandez 1939) but convulsant and lethal in rats above 0.2 mL/kg (Millet et al 1981). In rats, the highest ip dose producing no convulsions was 0.02 mL/kg (Sampson & Fernandez 1939). Both α- and β-thujone inhibit GABA$_A$ receptor-mediated responses (Hall et al 2004).

A number of essential oils contain substantial concentrations of thujones (Table 10.2). For example, boldo oil (21.5% total thujone) caused convulsions in rats at an oral dose of 70 mg/kg (Opdyke & Letizia 1982 p. 643–644). Other essential oils for which there are animal data or recorded cases of convulsions are outlined below.

Sage oil

Commercial Dalmatian sage oil typically consists of 13.1–48.5% α-thujone and 3.9-19.1% β-thujone. When administered ip to rats, cortical effects began to appear at single doses of 300 mg/kg ip, with convulsions at 500 mg/kg. The maximum non-lethal dose was 3.2 g/kg (Millet et al 1979, 1980). The summary of a Slovenian paper states that *Artemisia caerulescens* oil,

Table 10.1 Dermal and oral maxima for convulsant essential oil constituents

Constituent	Dermal	Oral
Camphor isomers	4.8%	2 mg/kg
Methyl salicylate	5%	5 mg/kg
Pinocamphone isomers	0.25%	0.1 mg/kg
β-Pulegone	1%	0.5 mg/kg
Thujone isomers	0.25%	0.1 mg/kg

Table 10.2 Potentially convulsant essential oils with dermal and oral maximum doses

Essential oil	Toxic constituent(s)	Concentration in oil	Dermal maximum[c]	Daily oral maximum[c]
Western red cedar	α- + β-Thujone	69–99%	0.25%	No safe dose
Wormwood (white)	α- + β-Thujone	<95%	0.25%	No safe dose
Genipi	α- + β-Thujone	90.2%	0.3%	No safe dose
Hyssop (pinocamphone CT)	Pinocamphone + isopinocamphone	62–82%	0.3%	No safe dose
Sage (Dalmatian)	α- + β-Thujone	17.0–67.6%	0.4%	No safe dose
Wormwood (sea)	α-Thujone	63.3%	0.4%	No safe dose
Wormwood (β-Thujone CT)	α- + β-Thujone	35.4–63.3%	0.4%	No safe dose
Thuja	α- + β-Thujone	61.4%	0.4%	No safe dose
Pennyroyal (all types)	(1R)-(+)- β-Pulegone + (−)-(E)-α-pulegone	61.3–86.7%	1.3%	No safe dose
Buchu (pulegone CT)	(1R)-(+)- β-Pulegone + (−)-(E)-α-pulegone + (+)-(Z)-α-pulegone	36–82%	1.4%	No safe dose
Calamint (lesser)	(1R)-(+)- β-Pulegone	17.6–76.1%	1.5%	No safe dose
Tansy	α- + β-Thujone	46.3%	0.5%	15 mg
Mugwort (great)	β-Thujone	34%	0.7%	20 mg
Lanyana	α- + β-Thujone	31.4%	0.8%	22 mg
Ho leaf (camphor CT)	Camphor[a]	42.0–84.1%	0.8%[b]	25 mg[b]
Boldo	α- + β-Thujone	21.5%	Prohibited for other reasons	
Wormwood (β-thujone / (Z)-epoxy-ocimene CT)	β-Thujone	20.9–21.7%	1.1%	32 mg
Mugwort (common, camphor/thujone CT)	Camphor, α-thujone	32.2%	2%	56 mg
Wintergreen	Methyl salicylate	96–99.5%	2.4%	175 mg
Birch (sweet)	Methyl salicylate	90.4%	2.5%	193 mg
Rosemary (verbenone CT)	Camphor[a] and isopinocamphone	12.5–17.8%	6.5%	192 mg
Yarrow (chamazulene CT)	α- + β-Thujone	2.9%	8.6%	241 mg
Lavender (Spanish)	(±)-Camphor	16.4–56.2%	8%	250 mg
Mugwort (common, chrysanthenyl acetate CT)	α- + β-Thujone	2.6%	9.6%	269 mg
Artemisia vestita	α- + β-Thujone	2.5%	10%	280 mg
Feverfew	Camphor[a]	28.0–44.2%	10%	318 mg
Buchu (diosphenol CT)	(1S)-(−)-β-Pulegone + isopulegone (E+Z)	1.0–9.1%	11%	384 mg
Sage (Spanish)	Camphor[a]	12.9–36.1%	12.5%	388 mg
Rosemary (camphor CT)	Camphor[a]	17.0–27.3%	16%	513 mg
Lavender (spike)	Camphor[a]	10.8–23.2%	19%	603 mg
Rosemary (α-pinene CT)	Camphor[a]	6.6–20.7%	22%	676 mg
Wormwood ((Z)-epoxy-ocimene CT)	α- + β-Thujone	1.0%	25%	700 mg

[a]Isomer not specified
[b]Restriction also accounts for safrole and methyleugenol content
[c]See Adjusting safe doses and concentrations (see Ch. 13, p. 189).

rich in camphor and α-thujone, produced generalized seizures in various test animals (Cvetko et al 1973).

Convulsions were induced in a 33-year-old man who accidentally ingested one 'swallow' of sage oil (Arditti et al 1978), and in two other adults who ingested 12 drops and at least one swallow (Burkhard et al 1999). In a fatal case, a 44-year-old woman ingested approximately 0.25 oz (∼7 mL) of Dalmatian sage oil, which was later found to be high in thujone. She suffered several episodes of convulsions in the hours between ingesting the oil and dying (Whitling 1908). She had chronic asthma, and this may have contributed to the fatal outcome.

Thuja oil

Commercial thuja oil typically consists of 50% α-thujone. There is one report of thuja oil causing convulsions. A 50-year-old woman ingested 20 drops twice a day for 5 days. She was advised to take it by a 'naturologist', but did not follow instructions to dilute the oil to 1% before taking the drops. Thirty minutes after her tenth dose she suffered a tonic seizure and fell, fracturing her skull (Millet et al 1981).

Wormwood oil

Commercial wormwood oil typically consists of 33.1–59.9% β-thujone. In perhaps the earliest formally recorded case, a male adult ingested "probably about half an ounce" of wormwood oil. Within minutes he was unconscious, convulsing, foaming at the mouth with his jaw clenched. After prompt medical intervention the man survived, but he could not remember taking the oil (Smith 1862). A 31-year-old man was hospitalized after ingesting 10 mL of wormwood oil. He had been found, by his father, in an agitated, incoherent and disoriented state. Paramedics noted tonic and clonic seizures with decorticate posturing (Weisbord et al 1997).

Camphor

The dose of subcutaneously injected camphor required to produce convulsions in mice was 600 mg/kg (Wenzel & Ross 1957). The camphor used is described as a 'commercial synthetic product'. 'Synthetic camphor' normally denotes (±)-camphor. Humans are more susceptible than rodents to camphor neurotoxicity.

Convulsions in children of 2 and 3 years of age were survived following ingestion of 9.5 mL and 700 mg camphor, respectively (Phelan 1976; Gibson et al 1989). In a fatal case, a 16-month-old boy ingested one teaspoon of camphorated oil (vegetable oil with 20% camphor). He experienced frequent fits, constricted pupils, rapid pulse and an extremely high respiratory rate (Smith & Margolis 1954). Two cases of intoxication were survived by a 19-year-old and a 72-year-old. Both ingested 1 oz of camphorated oil (∼6 g camphor) which caused generalized seizures with no serious consequences (Reid 1979). A 37-year-old man experienced prolonged tonic-clonic seizures after ingesting ∼90 mL of camphorated oil. He was given hemodialysis and survived (Kopelman et al 1979). A man attempted suicide by ingesting 150 mL of camphorated oil (∼30 g camphor). He suffered peripheral circulatory shock and severe, prolonged grand mal attacks, but he survived after intensive treatment (Vasey & Karayannoppoulos 1972). This is one of the highest doses of camphor to be survived.

Camphor does not have to be ingested to initiate convulsions. A 15-month-old child suffered loss of muscular coordination and seizures after crawling through camphorated oil spilled by his sibling. He recovered fully. This case may represent sensitivity to camphor in a near-epileptic (Skoglund et al 1977). A 9-month-old child had three seizures in the 24 hours after a dressing containing ∼15 g of camphor was administered to thoracic burns. The level of camphor in the blood was 2.6 mg/L at the time of the seizures. It is assumed that most of the camphor was percutaneously absorbed (Joly et al 1980).

Toxic effects may follow a pattern of CNS stimulation (delirium, seizures) followed by depression (lack of coordination, respiratory depression, coma (Budavari 1989)). Neurologic symptoms can include anxiety, depression, confusion, headache, dizziness and hallucinations (Siegel & Wason 1986; Committee on Drugs 1994). Initial symptoms of camphor toxicity may begin within 5 to 15 minutes of ingestion. Camphor presents a clear risk to humans, even from non-oral exposure in the case of infants.

Pulegone

Subcutaneously administered pulegone (isomer unspecified) induced seizures in mice at the lethal dose of 1,709 mg/kg (Wenzel & Ross 1957), but it is not clear whether the seizures and deaths were related. Since (1R)-(+)-β-pulegone is the major constituent of pennyroyal oil (61–87%), it was probably responsible for the seizures suffered in four cases of attempted abortion through pennyroyal oil ingestion (Wingate 1889; Kimball 1898; Holland 1902; Early 1961). The amounts taken were substantial, including one teaspoon (∼5 mL) in one case, and 30 mL in another, but there were no fatalities. The risk of seizures from pennyroyal oil is likely to be limited to oral overdose.

Eucalyptus oil

McPherson (1925) commented that seizures were an unusual but possible symptom of eucalyptus poisoning. Mack (1988) similarly stated that seizures were possible, and were more common in children than adults. Seizures are in fact very rare with eucalyptus, even after ingestion of large quantities. In a case reported by Witthauer (1922), a 39-year-old male had tonic-clonic seizures after swallowing 26 mL of eucalyptus oil. However, the report expresses reservations as to whether the liquid ingested was in fact eucalyptus oil, as there were symptoms unusual in eucalyptus oil poisoning, including dilated and fixed pupils, and cyanosis. The author commented that, in the previous 30 years, there had not been a reported case of eucalyptus oil causing convulsions.

In eleven early case reports, none had seizures. Five of these were adults (Myott 1906; Kirkness 1910; Winterbotham 1914; Gibbon 1927), four were children aged 6–16 years (Neale 1893; Benjamin 1906; Foggie 1911; Sewell 1925), and the remaining two were 20 months and 33 months (Orr & Edin 1906; Allan 1910). In four later cases, all in children of 3–7 years, none had seizures (Craig 1953; Patel & Wiggins 1980). Similarly, there were no seizures among nine cases of eucalyptus nose drop instillation in children aged 1–36 months, 42 cases of eucalyptus oil ingestion in children under 14 years, and 109 children aged from 2 weeks to 9 years (Mclis et al 1989; Webb & Pitt 1993; Tibballs 1995,).

Out of 14 further cases, including nine children, one suffered seizures with a fatal outcome: an 8-month-old child who ingested 30 mL of eucalyptus oil (Spoerke et al 1989). No description of the seizures is given. We could find only three further reports involving convulsions. In the first, an 11-month-old boy had 10–15 mL of eucalyptus oil spilled onto his face and into his mouth. On arrival at hospital he was given oxygen, and shortly after experienced a 'short-lived, generalized convulsion'. He eventually recovered (Hindle 1994). In the second, a 4-year-old girl, with no previous history of seizures, suffered a grand mal convulsion lasting less than 1 minute. Earlier that day her mother administered, for the first time, 40 mL of an OTC head lice treatment containing 11% eucalyptus oil, which was washed out after 10 minutes, as directed. A hair conditioner with 2.5% eucalyptus oil was then applied and left on the head. Three hours later the girl felt nauseated and lethargic, and the convulsion followed. She recovered rapidly after the conditioner was washed off (Waldman 2011).

Burkhard et al (1999) present the case of a healthy 12-month-old girl who was given five prolonged baths containing an unknown quantity of eucalyptus, pine and thyme oils over a 4-day period. Shortly after the last bath she had a tonic convulsion lasting for 1 minute, and two similar episodes occurred the same day. Over the following days the number of episodes increased to a maximum of 133 in 24 hours. After 4 weeks, seizure activity ceased while she was being treated with phenobarbital and phenytoin, but there were further episodes several months apart. If a large amount of essential oil was used, the frequency of the baths and the susceptible age of the child could possibly explain the seizure activity. It is not possible to determine what caused the seizures, but a strong predisposition seems likely.

In many of the above cases, very large quantities of eucalyptus oil were taken (up to 45 mL) and there were several fatalities. In spite of this, seizures were reported in only four of 192 cases (excluding the doubtful Witthauer case). All four were children of less than 5 years, and large amounts (10–15 mL and 30 mL) were ingested in two cases. Therefore, we might conclude that seizures can occur in 2% of young children after intensive exposure to eucalyptus oil. The Waldman (2011) case is atypical, but confirms that eucalyptus oil can cause CNS problems in young children.

If eucalyptus oil was convulsant, suspicion would naturally fall on its major constituent, 1,8-cineole. In in vitro studies, hyssop, sage, camphor, and thuja oils (Steinmetz et al 1985) as well as calamus oil (Dhalla et al 1961) and 1,8-cineole (Steinmetz et al 1987) were all shown to modulate the cellular respiration (calcium and potassium levels) of rat brain slices, 1,8-cineole slightly more so than camphor. This action is thought to possibly correlate with the potential to induce seizures. According to Burkhard et al (1999), the Steinmetz et al results demonstrate that both camphor and 1,8-cineole share the same potential to affect brain cell calcium and potassium levels as does the known convulsant, pentylenetetrazol (PTZ). However, in cat brain, during PTZ-induced seizures, potassium levels increased (Heinemann & Louvel 1983), while in the Steinmetz study they did not. In addition, the pathophysiology of PTZ-induced

seizures involves many more mechanisms than calcium and potassium gradients (Ahmed et al 2005) as does the pathophysiology of seizures in general (Kovacs et al 2005). Therefore the Steinmetz et al (1987) report is not evidence that 1,8-cineole is a convulsant.

It is notable that, while CNS depression and coma are seen in LD_{50} tests in rats given 1,8-cineole, convulsions are absent (Jenner et al 1964).

Seizures linked to eucalyptus have only been reported in young children who ingest or inhale substantial quantities. Therefore, eucalyptus oil may not present a general convulsant risk, whether to older children or adults. It is questionable whether a CNS depressant (such as 1,8-cineole) could even cause seizures. Anticonvulsant medications are generally CNS depressant. In a sense the matter is academic, since eucalyptus oil can clearly cause CNS disturbances in children.

Fennel oil

There is one report of fennel oil inducing an epileptic seizure. A 38-year-old woman developed a typical generalized tonic-clonic seizure lasting 45 minutes, 2 hours after eating five or six cakes containing an unknown quantity of fennel oil. She was an epileptic patient, and took 300 mg/day of lamictal (lamotrigine) to control her seizures (Skalli & Bencheikh 2011).

Sweet fennel oil contains 0.2–8.0% of (+)-fenchone, and Wenzel & Ross (1957) reported that subcutaneously injected fenchone (isomer unspecified) produced clonic convulsions in mice at 1,133 mg/kg. This is equivalent to a human sc injection of 79.3 g of fenchone, or >991 g of sweet fennel oil. The rat acute oral LD_{50} for (+)-fenchone was 6,160 mg/kg (equivalent human dose 431 g); even at this level, it did not cause seizures (Jenner et al 1964). This dose of fenchone is equivalent to human ingestion of at least 5.4 kg fennel oil, or 10,000 times the recommended maximum oral dose (Table 4.7). Sweet fennel oil also contains (E)-anethole, at 58.1–91.8%. In toxicity testing, no convulsions occurred in rodents given single, lethal doses of 3.2 or 5 g/kg, or ip doses of 300 mg/kg/day for 7 days (Newberne et al 1999). Similarly, there were no convulsions in rats given single oral doses of up to 1.5 mg/kg sweet fennel oil (Ostad et al 2001).

Since fennel oil appears to be devoid of convulsant activity, a likely cause of the seizures in the above case is drug interaction. Lamictal is metabolized by UDP-glucuronosyltransferase (UGT) enzymes, and (E)-anethole significantly enhances the activity of UGT (Rompelberg et al 1993). This could have the effect of metabolizing the drug and clearing it from the system too quickly, leaving the patient vulnerable to her seizures.

Turpentine oil

Craig (1953) reported 16 cases of turpentine oil ingestion, all in children of 5 years or under. There were convulsions in two of these cases, infants of 13 and 14 months, the older child having ingested 4 oz (~102 mL), and the younger child an unknown quantity. A fatal case involving convulsions was reported in a child of 11 months, who had been given two teaspoons of spirits of turpentine by her grandmother, who said she thought the baby had worms. The child was distressed before the turpentine was given, she had a temperature of 103 °F, and findings on post-mortem included an enlarged thymus and acute bronchitis. It is therefore possible that the turpentine was not the principal cause of either the convulsions or the fatal outcome (Harbeson 1936).

The only cases involving seizures appear to be in infants who ingested very large quantities of turpentine essential oil, but none of its constituents are known to be convulsant. Consequently turpentine oil should not be regarded as presenting a general convulsant risk.

Other reported cases

Convulsions are a frequent consequence of wintergreen oil or methyl salicylate poisoning, and there is a general CNS excitation, causing very rapid breathing and heartbeat (Adams et al 1957). In LD_{50} tests for methyl salicylate, convulsions have been seen in guinea pigs, but not in rats (Opdyke 1978 p. 821–825). Anise oil is reported to have caused seizures in a 12-day-old infant, who had been given 'multiple doses' by the parents as a treatment for colic. After admission to hospital the infant recovered rapidly, and had no further seizures (Tuckler et al 2002).[4]

Animal data

There are no recorded cases of seizures from peppermint oil, although it has produced convulsions in acute LD_{50} assays: at 3–5 mg/kg and 2–8 mL/kg (oral/rat), and at 0.5–2.0 mL/kg (ip/rat and ip/mouse) (Eickholt & Box 1965; Mengs & Stotzem 1989). However, there were no convulsions in rats dosed orally with up to 100 mg/kg/day for 90 days, or up to 500 mg/kg/day for 35 days (Mengs & Stotzem 1989; Spindler & Madsen 1992).

The maximum recommended human oral dose of peppermint oil is 1.2 mL (1.1 g), which is 116× less than the minimal dose causing convulsions in rats (assumed to be 2 mL/kg, though it could be greater, as the convulsant threshold in this study was not determined) and 32× less than the non-convulsant daily dose in rats given for 35 days. Since a peppermint oil with 1.1% (1R)-(+)-β-pulegone and 25% menthone had a 90-day oral NOAEL of 40 mg/kg/day in rats (Spindler & Madsen 1992), it is unlikely that peppermint oil will produce toxic effects from therapeutic use. In peppermint oil, the neurotoxic potential of pulegone and menthofuran may be mitigated by (–)-menthol, which potentiates $GABA_A$ receptor-mediated responses (Hall et al 2004).

It has been said that ketones in general are highly stimulant to the CNS, and therefore a risk to vulnerable groups (Franchomme & Pénöel 1990). Table 10.3 summarizes seizure data from Wenzel & Ross (1957), which may be the basis of this assertion. The constituents in the second (LD_{50}) column were convulsant, but were also lethal at about the same dose. Wenzel & Ross suggest that lethality in a group of terpenoid ketones correlates inversely with ease of conversion to less toxic alcohols and their glucuronides. However, this model would need to be refined if predictions were to be made about other ketones, and there are doubts about some of these findings.

Since this report concerned subcutaneous administration in mice, the convulsant doses and the relative risk of each

Table 10.3 CNS stimulant effects in albino mice on subcutaneous administration

Test substance	CD$_{50}$ mg/kg	Mouse sc LD$_{50}$ mg/kg[a]	Sleep duration (mins)
Control	–	–	40.7
Sesame oil	–	–	42.7
Pinocamphone[b]	585	–	18.7
α- + β-Thujone[c]	590	–	16.1
Camphor[b]	600	–	31.6
Fenchone[b]	1,133	–	19.4
Piperitone[b]	–	1,420	20.3
Pulegone[b]	–	1,709	32.0
Menthone[b]	–	2,180	22.0
α- + β-Ionone[c]	–	2,605	12.0
Carvone[b]	–	2,675	26.1
Dihydrocarvone[b]	–	2,900	17.5

Modified from Wenzel & Ross (1957)
[a]LD_{50} values were assessed for those compounds that were lethal at the convulsant dose.
[b]Isomer not specified
[c]Unknown ratio
CD_{50}, mean convulsant dose

compound cannot be extrapolated with confidence to human oral or inhalation use. For example, in oral LD_{50} testing, no convulsions occurred in rats administered lethal doses of carvone (isomer unspecified) (LD_{50} 1,640 mg/kg), piperitone (isomer unspecified) (LD_{50} 3,550 mg/kg), or α- + β-ionone (LD_{50} 4,590 mg/kg) (Jenner et al 1964, Opdyke 1978 p. 863–864). Therefore, oral administration of these compounds does not appear to cause seizures. Similarly, De Sousa et al (2007) found neither isomer of carvone to be convulsant in mice by ip administration, and (S)-(+)-carvone was anticonvulsant. While there is a known human convulsant potential for various isomers of pinocamphone, thujone, camphor and pulegone, we could find nothing to substantiate a convulsant effect for the other ketones listed in Table 10.3. In other research, thymoquinone protected mice against PTZ-induced seizures through a GABA-mediated mechanism (Hosseinzadeh & Parvardeh 2004), (Z)-jasmone potentiated $GABA_A$ receptor-mediated responses, and therefore is likely to be anticonvulsant (Hossain et al 2004), and valeranone is a CNS depressant, being sedative, hypotensive and hypothermic (Houghton 1988).

Discussion

In almost all the recorded cases where seizures have been induced by essential oils, most of them apparently in non-epileptics, the oils were taken orally, though in a few cases very young children have proved vulnerable to non-oral exposure. A review of olfactory stimulation of seizures in epileptics concluded that, 'Reflex epilepsy caused by scent in the narrowest sense of the word is very uncommon. It depends on the degree of oversensitivity of the individual to olfactory stimuli' (our translation from the original German) (Nedbal 1967). In addition to those who are known epileptics, there is a potential risk to those with a low convulsive threshold, i.e., a potential for epilepsy that has not yet declared itself. Essential oils with a convulsant potency requiring dose limitation are listed in Table 10.2. Most of these are also listed in Table 11.1, which addresses pregnancy, breast-feeding and infants.

In summarizing convulsant essential oils and the constituents responsible, Burkhard et al (1999) list 11 essential oils as 'powerful convulsants'. Six of these (hyssop, rosemary, sage, tansy, thuja and wormwood) contain camphor, pinocamphone and/or thujone, and so may present some risk. Pennyroyal oil is a risk if taken in overdose, as is wintergreen oil (not mentioned by Burkard et al). However, Burkhard et al make no reference to dose or mode of administration, and no consideration is given to chemotypes of, for example, hyssop or rosemary oils.

Although some evidence is presented for listing the other four oils (eucalyptus, fennel, savin and turpentine) this is often tenuous. For example, Spinner (1920) is cited as evidence of convulsions for both eucalyptus and savin oils, but this is a review paper, and no original cases are reported. Similarly, no hard evidence is presented for fennel oil. Turpentine and eucalyptus oils have already been discussed and only present a limited risk. It is noteworthy that anticonvulsant activity (against PTZ-induced seizures) has been documented for two essential oils with 1,8-cineole and α-pinene as major constituents: *Psidium guyanensis* (40.5% 1,8-cineole, 13.9% α-pinene) and *Laurus nobilis*, (typically ~40.8% 1,8-cineole, ~11.5% α-pinene) (Neto et al 1994; Santos et al 1997; Sayyah et al 2002a).

Many of the essential oils listed in Table 10.2 have not been tested for convulsant activity, but it is likely that, for example, Western red cedar oil presents a convulsant risk, since it contains 69–99% of α-+ β-thujone. On the other hand, lavandin and spike lavender oils contain greater quantities of (anticonvulsant) linalool than (convulsant) camphor, so risk here may be negligible. It is noteworthy that a methanol extract of *Lavandula stoechas* protected mice from PTZ-induced convulsions (Gilani et al 2000). This extract would contain the essential oil constituents camphor, fenchone, 1,8-cineole, and α-pinene (Ristorcelli et al 1998). *Lavandula stoechas* is listed as a 'well-known anticonvulsive drug' in Iranian medicine, along with clove oil, valerian oil, anise, fennel seed, caraway, calamus, rue, melissa and lovage (Gorji & Khaleghi Ghadiri 2001).

As in all areas of toxicology, there is an element of uncertainty in extrapolating the data for a single constituent to an essential oil containing it, since other constituents may interact in a positive or negative way. In one report, four eugenol-rich *Ocimum gratissimum* oils, one from each season, were tested against MES-induced seizures. The 'Spring' oil was the most effective, and this correlated with a higher content of each of the following sesquiterpene minor constituents: β-selinene, β-caryophyllene, α-selinene, β-elemene, germacrene A and germacrene D. However, there was no correlation with eugenol content (Freire et al 2006). Conversely, in a similar report on four *Salvia libanotica* oils, there was a strong correlation between degree of seizure activity and content of camphor and thujones (Farhat et al 2001).

People who are prone to epilepsy may have idiosyncratic reactions to essential oils, and this makes the prediction of adverse effects difficult. Epileptics should therefore exercise caution with essential oils, especially orally, if they suspect that they might react badly. It would be prudent for those with a strong family history of epilepsy to be cautious. The same applies to those who may be predisposed to epilepsy, for instance people who had seizures some time ago, and are now off medication. Anyone with a fever is also more prone to convulsions.

CNS depressant activity

Depression in physiology and medicine refers to a lowering or a reduction in a particular biological variable or the function of an organ. The CNS represents the largest part of the nervous system, including the brain and the spinal cord. Common effects of CNS depression include reductions in breathing rate, heart rate, blood pressure, temperature and alertness; other possible effects include analgesia, anxiolysis, sedation, anesthesia, memory impairment, partial loss of motor co-ordination, and anticonvulsant effects. Alcohol is a common example of a depressant exhibiting many of these.

Overdoses of depressant drugs may lead to loss of consciousness, coma and death. Because some essential oils depress the CNS, caution is needed in their application, particularly with regard to reducing alertness. CNS depression is a common sign of eucalyptus oil poisoning, and has been observed in high-dose animal testing with 1,8-cineole, estragole and safrole (see Constituent profiles, Chapter 14).

In an overdose incident, an otherwise healthy 47-year-old man was found unconscious in his home after he had unwisely ingested 10–15 mL of anise oil as an influenza preventative. He regained consciousness within several minutes, but was disoriented, did not recognize his wife, and his speech was incomprehensible. He had cramps and 'gastrointestinal symptoms', and en route to hospital he vomited explosively. A neurological examination showed no abnormalities, and within 24 hours he had fully recovered (Bang et al 2008). The amount ingested was 30–50 times the oral dose of 300 mg recommended by Blumenthal et al (1998).

Typical mechanisms of CNS depression include facilitation of GABA and/or opioid activity, and inhibition of adrenergic and/or acetylcholine activity. GABA is the principal inhibitory neurotransmitter in the CNS and has three receptor subtypes, $GABA_A$, $GABA_B$ and $GABA_C$. $GABA_A$ receptors are highly complex, with binding sites for diverse drugs, including benzodiazepines, barbiturates and anesthetics. These compounds are known as $GABA_A$ receptor modulators, and potentiate the response of GABA at the receptors. They typically cause anxiolytic, sedative and anticonvulsant effects. Essential oils and constituents that potentiate $GABA_A$ receptor-mediated responses are listed in (Box 10.1).

Anticonvulsants

Anticonvulsants are a sub-category of CNS depressant, and are used to treat epilepsy. An anticonvulsant constituent may inhibit the action of a convulsant one in the same essential oil. In anticonvulsant research, the degree to which a test substance inhibits convulsions induced by various agents is measured. The inducing agents include strychnine, nicotine, picrotoxin (PIC), PTZ and maximal electroshock (MES). MES-induced seizures are inhibited by substances that block glutamate excitation mediated by the NMDA receptor, while seizures induced by PTZ are inhibited by substances that either block calcium channels (calcium antagonists) or that stimulate GABA$_A$ receptors (Sayyah et al 2004). It is generally believed that substances effective in the PTZ model are protective against petit mal seizures, and those effective in the MES model prevent grand mal seizures.

GABA receptor antagonists, which tend to increase susceptibility to convulsions, include PIC and α-thujone. A compound that potentiates GABA receptor-mediated responses, therefore, is likely to exert an opposing effect to α-thujone. For example, bicuculline, a competitive GABA$_A$ receptor antagonist, diminished the GABA-mediated action of anise oil (Sahraei et al 2002). This action of anise oil is probably due to its high proportion (75.2–96.1%) of (E)-anethole. Thymol also potentiates GABA$_A$ receptor-mediated responses (Priestley et al 2003;

Garcia et al 2006), and so would be expected to have an anticonvulsant action at appropriate doses.

Multilateral action

Essential oils that inhibit both MES- and PTZ-induced seizures are presumed to act via multiple mechanisms, both increasing seizure threshold and inhibiting seizure spread, and may therefore possess the broadest therapeutic utility. For example, a tarragon oil containing 21.1% (E)-anethole, 20.6% α-(E)-ocimene, and 12.4% (+)-limonene demonstrated dose-dependent activity against both MES- and PTZ-induced seizures (Sayyah et al 2004). Anise oil showed a very similar activity (Pourgholami et al 1999; Karimzadeh et al 2012). These findings cast doubt on the report that anise oil was the cause of convulsions in an infant (see p. 137). Cumin oil was also effective against both types of seizure, and observed membrane effects suggest that cellular mechanisms are involved (Sayyah et al 2002b; Janahmadi et al 2006). Angelica root oil, which is rich in monoterpenes, inhibited both types of induced seizure (Pathak et al 2010). West Indian lemongrass oil was also multilaterally anticonvulsant (Blanco et al 2009). A Java type of citronella oil, with 27.4% citronellal and 10.5% (−)-citronellol, inhibited convulsions induced by PTZ, PIC (both GABA mediated) and strychnine (glycine receptors) in mice (Quintans-Júnior et al 2007). Citronellol (isomer unspecified) was multilaterally anticonvulsant, as was terpinen-4-ol (De Sousa et al 2006, 2009).

Unilateral action

Other essential oils have a unilateral action, either inhibiting seizure threshold or seizure spread. In tests on two eugenol-rich oils, clove bud and Russian basil, efficacy against PTZ-induced seizures was only minimal, but there were significant results for MES-induced seizures (Pourgholami et al 1999; Freire et al 2005). Taget oil offered no protection against strychnine-induced convulsions, but was effective for convulsions induced by MES and metrazol (Chandhoke & Ghatak 1969). β-Eudesmol was also anticonvulsant in relation to MES, but not to PTZ or PIC (Chiou et al 1997). Damask rose oil was effective against MES-induced seizures (Ramezani et al 2008).

In some early research, MES anticonvulsant activity was reported for two linalool-rich oils, lavender and clary sage (Atanassova-Shopova & Roussinov 1970a, 1970b). Neither essential oil inhibited strychnine-induced convulsions, and clary sage oil was not effective against PTZ (lavender oil was not tested). The anticonvulsant activity of linalool can be explained by its inhibition of glutamate binding, and a direct interaction with NMDA receptors in the brain (Elisabetsky et al 1995b, 1999; Silva Brum et al 2001a, 2001b). The inhibition of acetylcholine release by linalool, and potentiation of GABA$_A$-mediated effects provides further rationale for this effect (Re et al 2000; Hossain et al 2002).

PTZ seizures are inhibited by yarrow oil, bitter orange oil, (+)-limonene, β-myrcene and citral (Kudrzycka-Bieloszabska & Glowniak 1966; Viana et al 2000; Carvalho-Freitas & Costa 2002). Although there are similarities between different terpenoid ketone isomers for their effects on the CNS, clear differences have also been noted. For example, at a dose of 200 mg/kg ip in mice, (S)-$(+)$-carvone significantly delayed the onset of convulsions induced by PIC or PTZ, while (R)-$(-)$-carvone was ineffective (De Sousa et al 2007).

Seizure activity can be reduced by essential oil inhalation. Previous inhalation of lavender oil inhibited electroshock and PTZ seizures, had some effect on nicotine-induced seizures, but none on those caused by strychnine (Yamada et al 1994). Preinhalation of a β-asarone-rich calamus oil markedly inhibited PTZ convulsions, and there was significant potentiation of GABA and reduction of glutamate in the brain (Koo et al 2003). Preinhalation of an essential oil complex from 15 plants had a similar GABA-mediated effect on PTZ seizures, but little effect on those induced by PIC or strychnine (Koo et al 2004).

Sedatives

Sedatives, which are a second sub-category of CNS depressant, are commonly prescribed to treat anxiety. At low doses, they cause calmness, relaxation, drowsiness and reduced breathing rate. Higher doses may affect speech, gait judgment and reflexes, and in extreme cases, may lead to unconsciousness and death. Thus, sedation, if sufficiently potent, is relevant to a discussion of essential oil safety.

In animal research, sedation is measured by counting the number of spontaneous movements (motility), by an increase in the time of pentobarbital-induced sleep, by a reduction in sleep latency (time taken to fall asleep) or by similar observations. Sedative drugs often impair motor coordination, and this is assessed by the 'rota-rod' test, in which the length of time a rodent is able to balance on a rotating rod is measured. Table 10.4 summarizes the published research for these areas.

When given by the oral or intraperitoneal routes to rodents, high doses are sometimes required to produce sedation, suggesting a weak potency or bioavailability. For example, when mice were given 100 or 200 mg/kg ip of citral or β-myrcene, barbiturate-induced sleep duration more than doubled at the higher dose, but little effect was seen at the lower dose (Do Vale et al 2002). The 1,000 mg/kg used for bitter orange oil by Carvalho-Freitas & Costa (2002) is a massive dose, equivalent to adult human ingestion of 70 g. It is possible that anxiolytic activity occurs at much lower doses. In humans, ambient exposure to orange oil vapor (0.25 mL of orange oil vaporized in a dentist's waiting room) had a relaxant effect in women, decreasing 'state' anxiety and increasing calmness (Lehrner et al 2000).

In other animal studies, sedative effects are seen at low doses. For example, (E)-anethole dose-dependently increased sleep duration in mice when given ip at 12.5–75 mg/kg with pentobarbital (30 mg/kg ip), or 50–100 mg/kg with chloral hydrate (220 mg/kg ip) (Boissier et al 1967). At 20 mg/kg ip in mice, the nutmeg oil constituents elemicin and myristicin increased pentobarbital-induced sleep duration by 91% and 119%, respectively (Seto & Keup 1969).

Inhalation studies in mice have identified a sedative action (assessed as a reduction in motility) for essential oils of lavender, neroli, sandalwood and valerian, and for the constituents benzaldehyde, citronellal, geranyl acetate, isobornyl acetate, linalool, linalyl acetate, 2-phenylethyl acetate and α-terpineol. Some of these substances were also effective following treatment with the stimulant caffeine (Buchbauer et al 1991, 1992b, 1993). Also in mice, inhaled terpinyl acetate or 2-phenylethanol vapors significantly increased pentobarbital-induced sleep duration by 19%, while rose otto (only 1–2% 2-phenylethanol) had a slight, but statistically insignificant effect (Tsuchiya et al 1991). Therefore rose absolute, which contains 64.8–73.0% 2-phenylethanol, might have significant potency.

Some contradictory findings have been published, involving different routes of administration. For example, inhalation of lemon oil vapor (containing 56.6–76.0% $(+)$-limonene) was reported to significantly *reduce* pentobarbital-induced sleep duration in both rats and mice (Tsuchiya et al 1991; Komori et al 2006). However, at 200 mg/kg ip (but not at 100 mg/kg), limonene apparently *increased* pentobarbital-induced sleep duration in mice (Do Vale et al 2002).

Isomeric differences have also been noted. Both enantiomers of carvone have sedative actions, but slight differences were apparent in their effects on locomotor activity and pentobarbital sleep times in mice. Both (S)-$(+)$- and (R)-$(-)$-carvone caused significant decreases in locomotor activity when administered ip and via inhalation to mice, but exhibited slightly different time courses (Buchbauer et al 2005; De Sousa et al 2007). Both enantiomers potentiated pentobarbital sleep time, but showed different dose–response relationships between 100 and 200 mg/kg ip (De Sousa et al 2007).

Valerian oil

Herbal preparations of valerian roots are widely used to aid sleep, and valpotriates, which are not found in the essential oil, are considered active constituents. Reviews of the sedative effect of valerian roots often conclude that synergy must play a part. In an early inhalation study, even faint odors of valerian had a sedative effect on rats (Macht & Ting 1921). Komori et al (2006) reported that valerian oil vapor inhalation increased natural sleep duration in rats by 18%. Sedative constituents of the vapor include borneol, isoborneol and bornyl acetate (Buchbauer et al 1992a). The sedative effects of the constituents valeranone, valerenal and valerenic acid are regarded by researchers as especially potent following ip administration (Arora & Arora 1963; Hendriks et al 1981, 1985; Houghton 1988; Rücker et al 1978).

Lavender oil

Lavender oil has been the subject of much investigation. It was sedative in mice when administered by oral intubation at 10 µL/kg (equivalent to approximately 8.9 mg/kg), increasing pentobarbital sleep duration from 21 to 37 minutes, and reducing sleep latency (Guillemain et al 1989). Given ip to mice, 200 mg/kg of linalool increased pentobarbital sleep duration in mice, an effect comparable to diazepam at 2 mg/kg ip, but at 50 or 100 mg/kg, the effect was marginal (Elisabetsky et al 1995a).

The inhaled vapors of lavender oil, and its major constituents, linalool and linalyl acetate, had a sedative effect on mice, measured as a decrease in motility (Buchbauer et al 1991, 1993). In a similar study, an atmosphere saturated with 1% $(\pm)$-linalool did not affect mouse motility, but at 3% saturation linalool was

Table 10.4 Sedative actions of essential oils and their constituents

A. Essential oils

Essential oil	Animal	Dose	Action	Reference
Anise	Mouse	50 mg/kg ip	↑ PB-induced sleep duration	Marcus & Lichtenstein 1982
Basil	Mouse	50 mg/kg ip	↓ motility	Shipochliev 1968
Calamus	Mouse	50 mg/kg ip	↓ motility	Shipochliev 1968
Chamomile (Roman)	Rat	350 mg/kg ip	↓ motility	Rossi et al 1988
Citronella (Java)	Mouse	100–400 mg/kg ip	Dose-dependently ↓ motility; ↑ ptosis & ataxia	Quintans-Júnior et al 2007
Clary sage	Mouse	100 mg/kg ip	↑ ethanol- and epivan sodium-induced sleep duration	Atanassova-Shopova & Roussinov 1970a
	Mouse	50–200 mg/kg ip	Dose-dependently ↓ motility	Atanassova-Shopova & Roussinov 1970a
	Mouse	50 mg/kg ip	↓ motility	Shipochliev 1968
Fennel	Mouse	50 mg/kg ip	↓ motility	Shipochliev 1968
Geranium	Mouse	50 mg/kg ip	↓ motility	Shipochliev 1968
Lavender	Rat	200–1,000 mg/kg ip	↓ stimulant action of caffeine and aktedron; ↓ motility	Atanassova-Shopova & Roussinov 1970b
	Mouse	300–1,700 mg/kg ip	↓ stimulant action of caffeine and aktedron; ↓ motility	Atanassova-Shopova & Roussinov 1970b
	Mouse	ED_{50} 248 mg/kg ip	Caused loss of motor coordination	Atanassova-Shopova & Roussinov 1970b
	Mouse	10 µL/kg po	↑ PB-induced sleep duration	Guillemain et al 1989
	Mouse	Inhaled*	↓ motility	Buchbauer et al 1991
Lemongrass (W. Indian)	Rat	75 or 150 mg/kg ip	Dose-dependently ↑ PB-induced sleep duration	Seth et al 1976
	Mouse	500 or 1,000 mg/kg po	Dose-dependently ↑ PB-induced sleep duration	Blanco et al 2009
Marjoram	Mouse	50 mg/kg ip	↓ motility	Shipochliev 1968
Nutmeg	Chicken	200 mg/kg ip	↑ ethanol-induced sleep duration	Sherry & Burnett 1978
	Mouse	Inhaled[a]	↓ motility	Muchtaridi et al 2010
Orange (bitter)	Mouse	1,000 mg/kg po	↑ PB-induced sleep duration; no motor impairment	Carvalho-Freitas and Costa 2002
	Mouse	1,000 mg/kg po	No motor impairment	Pultrini et al 2006
Rose	Mouse	50 mg/kg ip	↓ motility	Shipochliev 1968
	Rat	Inhaled[a]	↑ PB-induced sleep duration	Komori et al 2006
Savory	Mouse	50 mg/kg ip	↓ motility	Shipochliev 1968
Valerian	Rat	Inhaled[a]	↑ natural and PB-induced sleep duration	Komori et al 2006
Yarrow	Mouse	100–600 mg/kg po	Dose-dependently ↓ motility	Kudrzycka-Bieloszabska et al 1966

B. Constituents

Constituent	Animal	Dose	Action	Reference
(E)-anethole	Rat	300–400 mg/kg ip	Induced sleep of dose-dependent duration	Boissier et al 1967
	Mouse	250–400 mg/kg ip	Induced sleep of dose-dependent duration	Boissier et al 1967
	Rat	50–200 mg/kg ip	Dose-dependently ↓ motility	Boissier et al 1967
	Mouse	200 mg/kg ip	↓ motility	Boissier et al 1967

Continued

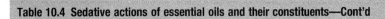

Table 10.4 Sedative actions of essential oils and their constituents—Cont'd

B. Constituents

Constituent	Animal	Dose	Action	Reference
(*E*)-anethole (*Cont'd*)	Mouse	50 mg/kg ip	↑ PB-induced sleep duration	Marcus & Lichtenstein 1982
	Mouse	12.5–75 mg/kg ip	↑ PB-induced sleep duration	Boissier et al 1967
	Mouse	50–100 mg/kg ip	↑ chloral hydrate-induced sleep duration	Boissier et al 1967
	Mouse	50–400 mg/kg ip	Did not impair motor function	Atanassova-Shopova and Roussinov 1970a
(*S*)-(+)-Carvone or (*R*)-(−)-Carvone	Mouse	100 + 200 mg/kg ip	Dose-dependently ↑ PB-induced sleep duration	De Sousa et al 2007
	Mouse	200 mg/kg ip	↓ motility	De Sousa et al 2007
α-Cedrol	Rat	Inhaled[a]	↑ PB-induced sleep duration; ↓ motility	Kagawa et al 2003
1,8-Cineole	Mouse	100–400 mg/kg ip	↑ PB-induced sleep duration; ↓ motility	Santos & Rao 2000
Citral	Mouse	100 and 200 mg/kg ip	Dose-dependently ↑ PB-induced sleep duration	Do Vale et al 2002
Elemicin	Mouse	20 mg/kg ip	↑ PB-induced sleep duration	Seto & Keup 1969
	Mouse	100 mg/kg ip	↑ ethanol-induced sleep duration	Seto & Keup 1969
(±)-Linalool	Mouse	1% inhaled	↑ PB-induced sleep duration	Linck et al 2009
	Mouse	3% inhaled	↑ PB-induced sleep duration; ↓ motility; no effect on motor coordination	Linck et al 2009
Linalool[b]	Mouse	Inhaled[a]	↓ motility	Buchbauer et al 1991
	Mouse	200 mg/kg ip	↑ PB-induced sleep duration	Elisabetsky et al 1995a
	Mouse	ED$_{50}$ 178 mg/kg ip	Dose-dependently impaired motor function	Atanassova-Shopova et al 1973
	Rat	100 mg/kg ip	↓ motility; ↑ sleep duration induced by hexobarbital	Atanassova-Shopova et al 1973
	Mouse	1–100 mg/kg po	Dose-dependently ↓ motility	Wagner and Sprinkmeyer 1973
Linalyl acetate[b]	Mouse	1–100 mg/kg po	Dose-dependently ↓ motility	Wagner and Sprinkmeyer 1973
	Mouse	Inhaled[a]	↓ motility	Buchbauer et al 1991
β-Myrcene	Mouse	200 mg/kg ip	↑ PB-induced sleep duration	Do Vale et al 2002
Myristicin	Mouse	20 mg/kg ip	↑ PB-induced sleep duration	Seto & Keup 1969
2-Phenylethanol	Mouse	Inhaled[a]	↑ PB-induced sleep duration	Tsuchiya et al 1991
α-Terpineol	Rat	50 or 100 mg/kg ip	↓ motility; ↑ sleep duration induced by hexobarbital	Atanassova-Shopova et al 1973
	Mouse	ED$_{50}$ 130 mg/kg ip	Dose-dependently impaired motor function	Atanassova-Shopova et al 1973
Terpinyl acetate[b]	Mouse	Inhaled[a]	↑ PB-induced sleep duration	Tsuchiya et al 1991
Valeranone	Mouse	100 mg/kg ip or 100 mg/kg po	↑ PB-induced sleep duration	Arora & Arora 1963
	Mouse	100 mg/kg ip	↓ motility; impaired motor function	Hendriks et al 1981
Valerenal	Mouse	50 mg/kg ip	↓ motility; impaired motor function	Hendriks et al 1981
Valerenic acid	Mouse	50 mg/kg ip	↓ motility; impaired motor function	Hendriks et al 1981
	Mouse	60 mg/kg ip	↑ PB-induced sleep duration	Hendriks et al 1985

PB, pentobarbital

[a]In these studies, ambient vapor concentrations were not measured

[b]Isomer not specified

sedative. In combination with pentobarbital, 1% linalool increased sleep duration by 201.2%, 3% linalool increased it by 236.5%, and this compared with a 213.5% increase from 1 mg/kg of ip diazepam. Neither concentration of linalool affected motor coordination (Linck et al 2009).

A bath with an unstated quantity of lavender oil added significantly increased the time spent in subsequent deep sleep by infants, aged 1–18 weeks. For three elderly human subjects, inhaled lavender oil vapor was as effective as their regular sleep medication (10 mg temazepam, 25 mg promazine or 192 mg heminevrine) in terms of number of hours slept at night (Hardy 1991). In two further pilot studies, one with insomnia patients, lavender oil inhalation resulted in improvements in sleep quality rather than duration (Goel et al 2005; Lewith et al 2005).

Mechanisms of action

The sedative effects of some essential oils are mediated via GABA receptors (see Box 10.1), and can follow inhalatory, oral or dermal administration (Aoshima & Hamamoto 1999). The potentiation of $GABA_A$ receptor-mediated responses by thymol is through a previously unidentified binding site, neither related to benzodiazepines nor steroids (Priestley et al 2003). Taget oil is tranquilizing in rats at 50 mg/kg ip, and tagetone is known to have a complex interaction with $GABA_A$ receptors (Chandhoke & Ghatak 1969; Perillo et al 1999). Sedative essential oils that act via GABA may also possess anticonvulsant or anxiolytic effects.

Inhaled blue chamomile oil vapor significantly decreased levels of plasma ACTH (corticotrophin) in ovariectomized rats that had been stressed by restricting their movement, demonstrating a sedative action. The effect was blocked by injected flumazenil (a benzodiazepine receptor antagonist) suggesting that one or more constituents of the oil were acting via benzodiazepine-sensitive (probably GABA) receptors (Yamada et al 1994).

The action of lavender oil in combination with sedatives has been described as 'real potentiation, and not [due to] any interference in the metabolism of the narcotic' (Atanassova-Shopova & Roussinov 1970b). Interestingly, however, when mice were treated with 1,000 mg/kg lavender oil ip for 5 days, they showed significantly increased motor activity compared to controls. This was accompanied by dose-dependent increases in dopamine D_3 receptor mRNA and protein expression in the olfactory bulb (Kim YK et al 2009). In humans, inhalation of lavender oil vapor reduced cortisol levels in the blood and in saliva (Atsumi & Tonosaki 2007; Shiina et al 2008).

The possibility of an olfactory mechanism has been suggested. In a study using rats with an intact olfactory system, inhalation of valerian oil vapor increased pentobarbital-induced sleep time by 46%. This was accompanied by a 39% reduction in GABA transaminase activity, supporting a GABA-mediated mechanism. However, the same treatment had no significant effect on either sleep duration or GABA transaminase activity in anosmic rats (Komori et al 2006). This might suggest olfactory involvement, but the authors were unable to give an explanation. Olfactory receptors are linked via nerve projections from the olfactory bulb to the neocortex, which is concerned with the perception of odor. They are also linked to the limbic system,[5]

which is supposedly involved in affective responses. In disagreement with the findings of Komori et al (2006), Kagawa et al (2003) found that inhaled α-cedrol produced marked sedation in both normal and anosmic rats, casting doubt on an olfactory mechanism.

Discussion

One concern with sedation is impairment of muscle coordination. This could feasibly be hazardous, for example, when driving or using other potentially dangerous machinery. Table 10.4 includes some motor coordination data in mice, from ip administration. The most potent substances of those tested were valerenal (50 mg/kg), valerenic acid (50 mg/kg) and valeranone (100 mg/kg), all constituents of valerian oil. These are the same doses required to induce sedation, which suggests that a sedative dose may affect muscle coordination.

Lavender oil has a motor impairment ED_{50} of 248 mg/kg ip in mice, implying that a very high oral dose would be required to interfere with muscle coordination. However, this is close to the ip dose of 300 mg/kg producing sedation in this species. In rodent studies, the separation of doses causing sedation and motor impairment is greater for clary sage than for any other essential oil or constituent. Doses of 100 mg/kg ip reduced motility and prolonged alcohol-induced sleep, but even 400 mg/kg ip did not affect motor coordination (Atanassova-Shopova & Roussinov 1970a).

Impairment of cognitive function (memory, alertness) is another potential concern, though this is not seen in clinical trials. Spanish sage oil has sedative effects, as do many of its constituents. They also inhibit acetylcholinesterase thus increasing the concentration of acetylcholine, which is likely to improve cognitive function. In a pilot open-label trial, daily oral doses ranging from 50–150 µl of the essential oil over 6 weeks resulted in an improvement in attention in 11 patients with probable Alzheimer's disease (Perry et al 2003). In another controlled trial, inhaled lavender oil was effective in the control of agitated behavior in patients with severe dementia (Holmes et al 2002). In a randomized controlled trial (RCT), subjects reported feeling more relaxed after three minutes of inhaling lavender oil vapor. The lavender group completed numerical computations faster and more accurately than the control group, suggesting a relaxed alertness rather than a stupefying effect (Diego et al 1998).

When inhaled or applied to the skin, essential oils may be absorbed in much lower amounts than those required to induce sedation in animal tests. However, anxiolytic effects may be largely responsible for improving sleep quality, and sometimes sleep duration, in humans, since inhaled lavender oil has anxiety-reducing effects (Itai et al 2000; Lehrner et al 2005). In a double-blind study, oral capsules of 0.2 mL (182 mg) lavender oil lowered anxiety, especially in women (Bradley et al 2009). This is 3.5 × less than the equivalent oral barbiturate-potentiating sedative dose in mice (Guillemain et al 1989). The combination of massage and essential oils is well known for its calming effect, and massage alone sometimes induces sleep. However, this does not mean that the individual, once awake, is not able to function normally.

Whether the sedative action of any essential oil is sufficiently potent to require warnings will depend on the dose and the route of administration. Caution is advised when using sedating oils in anyone receiving barbiturates, benzodiazepines or anesthetics, due to possible interactions with these drugs, a theoretical possibility even from essential oil inhalation. Of the essential oils studied, valerian seems to possess the strongest sedative activity, by any route of administration.

Psychotropic activity

A psychotropic (psychoactive) substance is one that affects the brain in such a way as to alter mood, behavior or mental function. Although psychotropic effects are arguably more relevant to pharmacology, toxicologists consider them a part of 'behavioral toxicology'. This is the study of changes in behavior caused by toxic substances, and due to their effects on both the PNS and CNS (Niesink 1996). These may include distortions of perception and judgment, and impairment of attention or mental processes.

Catnip oil

The herb is a well-known attractant of domestic cats, and has to be smelled, not ingested, to influence cat behavior. There have been accounts of a mild and transitory psychotropic effect in humans after smoking the dried herb. Four such cases were reported in 1969, with effects said to be similar to that of *Cannabis sativa*, i.e., euphoria, mood elevation, but less intense. Other effects included visual hallucinations, fascination with music, and a sense of unreality (Jackson & Reed 1969). There is one report of a 19-month-old child experiencing prolonged CNS depression after consuming a large quantity of the herb (Osterhoudt et al 1997). The constituent mainly responsible for the CNS effects of catnip is thought to be nepetalic acid, a metabolite of nepetalactone (Massoco et al 1995). There are no reports of the essential oil having CNS effects, but it contains 1.2–43.0% of nepetalic acid and 12.7–84.0% of nepetalactones.

Hemp oil

The substances that imbue *Cannabis sativa* with its psychotropic and hallucinogenic effects are the cannabinoids. These are present in quantity in the glandular hairs of the plant, where the essential oil originates (Malingré et al 1975). While strains producing essential oils with 1–2% of cannabinoids do exist (Malingré et al 1973, 1975), commercially available oils contain only traces, insufficient to cause a psychotropic effect.

Mexican marigold oil

The botanical name is *Tagetes lucida*, and 'lucida' derives from a psychotropic action dating back to the Aztecs, who threw the powdered leaves in the faces of captives about to be sacrificed, presumably to deaden their senses. There are numerous anecdotal reports of narcotic effects; the dried herb is smoked and is said to be mildly psychoactive (Emboden 1979). The active constituent is unknown, but neither estragole nor β-myrcene seems a likely candidate, so the essential oil may not be responsible.

Nutmeg oil

Many reports of essential oils with CNS activity relate to nutmeg and its constituents (Power & Salway 1908). A few of these describe hallucinogenic effects. Nutmeg has apparently been used as a hallucinogen since the 11th Century (Mack 1982). In 1576, the botanist Löbel described 'a pregnant English lady who, having eaten ten or twelve nutmegs, became deliriously inebriated'. Current knowledge suggests that ground nutmeg is moderately-to-strongly psychotropic when taken in high doses, and may occasionally cause hallucinations.

The effects of ingested whole nutmeg are subject to considerable individual variation. In one study, 6 g had no greater effect than placebo, supporting the author's hypothesis that any psychotropic effects of nutmeg were due to suggestion (Beattie 1968). However, this amount may be insufficient to produce psychotropic effects (Forrest & Heacock 1972). In two separate but almost identical cases, women ingested one whole ground nutmeg (~6 g) to correct irregular menstruation. Each was found in a state of collapse, with a feeble pulse, cold skin and irregular respiration, but recovered rapidly after strychnine sulfate injection (Hamond 1906, Reekie 1909).

Most commonly, subjects experience altered perceptions of reality and awareness. These are described as dreamlike states and feelings of unreality or incoherence. Moods vary from elation and euphoria to distress, anxiety, panic attacks and a sense of impending doom. Some individuals report agitation and excitement, while others become drowsy or fall into a stupor (Green 1959; Weiss 1960; McCord & Jervey 1962; Payne 1963; Åkesson & Wålinder 1965; Panayotopoulos & Chisholm 1970). Hallucinations occur at higher doses (15–30 g), and include visual and audible disturbances, such as flashing lights, 'melting walls', micropsia[6] and loud music (Åkesson & Wålinder 1965; Panayotopoulos & Chisholm 1970; Forrest & Heacock 1972; Abernethy & Becker 1992).

The largest reported amount of nutmeg ingested is 47 g, in prison inmates, who claim that it positively affects mood, sociability, perception and libido (Weiss 1960). The effects of nutmeg have been compared to those of cannabis, alcohol and heroin (Weiss 1960; Mann 1992). One case of apparent addiction to nutmeg was reported in a young man, who presented with psychosis and excessive thirst (Brenner et al 1993). Recovery from the effects of nutmeg intoxication can take up to seven days.

Nutmeg, deprived of its essential oil, may be devoid of psychotropic activity in both animals and humans (Power & Salway 1908). Two nutmeg oil constituents, myristicin (3.3–13.5%) and elemicin (0.1–4.6%) have been reported to reproduce many of the psychotropic characteristics of ground nutmeg in rats and mice (Truitt 1967). Myristicin is an inhibitor of monoamine oxidase especially MAO_A, an enzyme important in deactivating certain of the body's neurotransmitters, and this could partly explain nutmeg's euphoriant effects (Truitt et al 1963, Truitt & Ebersberger 1962). Myristicin also increases the levels of the neurotransmitter serotonin in rat brain (Truitt 1967), and this could cause psychotropic effects.

A metabolic pathway has been proposed which could lead to the conversion of myristicin and elemicin to 3,4,5-trimethoxyamphetamine (TMA) (Weil 1965, Weil 1966) or 3-methoxy-4,5-methylenedioxyamphetamine (MMDA) (Kalbhen 1971), both known hallucinogens. MMDA is similar in structure to MDMA, also known as Ecstasy (Shulgin 1966). However, in a case of suspected nutmeg abuse, no amphetamine derivatives were found in the urine, although metabolites of elemicin, myristicin and safrole were detected (Beyer et al 2006). When taken orally by humans, 400 mg myristicin (equivalent to ~40 g of whole nutmeg) appeared to have no psychotropic effects (Truitt et al 1961).

In a study conducted by one of us (RT), a subject ingested 1 mL of nutmeg oil (equivalent to ~10 g of whole nutmeg) but noticed no effects. When four subjects ingested 1.5 mL of the same oil, experiences ranged from euphoria lasting for 36 hours, to heavy-headedness, nausea, restlessness, proneness to laughter, a sense of unreality, heightened awareness, and clarity of thought and emotion. The only negative effect reported was a brief 'panic attack' in one subject the next morning.

On another occasion, one of the above subjects ingested 1 mL of parsleyseed oil, but experienced no psychotropic effects. This amount of parsleyseed oil contained four times as much myristicin as the amount in 1.5 mL of the nutmeg oil that did produce an effect. This lends support to the suggestion that myristicin is not psychotropic when taken alone, at least at these doses, and that other components of the essential oil probably act synergistically with myristicin and elemicin to produce the observed effects. Consequently, other oils rich in myristicin (e.g., parsley leaf and parsnip) may not be psychotropic, though mace oil may have similar effects to nutmeg oil as they have similar chemical compositions.

Thujone

The production of *absinthe* containing wormwood oil was banned in France in 1915. It was claimed that the oil acted as a narcotic in higher doses and was habit-forming. 'Absinthism', a syndrome of hallucinations, sleeplessness, tremors, convulsions and paralysis, was associated with long-term ingestion of the liqueur (Weisbord et al 1997). However, absinthes produced according to historical recipes are very low in thujone (0–4.3 mg/L) and a psychotropic effect from this amount is unlikely (Lachenmeier et al 2005).

It has been suggested that thujone and δ-9-tetrahydrocannabinol, the most active constituent of cannabis, interact with a common receptor in the CNS and so have similar psychotropic effects (Del Castillo et al 1975). However, thujone binds with relatively low affinity to cannabinoid CB_1 and CB_2 receptors and fails to mimic δ-9-tetrahydrocannabinol at appropriate doses (Meschler & Howlett 1999). Therefore thujone probably has a much weaker psychotropic effect than δ-9-tetrahydrocannabinol.

Discussion

The amounts of essential oils used externally in aromatherapy are unlikely to cause a psychotropic effect, no matter which oils are used. Some caution would be advisable with oral dosing of either mace or nutmeg oils, although normal oral doses may not be sufficient to produce any psychotropic effect. Thujone-containing oils are already restricted due to their neurotoxicity. Those with clinical psychological conditions, a history of psychotic episodes, or a history of use of cannabis and/or psychedelic drugs should be carefully monitored for their reactions to aromatherapy.

Summary

- A neurotoxic substance causes temporary (reversible) or permanent (irreversible) disruption by interfering with the structure and/or function of neural pathways, circuits and systems.
- Infants are especially susceptible to neurotoxicity and to convulsants.
- Wormseed oil is powerfully neurotoxic, and should be avoided by any route.
- Reversible disruption may temporarily affect motor coordination, mood, sleep, or cognitive function. Irreversible changes may cause similar, but permanent effects.
- CNS stimulants may reduce sleep duration, and/or lead to seizures.
- Sedatives and psychotropics also have functional CNS effects that may be detrimental to safety.
- The ketones α- and β-thujone, pinocamphone, (±)-camphor and (1R)-(+)-β-pulegone can all cause seizures, as can methyl salicylate. Essential oils with significant amounts of these compounds therefore present a dose-dependent risk.
- Some ketones do not cause seizures, and some are anticonvulsant.
- Eucalyptus and turpentine oils have caused seizures in a minority of children after substantial exposure from inhalation or oral ingestion. These may be idiosyncratic reactions with no dose–response relationship.
- An anticonvulsant constituent in an essential oil may counter the effect of a convulsant constituent, e.g., linalool (anticonvulsant) and camphor (convulsant) in lavandin oil.
- In animal testing, some essential oils have significant sedative effects. These oils are generally given orally or injected ip, often in high doses.
- Caution is advised when using sedating oils in anyone receiving barbiturates, benzodiazepines (or anesthetics), due to possible interactions with these drugs.
- In humans, inhaled sedative essential oils may be anxiolytic, without causing any impairment of cognitive or motor function.
- An unsafe psychotropic effect is unlikely from massage or inhalation with any essential oil, but may be possible from oral dosing with mace oil or nutmeg oil.
- Those with clinical psychological conditions, a history of psychotic episodes, or a history of use of psychedelic drugs should be carefully monitored for their reactions to aromatherapy.

Notes

1. The blood–brain barrier is not a physical structure as such. The relative lack of permeability of cerebral blood capillaries compared to peripheral capillaries is due to tight junctions between adjacent endothelial cells, which means that substances must pass through the cells if they are to reach the brain's nerve tissue. The result is to protect the brain from a wide range of potentially toxic chemicals. Substances bound to plasma proteins and those with a very low fat solubility do not readily pass through the barrier into the brain. Conversely, small, highly lipid-soluble compounds do.

2. There are three cresol isomers: o-cresol, m-cresol and p-cresol. p-Cresol is a constituent of birch tar and unrectified cade oils, and other cresol isomers may also be present in relatively small amounts. o-Cresol, which is also a metabolite of toluene, is a much more potent neurotoxin than p-cresol (http://www.oehha.org/air/chronic_rels/pdf/cresols.pdf accessed April 28th 2012).

3. Eugenol protected mouse cortical cells from neurotoxicity induced by NMDA, xanthine, or oxygen and glucose deprivation (Wie et al 1997). Bergamot oil protected human neuroblastoma cells from NMDA-induced neuronal damage in vitro (Corasaniti et al 2007) and at 0.1–0.5 mL/kg ip, it protected rats against induced cerebral ischemia (Amantea et al 2009). Turmeric oil was similarly neuroprotective in rats with induced cerebral ischemia, attenuating both nitrosative and oxidative stress (Dohare et al 2008). Greek sage oil, and its constituents α-caryophyllene and α-pinene, protected astrocytes from hydrogen peroxide-induced cell death in vitro (Elmann et al 2009).

4. There are a number of cases of neurotoxicity, many in infants, from the ingestion of star anise tea. However, toxicity is due to sesquiterpene lactones not found in the essential oil, and may also be due to contamination of *Illicium verum* with other, more neurotoxic species.

5. The limbic system consists of the hypothalamus, hippocampus, amygdaloid nuclei and basal ganglia. The hypothalamus is concerned with such processes as metabolism, growth, motivation, emotions, food and water intake, the immune system and homeostasis. The hippocampus is concerned with memory and spatial orientation.

6. Micropsia is a visual disorder in which objects appear much smaller than they actually are. It may be caused by a retinal disorder but is often associated with hallucination or an unconscious attempt to shrink the world to a less threatening size. Also referred to as 'Alice in Wonderland syndrome'.

The reproductive system

11

CHAPTER CONTENTS

Human reproduction is a long and complex process involving a series of events beginning with the production of ova in the female and sperm cells in the male through to birth and sustenance of the child in the early neonatal period. Each stage of this process is dependent on the co-ordinated synthesis and release of appropriate amounts of numerous endogenous hormones. Reproduction is therefore vulnerable to the influences of external factors, not least to exposure to exogenous chemicals presented as drugs, food constituents and products applied externally to the body.

Reproductive toxicology

Reproductive toxicology is the study of the harmful effects of xenobiotics on male and female reproductive functions and on the progeny. It encompasses fertility impairment, teratology, embryotoxicity, fetotoxicity, perinatal and postnatal toxicity, and is concerned with their causes, mechanisms, effects and prevention. These categories overlap, and substances may produce effects in several of them. One concern is that essential oil constituents may interfere with one or more of the processes involved in reproduction, for example, by mimicking or antagonizing the actions of reproductive hormones, thereby disrupting the finely controlled levels in the circulation.

Even when several reports are available on the effects of a substance in pregnancy, conflicting results are not unusual, and a complete absence of risk is impossible to demonstrate conclusively. However, dose is a critical feature of reproductive toxicity, and adverse effects will only occur when dose exceeds a certain threshold (Cragan et al 2006).

Xenobiotics in pregnancy and lactation

Few aspects of toxicology arouse such concern as the effects of chemical substances on the female reproductive system and the development of the fetus. A principal reason for this is a lack of information. Less is known about the effect of chemicals (from whatever source) on the reproductive system than in any other area of toxicology. As with carcinogens, there is no possibility of intentional human testing, and extrapolating from studies in pregnant animals is problematic (Neubert et al 1987).

Although human and animal reproductive physiologies share many similarities, there are also major differences. For example, one offspring per pregnancy, common in humans, is atypical of laboratory mammals, where there may be great variability in the toxic effects of an administered substance within and between litters. In rodents, a background of spontaneous malformations exists which makes it difficult to recognize weak fetotoxic effects. An observed effect may only occur under special conditions and in some species, and may be irrelevant to humans. Also, the distinction between gross abnormalities caused by toxic substances (teratogens) and normal structural 'variation' is a gray area.

A complicating factor of animal studies is that a compound may also induce adverse effects in the mother, and it can be difficult to distinguish between direct effects and indirect effects in the developing organism (Niesink et al 1996).

When thalidomide was tested on rats and mice, it did not cause the teratogenic effects later seen in humans.[1] On the other hand, drugs such as diflunisal were teratogenic in animal models but not in humans. While animal toxicology studies have been somewhat successful in identifying human teratogens, alert physicians and epidemiology studies have also made significant contributions. In vitro studies play a very minor role, although they are helpful in describing effects on cells or tissues (Brent 2004). For all these reasons, animal reproductive toxicity data must be extrapolated to the human situation with a degree of circumspection.

However, because toxicity testing in humans cannot be justified, considerable weight is normally given to animal tests for reproductive toxicity. Therefore we have to assume that substances which are reproductively toxic in animals should be either prohibited or restricted. Human case reports, such as those given below under Camphor are rare, but may provide useful information. Practitioners who use essential oils are encouraged to report cases in which pregnancy may have been adversely affected, as well as cases in which essential oils have apparently been safely used during pregnancy.

It is arguable that the human body will be able to metabolize and eliminate essential oil constituents more readily than synthetic pharmaceutical drugs, since they are found not only in many spices and herbs that have been consumed by humans for thousands of years, but also some common foods (Box 11.1). It is also a reasonable assumption that such substances are safe to consume, at least in very small amounts.

The safety of herbal preparations in pregnancy is frequently misrepresented. The American Pregnancy Association states, on its website: 'Unlike prescription drugs, natural herbs and vitamin supplements do not have to be tested to prove they work and are safe before they are sold.' (In the US, herbs are classified as dietary supplements, and manufacturers are therefore not required to provide proof of efficacy or safety.) In a review of herbs in pregnancy, Born & Barron (2005) comment: 'Few studies about the effects of herbs have been conducted in the general

population, and fewer still have been published about pregnancy use.' In a similar review, Marcus & Snodgrass (2005) comment: 'There are no rigorous scientific studies of dietary supplements [including herbs] during pregnancy, and the Teratology Society has stated that it should not be assumed that they are safe for the embryo or fetus.'

There are two major problems with these statements. First, there are in fact rigorous scientific studies of some herbs and essential oils during pregnancy in animals. Second, they smack of double standards, because they imply that all pharmaceutical drugs have passed through rigorous scientific studies for safety in pregnancy. They have not. The FDA classifies drugs into five categories, according to their assumed degree of safety in pregnancy (Box 11.2). Most drugs fall into category C, which means that either animal studies have revealed adverse effects, or that no studies have been done, whether in pregnant women or animals. (Less than 1% of pharmaceutical drugs are ever tested on pregnant women, for ethical and safety reasons.) If we apply the same standards to essential oils and pharmaceutical drugs, then either most drugs (whether prescription or over the counter) and most essential oils should never be used in pregnancy, or

---

Box 11.1

Examples of essential oil constituents found in common foods

Allyl isothiocyanate – arugula, broccoli, cabbage, cauliflower

Benzaldehyde – apricot, fig, apple, peach, tomato

Benzyl alcohol – apricot, papaya, peach

Benzyl isothiocyanate – papaya

β-Caryophyllene – carrot

p-Cymene – apricot, carrot

2-Decenal – beef, carrot, chicken, cranberry, fish, melon, milk, pork, potato, soy bean

Estragole – apple

Guaiacol – asparagus, celery, cloudberry, milk, passion fruit, tomato

Hexyl butyrate – apple, banana, grape, passion fruit, pear, strawberry

β-Ionone – apricot

Isoamyl isovalerate – banana, olive oil

(+)-Limonene – apricot, carrot, celery, citrus fruit, mango, peach

Linalool (isomer not stated) – apricot, papaya

β-Myrcene – carrot, celery

3-Octanol – banana, bilberry, citrus fruit, cranberry, grape, leek, mushroom, soy bean, strawberry

α-Pinene – carrot

γ-Terpinene – carrot

Terpinen-4-ol – papaya

Terpinolene – carrot

Velaraldehyde[a]– apple, asparagus, banana, bilberry, cabbage, carrot, celery, chicken, cranberry, citrus fruit, fish, grape, guava, milk, mushroom, pea, potato, soy bean, tomato, turkey, walnut

All of these constituents are profiled in Chapter 14, except for velaraldehyde

Information from Jennings & Sevenants 1964; Opdyke 1979a p. 761, p. 815, p. 881, p. 919; Opdyke and Letizia 1982 p. 697; Neudecker and Henschler 1985; Lawrence 1989 p. 157; Alasalvar et al 1999; Almora et al 2004; Guillot et al 2006

[a]A minor constituent of essential oils of clary sage, eucalyptus and rose

Box 11.2

FDA classification of drug safety during pregnancy

Category A

Controlled studies in women fail to demonstrate a risk to the fetus in the first trimester (and there is no evidence of risk in later trimesters), and the possibility of fetal harm appears remote.

Category B

Either animal reproduction studies have not demonstrated a fetal risk but there are no controlled studies in pregnant women, or animal reproduction studies have shown an adverse effect (other than a decrease in fertility) that was not confirmed in controlled studies in women in the first trimester (and there is no evidence of risk in later trimesters).

Category C

Either studies in animals have revealed adverse effects on the fetus (teratogenic or embryocidal or other) and there are no controlled studies in women, or studies in women and animals are not available. Drugs should be given only if the potential benefit justifies the potential risk to the fetus.

Category D

There is positive evidence of human fetal risk, but the benefits from use in pregnant women may be acceptable despite the risk (e.g., if the drug is needed in a life-threatening situation or for a serious disease in which safer drugs cannot be used or are ineffective).

Category X

Studies in animals or human beings have demonstrated fetal abnormalities or there is evidence of fetal risk based on human experience, and the risk of the use of the drug in pregnant women clearly outweighs any possible benefit. The drug is contraindicated in women who are or may become pregnant.

Information from Briggs et al 1998

we should continue with the status quo, meaning that most drugs and essential oils are considered safe to use, with some degree of caution, during pregnancy.

Fertility

Female Fertility

The female reproductive cycle includes a series of changes that take place in the uterus, ovaries and breasts, as well as the associated changes in regulatory hormone levels. Monthly pulses of gonadotropin-releasing hormone (GnRH) are secreted by the hypothalamus, and in turn, stimulate the release of follicle-stimulating hormone (FSH) and luteinizing hormone (LH) from the anterior pituitary gland. FSH and LH stimulate the growth and development of ovarian follicles and their release of estrogens and inhibin. A number of mechanisms operate to regulate circulating sex hormone levels. Increasing concentrations of estrogens in the blood inhibit the secretion of GnRH from the hypothalamus and FSH and LH from the pituitary by negative feedback. Inhibin also inhibits the secretion of FSH and LH. The result is a reduction in the secretion of estrogens.

The corpus luteum (yellow body), formed in the ovary on rupture of the ovarian follicle produces a number of hormones, including progesterone and estrogens. These hormones act together during the reproductive cycle to prepare the endometrium for implantation, and the mammary glands for the production of milk. After the menopause, the secretion of these two hormones declines, leading to changes in the sex organs, skin and bone, as well as emotional lability.

Endogenous mammalian estrogens comprise mainly 17β-estradiol, estriol and estrone, of which the first is the most important in premenopausal, non-pregnant women. Estrogens are responsible for the development of the female reproductive organs and secondary sex characteristics, and also protect the cardiovascular system, maintain bone integrity, cognition and behavior, and protect against skin aging. They also play an important role in glucose homeostasis, and modulate insulin sensitivity (Howes et al 2002; Ososki & Kennelly 2003).

Blood and tissue concentrations of estrogens are regulated by a complex series of steroidogenic metabolic pathways. Enzymes involved in these pathways, including aromatase and 17β-hydroxysteroid dehydrogenase, are inhibited by certain exogenous substances including some plant extracts. Alternatively, blood levels of 'free' estrogens may be altered by modulating the production of 'sex hormone binding globulins' (SHBGs). However, there is no clear evidence that essential oil constituents affect any of these mechanisms.

Two estrogen receptors, known as ERα and ERβ, have been identified. ERα is found in uterus, breast, ovary, testis, endometrium and hypothalamus; ERβ is found in ovary, breast, testis, prostate, thymus, spleen, adrenals, kidney, brain, bone, heart, lungs and intestines (Mosselman et al 1996; Brandenberger et al 1997; Kuiper et al 1996).

Citral impairs reproductive performance in female rats by reducing the number of normal ovarian follicles (Toaff et al 1979). The effect, however, was seen only after a series of six monthly ip injections at a dose of 300 mg/kg. This is equivalent to injecting ~25 mL of lemongrass oil into a woman's abdomen. Based on other research, we have restricted citral exposure in pregnancy.

Carrot seed oil has been reported to cause antigestational effects in rats and mice (Dong et al 1981). In a subsequent study, sc injection of 2.5–5 mL/kg of carrot seed oil into female rats or mice prevented implantation and blocked progesterone synthesis (Chu et al 1985). These are massive doses, although wild carrot has a traditional reputation as a contraceptive. Chinese zedoary oil terminated pregnancy in 90% of mice when administered as a 10% solution on days 4–6 of pregnancy. It was equally effective on pregnant rabbits when delivered as a vaginal tampon on days 2–4 of pregnancy (An et al 1983). Ethanol extracts and decoctions of zedoary rhizomes have antifertility effects (Kong et al 1986). We have contraindicated both of these essential oils in pregnancy.

Estrogenic activity

Substances with estrogen-like activity are widely distributed in the plant kingdom. Estrone has been found in potatoes, beets, yeast and palm kernel oil (Zondek & Bergmann 1938), and 17β-estradiol is a constituent of willow catkins and other plants

(Agarwal 1993). The hormonal actions of 17β-estradiol are mimicked by many plant constituents, known collectively as phytoestrogens. These include flavones, isoflavones, lignans and coumestans. Although the potency of many of these compounds is low compared to that of 17β-estradiol, their effects may be significant if ingested in sufficient quantities. For example, the isoflavone genistein in sweet clover was first recognized as being responsible for low fertility and abortion in grazing sheep (Hughes 1988). However, none of these compounds are likely to be found in essential oils because of their lack of volatility.

Epidemiological and animal studies suggest that the weak activity of estrogenic plant constituents may have beneficial effects, e.g., in breast and prostate cancers, cardiovascular disease and post-menopausal ailments (Dixon & Ferreira 2002). However, they may also disrupt the effects of endogenous hormones and cause developmental and reproductive disturbances (Diel et al 1999). The potential risks and benefits of these compounds may depend on whether they stimulate or block estrogen receptors, their relative potencies at the two receptors (ERα and ERβ), and local concentrations of 17β-estradiol.

A number of in vitro assays have been developed for estrogenic activity, focusing on binding to estrogen receptors, proliferation of estrogen-sensitive cells, stimulation of reporter gene transcription and estrogen-sensitive gene regulation in cell lines (Diel et al 1999). Some essential oil constituents have been found to bind to estrogen receptors, but with very low affinity. Citral, geraniol, nerol and eugenol displaced [^{3}H]17β-estradiol from isolated human ERα and ERβ receptors at concentrations some 4 to 5 orders of magnitude higher than estradiol. However, they lacked estrogenic or anti-estrogenic activity in both an estrogen-responsive human cell line (below cytotoxic concentrations) and a yeast screen for androgenic and anti-androgenic compounds. In yeast cell-expressed human estrogen receptors, citral, geraniol, nerol and (E)-anethole showed very weak agonist activity, while eugenol was anti-estrogenic (Howes et al 2002). α-Terpineol was anti-estrogenic in human breast cancer MCF-7 cells (Nielsen 2008).

Blair et al (2002) measured the binding affinity of 188 compounds for rat uterus estrogen receptors, including eight essential oil constituents: benzyl alcohol, 1,8-cineole, cinnamic acid, ethyl cinnamate, eugenol, isoeugenol, nerolidol and vanillin. No affinity could be measured for any of these compounds. In other research, Nishihara et al (2000) used a yeast screen to test 517 compounds for estrogenic activity, including eight essential oil constituents. Seven of these were considered inactive: benzoic acid, carvacrol, o-cresol, eugenol, isoeugenol, β-thujaplicin and thymol; p-cresol was considered active.

Geldof et al (1992) suggested that citral competes with 17β-estradiol for estrogen receptors and considered it estrogenic on the basis that it causes vaginal hyperplasia in rats. However, citral and geraniol failed to show any estrogenic effects in ovariectomized mice (Howes et al 2002). The in vivo action of citral seems to be species-specific, and under Male fertility we see evidence of strain-specificity. In early, poorly described research, very weak estrogenic activity was reported after injecting rats or mice with anise oil, fennel oil and (E)-anethole. No activity was seen with oils of bay, cinnamon bark, clove, dill, orange, pimento or thyme, nor with the constituents anisaldehyde,

estragole, methyleugenol, methyl isoeugenol, piperonal or vanillin (Zondek & Bergman 1938).

Albert-Puleo (1980) suggested that any estrogenic activity of (E)-anethole may be due to a polymer or a metabolite rather than to the compound itself. (A polymer is a chain of, in this case, anethole molecules.) The anethole metabolite, 4-hydroxy-1-propenylbenzene, weakly displaced 17β-estradiol from ERα receptors with an IC$_{50}$ value of 10^{-5} M, and promoted the proliferation of cultured human MCF-7 cells at 10^{-8}–10^{-6} M. In the latter assay, anethole had no effect up to 10^{-5} M (Nakagawa & Suzuki 2003). When given orally at 80 mg/kg/day for three days, (E)-anethole caused a significant increase in uterine weight in immature female rats (Dhar 1995), suggesting a hormonal action.

Anise, fennel and caraway oils demonstrated estrogenic effects in human MCF-7 cells, but did not stimulate the secretion of prolactin in vitro (Melzig et al 2003). In a yeast assay expressing human ERα receptors, oils from Pimpinella species were studied. Potencies were 5–8 orders of magnitude weaker than 17β-estradiol, and maximal responses ranged from 12.6–50.4% (Tabanca et al 2004). It was suggested that constituents other than (E)-anethole in these plants may contribute to their estrogenic activity.

Circulating 17β-estradiol levels were dose-dependently reduced in female rats by both bergapten and methoxsalen, when given in the diet at ~100 mg/kg and ~200 mg/kg. Enhanced metabolism of estrogens may partly explain the reproductive toxicity of bergapten and methoxsalen cited earlier, and this may be associated with a reduction in ovarian follicular function and ovulation (Diawara et al 1999; Diawara & Kulkosky 2003). These are extremely high doses compared to the amounts of bergapten or methoxsalen present in any essential oil.

It has been suggested that hop oil has estrogen-like properties (Franchomme & Pénöel 1990). However, although estrogenic substances have been found in the plant, notably 8-prenylnaringenin in the fruit (strobile) (Bradley 1992; Chadwick et al 2006), these are not found in the essential oil. Spanish sage oil (0.01 mg/mL) has been reported as estrogenic since it induced β-galactosidase activity in yeast cells (Perry et al 2001).

Although some essential oil constituents exhibit estrogen-like activity in various in vitro tests, their actions are extremely weak. Moreover, estrogenic activity data from single assays are insufficient to make confident predictions about their actions in vivo. For example, estrogen receptor binding assays measure only the affinity of a substance for its receptor, but give no information about whether it is an agonist or an antagonist (Diel et al 1999). Based on evidence available at this time, and with one exception, the case for contraindicating essential oils with potential estrogenic activity in pregnancy, in breastfeeding mothers or in patients with estrogen-sensitive cancers or endometriosis is not proven. The exception is (E)-anethole and we consider that there is sufficient evidence to contraindicate essential oils with high levels of this compound in these groups.

Dopaminergic activity

Chaste tree has been found to compensate for progesterone deficiency, and is used in traditional medicine for treating various gynecological problems. Alcoholic extracts of the plant have been found to stimulate dopamine D_2 receptors, leading to inhibition of prolactin release and normalization of the menstrual cycle (Caron 1986; Jarry et al 1991). Analysis of these extracts has led to the identification of diterpenes with dopaminergic activity (Hoberg et al 1999). Recent studies have reported similar benefits using the essential oils of chaste tree fruits and leaves (Lucks 2002, 2003), and a number of sesqui- and diterpene constituents have been reported (Senatore et al 1996; Zwaving & Bos 1996; Sørensen & Katsiotis 2000). Chaste tree oil, therefore, should be avoided in pregnancy.

Male Fertility

As in women, GnRH, FSH and LH play key roles in male reproductive processes. LH stimulates Leydig cells in the testes to secrete the principal androgen, testosterone. In some organs, including the prostate, testosterone may be converted to its more potent metabolite dihydrotestosterone (DHT). Androgens are also involved in the development and maintenance of male genitalia and of secondary sexual characteristics, and in the stimulation of anabolism.

FSH and testosterone stimulate spermatogenesis, beginning with germ cells called spermatogonia. These cells divide and differentiate first into primary spermatocytes, and ultimately into sperm cells. FSH and testosterone act together on Sertoli cells in the testes to stimulate the secretion of androgen-binding protein (ABP). This protein binds to testosterone and DHT, reducing their lipophilicity, and helps to maintain high local concentrations. Negative feedback mechanisms control the production of FSH and LH and their pro-secretory hormone, GnRH in the same way as in women.

The steroidogenic metabolic pathways important for regulating blood and tissue concentrations of estrogens also affect androgen levels, and it is worth noting that testosterone may be converted to 17β-estradiol by the enzyme aromatase. Although certain plant extracts are known to inhibit some of these enzymes, none of them appear to be essential oil constituents.

Estrogenic and androgenic activity

Three isolated cases of gynecomastia have been reported in prepubertal boys who used topical products alleged to contain either lavender or tea tree oil. This study has been criticized on a number of grounds, including that insufficient essential oil would penetrate the skin from wash-off products to cause such an effect, that no controls were introduced to exclude potential environmental chemicals such as phthalates, and that no relationship was established between the cases and the in vitro effects reported. Both essential oils did show a weak estrogenic action in human breast cancer (MCF-7) cells (Henley et al 2007).

Subsequent testing in an in vivo uterotrophic rat assay gave no indication that lavender oil had an estrogenic action when applied to the skin in occlusive patches at 4% and 20% in corn oil (Politano et al 2013). These concentrations are 5,000 to 1,000,000 times greater than the estimated exposure to lavender oil (0.0001–0.004 mg/kg/day) experienced by the

Henley et al boys. They are also more than 6,000 and 30,000 times greater than a conservative estimate of human skin exposure from multiple cosmetic products containing lavender oil.

Gynecomastia was reported in an embalmer who used an embalming cream containing geraniol. Abramovici & Sandbank (1988) proposed that geraniol had converted to citral in the liver, and that citral was estrogenic. However, as with the three cases above, no causality was established. The doctors who originally reported the case considered geraniol/citral to be an unlikely cause of their patient's gynecomastia.

When applied topically, citral induces malformations in chick embryos, causes selective oocyte degeneration and impaired fertility in rats. It was suggested that citral may affect tissue responses to sex hormones by inducing hyperplasia of sebaceous and prostate glands. It does not appear to be andromimetic (Abramovici 1972; Abramovici et al 1978; Toaff et al 1979).

Citral, applied in ethanol at a dose of 185 mg/kg/day to the shaved dorsal skin of male Wistar rats for three months, produced benign prostatic hyperplasia (BPH; Abramovici et al 1985). This may be testosterone dependent (Servadio et al 1986). In a later study, similar application of citral for only 30 days caused BPH in adolescent male Wistar rats. This was especially marked in rats with high serum testosterone levels, suggesting possible synergy between citral and testosterone (Engelstein et al 1996).

Both androgens and estrogens are capable of contributing to BPH (Wilson 1980). In these BPH studies, the amount of citral applied daily would be equivalent to ~10 mL for a human on a body weight basis. However, the morphology and function of the prostate exhibit marked species differences that make extrapolation to other animals and man difficult. It is apparent that the Wistar rat ventral prostate is reactive to citral. Further work demonstrated that the Wistar and Sprague-Dawley strains were the most susceptible to developing BPH, but that the F344 and Acl/Ztm rat strains remained resistant to treatment with citral (Scolnik et al 1994a). When applied to the rat ventral prostatic vascular bed, citral produced an effect resembling a classic inflammatory triple response. The ability of citral to cause BPH in some species may therefore be mediated via a non-specific inflammatory reaction modulated either by local release of neurotransmitters or through a direct effect on the endothelial cells (Scolnik et al 1994b).

Perillyl alcohol (a constituent of perilla oil) inhibits expression and function of the androgen receptor by inhibiting androgen-induced cell growth and androgen-stimulated secretion of prostate-specific antigen and human glandular kallikrein in human prostate cancer cell line LNCaP. This suggests that perillyl alcohol might be useful in treating some prostate cancers (Chung et al 2006). Eugenol is also an androgen receptor antagonist, with an IC_{50} of 19 µM in human breast cancer MDA-kb2 cells (Ogawa et al 2010).

Male rats given dietary bergapten or methoxsalen at 0, 1,250 or 2,500 ppm (corresponding to 0, ~75 or ~150 mg/kg) for eight weeks had significantly elevated levels of testosterone, and had smaller pituitary and prostate glands. Sperm counts were reduced in the high-dose group and more breeding attempts were required to impregnate females (Diawara et al 2001). These are extremely high doses, equivalent to 1,590 g or 3,180 g of bergamot oil in an adult human for bergapten.

Other actions

East Indian nutmeg oil has been found to reduce fertility in male mice (Pecevski et al 1981). The dose-dependent effect occurred at 60–400 mg/kg/day given 5 days per week for 8 weeks. The number of fertile mice was reduced from 95% (control) to 71% (lowest dose) and 32% (highest dose). Chromosomal damage was seen in some of the male offspring. It is difficult to draw any firm conclusions from this research. Even 60 mg/kg/day (equivalent to 4 g in an adult human) is a very high dose, especially when taken for 8 weeks, and effects on fertility are often species/strain-specific.

Eugenol caused degenerative changes in the secretory cells of rat seminal vesicles when given im at doses of 0.2–0.3 mg/kg/day for 10 days. The resemblance between eugenol and other polyphenolic compounds with estrogenic activity, such as anethole and diethylstilbestrol, was discussed (Vanithakumari et al 1998). Other effects on tissues of the reproductive system include that of thyme oil, which, unlike clove, caraway, sage and melissa oils, relaxed the isolated smooth muscle of rat seminal vesicles (Zarzuelo & Crespo 2002).

Conception

On fertilization, the nuclei of an ovum and a sperm combine to form a new cell possessing a unique combination of genes, known as an embryo, zygote or conceptus. This cell begins to divide and the embryo travels along the fallopian tube until, after about four days, it reaches the uterus. Cell differentiation (organization into different parts and functions) then takes place.

All oral contraceptives contain a synthetic form of progesterone. Some contain only progesterone (the progesterone-only pill) while others contain variable amounts of estrogens as well (the combined and phased pills). These drugs work mainly by negative feedback inhibition of the secretion of FSH and LH from the pituitary gland. Low FSH and LH concentrations prevent development of the dominant follicle and thus suppresses ovulation. The progesterone-only pill does not always suppress ovulation, and works mainly by making the cervical mucus impenetrable to sperm. It is somewhat less reliable than the estrogen-containing types.

Although some plants have contraceptive actions in males or females, there is no evidence for essential oils interfering with conception. (However, an anti-implantation effect has a similar result; see Implantation below.) It seems unlikely that estrogenic essential oils could interfere with orthodox oral contraceptives. Any estrogen-like effect of the oils would almost certainly be far weaker than the pill's hormonal action, especially after dermal application of the oil.

It is worth noting that latex condoms can be weakened by both vegetable oils and essential oils.[2]

Implantation

After conception, progesterone acts with estrogens to stimulate the uterus to form a spongy lining ready for implantation of the fertilized ovum. In humans, this begins 6 days after fertilization and is completed within the next 7 days. During and after implantation, the embryo becomes surrounded by a protective, fluid-filled capsule, which protects it from injury. It should be noted that the gestational period for rats and mice is three weeks, one week per trimester.

Subcutaneously administered savin oil, containing 50% sabinyl acetate, prevented implantation in mice at 45 and 135 mg/kg, but not at 15 mg/kg when given on gestational days 0–4. The same pattern was observed with sabinyl acetate given at 70 mg/kg. However, no anti-fertility effect was found when savin oil was given on gestational days 8–11, indicating that the abortifacient action of sabinyl acetate is due to inhibition of implantation (Pages et al 1996). Savin oil is contraindicated in pregnancy (Table 11.1).

Table 11.1 Essential oils that should be avoided by any route throughout pregnancy and lactation

Essential oil	Toxic constituent	Concentration in oil
Anise	(E)-Anethole	<96.1%
Anise (star)	(E)-Anethole	91.8%
Araucaria	β–Eudesmol	25.9%
Artemisia vestita	α- + β-Thujone	2.5%
Atractylis	β–Elemene + β-Eudesmol	44%
Birch (sweet)	Methyl salicylate	90.4%
Black seed	Thymoquinone	<54.8%
Buchu (diosphenol CT)	α- + β-Pulegone	<9.1%
Buchu (pulegone CT)	β-Pulegone	<73.2%
Calamint (lesser)	β-Pulegone	<76.1%
Carrot seed	Not identified	–
Cassia	Not identified	–
Chaste tree	Not identified	–
Cinnamon bark	Not identified	–
Costus	Costunolide + dehydrocostus lactone	17%
Cypress (blue)	β–Eudesmol	14.4%
Dill seed (Indian)	Apiole (dill)	<52.5%
Fennel (bitter)	(E)-Anethole	<84.3%
Fennel (sweet)	(E)-Anethole	<92.5%
Feverfew	Camphor	<44.2%
Genipi	α-Thujone	79.8%
Hibawood	β-Thujaplicin	Major constituent
Ho leaf (camphor CT)	Camphor	<84.1%
Hyssop (pinocamphone CT)	Pinocamphones	<80%
Lanyana	α- + β-Thujone	<32%
Lavender (Spanish)	Camphor	<56.2%

Continued

Table 11.1 Essential oils that should be avoided by any route throughout pregnancy and lactation—Cont'd

Essential oil	Toxic constituent	Concentration in oil
Mugwort (common, camphor/thujone CT)	α-Thujone	11.4%
Mugwort (common, chrysanthenyl acetate CT)	α- + β-Thujone	<2.6%
Mugwort (great)	β-Thujone	34.0%
Myrrh	β–Elemene + furanodiene	28.4%
Myrtle (aniseed)	(E)-Anethole	95.0%
Oregano	Not identified	–
Parsley leaf	Apiole (dill), possibly p-menthatriene	<50%
Parsleyseed	Apiole (parsley)	<67.5%
Pennyroyal	β-Pulegone	<86.7%
Rue	Not identified	–
Sage (Dalmatian)	α- + β-Thujone	<60%
Sage (Spanish)	Sabinyl acetate	<9.0%
Savin	Sabinyl acetate	<53.1%
Tansy	α- + β-Thujone	<46%
Thuja	α- + β-Thujone	<60%
Western red cedar	α- + β-Thujone	<99%
Wintergreen	Methyl salicylate	<99.5%
Wormwood (all chemotypes)	Thujones and sabinyl acetate	Varying amounts
Wormwood (sea)	α-Thujone	63.3%
Wormwood (white)	α- + β-Thujone + camphor	<95%
Yarrow (green)	Sabinyl acetate	3.7%
Zedoary	Not identified	–

Bergapten or methoxsalen were given in the diet to pregnant female rats for 39–49 days (until the day before expected parturition) at 0, 1,250 or 2,500 ppm, corresponding to 0, ~100 mg/kg and ~200 mg/kg. Bergapten, but not methoxsalen, caused a significant reduction in the number of implantation sites. The number of pups per female was significantly lower at both dose levels for bergapten, and in the high-dose group for methoxsalen. Uterine weight was significantly reduced in the high-dose group for bergapten, and in both dosed groups for methoxsalen. Enhanced metabolism of estrogens may explain the observed reproductive toxicity of bergapten and methoxsalen (Diawara et al 1999; Diawara & Kulkosky

2003). Extrapolating the bergapten study to a 50 kg woman suggests that 5 g bergapten orally could reduce implantation. Since this would be equivalent to consuming 1.5–3.0 kg lime oil, the findings have no relevance to essential oil use.

Doses of 50, 70 and 80 mg/kg/day po of (E)-anethole, given on days 1–10 of pregnancy, were reported to cause 33.3%, 66.6% and 100% reductions in implantation in female rats. When 80 mg/kg/day po of (E)-anethole was given on days 1–2 of pregnancy, there was no antifertility effect. When the same dose was given on days 3–5, pregnancy was prevented in all five rats. When given on days 6–10, pregnancy was prevented in three of five rats. It is suggested that this may be related to a disruption of hormonal balance (Dhar 1995). These results were not supported in an earlier study, in which female rats were given (E)-anethole at 25, 175 or 350 mg/kg by gavage for 7 days prior to mating and until day 4 of lactation. There was no reproductive toxicity at the lower doses, while some increase in mortality, stillbirths and reduction in body weight at birth was seen in the high-dose group. Body weight gain was reduced in the two higher dose groups during the pre-mating period, and this was attributed to palatability problems (ARL 1992, cited in Newberne et al 1999). There is no obvious reason for the inconsistency between these studies. The Dhar (1995) data suggest that in rats, (E)-anethole is only effective after day three of pregnancy, which might result from physiological changes leading to altered susceptibility to anethole.

Toxicity during gestation

This includes any toxic effect on the conceptus resulting from pre-natal exposure, including structural or functional abnormalities. (Developmental toxicity also includes postnatal manifestations of such effects.) Structural defects are mainly induced in the embryonic period, whereas functional defects are established during the fetal period and later stages of development (Niesink et al 1996). There are very few data on the distribution and fate of drugs within the human embryo because it is almost impossible to design safe experiments.

Some essential oil constituents could prove damaging to the development of the conceptus. That is, they could be teratogenic, or they could in some way disturb the normal outcome of the pregnancy, for instance by promoting resorption of the early embryo. Another concern is that any large or polar metabolites produced by the fetus might be unable to diffuse across the placenta to the maternal bloodstream, and may thereby become trapped inside it (Timbrell 2000). This, however, may not be important for essential oil constituents.

Some, such as (E)-anethole and eugenol, would be classed as toxic if they were not rapidly detoxified in the liver (see Table 12.2). The question of whether they are toxic to the fetus depends on the amount of the substance in the mother's circulation, and her metabolic status. Any unmetabolized compound would be expected to cross into the fetal circulation and may be toxic.

The developing child is particularly sensitive to chemical insult during the first three months of pregnancy. However, the fetus remains vulnerable throughout pregnancy, and different fetal systems are sensitive to different chemicals at specific times (Reynolds 1993).

Crossing the placenta

Any embryo fetotoxicity caused by an essential oil is dependent on one or more of its constituents crossing the placenta. It is often assumed that drug concentrations in the conceptus reach similar levels to those in the mother's blood. This is likely to be wildly inaccurate for general application and we do not know to what extent many foreign substances circulating in the mother's bloodstream reach the developing child (Neubert et al 1987). A recent review lists ethanol, nicotine, PCBs, and a number of pesticides, heavy metals, illicit drugs and pharmaceuticals (or their metabolites) as being unequivocally detected in the fetal environment (Barr et al 2007).

During pregnancy, the fetus receives oxygen and nutrients in its bloodstream from the mother via the placenta and umbilical cord, and its waste products are removed in the opposite direction. The fetus is vulnerable to drugs and other chemicals in the mother's body because the placenta does not provide a very effective barrier between maternal and fetal blood. In general, the placenta will carry any uncharged, un-ionized molecule with high lipid solubility and a molecular weight of less than 1000 (Baker 1960; Heikkila et al 1992; Gedeon & Koren 2007). This includes many drugs and essential oil constituents.

The passive diffusion of substances across the placenta, like the skin and cell membranes (see Chapter 4), is largely governed by lipophilicity and molecular size. It is believed that most pharmaceutical drugs cross the placenta to some degree, even those with relatively high molecular weights (Myllynen et al 2007). Essential oil constituents in general are likely to cross the placenta efficiently because of their favorable lipophilicity and low molecular weight. This does not indicate a hazard per se which, for any substance, is determined by plasma concentration and toxicity.

The fetal central nervous system (CNS), because it is still growing, is more susceptible to damage by chemicals than is the adult CNS. The blood–brain barrier is somewhat underdeveloped at and before birth, increasing the likelihood that compounds that do cross the placenta will reach the fetal CNS (Maickel & Snodgrass 1973).

1,8-Cineole crossed the placenta in sufficient quantity to affect the activity of fetal liver enzymes when given by sc injection to pregnant rats at a dose of 500 mg/kg for four days (Jori & Briatico 1973). Although this dose represents a vastly higher maternal blood level of 1,8-cineole than would be encountered in aromatherapy, the study demonstrates the ability of some essential oil constituents to reach the fetus. Eucalyptus oil (~75% 1,8-cineole) showed no embryotoxicity or fetotoxicity when tested on mice (injected sc at 135 mg/kg on gestational days 6–15) and had no effect on birth weight or placental size (Pages et al 1990). Niaouli oil (50.6% 1,8-cineole) was maternally toxic and fetotoxic when injected ip to pregnant rats for 18 days at 1,350 mg/kg (Laleye et al 2004).

Extrapolating from the above information, in pregnant rodents, 1,8-cineole at 101 mg/kg sc for 10 days had no adverse effect, at 500 mg/kg sc for 4 days it affected fetal liver enzymes

(i.e., it was fetotoxic), and at 682 mg/kg ip for 18 days it was both maternally toxic and fetotoxic.

Camphor is able to cross the placenta, as are at least some of the sulfur compounds found in garlic oil. Following accidental ingestion of camphorated oil by a pregnant woman, camphor was found to be present in the body of her stillborn baby (Riggs et al 1965). After crossing the placenta, camphor passes into fetal lung, liver, brain and kidney tissue. When taken in overdose, it also destroys the placenta, causing hemorrhage (Phelan 1976). The odor of garlic was detected in both maternal and fetal blood and in amniotic fluid in samples taken 100 minutes after a ewe was given garlic orally (Nolte et al 1992). Similarly, garlic imparts a pronounced odor to amniotic fluid after being ingested by pregnant women (Mennella et al 1995).

A 30-year-old woman, at 30 weeks of gestation, ingested several cookies made with 7 g of ground nutmeg, instead of the recommended eighth of a teaspoon (Lavy 1987). Four hours later, she experienced toxic effects. The fetal heartbeat rose to 160–170 bpm, and returned to a normal 120–140 bpm within 12 hours. The fetal response was attributed to the myristicin content of nutmeg oil, and its anticholinergic (i.e., sympathomimetic) effect. It is assumed that myristicin readily crosses the placenta. When safrole, a minor constituent of nutmeg oil, was given orally to pregnant mice at 120 mg/kg on four gestational days, kidney epithelial tumors occurred in 7% of offspring, compared to none of the control animals (Vesselinovitch et al 1979).

On transit through the placenta, essential oil constituents might be metabolized by local enzymes. Human term placental peroxidase (HTPP), in the presence of hydrogen peroxide, catalyzes the oxidation of eugenol to a quinone methide widely regarded as the compound responsible for its cellular toxicity. Safrole and estragole, however, which cannot form quinone methides, are not oxidized by HTPP. There is evidence that the activity of this enzyme is highest in the first trimester of pregnancy, and that it is present in human fetal tissues and possibly also in human intrauterine conceptual tissues in the organogenesis period (Zhang & Robertson 2000). This oxidation of eugenol by HTPP might explain the toxicity of clove bud oil to embryo cells described below.

Embryotoxicity

Essential oils of Dalmatian sage, thyme (thymol/carvacrol CT), clove bud and cinnamon bark (all at 375 mg/kg/day) and oregano (at 150 mg/kg/day) were fed to female mice for 2 weeks prior to mating. Thyme oil had no effect on embryo development, but oregano and clove oils significantly increased the rate of cell death. Cinnamon bark oil reduced the number of nuclei, and altered the distribution of embryos according to nucleus number. Dalmatian sage oil negatively influenced the distribution of embryos according to nucleus number (Domaracky et al 2007). The negative effects seen in this study may be due to the high doses used, but we do not know what a safe dose might be, except in the case of clove oil. We have therefore contraindicated oregano and cinnamon bark oils, as well as cassia oil, for its similarity to cinnamon bark (Table 11.1). Since oral administration of 100 mg/kg eugenol to pregnant mice throughout gestation caused no increase in resorption, and no detectable fetal defects (Amini et al 2003), and since eugenol constitutes 85% of clove oil, no contraindication is necessary for clove oils. Dalmatian sage oil is contraindicated in pregnancy anyway, because of its neurotoxicity.

Sweet fennel oil, containing 72% (E)-anethole, 12.0% fenchone and 5% estragole, was tested at various concentrations on a rat embryo limb bud culture. Compounds that inhibit differentiation of these cells by more than 50% have a high correlation with teratogenicity. At a concentration as low as 0.93 mg/mL, the oil produced a significant reduction (approximately 50%) in differentiated limb bud foci. However, this was due to cytotoxicity, resulting from exposing the cells directly to the essential oil. It was concluded that fennel oil, at certain concentrations, is toxic to fetal cells, but does not impact normal development (Ostad et al 2004). The relevance of testing essential oils in this way is limited, since there is no metabolism, but for other reasons, we have contraindicated fennel oils in pregnancy.

An essential requirement for the growth, development and normal functioning of body tissues is a vascular system capable of supplying oxygen and nutrients. During gestation, as tissues grow in the placenta and embryo, new blood vessels form from pre-existing ones by a process known as angiogenesis. Suppressing angiogenesis may be useful in preventing tumor growth, but if it is suppressed during gestation, adverse reproductive and developmental consequences are likely to occur such as preeclampsia, fetal growth restriction and fetal death (Chaiworapongsa et al 2010).

Evidence supporting a link between inhibition of angiogenesis and reproductive toxicity is provided by zedoary essential oil in rats. High oral doses of 100 and 200 mg/kg were embryotoxic in vivo, and adverse effects in rat embryos ex vivo were observed at 10 μg/mL and above. The authors suggested that curdione, curzerene, germacrone, β-elemene, γ-elemene and neocurdione (20%, 16%, 5%, 3%, 2% and 2% in their oil, respectively) may contribute to this toxicity (Zhou et al 2013). However of these, only β-elemene is known to be antiangiogenic. The use of Curcuma zedoaria in pregnant women is prohibited in China because it carries a high risk of inducing abortion (Chen et al 2011, Zhou et al 2013).

Several essential oil constituents have been shown to inhibit angiogenesis, and it is likely that they can pass through the placental barrier (see Crossing the placenta, above). These include costunolide, dehydrocostus lactone, β-elemene, β-eudesmol, furanodiene and thymoquinone. Of these, only thymoquinone is known to be fetotoxic. We have contraindicated the use of any essential oils that contain >10% of one or more of these constituents in pregnancy and breastfeeding in the appropriate oil profiles. Eugenol inhibits angiogenesis (Manikandan et al 2010). However, since it is not fetotoxic in mice, even when given maternally at 100 mg/kg/day throughout gestation (Amini et al 2003) we have not red-flagged eugenol containing oils.

Fetotoxicity

Fetal metabolism is undeveloped compared to that of an adult, and the fetus is usually less protected from xenobiotics. Consequently, first-pass metabolism is less effective, so some substances may

have higher oral bioavailability. However, substances that reach the fetus would only be expected to pose a risk if they are sufficiently toxic and reach high enough plasma concentrations. In other instances, reduced metabolic capacity may be protective; for example, in cases when the fetal liver might otherwise metabolize a compound into a more toxic one (Tenenbein 1990).

Camphor

Four cases have been reported of (usually accidental) camphorated oil ingestion by pregnant women. In one case, 45 mL of camphorated oil was ingested during the third month of pregnancy, and an apparently normal infant was born six months later (Blackmon & Curry 1957). In a second case, a woman, at 40 weeks gestation, swallowed 2 oz (~57 mL) of camphorated oil while in hospital. Although severely intoxicated by the camphor, she recovered fully after gastric lavage, but her baby did not survive. Other factors may have contributed to the death of this infant, but camphor likely played a major role; it was detected in the infant's liver, brain and kidneys (Riggs et al 1965).

In a third case, the baby was also a full-term infant, and the woman also ingested 2 oz of camphorated oil. Spontaneous labor commenced the following morning, and her baby, smelling distinctly of camphor, was born without complication (Weiss & Catalano 1973). The baby in this case was 1.5 kg heavier than the second case infant. A fourth case is outlined in the Camphor profile, Chapter 13.

Even at relatively high doses, there is little evidence in animal studies of camphor toxicity. No adverse fetal effects were seen from feeding pregnant rats at 1,000 mg/kg/day, or pregnant rabbits at 681 mg/kg/day. Maternal toxicity was seen in rats at 400 mg/kg/day, but not at 100 mg/kg/day (Leuschner 1997). However, camphor is thought to be more toxic to humans than experimental animals.

The neurotoxicity data suggest a human daily oral maximum dose of 2 mg/kg/day for camphor, or 140 mg per adult, equivalent to a dermal exposure of 4.5% (see Camphor profile). This dose is approximately 90 times less that the amount of camphor ingested in the second and third cases cited above (camphorated oil contains 20% camphor). However, essential oils with a high camphor content should be avoided in pregnancy (Table 11.2).

Sabinyl acetate

Sabinyl acetate is found in several commercial essential oils, including savin and most chemotypes of wormwood. It is also found in two essential oils which are not commercially available: Plectranthus fruticosus (> 60%) and Juniperus pfitzeriana (2–17%) (Fournier et al 1990). Oils rich in sabinyl acetate are among the most dangerous in pregnancy. There are anecdotal reports of savin oil being able to cross the placenta and causing abortion (Grieve 1978; Papavassiliou 1935).

Plectranthus oil is embryotoxic and fetotoxic in rodents. Strong abortifacient and/or fetotoxic effects were reported after administration of 5.0 mg/kg of plectranthus oil in pregnant rats (Fournier et al 1986). Plectranthus oil dramatically increased the rate of fetal resorption in pregnant rats after oral administration of 0.5, 2.5 or 5.0 mg/kg on gestational days 6–15. Fetal toxic

Table 11.2 Essential oils that should be restricted during pregnancy and lactation

Essential oil	Toxic constituent	Maximum dermal dose[a]	Maximum oral dose[c]
Basil (lemon)	Citral	1.4%[b]	99 mg
Boswellia papyrifera	Octyl acetate	1.7%	116 mg
Champaca (orange) absolute	2-Phenylethanol	17.5%	555 mg
Lemon balm (Australian)	Citral	3.4%[b]	238 mg
Lemon leaf	Citral	1.2%[b]	84 mg
Lemongrass	Citral	0.7%[b]	46 mg
May chang	Citral	0.8%[b]	56 mg
Melissa	Citral	0.9%[b]	65 mg
Myrtle (honey)	Citral	0.9%[b]	63 mg
Myrtle (lemon)	Citral	0.7%[b]	46 mg
Nasturtium absolute	Benzyl isothiocyanate	0.26%	8.7 mg
Tea tree (lemon-scented)	Citral	0.8%[b]	54 mg
Thyme (lemon)	Citral	3.7%[b]	258 mg
Verbena (lemon)	Citral	0.9%[b]	61 mg

[a]Calculated to allow for whole-body, once daily application (e.g. body oil or body lotion)
[b]This limit was determined for skin sensitization, and also a safe concentration in pregnancy
[c]See Adjusting safe doses and concentrations (see Ch. 13, p. 189)

but can present in different ways. Major malformations are thought to occur in 2% of all live births, but the proportion increases if observations are continued beyond childhood and on into adulthood. The term 'teratogen' is also now used in a broader sense, denoting any agent that interferes with normal embryonic development.

Apparently avoidable disasters such as those involving stilbestrol and thalidomide[1] have highlighted the fact that the reproductive process can be extremely sensitive to chemical agents. Stilbestrol (diethyl stilbestrol) is a drug that was used in the first trimester of pregnancy to prevent miscarriage, and also post-pregnancy to prevent lactation. It caused vaginal cancer in females born to women who had taken it, and was banned for these two uses in the 1970s. Stilbestrol is now used in men for the treatment of advanced prostate cancer.

Koren (1990) reported some 20 drugs and chemicals proven to be teratogenic. A more recent catalogue of teratogenic drugs, chemicals and other physical and biological agents lists over 2,000 agents (http://www.cehn.org/catalog_teratogenic_agents_shepards_catalog Accessed April 28th 2012). Although there is naturally concern that some essential oils may not be safe if used during pregnancy, few have thus far raised significant concerns.

Essential oils

Plectranthus, which is not commercially available, is the only essential oil known to be strongly teratogenic. Sabinyl acetate is thought to be responsible for these effects, and is present in higher concentrations in this oil than in any other oil. When plectranthus oil was administered to pregnant rats by directly applying to the tongue at 0.5, 2.5 or 5.0 mg/kg on gestational days 6–15, it was dose-dependently teratogenic. Signs of toxicity included microphthalmia (abnormally small eyeballs) and anophthalmia (lack of eyes) (Pages et al 1988). Plectranthus oil was embryotoxic and fetotoxic in mice, producing malformed embryos and an increased frequency of resorption. Its effects on mouse fetal development include kidney and heart defects, skeletal alterations and anophthalmia (Pages et al 1991).

Constituents

Salicylates cause dose-dependent congenital abnormalities in experimental animals (Wilson 1973). This is thought to involve oxygen free radicals, since superoxide dismutase, an antioxidant enzyme, reduced salicylate teratogenicity in rat embryos (Karabulut et al 2000). In rat studies using substantial ip, sc or gavage doses of methyl salicylate (200–1,750 mg/kg), teratogenic effects have included adverse effects on brain, liver, lung and kidney development (Kavlock et al 1982) as well as skeletal anomalies (Warkany & Takacs 1959; Pyun 1970).

However, when methyl salicylate was topically applied to pregnant rats at 3% in petrolatum at doses corresponding to 30, 60, 90 or 180 mg/kg/day methyl salicylate, there were no signs of maternal, developmental or embryo/fetotoxicity at any dose (Infurna et al 1990). In a two generation gavage dose mouse study, the reproductive toxicity NOAEL was 100 mg/kg/day (National Toxicology Program 1984a, 1984b), and in a three generation dietary dose rat study, it was 25 mg/kg/day (Collins et al 1971).

effects, which increased with dose, included cerebral hemorrhage and hydrocephalus (Pages et al 1988).

When pregnant mice were injected sc with 0, 15, 45 or 135 mg/kg of plectranthus oil on gestational days 6–15, toxicity increased with dose, and included a reduction in weight gain attributed to the number of fetal resorptions in the treated groups. Slight maternal toxicity was observed (Pages et al 1991). Savin oil caused an increase in the number of resorptions in pregnant mice when given at 15, 45 or 135 mg/kg on gestational days 6–15 (Pages et al 1989b).[3]

These findings do not indicate a NOAEL for sabinyl acetate. Since even 0.5 mg/kg of plectranthus oil was fetotoxic in rats, we advise complete avoidance of essential oils containing sabinyl acetate in pregnancy.

Teratogenicity

Teratology is the study of birth defects of a structural nature that arise during embryonic development. These most often appear as congenital malformations that are apparent at birth,

Octyl acetate, another ester, is much less toxic. It was administered by gavage to pregnant Sprague-Dawley rats on gestational days 6–15 at doses of 0, 100, 500, and 1,000 mg/kg. The number of litters with at least one malformed fetus and the mean percentage of the litter malformed were significantly elevated in the high-dose group only (Daughtrey et al 1989b).

Monoterpenes generally have very low reproductive toxicity (see alkenes, Table 11.3). Oral α-terpinene (89% pure) caused rat embryo/fetotoxicity above 30 mg/kg, in the form of reduced fetal body weight and minor skeletal malformations (Araujo et al 1996). However, the low purity of the α-terpinene used invalidates these findings.

Early fetal development is stimulated by endogenous retinoic acid, and citral (a mixture of neral and geranial) inhibits retinoic acid synthesis (Le Bouffant et al 2010). In an ex vivo study, citral interfered with tissue morphogenesis in animal embryos (Kronmiller et al 1995). Both citral and geranial have produced malformations in chick embryos when injected into fertilized hen's eggs (Abramovici 1972; Tanaka et al 1996). In rats, citral is non-teratogenic by inhalation (Gaworski et al 1992) but it is slightly teratogenic on oral dosing; the rat NOAEL is 60 mg/kg (Nogueira et al 1995).

Using chick embryos at 72 hours of incubation, Forschmidt (1979) determined the following relative teratogenic values: citral 60.1%, cinnamaldehyde 43.05%, cinnamyl alcohol 29.6%, citronellal 12.0%, nerol 11.9%, geraniol 11.3% octanol 6.45% and octanal 4.16%. The control group received olive oil, and came out at 7.9%. The skeletal system, mainly involving the limbs, was affected. If these data have any human relevance (and this is not known) they indicate a teratogenic potential for citral, cinnamaldehyde and cinnamyl alcohol.

Attempts have been made to find correlations between molecular structure and teratogenicity for fragrance additives (Abramovici & Rachmuth-Roizman 1983). Unsaturation (the presence of one or more carbon–carbon double bonds) and the presence of carbonyl or aldehyde groups may indicate an increased capacity to interact with lipid constituents of embryo cell membranes (Forschmidt 1979). This would implicate, for example, cinnamaldehyde, citral and β-pulegone. We know that there are reproductive toxicity problems with citral, though its inhibition of retinoic acid synthesis has not been seen with other aldehydes. We have also seen problems with cinnamon bark oil, which would implicate cinnamaldehyde. Teratogenic effects for both compounds were predicted by Forschmidt (1979). However, generalizing about structure/activity relationships in this area is risky without evidence.

Developmental toxicity

Developmental toxicity pertains to adverse effects induced prior to maturity as an adult; it includes effects induced or manifested either before birth or after birth. Teratogenicity is an important manifestation of developmental toxicity, and the two terms are often used synonymously. The Organisation for Economic Co-Operation and Development (OECD) guidelines list the following developmental toxicity endpoints: number and per cent of pre- and post-implantation loss, morphological alterations in fetuses, and decreased fetal weight (OECD 2001). Adverse effects on development from essential oil constituents are generally seen only with very high doses.

There was no effect on peri- and postnatal development when β-myrcene was given orally to pregnant rats at doses of up to 250 mg/kg from day 15 of pregnancy to postnatal day 21. Above 500 mg/kg, some adverse effect on birth weight, perinatal mortality and postnatal development was seen (Delgado et al 1993a, 1993b; Paumgartten et al 1998). When pregnant mice were fed 0.05%, 0.1% or 0.25% coumarin in the diet on gestational days 6–17, no abnormalities were found in the offspring, but the 0.25% dose level (~1,500 mg/kg) led to increased ossification (Roll & Bär 1967). When groups of pregnant mice were administered 591 or 2,363 mg/kg/day (+)-limonene by gavage on gestational days 7–12, developmental toxicity (increase in the number of fetuses with skeletal anomalies and delayed ossification) was seen only in the high-dose group (Kodama et al 1977a).

In mice, a single oral dose of β-thujaplicin caused retardation in growth and developmental parameters at 560 mg/kg, but not at 420 mg/kg (Ogata et al 1999). In rats, gavage dosing at 135 mg/kg on gestational days 6–15 resulted in a significant increase in postimplantation loss and fetal malformations. Based on decreases in maternal weight gain, and the weight of female fetuses at 45 mg/kg or higher, the NOAEL for both dams and fetuses was 15 mg/kg (Ema et al 2004). We have contraindicated hibawood oil in pregnancy, as it contains β-thujaplicin as a major constituent.

Developmental neurotoxicity

In humans, a period of rapid nerve cell growth in the brain extends from the sixth month of gestation to several years after birth. During this time, immature CNS neurons are highly sensitive to toxicity from environmental agents (Olney 2002). Developmental neurotoxicity is caused during pregnancy or lactation, most commonly by maternal exposure to certain industrial chemicals, heavy metals or pesticides. Developmental neurotoxins may not cause seizures, and may not be grossly fetotoxic to the embryo. Essential oil constituents that are known to be human developmental neurotoxins include benzyl alcohol, ethyl acetate and styrene (Grandjean & Landigran 2006). Ethyl acetate is a minor constituent of mustard essential oil, which anyway is highly toxic and is not used in therapy. Styrene can be found in styrax oil at 1.8%, and is unlikely to cause problems at 0.01% (1.8% of 0.6%, the IFRA maximum for styrax oil).

Benzyl alcohol is a major constituent of tolu balsam and benzoin. Sixteen cases of preterm neonatal death were associated with benzyl alcohol used as a bacteriostatic agent in isotonic saline used to flush intravascular catheters. The estimated daily intake of benzyl alcohol ranged from 99–405 mg/kg (Gershanik et al 1981; Brown et al 1982). In critically ill neonates receiving continuous infusions, the median benzyl alcohol exposure was 106 mg/kg/day (Shehab et al 2009). In two neonatal intensive care units there was a significant improvement in the survival rate of infants weighing less than 1 kg following the discontinuation of benzyl alcohol solutions (Menon et al 1984; Hiller et al 1986).

Table 11.3 Reproductive NOAEL or LOAEL values for some essential oil constituents

Constituent	NOAEL	LOAEL	Animal/route	Reference
Alkenes				
Camphene[a]	>250 mg/kg/day		Rat/oral	Hoechst AG 1992, cited in Environmental Protection Agency 2006
(+)-Limonene	250 mg/kg/day		Rabbit/oral	Kodama et al 1977b
	591 mg/kg/day		Mouse/oral	Kodama et al 1977a
β-Myrcene	250 mg/kg/day		Rat/oral	Delgado et al 1993a, 1993b
α-Pinene[a]	>260 mg/kg/day		Rat/oral	Environmental Protection Agency 1973
β-Pinene[a]	>43 mg/kg/day		Rat/oral	Morgareidge 1973c, cited in FFHPVC, 2006
	>93 mg/kg/day		Mouse/oral	Morgareidge 1973a, cited in FFHPVC, 2006
	>99 mg/kg/day		Hamster/oral	Morgareidge 1973b, cited in FFHPVC, 2006
Sabinene[a]	>105 mg/kg/day		Rat/oral	Morgareidge 1973c, cited in FFHPVC, 2006
	>224 mg/kg/day		Mouse/oral	Morgareidge 1973a, cited in FFHPVC, 2006
	>240 mg/kg/day		Hamster/oral	Morgareidge 1973b, cited in FFHPVC, 2006
Alcohols				
α-Bisabolol[a]	>1 mL/kg/day		Rat/oral	Habersang et al 1979
Cinnamyl alcohol[a]	53.5 mg/kg		Rat/oral	Zaitsev & Maganova 1975
Linalool	500 mg/kg/day		Rat/oral	Politano et al 2008
(−)-Menthol[a]	185 mg/kg/day		Mouse/oral	Nair 2001b
	218 mg/kg/day		Rat/oral	
	405 mg/kg/day		Hamster/oral	
	425 mg/kg/day		Rabbit/oral	
2-Phenylethanol	266 mg/kg/day		Rat/oral	Adams et al 2005a
Phenols				
Carvacrol[a]	>940 ppm		Rat/oral	Abdollahi et al 2003
Isoeugenol[b]		250 mg/kg/day	Rat/oral	George et al 2001
Aldehydes				
Citral	60 mg/kg/day		Rat/oral	Nogueira et al 1995
Ketones				
Camphor	681 mg/kg/day		Rabbit/oral	Leuschner 1997
β-Ionone		480 mg/kg	Hamster/oral	Willhite 1986
β-Thujaplicin	15 mg/kg/day		Rat/oral	Ema et al 2004
Thymoquinone	15 mg/kg		Rat/ip	AbuKhader et al 2013
Acids				
Benzoic acid	510 mg/kg		Rat/oral	Kimmel et al 1971
(E)-Cinnamic acid[a]	>50 mg/kg/day		Rat/oral	Zaitsev & Maganova 1975
Esters				
Benzyl acetate	500 mg/kg/day		Rat/oral	Ishiguro et al 1993
Benzyl benzoate[a]	>24 mg/kg/day		Rat/oral	Cosmetic Ingredient Review Expert Panel 2011
Octyl acetate	100 mg/kg/day		Rat/oral	Daughtrey et al 1989b
Methyl salicylate	25 mg/kg		Rat/oral	Collins et al 1971
	50 mg/kg		Mouse/oral	National Toxicology Program 1984a, 1984b
Sabinyl acetate		1 mg/kg/day	Rat/oral	Pages et al 1988

Continued

Table 11.3 Reproductive NOAEL or LOAEL values for some essential oil constituents—Cont'd

Constituent	NOAEL	LOAEL	Animal/route	Reference
Ethers				
(E)-Anethole		50 mg/kg/day	Rat/oral	Dhar 1995
α-Asarone		10 mg/kg/day	Mouse/oral	Chamorro et al 1998
1,8-Cineole[a]	>100 mg/kg/day		Mouse/sc	Pages et al 1990
Isoeugenol		250 mg/kg/day	Rat/oral	George et al 2001
Lactones				
Coumarin[a]	>25 mg/kg/day		Pig/oral	Grote et al 1977
Furanocoumarins				
Methoxsalen	20 mg/kg/day		Rat/oral	National Toxicology Program 1994a, 1994b
Sulfur compounds				
Benzyl isothiocyanate	12.5 mg/kg/day		Rat/oral	Adebiyi et al 2004

[a]The dose recorded was not reproductively toxic, but either higher doses were not studied or the only other dose used was more than ten times this one. Therefore, these are not meaningful NOAEL values; they are simply doses that were not toxic.
[b]The developmental toxicity NOAEL for isoeugenol was 500 mg/kg/day. There was minimal maternal toxicity at 250 mg/kg/day.

Toxic symptoms displayed by the infants included respiratory distress progressing to gasping respirations. Many infants had central neural depression, seizures or intracranial hemorrhage (Anon 1982). Benzyl alcohol has been associated with delayed mental development and other neurological deficits in low birth weight infants (Benda et al 1986; Sreenan et al 2001). Hippuric acid formation is deficient in preterm neonates, confirming that the benzyl alcohol/benzoic acid detoxification process is poorly developed in premature newborns (LeBel et al 1988). The ADI for benzyl alcohol is 5 mg/kg, and we support that limit. The benzyl alcohol findings highlight the risks of intensive essential oil administration to premature or low birth weight infants.

In cases of human fetal toxicity from camphor ingestion, camphor has been found in the fetal brain (Riggs et al 1965; Phelan 1976). In a fatal case, one teaspoon of camphorated oil was ingested by a 16-month-old boy, and gross CNS damage was noted on autopsy (Smith & Margolis 1954). Constituents (such as camphor) or essential oils known to cause seizures are all candidates for developmental toxicity, especially if they induce changes in the synaptic environment. Such changes may adversely affect brain development. Thujone and pinocamphone isomers, for example, inhibit GABA$_A$ receptor-mediated responses, and affect both pre- and post-synaptic mechanisms (Höld et al 2002; Hall 2004; Szczot et al 2012). We have prohibited many essential oils containing these toxic compounds in pregnancy and breastfeeding (Table 11.1), although camphor is less of a risk than thujone and pinocamphone isomers.

Termination of pregnancy

Normal pregnancy ends after 37–42 weeks of gestation. At this time a number of hormones, including progesterone, estrogens, oxytocin and relaxin, interact and trigger a series of events that cause the expulsion of the fetus through the vagina. Sometimes expulsion occurs prematurely, and if the fetus fails to survive it is referred to as a miscarriage or abortion. This may occur spontaneously or it may be induced. Koren (1990) estimates that approximately one fetus is aborted for every child born in Western countries, while Niesink et al (1996) postulate that only one quarter of all fertilizations lead to the birth of a child.[4]

One concern about essential oils is that some could cause abortion. There is a popular belief among aromatherapists that emmenagogic essential oils are unsafe during pregnancy, because they might lead to miscarriage. Since many essential oils have been labeled as emmenagogues in the popular literature this has led to some being flagged as dangerous in pregnancy. Whether or not these oils encourage menstruation, there is often no evidence that they are abortifacient in the amounts used in aromatherapy.

The term 'emmenagogue' is used to describe substances that promote menstrual bleeding. A large number of plants are classified in this way, although their mechanisms of action are not well understood. Potentially, they could involve mimicry or antagonism of one or more of the hormones discussed above.

Battaglia (1997 p. 132) lists cedarwood (type unspecified), clary sage, jasmine, juniper, marjoram, myrrh, peppermint, rose and rosemary as emmenagogues, and as being unsafe to use in pregnancy. Davis (1988) lists clary sage, cypress, lavender, marjoram, peppermint and rose. However, as will be seen below, only massive quantities of relatively toxic essential oils are able to induce abortion. Almost all of the alleged emmenagogic or uterine stimulant essential oils either do not have such an effect (there is often no basis for these claims) or if they do, it is not powerful enough to cause miscarriage. In some cases it is the whole herb that is classed as an emmenagogue, and an assumption has been made that the essential oil possesses the same activity.

Franchomme & Pénöel (1990) put forward the hypothesis that all essential oils containing ketones are both neurotoxic and abortifacient. Consequently, they cite dozens of essential oils as being abortifacient, and therefore unsafe in pregnancy, such as caraway (carvone), davana (davanone), peppermint eucalyptus (piperitone), rosemary verbenone CT (verbenone), taget (tagetone), turmeric (turmerone) and zdravetz (germacrone). The basis for the hypothesis is not clear, but may be due to the fact that, for example, pulegone is an abortifacient ketone, and that camphor, pinocamphone and thujone are all neurotoxic ketones. However, to deduce from this that all ketones are abortifacient has no scientific basis. A massive oral dose of β-ionone (1,000 mg/kg) did cause a high proportion of resorptions in rats. However, at 250, 500 or 750 mg/kg, it attenuated cyclophosphamide-induced embryolethality and teratogenicity (Gomes-Carneiro et al 2003).

Savin, tansy, juniper, pennyroyal and rue[5] have all been considered abortifacient at one time or another (Macht 1913), and the whole herbs may be active. However, work using the isolated human uterus shows that the essential oils of these plants have no direct action on uterine muscle (Macht 1913, 1921; Gunn 1921; Soares PM et al 2005). Furthermore, they do not tend to induce abortion by causing the death of the fetus (Datnow 1928; Renaux & La Barre 1941; Kong et al 1989). However, the fact that these oils do not stimulate the isolated human uterus does not in itself prove that they are not abortifacient. It is possible that constituents of the essential oils are metabolized in vivo to more toxic compounds. We know, for example, that (1R)-(+)-β-pulegone is metabolized to (6R)-(+)-menthofuran, increasing toxicity.

Juniper oil

Although an ethanolic extract of juniper berries has demonstrated clear abortifacient effects (Agrawal et al 1980), there is good reason to believe that the essential oil is not responsible. Historically, juniper has a reputation as an abortifacient. It is clear, however, that there has been confusion between juniper (*Juniperus communis*) and savin (*Juniperus sabina*), and it is our opinion that juniper oil presents no abortifacient risk (see Juniper profile, Chapter 13).

Parsley oil / parsley apiole

It is ironic that pennyroyal is widely known as an abortifacient, and parsley is assumed to be safe. In fact they are probably equally safe when taken in small enough doses. However, concentrated preparations made from parsley have been used to procure abortion for a great many years, and are still in use today, notably in Italy. Parsley apiole, a major constituent of most parsley leaf and seed oils, is thought to be the active constituent, and is also used in its own right as an abortifacient. Data is often difficult to obtain, partly because of the legal implications of patients admitting to illegal abortion, and in some cases because death followed abortion and there is no record of how much apiole was taken. The cases which have been recorded tend to be the worst ones, in which medical intervention has been urgently sought.

D'Aprile (1928) is the most prolific source of case data. Out of five cases, all of whom were between two and seven months pregnant, one aborted and later died, one did not abort but died, and three aborted and survived. In the case that did not abort, the fetus did not survive. Post-abortive vaginal bleeding, sometimes profuse, is a feature of these cases. A cumulative effect is apparent, apiole being taken daily for between 3 and 8 days before either death or abortion ensues. Other researchers have reported similar cases of parsley apiole intoxication, such as that of a woman who consumed 6 g of parsley apiole over 3 days, aborted, and later died, having suffered massive internal bleeding, convulsions, oliguria and pyrexia (Laederich et al 1932).

The lowest daily dose of parsley apiole that induced abortion was 900 mg taken for 8 consecutive days. This is approximately equivalent to 6 mL of parsley leaf oil, 1.5–6 mL of parsleyseed oil, or 5 mL of Indian dill oil. The inevitable conclusion is that all of these parsley apiole-rich essential oils present a high risk of abortion if taken in oral doses, and that external use is also inadvisable in pregnancy. In animal studies, considerably higher doses of parsley apiole appear to be tolerated. In pregnant guinea pigs, abortion generally did not occur except at lethal doses, around 2 g (D'Aprile 1928). Pregnant rabbits aborted following doses of 5–14 g, with severe hemorrhage (Patoir et al 1936). In both types of animal, the dosage is equivalent to approximately 100–200 g in a human. This is 20–40 times higher than the amount of parsley apiole inducing abortion in humans, and highlights the poor correlation between animals and humans in this area.

Pennyroyal oil

Pennyroyal has already been mentioned in regard to the effect that its pulegone content has on the liver (see Ch. 9, p. 127). The plant has enjoyed folk status as an emmenagogue (Girling 1887; Stephen & Rishton 1894) and as an abortifacient from ancient times (Flynn 1893; Gunby 1979).

In two separate cases, 7.5 mL of pennyroyal oil, taken orally, failed to induce miscarriage (Anon 1978). In another two cases, 5 mL and 10 mL, taken orally, also failed (Wingate 1889; Sullivan et al 1979). A more serious case was reported in *The Lancet* in 1955. It is not known how much oil was taken, but abortion did take place, and the woman died following massive urea leakage into the blood (Vallance 1955). This is the only reported case of abortion from the use of pennyroyal oil out of four recorded attempts (Anon 1978; Sullivan et al 1979). Two further fatalities have been reported from pennyroyal oil ingestion; one was an attempted abortion (but post-mortem examination revealed no pregnancy), the other was an attempt to induce menstruation (Allen 1897; Sullivan et al 1979). The quantities ingested in these instances were 'one tablespoon' and 1 oz, respectively. The toxicity of pennyroyal is due to its high content of the hepatotoxic constituents $(6R)$-$(+)$-menthofuran and $(1R)$-$(+)$-β-pulegone (see Constituent profiles, Chapter 14).

Pennyroyal oil, it seems, is not abortifacient, unless taken in such massive quantities that it causes acute hepatotoxicity in the mother. She miscarries only because she is so poisoned by pulegone that the pregnancy cannot be maintained (Macht 1921). Maximum exposure levels for pennyroyal and other pulegone-rich oils are given in the Essential oil profiles (Chapter 13), and these apply equally to pregnant and non-pregnant individuals.

Rue oil

There are isolated reports that rue oil has a direct stimulant action on the uterus, but the details of the research on which they are based are obscure (Papavassiliou et al 1937). Rue oil had no stimulant effect on the isolated uteri of pregnant and non-pregnant cats; in fact it had a spasmolytic action (Macht 1913). Used in massive amounts on pregnant rabbits (12 mL/kg) and guinea pigs (50 mL/kg) rue oil, not surprisingly, was toxic to both mother and fetus, causing widespread tissue damage and some fatalities (Patoir et al 1938a, 1938b). These dose levels are equivalent to human ingestion of approximately 800 mL and 3.2 L. Two pregnant guinea pigs, each fed 12 drops of rue oil, aborted; rue oil was found in the fetal tissue, and was considered toxic to it (Anon 1974). This is still a very high dose, around 3 mL/kg, and equivalent to human ingestion of some 200 mL. In teratology studies on rats and mice, at doses of rue oil up to 820 and 970 mg/kg, respectively, no significant maternotoxic, embryotoxic or teratogenic effects were observed (cited in Committee for Veterinary Medicinal Products 1999).

The plant is used as an abortifacient in South America (Ciganda & Laborde 2003) and constituents not present in the essential oil, such as pilocarpine, have been identified as abortifacients (Farnsworth et al 1975). However, this does not preclude the possibility that the essential oil could have a similar action. There are anecdotal reports that rue oil can cause abortion in humans. However, it is possible that any abortifacient activity that rue oil possesses is, like that of pennyroyal, due entirely to maternal toxicity associated with massive doses.

The FDA considers that rue oil is safe to humans as currently used in food flavorings, 'but not necessarily under different conditions of use'; in particular, further teratological research is recommended (Anon 1974). We suggest that rue oil is avoided altogether during pregnancy, at least until further data are available.

Sabinyl acetate

When either plectranthus oil (60% sabinyl acetate), or a fraction of Spanish sage oil containing 50% sabinyl acetate, was injected sc into pregnant mice on gestational days 6–15 at 15, 45 and 135 mg/kg, both were dose-dependently abortifacient (Pages et al 1991, 1992). In a similar study, a savin oil with 50% sabinyl acetate prevented implantation in mice when given on gestational days 0–4, but not when given on gestational days 8–11, suggesting that the abortifacient action of sabinyl acetate is due to inhibition of implantation (Pages et al 1996). It seems likely that sabinyl acetate-rich oils would be abortifacient in early pregnancy in humans, although the effective dose might not be the same as for rodents. No safe dose is known for sabinyl acetate.

Childbirth

Several essential oils reduce uterine contractions in isolated cat or rat uteri. These include black seed, caraway, fennel (sweet), ginger, kanuka, lavender, manuka, pennyroyal, rue, savin, tansy, tea tree, thorow-wax (*Bupleurum fruticosum*), thyme, *Zataria multiflora* (41.4% carvacrol, 21.2% thymol) and turpentine, in addition to the constituents parsley apiole, $(+)$-δ-3-carene, 1,8-cineole, citral, ligustilide, piperitone, $(1R)$-$(+)$-β-pulegone and α-terpineol (Macht 1913; Lorente et al 1989; Ocete et al 1989; Aqel & Shaheen 1996; Lis-Balchin and Hart 1999; Lis-Balchin et al 2000; Ostad et al 2001; Sadraei 2003; Soares PM et al 2005; Du et al 2006a; Buddhakala et al 2008; Ponce-Monter et al 2008).

To give some specifics, in an ex vivo rat study, sweet fennel oil showed a dose-dependent reduction in the intensity of uterine contractions induced by either oxytocin or prostaglandin E_2 (PGE_2). Some effect was seen at 25 μg/mL for oxytocin and 10 μg/mL for PGE_2; more significant effects were seen at 50 μg/mL for oxytocin and 20 μg/mL for PGE_2 (Ostad et al 2001). Black seed oil concentration-dependently inhibited the spontaneous movements of rat and guinea pig uterine smooth muscle and also the contractions induced by oxytocin stimulation (Aqel & Shaheen 1996). Similarly, an essential oil of *Bupleurum gibraltaricum* (33.0% δ-3-carene) and δ-3-carene antagonized oxytocin-induced contractions in rat uterus (Ocete et al 1989).

While some of these oils might have useful applications, such as in dysmenorrhea, it could be argued that they should not be used during labor that is not progressing well. However, we know nothing about the clinical relevance of these findings to human childbirth. Because of the varied constituents of the essential oils listed above, it seems likely that many others could demonstrate similar activity. Since there are no essential oils that have been found to stimulate uterine contractions, the antispasmodic action may be a non-specific action of almost all essential oils when tested ex vivo.

The use of aromatherapy during childbirth was an increasingly popular care option with mothers and midwives in an eight-year observational study at the John Radcliffe Hospital in Oxford, UK. Prospective data for a total of 8,058 mothers who delivered between 1990 and 1998 were analyzed, and contemporaneous data from the unit audit provided a comparison group of 15,799 mothers who did not use aromatherapy. Women were offered essential oils to relieve anxiety, pain, nausea and/or vomiting or to strengthen contractions. The essential oils were: chamomile (Moroccan), clary sage, eucalyptus, frankincense, jasmine absolute, lavender, lemon, mandarin, peppermint and rose absolute.

Aromatherapy was available to all women who presented on the delivery suite, irrespective of risk factors. The only exclusions were no consent, and women who had multiple allergies. Sixty per cent (4,834) of the sample were pregnant for the first time, and 32% (2,578) overall had their labor induced. The administration of aromatherapy in childbirth did appear to reduce the need for additional pain relief in a proportion of mothers. More than 8% (387) of those pregnant for the first time, and 18% (580) of those not, used no conventional pain relief during labor after using essential oils. During the years of the study, the use of pethidine in the study center declined from 6% to 0.2% of women. The findings suggested that aromatherapy may have the potential to augment contractions for women in dysfunctional labor. Adverse effects in those using aromatherapy were reported by 1.0% of women (100), and included nausea, rash, headache, and rapid labor, though it is not known whether any of these were caused by essential oils, and no information on adverse events was collected in the comparison group (Burns et al 2000).

In a pilot RCT, 251 women received aromatherapy during labor, with 262 controls. One of five essential oils was applied to each aromatherapy group participant: Roman chamomile, lavender, frankincense, mandarin or clary sage. Modes of application included acupressure, massage, taper (a drop of essential oil on an absorbent paper strip attached to clothing), compress, footbath or birthing pool. There were no significant differences for the following outcomes: cesarean section, ventouse, Kristeller maneuver, spontaneous vaginal delivery, first-stage augmentation, and second-stage augmentation. Significantly more babies born to control participants were transferred to a neonatal intensive care unit, 0 versus 6 (2%), and pain perception was reduced in the aromatherapy group for nulliparae (Burns et al 2007).

Inhalation of costus oil by women in labor is said to have minimized pain and anxiety, with no adverse effects on mother or fetus (Huntose et al 1999). These studies suggest that the benefits of aromatherapy during labor outweigh risk, at least when administered under the supervision of a qualified health practitioner.

Breastfeeding and lactation

The secretion of milk by the mammary glands (lactation) is promoted by the hormone prolactin, from the anterior pituitary gland. Oxytocin from the posterior pituitary gland promotes the release of milk into the mammary ducts, where it can be suckled by the infant. It is important to take account of the amount of milk ingested by an infant, which has been estimated to be typically 150 mL/kg/day. It should also be remembered that infants have an undeveloped capacity for metabolism and renal excretion, and so their ability to clear drugs is relatively impaired.

Most substances that pass from maternal plasma into breast milk do so by passive diffusion, and this is likely the case for most essential oil constituents (Hausner et al 2008). This process is determined by protein binding, lipid solubility, ionization and molecular size in a similar way to passage across the placenta. Nearly all drugs are secreted into breast milk to some extent (Atkinson et al 1998). Volatile compounds from the mother's diet affect the flavor of breast milk, and can positively influence breastfeeding (Mennella & Beauchamp 1993).

During lactation, the maximum proportion of a maternal dose of a drug considered safe for an infant has been arbitrarily set at 10%. However, it is cautioned that if a mother is taking drugs that are particularly toxic, or have the potential for severe adverse effects, breastfeeding should be avoided (Ilett et al 1997). Likely exposure in breast milk to most essential oil constituents is less than 1% of the maternal dose (Hausner et al 2008).

The risk to the infant must be considered in relation to the toxicity of the drug used, the dosage regimen and the area of application. When safrole was given to nursing mice at 120 mg/kg/bw po 12 times every second day following birth, 34% of male offspring developed hepatocellular tumors, compared to none of the female or control animals (Vesselinovitch et al 1979).

Constituents or metabolites of sandalwood oil pass via maternal milk in lactating mice, and affect hepatic metabolic enzymes (Chhabra & Rao 1993). Ingestion of garlic (Menella & Beauchamp 1991), (+)-carvone or (E)-anethole by nursing mothers resulted in peaks in breast milk at 2 hours after ingestion (Hausner et al 2008). However, 3-methylbutyl acetate could not be detected in breast milk, and concentrations of (−)-menthol plateaued, with no peak. Concentrations of constituents varied considerably between substance and individuals (1.56–108 μg/L). It was concluded that ingested flavor volatiles are transferred to breast milk selectively and in relatively low amounts (Hausner et al 2008).

Essential oils to be avoided or restricted during breastfeeding are listed in Tables 11.1 and 11.2, and Box 7.1.

Discussion

If present in the maternal circulation, most essential oil constituents would be expected to reach the fetus, where some have the potential to exert toxic effects. Parsley apiole and sabinyl acetate, and essential oils containing these compounds, present a clear risk of terminating pregnancy. However, while we know that apiole can cause late-term abortion in humans, the only data for sabinyl acetate is in rodents, and shows an anti-implantation effect in early pregnancy—preventing the implantation of the embryo into the wall of the uterus. This would be more correctly defined as an antifertility effect than an abortifacient one.

There is no clear evidence that any other essential oils present such a risk, *as they are used in aromatherapy*. Both the essential oils of pennyroyal and rue, and the constituents parsley apiole and camphor, are not abortifacient except in lethal or almost lethal doses. Although camphor is ubiquitous in essential oils, there is good evidence to support a safe dosage in pregnancy. However, there is sufficient evidence to be doubtful about the safety of a number of other essential oils, such as cinnamon bark, clove, carrot seed, chaste tree and others, and we have therefore contraindicated them (Table 1.1).

It is interesting that parsley apiole, pulegone, rue oil, savin oil and pennyroyal oil all inhibit uterine contractions (Macht 1921; Soares PM et al 2005), and yet, in maternally hepatotoxic doses, abortion may occur. Since this is not due to a direct contractile effect on the uterus, it may be due to an indirect effect through, for example, inducing placental hemorrhage. Severe hemorrhage has been observed in abortion from camphor, parsley apiole and pennyroyal (Patoir et al 1936; Phelan 1976; Vallance 1955).

In high doses, camphor is neurotoxic, and both (1R)-(+)-β-pulegone and sabinyl acetate are hepatotoxic, although exactly what mechanism might lead from either of these to abortion is not known. No evidence could be found for a uterine stimulant or abortifacient action for the convulsants pinocamphone, thujone, hyssop oil, or any thujone-rich oil.

Miscarriage in early pregnancy is very common, and women who use essential oils while they are pregnant and then miscarry may suspect that the essential oils contributed to or caused the miscarriage. In most cases no definite conclusion will be possible, but the overall risk from essential oils is very small. Perhaps the greater risk is that of physical malformation or developmental toxicity.

Safe levels of exposure

Although animal studies do not always extrapolate well to humans, some consideration should be given to the existing animal data. A summary of the known constituent animal data is given in Table 11.3, from which it is evident that at least one constituent from each of the principal chemical groups has been studied. The NOAEL values vary greatly, with sabinyl acetate being less than 1 mg/kg/day and linalool 500 mg/kg/day.

Essential oils that should be avoided completely throughout pregnancy are listed in Table 11.1, and those that should only be used in limited amounts are listed in Table 11.2. For essential oils in general, a maximum somewhere between 1% and 4% for whole-body topical application might be appropriate for safe dosing in pregnancy.

Summary

- Reproductive toxicology is the study of the harmful effects of exogenous chemicals on male and female reproductive functions and on the progeny.
- Studying the effects of xenobiotics during pregnancy is challenging. In animals, susceptibility to a substance may vary within a litter or between species, and spontaneous malformations make it difficult to recognize weak fetotoxic effects.
- One concern with essential oils is that some of their constituents may interfere with one or more of the processes involved in reproduction, for example, by mimicking or antagonizing the actions of reproductive hormones.
- Although positive safety information is not available for many essential oils during pregnancy, the same is true for many prescription and over the counter drugs.
- Although weak in vitro estrogenic activity has been shown for a few essential oils and constituents, this should not be taken as a definite indication of in vivo action.
- Essential oils high in (E)-anethole should be avoided in patients with estrogen-dependent cancers or endometriosis.
- Aromatherapy is unlikely to have any unwanted effect on oral contraception or hormone replacement therapy.
- In spite of reports concerning prepubertal gynecomastia, BPH and reduced fertility, there is currently no material evidence that any essential oils present a significant risk to the male human reproductive system.

- Many essential oil constituents probably cross the placenta and reach the embryo or fetus, but this does not indicate risk per se.
- Those essential oils which are potentially dangerous should be avoided throughout pregnancy, not just during the first trimester.
- It would be prudent to administer essential oils only with great caution orally, rectally or vaginally during pregnancy.
- There is no evidence that the external use of any essential oils presents an abortifacient risk.
- It should not be assumed that essential oils that are sometimes described as emmenagogues possess an abortifacient potential.
- All the essential oils that are reputed to be abortifacients inhibit, rather than induce, uterine contractions. In these cases, abortion is probably a consequence of maternal toxicity, and is due to the ingestion of toxic and often almost fatal doses.
- Pennyroyal oil does not present a high risk of abortion, but it is restricted due to its potential for hepatotoxicity.
- It could be argued that essential oils that inhibit uterine contractions should not be used during labor that is not progressing well. However, there is currently no clinical evidence that any essential oils, as used in aromatherapy, interfere with the progression of labor.
- Due to the many potential risks of reproductive toxicity, an overall limit for topical essential oil exposure should possibly be set somewhere in the 1–4% range.

Notes

1. Thalidomide was used as a sedative hypnotic for nausea in pregnancy. It caused gross limb deformities in the fetuses of women who took it. It is still prescribed in some parts of the world, and the problem continues, notably in South America. Thalidomide was sold as a mixture of S and R enantiomers. The S enantiomer is now known to be responsible for its teratogenic activity, while the R enantiomer has anti-inflammatory activity.

2. Corn oil has been shown to cause a loss of up to 77% of a condom's strength after only 15 minutes (Anon 1993). In either case it is important to avoid contact with essential or vegetable oils.

3. The situation with savin is complicated by the fact that the oil is frequently substituted by oils from other Juniperus species, notably J. thurifera and J. phoenica, neither of which contains much sabinyl acetate (Fournier et al 1989), and neither of which is teratogenic in mice (Pages et al 1989a).

4. The WHO uses the weight of the conceptus as a criterion and defines 'abortion' as the expulsion of a product of conception weighing 500 g or less (this may be after 20 weeks). The birth of a child weighing over 500 g before the 37th week of pregnancy is defined as a 'premature birth'.

5. In Mexico, cottonroot bark is used; in India, pulsatilla; and in the US, rue and sage are mentioned in herbal medicine textbooks (Gold & Gates 1980). However, it is not always easy to see how these plants have gained their reputations as abortifacients.

Cancer and the immune system

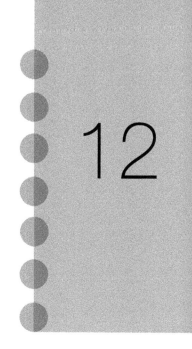

12

Cancer and carcinogens

Cancer is a complex, multi-step process. It is the result of uncontrolled cell division (neoplasia). Neoplasms are new growths and are classified as either benign or malignant, although in some instances the distinction is unclear. The most important differentiating feature is that a malignant tumor will invade surrounding structures and metastasize (spread) to distant sites whereas a benign tumor will not. Malignancies are composed of abnormal cells, and tend to show more rapid growth.

Causes of cancer include chemical carcinogens, radiant energy, and viruses such as the human papilloma and Epstein-Barr viruses. Factors that contribute to cancer risk include inherited genetic abnormalities, hormones, increasing age, chronic irritation, trauma and local environmental factors such as pollution and parasites. These operate in a secondary way to predispose an individual to cancer, they are not carcinogenic as such.[1]

It has been estimated that 70–90% of all human cancers can be attributed to environmental chemical causes (Tomatis 1979). Many of the known human carcinogens are products of the industrial revolution, such as diethylstilbestrol, benzene and asbestos. Today we are exposed to a greater number of industrial chemicals, often in complex combinations, than at any previous time, and these may include some as yet unidentified carcinogens. Some may be present in household products such as paints and cleaning agents, which often contain chemicals of unknown or dubious toxicity. Unidentified carcinogens possibly remain to be found in essential oils too.

Increased exposure to chemical carcinogens does increase risk. Fire fighters, who are exposed to high levels of carcinogens such as benzene, formaldehyde, soot and styrene, have elevated levels of some cancers (LeMasters et al 2006). According to the WHO, 30% of all cancer deaths are caused by cigarette smoking, which exposes smokers to many chemical carcinogens. Certain populations may be overexposed to known environmental carcinogens such as aflatoxins, dioxins or pesticides.

There are two basic types of carcinogen: those that react directly with DNA (DNA-reactive or genotoxic) and those that do not (epigenetic). Epigenetic carcinogens act in different ways, for example, by enhancing spontaneous mutation through stimulating cell proliferation, or increasing the amount of oxygen radicals in the cell (Williams 2001). They operate largely as promoters of cancer ('promotion' is explained below) and usually require high levels of sustained exposures. For example, dietary fat can act as an enhancer of cancer induction at about 40% of calories. The effects of epigenetic agents, unlike genotoxins, are reversible (Weisburger & Williams 2000).

Some essential oil constituents have been found to exhibit estrogen-like activity in vitro or in vivo (see Chapter 11). This may be a concern for patients with estrogen-sensitive cancers, since there is a theoretical possibility of exacerbating tumor growth and proliferation. However, these estrogen-like actions in animals are mainly weak or limited to certain experimental conditions, and their affinity for estrogen receptors is generally extremely weak compared with that of 17β-estradiol. With the exception of (E)-anethole, we do not consider that essential oils containing these constituents pose a significant risk to patients with estrogen-sensitive cancers.

DNA damage

The unregulated growth that characterizes most cancers is caused by damage to DNA, resulting in mutations to genes that encode for proteins controlling cell division. Many mutation events may be required to transform a normal cell into a malignant cell. Some chemicals, such as tobacco smoke carcinogens, directly form a bond with the chromosomal DNA of a cell, forming a DNA 'adduct', which can lead to gene mutations. For this reason they are described as being genotoxic. However, most genotoxic carcinogens, such as those found in foods and plants, require bioactivation to DNA-reactive products, usually via CYP enzymes (Weisburger & Williams 2000). Genotoxicity is a process that may or may not lead to cancer.

In order for cell division and tissue growth to take place, chromosomal DNA must produce exact copies of itself. This process is not without errors, and mutations commonly occur. It is estimated that approximately 800 DNA bases per hour are damaged in the human body, due to mechanisms such as oxidation and methylation (Vilenchik & Knudson 2000). This 'background' level of DNA mutation can also be expressed as one lesion per million (10^6) bases. Adduct levels of less than one in 10^8 bases can be regarded as of no biological significance (Williams 2008). In healthy individuals, efficient DNA repair enzymes ensure that these defects do not lead to the growth of abnormal cells. Cut-and-paste repair mechanisms have been elucidated in some detail (Fortini et al 2003; Huffman et al 2005). In certain inherited genetic diseases, the activity of one of the DNA repair enzymes is reduced, and this can predispose an individual to some forms of cancer.

DNA damage may be caused by highly reactive oxygen radicals (also known as reactive oxygen species, or ROS) and other intermediates of oxygen reduction. Oxygen radicals can attack DNA directly, or other cellular components such as lipids, leaving behind reactive species that in turn can bind with DNA bases (Valko et al 2004). Such oxidative processes, which may be either exogenous or endogenous in origin, can cause significant pre-carcinogenic changes. These include the mutation of oncogenes, tumor-suppressor genes and apoptosis-regulating genes, damage to mitochondrial DNA, and alteration of cell growth regulation pathways (Hursting et al 1999; Marnett 2000; Klaunig and Kamendulis 2004). The modification of gene expression by ROS has direct effects on cell proliferation and apoptosis.[2] Apoptosis is a normal cellular process involving a genetically programmed series of events leading to the death of a cell.

The involvement of ROS in the carcinogenic process highlights the importance of antioxidants as preventative agents, as well as the avoidance of pro-oxidants (Moller & Loft 2004). Essential oils with antioxidant properties are listed below, under Antioxidant activity.[3] Although DNA damage can be measured in cells, this does not accurately predict the risk of cancer nor correlate with its extent, as this varies greatly with factors such as adduct type, frequency, persistence and ease of repair. Rather, it should be considered one of many factors in assessment (Jarabek et al 2009).

For example, Table 12.1 shows the total of the two primary adducts detected for each test substance at three doses (Zhou et al 2007). Apart from high-dose dill apiole, the adduct levels for the apiole isomers are less than one in 10^8 bases, and so these molecules are very unlikely to be carcinogenic. The human hepatoma cells used here retain many of the phase I and phase II toxification and detoxification enzymes, but they have little or no CYP1A2, one of the most important enzymes for toxification of methyleugenol and estragole. One assay suggests that this enzyme is 53% more active in 1'-hydroxylating methyleugenol than estragole (Rietjens et al 2005a, 2005b). It is notable here that the formation of methyleugenol adducts is not dose related, neither is that for safrole at the high dose, and that the dose–response relationships for both apiole isomers have lower gradients than those for estragole and myristicin.

Initiation, promotion and progression

Carcinogenesis is classically considered to evolve in three consecutive stages: initiation, promotion and progression. During initiation, the potential carcinogen bonds with cellular DNA, forming a DNA adduct. However, this step may have no adverse consequence if the cell efficiently repairs the DNA damage, or if it leads to cell death. In either case, the DNA adduct is short-lived, and will not lead to initiation. This is an important point, because a substance may appear to be mutagenic in an in vitro study, due to the appearance of transient DNA adducts (Rietjens et al 2005a). However if these are stable, the mutation will become 'fixed' in the cell, and then passed on to 'initiated' daughter cells. At this point the cell has been irreversibly altered, but is not yet malignant (Niesink et al 1996).

Table 12.1 Relative adduct level (RAL) of some alkenylbenzenes in human hepatoma (HepG2) cells

Constituent	Dose (μM)	RAL × 10⁹ value for adducts 1 and 2
Methyleugenol	50	37.52
	150	31.76
	450	37.35
Estragole	50	23.66
	150	72.81
	450	209.99
Safrole	50	9.12
	150	27.66
	450	33.93
Myristicin	50	5.67
	150	16.27
	450	55.10
Dill apiole	50	6.00
	150	7.88
	450	11.65
Parsley apiole	50	1.95
	150	3.90
	450	5.66

(Data from Zhou G-D, Moorthy B, Bi J et al 2007 DNA adducts from alloxyallylbenzene herb and spice constituents in cultured human (HepG2) cells. Environmental & Molecular Mutagenesis 48:715-721)

Cancer promoters facilitate malignant growth by the selective, clonal expansion of initiated cells through an increase in cell proliferation. Promotion may involve altered gene expression enzyme activities, or the inhibition of DNA repair mechanisms. It is dose dependent and reversible upon removal of the tumor promotion stimulus. Progression, the third stage, involves processes such as abnormal cell growth, gene amplification (repeated copying of a segment of DNA), disruption of chromosome integrity, loss of tumor-suppressor activity, angiogenesis (the creation of a blood supply for a growing tumor), invasion and metastasis (Hursting et al 1999; Klaunig & Kamendulis 2004).

A chemical that is only a promoter or an initiator is not a 'complete carcinogen'. Initiated cells have to be subsequently and frequently exposed to doses of a promoter, over a certain period of time (which varies between chemicals) in order to induce malignant growth. A few essential oil constituents are clearly promoters but not initiators, as they only lead to neoplasia if administered subsequent to a known initiator. These include benzyl acetate, which promotes pancreatic tumors in rats, dodecyl acetate, α-phellandrene, and oxidation products of (+)-limonene, all of which promote skin tumors in mice

[(+)-limonene itself is anticarcinogenic].[4] Complete carcinogens are both initiators and promoters, and so are able to produce malignant changes by themselves.[5]

Carcinogenic essential oil constituents

The alkenylbenzenes α-asarone, β-asarone, estragole, methyleugenol and safrole are all carcinogenic in rodents (see Constituent profiles, Chapter 14). However, before they can produce malignant change, these complete carcinogens go through a two-stage process of enzyme-activated biotransformation. Estragole, for example, is activated to the 'proximate carcinogen' 1′-hydroxyestragole, which is further activated to the 'ultimate carcinogen', 1′-sulfooxyestragole (1′-hydroxyestragole sulfate).[6] The amount of ultimate carcinogen formed is dependent on the activity of the relevant metabolic enzymes. Activity can be increased by inducing enzyme synthesis, or decreased by inhibiting it. Factors that can affect this process of activation are discussed below under Carcinogenicity testing, and Genetic susceptibility.

Benzo[a]pyrene is also a carcinogen, though this is an artefact of dry distillation rather than a true essential oil constituent.

1′-Hydroxyelemicin has shown weak hepatocarcinogenicity in one species of male mouse (Wiseman et al 1987), but elemicin has shown anticarcinogenic activity in vitro (Ikeda et al 1998) and is not regarded as a carcinogen. Elemicin, (E)-anethole and eugenol may manifest very weak carcinogenicity at high doses in rodents, but at low doses in humans there is negligible risk, because epoxidation is much less prevalent in humans, and because low doses are more easily detoxified in all species (Solheim & Scheline 1980; Wiseman et al 1987; Smith et al 2002).

The three isothiocyanates found in essential oils (allyl, benzyl and phenylethyl) have all induced bladder cancer in male rats, but this is related to the irritancy of the compounds. It may also be gender- and species-specific since, in a two-year assay of allyl isothiocyanate, neither male or female mice, nor female rats, developed bladder tumors (Bechtel et al 1998). The isothiocyanates all show promise as therapeutic agents for lung cancer, as does phenylethyl isothiocyanate for colon cancer (see Constituent profiles, Chapter 14).

A few chemical carcinogens are so powerful that even a single exposure to a dangerous level is likely to result in cancer. Although it is difficult to grade levels of risk, we do know that in most of the studies reported for the carcinogens listed in Table 12.2, daily exposure to high oral doses over many months is required to induce cancer in rodents (neonates excepted). One reason for this is that only 1 in 1,000 or less preneoplastic lesions in the liver lead to tumor formation, and the continued presence of a carcinogen is required to enable it to overcome host resistance factors (Williams et al 2005b).

Defense mechanisms

Cancer is a disease that progresses very slowly, and at each stage there are natural defense mechanisms capable of preventing further progression. Understanding this is important since, while some essential oils contain carcinogenic constituents, most also

Table 12.2 Essential oil constituents for which carcinogenic activity has been reported

Constituent	Target organ	Gender, species	Route, duration	Doses used in study	Reference
Allyl isothiocyanate[a]	Bladder	Male rat	Oral, 2 years	12 or 25 mg/kg/day bw	Bechtel et al 1998
α-Asarone	Liver	Infant mouse	ip, single dose[c]	0.25 or 0.5 μmol/g bw	Kim SG et al 1999
	Liver	Male mouse[b]	ip, single dose[c]	0.75 μmol/g bw	Wiseman et al 1987
	Liver	Male mouse[b]	4 ip doses over 21 days[c]	4.8 μmol/g total dose[d]	
β-Asarone	Small intestine	Male rat	Oral, 2 years	20, 40 or 100 mg/kg/day bw	SCF 2002a
	Liver	Male mouse†	ip, single dose[c]	0.25 or 0.5 μmol/g bw	Wiseman et al 1987
	Liver	Male mouse†	4 ip doses over 21 days[c]	4.8 μmol/g total dose[d]	
Benzaldehyde[a]	Forestomach	Mouse	Oral, 2 years	200-400 mg/kg/day bw	National Toxicology Program 1990b
Benzyl acetate[a]	Pancreas	Male rat	Oral, 2 years	500 or 1,000 mg/kg/day bw	National Toxicology Program 1986
Benzyl isothiocyanate[a]	Bladder	Male rat	Oral, 32 weeks	0.1% of diet	Hirose et al 1998
Coumarin[a]	Liver	Rat	Oral, 2 years	25, 50 or 100 mg/kg/day bw	National Toxicology Program 1993a
	Lung	Mouse	Oral, 2 years	50, 100 or 200 mg/kg/day bw	
Estragole	Liver	Infant male mouse	4 sc doses over 21 days[c]	4.4 or 5.2 μmol total dose[d]	Drinkwater et al 1976
	Liver	Male mouse†	ip, single dose[c]	0.75 μmol/g bw	Wiseman et al 1987
	Liver	Infant mouse	4 ip doses over 21 days[c]	4.75 μmol total dose[d]	Miller et al 1983
	Liver	Infant male mouse	4 ip doses over 21 days[c]	9.45 μmol total dose[d]	
	Liver	Female mouse	Oral, 1 year	0.23% or 0.46% of diet	
Eugenol[a]	Liver	Male mouse	Oral, 2 years	3,000 or 6,000 ppm	National Toxicology Program 1983
Isoeugenol[a]	Liver	Male mouse	Oral, 2 years	75, 150 or 300 mg/kg/day	National Toxicology Program 2010a
(+)-Limonene[a]	Kidney	Male rat	Oral, 2 years	75 or 150 mg/kg/day bw	National Toxicology Program 1990a
Methyleugenol	Liver	Rat	Oral, 2 years	37, 75 or 150 mg/kg/day bw	National Toxicology Program 2000
	Glandular stomach	Male mouse	Oral, 2 years	10, 30, 100, 300 or 1,000 mg/kg/day bw	
β-Myrcene[a]	Liver	Male mouse	Oral, 2 years	250, 500 or 1,000 mg/kg/day bw	National Toxicology Program 2010b
	Kidney	Male rat			
Phenylethyl isothiocyanate[a]	Bladder	Male rat	Oral 48 weeks	0.1% of diet	Sugiura et al 2003
β-Pulegone[a]	Liver	Mouse	Oral, 2 years	37.5, 75 or 150 mg/kg/day	National Toxicology Program 2009
	Bladder	Female rat			

Continued

Table 12.2 Essential oil constituents for which carcinogenic activity has been reported—Cont'd

Constituent	Target organ	Gender, species	Route, duration	Doses used in study	Reference
Safrole	Liver	Rat	Oral, 2 years	0.25% or 0.5% of diet	Hagan et al 1967
	Liver	Rat	Oral, 2 years	0.1% or 0.5% of diet	Long et al 1963
	Liver	Mouse	Oral, 1 year	0.5% of diet	Wislocki et al 1977
	Liver	Female mouse	Oral, 1 year	0.25% or 0.5% of diet	Miller et al 1983
	Liver	Female mouse	Oral, 180 doses over 90 weeks	120 µg/g bw gavage study	Vesselinovitch et al 1979
	Liver	Mouse	Oral, 78 weeks	0.11% of diet	Innes et al 1969
	Liver	Mouse	Oral, 36–75 weeks	0.4% of diet	Lipsky et al 1981
	Liver	Infant male mouse	4 ip doses over 21 days[c]	9.45 µmol total dose[d]	Miller et al 1983
	Liver	Infant mouse	4 sc doses over 21 days[c]	0.66 or 6.6 mg total dose[d]	Epstein et al 1970
α- + β-Thujone[a]	Preputial gland	Male rat	Oral, 2 years	12.5, 25 or 50 mg/kg/day	National Toxicology Program 2011

[a]Species-specific carcinogens, some of which are also gender-specific and/or organ-specific
[b]Females not tested
[c]Tumors found at 10, 12, 15, or 18 months of age
[d]In the instances where 'total dose' is given, the doses administered were not equal.

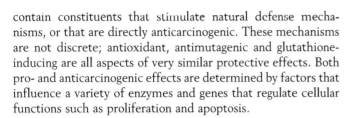

contain constituents that stimulate natural defense mechanisms, or that are directly anticarcinogenic. These mechanisms are not discrete; antioxidant, antimutagenic and glutathione-inducing are all aspects of very similar protective effects. Both pro- and anticarcinogenic effects are determined by factors that influence a variety of enzymes and genes that regulate cellular functions such as proliferation and apoptosis.

Induction of detoxifying enzymes

Cells have elaborate mechanisms for avoiding mutation, including DNA repair enzymes, and pathways that either regulate cell growth or suppress oxidative stress (Dixon & Kopras 2004). Detoxifying and antioxidant enzymes include glutathione S-transferase, glutathione peroxidase, glutathione reductase, superoxide dismutase, quinone reductase and UDP-glucuronyltransferase. Eugenol induces UDP-glucuronyltransferase (Yokota et al 1988; Yokota & Yuasa 1990), various sulfur compounds induce quinone reductase (Fukao et al 2004; Munday & Munday 2001), as do (+)-limonene, perillyl alcohol and phenylethyl isothiocyanate (Gerhäuser et al 2003) and thyme oil induces superoxide dismutase (Youdim & Deans 1999). Essential oils that induce glutathione S-transferase are shown in Box 4.1.[8] Melatonin inhibited safrole-DNA adducts in rat liver by 98.7%, possibly due to activation of protective enzymes such as glutathione peroxidase (Tan et al 1993).

Glutathione is central to one of the most important protective enzyme systems. Glutathione transferases, for example, catalyze the conjugation and detoxification of electrophiles, which are usually generated in response to free radical damage to lipids and to DNA (Ketterer 1988). Associations have been shown between glutathione depletion and cancers of the breast, stomach, colon, lung and prostate (Cai et al 2001; Perera et al 2002; Acevedo et al 2003; Saygili et al 2003; Todorova et al 2003). Glutathione depletion is associated with critical illness and with many chronic conditions such as emphysema, alcoholism, Crohn's disease, macular degeneration, Parkinsonism, Alzheimer's disease, HIV infection and chronic fatigue syndrome. It is also associated with old age (Samiec et al 1998). Consequently people with chronic disease, and older people, may be more susceptible to chemical carcinogenesis.

Antioxidant activity

The importance of antioxidants in the context of cancer has already been elaborated. Essential oils that scavenge 1,1-diphenyl-2-picrylhydrazyl (DPPH) radicals are shown in Table 12.3. Antioxidant constituents include benzyl alcohol, carvacrol, 1,8-cineole, eugenol, (−)-menthol, (6R)-(+)-menthofuran, (−)-menthyl acetate, methyl salicylate, γ-terpinene, thymol and thymoquinone (see Constituent profiles, Chapter 14). Some unsaturated aldehydes, including (E)-cinnamaldehyde, citral, perillaldehyde and safranal, activate the antioxidant responsive element (ARE), which regulates important cellular antioxidants (Masutani et al 2009). Antioxidants are also protective in many other ways, unrelated to cancer.

The use of antioxidant essential oils during chemotherapy or radiation is controversial. While it may protect normal cells

Table 12.3 Comparative activity of some DPPH radical scavenging essential oils

Essential oil	IC_{50} (μg/mL)	Reference
Oregano	0.17	Bozin et al 2006
Thyme (thymol/carvacrol CT)	0.19	Bozin et al 2006
Sage (Dalmatian)	1.78	Bozin et al 2007
Peppermint	2.53	Mimica-Dukic et al 2003
Rosemary	3.82	Bozin et al 2007
Pimento berry	4.82	Padmakumari et al 2011
Melissa	7.58	Mimica-Dukic et al 2004
Bay (W. Indian)	10.00	Jirovetz et al 2007
Tea tree	29.70	Tsai et al 2011
Palmarosa	51.42	Tsai et al 2011
Laurel leaf	53.50	Saab et al 2012b
Marjoram	58.67	Mossa & Nawwar 2011

from collateral damage, it may also protect the cancer cells that the treatment is designed to eliminate. Restriction on the use of essential oils would therefore seem appropriate (see final point of Summary).

Antimutagenesis

There are a variety of antimutagenic factors (often antioxidants) that occur naturally in the diet such as vitamin E, β-carotene, D-glucaric acid, selenium, ascorbic acid and uric acid. Like glutathione, these act either by directly reacting with the mutagens or by suppressing cellular mutagenesis (Azizan & Blevins 1995). They can also act synergistically to prevent tumor initiation, promotion and progression (Hanausek et al 2003).

Antioxidant and antimutagenic essential oils may therefore perform a valuable role in protecting against carcinogenesis. Essential oils that have demonstrated an antimutagenic action include those from blue chamomile (Hernandez-Ceruelos et al 2002), lavender (Evandri et al 2005), nut grass (Kilani et al 2005), rosemary (Fahim et al 1999), Dalmatian sage (Vuković-Gačić et al 2006), and turmeric rhizome (Jayaprakasha et al 2002). Many essential oil constituents are also antimutagenic. Perillyl alcohol, for example, effectively blocks the binding of the carcinogen DMBA with DNA, probably via enzyme inhibition (Chan et al 2006).

In addition to these effects, essential oils may act more directly, as anticarcinogens. This action is discussed below, under Chemoprevention.

The immune system

Several essential oils and essential oil constituents have been shown to stimulate immune responses. For example, eucalyptus oil induced morphological and functional activation of human monocyte-derived macrophages in vitro, dramatically stimulating their phagocytic response (Serafino et al 2008). Carvone and (+)-limonene increased the total number of white blood cells, and stimulated antibody production in spleen and bone marrow when administered to mice at 100 µmol/kg bw (Raphael & Kuttan 2003b). A feed additive containing the essential oil and dried plant parts of *Origanum vulgare* showed non-specific immune stimulant effects on porcine CD4 and CD8 immune cells, MHC class II antigen and non-T/non-B cells in peripheral blood lymphocytes compared to control animals (Walter & Bilkei 2004).

Immunity and cancer

For most of the 20th Century it was believed that the immune system was not able to protect against cancer development, but that view has now radically altered. In the 1980s evidence began accumulating that cells such as macrophages could kill cancer cells in vitro (Caignard et al 1985), but in vivo evidence was lacking until Shankaran et al (2001) demonstrated that lymphocytes and interferon-gamma (IFN-γ) collaborate to inhibit the development of carcinogen-induced sarcomas and spontaneous epithelial carcinomas, and that together they function as a tumor-suppressor system. We now know that cancer 'immunosurveillance' also involves, for example, other interferons, natural killer (NK) cells and T cells (Dunn et al 2004, 2006; Ghiringhelli et al 2006). NK cells act directly against tumor cells, and also secrete potent cytokines, such as IFN-γ (Miller 2001).[7]

There is evidence that immune stimulation is one mechanism through which essential oil constituents play a protective role. For example, benzaldehyde inhibited pulmonary metastasis in mice through an augmentation of NK cell activity (Ochiai et al 1986; Masuyama et al 1987, 1988). NK cell activity was enhanced in vitro by linalyl acetate (Standen et al 2006). A similar effect is reported for the essential oils of various trees native to Japan, including *Thujopsis dolobrata* stems and *Chamaecyparis obtusa* leaves, and for α-pinene, 1,8-cineole and (+)-limonene, all at concentrations of 0.05 or 0.1 ppm. This was partially mediated by induction of intracellular perforin, granzyme A and granulysin (Li et al 2006). The increased survival of mice with ascites tumors was associated with a restoration of NK cell activity to normal levels after four daily ip doses of β-caryophyllene at 20 mg/kg (Da Silva et al 2007).

Eugenol dose-dependently enhanced mouse NK cell activity in vitro between 0.25 and 2.5 µmol/kg bw. It also showed a biphasic effect on plaque-forming antibody responses of mouse splenocytes to sheep erythrocytes in vivo, inhibiting these responses at about 0.1 µmol/kg bw, and enhancing them at about 0.25 µmol/kg. In vitro, eugenol was cytotoxic above 1.0 mM (Vishteh et al 1986). Benzyl alcohol had an inhibitory effect on cell proliferation and on induction of lymphokine-activated killer cell activity. Dose-dependent reductions in cell proliferation were seen when lymphocytes were incubated with 4 µL/mL of benzyl alcohol in heparin salt solution or in saline (Marincola et al 1987).

It has been suggested that the anticarcinogenic activity of costus oil may be due to immune stimulation caused by the allergic skin response to the lactone content of the oil (Takanami et al 1987). The degree of dermal inflammation caused by costus oil correlated with the development stage of human breast, colon, lung and stomach cancers; the more virulent the reaction the higher the lymphocyte count, and the better the prognosis (Takanami et al 1983, 1984, 1985).

Lymphocyte proliferation is stimulated by (+)-limonene in vitro (Manuele et al 2008), and in vivo immune enhancement has also been seen. There were marked increases in both the number and the phagocytic activity of alveolar macrophages in rats fed (+)-limonene for eight days (Hamada et al 2002). In lymphoma-bearing mice fed (+)-limonene for 9 days, macrophage phagocytosis was restored to normal levels, and nitric oxide production in macrophages was increased (Del Toro-Arreola et al 2005). Concurrent treatment with diallyl disulfide significantly inhibited the depression in leukocyte count and spleen weight experienced by rats receiving chemotherapy with fluorouracil (Sundaram & Milner 1996).

Possible adverse effects

Since immune competence is important in relation to cancer, it would be prudent to avoid essential oils that compromise the immune response in people with cancers (though they may be helpful in other clinical conditions). This especially applies to T cells in patients receiving chemotherapy. For example in mice, ginger oil inhibited T lymphocyte proliferation, and decreased the number of total lymphocytes and T helper cells (Zhou et al 2006). Studies using mouse splenocytes show in vitro inhibition of T lymphocyte proliferation by (E)-anethole, eugenol and isoeugenol (Yea et al 2006; Park et al 2007). Black seed essential oil reduced the antibody titer and splenocyte and neutrophil counts in rats, while increasing peripheral lymphocytes and monocytes (Islam et al 2004).

At therapeutic doses in psoriasis patients, PUVA with methoxsalen caused some signs of mild immunosuppression characterized by reduced delayed-type hypersensitivity, changes to immunocompetent cells in the skin, and small reductions in the number and activity of circulating T lymphocytes. Reductions in T cell numbers were also found in healthy volunteers receiving the same treatment (Department of Health 1998).

The clinical relevance of these findings is not known, but they suggest that some essential oils might exacerbate lymphocyte depletion in patients receiving chemotherapy. Restriction on the use of essential oils would therefore seem appropriate (see final point of Summary).

Essential oils may cause systemic allergic reactions through involvement of the immune system. For example, a 60-year-old man suffered a widespread rash and had an elevated white blood cell count after ingesting about 3 mL of tea tree oil, although he had taken it three or four times before without any undesirable effects except for itchy palms (Elliott 1993).

Carcinogenicity testing

The main predictive assays for carcinogenicity are mutagenicity/genotoxicity tests and live rodent tests. Generally, only a substance that tests positive in both areas is classed as a potential human carcinogen. However, in addition to genotoxic carcinogens, there are non-genotoxic carcinogens and genotoxic non-carcinogens (Sakai et al 2002). There are also species-specific

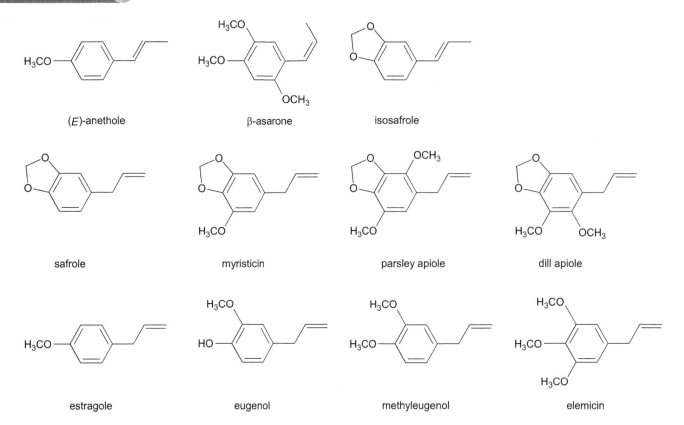

Figure 12.1 • Molecular structures of some alkenylbenzenes.

and gender-specific carcinogens, which only lead to cancer in one species, or in one gender of one species.

Types of molecular structure that give rise to suspicion of carcinogenicity are known as 'structural alerts'. Alkenylbenzenes are clearly a structural alert in essential oils, since several of them are carcinogenic (Figure 12.1). However, some are not, and it can take years of testing before a single substance can be classified with confidence.

In order to evaluate human risk, epidemiological data are helpful if available. No such data exist, however, for any essential oils or constituents, with two exceptions: furanocoumarins + UV light (see Ch. 5, p. 89), and safrole (see Betel quid: a case study below). When there are no epidemiological data, the comparative toxicokinetics of the chemical in rodents and humans may be studied. If there are no significant differences, this increases the likelihood that the rodent carcinogen is also a human carcinogen. Interspecies differences may mean the chemical is carcinogenic to rodents but not humans.

Even carcinogens have threshold levels, below which they are not toxic, so the amount and duration of exposure have great relevance. Finally, carcinogens are subject to the vagaries of synergy and antagonism, and in particular to the co-presence of antimutagens and anticarcinogens. These issues are discussed in more detail below.

Mutagenicity/genotoxicity tests

The main purpose of genotoxicity testing is to attempt accurate identification of carcinogens, in a way that is quicker and

cheaper than rodent testing. There are many types of assays, and it is not unusual for a substance to test positive in some and not in others. Weight of evidence is an important consideration, as is understanding the mechanisms of action. Any genotoxicity identified in a substance that is not in fact carcinogenic is considered a false positive.

Genetic mutations have already been described. They can be inherited across generations of cells, and may arise spontaneously or as a result of environmental factors. A genotoxic chemical can also be described as mutagenic. It has been postulated that mutagenesis plays a role in both the initiation and progression phases of carcinogenesis (Dixon & Kopras 2004). When an unfavorable DNA mutation occurs, repair mechanisms are engaged, and these have variable degrees of efficiency. Some carcinogens enhance mutagenesis through suppression of these mechanisms.

In somatic cells, surviving mutations may lead to the development of cancer, while in fetuses they can cause effects such as malformations and spontaneous abortions. It is notable that the frequency of human chromosomal aberrations in spontaneous abortions within 12 weeks is 61.4%, compared to 0.65% in surviving neonates (Niesink et al 1996). α-Asarone has caused fetal malformations when given to pregnant mice (Salazar et al 1992); kidney and liver tumors were found in the offspring of female mice given four small doses of safrole (Vesselinovitch et al 1979).

Many tests have been developed for detecting chemical mutagens. In vitro methods may employ bacteria, bacteriophages, human or other mammalian cells, while in vivo tests may be conducted in fruit flies or mammals. Tests for

Table 12.4 The action of potentially toxic epoxide metabolites

Constituent	Epoxide metabolite	Action of metabolite
(E)-anethole	Anethole 1′,2′-oxide	Possibly mutagenic, carcinogenic in rats, less is formed in humans, detoxified at low doses
α-Asarone	Asarone 1′,2′-oxide	Mutagenic, carcinogenic
Coumarin	Coumarin 3,4-oxide	Hepatotoxic in rats, much less is formed in humans
Estragole	Estragole 2′,3′-oxide	Mutagenic but not carcinogenic, rapidly detoxified, especially in human liver
Eugenol	Eugenol 2′,3′-oxide	Potentially mutagenic, rapidly detoxified, especially in human liver
Safrole	Safrole 2′,3′-oxide	Potentially mutagenic, rapidly detoxified

mutagenicity are carried out in non-mammalian cells or fruit flies, while tests for genotoxicity are carried out in mammalian cells, although the two terms are often used as if they were synonymous. Approximately 74% of carcinogenic chemicals are mutagenic in the Ames test, probably the best-known and most widely used assay. This is also known as the *Salmonella*/microsome assay or bacterial reversion assay, and was developed by Bruce Ames and others (Ames et al 1973; Mortelmans & Zeiger 2000). Various strains of the bacterium *Salmonella typhimurium* are used, each being sensitive to a different type of mutagenicity.

Many substances require bioactivation to become mutagenic, and since microorganisms and mammalian cells do not possess all the necessary enzymes (except for rat hepatocytes), enzyme extracts are sometimes added during testing. A mixture of microsomal enzymes taken from rodent liver, known as the S9 fraction, is frequently used. Even rat hepatocytes have predictive limitations as they are not a complete model of the intact liver, and also do not account for differences in metabolism between rodent and human.

Chromosomal aberrations (CA) can be detected using yeasts, fungi, bacteria, or mammalian cells, commonly Chinese hamster fibroblasts, lung or ovary cells. These aberrations are a sign of DNA damage. An in vivo mammalian test is the rat or mouse bone marrow micronucleus assay. This detects chromosome fragments that form so-called 'micronuclei' outside the nucleus in a daughter cell, and the number of these micronuclei reflects the extent of genotoxic damage. It is one of the more accurate predictors of carcinogenesis, but is mostly being phased out, as it is an animal test.

Alkylating chemicals, such as epoxides, form the largest group of mutagenic agents. (An alkylating agent is a reactive chemical that can irreversibly alter the structure of another, such as DNA, by attaching an alkyl group.) Epoxides are not often found as constituents of essential oils, but may be formed during oxidation or through bioactivation (Table 12.4). Since these are inactivated almost as soon as they are activated, they do not have sufficient time to cause mutations. They are inactivated more efficiently in humans than rodents (Guenthner & Luo 2001).

Although known carcinogens frequently test positive in genotoxicity assays, it has been recognized for over 20 years that there is a high proportion of false positives (Tennant et al 1987). Of 533 carcinogens, 93% were positive in at least one of three commonly used assays. However, 75–95% of non-carcinogens also tested positive in at least one assay, and this was not due to very high dosing. Surprisingly, tests using mammalian cells were more likely to give rise to false positives than the Ames test (Kirkland et al 2005). The high false-positive rate may be due to the failure of in vitro genotoxins to express their genetic toxicity in whole animals. Another possible factor is 'genetic drift' in rodent cell lines that have been cultured and sub-cultured innumerable times in multiple laboratories over decades (Tweats et al 2007).

Despite these difficulties, a positive finding in all of three specific tests suggests that the substance is more than three times more likely to be a rodent carcinogen, and three negative results suggest it is more than twice as likely to be a non-carcinogen. The tests used were the Ames test, the mouse lymphoma assay, and either an in vitro micronucleus or chromosomal aberration test (Kirkland et al 2005).

Essential oils and their constituents

Several essential oils have tested positive in mutagenicity tests. For example, both dill weed and European dill seed oils induced CA in human lymphocytes and also were genotoxic in fruit flies (Lazutka et al 2001). The major constituent in both oils, (+)-carvone, has been reported as both genotoxic and non-genotoxic, but it is not carcinogenic, suggesting that neither dill seed nor dill weed oil is either. Scots pine needle oil was genotoxic in fruit flies and weakly induced CA in human lymphocytes (Lazutka et al 2001). The oil contains no known carcinogens.

Peppermint oil was not mutagenic in the Ames test, but was marginally mutagenic in a CA test using Chinese hamster fibroblasts (Ishidate et al 1984). Lazutka et al (2001) reported that peppermint oil induced CA in human lymphocytes and also was genotoxic in fruit flies. Menthone (isomer not specified) has shown similar genotoxicity (Franzios et al 1997) and may be responsible for that of peppermint oil. However, it was not carcinogenic in mice (Stoner et al 1973). Peppermint oil was not mutagenic in a mouse lymphoma assay, and was not genotoxic in rat hepatocytes (Heck et al 1989).

Some constituents have one or more reports of mutagenicity, but these are outweighed by other data that suggest they are non-carcinogenic. Examples include benzyl acetate, citronellal, linalyl acetate, isoeugenol, diallyl disulfide and diallyl sulfide. In other cases, such as piperonal, there are insufficient data to make a judgement. Low levels of genotoxicity have been reported for the alkenylbenzenes myristicin, parsley apiole and dill apiole, but rodent testing has so far failed to show any carcinogenicity for these constituents. (E)-Anethole, benzyl alcohol, (+)-carvone, (E)-cinnamaldehyde, eugenol, geranyl acetate and guaiacol are non-carcinogens with some false-positive genotoxicity assays (see Constituent profiles, Chapter 14).

Thymol, carvacrol and γ-terpinene have demonstrated genotoxic activity in human lymphocytes in high concentrations, and antigenotoxic activity in low concentrations (Aydin et al 2005). All three compounds are notable antioxidants (see Constituent profiles, Chapter 14). Eugenol, another powerful antioxidant, has shown genotoxic, non-genotoxic and antigenotoxic properties in different tests, and is antioxidative in low doses and pro-oxidative in high doses (see Eugenol profile, Chapter 14). This apparent conflict is also seen in thymol, where a concentration of 0.2 mM was genotoxic to human lymphocytes when used on its own, but when combined with a mutagen at the same concentration was antigenotoxic (Aydin et al 2005). Both carvacrol and its isomer thymol prevented DNA strand breaks in human cells in vitro in the presence of the oxidant hydrogen peroxide (Slamenová et al 2007). Similarly, human colon and liver cancer cell lines treated with thymol or carvacrol at non-toxic doses showed significant resistance to DNA damage induced by hydrogen peroxide (Horváthová et al 2006). An *Origanum compactum* oil with 30.5% carvacrol and 27.5% thymol was genotoxic to mitochondrial DNA in *Saccharomyces cerevisiae*, but the absence of nuclear DNA damage suggests that long-term genotoxic risks are unlikely (Bakkali et al 2005).

In some cases, reactive metabolites are removed by scavenging systems, such as glutathione, before they can bind with DNA. For example, there are some potentially mutagenic metabolites of essential oil constituents, such as estragole 2′,3′-oxide and eugenol 2′,3′-oxide, that are rapidly and efficiently detoxified (Table 12.4). This process, known as 'inactivation', prevents the formation of mutagens, so long as the scavenging systems are operating well, which they may not be in the very old or in people with chronic disease. In an in vitro study of substances used in dental practice, eugenol, guaiacol and thymol induced CA in human dental pulp cells after 30 hours exposure, but were not genotoxic after 3 hours (Someya et al 2008). Metabolites such as eugenol 2′,3′-oxide were thought to be responsible for this toxicity, which would probably not occur in vivo, since they would be rapidly inactivated. The short half-life of essential oil constituents in vivo is also likely to be a protective factor.

Perhaps the most likely reason that the alkenylbenzenes eugenol, elemicin and (E)-anethole are positive in some tests for genotoxicity but are not carcinogenic, is that they only produce one mutation, one type of DNA adduct (in mouse liver) as do parsley apiole and dill apiole (Phillips et al 1984). However, at least two mutations are required to cause cancer, one in an oncogene and one in a tumor-suppressor gene, and in most cases a minimum of three or four mutations is needed before cells become malignant (Vogelstein & Kinzler 1993; Williams et al 2005b). Safrole, estragole and methyleugenol each produce four DNA adducts (Phillips et al 1984), though very low doses may only produce two adducts, as was seen in rats given 10 mg/kg of safrole orally (Daimon et al 1998).

A substance that produces only one DNA adduct could stimulate repair mechanisms that have antigenotoxic effects. The manifestation of both genotoxic and antigenotoxic effects would then make sense, especially in potent antioxidant substances such as eugenol or thymol. Two aldehydes, cinnamaldehyde and vanillin, cause a type of mutagenicity that elicits recombinational repair, which fixes not only the damage caused by aldehyde, but also other DNA damage, resulting in both mutagenic and antimutagenic findings (Shaughnessy et al 2006; King et al 2007).

Sekizawa & Shibamoto (1982) raised the issue of compound purity in mutagenesis testing. They found that estragole of 96% purity was weakly mutagenic in four *Salmonella* strains without S9, but 99.9% pure estragole was not mutagenic in these strains, with or without S9. They point out that compound purity for safrole has not always been specified.

Photomutagens are by definition only mutagenic in the presence of UV light, and this is covered in Chapter 5. Some photomutagenic furanocoumarins are antigenotoxic or anticarcinogenic in the absence of UV light (Lee et al 2003; Takeuchi et al 2003). Linear furanocoumarins such as imperatorin and isopimpinellin had a greater inhibitory effect on DMBA-DNA adduct formation in mouse mammary glands compared to simple coumarins such as coumarin and limettin (Prince et al 2006).

Live animal tests

Typically, groups of male and female rats and/or mice are used for this type of assay, and the test substance is normally given orally, either in the diet or by stomach tube (gavage), for periods ranging from 20 weeks to 2 years. The numbers of tumors in experimental groups of rodents, on different dosages, are compared to those of a control group. Dietary doses generally range from 0.01% to 5% of feed, and daily gavage doses from 10–1,000 mg/kg/day bw, but other protocols may be employed. Often there are both malignant and benign tumors, and the liver is the most common site.

In a less commonly used test, infant mice are injected ip or sc with test substance either on day one of life, or in four escalating doses over the first three weeks. They are checked for tumor growth at 10–18 months. This protocol was used in all the α-asarone tests, all but one of the estragole tests, and some of the safrole tests (Table 12.2). Questions have been raised about using this method for carcinogens that require metabolic activation, since infants have immature hepatic enzyme function. However, test results suggest that it is a method with high sensitivity to weak carcinogens. After allowing for differences in route of administration and body weight, Epstein et al (1970) calculated that infant mice develop liver tumors at doses of injected safrole 1,100 × lower than the oral dose needed to produce similar tumors in adult mice. The production of pulmonary tumors by safrole in infant mice is notable, since safrole does not produce these in adult mice (Epstein et al 1970). Clearly, infant mice are highly susceptible to injected carcinogens.

There are arguments to support the predictive value of rodent carcinogenicity testing. Most human carcinogens are also carcinogenic in more than one animal species. Experimental evidence of carcinogenicity has, in some cases, preceded human observation and there is a good correlation between animal and human target organ sites (Tomatis 1979). However, the relevance of the high doses used in many animal tests to actual human exposure has always been controversial (Zangouras et al 1981). 'There is little sound scientific basis for this type of extrapolation, in part due to our lack of knowledge about mechanisms of cancer induction, and it is viewed with great unease by many epidemiologists and toxicologists. Nevertheless, to be prudent in regulatory policy, and in the absence of good human data (almost always the case), some reliance on animal cancer tests is unavoidable' (Ames et al 1987).

Interspecies differences

A significant problem in extrapolating animal data to humans is the relatively high occurrence of spontaneous tumors in laboratory animals. These tumors are caused, to a significant extent, by genetic factors and/or viruses that do not exist in the human species (Toth 2001). For DNA-reactive carcinogens in general, at least one rodent species is equally responsive or more responsive than the most sensitive human group (Williams et al 2005b). In a review comparing DNA repair activity in different species relative to that of rats (rat = 1), mice were 0.9, and humans 5.3, suggesting that human DNA repair activity is 5–6 times more efficient than that of mice or rats (Cortopassi & Wang 1996).

In Europe, only data from rats (supported by other appropriate data) may now be used for the licensing of human medicines (Battershill & Fielder 1998). This means that live tests in mice for carcinogenicity are no longer regarded as useful (for pharmaceutical tests) by European regulatory authorities, although genetically bred mice may be used in future. The US has declined to support this position, and continues to test carcinogens in both species.

Benzaldehyde, (+)-limonene and coumarin are epigenetic, species-specific, organic-specific carcinogens (citral probably is too), that do not present any carcinogenic risk to humans, and all have been used as anticancer drugs (see Constituent profiles, Chapter 14). In spite of this, they are often referred to as being carcinogenic, notably on websites warning of carcinogens in common foods. Interspecies differences in metabolism are even seen in probable human carcinogens such as safrole and estragole. When safrole was orally administered to both rats and humans, 1'-hydroxysafrole and 3'-hydroxyisosafrole were found as conjugates in rat urine, but not in human urine (Benedetti et al 1977). However, since safrole produces a multitude of metabolites, this does not necessarily mean it is not carcinogenic in humans.

These interspecies differences strongly imply that rodents are more sensitive than humans to the carcinogens that we are concerned with here, and that tests in mice should be regarded with particular scepticism. However, regulatory agencies generally assume that humans are *more* at risk than rodents, and allow an uncertainty factor of 10 for interspecies differences. Effective in vitro assays for the prediction of mutagenic carcinogens are in early stages of development.

Risk factors

In assessing whether genotoxic or animal data indicate a risk to humans from essential oils, certain other factors need to be taken into account. These include exposure levels, individual susceptibility, and synergistic and antagonistic effects.

At-risk groups

There is insufficient information to specify different safe exposure levels for different groups of individuals, although some are undoubtedly at greater risk than others. At-risk groups include infants, the very old, smokers, heavy drinkers, people with an occupational exposure to carcinogens, people with a personal or family history of cancer, and those with genetic susceptibilities to specific carcinogens. Wild & Kleinjans (2003) have reviewed the question of increased susceptibility in children. Genetic susceptibilities do exist for essential oil constituents, but we do not know who these individuals are.

Genetic susceptibility

Pharmacogenetics was introduced on Ch. 4, p. 56, and is a new area of study attracting much interest. The capacity of individuals to metabolize a specific chemical can vary, because genetic differences can lead to the creation of different metabolizing enzymes. Such variations are known as polymorphisms and are often related to ethnic origin.[8]

In 13 human liver samples, the rate of methyleugenol 1'-hydroxylation varied by up to 27-fold, implying that methyleugenol toxicity is subject to wide variability in the population (Gardner et al 1997). Other research suggests a variation of only fivefold for methyleugenol, and CYP1A2 was identified as the most important enzyme for bioactivation to 1'-hydroxymethyleugenol, with CYP2C9, 2C19 and 2D6 playing lesser roles (Jeurissen et al 2006). A similar enzymatic profile has been elucidated for estragole, with CYP1A2 and 2A6 as the major players (Rietjens et al 2005a; Jeurissen et al 2007). In the case of safrole, CYP2A6, 2D6, 2C19 and 2E1 play a more or less equal role (Jeurissen et al 2004). Substances that inhibit these particular CYP enzymes, such as blue chamomile oil, may therefore afford some protection (Box 4.1). Estragole, methyleugenol and safrole compete for the catalytic sites of CYP1A2 and 2A6, the main enzymes responsible for bioactivation. 1'-Hydroxlation of equal concentrations of estragole and methyleugenol, for example, amounted to only 50% of the expected metabolism. Therefore a reduction of expected toxicity is likely when these constituents are both present in an essential oil (Jeurissen et al 2007).

Genetic polymorphisms may result in either increased or decreased sensitivity to these carcinogens. Lifestyle differences such as alcohol use (in the case of safrole), or smoking and barbiturate use (for safrole, estragole and methyleugenol) could increase sensitivity because they may increase the activity of the relevant CYP enzymes (Jeurissen et al 2004, 2006; Rietjens et al 2005a). Differences in diet, or interactions with prescribed drugs such as ibuprofen may lead to different capacities for detoxification of 1'-hydroxyestragole (Iyer et al 2003). Variations such as these suggest that caution is needed in setting safe levels for human consumption.

Exposure

As with all types of toxicity, carcinogenesis is dependent on level of exposure, and a variety of models exist to assess safety thresholds. Some essential oil constituents are only safe at very low concentrations, while others are not classed as carcinogens, since they only manifest a minimal toxic effect at elevated doses in rodents.

Detoxification and dosage

The metabolism of many chemicals is dose-dependent and this is of particular significance when biotransformation produces a carcinogenic metabolite. 'At low doses a compound may be safely disposed of metabolically whereas at higher doses these pathways become saturated and alternative routes become increasingly employed which lead to the formation of toxic metabolites' (Zangouras et al 1981).

Hepatotoxicity is seen, for example, with (E)-anethole in high doses. In female rats chronic hepatotoxicity and a low incidence of liver tumors were evident at a dietary intake of 550 mg/kg/day. At this dose, daily hepatic production of anethole 1',2'-epoxide (AE) exceeded 120 mg/kg body weight. However, there was no hepatotoxicity when the daily hepatic production of AE was below 30 mg/kg (Newberne et al 1999).

Methyleugenol, estragole, α-asarone, β-asarone and safrole cause liver tumors in rodents after repeated dosing, and two key factors contribute to tumor growth. Firstly, the degree of oxidative metabolism is increased due to the dose-related induction of a CYP enzyme. Secondly, dose-dependent hepatotoxicity occurs which seems to be a necessary precursor to cancer in the liver. At low doses, these factors are much diminished. CYP induction has not been observed in rats receiving oral doses of less than 10 mg/kg of estragole, methyleugenol or safrole for five days, and the formation of toxic 1'-hydroxy derivatives is greatly reduced. The dose of methyleugenol needed to cause hepatotoxicity in rodents is estimated to be in the range of 1–10 mg/kg/day (Smith et al 2002).

The formation of estragole or methyleugenol-DNA adducts depends on activation to the 1'-hydroxy metabolite, and on how much of it is formed (Gardner et al 1995). Adduct levels of at least 15 pmol/mg of DNA at 23 days are required for statistically significant tumor formation (Phillips et al 1984). At low doses, it is presumed that any reactive species formed from 1'-hydroxy derivatives are effectively inactivated by glutathione and other compounds. This is evidenced by the transience of adducts formed after low doses. A rapid drop in adduct formation occurred within 7 days following the ip administration of a 2 or 10 mg dose of estragole, methyleugenol or safrole (equivalent to 100 or 500 mg/kg) to mice (Randerath et al 1984). In mice given 12 µmol of $[2',3'-{}^3H]1'$-hydroxyestragole ip, the three adducts of estragole-deoxyribonucleoside were removed rapidly from mouse liver DNA (Phillips et al 1981a).

The percentage of 1'-hydroxyestragole excreted in urine after oral doses of estragole increased from 1.3% to 13.7% in rats, and from 1.3% to 9.4% in mice as the dose was increased from 0.05 mg/kg to 1,000 mg/kg (Anthony et al 1987). In humans, the amount of 1'-hydroxyestragole found in excreted urine was only 0.3% following ingestion of 100 µg of estragole (Sangster et al 1987).

Lower doses of estragole and methyleugenol are detoxified much more efficiently than higher doses, preventing hepatotoxicity and adduct formation. If detoxification is more efficient in humans than rodents, this should be factored into safety considerations. In a recent review of physiologically based biokinetic models for estragole, methyleugenol and safrole, it was concluded that in spite of differences in the rate of specific metabolic conversions, the overall bioactivation levels for all three are comparable, which is in line with their comparable carcinogenic potential (Martati et al 2011).

Thresholds

The idea that some carcinogens are more potent than others was first mooted in 1939 and eventually led, in 1984, to the proposal

Table 12.5 Comparison of carcinogenic potencies in rodent studies

Constituent	Rat TD$_{50}$	Mouse TD$_{50}$
Allyl isothiocyanate	96	No positive test results
Benzaldehyde	No positive test results	1,490
Benzo[a]pyrene	0.9	3.5
Benzyl acetate	No positive test results	1,440
Coumarin	39.2	103
Estragole	No tests done	51.8
(+)-Limonene	204	No positive test results
Methyleugenol	19.7	19.3
Safrole	441	51.3

The TD$_{50}$ is analogous to an LD$_{50}$, so a low number indicates higher toxicity. It is measured in mg/kg/day
(Data from The Carcinogenic Potency Project [http://potency.berkeley.edu/index.html accessed April 28th 2012]).

of a TD$_{50}$ for carcinogens; the criterion being the appearance of malignant tumors in 50% of animals within a fixed period (Sawyer et al 1984). The TD$_{50}$ is a useful measure of the relative carcinogenicity of substances, and takes data from many rodent studies. The information in Table 12.5 suggests that, in mice, estragole and safrole are equally potent, and methyleugenol is 2.6 times more potent than either. In rats, benzo[a]pyrene is almost 500 times more potent than safrole. While the TD$_{50}$ does not incorporate the notion of a threshold per se, it naturally gives rise to it. In 1990, the HADD (highest average daily dose) was proposed for carcinogens by an EPA researcher, on behalf of the CIPEMC (Nesnow 1990). The HADD is the highest dose administered in a cancer study that did not give rise to a statistical increase in tumors, and is analogous to a NOAEL.

Toxicity in relation to dosage (the dose–response relationship) is expressed in terms of one of three models – threshold, linear non-threshold (LNT) or hormetic. The threshold model is normally used for non-carcinogens, and assumes that below a certain dose (the NOAEL) there is no harmful effect at all. The LNT model is the one traditionally used for carcinogens and assumes that even very low doses can be harmful. In the counter-intuitive hormetic model, very low doses of carcinogens are not carcinogenic, and may even be beneficial since their biological action is totally different to that of larger doses.

The concept of hormesis was well established in toxicology 100 years ago, it fell out of favor in the 1930s, and has only re-emerged as a credible model since the 1980s (Calabrese 2002). Proponents of hormesis believe that it is erroneous to assume that the LNT model applies universally to carcinogens (Calabrese & Baldwin 2003). Hormesis applies to any situation in which a carcinogenic substance has completely different, often opposite, effects at different doses. Hormesis is more widely accepted in relation to epigenetic carcinogens than genotoxic ones. Evidence of hormesis was identified in 350 of 4,000 potentially relevant articles scanned by Calabrese & Baldwin (1998).

The finding of opposite effects at different doses is not uncommon in pharmacology, and is often referred to as 'biphasic'.

A separate, and more controversial challenge to the LNT model for carcinogens has come from proponents of the threshold model. Gaddum (1945) pointed out that dose needs to be plotted on a logarithmic scale to achieve a linear response. A linear (arithmetic) scale for the dose of a chemical obscures effects at doses below those used in the experiment, and distorts the effects seen over the range of doses used (Waddell 2003). Waddell contends that conventional approaches to carcinogen dose–response relationships have concealed the presence of thresholds in major studies, and that the 'Rozman scale' should be used, since it is continuous down to one molecule, and so permits the plotting of very small doses (Rozman et al 1996; Waddell et al 2004).[9] Research by others supports this idea. Williams et al (2005a) reported that very low levels of two carcinogens were not hepatocarcinogenic in rats, and that the appearance of DNA adducts was non-linear in respect to dose. They therefore cautioned against extrapolation from high-dose effects to potential carcinogenicity at low doses.

As an example of the Rozman scale, data from the NTP study on methyleugenol (National Toxicology Program 2000) and DNA adduct data (Carmichael et al 1999), shows a linear response for methyleugenol, and indicates that tumor formation closely follows adduct formation (Figure 12.2). The threshold dose for adduct formation in rats was $10^{20.07}$ molecules of methyleugenol/kg/day.[10] This is equivalent to 34.8 mg/kg/day, which is about 10 times less than the dose that produced tumors in rats (Waddell et al 2004). Using data from carcinogenesis assays, linear responses have also been found for allyl isothiocyanate, estragole and benzyl acetate, with thresholds of 4.14, 174 and 321 mg/kg/day, respectively. When compared to estimated levels of human daily exposure, these results suggest that considerable margins of safety exist for all these constituents.

The lack of risk at very low doses of carcinogens is often reflected in legislation, and is why maximum exposure levels for essential oil constituents such as safrole and methyleugenol

exist. It also explains why there are no restrictions on the sale and use of herbs such as basil and tarragon, which contain methyleugenol. Pesto, which contains concentrated basil, has been the subject of particular scrutiny. The evidence for threshold models suggests that we examine much more closely what happens in the body when carcinogens are present at very low levels. It is likely that millennia of exposure to naturally occurring carcinogens has given rise to protective cellular mechanisms to control genetic damage (Doak et al 2007; Jenkins et al 2010). A rationale for thresholds in genotoxic carcinogens is offered by Williams et al (2005b), and includes the following:

- only a percentage of the potential carcinogen is bioactivated into electrophilic compounds
- the only cells at risk are those that are replicating, usually less than 1% of the cell population
- before reaching the cell's nucleus, a carcinogen needs to escape the attentions of the numerous detoxifying enzymes such as glutathione
- a proportion of the ultimate carcinogen, perhaps 50–90%, will bind to sites that have no toxic consequence
- once it reaches the cell's DNA, the carcinogen is confronted with some 30,000 genes, only a few of which will lead to cancer if mutated.

Taking account of these and other factors, Williams et al (2005b) estimate that a lifetime dose of at least 90 g of a DNA-reactive carcinogen would need to be consumed, equivalent to a daily dose of ~1.3 mg/kg for a life expectancy of 70 years, in order to cause sufficient DNA mutations to cause cancer. In in vitro testing with human lymphoblastoid cells, concentrations of some DNA-reactive carcinogens below 1 µg/mL had no mutagenic effect, a clear indication of a NOAEL. This is reflected in a 'hockey stick' shaped graph, with increasing dose causing no response until a threshold dose is reached, and the subsequent genotoxic response is linear (Doak et al 2007, Johnson GE et al 2009).

Synergistic and antagonistic effects

When two or more carcinogenic constituents are present in an essential oil or in a mixture of essential oils, we have assumed such actions to be additive. For example, betel leaf oil, which contains estragole, safrole and methyleugenol. In such cases, we have reduced our estimates of maximum doses in proportion to the concentrations of all the relevant constituents. Although several oils contain more than one carcinogen, the possibility for such interactions has not yet been demonstrated. When an essential oil or a mixture of oils contains a minority of carcinogenic, and a majority of anticarcinogenic constituents, we have assumed that the principle of antagonism (see Ch. 3, p. 24) applies. Support for antagonism between different carcinogenic constituents has been observed by Ruediger (2006). See Adjusting safe doses and concentrations (see Ch. 13, p. 189) for dose adjustment when using more than one essential oil containing carcinogens.

Even if the carcinogenicity of an essential oil constituent in humans has been established beyond reasonable doubt, there remains the possibility that its metabolism and potential for toxicity will be modified by other constituents. These effects are seen in humans. Extracts of *Piper betle* L. containing both safrole

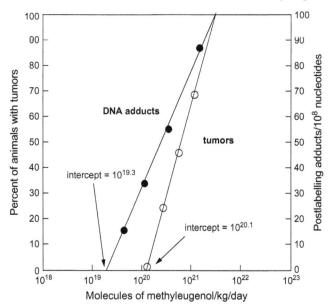

Figure 12.2 • Relationship between methyleugenol gavage dosing and the occurrence of DNA adducts and tumors in male F344 rats. Adapted from Figure 1 in Waddell et al 2004.

and anticarcinogenic constituents are not carcinogenic (antagonism) until the betel is mixed with areca nut (additivity or synergy) (see Betel quid: a case study below).

This antagonistic effect is not unexpected. It has been known for many years that, if hepatic sulfotransferases (enzymes that catalyze sulfate conjugation) are inhibited in mice, this significantly decreases the binding of safrole to hepatic DNA, and the formation of the ultimate carcinogen, 1′-sulfooxysafrole (Boberg et al 1983; Randerath et al 1984). The 1′-hydroxylation of methyleugenol in rat liver microsomes is inhibited by diallyl disulfide (Gardner et al 1997), suggesting that garlic oil may inhibit the carcinogenesis of methyleugenol. In human liver cells, basil extract inhibits estragole biotransformation at the sulfotransferase stage, preventing DNA adduct formation (Jeurissen et al 2008). Biokinetic modelling predicts that nevadensin inhibits the formation of 1′-sulfooxyestragole by almost 100% (Alhusainy et al 2010). Nevadensin is found in basil herb and not essential oil, but findings such as these establish the principal of antagonism in carcinogenesis.

The possibility of anticarcinogenic synergy also exists. β-Caryophyllene (an anticarcinogen) significantly increased the anticarcinogenic activity of α-humulene on human breast cancer MCF-7 cells (Legault & Pichette 2007). Similarly, a mixture of linalyl acetate, terpineol and camphor (isomers not specified) was significantly more active against cultured human colon cancer cells than linalyl acetate+terpineol, or linalyl acetate+camphor (Itani et al 2008).

Chemoprevention

This is defined as the use of natural, synthetic, or biologic chemical agents to reverse, suppress, or prevent carcinogenic progression to invasive cancer (Tsao et al 2004). For example, tamoxifen is recognized for its efficacy in the prevention of breast cancer, and the favorable modification of oxidative DNA adducts by dietary intervention has been demonstrated in clinical studies (Sharma & Farmer 2004; Tsao et al 2004). In addition to antioxidants such as tocopherol and vitamin C, epidemiological studies suggest that dietary isothiocyanates similar to those found in essential oils are chemopreventive, through the induction of phase II enzymes (Talalay & Fahey 2001).

Some dietary factors affect cell-signalling pathways in ways that inhibit carcinogenesis. These include substances not found in essential oils, such as resveratrol (grapes), catechins (green tea) and indole-3-carbinol (cruciferous vegetables), and some that are found in essential oils, including (E)-anethole, eugenol and (+)-limonene (Aggarwal & Shishodia 2006). Many essential oil constituents, and some essential oils, demonstrate chemopreventive effects in either animal or human cancer cell lines.[11]

Mechanisms

Monoterpenes such as (+)-limonene and geraniol, sulfur compounds such as diallyl disulfide, and other classes of essential oil constituent, act through multiple mechanisms in the chemoprevention and chemotherapy of cancer. These include enzyme modulation, the induction of apoptosis or cell differentiation, and the inhibition of cell proliferation, cell migration and angiogenesis.

The action of monoterpenes in the initiation phase of mammary carcinogenesis is in part due to the induction of phase I and phase II enzymes, resulting in a significant reduction in the formation of DNA adducts (Elegbede et al 1993; Crowell 1999). Both (+)-limonene and perillyl alcohol inhibit inducible nitric oxide synthase (iNOS) induction, which in turn protects against high nitric oxide levels and DNA adduct formation (Gerhäuser et al 2003). Garlic oil and phenylethyl isothiocyanate have similar effects in relation to iNOS (Chen YH et al 2003; Chiang et al 2006). Similarly, the anti-initiating properties of diallyl sulfide and diallyl disulfide in NDEA- or AFB1-induced rat liver carcinogenesis are thought to be associated with enzyme modulation (Haber-Mignard et al 1996). The role of glutathione in relation to cancer has already been discussed. Some essential oil constituents, including eugenol, α-humulene and diallyl disulfide, increase intracellular glutathione in normal cells (Wu et al 2001; Zheng et al 1992c), but decrease it in cancerous cells (Babich et al 1993; Sundaram & Milner 1993; Legault et al 2003).

Chemoprevention by monoterpenes during the promotion phase of mammary and hepatic carcinogenesis may be due to the inhibition of cell proliferation, the acceleration of apoptosis or, more rarely, the induction of tumor cell differentiation (Morse & Stoner 1993). (+)-Limonene, for example, inhibits rat liver carcinogenesis by suppressing cell proliferation and enhancing apoptosis (Kaji et al 2001). (+)-Limonene, perillyl alcohol, geraniol, carvone (isomer not specified), (±)-linalool and other monoterpenes act by selectively disrupting the action of cell-growth regulatory proteins (Crowell et al 1992, 1994b, 1996). Costunolide enhances the differentiation of leukemic cells into monocytes (Kim et al 2002).

The selective inhibition of cancer cell growth may take place during various phases of cell division. For example, perillyl alcohol caused cell cycle arrest in the G1 phase in cell lines for human head/neck and lung cancer (Elegbede et al 2003). The in vitro inhibitory effect of β-elemene on the proliferation of leukemic cells, and of diallyl disulfide on human hepatoma, colon cancer, and bladder cancer cells are associated with cell cycle arrest in the G2/M phase (Yang et al 1996; Knowles & Milner 1998; Lu HF et al 2004; Wu et al 2004b).

Apoptosis may be brought about through a variety of mechanisms. Sclareol induced apoptosis in human leukemia cells through a reduction of c-myc proto-oncogene levels (Dimas et al 2001). The induction of apoptosis in several blood-related cancer cell lines by citral was accompanied by the activation of caspase-3, an enzyme that plays a key role in apoptosis (Dudai et al 2005). Three further mechanisms have been observed in the apoptotic action of costunolide (Lee et al 2001; Park et al 2001; Choi et al 2002). Costunolide also acts via non-apoptotic mechanisms such as reducing telomerase activity and the impairment of cellular microtubules (Bocca et al 2004, Choi SH et al 2005). Jasmonates such as (Z)-jasmone and methyl jasmonate (isomer not specified) selectively kill cancer cells through a novel, non-apoptotic mechanism, targeting cells with mutant p53 genes. They were therefore effective where conventional chemotherapy was not, in in vitro tests (Fingrut et al 2005). Jasmonates act directly on mitochondria derived from cancer cells, by-passing pre-mitochondrial apoptotic blocks (Rotem et al 2005).

There are also data that relate to the progression phase. Diallyl sulfide greatly reduced DMBA-induced skin tumors in mice by regulating the cell cycle inhibiting proteins p53 and p21/WAF1 (Arora et al 2004). (Inhibition of the p53 enzyme has no effect on initiation or promotion in mouse skin cancer, but it enhances malignant progression [Kemp et al 1993].) Carcinogens can activate nuclear factor-kappa B (NF-κB), a protein controlling genes involved in cell growth. Blocking this activation helps protect against the late stages of aggressive cancers, since many of the target genes are those required for metastasis and angiogenesis (Dorai & Aggarwal 2004). NF-κB activation is blocked by *Eucalyptus globulus* oil, (E)-anethole, (E)-cinnamaldehyde, citral, costunolide, dehydrocostus lactone, eugenol, α-pinene, α-terpineol and thymoquinone (Chainy et al 2000; Koo et al 2001; Matsuda et al 2003; Zhou et al 2003; Kim DH et al 2007; Lin et al 2008; Banerjee et al 2009; Hassan et al 2010; Neves et al 2010; Manikandan et al 2011).

Both costunolide and mastic oil inhibited angiogenesis in vitro by blocking signalling pathways for vascular endothelial growth factor (VEGF) (Jeong SJ et al 2002; Loutrari et al 2006). Allyl isothiocyanate blocked angiogenesis, both in vivo and in vitro;

VEGF and nitric oxide were down-regulated, as were cytokines such as TNF-α (Thejass & Kuttan 2007a, 2007b; Kumar et al 2009). Antiangiogenic activity has also been reported for zedoary oil, β-eudesmol, perillyl alcohol and thymoquinone (Loutrari et al 2004; Tsuneki et al 2005; Yi et al 2008; Chen et al 2011).

Perillyl alcohol inhibited the migration of cultured breast cancer cells, and so could be expected to prevent metastasis (Wagner et al 2002b). Methyl jasmonate (isomer not specified) suppressed experimental lung metastasis of both normal and drug-resistant B16-F10 melanoma cells (Reischer et al 2007), and xanthorrhizol similarly inhibited lung metastasis of mouse colon cancer cells (Choi M-A et al 2005). Eugenol showed a dramatic anticarcinogenic action against malignant melanoma in female mice and completely prevented metastasis, resulting in no fatalities (Ghosh et al 2005).

In summary, there are varying degrees of evidence for a chemopreventive and/or chemotherapeutic effect for essential oils or their constituents in leukemia, and in cancers of the bladder, bone, brain, breast, cervix, colon, connective tissue, larynx, liver, lung, mouth, esophagus, ovary, pancreas, prostate, skin and stomach (Table 12.6).

Table 12.6 Essential oils and constituents for which chemopreventive/chemotherapeutic activity has been reported, either in vitro or in vivo

	Target organ/cell type	Species	Reference
Essential oil			
Basil (holy)	Stomach	Mouse	Aruna & Sivaramakrishnan 1996
Basil (pungent)	Skin	Mouse	Singh et al 1999
Black seed	Colon	Rat	Salim & Fukushima 2003
Caraway	Skin	Mouse	Shwaireb 1993
Cedarwood (Atlas)	Leukemia	Human	Saab et al 2012a
Cedarwood (Himalayan)	Leukemia	Human	Saab et al 2012a
Cumin	Stomach	Mouse	Aruna & Sivaramakrishnan 1996
Curry leaf	Breast	Human	Nagappan et al 2011
Fir needle (Canada)	Various cell lines	Human	Legault et al 2003
Frankincense	Bladder	Human	Frank et al 2009
Garlic	Skin	Mouse	Belman 1983, Sadhana et al 1988
	Cervix	Mouse	Rai & Ahujarai 1990
	Leukemia	Human	Seki et al 2000
Grapefruit	Lung, forestomach	Mouse	Wattenberg et al 1985
Laurel leaf	Kidney, skin	Human	Loizzo et al 2007
	Leukemia	Human	Saab et al 2012a
Lavender	Mouth	Human	Manosroi et al 2005
Lemon	Lung, forestomach	Mouse	Wattenberg et al 1985; Wattenberg & Coccia 1991
Lemongrass (E. Indian)	Cervix, lung, liver, colon, prostate, mouth, nerves	Human	Sharma et al 2009
Lemongrass (W. Indian)	Mouth	Human	Manosroi et al 2005
	Leukemia	Mouse	Manosroi et al 2005

Continued

Table 12.6 Essential oils and constituents for which chemopreventive/chemotherapeutic activity has been reported, either in vitro or in vivo—Cont'd

	Target organ/cell type	Species	Reference
Mastic	Leukemia	Human	Loutrari et al 2006
Melissa	Breast, colon, lung, leukemia	Human	De Sousa et al 2004
	Skin	Mouse	De Sousa et al 2004
Myrtle (bog)	Lung, colon	Human	Sylvestre et al 2005
Nut grass	Leukemia	Mouse	Kilani et al 2008
Onion	Skin	Mouse	Belman 1983
	Leukemia	Human	Seki et al 2000
Orange	Liver	Rat	Bodake et al 2002
	Breast	Rat	Maltzman et al 1989
	Lung, forestomach	Mouse	Wattenberg et al 1985; Wattenberg & Coccia 1991
Rosewood	Skin	Human	Sœur et al 2011
Salvia libanotica	Skin	Mouse	Gali-Muhtasib & Affara 2000
Sandalwood (E. Indian)	Skin	Mouse	Dwivedi & Abu-Ghazaleh 1997
Tangerine	Lung, forestomach	Mouse	Wattenberg et al 1985
Tea tree	Skin	Human	Calcabrini et al 2004
Constituent			
Alantolactone	Leukemia	Human	Lawrence et al 2001
	Stomach, uterus	Human	Konishi et al 2002
Allyl isothiocyanate	Various tissues	Rat	Chung et al 1984
	Lung (melanoma cells)	Mouse	Manesh & Kuttan 2003
Ascaridole	Colon, leukemia	Human	Bezerra et al 2009
	Breast, leukemia	Human	Efferth et al 2002b
Benzaldehyde	Various	Human	Kochi et al 1980
Benzyl isothiocyanate	Lung	Mouse	Hecht et al 2002
	Bladder	Rat	Okazaki et al 2002
	Ovary	Human	Pintao et al 1995
	Lung	Mouse	Yang et al 2002
	Breast	Mouse	Wattenberg 1983
Bergamottin	Breast	Human	Kleiner et al 2003
α-Bisabolol	Brain	Human	Cavalieri et al 2004
	Pancreas	Human	Darra et al 2008
Carvacrol	Breast	Human	Arunasree 2010
	Lung	Human	Koparal & Zeytinoglu 2003
	Leukemia	Human	Lampronti et al 2006
	Skin	Mouse	He et al 1997b
α-Cadinol	Colon	Human	He et al 1997a

Continued

Table 12.6 Essential oils and constituents for which chemopreventive/chemotherapeutic activity has been reported, either in vitro or in vivo—Cont'd

	Target organ/cell type	Species	Reference
α-Caryophyllene	Various cell lines	Human	Legault et al 2003
(E)-Cinnamaldehyde	Leukemia	Mouse	Moon & Pack 1983
	Melanoma	Human	Cabello et al 2009
	Colon	Human	Duessel et al 2008
Costunolide	Colon	Rat	Kawamori et al 1995
Coumarin	Various	Human	Cox et al 1989
Diallyl disulfide	Leukemia	Human	Efferth et al 2002a; Kwon et al 2002
	Breast	Human	Nakagawa et al 2001
	Colon	Human	Knowles & Milner 1998
	Lung, forestomach	Mouse	Wattenberg et al 1989
Diallyl sulfide	Breast	Rat	Ip et al 1992
	Liver	Rat	Tsuda et al 1994
	Lung	Mouse	Hong et al 1992
	Esophagus	Rat	Wargovich et al 1988
	Skin	Mouse	Singh and Shukla 1998
β-Elemene	Brain	Human	Tan et al 2000
	Lung	Human	Wang et al 2005
	Ovary	Human	Li et al 2005
	Larynx	Human	Tao et al 2006
β-Eudesmol	Liver	Human	Ma et al 2008
Eugenol	Liver	Human	Babich et al 1993
	Skin	Human, mouse	Ghosh et al 2005
	Forestomach	Mouse	Bhide et al 1991a
Farnesol[a]	Pancreas	Human, hamster	Burke et al 2002
	Leukemia	Human	Rioja et al 2000
Geraniol	Colon	Human	Carnesecchi et al 2001
	Skin	Mouse	Yu et al 1995a, He et al 1997b
	Skin, leukemia	Mouse	Shoff et al 1991
	Liver	Rat	Yu et al 1995a
	Breast	Rat	Zheng et al 1993a
β-Ionone	Breast	Rat	Yu et al 1995b
(Z)-Jasmone	Lung	Human	Yeruva et al 2006

Continued

Table 12.6 Essential oils and constituents for which chemopreventive/chemotherapeutic activity has been reported, either in vitro or in vivo—Cont'd

	Target organ/cell type	Species	Reference
(+)-Limonene	Breast	Rat	Elegbede et al 1984, 1986b; Elson et al 1988; Maltzman et al 1989; Russin et al 1989
	Liver	Rat	Kaji et al 2001
	Liver, lung, stomach	Human	Kim et al 2001
	Stomach	Human-mouse	Lu XG et al 2004b
	Stomach	Rat	Uedo et al 1999
	Lung (melanoma cells)	Mouse	Raphael & Kuttan 2003a
Linalool[a]	Kidney, skin	Human	Loizzo et al 2007
	Liver	Human	Usta et al 2009
	Lymphoma	Human	Chiang et al 2003
	Leukemia	Human	Gu et al 2010
(−)-Menthol	Breast	Rat	Russin et al 1989
	Bladder	Human	Li Q et al 2009
	Leukemia	Human	Lu et al 2006
Methoxsalen	Lung	Mouse	Takeuchi et al 2003
Methyl jasmonate[a]	Prostate	Human	Samaila et al 2004
	Skin	Human	Reischer et al 2007
	Breast	Human	Fingrut & Flescher 2002
Myristicin	Lung	Mouse	Zheng et al 1992a
Nerolidol[a]	Colon	Rat	Wattenberg 1991
Perillyl alcohol	Lung	Mouse	Lantry et al 1997
	Breast	Rat	Haag & Gould 1994
	Liver	Rat	Mills et al 1995
	Colon	Rat	Reddy et al 1997
	Pancreas	Hamster	Stark et al 1995
	Skin	Mouse	Lluria-Prevatt et al 2002
Phenylethyl isothiocyanate	Colon	Rat	Chung et al 2000
	Lung	Mouse, rat	Hecht 1995
	Lung	Mouse	Hecht et al 2000
α-Santalol	Skin	Mouse	Dwivedi et al 2003, 2006
Sclareol	Skin, lung	Human	Chinou et al 1994
	Leukemia	Human	Dimas et al 1999
	Breast	Human	Dimas et al 2006
	Colon	Human	Hatziantoniou et al 2006
Terpinen-4-ol	Liver Leukemia	Human	Hayes et al 1997
	Skin	Human	Calcabrini et al 2004

Continued

Table 12.6 Essential oils and constituents for which chemopreventive/chemotherapeutic activity has been reported, either in vitro or in vivo—Cont'd

	Target organ/cell type	Species	Reference
Thymoquinone	Forestomach	Mouse	Badary et al 1999
	Connective tissue	Mouse	Badary & Gamal El-Din 2001
	Skin	Mouse	Gali-Muhtasib et al 2004b
	Bone	Human	Roepke et al 2007
	Leukemia	Human	El-Mahdy et al 2005
	Prostate	Human	Yi et al 2008
	Colon	Human	El-Najjar et al 2010
ar-Turmerone	Connective tissue	Mouse	Itokawa et al 1985
Vanillin	Liver	Rat	Tsuda et al 1994
Xanthorrizol	Peritoneum	Mouse	Itokawa et al 1985

[a]Isomer not specified

Carcinogens and anticarcinogens

In assessing the biological action of an essential oil in relation to cancer, the presence of chemopreventive constituents should be taken into account just as much as the presence of carcinogenic ones. It is our view that the mere presence of a carcinogenic constituent in an essential oil does not necessarily constitute a risk, quantifiable according to its concentration in the oil, even though this is the approach currently taken by most regulatory agencies. While it seems logical to assume that an essential oil containing a carcinogen is itself carcinogenic, it is also possible that some of the essential oils consequently flagged as such are non-carcinogenic, or even anticarcinogenic.

Nutmeg oil, for example, contains safrole and methyleugenol, both carcinogens, but it also contains the anticarcinogens (+)-limonene and myristicin, and in greater quantity. The available data on nutmeg oil, even though inconclusive, point to a non-carcinogen or a chemopreventive, anticarcinogen. In vitro evidence suggests that nutmeg oil dose-dependently inhibits aflatoxin B_1-induced carcinogenesis (Hashim et al 1994). Nutmeg oil significantly induces glutathione *S*-transferase in mouse liver (Banerjee et al 1994), and it has demonstrated significant antioxidant activity (Deans et al 1993; Dorman et al 1995; Recsan et al 1997). Most significantly, although safrole produces CA in Chinese hamster lung cells, nutmeg oil is not mutagenic in the same test (Ishidate et al 1984, 1988).

A laurel leaf oil containing 2.5% methyleugenol, 7.1% linalool (isomer not specified) and 35.2% 1,8-cineole was cytotoxic to human melanoma and renal cell adenocarcinoma cells in vitro (Loizzo et al 2007). Holy basil oil (typically 9.7–12.0% estragole, 0.2–0.3% methyleugenol, 31.9–50.4% eugenol) significantly inhibited B[*a*]P-induced squamous cell stomach carcinoma in mice (Aruna & Sivaramakrishnan 1996) and was highly active against human mouth epidermal carcinoma and mouse leukemia cells (Manosroi et al 2005). Similarly, a basil oil containing 69.2% linalool, 2.4% estragole, 1.9% geraniol, 1.4% eugenol and no methyleugenol was antimutagenic in *S. typhimurium* strains TA98, TA100 and TA102. This was attributed to the antioxidant action of both the essential oil and linalool, and suggests that the linalool chemotype of basil oil is not carcinogenic (Berić et al 2007).

Other constituents, such as eugenol, 1,8-cineole and linalool, may block the action of the carcinogens in these instances, through an antioxidant/antimutagenic action. In other essential oils, the data are either equivocal or raise concerns. Tarragon oil (73–87% estragole, 0.1–1.5% methyleugenol, 0–3.5% (+)-limonene) was mutagenic in the *Bacillus subtilis* rec-assay, but not in the Ames test; DNA-damaging activity was found to reside in the estragole fraction of the oil (Zani et al 1991). Calamus oil (42.5–78.4% β-asarone) given orally at 500, 1,000, 2,500 and 5,000 ppm to rats for 59 weeks produced growth retardation and increased the likelihood of duodenal ulcer-related malignant tumors at all doses (Taylor et al 1967). Sassafras oil (61.7–92.9% safrole) is clearly carcinogenic in rodents (see Sassafras profile, Chapter 13).

It is very likely that the relative quantities of carcinogens and anticarcinogens, rather than simply the concentration of carcinogens, in an essential oil determine its action. Neither calamus nor sassafras oil contains any known protective compounds. In a test of genotoxicity using *Saccharomyces cerevisiae*, a tarragon oil with 61.0% estragole+methyleugenol and 0.3% linalool+eugenol was genotoxic, but a basil oil with 17.0% estragole+methyleugenol, and 52.5% linalool+eugenol was not (Tateo et al 1989).

Betel quid: a case study

Betel quid, or paan, is an addictive stimulant and psychoactive preparation chewed or sucked by some 600 million people in

Southeast Asia. It is composed of a mixture of areca nut (*Areca catechu* L.), slaked lime (calcium hydroxide) and various flavoring ingredients such as catechu (*Acacia catechu* Willd.), wrapped in the leaves or flowers of *Piper betle* L. In India and Pakistan, tobacco is often added, though not in Taiwan or Southern China.

Even without tobacco, betel quid is carcinogenic (Ko et al 1995; Wu MT et al 2004c). In Assam, India, cancer of the esophagus is the most commonly diagnosed cancer in males, and ranks second for females (Phukan et al 2001). In Taiwan, quid chewing is associated with 80% of oral cancer deaths, although this figure includes smokers (Kwan 1976, cited in Jeng et al 1994b). Betel quid chewing is also a risk factor for hepatocellular carcinoma (HC) especially among Taiwanese quid chewers (Tsai et al 2001, 2004; Chang et al 2004).

Safrole is a major constituent of betel, and the flowers have been reported to contain 15 mg/g (Liu et al 2000). Safrole-DNA adducts were detected in the liver of a Taiwanese man who had chewed betel quid for 32 years, and was diagnosed with HC (Liu et al 2000). Similar adducts were found in the liver tissue of two out of 28 Taiwanese with HC. They were the only patients who were betel quid chewers. Six were smokers, including one of the quid chewers, who had six times as many adducts as the non-smoker. Safrole-DNA adducts have been found in the white blood cells of 94.3% of quid-chewing male Taiwanese, compared to only 13.0% of non-chewers, and they have also been found in the tissues of Taiwanese oral or esophageal cancer patients with a betel quid habit (Chen et al 1999; Liu et al 2004).

Although it might seem reasonable to suspect safrole as the cause of the genotoxicity of betel quid, *Piper betle* is in fact antimutagenic, antigenotoxic and anticarcinogenic in human and animal models (Padma et al 1989a, 1989b; Azuine et al 1991; Bhide et al 1991a, 1991b, 1994; Jeng et al 1999a; Rao et al 1985; Trivedi et al 1994). The reason why many Taiwanese quid chewers develop cancers must therefore be due to one or more other carcinogens. Areca nut contains the alkaloids arecoline and arecaidine, both of which are genotoxic (Panigrahi & Rao 1984; Tsai et al 2008). Arecoline also depletes antioxidant enzymes, and is cytotoxic to human oral mucosal cells (Jeng et al 1999b; Miyazaki et al 2005a; Dasgupta et al 2006). Areca nut extract was genotoxic to human gingival keratinocytes (Jeng et al 1999b), and areca-derived carcinogenic nitrosamines have been found in the saliva of betel chewers (Stich et al 1986; Nair J et al 1987).

In 2012 an IARC report cited betel quid with or without tobacco, and areca nut, as carcinogenic to humans. It cited betel leaf as probably not carcinogenic in animals (http://monographs.iarc.fr/ENG/Monographs/vol100E/mono100E-10.pdf, accessed July 10th 2012).

Interestingly, while aqueous extracts of areca nut have been found to induce tumors in animals, aqueous betel leaf extracts either lacked tumorigenic activity or reversed tumorigenesis induced by known carcinogens (Bhide et al 1979; Rao 1984). The antimutagenic action of *Piper betle* is thought to be due to antioxidant constituents such as eugenol, chevibetol, hydroxychavicol, allyl pyrocatechol, α-tocopherol and β-carotene (Amonkar et al 1986; Azuine et al 1991; Chang et al 2002; Rathee et al 2006). It is likely, therefore, that antioxidant and antimutagenic constituents of betel leaf counteract the toxicity of areca nut alkaloids, and evidence of this can be found in the

antagonistic effect of arecoline in relation to the chemopreventive action of clocimum oil (85–90% eugenol) in mice (Singh A et al 2000). Moreover, in the context of oral cancer, safrole has shown in vitro and in vivo antitumoral activity through apoptosis of human oral cancer HSC-3 cells, and in a mouse solid tumor xenograft model of the same cancer type (Yu et al 2011).

The discussion above highlights a causal relationship between betel quid chewing and oral, esophageal and liver cancers. However, the levels of safrole-DNA adducts found in the liver were surprisingly low, suggesting that there may be no causal relationship between the safrole-DNA adducts and the cancers. Safrole-DNA adducts were found in the livers of mice who drank commercial cola drinks ad libitum for up to eight weeks, while they were not found in mice who drank non-cola soft drinks or water. The level of adducts increased to 1 in 10^8 (100 million) nucleotide bases by week eight (Randerath et al 1993). Cola contains very small amounts of safrole, presumed to be due to the presence of nutmeg oil.[12] However, there is no correlation between cola consumption and liver cancer in humans (Bosch et al 2004; http://www.thecoca-colacompany.com/ourcompany/ar/pdf/2009-per-capita-consumption.pdf accessed April 28th 2012).

Thus, despite the causal relationship between betel quid chewing and oral, esophageal and liver cancers, the presence of safrole-DNA adducts *per se* is not a cause for alarm. The above illustrates the possible interactions of carcinogenic and anticarginogenic constituents in relation to human risk.

Essential oils

We know little about the action of many essential oils containing both carcinogens and anticarcinogens, or indeed about the action of the majority of essential oils containing estragole and/or methyleugenol. The extent to which the rodent carcinogenicity data for a single constituent is relevant to a human using an essential oil containing it depends on factors such as interspecies differences in metabolism, exposure levels, the synergistic/antagonistic action of other constituents, and individual differences in bioactivation efficiency. There is no evidence that tumors in humans have ever been induced by the use of essential oils. Nevertheless, a few do contain potentially carcinogenic substances, and there is concern that these oils may not be safe to use in aromatherapy.

While it is likely that a single application of a potentially carcinogenic essential oil in an aromatherapy context will present a negligible risk, aromatherapy oils or other products containing significant concentrations of, for example, estragole-rich basil oil, might feasibly contribute to carcinogenesis if used on a regular basis. Therefore we recommend that the use of certain essential oils should be restricted on the basis of the current evidence.

In an aromatherapy massage, the recipient could be exposed to 1.5 mL of an essential oil per session (Table 4.2). If, for example, 87% of that dose is composed of methyleugenol, as would be possible in tarragon oil, then up to 0.13 mL of methyleugenol could be absorbed into the bloodstream in one session, assuming that 10% is transdermally absorbed. For an adult weighing 70 kg, this approximates to 1.8 mg/kg/day, which is close to the threshold of 5.91 mg/kg/day calculated for rodents. On the other hand, clove bud oil contains a maximum of 0.2% methyleugenol, and 1.5 mL of this oil would result in a dose of methyleugenol 350 times less than the threshold.

Since daily exposure to 1.5 mL of an essential oil is unlikely to occur for a prolonged period for a person receiving a typical course of massage, it could be argued that the use of tarragon oil would not pose a significant risk. However, individual susceptibility also needs to be considered, and the fact that the same individual may be concurrently exposed to other carcinogens. Practitioners administering essential oils are advised to minimize their exposure to carcinogenic constituents as a sensible precaution, since they are probably at greater risk than their clients. Maximum use levels for essential oils containing rodent carcinogens will be found in the appropriate essential oil profiles (see Chapter 13).

Some essential oil constituents have been found to exhibit estrogen-like activity in vitro or in vivo (see Chapter 11). This may be a concern for patients with estrogen-sensitive cancers, since there is a theoretical possibility of exacerbating the growth and proliferation of tumors. However, estrogen-like actions in animals were mainly weak or limited to certain experimental conditions, and estrogen receptor binding affinity was generally much weaker than that of 17β-estradiol. We therefore do not consider that essential oils containing these constituents pose any significant risk in patients with estrogen-sensitive cancers.

Current regulations

These are summarized in Table 14.1. At the time of writing, estragole has been neither banned nor restricted in Europe. It is simply listed by the Council of Europe under 'substances which are suspected to be genotoxic carcinogens'. It is listed as a carcinogen by the state of California, and IFRA has set a maximum use level of 0.01% for estragole in body lotions. IFRA and the EU have different standards for methyleugenol. For leave-on products the IFRA standard is 0.0004%, and the EU standard is 0.0002%. For rinse-off products the standards are 0.001% and 0.0005%, respectively. The EU standards are a legal requirement and apply to EU member states, and the IFRA standards constitute a voluntary code that applies universally. IFRA does not permit the use of α-asarone, β-asarone or safrole except as natural constituents of essential oils.

Summary

- The chemical induction of a malignant tumor is thought to occur in three stages: initiation, promotion and progression. During initiation, the potential carcinogen forms a bond with the chromosomal DNA of a cell, forming a DNA adduct. Promotion entails an increase in cell growth, and progression involves processes such as invasion and metastasis.
- Some essential oil constituents are promoters, but not initiators. Some, known as 'complete carcinogens', are capable of both initiation and promotion. The known complete carcinogens are α-asarone, β-asarone, estragole, methyleugenol and safrole.
- There are defense mechanisms in the body that protect against mutagenesis and carcinogenesis, such as antioxidants, detoxifying enzymes, and factors in the immune system. These are stimulated by certain essential oil constituents, which may therefore help protect the body against carcinogenic constituents.
- The two main predictive assays for carcinogenesis are mutagenicity/genotoxicity tests and live rodent tests. There are genotoxic carcinogens, non-genotoxic (epigenetic) carcinogens, genotoxic non-carcinogens and species-specific carcinogens.
- In vitro tests for mutagenicity may involve bacteria, bacteriophages or mammalian or human cells. In vivo tests may be conducted in fruit flies and mammals. The most widely used assay is the Ames test, but no single test can detect all mutagenic effects with a high degree of accuracy.
- There are valid arguments to support the predictive value of rodent carcinogenicity testing. However, the relevance to actual human exposure of the high doses often used in animal tests remains controversial, and rodents are generally more susceptible to carcinogens than humans.
- Some rodent carcinogens, such as benzaldehyde and coumarin, are species-specific in their action, and are not carcinogenic in humans.
- In some instances, carcinogenicity only occurs in rodents at high doses, when detoxification mechanisms become saturated.
- There are threshold levels for the carcinogens found in essential oils, below which they are not carcinogenic.
- The potency of carcinogens found in essential oils can be altered by other constituents, which may enhance or inhibit the development of neoplasia.
- Many essential oil constituents have a chemopreventive action, meaning that they inhibit one or more of the stages of carcinogenesis. Some essential oils containing carcinogens are non-mutagenic, and some are antimutagenic or anticarcinogenic. This may be because they also contain chemopreventive constituents.
- There may be differences between individuals, and sometimes between ethnic groups, in the way they metabolize carcinogens, resulting in significant differences in susceptibility to carcinogens.
- The extent to which the rodent carcinogenicity data for a single constituent is relevant to a human using an essential oil containing it depends on exposure level and frequency, interspecies differences in metabolism, individual differences in bioactivation efficiency, and the synergistic/antagonistic action of other constituents.
- Some essential oils containing carcinogens should not be used in therapy because they present a high level of risk. Others should be used only at restricted doses or concentrations.
- We do not consider that essential oils containing phytoestrogens pose any significant risk to people with estrogen-sensitive cancers.
- Because of possible and unpredictable effects on immune mechanisms, we recommend that essential oils are avoided from one week before to one month following a course of chemotherapy or radiotherapy, and in patients undergoing organ or tissue transplants who are taking conventional immunomodulatory drugs.

Notes

1. Malignant tumors may arise almost anywhere in the body. Those derived from epithelial tissue are called carcinomas, those derived from connective tissue or muscle, sarcomas. They may also arise in tissues of the immune system: myeloid tumors in the bone marrow, lymphoid tumors in lymphoid tissue. Even embryonic tissue may become malignant. One of the great problems facing medicine is the understanding of why such malignant changes should sometimes occur in previously normal tissues. There is undoubtedly no single reason.

2. A substance that selectively induces apoptosis in cancer cells is a candidate for the treatment of cancer. Various drugs used in cancer chemotherapy, such as cisplatin, Adriamycin and Taxol, have an apoptosis-inducing activity.

3. Paradoxically, ROS generation can also play a part in the death of cancer cells. Eugenol, for example, induced apoptosis in human leukemia cells via ROS generation, depleting intracellular glutathione (Yoo et al 2005).

4. One of the cancer initiators found in cigarette smoke (benzo[a]pyrene) was used in some of the tests where subsequent application of citrus oils leads to tumor development. Factors in the citrus oils, now believed to be oxidized components of the oils, were thus acting as promoters of tumor development. There is a theoretical possibility that oxidized citrus oils could act as promoters in people already initiated by constituents of cigarette smoke. The actual risk to smokers from using oxidized citrus oils is vanishingly small, and is not currently regarded as a risk by any regulatory agencies. However, the studies highlight the importance of using unoxidized citrus oils, which present no risk.

5. Some of the most notorious chemical carcinogens are the polycyclic aromatic hydrocarbons, such as benzo[a]pyrene, found in cigarette smoke. Burnt organic material very often contains these chemicals. They probably need to be converted to highly reactive intermediates (e.g., epoxides) by metabolic processes before cancer can result. With the exception of cade and birch tar oils, which are produced by burning during distillation (dry distillation) essential oils do not contain polycyclic aromatic hydrocarbons or other chemicals with similarly high carcinogenic potential. Indian 'choyas', used in perfumery, may present similar risks as they are also produced using dry distillation.

6. Ultimate carcinogens, usually electrophiles, form adducts with cellular electron-rich or nucleophilic sites (often sulfur, nitrogen or oxygen). If this occurs at the level of DNA or RNA, initiation of carcinogenesis may occur.

7. Cancer is an age-related disease. In the US, the Centers for Disease Control data for 2001 show male cancer mortality steadily increasing in each of 19 age groups, from 1.5 per 100,000 up to age 1, to 43.9 at age 40–44, and 2,571.1 per 100,000 (2.57%) for those over 85 years. Incidence rates are much higher, but show the same age-related tendency.

8. Other phase II proteins with protective functions include epoxide hydrolases, heme oxygenase, dihydrodiol dehydrogenase and ferritin (Talalay & Fahey 2001). Little is currently known about the action of essential oils in relation to these enzymes. The p53 enzyme system is often central to cellular response to DNA damage, and is involved in suppressing tumor growth and instigating apoptosis. It is able to detect many types of DNA damage and coordinate cellular response from multiple options (Liu and Kulesz-Martin 2001).

9. The debate among toxicologists concerning the existence or otherwise of thresholds for carcinogens goes far beyond essential oil constituents, and radically divides organizations such as the FDA (who favor thresholds for PCB-like chemicals, for instance) and the EPA (who do not).

10. $10^{20.07}$ is a very large number. It refers of 10 raised to the power 20.07. As a simpler example, 10^6 represents 10 to the power 6, or one million. According to Avogadro's law, 1 mole of any substance contains 6.02×10^{23} particles. For methyleugenol, 178.23 g (1 mole) contains 6.02×10^{23} molecules. So, 1 molecule of ME should weigh $178.23 \div (6.02 \times 10^{23})$ g, which is 2.96×10^{-22} g. According to the data, the threshold for methyleugenol is five times lower than that for estragole, so the difference in maximum use level should be about fivefold. It should be remembered that these are thresholds for rodents, and metabolic differences mean that in some cases, estragole for example, human thresholds may be higher.

11. Substances that are cytotoxic to cancer cells may also be cytotoxic to normal cells, which is of course a common problem in chemotherapy.

12. In a 1998 analysis of cola drinks in Taiwan, 20 of 25 contained three to five times more safrole than the regulated amount of 1 µg/mL (Choong & Lin 2001).

Essential oil profiles

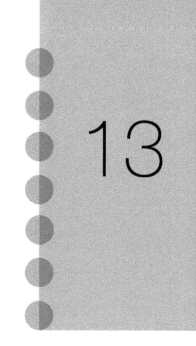

13

CHAPTER CONTENTS

Notes

This chapter consists of 400 safety profiles on essential oils, absolutes and resinoids. In cases where there are no toxicity data for an essential oil, but there are for its major constituents we have indicated the likely safety of the oil on this basis. Because of interactions between constituents, toxicity in the whole essential oil might be either greater or lesser than would be expected from the concentration of a particular constituent or constituents. However, in the absence of data on an essential oil, we feel that it is more useful to extrapolate constituent data than to take the view that nothing is known.

The aromatic raw materials profiled were selected because they are commercially available. We have no hard data for annual production, but if at least one supplier in the West is offering the material for sale on the open market, we have attempted to include it. However this has proved a daunting task, and no doubt there are omissions. A few profiles are included of essential oils that are not commercially available (such as plectranthus) because information about their toxicity sheds light on chemically similar, commercially available oils.

We have not attempted to restrict the materials covered in this section to those currently or most popularly used in aromatherapy, since there is no definitive list. Increasingly, practitioners, product formulators and private individuals seek out unusual aromatic materials.

Information given in the profiles

Common name: The essential oils are indexed under common name, not botanical name. This causes difficulties where there is no common name, or where common names are not widely known or used. However, it makes for ease of use by readers not familiar with botanical names, and more importantly, it facilitates the grouping of chemically and toxicologically similar essential oils, such as the various pennyroyal or sassafras oils, into one profile.

In some instances, such as cedarwood, chamomile, citronella, fir needle, lemongrass, lime and valerian, a different place of origin is consistent with a different species. For example, Mexican type lime, *Citrus x aurantifolia* Christm., and Persian type lime, *Citrus x latifolia* Tanaka. In such cases, the species was originally cultivated in that country or region, but is now also grown in other geographical locations. Therefore 'Mexican' lime may not come from Mexico.

Botanical name: We have tried to give preference to the most currently accepted botanical name and synonyms. When essential oils derive from more than one botanical source we have attempted to include all origins.

Family: Where there are alternative names for the same family, these are given in brackets.

Source: The part of the plant from which the essential oil, absolute or resinoid is distilled, expressed or solvent extracted.

Key constituents: Where they are known, constituents are listed in descending order of percentage down to the level of 1%, or lower for known toxic constituents such as carcinogens or phototoxins. We have not included most constituents occurring at less than 1% in the interests of space, and because these are likely to have little toxicological relevance. The percentages are given as ranges where possible and where appropriate. These ranges represent the types of essential oil commercially available. Occasionally we have given compositional data for oils of the same species but from different countries of origin, for example, ginger, patchouli and sweet orange. In these instances differences in composition are of little toxicological significance, but the data were included because they were readily available. In other cases, such as mace, nutmeg and tarragon, such differences are toxicologically significant.

In some instances, different chemotypes are described within a single profile (rosemary, wormwood) and in others, where the differences are more toxicologically significant, each chemotype has its own profile (basil, ho leaf, niaouli, thyme).

The abbreviation 'tr' denotes trace. Where isomeric compounds occur in an essential oil the quantities are often inversely proportional. For example, in *Thymus serpyllum* thymol/carvacrol CT, we find carvacrol 15.6–27.8% and thymol 16.7–25.9%. The highest likely amount of both compounds in a single oil is not 53.7% (27.8% + 25.9%), but 44.5% (e.g., 27.8% + 16.7%). In many cases, specific isomers of constituents were not reported, and unless stated, they are unspecified.

Hazards: Brief details are given here of why the substance may be hazardous. Note that 'hazard' denotes a potential for risk, not necessarily an actual risk.

Contraindications: When the oil should be avoided. The method of administration is also stated. Oral contraindications apply to the oral administration of essential oils as used in aromatic medicine. Oral contraindications do not apply to the use of essential oils in any other context, such as in foods, fragrances, personal care products or by inhalation.

Cautions: These are potential hazards that do not warrant contraindications, either because the evidence is flimsy or because the hazard is not especially worrying.

Maximum adult daily oral dose: Most of these values are extrapolated from our own safety guidelines. They are based on an average human weight of 70 kg (154 lb).

Maximum dermal use level: For many of the profiled oils a recommended maximum level for external use is given. This is often based on already established guidelines, and is intended to avoid skin reactions, carcinogenesis or other forms of toxicity. But, see EU allergens legislation and IFRA guidelines below. The maximum dermal use level is based on the maximum possible concentration in the essential oil of the toxic constituent(s). Therefore essential oils with lower concentrations of toxic constituents (in some cases zero) may require less restriction, or even no restriction.

Toxic constituents are assessed collectively, according to their action. So the effect of all known carcinogens is taken into account in a single essential oil, but this is not combined with the action of neurotoxins or allergens. In a few cases the maximum dermal use level depends on which type of toxic effect is considered, and in those cases we recommend the lowest concentration.

For carcinogens, we include a box showing the regulations that would be applied (a) in the EU, (b) by IFRA, and (c) our own recommendation, according to the maximum level of carcinogenic constituents shown in the profile. Note that

regulations change on a regular basis, and the ones shown may not be current. In the case of phototoxicity, maximum use levels can be exceeded if care is taken to avoid exposing the skin to UV rays for 12–18 hours after application. Note that, unless there is a separate guideline for pregnancy, maximum use levels include safety in pregnancy.

Our safety advice: The advice given in this section is from the authors of this book. Our own safety guidelines for specific constituents are often applied. We decided to do this because we felt strongly that regulatory guidelines are sometimes over- or under-precautionary. In addition to these specific guidelines, there are general ones that apply to children (Table 4.5).

Regulatory guidelines: This is discussed below, in a separate section.

Organ-specific effects: This section varies according to the information available. For example, if there is nothing on hepatotoxicity, then there is no section on hepatotoxicity.

Adverse skin reactions: For skin irritation in animals, the undiluted test materials are applied to the backs of hairless mice, to intact or abraded rabbit skin, or to other test animals. In humans irritation is tested by a 48-hour closed-patch test in 25–30 volunteers at the dilution given. Sensitization is tested by a maximation test, usually on 20–30 volunteers at the dilution given. Phototoxicity testing is generally carried out on pigs. In this particular test a strong correspondance has been established between the reaction of pig skin and human skin.

Systemic effects: As with organ-specific effects, the sub-sections included here vary according to the available information.

Acute toxicity: Details are given of the results of acute oral or dermal toxicity tests or, where relevant, of any known toxic constituents. In most cases more detail on the toxic constituents will be found in Constituent profiles, Chapter 14.

Carcinogenic/anticarcinogenic potential: Any positive or negative data are given here for genotoxicity and carcinogenicity.

Drug interactions: Much of the information included here is unique to this text. For space reasons, we could not list each drug involved, and some cross-referencing will need to be done with Appendix B.

Comments: Any further useful information or observations are given here.

In a few profiles, other headings such as hepatotoxicity, neurotoxicity and subacute toxicity are included.

Regulatory guidelines

Details are given here of safety guidelines from organizations concerned with safety.

GRAS

Some essential oils are flagged as having 'GRAS status'. GRAS is an acronym for 'generally recognized as safe.' It is an EPA list of substances considered safe to use in foods in the amounts normally used in food flavoring. Although these amounts are generally much lower than a therapeutic dose of essential oil, in some instances the GRAS listing fills a knowledge gap.

The list of GRAS essential oils, as of April 2011, may be found here: http://www.accessdata.fda.gov/scripts/cdrh/cfdocs/cfcfr/CFRSearch.cfm?fr=182.20 (accessed June 15th 2012) and an outline of the GRAS criteria can be found here: http://fda.gov/Food/GuidanceComplianceRegulatoryInformation/GuidanceDocuments/FoodIngredientsandPackaging/ucm061846.htm#Q3 (accessed June 15th 2012).

EU allergens legislation

This mandates a label declaration, and is not a legal restriction of the amount of an ingredient that is permitted. We do not believe that even the label declaration is justified in many cases, and we have not included this information in the essential oil profiles. A fuller explanation can be found in Chapter 5.

IFRA guidelines

We have not included many of the IFRA guidelines, or standards. This is partly because they are so complex: maximum use levels are divided into 11 product categories, and this level of detail is beyond the scope of this book. It is also because we do not agree with some of them. Where we have shown an IFRA standard, this is for category 4 body oils and lotions. A full explanation of our views on IFRA standards can be found in Chapter 5. The IFRA standards can be found at http://www.ifraorg.org.

Adjusting safe doses and concentrations

The amount applied

Our maximum dermal use levels are based on 30 mL, which we estimate to be the maximum amount of a single product application in one day. For local skin reactions (irritation, sensitization and phototoxicity) these maximum percentages should be adhered to, even if a smaller quantity of total product is used. Skin reactions depend on the concentration of toxic substance per square cm of skin, so even a small amount applied to a small area of skin can be problematic. For more general and systemic types of toxicity (carcinogenicity, hepatotoxicity, neurotoxicity, teratogenicity, drug interactions), when a smaller amount of product is applied topically, the maximum % can be increased proportionally, because toxicity is dependent on total dose, not dermal concentration. For example, the maximum dermal use level for Dalmatian sage oil is 0.4%. But if only 5 mL (approximately 5 g) of a product containing this oil is used, the maximum concentration could be increased to 2.4% (30/5 × 0.4). These calculations apply equally to leave-on and wash-off types of product. For infants and children, see (Ch. 4, p. 47).

Combinations of toxic essential oils

When essential oils are combined that contain the same toxic constituent, or different constituents that exhibit the same type of toxicity, this should be taken into account when considering maximum safe doses. This applies to skin irritants, allergens, phototoxins, neurotoxins, teratogens, carcinogens, hepatotoxins or drug interactors. In this book, we have assumed that such actions are additive. For example, lemongrass and lemon myrtle oils both contain citral, and both have limits of 0.7% for skin sensitization and teratogenicity. But if both essential oils were used

together, the limit would need to be 0.7% of the two oils combined. The same principle applies to oral dosing.

Phototoxic oils

If several phototoxic oils are used together, the risk is assumed to increase proportionally, as outlined above. For instance, bergamot and cumin oils both have maximum dermal use levels of 0.4%. If both are used in a product in equal proportions, the maximum safe percentage will be 0.2% for each, not 0.4% for each. Phototoxicity cautions apply to leave-on products and to steam inhalation, but they do not apply to wash-off products or to ambient inhalation. When using deterpenated (folded) citrus fruit oils, we recommend checking with the supplier for phototoxicity risk. Deterpenated citrus oils are generally produced from distilled oils, which possess zero or very low phototoxicity, but the process of deterpenation may increase the total percentage of phototoxic constituents.

Essential oils A–Z

African bluegrass

Synonyms: Giant turpentine grass, tambookie grass, tambuti
Botanical name: *Cymbopogon validus* Stapf.
Family: Poaceae (Gramineae)

Essential oil

Source: Leaves
Key constituents:

β-Myrcene	15.4–20.2%
(Z)-β-Ocimene	10.3–11.5%
Borneol	6.4–9.5%
Geraniol	1.7–3.2%
Germacrene D-4-ol	1.6–6.6%
Camphene	3.6–5.4%
γ-Terpinene	0.1–5.7%
α-Cadinol	1.9–4.2%
α-Pinene	3.0–3.9%
Bornyl acetate	2.8–3.1%
(E)-β-Ocimene	tr–2.8%
Elemicin	1.8–2.7%
Germacrene A	1.9–2.1%
β-Cadinol	1.1–1.9%
T-Muurolol	1.0–1.9%
Neral	0.1–1.4%
Linalool	1.3%
α-Caryophyllene	0.5–1.2%
Methyleugenol	0.2–0.3%

(Teubes, private communication, 2003)

Safety summary

Hazards: Potentially carcinogenic, based on methyleugenol content.

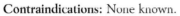

Contraindications: None known.
Maximum adult daily oral dose: 233 mg
Maximum dermal use level:

EU	0.07%
IFRA	0.13%
Tisserand & Young	6.7%

Our safety advice

Our oral and dermal restrictions are based on 0.3% methyleugenol content with dermal and oral limits of 0.02% and 0.01 mg/kg (see Methyleugenol profile, Chapter 14).

Regulatory guidelines

IFRA recommends that the maximum concentration of methyleugenol for leave-on products such as body lotion should be 0.0004% (IFRA 2009). The equivalent SCCNFP maximum is 0.0002% (European Commission 2002).

Organ-specific effects

Adverse skin reactions: No information found for African bluegrass oil, but judging from its composition the risk of skin reactions is likely to be low.
Reproductive toxicity: Oral β-myrcene was reproductively toxic in pregnant rats at 500 mg/kg, but not at 250 mg/kg (Delgado et al 1993a, 1993b; Paumgartten et al 1998). This does not suggest any dose limitation for African bluegrass oil.

Systemic effects

Acute toxicity: No information found
Carcinogenic/anticarcinogenic potential: No information found for African bluegrass oil. Methyleugenol is a rodent carcinogen if exposure is sufficiently high. Geraniol and α-caryophyllene display anticarcinogenic activity (see Constituent profiles, Chapter 14), and α-cadinol is active against the human colon cancer cell line HT-29 (He et al 1997a).

Comments

Limited availability.

Agarwood

Synonyms: Agar, aloes wood, eaglewood, lignum aloe, ood
Botanical name: *Aquilaria malaccensis* Lamk
Botanical synonyms: *Aquilaria agallocha* Roxb., *Agallochum malaccense* (Lamk) Kuntze, *Aquilariella malaccensis* (Lamk) v. Tieghem
Family: Thymelaeaceae

Essential oil

Source: Wood
Key constituents:

Vietnamese

2-(2-(4-Methoxyphenyl)ethyl) chromone	21.2–33.0%
2-(2-Phenylethyl) chromone	16.1–23.6%
Oxo-agarospirol	1.4–5.3%
Guaia-1(10),11-dien-15-oic acid	<4.7%
6-Methoxy-2-(4-methoxyphenyl)ethyl) chromone	2.0–3.7%
Guaia-1(10),11-dien-15-al	0.4–3.4%
Selina-3,11-dien-9-ol	0.4–2.8%
Selina-3,11-dien-9-one	0.2–2.1%

(Lawrence 1998e p. 62–66)

Safety summary

Hazards: None known.
Contraindications: None known.

Organ-specific effects

Neurotoxicity: Agarwood oil vapors are sedative to mice (Takemoto et al 2008).

Systemic effects

Acute toxicity: No information found.
Carcinogenic/anticarcinogenic potential: No information found, but agarwood oil contains no known carcinogens.

Comments

Agarwood essential oil is one of the most expensive aromatic raw materials, being 10–15 times the cost of jasmine absolute. The oil is extracted only from fungus-infected wood. Other analyses, showing quite different constituents, have been published by Näf et al (1995) for Indian agarwood oil, and by Bhuiyan et al (2009) for agarwood oil from Bangladesh. Agarwood oil may also derive from *Aquilaria sinensis* (Lour.) Gilg. *Aquilaria malaccensis* is classed by CITES under their Appendix II: 'species that are not necessarily now threatened with extinction but that may become so unless trade is closely controlled.' CO_2 extracts are also produced.

Ahibero

Botanical name: *Cymbopogon giganteus* (Hochst.) Chiov.
Family: Poaceae (Gramineae)

Essential oil

Source: Leaves
Key constituents:

(*E*)-*p*-Mentha-1(7),8-dien-2-ol	24.0–35.2%
(*Z*)-*p*-Mentha-1(7),8-dien-2-ol	16.0–24.0%
(*E*)-*p*-Mentha-2,8-dien-1-ol	13.3–16.2%
(+)-Limonene	0.5–13.2%
(*Z*)-*p*-Mentha-2,8-dien-1-ol	8.2–10.2%
p-Methylacetophenone	3.2–6.0%

Piperitenol	1.3–3.8%
(E)-Carveol	2.6–3.7%
Carvone*	0.1–2.9%
(Z)-Dihydrocarvone	0.2–2.0%
p-Mentha-1,3,8-triene	0.4–1.6%
Myrtenol	0.1–1.6%
(E)-Limonene oxide	0.7–1.2%
Cuminyl alcohol	tr–1.2%
1,8-Cineole	0.1–1.1%

(Sidibé et al 2001)

Safety summary

Hazards: None known.
Cautions: Unknown toxicity.

Organ-specific effects

Adverse skin reactions: No information found.

Systemic effects

Acute toxicity: No information found.
Carcinogenic potential: No information found. (+)-Limonene displays anticarcinogenic activity (see (+)-Limonene profile, Chapter 14).

Comments

The plant grows in many parts of Africa, and essential oil composition does not vary greatly. The composition above is for Mali.

Ajowan

Synonyms: Ajwain, bishop's weed, sprague
Botanical name: *Trachyspermum ammi* L.
Botanical synonyms: *Carum copticum* L., *Trachyspermum copticum* L.
Family: Apiaceae (Umbelliferae)

Essential oil

Source: Seeds
Key constituents:

Thymol	36.9–53.8%
γ-Terpinene	14.6–35.0%
p-Cymene	20.8–24.0%
Carvacrol	1.0–16.4%
(+)-Limonene	0.25–5.1%
β-Pinene	1.2–3.5%
α-Pinene	0.3–1.8%

(Lawrence 1981 p. 5, 1995g p. 143–144)

Safety summary

Hazards: Drug interaction; may inhibit blood clotting; skin irritation (low risk); mucous membrane irritation (moderate risk).

Cautions (oral): Anticoagulant medication, major surgery, peptic ulcer, hemophilia, other bleeding disorders (Box 7.1).
Maximum dermal use level: 1.4%

Our safety advice

Our dermal maximum is based on 70.2% total thymol and carvacrol content and a dermal limit of 1% for carvacrol and thymol to avoid skin irritation (see Carvacrol and Thymol profiles, Chapter 14).

Organ-specific effects

Adverse skin reactions: No information found for ajowan oil. In a 48 hour occlusive patch test on 50 volunteers, the highest concentration of thymol producing no adverse reaction was 5% (Meneghini et al 1971).
Cardiovascular effects: Thymol and carvacrol inhibit platelet aggregation (Enomoto et al 2001), an essential step in the blood clotting cascade.
Gastrointestinal toxicity: No information found for ajowan oil. Because of its thymol content, ajowan oil may possess some degree of mucous membrane irritancy.

Systemic effects

Acute toxicity: No information found
Carcinogenic/anticarcinogenic potential: No information found, but ajowan oil contains no known carcinogens. (+)-Limonene, carvacrol and thymol display antitumoral activity (see Constituent profiles, Chapter 14).
Drug interactions: Anticoagulant medication, because of cardiovascular effects, above. See Table 4.10B.

Comments

A type of ajowan oil devoid of thymol does exist, containing 46% carvone and 38% limonene. Ajowan oil is rarely found outside India, the Seychelles and the West Indies.

Almond (bitter, FFPA)

Botanical name: *Prunus dulcis* (Mill.) var. *amara*
Botanical synonyms: *Prunus communis* L. var. *amara*, *Prunus amygdalus* Batsch. var. *amara*, *Amydalus communis* L. var. *amara*, *Amygdalus dulcis* Mill. var. *amara*
Family: Rosaceae

Essential oil

Source: Kernels
Key constituents:

Benzaldehyde	~98%

Quality: Benzaldehyde may be used as an adulterant of, or a complete substitute for bitter almond oil (Burfield 2003). Benzaldehyde is susceptible to autoxidation.

*Isomer not specified

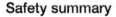

Safety summary

Hazards: None known.
Cautions: Old or oxidized oils should be avoided.
Maximum adult daily oral dose: 357 mg

Our safety advice

Our oral maximum of is based on 98% benzaldehyde and a benzaldehyde limit of 5 mg/kg/day. Oxidation of bitter almond oil should be avoided by storage in a dark, airtight container in a refrigerator. The addition of an antioxidant to preparations containing it is recommended.

Regulatory guidelines

Has GRAS status. A group ADI of 0–5 mg/kg body weight for benzoic acid, the benzoate salts (calcium, potassium and sodium), benzaldehyde, benzyl acetate, benzyl alcohol and benzyl benzoate, expressed as benzoic acid equivalents, was established by JECFA in 1996.

Organ-specific effects

Adverse skin reactions: Undiluted bitter almond oil FFPA produced hyperkeratosis and dry desquamation when applied to mice or pigs; tested at 4% on 25 volunteers, the oil was neither irritating nor sensitizing. It is non-phototoxic (Opdyke 1979a p. 707).

Systemic effects

Acute toxicity: Bitter almond oil FFPA acute oral LD_{50} in rats 1.49 mL/kg; acute dermal LD_{50} in rabbits >3 g/kg (Opdyke 1979a p. 707).
Carcinogenic/anticarcinogenic potential: No information was found for bitter almond oil FFPA, but it contains no known carcinogens. Benzaldehyde is anticarcinogenic in humans (see Benzaldehyde profile, Chapter 14).

Comments

FFPA denotes 'free from prussic acid'. Prussic acid, or hydrocyanic acid (HCN) is highly toxic, and is formed during the distillation of the essential oil. The HCN is removed by treatment with calcium hydroxide and ferrous sulfate in order to make the oil safe for human use. A maximum of 0.01% HCN is permitted (Annexes 1 & 2, EEC directive 88/388, http://whqlibdoc.who.int/publications/2012/9789241660655_eng.pdf). The benzaldehyde in bitter almond oil has a tendency to oxidize to benzoic acid (Budavari 1989).

Almond (bitter, unrectified)

Botanical name: *Prunus dulcis* (Mill.) var. *amara*
Botanical synonyms: *Prunus communis* L. var. *amara*, *Prunus amygdalus* Batsch. var. *amara*, *Amydalus communis* L. var. *amara*, *Amygdalus dulcis* Mill. var. *amara*
Family: Rosaceae

Essential oil

Source: Kernels
Key constituents:

Benzaldehyde	95%
Hydrocyanic acid	2.0–4.0%

(Budavari 1989 p. 6689)

Safety summary

Hazards: Toxicity.
Contraindications: Should not be used, either internally or externally.

Regulatory guidelines

Because of its hydrocyanic acid (HCN) content this essential oil is not commercially available.

Organ-specific effects

Adverse skin reactions: When patch tested at 25% on a panel of 25 volunteers, unrectified bitter almond oil was neither irritating nor sensitizing (Opdyke 1979a p. 705–706).

Systemic effects

Acute toxicity, human: There are many recorded cases of poisoning from the 19th century when unrectified bitter almond oil was widely available. A 'druggist', who ingested ~2 g of the oil, having mistaken it for another substance, survived. A colleague of his induced vomiting within 20 minutes, and observed delirium, difficulty breathing, feeble pulse, cold skin, and slight convulsions at different times during the episode (Chavasse 1939). An 8-year-old girl survived after ingesting a flavoring containing 1–2 drops of unrectified bitter almond oil. She appeared unconscious, and had no detectable pulse. Her jaw had to be forced open, and the two doctors present induced emesis, which smelled strongly of bitter almonds (Smith 1844).

A 57 year-old man ingested two drachms (3.5 g) of unrectified bitter almond oil, it was believed to be done intentionally, and was hospitalized shortly after. About 35 minutes later a stomach pump was administered, but 3 hours after the ingestion he died. On post-mortem, no abnormalities were seen in the liver, kidneys or abdominal viscera, but signs of toxicity were apparent in the heart, stomach and brain, the last two smelling of bitter almonds (Barclay 1866). In another fatal case, a 36-year-old female ingested at least two drachms of unrectified bitter almond oil, and died within 25 minutes. Post-mortem findings included an intense odor of bitter almonds in the stomach, lungs and chest cavity, black blood in the lungs, and almost no blood in the heart; the kidneys and spleen appeared normal, but the liver was slightly congested (Ellis 1863).

A feature of bitter almond oil poisoning is a lack of radial pulse and cold, clammy extremities. Survival was invariably linked to immediate medical intervention. HCN has an estimated adult human lethal dose of 50 mg, which equates to ~0.7 mg/kg (Reynolds 1993).

Acute toxicity, animal: Unrectified bitter almond oil acute oral LD$_{50}$ in rats 960 mg/kg, acute dermal LD$_{50}$ in rabbits 1,220 mg/kg (Opdyke 1979a p. 705–706).

Carcinogenic/anticarcinogenic potential: No information was found for unrectified bitter almond oil, but it contains no known carcinogens. Benzaldehyde is anticarcinogenic in humans (see Constituent profiles, Chapter 14).

Comments

The animal LD$_{50}$ results cited above seem remarkably high compared with known human toxicity (also cited above), and to animal toxicity for HCN (see Constituent profiles, Chapter 14). It also seems surprising that RIFM would carry out human skin sensitization tests using 25% unrectified bitter almond oil. Presumably the oil used in the tests reported by RIFM contained very little HCN.

HCN is not present in the nuts in their natural state. Prior to distillation, the nuts are comminuted and reduced to a press-cake. This is macerated in warm water for 12–24 hours, during which time the HCN is formed by the decomposition of amygdalin, a naturally occurring glycoside. It is interesting that HCN has a similar odor to benzaldehyde, even though the two compounds are chemically unrelated. This makes it impossible to tell the rectified from the unrectified oil by smell. Rectified bitter almond oil is referred to as bitter almond oil FFPA. It was introduced by some manufacturers as a safer option in the 1850s, but the use of the unrectified oil continued until 1890, and was even available over the counter. In the mid-19th century an estimated 8,000 lb of the unrectified oil was used annually as a food flavoring in Britain (Anon 1857).

Ambrette

Synonyms: Ambrette seed, musk seed
Botanical name: *Abelmoschus moschatus* Medik.
Botanical synonym: *Hibiscus abelmoschus* L.
Family: Malvaceae

Essential oil

Source: Seeds
Key constituents:

(E,E)-Farnesyl acetate	30.0–65.3%
(E,E)-Farnesol	3.4–39.0%
Ambrettolide	7.6–14.7%
(Z,E)-Farnesyl acetate	2.6–5.8%
Decyl acetate	0–5.6%
Dodecyl acetate	0.2–4.0%
(Z,E)-Farnesol	0.3–3.3%
(E)-Nerolidol	0.1–2.0%
(Z)-Tetradecen-14-olide	0–1.8%
Tetradecenyl acetate	0–1.6%
Hexadecanoic acid	0–1.4%
Decanol	tr–1.0%

(Lawrence 1993 p. 177–178, 1996d p. 58)
Quality: Prone to oxidation

Safety summary

Hazards: None known.
Contraindications: None known.

Our safety advice

Oxidation of ambrette oil should be avoided by storage in a dark, airtight container in a refrigerator. The addition of antioxidants is recommended.

Regulatory guidelines

Has GRAS status.

Organ-specific effects

Adverse skin reactions: Undiluted ambrette seed oil was not irritating either to rabbits or to mice; tested at 1% on 25 volunteers it was neither irritating nor sensitizing. It was non-phototoxic (Opdyke 1975 p. 705).

Systemic effects

Acute toxicity: Ambrette seed oil acute oral LD$_{50}$ in rats >5 g/kg; acute dermal LD$_{50}$ in rabbits >5 g/kg (Opdyke 1975 p. 705).
Carcinogenic/anticarcinogenic potential: Ambrette seed oil residues significantly induced glutathione *S*-transferase activity in mouse tissues (Lam & Zheng 1991). The essential oil contains no known carcinogens. Farnesol displays anticarcinogenic activity (see Farnesol profile, Chapter 14).

Comments

Ambrette absolutes and CO$_2$ extracts are also produced.

Amyris

Synonyms: West Indian sandalwood, balsam torchwood
Botanical name: *Amyris balsamifera* L.
Family: Rutaceae

Essential oil

Source: Wood
Key constituents:

Valerianol	15.1–21.5%
α-Eudesmol	4.4–16.2%
7-*epi*-α-Eudesmol	0–10.7%
10-*epi*-γ-Eudesmol	5.3–9.7%
Elemol	6.6–9.1%
β-Sesquiphellandrene	1.5–8.6%
γ-Eudesmol	6.6–8.0%
β-Eudesmol	3.2–7.9%
α-Zingiberene	0–5.2%
Amorpha-4,11-diene	0–3.5%
Drimenol	1.1–3.3%
ar-Curcumene	1.3–2.5%
Selina-3,7(11)-diene	1.3–2.5%
γ-Curcumene	0–2.3%

Cadina-4,11-diene	0–1.5%	β-Pinene	0.2–1.2%
β-Dihydroagarofuran	0.2–1.3%	α-Muurolene	0–1.2%
α-Agarofuran	0.3–1.2%	(Lawrence 1979 p. 17, 1989 p. 10)	
(E)-Nerolidol	0.4–1.1%		
α-Acoradiene	0–1.0%		

(Pappas, private communication, 2004; Tucker, private communication, 2003; Van Beek et al 1989)

Safety summary

Hazards: None known.
Contraindications: None known.

Organ-specific effects

No information found for amyris oil or any of its constituents.

Systemic effects

Acute toxicity: Amyris oil acute oral LD_{50} in rats 5.58 g/kg (Jenner et al 1964).
Carcinogenic/anticarcinogenic potential: No information found, but amyris oil contains no known carcinogens. γ-Eudesmol and β-sesquiphellandrene display anticarcinogenic properties (see Constituent profiles, Chapter 14).

Comments

Amyris balsamifera is listed as an endangered species by the state of Florida, USA. The essential oil is primarily produced in Haiti, with some production in the Dominican Republic, Jamaica and Venezuela.

Angelica root

Botanical name: *Angelica archangelica* L.
Family: Apiaceae (Umbelliferae)

Essential oil

Source: Roots
Key constituents:

β-Phellandrene	10.0–24.0%
α-Pinene	4.4–24.0%
α-Phellandrene	7.5–20.0%
(+)-Limonene	6.0–13.2%
δ-3-Carene	4.5–13.0%
p-Cymene	3.5–9.8%
β-Myrcene	1.6–5.5%
(E)-β-Ocimene	2.4–4.9%
Pentadecanolide	0.4–2.4%
Terpinolene	0.7–2.2%
(Z)-β-Ocimene	1.0–1.9%
α-Copaene	0–1.9%
Camphene	0.2–1.3%
Sabinene	0.4–1.2%

Non-volatile compounds

Angelicin	0.023%
Psoralen	0.0112%
Bergapten	0.0078%

(SCCP 2005b)
Quality: Angelica seed oil is less expensive than the root oil, and is a known adulterant of it.

Safety summary

Hazards: Phototoxicity.
Contraindications (dermal): If applied to the skin at over maximum use level, skin must not be exposed to sunlight or sunbed rays for 12 hours.
Maximum dermal use level: 0.8% to avoid phototoxicity.

Our safety advice

Because of its (+)-limonene, α-pinene and δ-3-carene content, we recommend that oxidation of angelica root oil is avoided by storage in a dark, airtight container in a refrigerator. The addition of an antioxidant to preparations containing it is recommended.

Regulatory guidelines

Has GRAS status. IFRA recommends that for application to areas of skin exposed to sunshine, angelica root oil be limited to a maximum of 0.8% in products applied to the skin except for bath preparations, soaps and other wash-off products (IFRA 2009).

Organ-specific effects

Adverse skin reactions: Undiluted angelica root oil was not irritating to rabbit or mouse skin; tested at 1% on 25 volunteers it was neither irritating nor sensitizing (Opdyke 1975 p. 713–714). In a modified Draize procedure on guinea pigs, angelica root oil was non-sensitizing when used at 1% in the challenge phase (Sharp 1978). In a study of 200 consecutive dermatitis patients, two (1%) were sensitive to 2% angelica root oil on patch testing (Rudzki et al 1976). Autoxidation products of (+)-limonene, α-pinene and δ-3-carene can cause skin sensitization (see Constituent profiles, Chapter 14). In phototoxicity tests, distinct positive results were obtained with concentrations of 100%, 50%, 25%, 12.5%, 6.25% and 3.125%. A doubtful reaction was obtained with 1.56%, and a negative result with 0.8% (Opdyke 1975 p. 713–714).

Systemic effects

Acute toxicity: Angelica root oil acute oral LD_{50} reported as 1.116 g/kg in rats and 2.2 g/kg in mice; acute dermal LD_{50} in rabbits >5 g/kg (Opdyke 1975 p. 713–714).
Subacute & subchronic toxicity: Angelica root oil was given orally to rats for eight weeks at 0.5, 1.0, 2.0 or 3.0 g/kg; the

NOAEL was 1.5 g/kg. At the higher two doses there was weight loss and decreased activity, and there were fatalities associated with severe liver and kidney damage (von Skramlik 1959). These are very high doses, and subacute toxicity for angelica root oil is not a concern.

Carcinogenic/anticarcinogenic potential: Angelica root oil significantly induced glutathione *S*-transferase activity in mouse tissues (Lam & Zheng 1991). (+)-Limonene displays anticarcinogenic activity (see (+)-Limonene profile, Chapter 14).

Comments

Angelica root oil contains a small proportion of non-volatile constituents, in spite of the fact that is it extracted by steam distillation. The reasons for this are explained on Ch. 2, p. 6.

Angelica root (Himalayan)

Synonym: Smooth angelica
Botanical name: *Angelica glauca* Edgew.
Family: Apiaceae (Umbelliferae)

Essential oil

Source: Roots
Key constituents:

(*Z*)-3-Butylidene phthalide	11.3–20.5%
(*Z*)-Ligustilide	5.2–20.4%
3-Methyl oct-2-ene	6.0–13.8%
(*E*)-Ligustilide	0.5–12.4%
Camphene	3.0–6.0%
β-Pinene	2.0–5.3%
β-Phellandrene	0.8–4.6%
β-Caryophyllene oxide	2.0–4.0%
Citronellyl acetate	2.2–3.4%
Citronellol	1.5–3.0%
γ-Terpinene	1.0–2.5%
(*E*)-3-Butylidene phthalide	0.4–2.3%
Spathulenol	0.2–2.0%
Sabinene	1.5–1.9%
ar-Curcumene	1.2–1.5%
(+)-Limonene	1.2–1.5%
p-Cymene	1.0–1.5%
Terpinen-4-ol	0.8–1.0%
α-Phellandrene	0.5–1.0%

(Thappa et al 2005)

Safety summary

Hazards: None known.
Contraindications: None known.

Organ-specific effects

Adverse skin reactions: No information found for Himalayan angelica root oil. Tested at 2% on the skin of 25 volunteers,

3-butylidene phthalide was neither irritant nor sensitizing (Opdyke & Letizia 1983 p. 659–660).

Systemic effects

Acute toxicity: No information found for Himalayan angelica root oil. The acute oral LD_{50} in rats for 3-butylidene phthalide has been reported as 1.85 g/kg and 2.42 g/kg (Opdyke & Letizia 1983 p. 659–660).

Carcinogenic/anticarcinogenic potential: No information found, but the oil contains no known carcinogens. 3-Butylidene phthalide and (*Z*)-ligustilide are cytotoxic to human colon cancer cells in vitro (Kan et al 2008).

Comments

There are several reports of neuroprotective effects for (*Z*)-ligustilide. Limited availability.

Angelica seed

Botanical name: *Angelica archangelica* L.
Family: Apiaceae (Umbelliferae)

Essential oil

Source: Seeds
Key constituents:

β-Phellandrene	35.4–72.1%
(+)-Limonene	2.3–38.7%
α-Pinene	8.8–9.2%
β-Caryophyllene	0.1–3.3%
β-Myrcene	1.5–2.9%
α-Phellandrene	2.7–2.8%
α-Caryophyllene	0.7–1.1%

(Formacek and Kubeczka 1982, Kubeczka 2002)
Quality: (+)-Limonene and β-phellandrene may polymerize when the oil is improperly stored (Kubeczka 2002).

Safety summary

Hazards: None known.
Cautions: Old or oxidized oils should be avoided.

Our safety advice

Because of the (+)-limonene content, oxidation of angelica seed oil should be avoided by storing the oil in a dark, airtight container in a refrigerator. The addition of an antioxidant to preparations containing it is recommended.

Regulatory guidelines

Has GRAS status. IFRA recommends that essential oils rich in limonene should only be used when the level of peroxides is kept to the lowest practical level, for instance by adding antioxidants at the time of production (IFRA 2009).

Organ-specific effects

Adverse skin reactions: Undiluted angelica seed oil was mildly irritating to rabbits, but not to mice or pigs; tested at 1% on 25 volunteers it was neither irritating nor sensitizing. It is non-phototoxic (Opdyke 1974 p. 821). Autoxidation products of (+)-limonene can cause skin sensitization (see (+)-Limonene profile, Chapter 14).

Systemic effects

Acute toxicity: Angelica seed oil acute oral LD_{50} in rats >5 g/kg; acute dermal LD_{50} in rabbits >5 g/kg (Opdyke 1974 p. 821).
Antioxidant/pro-oxidant activity: Angelica seed oil showed moderate antioxidant activity as a DPPH radical scavenger and in the aldehyde/carboxylic acid assay (Wei and Shibamoto 2007a).
Carcinogenic/anticarcinogenic potential: Two angelica seed oils, one with 0% β-phellandrene and 41.4% α-pinene, and the other with 55.2% β-phellandrene and 14.4% α-pinene, were cytotoxic to both human pancreas and mouse breast cancer cell lines (Sigurdsson et al 2005). (+)-Limonene displays anticarcinogenic activity (see Constituent profiles, Chapter 14).

Comments

Six psoralens have been found in the seeds of *Angelica archangelica*, at least three of which (bergapten, imperatorin and methoxsalen) are phototoxic (Müller et al 2004). However, none of these have been reported as constituents of the essential oil.

Anise

Synonym: Aniseed
Botanical name: *Pimpinella anisum* L.
Family: Apiaceae (Umbelliferae)

Essential oil

Source: Seeds
Key constituents:

(*E*)-Anethole	75.2–96.1% (87–94%)*
(+)-Limonene	tr–4.9%
Estragole	0.3–4.0% (0.5–5.0%)*
Anisyl alcohol	0–3.5%
γ-Himachalene	~2.2%
Anisaldehyde	0.6–2.0% (0.1–1.4%)*
ψ-Isoeugenyl 2-methylbutyrate	~1.4% (0.3–2.0%)*
(*Z*)-Anethole	tr–0.5% (0.1–0.4%)*

(Tabacchi et al 1974; Lawrence 1995g p. 199; Kubeczka 2002)
Quality: Prone to oxidation. May be adulterated with the cheaper star anise oil or technical grade anethole (Kubeczka 2002; Burfield 2003).

Safety summary

Hazards: Potentially carcinogenic, based on estragole content; reproductive hormone modulation; may inhibit blood clotting.

Contraindications (all routes): Pregnancy, breastfeeding, endometriosis, estrogen-dependent cancers, children under five years of age.
Cautions (oral): Diabetes medication. Diuretic medication, renal insufficiency, edematous disorders. Anticoagulant medication, major surgery, peptic ulcer, hemophilia, other bleeding disorders (Box 7.1).
Maximum adult daily oral dose: 70 mg
Maximum dermal use level:

EU	No limit
IFRA	0.2%
Tisserand & Young	2.4%

Our safety advice

We recommend a dermal maximum of 2.4% and a daily oral maximum of 70 mg for anise oil based on 5.0% estragole content and dermal and oral limits of 0.12% and 0.05 mg/kg (see Estragole profile, Chapter 14). We recommend that oxidation of anise oil is avoided by storage in a dark, airtight container in a refrigerator. The addition of an antioxidant to preparations containing it is recommended.

Regulatory guidelines

IFRA recommends a maximum dermal use level for estragole of 0.01% in leave-on or wash-off preparations for body and face (IFRA 2009). The EU does not restrict estragole.

Organ-specific effects

Adverse skin reactions: Anise oil produced no irritation when tested at 2% on 25 volunteers (Opdyke 1973 p. 865–866); one source states that anise oil is not a primary irritant to normal skin (Harry 1948). When tested at 2% it produced no sensitization reactions; several cases of sensitivity to anise oil have been reported, due to the (*E*)-anethole content (Opdyke 1973 p. 865–866). (*E*)-Anethole is prone to oxidation, and one or more of its oxidation products (anisaldehyde and anisic ketone) may be skin sensitizing (see (*E*)-Anethole profile, Chapter 14). In a clinical trial for head lice, a preparation containing unknown concentrations of ylang-ylang oil and anise oil was applied to the heads of 70 children aged 6–14 years, three times over 2 weeks. No clinically detectable adverse reactions were seen (Mumcuoglu et al 2002).
Cardiovascular effects: (*E*)-Anethole inhibits platelet aggregation (Yoshioka & Tamada 2005), an essential step in the blood clotting cascade. Anise oil significantly enhanced the absorption of glucose in rat jejunum (Kreydiyyeh et al 2003) and so may alter blood sugar levels in diabetes.
Urinary effect: When freshly distilled anise oil was added to the drinking water of rats at 0.05%, it exerted a significant antidiuretic effect but did not affect water intake. The oil increased the activity of renal Na^+/K^+ ATPase, an enzyme which increases the tubular reabsorption of sodium and therefore water retention, at concentrations as low as 0.025 nL/L, peaking at 250 nL/L (Kreydiyyeh et al 2003).

*European Pharmacopoeia Standards (5th edition)

Neurotoxicity: One case of seizures in a 12-day-old infant has been reported, with anise oil the presumed cause. The infant had been given 'multiple doses' of anise oil by the parents as a treatment for colic. After admission to hospital the infant recovered rapidly, and had no further seizures (Tuckler et al 2002).

Reproductive toxicity: Both anise oil and (E)-anethole have tested positive in one or more in vitro assays for estrogenic activity (Albert-Puleo 1980; Howes et al 2002; Melzig et al 2003). Sweet fennel tea (containing (E)-anethole) has shown in vivo estrogenic effects in humans (Türkyilmaz et al 2008).

Hepatotoxicity: No information found for anise oil. (E)-Anethole shows a dose-dependent hepatotoxicity that is due to a metabolite, anethole 1',2'-epoxide (AE) and different amounts of AE are produced in different species. However, the amounts of (E)-anethole-rich essential oils used in aromatherapy pose no risk to humans (see (E)-Anethole profile, Chapter 14). High doses of (E)-anethole or AE deplete glutathione (Marshall & Caldwell 1992, 1993) but sweet fennel oil, which has a very similar composition to anise, significantly induced glutathione S-transferase activity in mouse tissues (Lam & Zheng 1991).

Systemic effects

Acute toxicity: Anise oil acute oral LD_{50} in rats 2.25 g/kg; acute dermal LD_{50} in rabbits >5 g/kg (Opdyke 1973 p. 865–866).

Carcinogenic/anticarcinogenic potential: No information found for anise oil. (E)-Anethole is not a rodent carcinogen. Estragole is carcinogenic, depending on dose; both (+)-limonene and anisaldehyde display anticarcinogenic activity (see Constituent profiles, Chapter 14).

Drug interactions: Antidiabetic, anticoagulant or diuretic medication, because of urinary and cardiovascular effects, above. See Table 4.10B.

Comments

According to Davis (1999 p. 33) 'The essential oil of aniseed is seldom used, on account of its relatively high toxicity. In high doses, or taken over a long period of time, it is a narcotic which slows the circulation, damages the brain and is addictive.' These comments, none of which seem to have any foundation, are the apparent source of a belief among some aromatherapists that anise oil is highly toxic. A concern about estragole content would be understandable, but the same book gives no warning about basil oil, a richer source of estragole. Safrole has been reported in anise oil at 0.58%, but the purity of this oil was doubtful, and therefore the safrole could have been an adulterant (Lawrence 1989 p. 72–73).

Anise (star)

Botanical name: *Illicium verum* J.D. Hook.
Family: Illiciaceae

Essential oil

Source: Fruits
Key constituents:

(E)-Anethole	71.2–91.8%
Foeniculin	0.5–14.6%
Estragole	0.3–6.6%
(+)-Limonene	0.7–5.0%
Linalool	0.4–2.3%
α-Pinene	tr–2.1%
β-Caryophyllene	0.5–2.0%
Safrole	0–0.1%
(Z)-Anethole	tr–0.4%

(Lawrence 1995g p. 18, p. 199)

Quality: Prone to oxidation. Star anise oil is frequently adulterated with technical anethole, which can contain high concentrations of the relatively toxic (Z)-anethole (Kubeczka 2002).

Safety summary

Hazards: Potentially carcinogenic, based on estragole and safrole content; reproductive hormone modulation; may inhibit blood clotting.

Contraindications (all routes): Pregnancy, breastfeeding, endometriosis, estrogen-dependent cancers, children under five years of age.

Cautions (oral): Diabetes medication, anticoagulant medication, major surgery, peptic ulcer, hemophilia, other bleeding disorders (Box 7.1).

Cautions (dermal): Old or oxidized oils should be avoided.

Maximum adult daily oral dose: 53 mg

Maximum dermal use level:

EU	10%
IFRA	0.15%
Tisserand & Young	1.75%

Our safety advice

We recommend a dermal maximum of 1.75%, based on 6.6% estragole and 0.1% safrole content, and dermal limits of 0.12% for estragole and 0.05% for safrole. We recommend a daily oral maximum of 53 mg based on oral limits of 0.05 mg/kg for estragole and 0.025 mg/kg for safrole (see Constituent profiles, Chapter 14).

Regulatory guidelines

IFRA and the EU recommend a maximum exposure level of 0.01% of safrole from the use of safrole-containing essential oils in cosmetics. IFRA recommends a dermal maximum for estragole of 0.01% in leave-on or wash-off preparations for body and face (IFRA 2009). The EU does not restrict estragole.

Organ-specific effects

Adverse skin reactions: Undiluted star anise oil was not irritating to rabbit or mouse skin; tested at 4% on 25 volunteers it was neither irritating nor sensitizing (Opdyke 1975 p. 715–716). In skin sensitization tests on 100 dermatitis patients, 1.0% or 2.0% star anise oil elicited positive reactions in five test subjects, but none of the same group reacted to a 0.5% concentration (Rudzki & Grzywa 1976). Star anise oil is non-phototoxic (Opdyke 1975 p. 715–716). (E)-Anethole is prone to oxidation, and one or more of its oxidation products (anisaldehyde and anisic ketone) may be skin sensitizing (see (E)-Anethole profile, Chapter 14).

Cardiovascular effects: (*E*)-Anethole inhibits platelet aggregation (Yoshioka & Tamada 2005), an essential step in the blood clotting cascade. Anise oil (which is very similar to star anise oil in composition) significantly enhanced the absorption of glucose in rat jejunum (Kreydiyyeh et al 2003) and so may alter blood sugar levels in diabetes.

Neurotoxicity: There are a number of cases of neurotoxicity, many in infants, resulting from the ingestion of star anise tea. However, causation is due to sesquiterpene lactones not found in the essential oil. Neurotoxicity is often due to contamination of *I. verum* with other, more neurotoxic species.

Reproductive toxicity: (*E*)-Anethole is weakly estrogenic in in vitro yeast assays (Albert-Puleo 1980; Howes et al 2002) and sweet fennel tea (containing (*E*)-anethole) has shown in vivo estrogenic effects in humans (Türkyilmaz et al 2008).

Hepatotoxicity: (*E*)-Anethole shows a dose-dependent hepatotoxicity which is due to a metabolite, anethole 1',2'-epoxide (AE) and different amounts of AE are produced in different species. However, the amounts of (*E*)-anethole-rich essential oils used in aromatherapy pose no risk to humans (see (*E*)-Anethole profile, Chapter 14). High doses of (*E*)-anethole or AE deplete glutathione (Marshall & Caldwell 1992, 1993) but sweet fennel oil, which has a very similar composition to star anise oil, significantly induced glutathione *S*-transferase activity in mouse tissues (Lam & Zheng 1991).

Systemic effects

Acute toxicity: Star anise oil acute oral LD_{50} in rats 2.57 g/kg; acute dermal LD_{50} in rabbits >5 g/kg (Opdyke 1975 p. 715–716).

Carcinogenic/anticarcinogenic potential: No information found for star anise oil. Estragole and safrole are rodent carcinogens when oral exposure is sufficiently high. (*E*)-Anethole is not a rodent carcinogen, and (+)-limonene is anticarcinogenic (see Constituent profiles, Chapter 14).

Drug interactions: Antidiabetic or anticoagulant medication, because of cardiovascular effects, above. See Table 4.10B.

Comments

Caution is needed, because of the risks of adulteration and oxidation, in addition to the presence of carcinogens. The Commission E Monograph 'average daily dose' of star anise oil is 300 mg (Blumenthal et al 1998). We consider this an unsafe dose.

Araucaria

Botanical name: *Neocallitropsis pancheri* (Carrière) de Laub.
Botanical synonyms: *Callitropsis araucarioides* Compton, *Neocallitropsis araucarioides* (Compton) Florin
Family: Cupressaceae

Essential oil

Source: Wood
Key constituents:

β-Eudesmol	25.9%
γ-Eudesmol	19.0%
α-Eudesmol	13.3%
Guaiol	6.0%
Elemol	5.0%
β-Bisabolenol	4.9%
Bulnesol	3.7%
Carissone	2.4%
β-Acoradienol	2.0%
β-Bisabolene	1.4%
β-Selinene	1.4%
β-Bisabolenal	1.0%

(Raharivelomanana et al 1993)

Safety summary

Hazards: Drug interaction; may be fetotoxic (based on β-eudesmol content); may inhibit blood clotting.
Contraindications (all routes): Pregnancy and lactation.
Cautions (oral): Low blood pressure, anticoagulant medication, major surgery, peptic ulcer, hemophilia, other bleeding disorders (Box 7.1).

Organ-specific effects

Cardiovascular effects: β-Eudesmol inhibits platelet aggregation (Wang et al 2000), an essential step in the blood clotting cascade. Guaiol and β-eudesmol are hypotensive (Arora et al 1967).

Reproductive toxicity: Since β-eudesmol is antiangionenic (Tsuneki et al 2005), and in view of the probable link between antiangiogenic effects and reproductive toxicity (Chaiworapongsa et al 2010; Zhou et al 2013), we have contraindicated araucaria oil in pregnancy and lactation.

Systemic effects

Acute toxicity: No information found for araucaria oil. β-Eudesmol has an acute oral LD_{50} in mice of >2 g/kg (Chiou et al 1997).

Carcinogenic/anticarcinogenic potential: No information found, but araucaria oil contains no known carcinogens. γ-Eudesmol has anticarcinogenic, and β-eudesmol antiangiogenic activity (Hsieh et al 2001; Tsuneki et al 2005).

Drug interactions: Anticoagulant medication, because of cardiovascular effects, above. See Table 4.10B.

Comments

The tree is native to New Caledonia, and is on the IUCN (International Union for Conservation of Nature) list of threatened species. Limited availability.

Arina

Synonym: Iary
Botanical name: *Psiadia altissima* Benth. & J.D. Hook.
Family: Asteraceae (Compositae)

Essential oil

Source: Leaves
Key constituents:

β-Pinene	39.7%
(*E*)-β-Ocimene	7.0%

α-Caryophyllene	4.9%
Terpinen-4-ol	4.9%
(+)-Limonene	3.8%
δ-Cadinene	3.7%
β-Selinene	3.7%
α-Pinene	3.5%
Cyperene*	3.4%
1(10)-Aromadendrene	3.0%
β-Eudesmol	2.2%
β-Elemene	2.1%
α-Muurolene	1.6%
β-Myrcene	1.6%
δ-Cadinol	1.2%
Germacrene D	1.0%

(Ramanoelina et al 1994b)

Safety summary

Hazards: None known.
Contraindications: None known.

Organ-specific effects

Adverse skin reactions: No information found for arina oil, but β-pinene is not especially skin reactive (see β-Pinene profile, Chapter 14).

Systemic effects

Acute toxicity: No information found for arina oil. β-Pinene is non-toxic (Opdyke 1978 p. 859–861).
Carcinogenic/anticarcinogenic potential: No information found, but arina oil contains no known carcinogens. β-Pinene was not mutagenic in the Ames test (Florin et al 1980). α-Caryophyllene, (+)-limonene and β-elemene display anticarcinogenic activity (see Constituent profiles, Chapter 14).

Comments

Produced in Madagascar in limited quantities.

Artemisia vestita

Botanical name: *Artemisia vestita* Wallich
Family: Asteraceae (Compositae)

Essential oil

Source: Aerial parts
Key constituents:

β-Himachalene	10.1%
(E)-γ-Atlantone	6.8%
1,8-Cineole	5.3%
Himachalol	5.0%
Artemisia alcohol	4.5%
α-Himachalene	3.5%
Santolina alcohol	3.1%
allo-Himachalol	3.0%

Artemisyl acetate	3.0%
Santolinyl acetate	2.9%
γ-Himachalene	2.8%
Yomogi alcohol	2.6%
Caryophyllene	2.3%
α-Thujone	1.8%
Germacrene D	1.5%
(Z)-γ-Atlantone	1.5%
(Z)-Chrysanthenyl acetate	1.2%
Deodarone	1.1%
(E)-Thujanol	1.1%
β-Himachalene oxide	1.1%
Camphor	1.1%
β-Eudesmol	1.0%
β-Thujone	0.7%

(Lawrence 1989 p. 233)

Safety summary

Hazards: Slight neurotoxicity
Contraindications (all routes): Pregnancy, breastfeeding
Maximum adult daily oral dose: 280 mg
Maximum dermal use level: 10%

Our safety advice

Our oral and dermal restrictions are based on 2.5% total thujone content with dermal and oral thujone limits of 0.25% and 0.1 mg/kg (see Thujone profile, Chapter 14).

Organ-specific effects

Neurotoxicity: No information found. There is a risk of convulsions with moderately high doses of thujone. The thujone NOAEL for convulsions was reported to be 10 mg/kg in male rats and 5 mg/kg in females (Margaria 1963).

Systemic effects

Acute toxicity: No information found for the oil. Both α- and β-thujone are moderately toxic, with reported oral LD_{50} values ranging from 19–500 mg/kg for different species (see Thujone profile, Chapter 14). There is a risk of convulsions with moderately high doses of thujone.
Carcinogenic/anticarcinogenic potential: No information found, but *Artemisia vestita* oil contains no known carcinogens.

Comments

In the EU SCF report on thujone it was concluded that the available data were inadequate to establish a TDI/ADI (SCF 2003b). Limited availability, produced in India.

Asafoetida

Botanical name: *Ferula asa-foetida* L.
Family: Apiaceae (Umbelliferae)

Essential oil

Source: Gum resin
Key constituents:

1-(Methylthio)propyl (*E*)-1-propenyl disulfide	2.7–37.9%
2-Butyl (*E*)-1-propenyl disulfide	11.2–22.8%
1-(Methylthio)propyl (*Z*)-1-propenyl disulfide	2.6–18.5%
α-Pinene	tr–11.9%
2-Butyl (*Z*)-1-propenyl disulfide	0–11.1%
Isobutanol	0–7.7%
β-Pinene	0.2–7.1%
(*Z*)-β-Ocimene	0–6.1%
(*E*)-β-Ocimene	0–3.6%
Methyl (*E*)-1-propenyl trisulfide	0–2.6%
Dibutyl trisulfide	0.2–1.8%
Methyl (*E*)-1-propenyl disulfide	tr–1.7%
Methyl (*Z*)-1-propenyl trisulfide	0–1.3%
α-Fenchyl acetate	tr–1.2%
Dimethyl trisulfide	tr–1.1%

(Noleau et al 1991)

Safety summary

Hazards: Possible skin sensitizer.
Cautions: Its richness in sulfur compounds may imbue asafoetida oil with a degree of sensitization or irritancy.

Regulatory guidelines

Has GRAS status.

Organ-specific effects

Adverse skin reactions: No information found for asafoetida oil, but sulfur compounds have a tendency to cause skin reactions.

Systemic effects

Acute toxicity: No information found for asafoetida oil. Some sulfur compounds are moderately toxic.
Carcinogenic/anticarcinogenic potential: No information found but asafoetida oil contains no known carcinogens.

Comments

Other essential oils rich in sulfur compounds carry some risks, so caution in the use of asafoetida oil is recommended. See Garlic profile.

Atractylis

Synonym: Cang-zhu atractylodes
Botanical name: *Atractylodes lancea* (Thunb.) DC
Family: Asteraceae (Compositae)

Essential oil

Source: Roots
Key constituents:

β-Eudesmol	26.0%
β-Elemene	18.0%
Hinesol	10.0%
Elemol	6.0%
δ-Cadinene	2.0%
β-Caryophyllene	2.0%
β-Selinene	2.0%
Muurolenes	2.0%
Valencene	2.0%
α-Pinene	1.5%
Borneol	1.0%
Camphene	1.0%
δ-3-Carene	1.0%
p-Cymene	1.0%
β-Myrcene	1.0%
(*E*)-β-Ocimene	1.0%
(*Z*)-β-Ocimene	1.0%
α-Phellandrene	1.0%
β-Pinene	1.0%
Sabinene	1.0%
α-Terpinene	1.0%
Terpinolene	1.0%

(Bruns et al 1982)

Safety summary

Hazards: Drug interaction; may be fetotoxic (based on β-elemene and beta-eudesmol content); may inhibit blood clotting.
Contraindications (all routes): Pregnancy and lactation.
Cautions (oral): Anticoagulant medication, major surgery, peptic ulcer, hemophilia, other bleeding disorders (Box 7.1).

Organ-specific effects

Adverse skin reactions: No information found for atractylis oil, but there is nothing in its composition that would make it a likely cause of skin reactions.
Cardiovascular effects: β-Eudesmol inhibits platelet aggregation (Wang et al 2000), an essential step in the blood clotting cascade.
Reproductive toxicity: Since β-elemene and β-eudesmol are antiangionenic (Tsuneki et al 2005; Yan et al 2013), and in view of the probable link between antiangiogenic effects and reproductive toxicity (Chaiworapongsa et al 2010; Zhou et al 2013), we have contraindicated atractylis oil in pregnancy and lactation.

Systemic effects

Acute toxicity: No information found. Although the toxicity of some constituents is unknown, it seems unlikely that this oil would present any risk.

Carcinogenic/anticarcinogenic potential: No information found for atractylis oil, but β-elemene is antitumoral (see β-Elemene profile, Chapter 14) and β-eudesmol displays anti-angiogenic activity (Tsuneki et al 2005).
Drug interactions: Anticoagulant medication, because of cardiovascular effects, above. See Table 4.10B.

Comments

Limited availability.

Bakul

Synonyms: Bakula, vakul, vakula
Botanical name: *Mimusops elengi* L.
Family: Sapotaceae

Absolute

Source: Flowers
Key constituents:

2-Phenylethanol	38.8%
(*E*)-Cinnamyl alcohol	13.7%
3-Hydroxy-4-phenyl-2-butanone	4.7%
Methyl benzoate	3.8%
(*E*)-Methyl cinnamate	3.6%
Nerolidol	3.2%
2-Phenylethyl acetate	2.6%
Ethyl benzoate	2.4%
(*E*)-Ethyl cinnamate	1.9%
Methyl salicylate	1.9%
Benzyl alcohol	1.6%
4-Allyl-2,6-dimethoxyphenol	1.5%
Ethyl butanoate	1.4%
(*E*)-Cinnamaldehyde	1.3%
p-Methylanisole	1.3%
p-Methylguaiol	1.3%
o-Xylene*	1.3%
(*E*)-Cinnamyl acetate	1.2%
Benzyl benzoate	1.1%
1-Phenyl-2,3-butanedione	1.1%
2-Phenylethyl benzoate	1.1%

(Wong & Teng 1994)

Safety summary

Hazards: Skin sensitization (low risk).
Contraindications: None known.
Maximum dermal use level: 2.9% (see Regulatory Guidelines).

Regulatory guidelines

Cinnamyl alcohol should not be used such that the level in consumer products exceeds 0.4% for category five (women's facial creams, hand creams) and category four (body creams, oils, lotions) (IFRA 2009).

Organ-specific effects

Adverse skin reactions: No information found. Some skin sensitization is possible due to the cinnamaldehyde content.

Systemic effects

No information found.

Comments

The concentration of methyl salicylate is not sufficient to justify any restrictions. A restriction based on cinnamaldehyde content would be 3.8%. In addition to absolutes, CO_2 extracts are available, as is an attar produced by co-distillation with sandalwood. This is reputedly used as a stimulant, and *Mimusops elengi* flowers are used as a treament for diarrhea in Java (Wong & Teng 1994).

Balsamite

Synonyms: Costmary, alecost
Botanical name: *Chrysanthemum balsamita* L.
Botanical synonyms: *Balsamita major* Desf., *Pyrethrum majus* Desf.
Family: Asteraceae (Compositae)

Essential oil

Source: Aerial parts
Key constituents:

(−)-Carvone	51.5%
β-Cubebene	4.7%
(+)-Limonene	2.6%
α-Thujone	0.8%
β-Thujone	0.2%

(Bestmann et al 1984)

Safety summary

Hazards: May be slightly neurotoxic, based on thujone content skin sensitization (low risk).
Contraindications: None known.
Maximum adult daily oral dose: 700 mg
Maximum dermal use level: 2.3%

Our safety advice

We recommend a dermal maximum of 2.3%, based on 51.5% (−)-carvone content with a dermal limit of 1.2%, and a maximum oral dose of 700 mg, based on 1.0% total thujone content with an oral limit of 0.1 mg/kg. Our oral maximum for carvone isomers is 12.5 mg/kg, and so does not apply (see Carvone profile, Chapter 14).

*Environmental contaminant or artifact

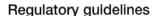

Regulatory guidelines

The IFRA standard for either isomer of carvone in leave-on products such as body lotions is 1.2% for skin sensitization. The Council of Europe (1992) has set an oral ADI of 1 mg/kg for carvone (isomer not specified). This is equivalent to a daily dose of 136 mg of balsamite oil for an adult, or approximately two drops.

Organ-specific effects

Adverse skin reactions: No information found.

Systemic effects

Carcinogenic/anticarcinogenic potential: No information found for balsamite oil. Carvone and (+)-limonene display anticarcinogenic activity (see Constituent profiles, Chapter 14).

Comments

Limited availability. There is also a camphor chemotype, which is not commercially available.

Balsam poplar

Synonyms: Hackmatack, tacamahac, black poplar
Botanical name: *Populus balsamifera* L.
Family: Salicaceae

Essential oil

Source: Flower buds
Key constituents:

α-Bisabolol	27.4%
δ-Cadinene	6.9%
(*E*)-Nerolidol	5.8%
γ-Curcumene	4.6%
α-Eudesmol	3.5%
δ-Amorphene	3.3%
γ-Muurolene	3.1%
γ-Eudesmol	2.4%
β-Curcumene	2.3%
(*E*)-α-Bergamotene	2.2%
Selina-3,7(11)-diene	2.2%
γ-Amorphene	1.9%
(*E*)-β-Farnesene	1.9%
ar-Curcumene	1.8%
1,8-Cineole	1.5%
epi-Cubenol	1.1%
epi-Zonarene	1.0%
α-Muurolene	1.0%

(Manguy, private communication)

Safety summary

Hazards: Drug interaction.
Cautions (all routes): Drugs metabolized by CYP2D6 (Appendix B).

Organ-specific effects

Adverse skin reactions: No information found.
Reproductive toxicity: Since α-bisabolol was not teratogenic in rats at 1 mL/kg (Habersang et al 1979), adverse effects in pregnancy for balsam poplar oil are unlikely.

Systemic effects

Acute toxicity: No information found.
Carcinogenic/anticarcinogenic potential: No information found for balsam poplar oil. α-Bisabolol and (*E*)-nerolidol demonstrate antitumoral activity (see Constituent profiles, Chapter 14).
Drug interactions: Since farnesene and α-bisabolol inhibit CYP2D6 (Table 4.11B), there is a theoretical risk of interaction between balsam poplar oil and drugs metabolized by this enzyme (see Appendix B).

Comments

The species epithet 'balsamifera', means 'balsam bearing' and derives from the sticky, resinous aromatic buds from which the essential oil is obtained. Also called Balm of Gilead in North America, though in Europe this traditionally refers to *Commiphora opobalsamum*.

Basil (estragole CT)

Botanical name: *Ocimum basilicum* L.
Family: Lamiaceae (Labiatae)

Essential oil

Source: Leaves
Key constituents:

Estragole	73.4–87.4%
Linalool	tr–8.6%
1,8-Cineole	0.6–6.0%
β-Caryophyllene	tr–4.0%
(+)-Limonene	0.1–3.0%
Methyleugenol	0–4.2%
(*E*)-β-Ocimene	0–2.2%
Terpinen-4-ol	0–2.2%
10-*epi*-α-Cadinol	0–1.3%
Eugenol	tr–1.2%
Bornyl acetate	0–1.1%
Camphor	tr–1.0%

(Lawrence 1993 p. 70–74, 1995 g p. 201, 1998f p. 35–48)
Quality: May be adulterated with added estragole.

Safety summary

Hazards: Potentially carcinogenic, based on estragole and methyleugenol content; may inhibit blood clotting.
Contraindications: Should not be taken in oral doses.
Maximum dermal use level:

EU	0.005%
IFRA	0.005%
Tisserand & Young	0.1%

Our safety advice

We recommend a dermal maximum of 0.1% based on 87.4% estragole and 4.2% methyleugenol content, and dermal limits of 0.12% for estragole and 0.02% for methyleugenol (see Constituent profiles, Chapter 14).

Regulatory guidelines

The Commission E Monograph for basil oil includes the following: 'Due to the high estragole content, basil oil preparations should not be used during pregnancy, nursing, by infants and small children, or over extended periods of time' (Blumenthal et al 1998). IFRA recommends a maximum dermal use level for estragole of 0.01% in leave-on or wash-off preparations for body and face (IFRA 2009). IFRA also recommends a maximum concentration of 0.0004% of methyleugenol for leave-on products such as body lotion (IFRA 2009). The equivalent SCCNFP maximum for methyleugenol is 0.0002% (European Commission 2002).

Organ-specific effects

Adverse skin reactions: Undiluted basil oil (estragole CT) was mildly irritating to mice; tested at 4% on 25 volunteers it was neither irritating nor sensitizing. It is non-phototoxic (Opdyke 1973 p. 867–868). A 65-year-old aromatherapist with multiple essential oil sensitivities reacted to both 1% and 5% basil oil (Selvaag et al 1995).
Cardiovascular effects: Estragole inhibits platelet aggregation (Yoshioka & Tamada 2005), an essential step in the blood clotting cascade.

Systemic effects

Acute toxicity: Basil oil (estragole CT) acute oral LD$_{50}$ in rats 1.4 mL/kg; acute dermal LD$_{50}$ in rabbits >5 mL/kg (Opdyke 1973 p. 867–868).
Carcinogenic/anticarcinogenic potential: A basil oil consisting of 88.2% estragole showed a very similar degree of genotoxicity to estragole in a rat liver DNA repair test (Müller et al 1994). Basil oil (estragole CT) showed moderate chemopreventive activity against human mouth epidermal carcinoma (KB) cells and significant activity against mouse leukemia (P388) cells, with respective IC$_{50}$ values of 303 and 36 µg/mL (Manosroi et al 2005). Estragole and methyleugenol are rodent carcinogens when oral exposure is sufficiently high (see Constituent profiles, Chapter 14).

Comments

The Müller et al (1994) data show that the other constituents of basil oil (estragole CT) have no effect on the genotoxicity of the estragole in the oil.

Basil (hairy)

Synonym: Hoary basil
Botanical name: *Ocimum americanum* L. var. *pilosum* (Willd.) A.J. Paton

Botanical synonym: *Ocimum canum* Sims
Family: Lamiaceae (Labiatae)

Essential oil

Source: Leaves
Key constituents:

Linalool	31.7–50.1%
Terpinen-4-ol	7.5–26.8%
β-Caryophyllene	4.3–10.0%
(E)-α-Bergamotene	3.5–7.6%
Sabinene hydrate	2.2–6.1%
γ-Terpinene	0.6–4.8%
Germacrene D	0.4–2.1%
(+)-Limonene	0.5–2.0%
Estragole	0.3–0.4%

(Yayi et al 2001)

Safety summary

Hazards: Contains estragole.
Contraindications: None known.
Maximum dermal use level:

EU	No limit
IFRA	2.5%
Tisserand & Young	30%

Our safety advice

We recommend a dermal maximum of 30%, based on 0.4% estragole content with a dermal limit of 0.12% (see Estragole profile, Chapter 14).

Regulatory guidelines

IFRA recommends a dermal maximum for estragole of 0.01% in leave-on or wash-off preparations for body and face (IFRA 2009). According to IFRA, essential oils rich in linalool should only be used when the level of peroxides is kept to the lowest practical value. The addition of antioxidants such as 0.1% BHT or α-tocopherol at the time of production is recommended (IFRA 2009).

Organ-specific effects

Adverse skin reactions: No information found. Oxidation products of linalool may be skin sensitizing.

Systemic effects

Acute toxicity: No information found.
Carcinogenic/anticarcinogenic potential: Hairy basil oil showed significant chemopreventive activity against human mouth epidermal carcinoma (KB) and mouse leukemia (P388) cell lines, with respective IC$_{50}$ values of 65 and 52 µg/mL. The oil was more effective than three of the four positive control drugs (Manosroi et al 2005). Estragole is a rodent hepatocarcinogen when oral exposure is sufficiently high;

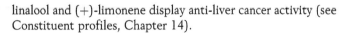
linalool and (+)-limonene display anti-liver cancer activity (see Constituent profiles, Chapter 14).

Comments

It is likely that any potentially carcinogenic action of estragole would be counteracted by other constituents of hairy basil oil. Concentrations of linalool and terpinen-4-ol are approximately inversely proportional in the oil, and the combination of these as major constituents is unusual.

Basil (holy)

Synonyms: Sacred basil, tulsi
Botanical name: *Ocimum tenuiflorum* L.
Botanical synonym: *Ocimum sanctum* L.
Family: Lamiaceae (Labiatae)

Essential oil

Source: Leaves
Key constituents:

Eugenol	31.9–50.4%
1,8-Cineole	12.6–16.5%
Estragole	9.7–12.9%
β-Bisabolene	9.7–10.5%
(Z)-α-Bisabolene	6.5–6.8%
(E)-β-Ocimene	3.4–6.2%
Chavicol	0.7–2.0%
β-Caryophyllene	1.3–1.5%
Camphene	0.9–1.5%
α-Caryophyllene	0.4–1.5%
β-Pinene	1.2–1.3%
Germacrene D	0.8–1.2%
(E)-α-Bergamotene	0.9–1.1%
Methyleugenol	0.2–0.3%

(Lawrence 1993 p. 200–201)

Safety summary

Hazards: May contain methyleugenol; drug interaction; may inhibit blood clotting; skin sensitization (moderate risk); mucous membrane irritation (low risk).
Cautions (oral): May interact with pethidine, MAOIs or SSRIs. Anticoagulant medication, major surgery, peptic ulcer, hemophilia, other bleeding disorders (Box 7.1).
Maximum dermal use level:

EU	0.07%
IFRA	0.05%
Tisserand & Young	1.0%

Our safety advice

We recommend a maximum dermal use level of 1.0%, based on 50.4% eugenol content with a dermal limit of 0.5% (see Eugenol profile, Chapter 14).

Regulatory guidelines

IFRA recommends a maximum dermal use level for eugenol of 0.5% for most product types, in order to avoid skin sensitization (IFRA 2009). IFRA recommends a dermal maximum for estragole of 0.01% in leave-on or wash-off preparations for body and face (IFRA 2009). IFRA recommends a methyleugenol maximum of 0.0004% for leave-on products such as body lotion (IFRA 2009). The equivalent SCCNFP maximum is 0.0002% (European Commission 2002).

Organ-specific effects

Adverse skin reactions: No information found. Eugenol is a potential cause of skin sensitization in dermatitis patients.
Cardiovascular effects: Eugenol and estragole inhibit platelet aggregation, an essential step in the blood clotting cascade (see Constituent profiles, Chapter 14).

Systemic effects

Acute toxicity: No information found.
Antioxidant/pro-oxidant activity: A holy basil oil with 59.4% eugenol and no estragole was a potent DPPH radical scavenger (IC$_{50}$ 0.26 μL/mL); this could not be correlated with phenol content (Salles Trevisan et al 2006).
Carcinogenic/anticarcinogenic potential: Holy basil oil increased glutathione *S*-transferase activity in the stomach, liver and esophagus of mice by more than 78%, and significantly inhibited B[*a*]P-induced squamous cell stomach carcinoma (Aruna & Sivaramakrishnan 1996). Holy basil oil showed significant chemopreventive activity against human mouth epidermal carcinoma (KB) and mouse leukemia (P388) cell lines, with respective IC$_{50}$ values of 95 and 85 μg/mL. The oil was more effective than three of the four positive control drugs (Manosroi et al 2005). Eugenol powerfully induces glutathione *S*-transferase in mice and displays antitumoral activity. Estragole and methyleugenol are rodent carcinogens when oral exposure is sufficiently high (see Constituent profiles, Chapter 14).
Drug interactions: Anticoagulant medication, because of cardiovascular effects, above. Since eugenol significantly inhibits human MAO (monoamine oxidase)-A (Tao et al 2005), oral doses of eugenol-rich essential oils may interact with pethidine, indirect sympathomimetics, MAOIs or SSRIs (Table 4.10B).

Comments

Although holy basil oil contains two carcinogens, it demonstrates significant anticarcinogenic and antioxidant activity, and therefore no maximum use levels are required, in our opinion, in regard to carcinogenesis. (Purely on the basis of its estragole and methyleugenol content, our dermal maximum would be 0.7%.) The potentially carcinogenic action of estragole and methyleugenol is presumably counteracted by other constituents of holy basil oil, such as eugenol. There are other chemotypes of holy basil oil, notably a methyleugenol one, but at the time of writing only the eugenol chemotype is commercially available. According to Kothari et al (2005a) an *Ocimum tenuiflorum* CT with >70% methyleugenol 'is being released for commercial cultivation.'

Basil (lemon)

Botanical name: *Ocimum* x *citriodorum* Vis.
Family: Lamiaceae (Labiatae)

Essential oil

Source: Leaves
Key constituents:

Geranial	23.3–25.1%
Neral	16.0–17.1%
Nerol	13.0–15.3%
Linalool	5.0–7.8%
(*E*)-α-Bisabolene	5.3–6.2%
Geraniol	4.3–4.7%
(*E*)-β-Caryophyllene	3.8–4.5%
Menthol	3.8–4.4%
Borneol	1.7–2.7%
Germacrene D	2.4–2.6%
Isopulegol + 2-undecanone	2.2–2.3%
(*E*)-α-Bergamotene	1.5–2.0%
Methyl heptenone	1.0–1.9%

(Fakhry, private communication, 2002)

Safety summary

Hazards: Drug interaction; teratogenicity; skin sensitization (low risk).
Cautions (oral): Diabetes medication, drugs metabolized by CYP2B6 (Appendix B), pregnancy.
Cautions (dermal): Hypersensitive, diseased or damaged skin, children under 2 years of age.
Maximum daily oral dose in pregnancy: 99 mg
Maximum dermal use level: 1.4%

Our safety advice

We recommend a dermal maximum of 1.4% to avoid skin sensitization, and a daily oral maximum in pregnancy of 99 mg. These are based on 42.2% citral content, with dermal and oral citral limits of 0.6% and 0.6 mg/kg (see Citral profile, Chapter 14).

Regulatory guidelines

IFRA recommends a maximum dermal use level for citral of 0.6% for body oils and lotions, in order to avoid skin sensitization (IFRA 2009).

Organ-specific effects

Adverse skin reactions: No information was found for lemon basil oil, but it may present some risk of sensitization due to the high citral (geranial + neral) content. Citral can induce sensitization reactions on patch testing at concentrations above 0.5% (see Constituent profiles, Chapter 14).
Cardiovascular effects: Gavage doses of 10, 15 or 20 mg/kg/day citral for 28 days, dose-dependently lowered plasma insulin

levels and increased glucose tolerance in obese rats (Modak & Mukhopadhaya 2011).
Reproductive toxicity: Citral is dose-dependently teratogenic because it inhibits retinoic acid synthesis, and this can affect fetal development (see Citral profile, Chapter 14).

Systemic effects

Acute toxicity: No information was found for lemon basil oil, but no significant acute toxicity is suspected.
Carcinogenic/anticarcinogenic potential: No information found. Citral and geraniol display anticarcinogenic activity (see Constituent profiles, Chapter 14).
Drug interactions: Antidiabetic medication, because of cardiovascular effects, above. Since citral and geraniol inhibit CYP2B6 (Table 4.11B), there is a theoretical risk of interaction between lemon basil oil and drugs metabolized by this enzyme (Appendix B).

Comments

Limited availability.

Basil (linalool CT)

Botanical name: *Ocimum basilicum* L.
Family: Lamiaceae (Labiatae)

Absolute

Source: Leaves
Key constituents:

Linalool	34.4%
Eugenol	33.7%
Linoleic & linolenic acids	9.7%
1,8-Cineole	3.1%
T-Cadinol	1.9%
Palmitic acid	1.6%
(*E*)-α-Bergamotene	1.4%
Germacrene D	1.2%
Estragole	1.0%

(Fakhry, private communication, 2002)

Safety summary

Hazards: Skin sensitization (low risk)
Contraindications: None known
Maximum dermal use level (based on estragole content):

EU	No limit
IFRA	1.0%
Tisserand & Young	No limit

Maximum dermal use level (based on eugenol content):

EU	No legal limit
IFRA	1.5%
Tisserand & Young	1.5%

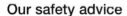

Our safety advice

We recommend a dermal maximum of 1.5% based on 33.7% eugenol and a dermal limit of 0.5%. As with the essential oil (see below) no restrictions are required, in our opinion, with regard to carcinogenesis.

Regulatory guidelines

IFRA recommends a maximum dermal use level for eugenol of 0.5% for most product types, in order to avoid skin sensitization (IFRA 2009). IFRA recommends a maximum dermal use level for estragole of 0.01% in leave-on or wash-off preparations for body and face (IFRA 2009). According to IFRA, essential oils rich in linalool should only be used when the level of peroxides is kept to the lowest practical value. The addition of antioxidants such as 0.1% BHT or α-tocopherol at the time of production is recommended (IFRA 2009).

Organ-specific effects

Adverse skin reactions: No information found. Oxidation products of linalool may be skin sensitizing, but eugenol is strongly antioxidant.

Systemic effects

Acute toxicity: No information was found for basil absolute (linalool CT) but toxicity data are known for the majority of the constituents and acute toxicity is not likely to be an issue.
Carcinogenic/anticarcinogenic potential: No information found. Estragole is a rodent carcinogen when oral exposure is sufficiently high; anticarcinogenic activity has been reported for eugenol (see Eugenol profile, Chapter 14).

Comments

No methyleugenol was detected at a level of 0.01%.

Essential oil

Source: Leaves
Key constituents:

Linalool	53.7–58.3%
Eugenol	9.4–15.2%
1,8-Cineole	6.0–6.7%
(E)-α-Bergamotene	2.0–3.8%
Germacrene D	2.0–3.0%
T-Cadinol	2.6–3.0%
Estragole	0.2–2.0%
α-Bulnesene	1.3–1.8%
β-Elemene	0.9–1.5%
δ-Cadinene	0.9–1.4%
(E)-β-Ocimene	1.0–1.3%
Bornyl acetate	0.8–1.2%
Methyleugenol	tr–0.1%

(Fakhry, private communication, 2002)
Quality: May be adulterated with added linalool.

Safety summary

Hazards: May contain estragole and methyleugenol; skin sensitization (low risk)
Contraindications: None known
Maximum dermal use level (based on carcinogen content):

EU	0.2%
IFRA	0.2%
Tisserand & Young	No limit

Maximum dermal use level (based on eugenol content):

EU	No legal limit
IFRA	3.3%
Tisserand & Young	3.3%

Our safety advice

We recommend a dermal maximum of 3.3%, based on 15.2% eugenol content with a dermal limit of 0.5% (see Eugenol profile, Chapter 14). Since this essential oil is antimutagenic, non-genotoxic, antioxidant and induces glutathione, it is likely that constituents such as linalool and eugenol counteract the potentially carcinogenic action of estragole and methyleugenol. Therefore, no restrictions are required, in our opinion, with regard to carcinogenesis.

Regulatory guidelines

IFRA recommends a maximum dermal use level for eugenol of 0.5% for most product types, in order to avoid skin sensitization (IFRA 2009). According to IFRA, essential oils rich in linalool should only be used when the level of peroxides is kept to the lowest practical value. The addition of antioxidants such as 0.1% BHT or α-tocopherol at the time of production is recommended (IFRA 2009). IFRA recommends a dermal maximum for estragole of 0.01% in leave-on or wash-off preparations for body and face (IFRA 2009). IFRA recommends that the maximum concentration of methyleugenol for leave-on products such as body lotion should be 0.0004% (IFRA 2009). The equivalent SCCNFP maximum is 0.0002% (European Commission 2002).

Organ-specific effects

Adverse skin reactions: In a mouse local lymph node assay, unoxidized basil oil linalool CT was a moderate skin sensitizer (Lalko & Api 2006). The dermal toxicity of linalool, eugenol and 1,8-cineole has been well studied, and eugenol is a potential cause of skin sensitization in dermatitis patients. Oxidation products of linalool may be skin sensitizing, but eugenol and 1,8-cineole are antioxidants.

Systemic effects

Acute toxicity: No information found.
Antioxidant/pro-oxidant activity: Basil oil linalool CT displayed potent DPPH radical scavenging activity, with an IC_{50} of 0.26 μL/mL (Tomaino et al 2005).
Carcinogenic/anticarcinogenic potential: A basil oil containing 69.2% linalool, 2.4% estragole, 1.9% geraniol, 1.4% eugenol and

no methyleugenol was antimutagenic in *S. typhimurium* strains TA98, TA100 and TA102. This was attributed to the antioxidant action of the essential oil, notably the linalool content (Berić et al 2007). Neither of two linalool CT basil oils was genotoxic in *Saccharomyces cerevisiae*. The oils contained linalool 46.0%, 50.0%, estragole 8.1%, 16.5%, methyleugenol 1.6%, 0.5%, and eugenol 2.5%, 2.5% (Tateo et al 1989). This is significant, since methyleugenol is genotoxic in *S. cerevisiae* (Schiestl et al 1989).

Basil oil (linalool CT) induced glutathione *S*-transferase activity to more than 2.5 times control level in mouse tissues (Lam & Zheng 1991). Eugenol powerfully induces glutathione *S*-transferase in mice and demonstrates anticarcinogenic activity. Estragole and methyleugenol are rodent carcinogens when oral exposure is sufficiently high (see Constituent profiles, Chapter 14).

Comments

Due to the absence of any human data, basil oil linalool CT has been classed here as a weak skin sensitizer, rather than a moderate one.

Basil (Madagascan)

Synonyms: Romba, ramy
Botanical name: *Ocimum gratissimum* L.
Botanical synonym: *Ocimum viride* Willd.
Family: Lamiaceae (Labiatae)

Essential oil

Source: Leaves
Key constituents:

Estragole	45.0–50.0%
Camphor	24.0–30.0%
(+)-Limonene	2.0–6.0%
β-Caryophyllene	1.0–4.0%
α-Caryophyllene	1.0–4.0%
Camphene	1.0–3.0%
(*E*)-β-Ocimene	0.5–3.0%
α-Pinene	tr–1.0%
1,8-Cineole	tr–1.0%

(Behra, private communication, 2003)

Safety summary

Hazards: Potentially carcinogenic; may inhibit blood clotting.
Contraindications: Should not be taken in oral doses.
Maximum dermal use level:

EU	No limit
IFRA	0.02%
Tisserand & Young	0.2%

Our safety advice

We recommend a dermal maximum of 0.2% based on 50.0% estragole content with a dermal limit of 0.12% (see Estragole profile, Chapter 14).

Regulatory guidelines

IFRA recommends a maximum dermal use level for estragole of 0.01% in leave-on or wash-off preparations for body and face (IFRA 2009). The EU does not restrict estragole.

Organ-specific effects

Cardiovascular effects: Estragole inhibits platelet aggregation (Yoshioka & Tamada 2005), an essential step in the blood clotting cascade.

Systemic effects

Acute toxicity: No information found. Camphor is potentially neurotoxic (see Camphor profile, Chapter 14).
Carcinogenic/anticarcinogenic potential: No information found. Estragole is a rodent hepatocarcinogen when exposure is sufficiently high; both (+)-limonene and α-caryophyllene display anticarcinogenic activity (see Constituent profiles, Chapter 14).

Comments

This chemotype of *Ocimum gratissimum* oil is produced in Madagascar. The eugenol chemotype is pungent basil (see below)

Basil (methyl cinnamate CT)

Synonym: Cinnamon basil
Botanical name: *Ocimum basilicum* L.
Family: Lamiaceae (Labiatae)

Essential oil

Source: Leaves
Key constituents:

Methyl cinnamate	58.0–63.1%
Linalool	17.3–27.3%
α-Cadinol	2.4–2.9%
δ-Cadinene	tr–2.4%
1,8-Cineole	0.4–1.8%
γ-Cadinene	1.2–1.6%
Zingiberene	1.1–1.3%
Estragole	tr–0.8%

(Telci et al 2006)

Safety summary

Hazards: May contain estragole.
Contraindications: None known.
Maximum dermal use level:

EU	No limit
IFRA	1.25%
Tisserand & Young	15%

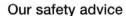

Our safety advice

We recommend a dermal maximum of 15% based on 0.8% estragole content and an estragole limit of 0.12% (see Estragole profile, Chapter 14).

Regulatory guidelines

IFRA recommends a maximum dermal use level for estragole of 0.01% in leave-on or wash-off preparations for body and face (IFRA 2009). The EU does not restrict estragole.

Organ-specific effects

Adverse skin reactions: No information found.

Systemic effects

Acute toxicity: No information found.
Carcinogenic/anticarcinogenic potential: No information found. Neither linalool nor methyl cinnamate is genotoxic. Estragole is a rodent carcinogen when exposure is sufficiently high.

Comments

Basil oils rich in methyl cinnamate are occasionally produced. Methyl cinnamate chemotypes also exist for *O. canum* and *O. minimum* (Viña & Murillo 2003).

Basil (pungent)

Synonyms: Shrubby basil, tree basil, Russian basil, East Indian basil, clocimum
Botanical name: *Ocimum gratissimum* L.
Botanical synonym: *Ocimum viride* Willd.
Family: Lamiaceae (Labiatae)

Essential oil

Source: Leaves
Key constituents:

Eugenol	62.9%
(*E*)-β-Ocimene	20.6%
Isoeugenol	2.4%
β-Caryophyllene	1.3%
Methyleugenol	0.4%
Estragole	0.2%

(Kothari et al 2005b)

Safety summary

Hazards: Drug interaction; may inhibit blood clotting; potentially carcinogenic, based on estragole and methyleugenol content; skin and mucous membrane irritant/sensitizer (low–moderate risk).
Cautions (oral): May interact with pethidine, MAOIs or SSRIs. Anticoagulant medication, major surgery, peptic ulcer, hemophilia, other bleeding disorders (Box 7.1), low blood pressure.
Maximum adult daily oral dose: 159 mg

Maximum dermal use level (based on methyleugenol content):

EU	0.05%
IFRA	0.1%
Tisserand & Young	4.6%

Maximum dermal use level (based on eugenol content):

EU	No legal limit
IFRA	0.8%
Tisserand & Young	0.8%

Our safety advice

We recommend a maximum adult daily oral dose of 159 mg, based on 0.4% methyleugenol and 0.2% estragole, with respective oral limits of 0.01 mg/kg/day and 0.05 mg/kg/day. We recommend a dermal limit of 0.8% based on 62.9% eugenol content, and a limit of 0.5% (see Eugenol profile, Chapter 14).

Regulatory guidelines

IFRA recommends a dermal maximum for eugenol of 0.5% for most product types, to avoid skin sensitization (IFRA 2009). Isoeugenol should not be used such that the level in finished products exceeds 0.02% (IFRA 2009, SCCNFP 2001a). IFRA has a dermal maximum of 0.01% for estragole and 0.0004% for methyleugenol (IFRA 2009). The SCCNFP dermal limit for methyleugenol in leave-on products is 0.0002% (European Commission 2002).

Organ-specific effects

Adverse skin reactions: No information found. Eugenol is a potential cause of skin sensitization in dermatitis patients.
Cardiovascular effects: Eugenol inhibits platelet aggregation (Janssens et al 1990), an essential step in the blood clotting cascade. Intravenous pungent basil oil reduced blood pressure in hypertensive rats (Interaminense et al 2005).

Systemic effects

Acute toxicity: No information found.
Antioxidant/pro-oxidant activity: An *Ocimum gratissimum* oil with 54.0% eugenol and 21.6% 1,8-cineole was a potent free radical scavenger, although this could not be correlated precisely to phenol content (Salles Trevisan et al 2006).
Carcinogenic/anticarcinogenic potential: Clocimum oil had a modest chemopreventive effect on murine DMBA-induced skin papilloma genesis. The oil increased hepatic levels of glutathione *S*-transferase, sulfhydryl and cytochrome b5 (Singh et al 1999, 2000). Eugenol powerfully induces glutathione *S*-transferase in mice and demonstrates anticarcinogenic activity (see Eugenol profile, Chapter 14).
Drug interactions: Anticoagulant medication, because of cardiovascular effects, above. Since eugenol significantly inhibits human MAO-A (Tao et al 2005), oral doses of eugenol-rich essential oils may interact with pethidine, indirect sympathomimetics, MAOIs or SSRIs (Table 4.10B).

Comments

The plant is grown in many parts of the world, but essential oil production is almost exclusively in India. A hybrid strain containing 85–90% eugenol and known as 'clocimum oil' (clove-scented ocimum) has been developed by the Regional Research Laboratory, Jammu, India. The estragole/camphor chemotype of *O. gratissimum* is Madagascan basil. Several other chemotypes exist, rich in geraniol, thymol, *p*-cymene, or ethyl cinnamate, though oils from these are not produced.

Bay (West Indian)

Botanical name: *Pimenta racemosa* var. *racemosa* (Miller) J. Moore
Botanical synonym: *Pimenta acris* Wight
Family: Myrtaceae

Essential oil

Source: Leaves
Key constituents:

Eugenol	44.4–56.2%
β-Myrcene	6.4–25.0%
Chavicol	9.3–21.6%
Linalool	1.7–6.0%
(+)-Limonene	0.8–3.9%
1-Octen-3-ol	0.9–2.0%
1,8-cineole	0.2–1.4%
Methyleugenol	0–1.4%
(*E*)-β-Ocimene	0–1.4%
Terpinen-4-ol	0.3–1.2%
3-Octanone	0.8–1.1%
δ-Cadinene	0.6–1.0%
3-Octanol	0.6–1.0%
p-Cymene	0.1–1.0%
Estragole	tr–0.1%

(McHale et al 1977; Tucker et al 1991a; Abaul & Bourgeois 1995; Jirovetz et al 2007)

Safety summary

Hazards: Drug interaction; may contain estragole and methyleugenol; may inhibit blood clotting; skin sensitization (low risk); mucous membrane irritation (low risk).
Cautions (oral): May interact with pethidine, MAOIs or SSRIs. Anticoagulant medication, major surgery, peptic ulcer, hemophilia, other bleeding disorders (Box 7.1).
Maximum adult daily oral dose: 50 mg
Maximum dermal use level (based on methyleugenol content):

EU	0.01%
IFRA	0.02%
Tisserand & Young	1.4%

Maximum dermal use level (based on eugenol content):

EU	No legal limit
IFRA	0.9%
Tisserand & Young	0.9%

Our safety advice

We recommend a dermal maximum of 0.9%, based on 56.2% eugenol content and a limit of 0.5% (see Eugenol profile, Chapter 14). Our oral maximum is based on 1.4% methyleugenol, and a limit of 0.01 mg/kg/day (see Methyleugenol profile, Chapter 14).

Regulatory guidelines

IFRA recommends that the maximum concentration of methyleugenol for leave-on products such as body lotion should be 0.0004% (IFRA 2009). The equivalent SCCNFP maximum is 0.0002% (European Commission 2002).

Organ-specific effects

Adverse skin reactions: Tested at 10% on 25 volunteers West Indian bay oil was neither irritating nor sensitizing (Opdyke 1973 p. 869–870). Eugenol is a potential cause of skin sensitization in dermatitis patients.
Cardiovascular effects: Eugenol inhibits platelet aggregation (Janssens et al 1990), an essential step in the blood clotting cascade.

Systemic effects

Acute toxicity: West Indian bay oil acute oral LD_{50} in rats 1.8 g/kg; acute dermal LD_{50} in rabbits >5 mL/kg (Opdyke 1973 p. 869–870).
Antioxidant/pro-oxidant activity: West Indian bay oil inhibited lipid peroxidation, and scavenged both DPPH radicals (IC_{50} 10 µg/mL) and OH radicals (0.6 µg/mL), almost as efficiently as eugenol (Jirovetz et al 2007). Eugenol and chavicol are potent antioxidants in lipid systems (Lee SJ et al 2005c).
Carcinogenic/anticarcinogenic potential: No information found. Methyleugenol is a rodent hepatocarcinogen when exposure is sufficiently high; eugenol, (+)-limonene and linalool display anti-liver cancer activity in vitro, and in vivo for (+)-limonene in rats (see Constituent profiles, Chapter 14).
Drug interactions: Anticoagulant medication, because of cardiovascular effects, above. Since eugenol significantly inhibits human MAO-A (Tao et al 2005), oral doses of eugenol-rich essential oils may interact with pethidine, indirect sympathomimetics, MAOIs or SSRIs (Table 4.10B).

Comments

There are few published analyses of West Indian bay oil, and since the methyleugenol content is a critical safety issue, it is worthy of some detailed remarks. There are five varieties of *Pimenta racemosa*, and there are three chemotypes of the *racemosa* variety: the commercial 'clove' type, rich in eugenol, a 'lemon' (citral) type, and an 'anise' type with, in one analysis, 32.8% estragole, and 48.1% methyleugenol (Abaul & Bourgeois 1995). Only the eugenol type is produced commercially.

The oil is distilled in the West Indies, primarily Dominica. In 1933, a commercial oil from the Virgin Islands was said to contain little, if any, methyleugenol, and in 1977 a Dominican oil was reported to contain only traces (Palkin & Wells 1933; McHale et al 1977). In 1991, no methyleugenol was detected

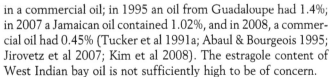

in a commercial oil; in 1995 an oil from Guadaloupe had 1.4%; in 2007 a Jamaican oil contained 1.02%, and in 2008, a commercial oil had 0.45% (Tucker et al 1991a; Abaul & Bourgeois 1995; Jirovetz et al 2007; Kim et al 2008). The estragole content of West Indian bay oil is not sufficiently high to be of concern.

West Indian bay oil is hydrodistilled, and separates into two fractions, one lighter and one heavier than water. These are re-combined to form the normal oil of commerce. This oil should not be confused with laurel leaf oil, which is also known as bay leaf.

Bee balm

Synonyms: Oswego tea, scarlet monarda, red bergamot
Botanical name: *Monarda didyma* L.
Family: Lamiaceae (Labiatae)

Essential oil

Source: Flowering plant
Key constituents:

Linalool	64.5–74.2%
p-Cymene	2.1–11.0%
Bornyl acetate	1.5–5.7%
Germacrene D	3.2–5.3%
γ–Terpinene	0.9–5.3%
Sabinene	1.4–5.0%
1-Octen-3-ol	0.3–2.8%
Camphene	0.3–1.3%

(Carnat et al 1991)

Safety summary

Hazards: None known.
Contraindications: None known.

Regulatory guidelines

According to IFRA, essential oils rich in linalool should only be used when the level of peroxides is kept to the lowest practical value. The addition of antioxidants such as 0.1% BHT or α-tocopherol at the time of production is recommended (IFRA 2009).

Organ-specific effects

Adverse skin reactions: No information found. Oxidation products of linalool may be skin sensitizing.
Reproductive toxicity: The virtual absence of reproductive toxicity for linalool (Politano et al 2008) suggests that pine oil is not hazardous in pregnancy.

Systemic effects

Acute toxicity: No information was found for bee balm oil, but some 83% of its constituents are known to possess low toxicity.
Carcinogenic/anticarcinogenic potential: No information found, but bee balm oil contains no known carcinogens. Linalool displays antitumoral activity (see Linalool profile, Chapter 14).

Comments

Limited availability.

Benzoin

Synonym: Gum Benjamin
Botanical names: *Styrax benzoin* Dryand (Sumatra benzoin), *Styrax paralleloneurus* Perkins (Sumatra benzoin), *Styrax tonkinensis* Pierre (Siam benzoin)
Family: Styracaceae

Resinoid

Source: Gum oleoresin
Key constituents:

Sumatra benzoin volatile compounds

Benzyl benzoate	50.7%
Benzyl alcohol	43.4%
(*Z*)-Cinnamyl (*E*)-cinnamate	1.5%
Cinnamic acid	1.4%
Ethyl cinnamate	1.0%
Benzoic acid	0.1%

(Moyler 1998)

Siam benzoin volatile compounds

Benzyl benzoate	39.3%
Benzyl alcohol	38.8%
Benzoic acid	18.4%
Ethyl cinnamate	0.8%

(Moyler 1998)

Quality: Benzoin resinoid is a sticky solid. To render it pourable, it is diluted to 50% in benzyl alcohol, benzyl benzoate, dipropylene glycol, or other solvent. Diethyl phthalate is less commonly used today as a diluent due to toxicity concerns (Burfield 2000). Small amounts of benzoic acid, benzyl cinnamate, ethyl cinnamate and vanillin may be added as odorous adulterants (Burfield 2003).

Safety summary

Hazards: Skin sensitization (low risk).
Cautions (dermal): Hypersensitive, diseased or damaged skin, children under 2 years of age.
Maximum adult daily oral dose: 368 mg
Maximum dermal use level: 2%

Our safety advice

Our oral maximum is based on a limit of 5 mg/kg for 'benzoic acid equivalents', which constitute up to 95% of benzoin. Our dermal maximum is a best-practice estimate for skin safety.

Regulatory guidelines

A group ADI of 0–5 mg/kg body weight for benzoic acid, the benzoate salts (calcium, potassium and sodium), benzaldehyde, benzyl acetate, benzyl alcohol and benzyl benzoate, expressed as benzoic acid equivalents, was established by JECFA in 1996. The CIR Expert Panel considers that benzoic acid is safe to use in cosmetic formulations at concentrations up to 5% (Nair 2001a).

Organ-specific effects

Adverse skin reactions: In a modified Draize procedure on guinea pigs, benzoin 'oil' was skin sensitizing when used at 10% in the challenge phase (Sharp 1978). Benzoic acid and cinnamic acid have produced some allergic reactions. Benzyl benzoate and benzyl alcohol are listed in the EU as allergens, but the risk of allergy from either is negligible (Tables 5.9 and 5.10). In patch tests of 477 dermatitis patients, 45 (9.2%) had a positive reaction to compound tincture of benzoin. Of the 45, 14 had strong positive reactions, and 28 had cross-reactions to similar allergens (fragrance mix, balsam of Peru, colophony and tea tree oil) (Scardamaglia et al 2003). Up to 80% of patients sentitive to Peru balsam reacted positively to Siamese benzoin (Hjorth 1961). Since both raw materials contain coniferyl benzoate this may be responsible, but it is not known to be present in benzoin resinoids.

Reproductive toxicity: The reproductive toxicity data for benzyl benzoate, benzyl alcohol, benzoic acid and cinnamic acid (Table 11.3) do not suggest any restrictions in the use of benzoin resinoid in pregnancy beyond those outlined above.

Systemic effects

Acute toxicity: No information found for benzoin. Benzyl alcohol and benzyl benzoate possess low acute toxicity (see Constituent profiles, Chapter 14).

Carcinogenic/anticarcinogenic potential: Gum benzoin was mutagenic in a mouse lymphoma assay (MLA), but not in Chinese hamster ovary cells (Oberly et al 1993). Gum benzoin produced CA in Chinese hamster lung (CHL) cells (Ishidate et al 1988), but was not genotoxic in a mouse micronucleus test (Shelby et al 1993) or in the *S. typhimurium* TA135/pSK1002 umu test (Nakamura et al 1987). It was not carcinogenic when fed to male rats at 125 or 250 ppm, to female rats at 250 or 500 ppm, and to male and female mice at 2,500 or 5,000 ppm for 104 weeks (National Toxicology Program 1980). The resinoid contains no known carcinogens, and the MLA and CHL results are false positives (Kirkland et al 2005).

Comments

Analysis of the volatile compounds reveals little significant difference between the two types of benzoin, except for benzoic acid. Coniferyl benzoate, a non-volatile constituent of the raw gum (up to 75%), may contribute slightly to skin sensitization in some preparations of benzoin. Resinoids, and occasionally absolutes, are used in aromatherapy, though neither is soluble in fixed oil. There is no benzoin essential oil. Benzoin Siam mostly comes from Laos, from the Luang Probang area which used to be partly in Thailand. It is also grown in Cambodia and China. Because of its botanical name (Styrax species), benzoin is sometimes confused with styrax (Liquidambar species).

Bergamot (expressed)

Synonym: Unrectified bergamot
Botanical name: *Citrus bergamia* Risso & Poit.
Botanical synonym: *Citrus aurantium* subsp. *bergamia* Risso & Poit.
Family: Rutaceae

Essential oil

Source: Fruit peel, by expression
Key constituents:

(+)-Limonene	27.4–52.0%
Linalyl acetate	17.1–40.4%
Linalool	1.7–20.6%
Sabinene	0.8–12.8%
γ-Terpinene	5.0–11.4%
β-Pinene	4.4–11.0%
α-Pinene	0.7–2.2%
β-Myrcene	0.6–1.8%
Neryl acetate	0.1–1.2%

Non-volatile compounds

Bergamottin 0.68–2.75%
5-Geranyloxy-7-methoxycoumarin 0.08–0.68%
Citropten 0.01–0.35%
Bergapten 0.11–0.33%
Bergaptol 0–0.19%
5-Methoxy-7-geranoxycoumarin 0.04–0.15%
Psoralen 0–0.0026%

(Lawrence 1989 p. 39–40, 1993 p. 7, p. 175; Verzera et al 1998; Dugo et al 1999b; SCCP 2005b)

Quality: Bergamot oil may be adulterated with synthetic linalool, limonene and linalyl acetate, and with other citrus oils or their residues, usually orange or lime. Bergamot oils sold through the 'Consorzio di Bergamotto' are guaranteed to be unadulterated (Kubeczka 2002). Other adulterants include rectified or acetylated ho oil (Burfield 2003).

Safety summary

Hazards: Phototoxic (moderate risk); may be photocarcinogenic.
Contraindications (dermal): If applied to the skin at over maximum use level, skin must not be exposed to sunlight or sunbed rays for 12 hours.
Cautions: Old or oxidized oils should be avoided.
Maximum dermal use level: 0.4% to avoid phototoxicity (see Regulatory Guidelines).

Our safety advice

Because of its limonene content, oxidation of bergamot oil should be avoided by storage in a dark, airtight container in a refrigerator. The addition of an antioxidant to preparations containing it is recommended.

Regulatory guidelines

Has GRAS status. IFRA recommends that, for application to areas of skin exposed to sunshine, bergamot oil be limited to a maximum of 0.4% in the final product, except for bath preparations, soaps and other wash-off products (IFRA 2009). In Europe, essential oils containing furanocoumarins must be used so that the total level of bergapten will not exceed: (a) 15 ppm in finished cosmetic products intended for application to skin areas likely to be exposed to sunshine, excluding rinse-off products; or (b) 1 ppm in sun protection and in bronzing products. In the presence of other phototoxic ingredients, the sum of their concentrations (expressed as % of the respective maximum levels) shall not exceed 100% (SCCNFP 2000). IFRA recommends that essential oils rich in limonene should only be used when the level of peroxides is kept to the lowest practical level, for instance by adding antioxidants at the time of production (IFRA 2009).

Organ-specific effects

Adverse skin reactions: No irritation was observed when 2% bergamot oil was patch tested in 1,200 dermatitis patients (Santucci et al 1987). In a 48 hour occlusive patch test on 50 Italian volunteers, the highest concentration of bergamot oil producing no adverse reaction was 30%. When similarly tested at 10%, it produced three reactions in 590 eczema patients (0.5%) (Meneghini et al 1971). Tested at 30% on 25 volunteers, bergamot oil was not sensitizing. Of 1,200 dermatitis patients patch tested, two (0.17%) were sensitive to 2% bergamot oil (Santucci et al 1987). In a study of 200 consecutive dermatitis patients, three (1.5%) were sensitive to 2% bergamot oil on patch testing (Rudzki et al 1976). Autoxidation products of (+)-limonene can cause skin sensitization (see (+)-Limonene profile, Chapter 14).

Severe phototoxic effects have been reported for bergamot oil in hairless mice, pigs and man using simulated sunlight, and in man using natural sunlight (Opdyke 1973 p. 1031–1033). Phototoxicity is due to the presence of bergapten and other furanocoumarins (Lawrence 1989 p. 39–45). Chronic skin pigmentation to exposed areas can be caused by bergamot oil phototoxicity. This is called berloque dermatitis, bergapten dermatitis, or photophytodermatitis. A more acute problem can be caused through an increase in the burning effects of UV light, which can lead to serious burns.

Full-thickness burns were sustained following a 20-minute session on a sunbed, which followed bergamot oil self-application in a female adult (private communication, 1993). In this instance, a few drops of undiluted bergamot oil were rubbed on both arms and both legs; 15 minutes later, the woman showered, and went on to the sunbed. (The shower was an attempt to remove any bergamot oil, much of which, by that time, would have crossed the epidermis.) Burns steadily developed during the following 48 hours, at which time she was admitted to hospital where she remained for 7 days. The skin on her arms and legs had a roasted appearance, and some blisters were 10 cm in diameter.

In a second case, a 10-year-old girl spilt an unknown quantity of undiluted bergamot oil on her hands and into the water while adding the oil to her bathwater. It was a sunny day, and following her bath she spent most of her time outside. The following morning she awoke with a blistering eruption on her hands and in a linear pattern along her forearms. Her thighs and lower legs were also affected, with a clear cut-off margin at mid-thigh level (she had knelt in the bath). The parts of her body that had not come in contact with the water were not affected. She was treated with oral prednisolone and a potent corticosteroid was applied twice daily. After one week the eruption had settled completely (Clark & Wilkinson 1998). Despite numerous documented accounts of the hazards of exposing the skin to UV light after applying bergamot oil, distressing phototoxic skin lesions and burns continue to be reported following self-administration (e.g., Nettelblad et al 1996; Cocks and Wilson 1998; Kaddu et al 2001).

Several studies demonstrate a carcinogenic action for bergamot oil when applied to mice which is then irradiated with UV light (Zajdela & Bisagni 1981; Young et al 1983, 1990). A comparison of berpaten in bergamot oil and bergapten prepared from pure bergapten crystals shows identical results, indicating that the active phototumorigenic agent in bergamot oil is bergapten (Young et al 1990). Bergamot oil, in the absence of UV light, is not carcinogenic, and even low concentration sunscreens can completely inhibit bergapten-enhanced phototumorigenesis (Young et al 1990). There is one report of bergamot oil production workers with 'keratomas or epitheliomas' of the skin, but possible confounding effects of age, gender and outdoor employment were not taken into account (IARC 1986b).

Reproductive toxicity: The low developmental toxicity of (+)-limonene and linalool (see Constituent profiles, Chapter 14) suggests that bergamot oil is not hazardous in pregnancy.

Systemic effects

Acute toxicity: No information found for unrectified bergamot oil, though rectified bergamot oil is distinctly non-toxic.

Carcinogenic/anticarcinogenic potential: Bergamot oil was not mutagenic in either a *Bacillus subtilis rec*-assay or an Ames test (Zani et al 1991). Bergamot terpenes induced glutathione *S*-transferase activity to more than 2.5 times control level in mouse tissues (Lam & Zheng 1991). Bergamot oil is cytotoxic to neuroblastoma (brain cancer) cells (Berliocchi et al 2011). Bergamot oil inhibited formation of the carcinogen NDMA in vitro by more than 70% (Sawamura 2010). (+)-Limonene displays anticarcinogenic activity (see (+)-Limonene profile, Chapter 14). Bergamot oil, however, may be photocarcinogenic (see above).

Comments

There is a need to raise public awareness to the phototoxic dangers of bergamot oil by adequate labeling and additional information. Assuming a maximum bergapten content of 0.33%, and to comply with the 15 ppm (0.0015%) SCCNFP guideline for bergapten, expressed bergamot oil should not be used at more than 0.45%, which correlates with the IFRA recommended maximum use level of 0.4%. A treated oil, sometimes rectified by distillation, is obtainable as bergapten-free. This oil is also known as rectified bergamot, furanocoumarin-free bergamot, or bergamot FCF (see below).

Bergamot (FCF)

Synonyms: Rectified bergamot, furanocoumarin-free bergamot
Botanical name: *Citrus bergamia* Risso & Poit.
Botanical synonym: *Citrus aurantium* subsp. *bergamia* Risso & Poit.
Family: Rutaceae

Essential oil

Source: Fruit peel, by expression
Key constituents:

(+)-Limonene	28.0–45.0%
Linalyl acetate	18.0–28.0%
Linalool	4.0–20.0%
γ-Terpinene	3.0–12.0%
β-Pinene	4.0–11.0%
α-Pinene	1.0–1.8%

Non-volatile compounds

Bergamottin	0–1.625%	
5-Geranyloxy-7-methoxycoumarin	0–0.19%	
Citropten	0–0.0052%	
Bergapten	0–0.0091%	

(Lawrence 1989 p. 41–42; Dugo et al 1999b)

Safety summary

Hazards: None known.
Cautions: Old or oxidized oils should be avoided.

Our safety advice

Because of its limonene content, oxidation of rectified bergamot oil should be avoided by storage in a dark, airtight container in a refrigerator. The addition of an antioxidant to preparations containing it is recommended.

Regulatory guidelines

IFRA recommends that essential oils rich in limonene should only be used when the level of peroxides is kept to the lowest practical level, for instance by adding antioxidants at the time of production (IFRA 2009). In Europe, essential oils containing furanocoumarins must be used so that the total level of bergapten will not exceed: (a) 15 ppm in finished cosmetic products intended for application to skin areas likely to be exposed to sunshine, excluding rinse-off products; or (b) 1 ppm in sun protection and in bronzing products. In the presence of other phototoxic ingredients, the sum of their concentrations (expressed as % of the respective maximum levels) shall not exceed 100% (SCCNFP 2000).

Organ-specific effects

Adverse skin reactions: Undiluted rectified bergamot oil was mildly irritating to rabbits. Tested at 30% on 25 volunteers it was not sensitizing. Rectified bergamot oil was non-phototoxic (Opdyke 1973 p. 1035). Autoxidation products of (+)-limonene can cause skin sensitization (see (+)-Limonene profile, Chapter 14).
Reproductive toxicity: The low developmental toxicity of (+)-limonene and linalool (see Constituent profiles, Chapter 14) suggests that rectified bergamot oil is not hazardous in pregnancy.

Systemic effects

Acute toxicity: Rectified bergamot oil acute oral LD_{50} in rats >10 g/kg; acute dermal LD_{50} in rabbits >20 g/kg (Opdyke 1973 p. 1035).
Carcinogenic/anticarcinogenic potential: No information found for rectified bergamot oil. Expressed bergamot oil is not mutagenic (see above). (+)-Limonene displays anticarcinogenic activity (see (+)-Limonene profile, Chapter 14).

Comments

To comply with the SCCNFP regulation, it would be safe to use bergamot (FCF) at up to 16.6%. The odor of bergamot FCF is inferior to that of the untreated, cold-pressed oil, but it is not phototoxic or photocarcinogenic. Bergamot (FCF) is more effective against *Candida* species than natural, expressed bergamot oil (Romano et al 2005).

Bergamot (wild)

Synonym: Horsemint
Botanical name: *Monarda fistulosa* L. var. *menthaefolia* J. Graham
Botanical synonyms: *Monarda menthaefolia* L.
Family: Lamiaceae (Labiatae)

Essential oil

Source: Flowering plant
Key constituents:

Geraniol	86.8–93.2%
Linalool	0.8–3.1%
Neral	1.4–2.0%
γ-Terpinene	0–1.8%
Geranial	1.2–1.6%
Nerol	0.8–1.4%
β-Myrcene	0–1.3%
1-Octen-3-ol	0.2–1.1%

(Lawrence 1981 p. 68–76, Mazza et al 1987)

Safety summary

Hazards: Drug interaction; skin sensitization (low risk).
Cautions (oral): Drugs metabolized by CYP2B6 (Appendix B).
Maximum dermal use level: 5.7%

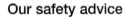

Our safety advice

Our dermal maximum is based on 93.2% geraniol content and a geraniol limit of 5.3% (see Geraniol profile, Chapter 14).

Organ-specific effects

Adverse skin reactions: No information found.

Systemic effects

Acute toxicity: No information found for the oil. Geraniol shows no signs of acute or subchronic toxicity (see Geraniol profile, Chapter 14).

Carcinogenic/anticarcinogenic potential: No information found, but wild bergamot oil contains no known carcinogens. Geraniol and citral (geranial + neral) display anticarcinogenic activity (see Constituent profiles, Chapter 14).

Drug interactions: Since citral and geraniol inhibit CYP2B6 (Table 4.11B), there is a theoretical risk of interaction between wild bergamot oil and drugs metabolized by this enzyme (Appendix B).

Comments

Limited availability.

Betel

Botanical name: *Piper betle* L.
Family: Piperaceae

Essential oil

Source: Leaves
Key constituents:

Safrole	6.5–45.3%
Eugenol	20.5–33.2%
α-Terpinyl acetate	6.8–11.0%
Isoeugenol	0–10.6%
(E)-Anethole	0–7.8%
β-Caryophyllene	0–7.8%
Dodecanal	0–7.1%
β-Selinene	0–6.4%
Sabinene	0–6.1%
Estragole	0–4.8%
α-Cubebene	0–4.4%
Camphene	0–3.7%
α-Pinene	0–3.2%
Decanal	0–2.9%
1,8-Cineole	0–2.8%
Octadecanal	0–2.7%
β-Elemene	0–2.6%
Geraniol	0–2.5%
α-Terpineol	0.3–2.3%
β-Myrcene	0–2.2%

α-Thujene	0–1.9%
γ-Elemene	0.9–1.8%
Methyleugenol	0.3–1.7%
γ-Terpinene	0.5–1.6%
Caryophyllene oxide	0–1.6%
Linalool	0.2–1.5%
Terpinen-1-ol	0–1.5%
β-Phellandrene	0–1.3%
Bornylene	0–1.2%
δ-Cadinene	0–1.2%
α-Muurolol	0–1.2%
γ-Cadinene	0–1.1%

(Lawrence 2005)

Safety summary

Hazards: Potentially carcinogenic, based on estragole, safrole and methyleugenol content; skin sensitization (low risk); mucous membrane irritation (low risk).

Contraindications: Should not be taken in oral doses.

Maximum dermal use level:

EU	0.008%
IFRA	0.01%
Tisserand & Young	0.1%

Our safety advice

We recommend a dermal maximum of 0.1%, based on a content of 45.3% safrole, 4.8% estragole and 1.7% methyleugenol with respective dermal limits of 0.05%, 0.12% and 0.02% (see Constituent profiles, Chapter 14).

Regulatory guidelines

IFRA recommends a maximum dermal use level for estragole of 0.01% in leave-on or wash-off preparations for body and face (IFRA 2009). IFRA and the EU recommend a maximum exposure level of 0.01% of safrole from the use of safrole-containing essential oils in cosmetics. IFRA recommends that the maximum concentration of methyleugenol for leave-on products such as body lotion should be 0.0004% (IFRA 2009). The equivalent SCCNFP maximum is 0.0002% (European Commission 2002).

Organ-specific effects

Adverse skin reactions: No information found.

Systemic effects

Acute toxicity: No information found.
Carcinogenic/anticarcinogenic potential: Betel leaf oil showed no chemopreventive activity against human mouth epidermal carcinoma (KB) or mouse leukemia (P388) cell lines, and in fact enhanced proliferation to a small degree (Manosroi et al 2005). Safrole, estragole and methyleugenol are rodent carcinogens when exposure is sufficiently high; β-elemene and geraniol display anticarcinogenic activity; there is evidence of both

antimutagenic and anticarcinogenic activity for eugenol (see Eugenol profile, Chapter 14). Several studies show extracts of betel leaf to be antimutagenic and anticarcinogenic, for example Bhide et al (1991a, 1991b, 1994) and Padma et al (1989a, 1989b). Although aqueous extracts were used in these studies, ethanol was used in part to extract the leaves, so the extracts would almost certainly contain safrole.

Comments

Other constituents of betel leaf oil may counter the carcinogenic action of the three known carcinogens, and there is tentative evidence to support this for betel leaf extracts. However, there is also evidence to the contrary for the essential oil, and there is great variation in the composition of betel leaf oils. There are numerous cultivars of betel leaf, many of which contain eugenol as a major constituent; these are the ones generally distilled for commercial use. Other cultivars have chavibetol, chavicol, iso-eugenol, or eugenyl acetate as major constituents (Lawrence 2005 p. 54).

Birch (sweet)

Synonyms: Black birch, cherry birch, mahogany birch, southern birch
Botanical name: *Betula lenta* L.
Family: Betulaceae

Essential oil

Source: Bark
Key constituents:

Methyl salicylate	90.4%
Ethyl salicylate	5.5%
Linalyl acetate	1.1%

(Pappas, private communication, 2003)

Safety summary

Hazards: Drug interaction; inhibits blood clotting; toxicity; high doses may be teratogenic
Contraindications (all routes): Anticoagulant medication, major surgery, hemophilia, other bleeding disorders (Box 7.1). Pregnancy, breastfeeding. Should not be used on or given to children. Should not be given to people with salicylate sensitivity (often applies in ADD/ADHD).
Contraindications (oral): Gastroesophageal reflux disease (GERD).
Maximum adult daily oral dose: 182 mg
Maximum dermal use level: 2.5%

Our safety advice

Our oral and dermal restrictions are based on a total of 95.9% total salicylate and methyl salicylate limits of 2.5 mg/kg/day and 2.4% (see Methyl salicylate profile, Chapter 14). Oral use of methyl salicylate-rich essential oils should be avoided in GERD, and salicylates are contraindicated in children due to the risk of developing Reye's syndrome. Essential oils with a high methyl salicylate content should be avoided in pregnancy and lactation, and by anyone concurrently taking anticoagulant drugs. Caution is advised in those with hypersensitivity to salicylates, or dermatological conditions where the integrity of the skin is impaired.

Regulatory guidelines

An ADI for methyl salicylate was set at 0.5 mg/kg bw by the Joint FAO/WHO Expert Committee on Food Additives (JECFA) in 1967 based on a dog NOAEL of 50 mg/kg and an uncertainty factor of 100. The same ADI, based on a two year rat study in 1963, was adopted by the Council of Europe Committee of Experts on Flavoring Substances. The Health Canada maximum for methyl salicylate is 1% in topical products (Health Canada Cosmetic Ingredient Hotlist, March 2011).

Organ-specific effects

Adverse skin reactions: Undiluted sweet birch oil was moderately irritating to rabbits and was irritating to both mice and pigs; tested at 4% on 25 volunteers it was neither irritating nor sensitizing. It is non-phototoxic (Opdyke 1979a p. 907).
Cardiovascular effects: Methyl salicylate inhibits platelet aggregation (Tanen et al 2008), an essential step in the blood clotting cascade.
Reproductive toxicity: Methyl salicylate is reproductively toxic in rodents at certain doses (see Methyl salicylate profile, Chapter 14).

Systemic effects

Acute toxicity (human): Numerous cases of poisoning have been reported from ingestion of wintergreen oil or methyl salicylate, with a 50–60% mortality rate; 4–8 mL is considered a lethal dose for a child (Opdyke 1978 p. 821–825). Methyl salicylate could be 1.5–4.5 times more toxic in humans than in rodents (see Ch. 3, p. 32). In the years 1926, 1928 and 1939–1943, 427 deaths occurred in the US from methyl salicylate or wintergreen oil poisoning (Davison et al 1961). Common signs of methyl salicylate poisoning are: CNS excitation; rapid breathing; fever; high blood pressure; convulsions; coma. Death results from respiratory failure after a period of unconsciousness (Opdyke 1978 p. 821–825). Methyl salicylate can be absorbed transdermally in sufficient quantities to cause poisoning in humans (Heng 1987).
Acute toxicity (animal): Sweet birch oil acute oral LD_{50} in rats 1.7 g/kg; acute dermal LD_{50} in rabbits >5 g/kg (Opdyke 1979a p. 907).
Chronic toxicity: In a two year study, sweet birch oil was included in the dry diet of rats at 700 and 2,100 ppm. Growth, survival, food usage, and general physical condition was comparable to that of control animals. Routine blood and urine studies were normal, and no adverse effects were observed on histology (Packman et al 1961).
Carcinogenic/anticarcinogenic potential: No information found for sweet birch oil. Methyl salicylate is not genotoxic,

and does not appear to be carcinogenic (see Methyl salicylate profile, Chapter 14).

Drug interactions: Topically applied methyl salicylate can potentiate the anticoagulant effect of warfarin, causing side effects such as internal hemorrhage (Le Bourhis & Soenen 1973). It is likely that methyl salicylate administered by other routes would result in a similar potentiation. A similar interaction is possible, but by no means certain, with other anticoagulants such as aspirin and heparin.

Comments

The ethyl salicylate content probably also contributes to the toxicity of the oil. The oil does not pre-exist in the bark, but is formed by the interaction of a glucoside, gaultherin, and an enzyme, betulase. Many 'sweet birch oils' are in fact synthetic methyl salicylate. Many liniments, mouthwashes, inhalants and soft drink flavorings contain methyl salicylate. Knowing that the LD_{50} in rodents is 1.0 g/kg, and assuming that methyl salicylate is five times more toxic in humans, this would give a human LD_{50} of 200 mg/kg, which is equivalent to 13 g in an adult or 4–8 g in a child.

Birch tar

Botanical names: *Betula lenta* L. (sweet birch); *Betula pendula* Roth. (European white birch); *Betula pubescens* Ehrh. (synonym: *Betula alba* L.) (white birch)
Family: Betulaceae

Essential oil

Source: Bark and wood, by destructive distillation
Key constituents:

Cresol*	Major constituent
Guaiacol	Major constituent
Creosol	Undetermined
Pyrocatechol	Undetermined
Xylenol	Undetermined

(Guenther 1949–1952 vol 6 p. 17)

Safety summary

Hazards: Toxicity; unrectified oils may be carcinogenic.
Contraindications: Should not be taken in oral doses; unrectified oils should not be used.

Our safety advice

We recommend that birch tar oil is not taken in oral doses due to the toxicity of cresol isomers (see Cresol profile, Chapter 14).

Regulatory guidelines

The IFRA Code of Practice requires that *crude* birch wood pyrolysate (birch tar oil) should not be used as fragrance ingredient. Only *rectified* (purified) birch tar oils may be used. Whether used alone or used in conjunction with cade oil, the final product may not contain more than 1 ppb of PAHs (polynuclear aromatic hydrocarbons), which may include benzo[*a*] pyrene and 1,2-benzanthracene (IFRA 2009). Cresols are prohibited as cosmetic ingredients in Canada.

Organ-specific effects

Adverse skin reactions: Undiluted birch tar oil was irritating to rabbits, but was not irritating to mice; tested at 2% on 25 volunteers it was neither irritating nor sensitizing. It is non-phototoxic (Opdyke 1973 p. 1037).
Hepatotoxicity: No information found for birch tar oil. *p*-Cresol rapidly depletes hepatic intracellular glutathione in rat liver ex vivo (Thompson et al 1994, 1996). Since birch tar oil contains *p*-cresol as a major constituent, it probably has a potential for glutathione depletion.

Systemic effects

Acute toxicity: Birch tar oil acute oral LD_{50} in rats >5 g/kg; acute dermal LD_{50} in rabbits >2 g/kg (Opdyke 1973 p. 1037). It is probable that guaiacol is more toxic in humans than other species (see Guaiacol profile, Chapter 14), so the rodent LD_{50} for birch tar oil may be misleading. *p*-Cresol is toxic when administered by the oral, dermal, subcutaneous, intravenous or intraperitoneal routes. Exposure can cause irritation to the eyes, nose and throat, severe eye damage, vomiting, sleeplessness and damage to the lungs, liver, kidneys, blood, nervous system and respiratory system. It can cause corrosion of all tissues (Lesaffer et al 2001). The acute oral LD_{50} for *p*-cresol is 207 mg/kg in rats, and in mice is 344 mg/kg (National Toxicology Program 2000). This suggests that rectified birch tar oil should only contain a low concentration of *p*-cresol.
Carcinogenic/anticarcinogenic potential: No information found for birch tar oil. Unrectified birch tar oils contain carcinogenic PAH see below. Guaiacol is not a rodent carcinogen (see Guaiacol profile, Chapter 14).

Comments

The oil is a dark, viscous liquid. Guaiacol and cresol are the major constituents, and the oil may also contain traces of phenol. Cade, the only other essential oil produced by destructive (dry) distillation contains similar constituents and carcinogenic polynuclear hydrocarbons.

Blackcurrant bud

Synonym: Cassis
Botanical name: *Ribes nigrum* L.
Family: Grossulariaceae

Essential oil

Source: Flower buds

---

*Isomer not specified, but likely to be a mixture of cresol isomers.

Key constituents:

δ-3-Carene	15.0–35.0%
β-Pinene	0.2–24.0%
β-Phellandrene	1.6–11.0%
(+)-Limonene	0.8–10.0%
Terpinolene	0–9.0%
α-Pinene	4.0–6.0%
γ-Terpinene	0–1.5%
Ocimene	0–1.5%
p-Cymene	0.7–1.4%

(Lawrence 1989 p. 234–236)

Absolute

Source: Flower buds
Key constituents:

δ-3-Carene	12.6–19.0%
p-Cymene	1.9–15.4%
Sabinene	1.8–15.4%
β-Caryophyllene	9.0–14.0%
Terpinolene	3.9–11.6%
β-Phellandrene	3.2–10%
(E)-β-Ocimene	0.6–6.7%
Terpinen-4-ol	0.5–6.3%
(+)-Limonene	3.2–4.9%
α-Caryophyllene + citronellyl acetate	1.5–4.5%
α-Terpinene	0.7–3.9%
β-Myrcene	2.2–3.8%
α-Terpineol	0–3.8%
γ-Terpinene	0.8–2.8%
Germacrene D	0–2.6%
(Z)-β-Ocimene	0–2.5%
α-Pinene	0.3–2.4%
β-Terpinyl acetate	0–1.9%
3-Octanone	0.7–1.8%
(Z)-β-Ocimene	1.3–1.6%

(Lawrence 1989 p. 235)

Safety summary

Hazards: Skin sensitization if oxidized.
Cautions: Old or oxidized essential oils and absolutes should be avoided.

Our safety advice

Because of their δ-3-carene content, oxidation of blackcurrant bud essential oil or absolute should be avoided by storage in a dark, airtight container in a refrigerator. The addition of an antioxidant to preparations containing either is recommended.

Organ-specific effects

Adverse skin reactions: No information found for blackcurrant bud essential oil or absolute. Autoxidation products of δ-3-

carene can cause skin sensitization (see δ-3-Carene profile, Chapter 14).
Reproductive toxicity: The low reproductive toxicity of β-pinene, α-pinene, sabinene, (+)-limonene (see Constituent profiles, Chapter 14) and the structural similarity of other monoterpenes suggests that neither blackcurrant bud oil or absolute is hazardous in pregnancy.

Systemic effects

Acute toxicity: No information found for blackcurrant bud essential oil or absolute, but the great majority of constituents are non-toxic.
Carcinogenic/anticarcinogenic potential: No information found for the essential oil or absolute, but neither contains any known carcinogens. (+)-Limonene and α-caryophyllene display anticarcinogenic activity (see Constituent profiles, Chapter 14).

Comments

Absolutes of blackcurrant bud are more commonly encountered than essential oils. It is unusual for an absolute to be rich in monoterpenes.

Black seed

Synonyms: Black cumin, black caraway, Roman coriander, fennel flower, nutmeg flower
Botanical name: *Nigella sativa* L.
Family: Ranunculaceae

Essential oil

Source: Seeds
Key constituents:

Thymoquinone	26.8–54.8%
p-Cymene	14.7–38.0%
Longifolene	1.2–10.2%
α-Thujene	1.3–10.1%
Carvacrol	0.5–4.2%
α-Cubebene	0.4–3.0%
α-Pinene	0.2–2.4%
(+)-Limonene	0.7–2.3%
β-Pinene	0.4–3.0%
Sabinene	0.2–1.6%

(Mozaffari et al 2000)

Safety summary

Hazards: Drug interaction; fetotoxic, based on thymoquinone content; skin sensitization (moderate risk).
Contraindications (all routes): Pregnancy, breastfeeding
Cautions (oral): Diabetes medication.
Cautions (dermal): Hypersensitive, diseased or damaged skin, children under 2 years of age.

Organ-specific effects

Adverse skin reactions: Of 240 consecutive dermatitis patients in Saudi Arabia, two presented with dermatitis caused by the topical application of black seed oil. One had pigmented dermatitis on the face, while the other had generalized reactions (El-Rab & Al-Sheikh 1995). Repeated applications of an ointment containing black seed oil caused ACD in a 31-year-old woman with preexisting eczema (Zedlitz et al 2002). Another case of ACD was reported in a 28-year-old man; patch testing confirmed black seed oil as the causative agent (Steinmann et al 1997). Two similar severe cases of systemic adverse reaction to black seed oil were diagnosed as generalized erythema multiforme (Nosbaum et al 2011) and bullous eruption (Gelot et al 2012). In the first case, capsules containing 500 mg of black seed oil were taken, and patch testing was positive for the same oil. The second case involved both oral ingestion and dermal application.

It was later established that in the Nosbaum et al (2011) case, black seed fixed oil was used, not the essential oil, and the same may well be true of some of the other reports. However, the fixed oil naturally contains up to 0.5% essential oil, and therefore essential oil constituents such as *p*-cymene and thymoquinone could still be causative.

It is almost certain that in some of these cases black seed fixed oil was used, and not black seed essential oil. However, the fixed oil contains up to 0.5% thymoquinone, and in either case it is the most likely cause of the adverse reactions. Thymoquinone is a relatively potent contact allergen (see Thymoquinone profile, Chapter 14).

Cardiovascular effects: In rabbits, 50 mg/kg ip of black seed essential oil reduced blood glucose in fasting normal and alloxan-diabetic animals (Al-Hader et al 1993).

Reproductive toxicity: The thymoquinone NOAEL for reproductive toxicity is 15 mg/kg from ip administration in rats. Since no safe oral or dermal guideline can be extrapolated from an ip dose, black seed oil containing thymoquinone should be avoided in pregnancy and breastfeeding. The strong antiangiogenic action of thymoquinone (Yi et al 2008) also suggests great caution in pregnancy. A freshly prepared infusion of *Nigella sativa* seeds, ingested shortly after childbirth by three women, had no stimulant effect on the uterus, while six of the total of nine herbs tested were uterine stimulants (Kapur 1948). Black seed oil concentration-dependently inhibited the spontaneous movements of rat and guinea pig uterine smooth muscle and also the contractions induced by oxytocin stimulation (Aqel & Shaheen 1996). This suggests that the oil may possess some anti-oxytocin potential, and that it could slow the progression of labor.

Immunotoxicity: When rats were injected im with 2.5 μL of black seed oil twice weekly for 4 weeks, there was a decrease in splenocytes and neurophils, but an increase in peripheral lymphocytes and monocytes (Islam et al 2004).

Hepatotoxicity: Injected black seed essential oil afforded protection against induced hepatotoxicity in rats (Turkdogan et al 2003).

Systemic effects

Acute toxicity: No information found. The acute oral LD_{50} of thymoquinone in mice was 2.4 g/kg (Badary et al 1998). *p*-Cymene acute oral LD_{50} in rats 4.75 g/kg (Jenner et al 1964).

Subacute & subchronic toxicity: When black seed oil was fed to rats at 0.3% of the diet for 8 weeks, there were no significant deviations in organ to body-weight ratios compared to controls for heart, liver, pancreas, lungs, spleen, left kidney and right kidney. Indices of red and white blood cells remained within normal limits, as did cardiac enzymes, liver function tests, urea, creatinine, albumin, globulins, A/G ratio and total proteins (Sultan et al 2009). As part of an experimental protocol to assess chemopreventive activity, male rats were dosed with 200 mg/kg/day of black seed oil for 14 weeks. Gross and microscopic examination of the liver, kidneys, spleen, lungs, stomach, intestine, testes and accessory organs, and thyroid gland, revealed no histopathological changes (Salim & Fukushima 2003).

Antioxidant/pro-oxidant activity: Black seed oil is an effective OH radical scavenger (Burits & Bucar 2000) and protects against lipid peroxidation (Hosseinzadeh et al 2007). In male rats, black seed oil offered significant protection against free radical damage from aflatoxins. These are mycotoxins which are potentially mutagenic, carcinogenic, hepatotoxic and teratogenic (Abdel-Wahhab & Aly 2005).

Carcinogenic/anticarcinogenic potential: Black seed oil had a significant antiproliferative activity against 1,2-dimethylhydrazine-induced colon carcinogenesis in male rats when administered at 200 mg/kg/day po for 14 weeks. The effect was evident in both initiation and post-initiation stages, especially in the latter, and there was no evidence of adverse effects (Salim & Fukushima 2003). Black seed oil showed both in vitro and in vivo antitumor activity, significantly inhibiting solid tumor development and metastasis in mice, and reducing mortality from 83% to 0% when injected into the tumor site (Ait M'barek et al 2007a). Black seed oil showed moderate lethality towards four human stomach cancer cell lines, with LC_{50} values of 120.4–384.5 μg/mL, but the LC_{50} for fibroblasts was 286.8 μg/mL (Islam et al 2004).

Drug interactions: Antidiabetic medication, because of cardiovascular effects, above. See Table 4.10B.

Comments

The plant is grown in India and Middle Eastern countries, but few currently produce the essential oil. The compositional data above are for oils steam distilled from Iranian seeds. In oils produced by microwave distillation from five different countries, thymoquinone content varied from 6.2 to 18.4% (Lawrence 2008). A high thymoquinone content is desirable for therapeutic applications. It is difficult to assess the allergenicity of black seed oil from the known data. There is also a fixed oil of *Nigella sativa*, and this is also referred to as 'black seed oil.'

Boldo

Botanical name: *Peumus boldus* Molina
Botanical synonym: *Boldoa fragrans* Gay
Family: Monimiaceae

Essential oil

Source: Dried leaves

Key constituents:

Ascaridole	21.3%
1,8-Cineole	21.1%
α-Thujone	14.3%
(Z)-Verbenol	9.9%
Guaiazulene	8.8%
p-Cymene	8.6%
β-Thujone	7.2%
Sabinyl acetate	2.4%

(Miraldi et al 1996)

Safety summary

Hazards: Toxicity; neurotoxicity.
Contraindications: Should not be used, either internally or externally.

Organ-specific effects

Adverse skin reactions: Undiluted boldo oil was moderately irritating to rabbits, and was irritating to mice; tested at 4% on 25 volunteers it was neither irritating nor sensitizing. It is non-phototoxic (Opdyke & Letizia 1982 p. 643–644).
Neurotoxicity: Boldo oil produced convulsions in rats at an oral dose of 70 mg/kg (Opdyke & Letizia 1982 p. 643–644). The thujone NOAEL for convulsions was reported to be 10 mg/kg in male rats and 5 mg/kg in females (Margaria 1963).

Systemic effects

Acute toxicity: Very toxic. The animal data show boldo oil to be only moderately toxic: acute oral LD_{50} in rats 130 mg/kg, convulsions being produced at doses of 70 mg/kg; acute dermal LD_{50} in rabbits 940 mg/kg (Opdyke & Letizia 1982 p. 643–644). However, the human data for wormseed oil indicate a fatal dose somewhere in the 10–40 mg/kg range, compared to rodent toxicity of 255–380 mg/kg, suggesting that ascaridole is many times more toxic to humans than rodents (see Wormseed profile, Chapter 14). Therefore boldo oil should also be classed as 'very toxic'. Both α- and β-thujone are moderately toxic, with reported oral LD_{50} values ranging from 190 to 500 mg/kg for different species (see Thujone profile, Chapter 14).
Carcinogenic/anticarcinogenic potential: No information found. Ascaridole is cytotoxic towards certain human cancer cell lines (see Ascaridole profile, Chapter 14).

Comments

The toxicity of boldo leaf oil is presumed to be due to its content of ascaridole. Our dermal maximum for ascaridole is 0.12%, and for thujone isomers 0.25%. We could, on this basis, allow 0.37% of boldo oil. However, on a risk/benefit basis, there would be no point. Some types of *Peumus boldus* contain very little ascaridole, though these are not commercially available.

Boronia

Botanical name: *Boronia megastigma* Nees ex Bartt.
Family: Rutaceae

Absolute

Source: Flowers
Key constituents:

(E)-β-Ionone	14.9%
Heptadecene	14.6%
(Z)-Methyl cinnamate + N-tiglamide	9.3%
(E)-Methyl cinnamate	6.7%
(E)-Cinnamic acid	4.3%
Dodecyl acetate	3.8%
Acetoxylinalool	2.4%
Hydroxymegastimenone	2.4%
Hydroxylinalyl decanoate	2.2%
(Z)-Cinnamic acid	1.9%
Hydroxylinalyl octanoate	1.8%
Hydroxylinalyl tridecanoate	1.4%
Dihydro-β-ionone	1.3%
Methyl jasmonate	1.2%
Sesquicineole	1.2%

(Weyerstahl et al 1995)

Safety summary

Hazards: None known.
Contraindications: None known.

Organ-specific effects

Adverse skin reactions: No information found. Ionones tend to be non-reactive on the skin (see Constituent profiles, Chapter 14).

Systemic effects

Acute toxicity: No information found. The acute oral LD_{50} in rats was 4.59 g/kg for 'ionone standard' (60% α-ionone, 40% β-ionone) (Jenner et al 1964).
Carcinogenic/anticarcinogenic potential: No information found. Methyl jasmonate displays anticarcinogenic activity (see Methyl jasmonate profile, Chapter 14).

Comments

This expensive absolute is not likely to be used in significant quantities in any capacity. There may be three distinct chemotypes.

Broom

Synonyms: Spanish broom, weaver's broom, genet
Botanical name: *Spartium junceum* L.
Family: Fabaceae (Leguminosae)

Absolute

Source: Flowers

Key constituents:

Linolenic acid	15.8–26.0%
Palmitic acid	20.9–24.0%
Ethyl palmitate	1.9–14.6%
Linalool	1.7–10.9%
Methyl linoleate	0–7.1%
Oleic acid	5.9–6.0%
Ethyl oleate	0–4.9%
Linoleic acid	4.0–4.7%
Capric acid	0–4.1%
Ethyl stearate	0–3.7%
Myristic acid	2.9–3.5%
Stearic acid	0–3.5%
Linalyl acetate	0–3.4%
1-Octen-3-ol	1.2–3.3%
Ethyl myristate	0–1.9%
(E,E)-α-Farnesene	0–1.8%
β-Farnesene	0–1.7%
Methyl linolenate	0.7–1.5%
2-Phenylethanol	0.5–1.3%
Estragole	0–0.01%
Safrole	0–0.01%

(Lawrence 1989 p. 7, 1995g p. 83–84)

Safety summary

Hazards: None known.
Contraindications: None known.

Organ-specific effects

Adverse skin reactions: Undiluted broom absolute was moderately irritating to rabbits, but was not irritating to mice or pigs; tested at 12% on 25 volunteers it was neither irritating nor sensitizing. It was non-phototoxic (Opdyke 1976 p. 779).

Systemic effects

Acute toxicity: Broom absolute acute oral LD_{50} in rats >5 g/kg; acute dermal LD_{50} in rabbits >5 g/kg (Opdyke 1976 p. 779).
Carcinogenic/anticarcinogenic potential: No information found. Estragole and safrole are carcinogenic if present in sufficient concentration (see Constituent profiles, Chapter 14).

Comments

The estragole and safrole contents are not high enough to be of concern, especially since this expensive absolute is only likely to be used in very small concentrations.

Buchu (diosphenol CT)

Botanical name: *Agathosma betulina* Bergius
Botanical synonym: *Barosma betulina* Bergius
Family: Rutaceae

Essential oil

Source: Leaves
Key constituents:

Isomenthone	4.6–29.1%
(+)-Limonene	11.6–28.2%
Disophenol	12.0–26.3%
Menthone	2.5–25.0%
ψ-Diosphenol	10.3–23.3%
8-Mercapto-*p*-menthan-3-one (*cis* + *trans*)	0.7–6.6%
α-Pulegone [(E)- + (Z)-]	0.4–4.6%
(1S)-(−)-β-Pulegone	0.6–4.5%
1,8-Cineole	tr–4.4%
β-Myrcene	0.2–2.8%
Sabinene	tr–1.2%

(Collins et al 1996)
Quality: May be adulterated with monoterpene sulfides, such as *p*-mentan-8-thiol-3-one (Burfield 2003).

Safety summary

Hazards: Hepatotoxic (low risk); skin sensitization if oxidized.
Contraindications (all routes): Pregnancy, breastfeeding.
Cautions: Use with caution due to uncertain toxicity; old or oxidized oils should be avoided.
Maximum adult daily oral dose: 384 mg
Maximum dermal use level: 11%

Our safety advice

Best avoided in pregnancy and breastfeeding due to uncertain toxicity and pulegone content. Our oral and dermal restrictions are based on 9.1% total pulegone content with limits of 0.5 mg/kg/day and 1% (see β-Pulegone profile, Chapter 14). Because of its limonene content, oxidation of *A. betulina* oil should be avoided by storage in a dark, airtight container in a refrigerator. The addition of an antioxidant to preparations containing it is recommended.

Regulatory guidelines

The CEFS of the Council of Europe identifies pulegone as a hepatotoxic compound, and has set a group TDI of 0.1 mg/kg for pulegone and menthofuran (Anon 1992b). IFRA recommends that essential oils rich in limonene should only be used when the level of peroxides is kept to the lowest practical level, for instance by adding antioxidants at the time of production (IFRA 2009).

Organ-specific effects

Adverse skin reactions: No information found. Autoxidation products of (+)-limonene can cause skin sensitization (see (+)-Limonene profile, Chapter 14).
Hepatotoxicity: Pulegone is toxic to the liver because it is metabolized to epoxides. It is especially toxic by mouth (see β-Pulegone profile, Chapter 14).

Systemic effects

Acute toxicity: No information found for *A. betulina* oil, isomenthone or diosphenol.
Carcinogenic/anticarcinogenic potential: No information found. Menthone is mutagenic; (+)-limonene displays anticarcinogenic activity (see Constituent profiles, Chapter 14).

Comments

The *British Herbal Compendium* gives pregnancy as a contraindication for buchu leaves (Bradley 1992). Very few data exist on the biological effects of buchu oils. This species is the more common source of buchu leaves or essential oil. In addition to the two principal taxa, two other types of buchu are occasionally available. One of these is a hybrid between these two, and the other is an isomenthone chemotype (39–49%) of *A. betulina* (Collins et al 1996).

Buchu (pulegone CT)

Botanical name: Agathosma crenulata L.
Botanical synonym: Barosma crenulata L.
Family: Rutaceae

Essential oil

Source: Leaves
Key constituents:

(1R)-(+)-β-Pulegone	31.6–73.2%
Isomenthone	3.6–27.6%
(+)-Limonene	2.1–17.2%
(E)-8-Acetylthio-p-menthan-3-one	0.4–10.4%
Menthone	1.3–7.0%
(−)-(E)-α-Pulegone	1.8–4.8%
8-Hydroxymenthone	0–4.7%
(+)-(Z)-α-Pulegone	2.2–3.9%
(Z)-8-Mercapto-p-menthan-3-one	0–3.1%
β-Myrcene	0.1–2.6%
(E)-β-Ocimene	0.1–2.6%
(E)-8-Mercapto-p-menthan-3-one	0–2.5%
α-Pinene	0.5–2.0%
1,8-Cineole	tr–1.9%
Sabinene	tr–1.8%
(Z)-8-Acetylthio-p-menthan-3-one	0.1–1.6%
β-Pinene	0.2–1.3%
8-Hydroxy-4-menthen-3-one	1.0%

(Collins et al 1996, Posthumus et al 1996)
Quality: May be adulterated with monoterpene sulfides, such as *p*-mentan-8-thiol-3-one (Burfield 2003).

Safety summary

Hazards: May be abortifacient; hepatotoxicity.
Contraindications (all routes): Pregnancy, breastfeeding.
Contraindications: Should not be taken in oral doses.
Maximum dermal use level: 1.4%

Our safety advice

Our dermal maximum is based on 81.9% total pulegone content and a pulegone limit of 1.2% (see β-Pulegone profile, Chapter 14).

Regulatory guidelines

The CEFS of the Council of Europe identifies pulegone as hepatotoxic, and has set a TDI of 0.1 mg/kg. Both the UK and EC 'standard permitted proportion' of pulegone in food flavorings is 25 mg/kg of food (Anon 1992b, European Community Council 1988).

Organ-specific effects

No information found.

Systemic effects

Acute toxicity: No information found for *Agathosma crenulata* oil. It is presumed to be toxic because of its content of pulegone, and is likely to present a risk similar to that of pennyroyal oil. Pulegone is hepatotoxic because it is metabolized to epoxides. It is especially toxic by mouth; rat acute oral LD_{50} 500 mg/kg (Opdyke 1978 p. 867–868).
Carcinogenic/anticarcinogenic potential: No information found, but *A. crenulata* oil contains no known carcinogens. (+)-Limonene displays anticarcinogenic activity (see (+)-Limonene profile, Chapter 14).

Comments

Our oral maximum for pulegone is 0.5 mg/kg/day, which would extrapolate to an adult oral dose of 43 mg. However, since there is no significant benefit from using *A. crenulata* oil medicinally, on a risk/benefit basis, it is best avoided. Very few data exist on the biological effects of buchu oils. This species is a less common source of buchu leaves or essential oil. The *British Herbal Compendium* gives pregnancy as a contraindication for buchu leaves (Bradley 1992).

Buddha wood

Synonyms: Desert rosewood
Botanical name: *Eremophila mitchellii* Benth.
Family: Myoporaceae

Essential oil

Source: Heartwood
Key constituents:

Eremophilone	43.0%
9-Hydroxy-7(11),9eremophiladien-8-one	18.0%
Santalcamphor	17.5%
β-Selenene	1.7%
9-Hydroxy-1,7(11),9eremophilatrien-8-one	1.0%

(Beattie et al 2011)
Quality: The oil has a tendency to polymerize.

Safety summary

Hazards: None known.
Contraindications: None known.

Organ-specific effects

No information found.

Systemic effects

Acute toxicity: No information found for Buddha wood oil or any of its known constituents.
Carcinogenic/anticarcinogenic potential: Buddha wood oil showed in vitro activity against mouse lymphoblast P388D1 cells, with an IC_{50} of 70 μg/mL. Eremophilone was more active, with an IC_{50} of 19 μg/mL (Beattie et al 2011).

Comments

The compositional data given here are averages. There are many sesquiterpenoids present in the oil that are yet to be fully characterized (Cornwell, private communication, 2004). The oil is either steam distilled or extracted with hexane followed by high vacuum distillation (Burfield 2000).

Cabreuva

Synonym: Cabureicica
Botanical name: *Myrocarpus fastigiatus* Allemão
Family: Fabaceae (Leguminosae)

Essential oil

Source: Wood
Key constituents:

(Z)-Nerolidol	c65–80%
Farnesol	2.5%

(Lawrence 1989 p. 63, 1995g p. 90–91)

Safety summary

Hazards: None known.
Contraindications: None known.

Organ-specific effects

Adverse skin reactions: Undiluted cabreuva oil was moderately irritating to rabbits, but was not irritating to mice or pigs; tested at 6% on 25 volunteers it was neither irritating nor sensitizing. The oil is non-phototoxic (Opdyke & Letizia 1982 p. 645).

Systemic effects

Acute toxicity: Cabreuva oil acute oral LD_{50} in rats >5 g/kg; acute dermal LD_{50} in rabbits >5 g/kg (Opdyke & Letizia 1982 p. 645).
Carcinogenic/anticarcinogenic potential: No information found, but cabreuva oil contains no known carcinogens.

Nerolidol and farnesol exhibit anticarcinogenic properties (see Constituent profiles, Chapter 14).

Comments

The tree, which produces a very hard wood, grows wild in Brazil and Argentina, and the oil is distilled from waste chippings and sawdust in Brazil. *Myrocarpus frondosus*, the source of Caboré oil, may also be a source of cabreuva oil, so there appears to be some confusion between the two oils.

Cade (rectified)

Synonym: Juniper tar
Botanical name: *Juniperus oxycedrus* L.
Family: Cupressaceae (Coniferae)

Essential oil

Source: Wood, by destructive distillation
Key constituents:

δ-Cadinene	24.2%
Torreyol (+ 3 other alcohols)	9.3%
Epicubenol	8.7%
Zonarene	8.1%
β-Caryophyllene	6.1%
(E)-Calamenene	5.1%
α-Caryophyllene	4.3%
14-Hydroxy-α-caryophyllene	2.8%
Gleenol	0.4%
α-Calacorene	2.3%
α-Muurolene	2.3%
Cadalene	1.3%
α-Selinene	1.2%
14-Oxo-α-caryophyllene	1.1%
14-Hydroxy-δ-cadinene	1.0%

(Abisset, private communication, 2004)

Safety summary

Hazards: Toxicity.
Contraindications: Should not be taken in oral doses.

Regulatory guidelines

The IFRA Code of Practice requires that crude cade oil should not be used as fragrance ingredient. Only rectified (purified) cade oils may be used. Whether used alone or in conjunction with birch tar oil, the final product may not contain more than 1 ppb of PAHs. PAHs may include benzo[a]pyrene and 1,2-benzanthracene (IFRA 2009).

Organ-specific effects

Adverse skin reactions: Undiluted rectified cade oil was not irritating to rabbit or mouse skin; tested at 2% on 25 volunteers it was neither irritating nor sensitizing. It is non-phototoxic

(Opdyke 1975 p. 733–734). A 3% concentration of rectified cade oil produced two mild irritation reactions in 25 volunteers (Bouhlal et al 1988a).

Systemic effects

Acute toxicity (human): See Cade oil (unrectified) below.
Acute toxicity (animal): Rectified cade oil acute oral LD_{50} in rats reported as 8.0 g/kg (Jenner et al 1964) and >5 g/kg; acute dermal LD_{50} in rabbits >5 g/kg (Opdyke 1975 p. 733–734).
Carcinogenic/anticarcinogenic potential: No information found. Benzo[a]pyrene, a polynuclear hydrocarbon, is a well-known carcinogen (Budavari 1989). It is present in rectified cade oil at up to 20 ppb, less than the concentration found in some foodstuffs (Bouhlal et al 1988a).

Comments

Cade is the name of the oil, but the plant it comes from is known as prickly juniper. Cade oil is generally prepared by dry distillation, without water or steam. This causes the wood to burn, which in turn leads to the formation of the PAHs found in the commercial oil. As the essential oil in the wood distils over, it is followed by a tar-like material which dissolves in the essential oil. Commercial cade oil is a mixture of both. Burning organic material, such as (juniper) wood or (tobacco) leaves generally produces carcinogenic PAHs. Benzo[a]pyrene is one of the carcinogenic compounds found in cigarette smoke. Since unrectified cade oil is potentially carcinogenic and the rectified oil is not, it is clearly important to distinguish between the two, as with birch tar oil.

Cade (unrectified)

Synonym: Juniper tar
Botanical name: *Juniperus oxycedrus* L.
Family: Cupressaceae (Coniferae)

Essential oil

Source: Wood, by destructive distillation
Key constituents:

δ-Cadinene	Principal constituent
α-Cedrene	<15.0%
β-Caryophyllene	Undetermined
γ-Muurolene	Undetermined
Cresols	<2.5%
Guaiacol	<1.5%
Phenol	<0.7%

(Burfield 2000)

Safety summary

Hazards: Potentially carcinogenic, based on benzo[a]pyrene content.
Contraindications: Should not be used, either internally or externally.

Regulatory guidelines

The IFRA Code of Practice requires that crude cade oil should not be used as fragrance ingredient. Only rectified (purified) cade oils may be used. Whether used alone or in conjunction with birch tar oil, the final product may not contain more than 1 ppb of PAHs. PAHs may include benzo[a]pyrene and 1,2-benzanthracene (IFRA 2009).

Organ-specific effects

Adverse skin reactions: Unrectified cade oil, tested at 3%, produced one mild irritation reaction in 25 volunteers (Bouhlal et al 1988a). Unrectified cade oil produced a worrying level of (potentially carcinogenic) DNA adducts in the skin of psoriasis patients receiving cade oil therapy (Schoket et al 1990).

Systemic effects

Acute toxicity (human): A case is reported of a previously healthy man who ingested a 'spoonful' of home-made extract of *Juniperus oxycedrus*. The poisoning caused fever, severe hypotension, renal failure, hepatotoxicity, and severe cutaneous burns on the face. After supportive and symptomatic treatment, the patient improved and was discharged in a good condition on the eleventh day (Koruk et al 2005). A 1-month-old Moroccan child had cade oil liberally applied to patches of atopic dermatitis on his face, neck and arms. Thirty minutes later he began convulsing and experiencing respiratory distress. Other signs and symptoms of poisoning included tachycardia, unrecordably low blood pressure, acute pulmonary edema, renal failure and hepatotoxicity. He recovered fully after 11 days of intensive care (Achour et al 2011). An infant of four months experienced a similar pattern of symptoms immediately following the administration by his mother of a traditional medicine based on cade oil, by intrarectal instillation to treat seborrheic dermatitis. He recovered after 3 days in intensive care (Rahmani et al 2004).
Carcinogenic/anticarcinogenic potential: Unrectified cade oil was mutagenic in two assays (Takizawa et al 1985), and was classified as weakly genotoxic (Ueno et al 1984, cited in Anon 2001b). Genotoxicity has been demonstrated in excised human skin, following application of cade oil (Phillips et al 1990; Schoket et al 1990). Benzo[a]pyrene, a polynuclear hydrocarbon, is a well-known carcinogen (Budavari 1989). It is present in unrectified cade oil at 8 ppm.

Comments

Unrectified cade oil may contain 8 ppm benzo[a]pyrene. Unrectified cade oil is still produced in the Atlas mountains of Morocco, where it has been used in traditional medicine for centuries, notably for skin lesions. 'Medicinal tar' is produced from *J. oxycedrus*, *J. phoenicea*, *J. thurifera* and several other plant species (www.ibg.uu.se/digitalAssets/106/106208_julin-madeleine.pdf accessed August 30th 2012). Also see cade (rectified).

Cajuput

Synonyms: Cajeput, river tea tree, swamp tea tree, weeping tea tree, punk tree

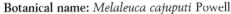

Botanical name: *Melaleuca cajuputi* Powell
Botanical synonym: *Melaleuca leucadendron* var. *cajuputi* Roxb.
Family: Myrtaceae

Essential oil

Source: Leaves and twigs
Key constituents:

Vietnamese

1,8-Cineole	41.1–70.8%
α-Terpineol	6.5–8.7%
p-Cymene	0.7–6.8%
Terpinolene	0–5.9%
γ-Terpinene	1.2–4.6%
(+)-Limonene	3.8–4.1%
Linalool	2.7–3.6%
α-Pinene	2.1–3.2%
β-Caryophyllene	0.7–2.5%
β-Myrcene	0.9–2.0%
α-Caryophyllene	0.5–1.6%
β-Pinene	0.8–1.5%
Terpinen-4-ol	0.6–1.5%
β-Selinene	0–1.5%
α-Selinene	0–1.5%
Guaiol	0–1.2%

(Motl et al 1990; Milchard et al 2004)
Quality: Eucalyptus oil may be added or substituted, as may oils from *M. quinquenervia* or *M. symphyocarpa*. Fixed oils or kerosene are occasionally used as adulterants (Oyen & Dung 1999).

Safety summary

Hazards: Essential oils high in 1,8-cineole can cause CNS and breathing problems in young children.
Contraindications: Do not apply to or near the face of infants or children.

Organ-specific effects

Adverse skin reactions: Undiluted cajuput oil was not irritating to the skin of rabbits, mice or pigs; tested at 4% on 25 volunteers it was neither irritating nor sensitizing. It is non-phototoxic (Opdyke 1976 p. 701). 1,8-Cineole presents a low risk of both skin irritation and sensitization (see 1,8-Cineole profile, Chapter 14).
Reproductive toxicity: The low reproductive toxicity of 1,8-cineole, (+)-limonene, linalool and α-pinene (see Constituent profiles, Chapter 14) suggests that cajuput oil is not hazardous in pregnancy.

Systemic effects

Acute toxicity (human): 1,8-Cineole has been reported to cause serious poisoning in young children when accidentally instilled into the nose (Melis et al 1989).

Acute toxicity (animal): Cajuput oil acute oral LD_{50} in rats 3.87 g/kg; acute dermal LD_{50} in rabbits >5 g/kg (Jenner et al 1964).
Carcinogenic/anticarcinogenic potential: No information found. 1,8-Cineole is non-mutagenic and shows no evidence of carcinogenesis in rodents (see 1,8-Cineole profile, Chapter 14).

Comments

Cajuput oil was formerly thought to originate from *Melaleuca leucadendra* L. It is commercially produced in Vietnam, China and Indonesia.

Calamint (lesser)

Synonyms: Cuckoo flower, field balm, nepitella
Botanical name: *Calamintha nepeta* L. subsp. *glandulosa* Req.
Botanical synonym: *Calamintha officinalis* Moench.
Family: Lamiaceae (Labiatae)

Essential oil

Source: Aerial parts
Key constituents:

(1*R*)-(+)-β-Pulegone	17.6–76.1%
Menthone	7.0–55.8%
Piperitenone	0–7.3%
Piperitone oxide	0–12.4%
Piperitone	0–7.4%
(+)-Limonene	0.6–7.2%
Terpinen-4-ol	0–6.8%
(*E*)-Sabinene hydrate	0–3.5%
Isomenthone	0–2.8%
3-Octanol	1.0–2.1%
Piperitenone oxide	0–1.1%

(Ristorcelli et al 1996)

Safety summary

Hazards: May be abortifacient; hepatotoxicity.
Contraindications (all routes): Pregnancy, breastfeeding.
Contraindications: Should not be taken in oral doses.
Maximum dermal use level: 1.5%

Our safety advice

Our dermal maximum is based on 76.1% β-pulegone content and a dermal limit of 1.2% (see β-Pulegone profile, Chapter 14).

Regulatory guidelines

The CEFS of the Council of Europe identifies pulegone as hepatotoxic, and has set a TDI of 0.1 mg/kg bw. Both the UK and EC 'standard permitted proportion' of pulegone in food flavorings is 25 mg/kg of food (Anon 1992b, European Community Council 1988).

Organ-specific effects

Hepatotoxicity: No information found. In rats, $(1R)$-$(+)$-β-pulegone depletes hepatic glutathione (Thomassen et al 1990), and in doses of >200 mg/kg, it destroys hepatic CYP (Moorthy et al 1989a).

Systemic effects

Acute toxicity: No information found. Pulegone is toxic to the liver because it is metabolized to epoxides. It is especially toxic by mouth; acute oral LD_{50} 500 mg/kg in rats (Opdyke 1978 p. 867–868).
Carcinogenic/anticarcinogenic potential: No information found for lesser calamint oil, but it contains no known carcinogens. Limonene exhibits anticarcinogenic activity (see $(+)$-Limonene profile, Chapter 14).

Comments

Our oral maximum for pulegone is 0.5 mg/kg/day, which would extrapolate to an adult oral dose of 46 mg. However, since there is no significant benefit from using lesser calamint oil medicinally, on a risk/benefit basis, it is best avoided. There are two subspecies, and the other one, *Calamintha nepeta* subsp. *nepeta*, has two chemotypes, a pulegone and a piperitone oxide. The *glandulosa* subspecies has piperitone oxide and piperitenone oxide chemotypes in addition to the commercially available pulegone chemotype, which most commonly contains ~40% of the ketone. This essential oil is sometimes confused with catnep oil (*Nepeta cataria*). Limited availability.

Calamus (diploid form)

Synonyms: North American calamus, sweet flag
Botanical name: *Acorus calamus* L. var. *americanus* (Raf.) Wulff
Family: Araceae

Essential oil

Source: Rhizomes
Key constituents:

Shyobunones	13.0–45.0%
Acorenone	9.0–13.0%
Preisocalamendiol	7.0–12.0%
Acorone + isoacarone	8.0–10.0%
Isocalamendiol	2.0–3.0%
β-Sesquiphellandrene	0–3.0%
Calamendiol	1.0%
α-Cadinol	1.0%
δ-Cadinene	1.0%

(Lawrence 1981 p. 47–48, 1989 p. 77–78)

Safety summary

Hazards: None known.
Contraindications: None known.

Organ-specific effects

Adverse skin reactions: No information found for diploid calamus oil, or any of its major constituents.

Systemic effects

Acute toxicity: No information found for diploid calamus oil, or any of its major constituents.
Carcinogenic/anticarcinogenic potential: No information found for diploid calamus oil, but it contains no known carcinogens. α-Cadinol is active against the human colon cancer cell line HT-29 (He et al 1997a).

Comments

The diploid form of calamus is found in North America and Siberia. This cytotype of *Acorus calamus*, which contains no β-asarone, has been identified by DNA sequencing (Bertea et al 2005). However, the toxicology of this type of oil and its major constituents remains unknown.

Calamus (tetraploid or hexaploid form)

Synonyms: East Asian calamus, Jammu calamus, sweet flag
Botanical name: *Acorus calamus* L. var. *angustatus* Bess.
Family: Araceae

Essential oil

Source: Rhizomes
Key constituents:

β-Asarone	42.5–78.4%
Isoeugenol	2.3–25.0%
Calamenene	3.8–5.0%
Calamene	3.8%
Calamol	3.2–7.8%
Asaronaldehyde	tr–5.7%
Methyl isoeugenol	tr–2.8%
Methyleugenol	tr–2.0%
α-Asarone	1.3–6.8%

(Lawrence 1981 p. 47–48, 1989 p. 183–184)

Safety summary

Hazards: Toxic (moderate); hepatotoxic; carcinogenic.
Contraindications: Should not be taken in oral doses.
Maximum dermal use level:

EU	0.01%
IFRA	0.007%
Tisserand & Young	0.2%

Our safety advice

We recommend a dermal maximum of 0.2% for calamus oil, based on a 78.4% β-asarone, 6.8% α-asarone and 2% methyleugenol, with dermal limits of 0.22%, 0.33% and 0.02%, respectively (see Constituent profiles, Chapter 14).

Regulatory guidelines

β-Asarone is not permitted in the US as a pharmaceutical ingredient, while α-asarone is permitted (Harborne & Baxter 1993). Both the UK and EC 'standard permitted proportion' of β-asarone in food flavorings is 0.1 mg/kg of food (Anon 1992b; European Community Council 1988). IFRA recommends that asarone should not be used as a fragrance ingredient, and that its level in consumer products containing calamus oil should not exceed 0.01% (IFRA 2009). IFRA recommends that the maximum concentration of methyleugenol in leave-on products such as body lotion should be 0.0004% (IFRA 2009). The equivalent SCCNFP maximum is 0.0002% (European Commission 2002). *Acorus calamus* is one of 30 herbs listed as unsafe by the FDA (Anon 1975).

Organ-specific effects

Adverse skin reactions: Undiluted calamus oil was not irritating to the skin of mice, guinea pigs, rabbits or pigs; tested at 4% on 25 volunteers it was neither irritating nor sensitizing (Opdyke 1977a p. 623–626). In a study of 200 consecutive dermatitis patients, none were sensitive to 2% calamus oil on patch testing (Rudzki et al 1976). Calamus oil is non-phototoxic (Opdyke 1977a p. 623–626).

Systemic effects

Acute toxicity: Calamus oil acute oral LD_{50} in rats 777 mg/kg (Jenner et al 1964); acute ip LD_{50} in rats 221 mg/kg; acute dermal LD_{50} in guinea pigs >5 g/kg (Opdyke 1977a p. 623–626); severe liver and kidney damage were found on investigation (Von Skramlik 1959).

Subacute & subchronic toxicity: Rats were given calamus oil in the diet at 2,500, 5,000 and 10,000 ppm for 18 weeks, equivalent to 100, 250 and 1,000 mg/kg. At 250 mg/kg and above, numerous gross and microscopic changes in the liver were seen; dose-related growth depression and slight myocardial degeneration were evident in all dosed groups (Hagan et al 1967). Atrophy of cardiac muscle was seen in rats fed 1 g/kg of Jammu calamus oil for 9–14 weeks (JECFA 1981). A NOAEL for cardiac adverse effects of the oil has been estimated at 5 mg/kg/day (SCF 2002a,b). In rats fed 0.1% calamus oil in the diet for 13 weeks (equivalent to 71 mg/kg bw), growth was depressed, but there were no adverse effects on clinical chemistry, hematology, urinalysis or organ weights (unpublished report, cited in JECFA 1981).

Carcinogenic/anticarcinogenic potential: Given daily in the diet at 0.005 mL/kg/bw to mice for 35 days, calamus oil was genotoxic, producing a high frequency of CA in bone marrow (Balachandran et al 1991). Jammu calamus oil given at 500, 1,000, 2,500 and 5,000 ppm to rats for 59 weeks produced growth retardation and increased the likelihood of malignant duodenal tumors at all doses, equivalent to 25, 50, 125 and 250 mg/kg/day (Taylor et al 1967). Methyleugenol and β-asarone are genotoxic carcinogens (see Constituent profiles, Chapter 14).

Comments

The tetraploid form is the type of calamus oil generally offered commercially, originating in India.

Calamus (triploid form)

Synonyms: European calamus, sweet flag
Botanical name: *Acorus calamus* L. var. *calamus*
Botanical synonym: *Acorus calamus* L. var. *vulgaris*
Family: Araceae

Essential oil

Source: Rhizomes
Key constituents:

Shyobunones	23.0–32.0%
β-Asarone	8.0–19.0%

(Lawrence 1981 p. 47–48)

Safety summary

Hazards: Potentially carcinogenic, based on β-asarone content.
Contraindications: None known.
Maximum adult oral daily dose: 37 mg
Maximum dermal use level:

EU	No limit
IFRA	0.05%
Tisserand & Young	1.1%

Our safety advice

We recommend a daily oral maximum of 37 mg and a maximum dermal use level of 1.1%, based on a 19% β-asarone content with an oral maximum of 0.1 mg/kg/day and a dermal limit of 0.22% (see β-Asarone profile, Chapter 14).

Regulatory guidelines

β-Asarone is banned in the US as a pharmaceutical ingredient. Both the UK and EC 'standard permitted proportion' of β-asarone in food flavorings is 0.0001 g/kg (European Community Council 1988, Anon 1992b). IFRA recommends that β-asarone should not be used as a fragrance ingredient, and that the level of asarone in consumer products containing calamus oil should not exceed 0.01% (IFRA 2009).

Organ-specific effects

No information found.

Systemic effects

Acute toxicity: A European calamus oil with ~5% β-asarone had a rat oral LD_{50} of 3,497 mg/kg (JECFA 1981).
Subacute & subchronic toxicity: For 5 days, pre-weaning rats were given ip doses of European calamus oil at 100 or 250 mg/kg. There were no deaths, but weight loss and decreased food consumption were noted, as were increases in adrenal weights, and reductions in heart and thymus weights. There was no effect on hematology, nor on liver enzyme levels (Ramos-Ocampo & Hsia 1987). Atrophy of cardiac muscle was seen in rats fed 1 g/kg of European calamus oil for 9–14 weeks (JECFA 1981).
Carcinogenic/anticarcinogenic potential: Calamus oil (triploid form) was not mutagenic in any of four concentrations, in six

S. typhimurium strains, with or without metabolic activation, and did not induce UDS in isolated rat hepatocytes (Ramos-Ocampo & Hsia 1988). Male and female rats were fed European calamus oil in the diet for 2 years, equivalent to doses of 50, 250, 500 and 1,000 mg/kg/day. In the higher two dose groups, there was increased incidence of malignant tumors in the liver and duodenum (unpublished study, cited by JECFA 1981).

Comments

This form of calamus is found in Eurasia.

Camphor (Borneo)

Synonyms: Barus camphor, Malay camphor, Sumatra camphor
Botanical name: *Dryobalanops aromatica* Gaertn.
Botanical synonym: *Dryobalanops camphora* Colebr.
Family: Dipterocarpaceae

Essential oil
Source: Wood
Key constituents:

α-Pinene	54.3%
β-Caryophyllene	18.1%
Borneol	8.3%
α-Caryophyllene	4.3%
α-Terpineol	3.0%
β-Pinene	2.5%
(+)-Limonene	2.5%

(Cornwell, private communication, 2004)

Safety summary

Hazards: Skin sensitization if oxidized.
Cautions: Old or oxidized oils should be avoided.

Our safety advice

Because of its high α-pinene content we recommend that oxidation of Borneo camphor oil is avoided by storage in a dark, airtight container in a refrigerator. The addition of an antioxidant to preparations containing it is recommended.

Organ-specific effects

Adverse skin reactions: No information found. Autoxidation products of α-pinene can cause skin sensitization (see α-Pinene profile, Chapter 14).

Systemic effects

Acute toxicity: No information found. α-Pinene acute oral LD_{50} in rats reported as 2.1, 3.2 and 3.7 g/kg; acute dermal LD_{50} in rabbits <5 g.kg (Opdyke 1978 p. 853–857).
Carcinogenic/anticarcinogenic potential: No information found for Borneo camphor oil, but it contains no known carcinogens.

β-Caryophyllene, (+)-limonene and α-caryophyllene display anticarcinogenic activity (see Constituent profiles, Chapter 14).

Comments

The compositional data given here are averages.

Camphor (brown)

Synonym: Camphor (red)
Botanical name: *Cinnamomum camphora* L.
Botanical synonym: *Laurus camphora* L.
Family: Lauraceae

Essential oil

Source: Wood and branches
Note: See camphor (white) profile for comments on camphor and camphor oils.
Key constituents:

Safrole	50–60%
Camphor	<3.0%

(Guenther 1949–1952 vol. 4 p. 301)

Safety summary

Hazards: Potentially carcinogenic, based on safrole content.
Contraindications: Should not be used, either internally or externally.

Our safety advice

Due to its high safrole content we recommend that brown camphor oil is not used in therapy.

Regulatory guidelines

IFRA and the EU recommend a maximum exposure level of 0.01% of safrole from the use of safrole-containing essential oils in cosmetics.

Organ-specific effects

Adverse skin reactions: Undiluted brown camphor oil was not irritating to rabbit, pig or mouse skin; tested at 4% on 25 volunteers it was neither irritating nor sensitizing. It is non-phototoxic (Opdyke 1976 p. 703).

Systemic effects

Acute toxicity: Brown camphor oil acute oral LD_{50} in rats 2.53 mL/kg; acute dermal LD_{50} in rabbits >4 mL/kg (Opdyke 1976 p. 703). The minimum lethal oral dose of safrole in the rabbit is 1.0 g/kg (Spector 1956).
Carcinogenic/anticarcinogenic potential: No information found. Safrole and its 2′,3′-epoxy, 1′-hydroxy and 1′-sulfate metabolites can form adducts with DNA and other macromolecules in the liver, and safrole is a weak carcinogen in rodents.

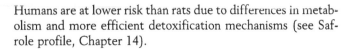

Humans are at lower risk than rats due to differences in metabolism and more efficient detoxification mechanisms (see Safrole profile, Chapter 14).

Comments

Brown camphor oil is not normally available commercially, as it is commonly used for the isolation of safrole or 1,8-cineole. Brown camphor oil is sometimes sold as 'Chinese sassafras oil'. See comments under Camphor (white).

Camphor (white)

Synonym: Hon-sho (true camphor)
Botanical name: *Cinnamomum camphora* L.
Botanical synonym: *Laurus camphora* L.
Family: Lauraceae

Essential oil

Source: Wood and branches
Key constituents:

(+)-Limonene	44.2%
p-Cymene	24.2%
α-Pinene	8.9%
1,8-Cineole	6.5%
Sabinene	4.2%
β-Pinene	4.0%
Camphene	3.0%
Camphor	2.4%
Safrole	tr

(Burfield, private communication, 2003)
Quality: White camphor oil is not subject to adulteration (Burfield 2003).

Safety summary

Hazards: Skin sensitization if oxidized.
Cautions: Old or oxidized oils should be avoided.

Our safety advice

Because of its (+)-limonene and α-pinene content we recommend that oxidation of white camphor oil is avoided by storage in a dark, airtight container in a refrigerator. The addition of an antioxidant to preparations containing it is recommended.

Regulatory guidelines

IFRA recommends that essential oils rich in limonene should only be used when the level of peroxides is kept to the lowest practical level, for instance by adding antioxidants at the time of production (IFRA 2009).

Organ-specific effects

Adverse skin reactions: In a modified Draize procedure on guinea pigs, white camphor oil was non-sensitizing when used at 30% in the challenge phase (Sharp 1978). Undiluted white camphor oil was mildly irritating to rabbits; tested at 20% on 25 volunteers it was neither irritating nor sensitizing (Opdyke 1973 p. 1047). Autoxidation products of (+)-limonene and α-pinene can cause skin sensitization; 1,8-cineole has antioxidant properties (see Constituent profiles, Chapter 14).
Reproductive toxicity: The low reproductive toxicity of (+)-limonene, α-pinene and 1,8-cineole (see Constituent profiles, Chapter 14) suggests that white camphor oil is not hazardous in pregnancy.

Systemic effects

Acute toxicity: White camphor oil acute oral LD_{50} in rats 5.1 mL/kg; acute dermal LD_{50} in rabbits >5 mL/kg (Opdyke 1973 p. 1047).
Carcinogenic/anticarcinogenic potential: No information found. Safrole is a rodent carcinogen, and (+)-limonene displays anticarcinogenic activity (see Constituent profiles, Chapter 14).

Comments

The presence in white camphor oil of traces of safrole is not a cause for concern. Camphor is the name of a tree, the name of its essential oil, and the name of a chemical constituent found in this, and other essential oils. The crude exudate from the tree contains around 50% of camphor. Camphor oil is separated into four distinct 'essential oils' by fractional distillation, after the crude camphor crystals are removed by filtration. These fractions are known as white camphor oil (a light fraction), brown camphor oil (a medium fraction), yellow camphor oil (another medium fraction) and blue camphor oil (a heavy fraction). Because of this fractionation process, none of these can be classed as true essential oils. White camphor oil, the most widely used therapeutically of these, contains very little camphor. In addition, the camphor plant exists in five chemotypes - borneol, nerolidol, camphor, 1,8-cineole and linalool. Only the last three are commercially available. Oils from the leaves of these plants are known as ho leaf oils.

Camphor (yellow)

Botanical name: *Cinnamomum camphora* L.
Botanical synonym: *Laurus camphora* L.
Family: Lauraceae

Essential oil

Source: Wood and branches
Key constituents:

Safrole	20%

(Guenther 1949–1952 vol. 4 p. 303)

Safety summary

Hazards: Potentially carcinogenic, based on safrole content.
Contraindications: Should not be taken in oral doses.

Maximum dermal use level:

EU	0.05%
IFRA	0.05%
Tisserand & Young	0.25%

Our safety advice

We recommend a dermal maximum of 0.25%, based on 20% safrole content with a dermal limit of 0.05% (see Safrole profile, Chapter 14).

Regulatory guidelines

IFRA and the EU recommend a maximum exposure level of 0.01% of safrole from the use of safrole-containing essential oils in cosmetics.

Organ-specific effects

Adverse skin reactions: Undiluted yellow camphor oil was slightly irritating to rabbits, but was not irritating to mice; tested at 4% on 25 volunteers it was neither irritating nor sensitizing. It is non-phototoxic (Opdyke 1975 p. 739–740).

Systemic effects

Acute toxicity: Yellow camphor oil acute oral LD_{50} in rats 3.73 g/kg; acute dermal LD_{50} in rabbits >5 g/kg (Opdyke 1975 p. 739–740).
Carcinogenic/anticarcinogenic potential: No information found. Safrole and its 2′,3′-epoxy, 1′-hydroxy and 1′-sulfate metabolites can form adducts with DNA and other macromolecules in the liver, and safrole is a weak carcinogen in rodents. Humans are at lower risk than rats due to differences in metabolism and more efficient detoxification mechanisms (see Safrole profile, Chapter 14).

Comments

See camphor (white) profile for comments on camphor and camphor oils. Yellow camphor oil may be carcinogenic, due to its safrole content. Yellow camphor oil is not normally available commercially, as it is commonly used for the isolation of safrole or 1,8-cineole. See comments under camphor (white).

Cananga

Botanical name: *Cananga odorata* (Lam.) J. D. Hook and T. Thompson f. *macrophylla* Koolhaas
Botanical synonym: *Canangium odoratum* f. *macrophylla*
Family: Annonaceae

Essential oil

Source: Flowers
Key constituents:

β-Caryophyllene	38.2%
α-Caryophyllene	9.2%
Germacrene D	8.3%
δ-Cadinene	6.0%
Linalool	5.6%
(Z,Z)-α-Farnesene	4.4%
(E,E)-α-Farnesene	3.8%
γ-Muurolene	2.7%
p-Cresyl methyl ether	2.6%
Benzyl benzoate	2.0%
α-Copaene	1.8%
Geraniol	1.5%
Geranyl acetate	1.5%
α-Muurolene	1.5%
Bicyclosesquiphellandrene	1.1%
α-Cadinol	1.1%
Methyleugenol	0.07%

(Kubeczka 2002)

Safety summary

Hazards: May contain methyleugenol; skin sensitization (moderate risk).
Contraindications: None known.
Maximum dermal use level (based on methyleugenol content):

EU	0.3%
IFRA	0.6%
Tisserand & Young	28%

Maximum dermal use level (based on skin sensitization):

EU	No legal limit
IFRA	0.8%
Tisserand & Young	0.8%

Our safety advice

We recommend the IFRA dermal maximum of 0.8% for skin sensitization. (The IFRA limit of 0.8% does not seem to account for as much as 0.07% methyleugenol, which would suggest a lower limit according to the IFRA standard for methyleugenol.)

Regulatory guidelines

Has GRAS status. Maximum dermal use level of 0.8% based on IFRA guidelines for cananga oil (IFRA 2009). IFRA recommends that the maximum concentration of methyleugenol for leave-on products such as body lotion should be 0.0004% (IFRA 2009). The equivalent SCCNFP maximum is 0.0002% (European Commission 2002).

Organ-specific effects

Adverse skin reactions: In a modified Draize procedure on guinea pigs, cananga oil was non-sensitizing when used at 10% in the challenge phase (Sharp 1978). Undiluted cananga oil was irritating to rabbits; tested at 10% on 25 volunteers it was neither irritating nor sensitizing (Opdyke 1973 p. 1049). In a study of 200 consecutive dermatitis patients, one was sensitive to 2% cananga oil on patch testing (Rudzki et al 1976). From 1990 to 1998 the average patch test positivity rate to 5% cananga oil in

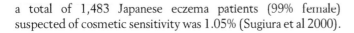

a total of 1,483 Japanese eczema patients (99% female) suspected of cosmetic sensitivity was 1.05% (Sugiura et al 2000).

Systemic effects

Acute toxicity: Acute oral LD_{50} in rats >5 g/kg; acute dermal LD_{50} in rabbits >5 g/kg (Opdyke 1973 p. 1049).
Carcinogenic/anticarcinogenic potential: No information found. Methyleugenol is a rodent hepatocarcinogen when exposure is sufficiently high. β-Caryophyllene and α-caryophyllene display anticarcinogenic activity, and linalool and geraniol display anti-hepatocarcinogenic activity (see Constituent profiles, Chapter 14). α-Cadinol is active against the human colon cancer cell line HT-29 (He et al 1997a).

Comments

It is possible that the anticarcinogenic activity of β-caryophyllene and α-caryophyllene would prevent any carcinogenic effect from the methyleugenol. Unlike ylang-ylang oil, the other commercial form of *Cananga odorata*, cananga oil is not fractionated on distillation.

Cangerana

Botanical name: *Cabralea cangerana* Saldanha
Botanical synonym: *Cabralea canjerana* Saldanha
Family: Meliaceae

Essential oil

Source: Wood
Key constituents:

β-Caryophyllene	28.6%
Germacrene D	9.3%
δ-Cadinene	7.4%
Germacrene B	6.2%
γ-Muurolene	5.0%
α-Calacorene	2.9%
γ-Cadinene	2.7%
α-Muurolene	2.4%
γ-Elemene	2.4%
δ-Elemene	2.3%
α-Copaene	2.1%
Caryolan-8-ol	1.8%
α-Caryophyllene	1.8%
γ-Amorphene	1.4%
β-Elemene	1.3%
(+)-Aromadendrene	1.1%
Safrole	0.5%

(Weyerstahl et al 1996)

Safety summary

Hazards: Potentially carcinogenic, based on safrole content.
Contraindications: None known.
Maximum adult daily oral dose: 350 mg

Maximum dermal use level:

EU	2.0%
IFRA	2.0%
Tisserand & Young	10.0%

Our safety advice

We recommend a dermal maximum of 10.0% and a daily oral maximum of 350 mg for cangerana oil based on 0.5% safrole content, with dermal and oral limits of 0.05% and 0.025 mg/kg/day for safrole (see Safrole profile, Chapter 14).

Regulatory guidelines

IFRA and the EU recommend a maximum exposure level of 0.01% of safrole from the use of safrole-containing essential oils in cosmetics.

Organ-specific effects

Adverse skin reactions: No information found for cangerana oil, but it contains no constituents known to be skin irritants or sensitizers.

Systemic effects

Acute toxicity: No information found. The majority of the constituents are non-toxic.
Carcinogenic/anticarcinogenic potential: No information found. Safrole is a rodent carcinogen when exposure is sufficiently high. β-Caryophyllene, α-caryophyllene and β-elemene exhibit anticarcinogenic activity (see Constituent profiles, Chapter 14).

Comments

Limited availability.

Cape May

Botanical name: *Coleonema album* (Thunb.) Bartl. & J.C. Wendl.
Family: Rutaceae

Essential oil

Source: Leaves and stem
Key constituents:

β-Myrcene	43.8%
β-Phellandrene + (+)-limonene	32.5%
(Z)-β-Ocimene	4.0%
Germacrene D	3.3%
α-Pinene	2.9%
Bicyclogermacrene	1.7%
β-Caryophyllene	1.7%
α-Phellandrene	1.6%
Sabinene	1.3%
Linalool	1.1%

(Graven, private communication, 1999)
Quality: Cape may oil polymerizes on ageing.

Safety summary

Hazards: None known.
Contraindications: None known.

Our safety advice

We recommend that degradation of Cape may oil is avoided by storage in a dark, airtight container in a refrigerator. The addition of an antioxidant to preparations containing it is recommended.

Organ-specific effects

Adverse skin reactions: No information found for Cape may oil or β-phellandrene. Little is known about the action of β-myrcene on the skin.
Reproductive toxicity: Oral β-myrcene was reproductively toxic in pregnant rats at 500 mg/kg, but not at 250 mg/kg (Delgado et al 1993a, 1993b; Paumgartten et al 1998). This does not suggest any dose limitation for Cape may oil.

Systemic effects

Acute toxicity: No information found for Cape may oil or β-phellandrene. β-Myrcene is non-toxic (see β-Myrcene profile, Chapter 14).
Carcinogenic/anticarcinogenic potential: No information found. β-Myrcene is not genotoxic and demonstrates antigenotoxic activity; it is a male mouse-specific hepatocarcinogen (see β-Myrcene profile, Chapter 14).

Comments

Limited availability.

Caraway

Botanical name: *Carum carvi* L.
Family: Apiaceae (Umbelliferae)

Essential oil

Source: Seeds
Key constituents:

(+)-Carvone	47.3–59.5%
(+)-Limonene	36.9–48.8%
β-Myrcene	0.2–1.0%

(Lawrence 1995g p. 202, 2002c p. 58–59)
Quality: Caraway oil may be adulterated with synthetic carvone and limonene (Kubeczka 2002).

Safety summary

Hazards: Skin sensitization if oxidized.
Cautions: Old or oxidized oils should be avoided.

Our safety advice

We agree with the IFRA guideline of 1.2% for skin sensitization, but only for (−)-carvone. Our dermal limit for (+)-carvone is 23%, for toxicity. We recommend a human daily oral maximum dose of 12.5 mg/kg for carvone isomers (see Carvone profile, Chapter 14). Therefore, caraway oil requires no restriction. Because of its limonene content, we recommend that oxidation of caraway oil is avoided by storage in a dark, airtight container in a refrigerator. The addition of an antioxidant to preparations containing it is recommended.

Regulatory guidelines

Has GRAS status. The IFRA standard for either isomer of carvone in leave-on products such as body lotions is 1.2%, for skin sensitization. The Council of Europe (1992) has set an ADI of 1 mg/kg for carvone (isomer not specified). This is equivalent to a daily adult dose of 100–135 mg of caraway oil (depending on carvone content). IFRA recommends that essential oils rich in limonene should only be used when the level of peroxides is kept to the lowest practical level, for instance by adding antioxidants at the time of production (IFRA 2009).

Organ-specific effects

Adverse skin reactions: Undiluted caraway oil was irritating to rabbits, but was not irritating to mice or pigs; tested at 4% on 25 volunteers it was neither irritating nor sensitizing. Low-level phototoxic effects have been found for caraway oil, but these are not considered significant (Opdyke 1973 p. 1051). Autoxidation products of (+)-limonene can cause skin sensitization (see (+)-Limonene profile, Chapter 14).

Systemic effects

Acute toxicity: Caraway oil acute oral LD_{50} in rats 3.5 mL/kg; acute dermal LD_{50} in rabbits 1.78 g/kg (Opdyke 1973 p. 1051). A 1-month-old rabbit was given 60 drops of caraway oil over a few minutes. It died after being seized with convulsions (Anon 1857).
Carcinogenic/anticarcinogenic potential: Whether supplemented in the diet or applied to the skin, caraway oil inhibited DMBA-induced and croton oil-induced skin tumors in female mice, and caused regression in established papillomas (Shwaireb 1993). Caraway oil significantly induced glutathione S-transferase activity in mouse tissues (Lam & Zheng 1991). Dietary caraway oil at 0.01% or 0.1% significantly inhibited the development of pre-malignant colon cancer lesions in rats, partly through maintaining a healthy level of hepatic glutathione and CYP1A1 (Dadkhah et al 2011). (+)-Carvone is not a rodent carcinogen, and both carvone and (+)-limonene display anticarcinogenic activity (see Constituent profiles, Chapter 14).

Comments

Caraway oil capsules are used in the treatment of gastrointestinal complaints, often in conjunction with peppermint oil.

Cardamon

Botanical name: *Elettaria cardamomum* L.
Family: Zingiberaceae

Essential oil

Source: Seeds
Key constituents:

1,8-Cineole	26.5–44.6%
α-Terpinyl acetate	29.2–39.7%
Linalyl acetate	0.7–7.7%
(+)-Limonene	1.7–6.0%
Linalool	0.4–5.9%
α-Terpineol	0.8–4.3%
Sabinene	2.5–3.8%
Terpinen-4-ol	0.9–3.2%
(*E*)-Nerolidol	0.1–2.7%
β-Myrcene	0.2–2.2%
α-Pinene	0.6–1.5%
Geraniol	0.3–1.1%

(Lawrence 1995g p. 199)
Quality: Cardamon oil may be adulterated by the addition of 1,8-cineole, α-terpinyl acetate or linalyl acetate (Burfield 2003).

Safety summary

Hazards: Essential oils high in 1,8-cineole can cause CNS and breathing problems in young children.
Contraindications: Do not apply to or near the face of infants or children.

Regulatory guidelines

Has GRAS status.

Organ-specific effects

Adverse skin reactions: Undiluted cardamon oil was not irritating to the skin of either rabbits or mice; tested at 4% on 25 volunteers it was neither irritating nor sensitizing. It is non-phototoxic (Opdyke 1974 p. 837–838). 1,8-Cineole presents a low risk of both skin irritation and sensitization (see 1,8-Cineole profile, Chapter 14).
Reproductive toxicity: 1,8-Cineole shows no evidence of teratogenesis in mice at 100 mg/kg/day sc (Pages et al 1990).

Systemic effects

Acute toxicity: Cardamon oil acute oral LD_{50} in rats ~5 g/kg; acute dermal LD_{50} in rabbits >5 g/kg (Opdyke 1974 p. 837–838). 1,8-Cineole has been reported to cause serious poisoning in young children when accidentally instilled into the nose (Melis et al 1989).
Carcinogenic/anticarcinogenic potential: Cardamon oil dose-dependently inhibited aflatoxin B_1-induced adducts in calf thymus DNA, in the presence of rat liver microsomes (Hashim et al 1994). Cardamon oil significantly induced glutathione *S*-transferase in mouse liver, but significantly reduced levels of CYP (Banerjee et al 1994).

Comments

Cardamon oil significantly inhibited gastric irritation and ulcerative lesions induced by ethanol and aspirin in rats (Jamal et al 2006).

Cardamon (black)

Synonyms: Large cardamon, Nepalese cardamon, greater Indian cardamon
Botanical name: *Amomum subulatum* Roxb.
Family: Zingiberaceae

Essential oil

Source: Seeds
Key constituents:

1,8-Cineole	61.3%
β-Pinene	8.9%
α-Terpineol	7.9%
α-Pinene	3.8%
(−)-*allo*-Aromadendrene	3.2%
γ-Terpinene	2.0%
δ-Terpineol	1.6%
Terpinen-4-ol	1.3%
δ-Elemene	1.2%
β-Myrcene	1.2%

(Gurudut et al 1996)

Safety summary

Hazards: Essential oils high in 1,8-cineole can cause CNS and breathing problems in young children.
Contraindications: Do not apply to or near the face of infants or children.

Organ-specific effects

Adverse skin reactions: No information found. 1,8-Cineole presents a low risk of both skin irritation and sensitization (see 1,8-Cineole profile, Chapter 14).
Reproductive toxicity: The low reproductive toxicity of 1,8-cineole and α-pinene (see Constituent profiles, Chapter 14) suggests that black cardamon oil is not hazardous in pregnancy.

Systemic effects

Acute toxicity: No information found. Only negligible toxicity results from subchronic dosing in rodents at under 500 mg/kg (Kristiansen & Madsen 1995). 1,8-Cineole has been reported to cause serious poisoning in young children when accidentally instilled into the nose (Melis et al 1989).
Carcinogenic/anticarcinogenic potential: No information found for black cardamon oil, but it contains no known carcinogens.

Comments

Limited availability.

Carnation

Synonym: Clove pink
Botanical name: *Dianthus caryophyllus* L.
Family: Caryophyllaceae

Absolute

Source: Flowers
Key constituents:

Benzyl benzoate	5.0–14.6%
Pentacosene	8.1%
Benzyl salicylate	3.9%
Eugenol	1.7–3.6%
Heptacosene	2.7%
Methyl linoleate	2.3%
Tricosene	1.4%

(Anonis 1993, Lawrence 1989 p. 132–134)

Safety summary

Hazards: None known.
Contraindications: None known.
Maximum dermal use level: 13.9%

Our safety advice

We recommend a maximum dermal use level of 13.9%, based on 3.6% eugenol content with a dermal maximum of 0.5% (see Eugenol profile, Chapter 14).

Organ-specific effects

Adverse skin reactions: No information found.

Systemic effects

Acute toxicity: No information found for carnation absolute, but benzyl benzoate appears to be non-toxic (see Benzyl benzoate profile, Chapter 14).
Carcinogenic/anticarcinogenic potential: No information found. Neither benzyl benzoate nor benzyl salicylate is mutagenic (Florin et al 1980; Zeiger et al 1987). Eugenol exhibits anticarcinogenic activity (see Eugenol profile, Chapter 14).

Comments

Although benzyl benzoate and benzyl salicylate are listed as allergens by the EU, they are allergens of negligible risk (see Constituent profiles, Chapter 14). The compositional data are for the Egyptian absolute. Limited availability. Due to its high cost it is unlikely that carnation absolute would be used at a concentration sufficient to cause adverse skin reactions.

Carrot seed

Botanical name: *Daucus carota* L. subsp. *sativus* Hoffm.
Family: Apiaceae (Umbelliferae)

Essential oil

Source: Seeds
Key constituents:

Carotol	36.1–73.1%
α-Pinene	0.9–11.2%
Dauca-4,8-diene	1.6–5.9%
β-Caryophyllene	0.7–5.6%
(E)-Dauc-8-en-4β-ol	1.7–4.1%
Sabinene	0–3.9%
Geranyl acetate	0–3.7%
β-Bisabolene	1.5–3.1%
Caryophyllene oxide	0.3–2.8%
(E)-β-Farnesene	1.6–2.5%
Geraniol	0–2.2%
(E)-α-Bergamotene	0.9–1.9%
Daucol	1.2–1.7%
(−)-Limonene	0.4–1.5%
β-Pinene	0.3–1.5%
β-Myrcene	0.4–1.3%
(Z)-α-Bergamotene	0–1.1%
β-Selinene	0–1.1%

(Mazzoni et al 1999)

Safety summary

Hazards: May interfere with gestation.
Contraindications (all routes): Pregnancy, breastfeeding.

Regulatory guidelines

Has GRAS status.

Organ-specific effects

Adverse skin reactions: Undiluted carrot seed oil was very slightly irritating to rabbits, but was not irritating to mice or pigs; tested at 4% on 25 volunteers it was neither irritating nor sensitizing. It is non-phototoxic (Opdyke 1976 p. 705–706).
Reproductive toxicity: Carrot seed oil has been reported to cause antigestational effects in rats and mice (Dong et al 1981). In a subsequent study, sc injection of 2.5–5 mL/kg of carrot seed oil to female rats or mice prevented implantation and blocked progesterone synthesis (Chu et al 1985). Wild carrot has a traditional reputation as a contraceptive.

Systemic effects

Acute toxicity: Carrot seed oil acute oral LD_{50} in rats >5 g/kg; acute dermal LD_{50} in rabbits >5 g/kg (Opdyke 1976 p. 705–706).

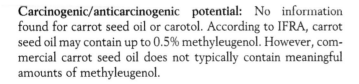

Carcinogenic/anticarcinogenic potential: No information found for carrot seed oil or carotol. According to IFRA, carrot seed oil may contain up to 0.5% methyleugenol. However, commercial carrot seed oil does not typically contain meaningful amounts of methyleugenol.

Comments

On the basis of Chinese research, we advise avoidance of carrot seed oil during pregnancy. However the quantities of essential oil used were very high, and an NOAEL for reproductive toxicity may yet be established. Carrot seed absolutes and CO_2 extracts are also produced.

Cascarilla

Synonym: Sweet-wood
Botanical names: *Croton eluteria* (L.) Sw. (Bahamas), *Croton reflexifolius* Homb., Bonpl. & Kunth (El Salvador)
Family: Euphorbiaceae

Essential oil

Source: Bark
Key constituents:

Bahamian

p-Cymene	10.0–18.0%
Cascarilladiene	4.6–6.0%
Linalool	1.9–5.1%
α-Pinene	2.6–4.6%
Cuparene	0.9–3.8%
(+)-Limonene + 1,8-cineole	0.9–3.6%
α-Thujene	2.1–3.5%
β-Myrcene	0.7–3.4%
β-Eudesmol	<3.0%
β-Selinene	0.6–2.4%
Geranyl acetone	<2.2%
β-Elemene	1.6–2.0%
Cuparophenol	0.4–1.9%
β-Copaene	<1.8%
Terpinen-4-ol	1.0–1.7%
Cascarilla hydroxyketone	<1.3%
Camphene	0.4–1.3%
Cascarilladienone	0.4–1.3%
β-Cederen-10-ol	<1.3%
α-Terpineol	0.6–1.1%
Borneol	0.4–1.1%
β-Caryophyllene	0.3–1.1%
β-Pinene	0.4–1.0%
Methyleugenol	0–0.2%

(Lawrence 1995g p, 128–131)

El Salvadorian

α-Pinene	14.7%
β-Pinene	9.5%
α-Copaene	6.2%
β-Myrcene	4.6%
Camphene	4.5%
β-Selinene	3.0%
1,8-Cineole	2.9%
p-Cymene	2.4%
Germacrene D	2.4%
(+)-Limonene	2.0%
Caryophyllene oxide	1.9%
Linalool	1.8%
γ-Cadinene	1.7%
Spathulenol	1.6%
Cascarilladiene	1.6%
Borneol	1.5%
Cascarillone	1.5%
β-Caryophyllene	1.1%
β-Elemene	1.0%
β-Phellandrene	1.0%

(Shapiro & Frances 2001)

Safety summary

Hazards: May contain methyleugenol.
Contraindications: None known.
Maximum adult daily oral dose (Bahamian cascarilla oil): 350 mg
Maximum dermal use level (Bahamian cascarilla oil):

EU	0.1%
IFRA	0.2%
Tisserand & Young	10.0%

Our safety advice

We recommend a maximum dermal use level of 10.0% and a daily oral maximum of 350 mg for Bahamian cascarilla oil based on 0.2% methyleugenol, with a dermal and oral limits of 0.02% and 0.01 mg/kg/day (see Methyleugenol profile, Chapter 14).

Regulatory guidelines

IFRA recommends that the maximum concentration of methyleugenol for leave-on products such as body lotion should be 0.0004% (IFRA 2009). The equivalent SCCNFP maximum is 0.0002% (European Commission 2002).

Organ-specific effects

Adverse skin reactions: Undiluted Bahamian cascarilla oil was not irritating to rabbit, pig or mouse skin; tested at 4% on 25 volunteers it was neither irritating nor sensitizing. It is non-phototoxic (Opdyke 1976 p. 707).

Systemic effects

Acute toxicity: Bahamian cascarilla oil acute oral LD_{50} in rats >5 g/kg; acute dermal LD_{50} in rabbits >5 g/kg (Opdyke 1976 p. 707).

Carcinogenic/anticarcinogenic potential: No information found. Methyleugenol is a rodent carcinogen if exposure is sufficiently high; both (+)-limonene and β-elemene exhibit anticarcinogenic activity (see Constituent profiles, Chapter 14).

Comments

The oil from El Salvador has only become available recently, and the toxicity data were established using the Bahamian oil.

Cassia

Synonyms: Chinese or false cinnamon
Botanical name: *Cinnamomum cassia* Blume
Botanical synonym: *Cinnamomum aromaticum* Nees

Essential oil

Family: Lauraceae
Source: Leaves, terminal branches, bark
Key constituents:

Bark oil

(E)-Cinnamaldehyde	73.2–89.4%
(Z)-Cinnamaldehyde	0.8–12.3%
(E)-Cinnamyl acetate	0.1–5.4%
Benzaldehyde	0.4–2.3%
2-Phenylethyl acetate	0–2.3%
α-Terpineol	tr–2.0%
Coumarin	tr–1.9%
Salicylaldehyde	0.04–1.8%
Borneol	tr–1.3%
Benzyl benzoate	tr–1.0%
Cinnamyl alcohol	0–0.04%

(Lawrence 1979 p. 13, 1995g p. 163, p201, 2001f p. 48–52)

Leaf oil

(E)-Cinnamaldehyde	54.6–90.1%
(E)-Cinnamyl acetate	1.4–12.5%
(Z)-Cinnamaldehyde	0.4–10.5%
Benzaldehyde	1.1–6.3%
Salicylaldehyde	0.05–3.1%
Benzyl benzoate	tr–2.9%
Coumarin	0.03–2.5%
α-Copaene	tr–2.2%
Phenylpropanal	tr–1.6%
Anisaldehyde	0–1.0%
Cinnamyl alcohol	0–0.2%
Methyleugenol	tr–0.1%

(Lawrence 1979 p. 13, 1995g p. 163, p201, 2001f p. 48–52)
Quality: May be adulterated with synthetic cinnamaldehyde, methyl cinnamic aldehyde and coumarin (Burfield 2003).

Safety summary

Hazards: May contain methyleugenol; drug interaction; may inhibit blood clotting; embryotoxicity; skin sensitization (high risk); mucous membrane irritation (low risk).
Contraindications (all routes): Pregnancy, breastfeeding.
Cautions (oral): Diabetes medication, anticoagulant medication, major surgery, peptic ulcer, hemophilia, other bleeding disorders (Box 7.1).
Cautions (dermal): Hypersensitive, diseased or damaged skin, children under 2 years of age.
Maximum adult daily oral dose: 200 mg
Maximum dermal use level:

EU	0.1%
IFRA	0.05%
Tisserand & Young	0.05%

Our safety advice

We recommend a dermal maximum of 0.05% for cassia leaf and bark oils based on 100% (E)- and (Z)-cinnamaldehyde content, and a dermal limit of 0.05% for cinnamaldehyde (see Regulatory Guidelines). We agree with the Commission E Monographs daily oral maximum of 200 mg for the oil.

Regulatory guidelines

The Council of Europe (1992) has set an ADI of 1.25 mg/kg for cinnamaldehyde, which is equivalent to an adult dose of approximately 90 mg of cassia oil. The Commission E Monographs recommend an oral dose range of 50–200 mg for cassia oil (Blumenthal et al 1998). IFRA recommends a maximum dermal use level for cinnamaldehyde of 0.05% for most product types (IFRA 2009). According to the SCCNFP (2001a) the concentration of cinnamaldehyde in any finished product should not exceed 0.1%. IFRA recommends that the maximum concentration of methyleugenol for leave-on products such as body lotion should be 0.0004% (IFRA 2009). The equivalent SCCNFP maximum is 0.0002% (European Commission 2002).

Organ-specific effects

Adverse skin reactions: Cassia oil is non-phototoxic. The undiluted oil was severely irritating to rabbits, and was mildly irritating to mice. Tested at 4% on 25 volunteers for 48 hours it was not irritating, but when patch tested at 100% for 24 hours there were two positive reactions of 24 test subjects. In a maximization test at 4%, cassia oil produced positive reactions in two out of 25 test subjects. A girl employed in dipping toothpicks in cassia oil had a skin reaction affecting her hands, face and abdomen (cited in Opdyke 1975 p. 109–110). In a study of 200 consecutive dermatitis patients, two were sensitive to 2% cassia oil on patch testing (Rudzki et al 1976). Of 750 consecutive dermatitis patients, five were sensitive to 2% cassia oil (Rudzki & Grzywa 1985). Sensitization is also seen with cinnamaldehyde (Guin et al 1984). This can allegedly be quenched by (+)-limonene and by eugenol. In ten people who developed urticaria after cinnamaldehyde had been applied to the skin, six had a

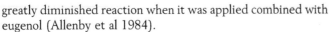

greatly diminished reaction when it was applied combined with eugenol (Allenby et al 1984).

Cardiovascular effects: Cinnamaldehyde inhibits platelet aggregation (Huang et al 2007a), an essential step in the blood clotting cascade. Cinnamaldehyde, at oral doses of 5, 10 or 20 mg/kg/day for 45 days, dose-dependently decreased plasma glucose concentrations in streptozotocin-diabetic male rats (Babu et al 2007).

Reproductive toxicity: In tests using cinnamaldehyde, there are inconclusive signs of reproductive toxicity (see Cinnamaldehyde profile, Chapter 14). When cinnamon bark oil (0.25%, 375 mg/kg) was fed to pregnant mice for two weeks it significantly reduced the number of nuclei and altered the distribution of embryos according to nucleus number (Domaracky et al 2007).

Hepatotoxicity: At 25 or 50 mg/kg ip in rats, both cinn-amaldehyde and cassia oil reduced the activity of glutathione S-transferase, but did not deplete glutathione, which slightly increased (Choi et al 2001).

Systemic effects

Acute toxicity: Cassia oil acute oral LD_{50} in rats 2.8 mL/kg; acute dermal LD_{50} in rabbits 0.32 mL/kg (Opdyke 1975 p. 109–110).

Carcinogenic/anticarcinogenic potential: Cassia oil was significantly cytotoxic to 3LL mouse Lewis lung cancer cells. Both glutathione depleting and anticarcinogenic actions are due to conjugation with sulfhydryl biomolecules (Choi et al 2001). Methyleugenol is a rodent carcinogen, but cinnamaldehyde is not; benzaldehyde and coumarin display anticarcinogenic activity in humans (see Constituent profiles, Chapter 14).

Drug interactions: Antidiabetic or anticoagulant medication (see Table 4.10B and Cardiovascular effects above).

Comments

Cassia is one of the few essential oils that contains coumarin. Any restriction for the very small content of methyleugenol in cassia leaf oil is irrelevant in light of the 0.05% maximum use level to avoid skin sensitization. Both cassia oil and cinnamalde-hyde are significantly more toxic dermally (rabbits) than orally (rats). Cassia oil is most commonly said to derive from the leaves and terminal branches of the plant (Opdyke 1975 p. 109–110). The bark may also be distilled along with the leaves, stalks and twigs (Arctander 1960) although both leaf and bark oils have a similar composition. There is a commercial oil produced from the bark of *Cinnamomum loureirii* Nees. in Vietnam, known as Saigon cinnamon, or Vietnamese cinnamon. The composition of this oil is said to be similar to that of cassia bark, and it is traded in the West in limited quantities.

Cassie

Botanical name: *Acacia farnesiana* L.
Family: Mimosaceae

Absolute

Source: Flowers
Key constituents:

Major constituents
Methyl salicylate   <5.0% (EFFA)
p-Anisaldehyde
Benzyl alcohol
Farnesol
Geraniol

Minor constituents
Benzaldehyde
Benzoic acid
Geranyl acetate
α-Ionone
β-Ionone
Linalool
Linalyl acetate
Nerolidol

(Lawrence 1989 p. 108–109, Leung & Foster 2003 p 131)
Quality: May be adulterated with mimosa absolute and with synthetic materials (Oyen & Dung 1999). Contains about 25% volatile constituents.

Safety summary

Hazards: None known.
Contraindications: None known.

Regulatory guidelines

An ADI for methyl salicylate was set at 0.5 mg/kg JECFA in 1967 based on a 2-year feeding study in dogs and using a safety factor of 100. The same ADI, based on a 2-year rat study in 1963, was adopted by the Council of Europe Committee of Experts on Flavoring Substances. The Health Canada maximum for methyl salicylate is 1% in topical products (Health Canada Cosmetic Ingredient Hotlist, March 2011).

Organ-specific effects

Adverse skin reactions: Undiluted cassie absolute was moderately irritating to rabbits; tested at 4% on 25 volunteers it was neither irritating nor sensitizing. It is non-phototoxic (Letizia et al 2000 p. 27–29).

Systemic effects

Acute toxicity: Cassie absolute acute oral LD_{50} in rats >5 g/kg; acute dermal LD_{50} in rabbits >5 g/kg (Letizia et al 2000 p. 27–29).
Carcinogenic/anticarcinogenic potential: No information found. Methyl salicylate is not mutagenic; *p*-anisaldehyde, benzaldehyde, geraniol and β-ionone display anticarcinogenic activity (see Constituent profiles, Chapter 14).

Comments

This costly absolute is not likely to be used in significant quantities. The 5% methyl salicylate content does not suggest any restriction.

Catnip

Synonyms: Catmint, catnep
Botanical name: *Nepeta cataria* L.
Family: Lamiaceae (Labiatae)

Essential oil

Source: Aerial parts
Key constituents:

Nepetalactone isomers	12.7–84.0%
Nepetalic acid	1.2–43.0%
Dihydronepetalactone	0–25.0%
β-Caryophyllene	6.2–24.6%
Caryophyllene oxide	14.3–19.4%
(E)-β-Farnesene	0–2.1%
Humulene oxide	1.0–1.6%
Piperitone	0–1.5%
α-Caryophyllene	0–1.3%
β-Elemene	0–1.2%
3-Hexenyl ester	0–1.2%

(Bourrel et al 1993a; Malizia et al 1996; Handjieva & Popov 1996)

Safety summary

Hazards: Skin sensitization (low risk); may be psychotropic.
Cautions: Oral administration.

Organ-specific effects

Adverse skin reactions: No information found.
Neurotoxicity: Given to mice as 10% of the diet for one day, dried catnip leaves caused increased susceptibility to seizures, decreased sleep duration, and increased stereotyped behavior. When given for seven days, it induced tolerance to stereotypic behavior, catalepsy and sleeping time, and increased susceptibility to seizures. The constituent mainly responsible for its CNS effects is thought to be nepetalic acid, the major metabolite of nepetalactone (Massoco et al 1995). However in rodents, epinepetalactone, a stereoisomer of nepetalactone, inhibited seizures induced by PTZ (Galati et al 2004). Therefore, there is no certainty that catnip oil is neurotoxic.

The herb is a well-known attractant of domestic cats, and has to be smelled (not ingested) to influence cat behavior. There are reports of a mild and transitory psychotropic effect in humans after smoking the dried herb. Four cases were reported in 1969, in each the effect was said to be similar to that of marijuana (euphoria, mood elevation) but less intense. Other effects included a sense of unreality, visual hallucinations and fascination with music (Jackson & Reed 1969). There is one report of a 19 month-old child experiencing prolonged CNS depression after apparently consuming a large quantity of the herb (Osterhoudt et al 1997).

Systemic effects

Acute toxicity: The acute ip LD_{50} of a catnip oil containing 40% nepetalactone and 43% nepetalic acid was 1.3 g/kg in mice (Harney et al 1978). This almost certainly equates to a non-toxic oral LD_{50}.

Carcinogenic/anticarcinogenic potential: No information found for catnip oil, but it contains no known carcinogens. β-Caryophyllene, α-caryophyllene and β-elemene display antitumoral activity (see Constituent profiles, Chapter 14).

Our safety advice

Since sesquiterpene lactones have a tendency to skin sensitization, some caution in this area is warranted.

Comments

There have been no studies using catnip essential oil except as an insect repellent. Catnip's traditional medicinal uses include treatment of restlessness, nervous headache, nervousness and hysteria, and it is said to induce sleep (Grieve 1978). The compositional data above seem to indicate the existence of at least two chemotypes, a nepatalic acid CT, and a β-caryophyllene CT, both nepetalactone-rich. Commercial catnip oils contain two isomers of nepetalactone, (Z,E)- and (E,Z)-. Other chemotypes exist, rich in different nepetalactones.

Cedarwood (Atlas)

Synonyms: Atlantic cedar, Moroccan cedar
Botanical name: *Cedrus atlantica* G. Manetti
Family: Pinaceae

Essential oil

Source: Wood
Key constituents:

β-Himachalene	30.8–40.4%
α-Himachalene	10.3–16.4%
(E)-α-Atlantone	5.2–13.4%
γ-Himachalene	6.7–9.7%
Deodarone	1.2–6.7%
(E)-γ-Atlantone	1.2–3.9%
Himachalol	1.7–3.7%
Isocedranol	1.2–3.1%
(Z)-α-Atlantone	1.0–2.8%
δ-Cadinene	0.5–2.6%
1-epi-Cubenol	1.1–2.5%
(Z)-trans-α-Bergamotol	0–2.0%
Cedranone	0.7–1.7%
α-Calacorene	0.5–1.6%
β-Himachalene oxide	0–1.6%
γ-Curcumene	1.0–1.5%
β-Vetivenene	0.2–1.4%
Cadalene	0–1.4%
α-Dehydroar himachalene	0.7–1.2%
Oxydohimachalene	0.6–1.0%

(Aberchane & Fechtal 2004)

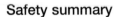

Safety summary

Hazards: None known.
Contraindications: None known.

Organ-specific effects

Adverse skin reactions: Undiluted Atlas cedarwood oil was slightly irritating to rabbits, but was not irritating to mice or pigs; tested at 8% on 25 volunteers it was neither irritating nor sensitizing. It is non-phototoxic (Opdyke 1976 p. 709).

Systemic effects

Acute toxicity: Atlas cedarwood acute oral LD_{50} in rats $>$5 g/kg; acute dermal LD_{50} in rabbits $>$5 g/kg (Opdyke 1976 p. 709).
Carcinogenic/anticarcinogenic potential: Atlas cedarwood oil showed in vitro growth-inhibiting action against human K562 myelogenous leukemia cells with an IC_{50} of 59.37 μg/mL (Saab et al 2012a).

Comments

Atlas and Himalayan cedars are members of the Pinaceae family, while all the other cedars are Cupressaceae.

Cedarwood (Chinese)

Synonyms: Chinese weeping cypress, mourning cypress
Botanical name: *Chamaecyparis funebris* (Endl.) Franco
Botanical synonym: *Cupressus funebris* Endl.
Family: Cupressaceae

Essential oil

Source: Wood
Key constituents:

Iso-α-cedrene	32.0%
Thujopsene	21.6%
Cedrenol	6.1%
Cuparene	4.9%
Longifolene	4.2%
α-Cedrene	2.1%

(Zhu et al 1993)

Safety summary

Hazards: None known.
Contraindications: None known.

Organ-specific effects

Adverse skin reactions: No information found for Chinese cedarwood oil. Little is known about most of its constituents, although α-cedrene appears to be non-reactive on healthy skin. Texas cedarwood oil, which has a similar composition, also seems to be relatively safe for dermal use.

Systemic effects

Acute toxicity: No information found for Chinese cedarwood oil or most of its constituents. Texas cedarwood oil seems to be non-toxic.
Carcinogenic/anticarcinogenic potential: No information found for Chinese cedarwood oil, but it contains no known carcinogens.

Comments

Produced in large quantities. Sometimes used as an adulterant of Virginian or Texan cedarwod oils.

Cedarwood (Himalayan)

Synonym: Deodar cedarwood
Botanical name: *Cedrus deodara* Roxb. Ex D. Don
Family: Pinaceae

Essential oil

Source: Wood
Key constituents:

α-Himachalene	20.0–30.0%
α-Cedrene	12.0–16.0%
β-Himachalene	8.0–13.0%
(*E*)-α-Atlantone	5.0–7.0%
Deodarone	4.0–6.0%
(*Z*)-α-Atlantone	2.0–3.0%
β-Cedrene	0.5–1.5%
allo-Himachalol	0.5–1.5%
Cedrol	1.0–2.0%
Himachalol	1.0–2.0%

(Lawrence 2012)

Safety summary

Hazards: May be moderately toxic.
Contraindications: None known.

Organ-specific effects

Adverse skin reactions: Tested at 15% in castor oil, Himalayan cedarwood oil was not irritating to the skin of rabbit or sheep (Chandra et al 1989). In a study of 200 consecutive dermatitis patients, three (1.5%) were sensitive to 2% Himalayan cedarwood oil on patch testing (Rudzki et al 1976). Himalayan cedarwood oil has anti-inflammatory effects, preventing histamine release and inhibiting type IV hypersensitivity (Shinde et al 1999a, 1999b).

Systemic effects

Acute toxicity: Himalayan cedarwood oil acute oral LD_{50} in mice was 500 mg/kg (Dhar et al 1968).
Subacute & subchronic toxicity: In rabbits exposed daily for 21 days by dermal application of 15% Himalayan cedarwood oil in castor oil, no significant changes were observed in the body weight, organ weight, or organ/body weight ratios of the treated

animals. Serum oxaloacetic transaminase and pyruvic transaminase levels remained unaltered, as did blood glucose and blood urea nitrogen values. Neither spontaneous nor treatment-related histopathological changes were observed. These data suggest that the oil was devoid of any adverse effect on skin or on liver and kidney functions of rabbits (Tandan et al 1989). **Carcinogenic/anticarcinogenic potential:** Himalayan cedarwood oil showed in vitro growth-inhibiting action against human K562 myelogenous leukemia cells with an IC_{50} of 37.09 μg/mL (Saab et al 2012a). Limonene exhibits anticarcinogenic activity (see (+)-Limonene profile, Chapter 14).

Comments

Since terpenes do not tend to be acutely toxic, since the subchronic data in rabbits did not show any toxicity, and since Atlas cedarwood, with very similar constituents, has a low toxicity, there must be some doubt about the LD_{50} of 500 mg/kg for this oil. The acute oral LD_{50} for α-cedrene has been reported as >5 g/kg (Opdyke 1978 p. 679–680).

Cedarwood (Port Orford)

Synonyms: Rose of cedar, Oregon cedar
Botanical name: *Chamaecyparis lawsoniana* (Andr. Murray) Parl.
Family: Cupressaceae

Essential oil

Source: Wood
Key constituents:

α-Terpineol	14.3%
δ-Cadinene	8.2%
α-Pinene	6.5%
Camphor	5.9%
α-Fenchol	5.5%
α-Cadinol	5.3%
Fenchone	4.7%
α-Muurolene	4.2%
T-Cadinol	3.4%
β-Terpineol	3.3%
(+)-Limonene	2.7%
T-Muurolol	2.7%
Citronellol	2.3%
α-Amorphene	1.9%
Terpinolene	1.6%
Isopulegol	1.4%
Borneol	1.3%
Camphene	1.3%
1,4-Cineole	1.3%
p-Cymene	1.3%
p-Cymenene	1.0%
β-Elemene	1.0%
Myrtenol	1.0%

(Tucker et al 2000)

Safety summary

Hazards: None known.
Contraindications: None known.

Organ-specific effects

Adverse skin reactions: In a local lymph node assay in mice, Port Orford cedarwood oil did not induce a hypersensitivity response at 0.5%, 5% or 50%, and is therefore not likely to be a sensitizer in humans. In a dermal irritation study on rabbits, the oil showed concentration-dependent irritation, with the undiluted oil being strongly irritant, and 5% being slightly irritant (Craig et al 2004). α-Terpineol is notably non-reactive dermally (see α-Terpineol profile. Chapter 14).

Systemic effects

Acute toxicity: No information found. α-Terpineol appears to be non-toxic (see α-Terpineol profile, Chapter 14).
Carcinogenic/anticarcinogenic potential: No information found for Port Orford cedarwood oil, but it contains no known carcinogens. (+)-Limonene and β-elemene display anticarcinogenic activity (see Constituent profiles, Chapter 14). α-Cadinol is active against the human colon cancer cell line HT-29 (He et al 1997a).

Comments

Limited availability. In a report on trees it has been proposed by UNEP-WCMC that CITES add *Chamaecyparis lawsoniana* to its list of threatened plant species.

Cedarwood (Texan)

Synonyms: Mexican cedar, Mexican juniper, mountain cedar, rock cedar
Botanical name: *Juniperus ashei* Buchholz
Botanical synonym: *Juniperus mexicana* Spreng.
Family: Cupressaceae (Coniferae)

Essential oil

Source: Wood
Key constituents:

Thujopsene	25.0–46.8%
α-Cedrene	22.6–30.7%
Cedrol	12.2–19.1%
β-Cedrene	5.5%
Cuparene	1.7–1.9%
Widdrol	1.1–1.6%
α-Chamigrene	1.2–1.5%
α-Selinene	0–1.5%
β-Himachalene	1.1–1.4%
β-Chamigrene	0–1.1%

(Lawrence 1998e p. 67–68)
Quality: May be adulterated with Chinese cedarwood oil.

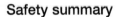

Safety summary

Hazards: None known.
Contraindications: None known.

Organ-specific effects

Adverse skin reactions: Undiluted Texan cedarwood oil was not irritating to rabbit, pig or mouse skin; tested at 8% on 25 volunteers it was neither irritating nor sensitizing. The oil is non-phototoxic (Opdyke 1976 p. 711–712). One case has been reported of an eczematous reaction to traces of cedarwood oil, probably a mixture of oils of *Juniperus ashei* and *Juniperus virginiana* (Franz et al 1998).

Systemic effects

Acute toxicity: Texan cedarwood acute oral LD_{50} in rats >5 g/kg; acute dermal LD_{50} in rabbits >5 g/kg (Opdyke 1976 p. 711–712).
Carcinogenic/anticarcinogenic potential: No information found for Texan cedarwood oil, but it contains no known carcinogens.

Comments

Millions of acres of farmland have been invaded by this opportunistic species. Cedar trees and stumps discarded by local ranchers as by-products of their land clearing operations are used for oil extraction. The tree also grows in Mexico and South America.

Cedarwood (Virginian)

Synonyms: Red cedar, Eastern red cedar
Botanical name: *Juniperus virginiana* L.
Family: Cupressaceae (Coniferae)

Essential oil

Source: Wood
Key constituents:

α-Cedrene	21.1–38.0%
Thujopsene	21.3–23.4%
Cedrol	12.3–22.2%
β-Cedrene	8.2–9.2%
α-Selinene	3.0%
Widdrol	1.9–2.3%
β-Himachalene	2.1%
β-Chamigrene	1.4–1.8%
α-Chamigrene	1.6%
Cuparene	0.9–1.6%

(Lawrence 1998e p. 67–68)
Quality: May be adulterated with Chinese cedarwood oil (Burfield 2003).

Safety summary

Hazards: None known.
Contraindications: None known.

Organ-specific effects

Adverse skin reactions: Undiluted Virginian cedarwood oil was moderately irritating to rabbits but was not irritating to mice; tested at 8% on 25 volunteers it was neither irritating nor sensitizing. It is non-phototoxic (Opdyke 1974 p. 845–846). In an in vitro assay, cedarwood oil (type unspecified) was non-phototoxic (Placzek et al 2007). Cedarwood oil (type unspecified) tested at 10%, induced allergic responses in 10 (0.6%) of 1,606 consecutive dermatitis patients (Frosch et al 2002b). There were no irritant or allergic reactions in a group of 100 consecutive dermatitis patients tested with 5% cedarwood oil (type unspecified) (Frosch et al 1995a). Five out of 747 dermatitis patients suspected of fragrance allergy (0.67%) reacted to 10% cedarwood oil (type unspecified) (Wöhrl et al 2001). In a multicenter study, Germany's IVDK reported that 48 of 6,223 dermatitis patients (0.77%) suspected of fragrance allergy tested positive to 10% Virginian cedarwood oil (Uter et al 2010). One case has been reported of an eczematous reaction to traces of cedarwood oil, probably a mixture of oils of *Juniperus ashei* and *Juniperus virginiana* (Franz et al 1998).

Systemic effects

Acute toxicity: Virginian cedarwood oil acute oral LD_{50} in rats >5 g/kg; acute dermal LD_{50} in rabbits >5 g/kg (Opdyke 1974 p. 845–846).
Carcinogenic/anticarcinogenic potential: No information found for Virginian oil, but it contains no known carcinogens.

Comments

The tree grows in many parts of the eastern and central United States.

Cedrela

Synonyms: Spanish cedar, West Indian cedar, cigar-box cedar, red cedar, stinking mahogany
Botanical name: *Cedrela odorata* L.
Botanical synonym: *Cedrela mexicana* M. Roem.
Family: Meliaceae

Essential oil

Source: Wood
Key constituents:

α-Copaene	15.6%
δ-Cadinene	11.7%
α-Cubebene	8.0%
(*E*)-Nerolidol	8.0%
β-Curcumene	6.8%
Calarene	3.4%
β-Cubebene	3.2%
Germacrene D	2.6%
α-Caryophyllene	2.1%
β-Farnesene	1.8%
epi-Cubenol	1.4%

Cadina-1,4-diene	1.3%
Caryophyllene	1.2%
Cubenol	1.0%
α-Muurolene	1.0%

(Lawrence, 1989 p. 219)

Safety summary

Hazards: None known.
Contraindications: None known.

Organ-specific effects

No information found.

Systemic effects

Carcinogenic/anticarcinogenic potential: No information found for cedrela oil, but it contains no known carcinogens. Nerolidol and α-caryophyllene display anticarcinogenic activity (see Constituent profiles, Chapter 14).

Comments

The oil is produced in Brazil, and the wood is listed by CITES under their Appendix III (prevention of unsustainable or illegal exploitation). The tree is listed by IUCN as a threatened species.

Celery leaf

Botanical name: *Apium graveolens* L.
Family: Apiaceae (Umbelliferae)

Essential oil

Source: Leaves and stems
Key constituents:

β-Myrcene	33.6%
(+)-Limonene	26.3%
(Z)-β-Ocimene	14.1%
3-Butyl phthalide	6.2%
β-Selinene	3.7%
3,4-Dehydroisobutylidene phthalide	3.2%
n-Pentylcyclohexadiene	1.0%

(Lawrence 1989 p. 157)

Safety summary

Hazards: Skin sensitization if oxidized.
Cautions: Old or oxidized oils should be avoided.

Our safety advice

Because of its high limonene content we recommend that oxidation of celery leaf oil is avoided by storage in a dark, airtight container in a refrigerator. The addition of an antioxidant to preparations containing it is recommended.

Organ-specific effects

Adverse skin reactions: No information found. Autoxidation products of (+)-limonene can cause skin sensitization (see (+)-Limonene profile, Chapter 14).
Reproductive toxicity: Oral β-myrcene was reproductively toxic in pregnant rats at 500 mg/kg, but not at 250 mg/kg (Delgado et al 1993a, 1993b; Paumgartten et al 1998). This does not suggest any dose limitation for celery leaf oil.

Systemic effects

Acute toxicity: No information found. β-Myrcene and (+)-limonene are non-toxic (see Constituent profiles, Chapter 14).
Carcinogenic/anticarcinogenic potential: No information found for celery leaf oil. β-Myrcene is not genotoxic and demonstrates antigenotoxic activity; it is a male mouse-specific hepatocarcinogen (see β-Myrcene profile, Chapter 14). 3-Butyl phthalide and (+)-limonene display anticarcinogenic activity (see Constituent profiles, Chapter 14).

Comments

May be used as an adulterant for celery seed oil.

Celery seed

Botanical name: *Apium graveolens* L.
Family: Apiaceae (Umbelliferae)

Essential oil

Source: Seeds
Key constituents:

(+)-Limonene	68.0–75.0%
β-Selinene	2.0–12.5%
α-Selinene	2.0–12.1%
Butylidene phthalide	2.3–8.0%
Sedanolide	2.3–3.8%
3-Butyl phthalide	2.1–3.0%
Ligustilide	0–2.4%
Sedanenolide	2.2–2.3%
Pentylbenzene	1.7–2.0%
Linalool	0–1.5%
β-Myrcene	1.0–1.2%
α-Pinene	0.1–1.0%

(Lawrence 1989 p. 157, 1993 p. 74–75)
Quality: Limonene is the most common adulterant found in commercial celery seed oils (Kubeczka 2002).

Safety summary

Hazards: Skin sensitization if oxidized
Cautions: Old or oxidized oils should be avoided

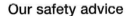

Our safety advice

Because of its limonene content we recommend that oxidation of celery seed oil is avoided by storage in a dark, airtight container in a refrigerator. The addition of an antioxidant to preparations containing it is recommended.

Regulatory guidelines

Has GRAS status. IFRA recommends that essential oils rich in limonene should only be used when the level of peroxides is kept to the lowest practical level, for instance by adding antioxidants at the time of production (IFRA 2009).

Organ-specific effects

Adverse skin reactions: Undiluted celery seed oil was not irritating either to rabbits or to mice; tested at 4% on 25 volunteers it was neither irritating nor sensitizing. It is non-phototoxic (Opdyke 1974 p. 849–850). Autoxidation products of (+)-limonene can cause skin sensitization (see (+)-Limonene profile, Chapter 14).

Reproductive toxicity: The low developmental toxicity of (+)-limonene in rabbits and mice (Kodama et al 1977a, 1977b) suggests that celery seed oil is not hazardous in pregnancy.

Systemic effects

Acute toxicity: Celery seed oil acute oral LD_{50} in rats >5 g/kg; acute dermal LD_{50} in rabbits >5 g/kg (Opdyke 1974 p. 849–850).
Antioxidant/pro-oxidant activity: Celery seed oil showed moderate antioxidant activity as a DPPH radical scavenger and high activity in the aldehyde/carboxylic acid assay (Wei & Shibamoto 2007a).
Carcinogenic/anticarcinogenic potential: Celery seed oil dose-dependently inhibited aflatoxin B_1-induced adducts in calf thymus DNA, in the presence of rat liver microsomes (Hashim et al 1994). Celery seed oil significantly induced glutathione S-transferase activity in mouse tissues (Lam & Zheng 1991; Banerjee et al 1994). (+)-Limonene displays anticarcinogenic activity (see (+)-Limonene profile, Chapter 14). Sedanolide and 3-butyl phthalide reduced the incidence of forestomach cancer in mice (Zheng et al 1993b).

Comments

Mainly produced in France, India and the Netherlands. The French oil is preferred in perfumery.

Chamomile (blue)

Synonyms: German chamomile, Hungarian chamomile, sweet false chamomile
Botanical name: *Matricaria recutita* L.
Botanical synonyms: *Chamomilla recutita* (L.) Rauschert, *Matricaria chamomilla* L.
Family: Asteraceae (Compositae)

Essential oil

Source: Aerial parts of flowering plant
Key constituents:

α-Bisabolol oxide A/(F)-β-farnesene CT (Egyptian)

α-Bisabolol oxide A	38.7%
(E)-β-Farnesene	25.7%
α-Bisabolol	5.0%
α-Bisabolol oxide B	4.4%
Chamazulene	3.4%
α-Bisabolone oxide	1.6%
Germacrene D	1.6%
Decanoic acid	1.3%

(Shaath & Azzo 1993)

α-Bisabolol oxide A CT (Egyptian, German, Dutch)

α-Bisabolol oxide A	44.7–53.6%
α-Bisabolol oxide B	9.5–13.5%
α-Bisabolone oxide	8.5–12.0%
(E)-β-Farnesene	7.7–8.9%
Chamazulene	2.7–7.6%
(Z) & (E)-Spiroethers	5.9–7.0%
α-Bisabolol	1.6–2.9%

(Piccaglia & Marotti 1993)

α-Bisabolol oxide A/α-bisabolol oxide B CT (Brazilian)

α-Bisabolol oxide B	23.5%
α-Bisabolol oxide A	16.9%
(Z)-β-Farnesene	16.0%
α-Bisabolol	13.2%
Chamazulene	8.2%
α-Bisabolone oxide	5.2%
en-yn-Dicycloether isomers	4.7%

(Matos et al 1993)

Farnesene/chamazulene CT (Bulgarian)

Farnesene	27.7%
Chamazulene	17.6%
α-Bisabolol oxide B	11.2%
α-Bisabolol	9.6%
α-Bisabolol oxide A	8.9%
δ-Cadinene	5.2%
α-Muurolene	3.4%
(E)-β-Ocimene	1.7%
γ-Muurolene	1.3%

(Tsutsulova & Antonova 1984)

α-Bisabolol/(E)-β-farnesene CT (Finnish)

α-Bisabolol	32.4–60.1%
(E)-β-Farnesene	11.6–43.8%
Chamazulene	10.8–21.8%
α-Bisabolol oxide B	0–7.5%
α-Bisabolol oxide A	0–6.2%

(Hyvönen et al 1991)

α-Bisabolol oxide A/chamazulene CT (German)

α-Bisabolol oxide A	57.7%
Chamazulene	23.4%
α-Bisabolol oxide B	4.4%
α-Bisabolone oxide	4.1%
(E)-β-Farnesene	2.9%
Germacrene D	1.5%

(Brunke et al 1992)

Quality: Blue chamomile oil is prone to oxidation, and should be stored in light-tight, cold conditions. Blue chamomile oil may be adulterated with synthetic and natural mixtures containing bisabolol and azulenes (Kubeczka 2002).

Safety summary

Hazards: Drug interaction.
Cautions (all routes): Drugs metabolized by CYP2D6 (Appendix B).
Cautions (oral): Drugs metabolized by CYP1A2, CYP2C9 or CYP3A4 (Appendix B).

Regulatory guidelines

Has GRAS status.

Organ-specific effects

Adverse skin reactions: Undiluted blue chamomile oil was moderately irritating to rabbits, but was not irritating to mice; tested at 4% on 25 volunteers it was neither irritating nor sensitizing. It is non-phototoxic (Opdyke 1974 p. 851–852). In a study of 200 consecutive dermatitis patients, one (0.5%) was sensitive to 2% blue chamomile oil on patch testing (Rudzki et al 1976).
Reproductive toxicity: Since α-bisabolol was not teratogenic in rats at 1 mL/kg (Habersang et al 1979), adverse effects in pregnancy for chamomile oils high in α-bisabolol are unlikely.

Systemic effects

Acute toxicity: Blue chamomile oil acute oral LD_{50} in rats >5 g/kg; acute dermal LD_{50} in rabbits >5 g/kg (Opdyke 1974 p. 851–852). Mouse LD_{50} 3.5 g/kg oral, 2.95 g/kg ip (Kudrzycka-Bieloszabska & Glowniak 1966).
Antioxidant/pro-oxidant activity: An Iranian blue chamomile oil, high in (E)-β-farnesene, chamazulene and guaiazulene, was an efficient inhibitor of lipid peroxidation (Owlia et al 2007).
Carcinogenic/anticarcinogenic potential: Blue chamomile oil was cytotoxic to human prostate, lung and breast cancer cells with an IC_{50} of 0.07% (Zu et al 2010). Blue chamomile oil is antimutagenic. It demonstrated a dose-dependent inhibitory effect on SCE formed by daunorubicin and methyl methanesulfonate with no toxic effects (Hernandez-Ceruelos et al 2002). Chamomile oil (type unspecified) significantly induced glutathione S-transferase activity in mouse tissues (Lam & Zheng 1991). The oil contains no known carcinogens.
Drug interactions: Since chamazulene, farnesene and α-bisabolol inhibit CYP2D6 (Table 4.11B), there is a theoretical risk of interaction between all blue chamomile oil CTs and drugs metabolized by this enzyme. The α-bisabolol/(E)-β-farnesene CT may also inhibit CYP1A2, CYP2C9 or CYP3A4. The α-bisabolol oxide A CT may inhibit CYP1A2 (see Appendix B).

Comments

Blue chamomile oils are produced in many parts of the world, and with greatly varying composition. The data above are given as six examples of this variation, which may represent chemotypes. The countries of origin are given for interest, but it should not be assumed that only one type of chamomile oil is available from each origin. They are ordered according to percentage of chamazulene. Chemotypes high in α-bisabolol are generally preferred for therapy.

Chamomile (Cape)

Botanical name: *Eriocephalus punctulatus* DC
Family: Asteraceae (Compositae)

Essential oil

Source: Aerial parts of flowering plant
Key constituents:

2-Methylbutyl 2-methylpropanoate	23.7%
Linalyl acetate	14.1%
2-Methylpropyl 2-methylpropanoate	8.1%
2-Methylbutyl 3-methylbutanoate	6.1%
3-Methylbutyl angelate	2.9%
3-Methylbutyl 2-methylpropanoate	2.3%
α-Copaene	2.1%
p-Cymene	1.6%
Terpinen-4-ol	1.5%
2-Methylpropyl 2-methylbutanoate	1.4%
Borneol	1.1%
2-Methylpropyl angelate	1.0%

(Graven, private communication, 1999)

Quality: Cape chamomile oil is prone to oxidation, and should be stored in light-tight, cold conditions.

Safety summary

Hazards: None known.
Contraindications: None known.

Organ-specific effects

No information found for Cape chamomile oil or most of its constituents.

Systemic effects

Acute toxicity: No information found for Cape chamomile oil or most of its constituents.
Carcinogenic/anticarcinogenic potential: No information found for Cape chamomile oil, but it contains no known carcinogens.

Comments

Approximately 80% of the oil is composed of esters which are similar to those found in Roman chamomile oils. It seems likely that this oil would present a similar degree of (low) toxicity. Limited availability.

Chamomile (Moroccan)

Synonym: Wild chamomile
Botanical names: *Ormenis mixta* Dumort; *Ormenis multicaulis* Braun-Blanw. & Maire
Family: Asteraceae (Compositae)

Essential oil

Source: Aerial parts of flowering plant
Key constituents:

Ormensis mixta

Santolina alcohol	32.0%
α-Pinene	15.0%
Germacrene	5.0%
(*E*)-Pinocarveol	3.0%
Bisabolene	2.5%
Yomogi alcohol	2.4%
Artemisia alcohol	2.3%
Bornyl acetate	2.2%
β-Caryophyllene	1.5%
Bornyl butyrate	1.3%
Borneol	1.0%
β-Myrcene	1.0%

(Toulemonde & Beauverd 1984)

Safety summary

Hazards: None known.
Contraindications: None known.

Organ-specific effects

No information found for any Moroccan chamomile oil.

Systemic effects

No information found for any Moroccan chamomile oil.

Comments

Commercial reconstructions are common (Burfield 2000). No reliable data was found for *Ormenis multicaulis* oil composition.

Chamomile (Roman)

Botanical name: *Chamaemelum nobile* (L.) All.
Botanical synonym: *Anthemis nobilis* L.
Family: Asteraceae (Compositae)

Essential oil

Source: Aerial parts of flowering plant
Key constituents:

Isobutyl angelate	0–37.4%
Butyl angelate	0–34.9%
3-Methylpentyl angelate	0–22.7%
Isobutyl butyrate	0–20.5%
Isoamyl angelate	8.4–17.9%
2-Methyl-2-propenyl angelate	0–13.1%
3-Methylpentyl isobutyrate	0–12.5%
2-Methyl-2-propyl angelate	0–7.4%
Camphene	0–6.0%
Borneol	0–5.0%
α-Pinene	1.1–4.5%
α-Terpinene	0–4.5%
Chamazulene	0–4.4%
(*E*)-Pinocarveol	0–4.4%
α-Thujene	0–4.1%
Hexyl butyrate	0–3.9%
Terpinolene	0–3.9%
Isobutyl isobutyrate	0–3.7%
Anthemol	0–3.2%
γ-Terpinene	0–3.2%
Isoamyl isobutyrate	0–3.1%
δ-3-Carene	0–2.8%
Isoamyl 2-methylbutyrate	0–2.8%
2-Methylbutyl 2-methylbutyrate	0–2.7%
Isoamyl butyrate	0–2.6%
Pinocarvone	0–2.4%
β-Myrcene	0–2.1%
p-Cymene	0–2.0%
β-Pinene	0.2–1.6%
Isoamyl methacrylate	0–1.5%
β-Phellandrene	0–1.4%
Propyl angelate	0–1.1%

(Chialva et al 1982; Srinivas 1986; Zani et al 1991; Lawrence 1998f p. 49)
Quality: Roman chamomile oil is prone to oxidation, and should be stored in light-tight, cold conditions. May be adulterated with isobutyl angelate and bisabolols (Burfield 2003).

Safety summary

Hazards: None known.
Contraindications: None known.

Regulatory guidelines

Has GRAS status. In a 2003 report, JECFA stated that the committee had "no safety concern" about isobutyl angelate, based on current intake as a food flavoring (http://www.inchem.org/documents/jecfa/jecmono/v52je27.htm accessed August 8th 2011).

Organ-specific effects

Adverse skin reactions: In a 48 hour occlusive patch test on 50 Italian volunteers, undiluted chamomile oil (assumed to be Roman) produced no adverse reactions. When similarly tested at 5%, it produced one reaction in 290 eczema patients (Meneghini et al 1971). Undiluted Roman chamomile oil was moderately irritating to rabbits, but was not irritating to mice; tested at 4% on 25 volunteers it was neither irritating nor sensitizing. It is non-phototoxic (Opdyke 1974 p. 853).

Urinary effect: Administration of 350 mg/kg of Roman chamomile oil to rats by sc or ip injection resulted in decreases in water elimination from 93.04% (controls) to 46.85% (sc) and 28.10% (ip) of the water administered. The major constituents of this oil were butyl angelate and isoamyl angelate (Rossi et al 1988). Nothing meaningful can be extrapolated from the massive dose used here.

Systemic effects

Acute toxicity: Roman chamomile oil acute oral LD_{50} in rats >5 g/kg; acute dermal LD_{50} in rabbits >5 g/kg (Opdyke 1974 p. 853).

Antioxidant/pro-oxidant activity: Roman chamomile oil showed moderate antioxidant activity as a DPPH radical scavenger and low activity in the aldehyde/carboxylic acid assay (Wei and Shibamoto 2007a).

Carcinogenic/anticarcinogenic potential: Roman chamomile oil was not mutagenic in either a *Bacillus subtilis rec*-assay or an Ames test (Zani et al 1991). Chamomile oil (type unspecified) significantly induced glutathione-*S*-transferase activity in mouse tissues (Lam & Zheng 1991). Roman chamomile oil contains no known carcinogens.

Comments

There is wide variation in the reported constituents of Roman chamomile oil, although the majority of the oil always consists of angelate and butyrate esters. On the basis of current knowledge, unlikely to present any hazard in aromatherapy.

Champaca (orange)

Synonyms: Golden champa, champak
Botanical name: *Michelia champaca* L.
Family: Magnoliaceae

Absolute

Source: Flowers
Key constituents:

2-Phenylethanol	25.0–34.0%
Methyl linoleate	10.0–18.0%
Indole	2.9–12.0%
Methyl anthranilate	2.1–9.0%
Methyl benzoate	1.0–5.0%
Phenylacetonitrile	1.2–4.3%
Benzyl acetate	0.1–4.0%
β-Ionone	0.2–3.4%
Methyl palmitate	2.0–3.0%
Ionone oximes	0–3.0%
(Z)-Linalool oxide (pyranoid)	0.2–2.5%
2-Phenylethyl acetate	0.4–2.0%
Benzyl alcohol	0.3–2.0%
Linalool	0.2–2.0%
α-Farnesene	0.6–1.6%
α-Ionone	0.1–1.6%
Dihydro-β-ionone	0.3–1.4%
Dihydro-β-ionol	0.3–1.1%
Phenylaldoxime	0.5–1.0%

(Kaiser 1991; Lawrence 2000d p. 55–60)

Quality: May be co-extracted with (cheaper) ylang-ylang flowers (Oyen & Dung 1999).

Safety summary

Hazards: None known.
Contraindications: None known.
Maximum daily oral dose in pregnancy and breastfeeding: 555 mg
Maximum dermal use level in pregnancy and breastfeeding: 17.5%

Our safety advice

Our restrictions for pregnancy and breastfeeding are based on 34.0% 2-phenylethanol, with an oral limit of 2.7 mg/kg/day, and a champaca absolute specific gravity of 0.96.

Organ-specific effects

Adverse skin reactions: No information found. 2-Phenylethanol is a very low risk skin sensitizer (see 2-Phenylethanol profile, Chapter 14).

Systemic effects

Acute toxicity: No information found.
Carcinogenic/anticarcinogenic potential: No information found for orange champaca absolute, but it contains no known carcinogens.

Comments

The plant is commonly found in S.E Asia, and the absolute is produced in India and Thailand. A CO_2 extract is also made.

Champaca (white)

Botanical name: *Michelia alba* DC
Family: Magnoliaceae

Absolute

Source: Flowers
Key constituents:

Linalool	76.3%
2-Phenylethanol	6.4%
9,12-Octadecadienal	2.3%
Methyleugenol	2.3%
Methyl hexanoate	1.0%

(Zhu et al 1993)

Safety summary

Hazards: Potentially carcinogenic, based on methyleugenol content
Contraindications: None known
Maximum dermal use level:

EU	0.01%
IFRA	0.02%
Tisserand & Young	0.9%

Our safety advice

We recommend a dermal maximum of 0.9%, based on 2.3% methyleugenol with a dermal limit of 0.02% (see Methyleugenol profile, Chapter 14).

Regulatory guidelines

According to IFRA, essential oils rich in linalool should only be used when the level of peroxides is kept to the lowest practical value. The addition of antioxidants such as 0.1% BHT or α-tocopherol at the time of production is recommended (IFRA 2009). IFRA recommends a maximum concentration of 0.0004% methyleugenol in leave-on products such as body lotions (IFRA 2009). The equivalent SCCNFP maximum is 0.0002% (European Commission 2002).

Organ-specific effects

Adverse skin reactions: No information found. Oxidation products of linalool may be skin sensitizing.

Systemic effects

Acute toxicity: No information found.
Carcinogenic potential. No information found for white champaca absolute. Methyleugenol is a rodent carcinogen when oral exposure is sufficiently high (see Methyleugenol profile, Chapter 14).

Comments

Limited availability. Magnolia leaf and flower oils are distilled from the same plant.

Chaste tree

Synonym: Monk's pepper
Botanical name: *Vitex agnus castus* L.
Family: Verbenaceae

Essential oil

Source: Leaves
Key constituents:

1,8-cineole	15.6–35.2%
Sabinene	6.9–17.1%
α-Pinene	1.0–13.9%
α-Terpineol	1.4–9.2%
γ-Elemene	0–9.1%
β-Selinene	0–9.0%
β-Caryophyllene	2.3–8.9%
(Z)-β-Farnesene	0–8.6%
Citronellyl acetate	0.3–7.8%
Citronellic acid	0–6.6%
(+)-Limonene	0.1–4.1%
Terpinen-4-ol	1.4–3.7%
β-Myrcene	0–3.5%
α-Bisabolol	0–2.7%
(E)-β-Farnesene	0–2.6%
(E)-Nerolidol	0–2.5%
β-Pinene	1.4–2.4%
(Z)-β-Ocimene	0.01–2.2%
(−)-*allo*-Aromadendrene	0–2.0%
Spathulenol	0.4–1.8%
(E)-Dihydroterpineol	0–1.8%
γ-Terpinene	0.8–1.6%
α-Gurjunene	0.4–1.6%
Guaiol	0–1.3%
Manool	0–1.3%
α-Guaiaiene	0–1.2%
T-Cadinol	0–1.2%
Dodecane	0–1.0%
Thymol	0–1.0%

(Senatore et al 1996; Valentini et al 1998)
Source: Seeds
Key constituents:

Sabinene	7.1–44.1%
1,8-Cineole	8.4–23.3%
α-Pinene	1.2–23.1%
γ-Elemene	0–17.0%
(E)-β-Farnesene	0–10.3%
β-Caryophyllene	0.8–9.3%
α-Terpineol	0.2–9.3%
(+)-Limonene	0.5–7.4%
(Z)-β-Farnesene	0–6.9%
Citronellyl acetate	0.2–6.0%
β-Selinene	0–6.0%
β-Myrcene	0–5.6%
α-Terpinyl acetate	0.1–4.6%
Linalyl acetate	0–3.6%
Linalool	0–3.0%
Thymol	0–2.7%
Caryophyllene oxide	0–2.5%

Terpinen-4-ol	tr–2.2%
(−)-*allo*-Aromadendrene	0–2.1%
Spathulenol	0.2–2.0%
α-Bisabolol	0–1.8%
γ-Terpinene	0.5–1.7%
T-Cadinol	0–1.6%
β-Pinene	0.8–1.5%
Methyleugenol	0–1.5%
(*E*)-Dihydroterpineol	0–1.3%
α-Gurjunene	0–1.2%
Piperitone	0–1.2%
Citronellol	0.2–1.0%
α-Guaiaiene	0–1.0%
Guaiol	0–1.0%
(*Z*)-β-Ocimene	0–1.0%
Germacrene D	0–1.0%

(Senatore et al 1996; Valentini et al 1998; Sørensen & Katsiotis 2000)

Safety summary

Hazards: Drug interaction; reproductive hormone modulation; may contain methyleugenol.
Contraindications (all routes): Progesterone therapy, pregnancy, breastfeeding, prepubertal children.
Cautions (all routes): May cause unpleasant side effects in some women.
Cautions (oral): Drugs metabolized by CYP2D6 (Appendix B), estrogen replacement therapy, oral contraceptives.

Regulatory guidelines

Because of its probable hormonal action, we recommend that chaste tree oil is not used during pregnancy or breastfeeding. IFRA recommends that the maximum concentration of methyleugenol for leave-on products such as body lotion should be 0.0004% (IFRA 2009). The equivalent SCCNFP maximum is 0.0002% (European Commission 2002).

Organ-specific effects

Adverse skin reactions: Of 13 women applying varying but unknown concentrations of chaste tree leaf oil, one found it to be a skin sensitizer and discontinued use (Lucks 2002). Of 52 women using a 1.5% concentration of an essential oil distilled from the fruiting plant (incorporating both leaf and seed) in a lotion base, one experienced a rash and one a prickling sensation (Lucks 2003).
Reproductive toxicity: In a pilot study involving 23 women to evaluate the effects of chaste tree leaf and seed oil on menopause, 13 used the leaf oil and 9 the seed oil. Methods of use were varied, but were mostly external. Two subjects discontinued the seed oil after experiencing hot flashes, something neither had experienced previously (Lucks 2002).

In a study with 52 participants, 2.5 mL of a 1.5% concentration of an essential oil distilled from the fruiting plant (incorporating both leaf and seed) was used topically, once daily, 5–7 days per week for 3 months. The subjects included 31 perimenopausal women, 11 postmenopausal, and 10 recent hysterectomies. There was no control group. Of the 52 participants, 12 (23.2%) experienced exacerbation of symptoms. 'Emotional decline' was reported by six subjects, five noted increased bleeding and three reported increased hot flashes/night sweats. Several other effects were noted by either one or two subjects. Side effects disappeared on discontinuing the oil. Subjects who used chaste tree oil concurrently with any form of progesterone (including progesterone cream) consistently experienced breakthrough bleeding (Lucks 2003).

Systemic effects

Acute toxicity: No information found.
Carcinogenic/anticarcinogenic potential: No information found. Methyleugenol is a rodent carcinogen if exposure is sufficiently high; both (+)-limonene and nerolidol display anticarcinogenic activity (see Constituent profiles, Chapter 14).
Drug interactions: Since farnesene and α-bisabolol inhibit CYP2D6 (Table 4.11B), there is a theoretical risk of interaction between chaste tree leaf or seed oil and drugs metabolized by this enzyme (Appendix B).

Comments

Chaste tree extract exhibits dopaminergic activity. It lowers serum estrogen and increases progesterone levels, and this activity may partly reside in the essential oil (Lucks 2002). Referring to the extract, Mills and Bone (2000) observe: 'Although the dopaminergic activity might suggest that chaste tree is best avoided during lactation, clinical trials have demonstrated its positive activity, albeit at low doses'. Methyleugenol has been found in non-commercial oils in Italy and Cyprus (Valentini et al 1998) but not in oils from Croatia (Males et al 1998) which is the main source of commercial chaste tree oil. The oil is also produced in Turkey. Chaste tree oils containing methyleugenol may need some restriction. This genus was formerly in the Verbenaceae. There are several varieties of *Vitex negundo* (Chinese chaste tree) grown in China, and essential oils may be produced from these. None of them are toxicologically significant, and β-caryophyllene is typically the major constituent.

Chervil

Botanical name: *Anthriscus cerefolium* (L.) Hoffm.
Family: Apiaceae (Umbelliferae)

Essential oil

Source: Leaves
Key constituents:

Estragole	49.9–81.3%
l-Allyl 2,4-dimethoxybenzene	13.4–31.9%
Nonanal	0.1–3.9%
l-Allyl 3,4-dimethoxybenzene	0.6–1.4%
Undecane	0.8–1.3%
1-Octadecanol	0–1.3%

(Fakhry, private communication, 2002)

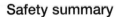

Safety summary

Hazards: Potentially carcinogenic; may inhibit blood clotting.
Contraindications: Should not be taken in oral doses.
Maximum dermal use level:

EU	No limit
IFRA	0.01%
Tisserand & Young	0.15%

Our safety advice

We recommend a dermal maximum of 0.15% based on 81.3% estragole content with an estragole limit of 0.12% (see Estragole profile, Chapter 14).

Regulatory guidelines

IFRA recommends a maximum dermal use level for estragole of 0.01% in leave-on or wash-off preparations for body and face (IFRA 2009).

Organ-specific effects

Cardiovascular effects: Estragole inhibits platelet aggregation (Yoshioka & Tamada 2005), an essential step in the blood clotting cascade.

Systemic effects

Acute toxicity: No information found for chervil oil. Estragole acute oral LD_{50} in mice 1.25 g/kg, in rats 1.82 g/kg (Opdyke 1976 p. 603).
Carcinogenic/anticarcinogenic potential: No information found for chervil oil. Estragole is a rodent carcinogen when oral exposure is sufficiently high (see Estragole profile, Chapter 14).

Comments

Limited availability.

Cinnamon bark

Botanical name: *Cinnamomum verum* J. Presl.
Botanical synonym: *Cinnamomum zeylanicum* Blume
Family: Lauraceae

Essential oil

Source: Dried inner bark of young trees
Key constituents:

(*E*)-Cinnamaldehyde	63.1–75.7%
Eugenol	2.0–13.3%
(*E*)-Cinnamyl acetate	0.3–10.6%
Linalool	0.2–7.0%
β-Caryophyllene	1.3–5.8%
p-Cymene	1.7–2.5%
1,8-Cineole	0.4–2.3%
Benzaldehyde	tr–2.2%
β-Phellandrene	<1.5%
α-Terpineol	0.4–1.4%
Camphor	tr–1.4%
Terpinen-4-ol	0.4–1.1%
Benzyl benzoate	tr–1.0%
α-Caryophyllene	0–1.0%
Safrole	0–0.04%

(Lawrence 1995 g p. 201; Tateo & Chizzini 1989; Kubeczka 2002)
Quality: Cinnamon bark oil is frequently adulterated with synthetic cinnamaldehyde and natural eugenol. Occasionally cassia oil or artificially reconstituted oils are sold as cinnamon bark oil (Kubeczka 2002). Reconstitutions may include cinnamon leaf oil and synthetic cinnamaldehyde (Burfield 2000).

Safety summary

Hazards: Drug interaction; may inhibit blood clotting; embryotoxicity; skin sensitization (high risk); mucous membrane irritation (low risk).
Contraindications (all routes): Pregnancy, breastfeeding.
Cautions (oral): Diabetes medication, anticoagulant medication, major surgery, peptic ulcer, hemophilia, other bleeding disorders (Box 7.1).
Maximum adult daily oral dose: 200 mg
Maximum dermal use level: 0.07%

Our safety advice

Our dermal maximum is based on 75.7% cinnamaldehyde content with a dermal limit of 0.05% (see Cinnamaldehyde profile, Chapter 14). We agree with the Commission E Monographs daily oral maximum of 200 mg for the oil.

Regulatory guidelines

Has GRAS status. The Council of Europe (1992) has set an ADI of 1.25 mg/kg for cinnamaldehyde, which is equivalent to an adult dose of 115 mg of cinnamon bark oil. The Commission E Monographs recommend an oral dose range of 50–200 mg for cinnamon bark oil (Blumenthal et al 1998). IFRA recommends a maximum dermal use level for cinnamaldehyde of 0.05% for most product types (IFRA 2009). According to the SCCNFP (2001a) the concentration of cinnamaldehyde in any finished product should not exceed 0.1%.

Organ-specific effects

Adverse skin reactions: The undiluted oil was severely irritating to rabbits, and was mildly irritating to mice; tested at 8% on two panels of 25 volunteers it was not irritating. In sensitization tests carried out on two panels, 8% cinnamon bark oil produced positive reactions in 18/25 and 20/25 volunteers (Opdyke 1975 p. 111–112). In another test, the lowest concentration causing positive reactions in patch tests was 0.01% (Mathias et al 1980). Of six dermatitis patients who developed ACD from the use of a proprietary skin ointment containing cinnamon oil two were positive to cinnamaldehyde on patch testing, and four were not (Calnan 1976). Undiluted cinnamon oil (type unspecified) caused severe burns in an 11-year-old boy after remaining in contact with the skin for 48 hours, when a vial broke in his pocket (Sparks 1985). Contact with the skin by undiluted cinnamon oil (type unspecified) is frequently associated with a burning sensation, and occasional blistering (Perry et al 1990). Sensitization is also seen with cinnamaldehyde, which is a frequent cause of contact dermatitis (see Cinnamaldehyde profile, Chapter 14).

Low-level phototoxic effects were reported for cinnamon bark oil, but these were not considered to be significant (Opdyke 1975 p. 111–112). In an in vitro assay, cinnamaldehyde showed phototoxic effects, but cinnamon bark oil did not (Placzek et al 2007).

Cardiovascular effects: Gavage doses of 25, 50 or 100 mg/kg/day of cinnamon bark oil for 35 days decreased plasma glucose concentrations in KK-A^y diabetic mice (Ping et al 2010). Cinnamaldehyde inhibits platelet aggregation (Huang J et al 2007a), an essential step in the blood clotting cascade.

Reproductive toxicity: When cinnamon bark oil (0.25%, 375 mg/kg) was fed to pregnant mice for two weeks it significantly reduced the number of nuclei and altered the distribution of embryos according to nucleus number (Domaracky et al 2007). In tests using cinnamaldehyde, there are inconclusive signs of reproductive toxicity (see Cinnamaldehyde profile, Chapter 14).

Hepatotoxicity: At 25 or 50 mg/kg ip in rats, cinnamaldehyde reduced the activity of glutathione S-transferase, but did not deplete glutathione, which slightly increased (Choi et al 2001).

Systemic effects

Acute toxicity, human: Cinnamon oil (type not known) caused poisoning after the ingestion of approximately 60 mL by a 7-year-old boy who drank the oil when dared to by a friend. Symptoms included a burning sensation in the mouth, chest and stomach, dizziness, double vision and nausea. There was also vomiting and later collapse. The doctors involved considered that had vomiting not occurred the dose could have been fatal, but there were no serious consequences (Pilapil 1989).

Acute toxicity, animal: Cinnamon bark oil acute oral LD$_{50}$ in rats 3.4 mL/kg; acute dermal LD$_{50}$ in rabbits 0.69 mL/kg (Opdyke 1975 p. 111–112). In mice, cinnamon bark oil has caused edema and variable changes in blood pressure after ip dosing at 100 mg/kg (Powers et al 1961). This dose is 5–10 times higher than the amount which would be absorbed from even oral administration.

Antioxidant/pro-oxidant activity: Cinnamon bark oil displayed powerful antioxidant activity in two in vitro models, of nitration and lipid peroxidation, decreasing 3-nitrotyrosine formation with an IC$_{50}$ value of 18.4 µg/mL. The same tests failed to reveal any antioxidant activity for cinnamaldehyde (Chericoni et al 2005). Cinnamon bark oil significantly scavenges DPPH and hydroxyl radicals (Singh G et al 2007). In another DPPH assay, an IC$_{50}$ of 0.065 µL/mL was determined (Tomaino et al 2005).

Carcinogenic/anticarcinogenic potential: Cinnamon bark oil was cytotoxic to human prostate, lung and breast cancer cells with IC$_{50}$ values of 0.01%, 0.01% and 0.07% respectively (Zu et al 2010). Cinnamon bark oil was not mutagenic in the Ames test and was marginally mutagenic in Chinese hamster fibroblasts (Ishidate et al 1984). Cinnamaldehyde is not a rodent carcinogen (National Toxicology Program 2004).

Drug interactions: Antidiabetic or anticoagulant medication, because of cardiovascular effects, above. See Table 4.10B.

Comments

The maximum dermal use level is based on cinnamaldehyde content as there are insufficient cinnamon bark oil data to make a determination. The maximum level of safrole present in cinnamon bark oil would not be dose-limiting. There is an unusual safrole chemotype of *Cinnamomum verum*, which contains 11% in the bark oil, and 52% in the leaf oil (Wijesekera 1978). These safrole-containing oils will present a carcinogenic risk. Two qualities of cinnamon bark oil are produced in Sri Lanka, a premium quality distilled from the inner bark, and a second quality from the chippings and the bark from shoots and twigs. This oil may have a reduced cinnamaldehyde content, and up to 20% eugenol (Burfield 2000).

Cinnamon leaf

Botanical name: *Cinnamomum verum* J. Presl.
Botanical synonym: *Cinnamomum zeylanicum* Blume
Family: Lauraceae

Essential oil

Source: Leaves
Key constituents:

Eugenol	68.6–87.0%
Eugenyl acetate	1.0–8.1%
Linalool	2.0–5.0%
(*E*)-Cinnamyl acetate	0.8–4.6%
Benzyl benzoate	tr–4.1%
β-Caryophyllene	1.9–3.7%
(*E*)-Cinnamaldehyde	0.6–1.1%
Safrole	0–1.0%
Cinnamyl alcohol	0–0.6%

(Lawrence 1979 p. 29, 1995g p. 148, p. 201)
Quality: Cinnamon leaf oil may be adulterated by the addition of clove fractions, eugenol or cinnamic aldehyde (Burfield 2003).

Safety summary

Hazards: Drug interaction; may inhibit blood clotting; may contain safrole; skin sensitization (moderate risk); mucous membrane irritation (low risk).
Cautions (oral): May interact with pethidine, MAOIs or SSRIs. Anticoagulant medication, major surgery, peptic ulcer, hemophilia, other bleeding disorders (Box 7.1).
Maximum adult daily oral dose: 175 mg
Maximum dermal use level (based on safrole content):

EU	1.0%
IFRA	1.0%
Tisserand & Young	5.0%

Maximum dermal use level (based on eugenol content):

EU	No legal limit
IFRA	0.6%
Tisserand & Young	0.6%

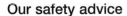
Our safety advice

We recommend a dermal maximum of 0.6% based on 87% eugenol content with a limit of 0.5% (see Eugenol profile, Chapter 14). Our oral maximum is based on 1.0% safrole, with a limit of 0.025 mg/kg/day (see Safrole profile, Chapter 14).

Regulatory guidelines

Has GRAS status. IFRA and the EU recommend a maximum exposure level of 0.01% of safrole from the use of safrole-containing essential oils in cosmetics. IFRA recommends a maximum dermal use level for eugenol of 0.5% for most product types, in order to avoid skin sensitization (IFRA 2009).

Organ-specific effects

Adverse skin reactions: Undiluted cinnamon leaf oil was moderately irritating to mice, and strongly irritating to rabbits; tested at 10% on 25 volunteers it was neither irritating nor sensitizing. It is non-phototoxic (Opdyke 1975 p. 749). Contact with the skin by undiluted cinnamon oil (type unspecified) is frequently associated with a burning sensation, and occasional blistering (Perry et al 1990). Undiluted cinnamon oil (type unspecified) caused severe burns in an 11-year-old boy after remaining in contact with the skin for 48 hours, when a vial broke in his pants pocket (Sparks 1985). In a case of extensive and long-lasting dermatitis following a mud bath containing cinnamon oil, patch testing confirmed allergy to cinnamon oil in a 74-year-old woman (García-Abujeta et al 2005). Several cases of occupational ACD to cinnamon oil have been reported, one of them through airborne contact (Ackermann et al 2009; Sánchez-Pérez & García-Díez 1999).

Cardiovascular effects: Eugenol inhibits platelet aggregation (Janssens et al 1990), an essential step in the blood clotting cascade.

Systemic effects

Acute toxicity, human: See Cinnamon bark oil, above.

Acute toxicity, animal: Cinnamon leaf oil acute oral LD_{50} in rats 2.65 g/kg; acute dermal LD_{50} in rabbits >5 g/kg (Opdyke 1975 p. 749).

Antioxidant/pro-oxidant activity: Cinnamon leaf oil was moderately active in scavenging activity against DPPH and hydroxyl radicals (Singh G et al 2007).

Carcinogenic/anticarcinogenic potential: No information found. Safrole is a rodent carcinogen when exposure is sufficiently high; anticarcinogenic activity has been reported for eugenol (see Eugenol profile, Chapter 14).

Drug interactions: Anticoagulant medication, because of cardiovascular effects, above. Since eugenol significantly inhibits human MAO-A (Tao et al 2005), oral doses of eugenol-rich essential oils may interact with pethidine, indirect sympathomimetics, MAOIs or SSRIs (Table 4.10B).

Comments

The safrole content of cinnamon leaf oil would mean that 1.0% or more of the oil could be used for dermal application. However, a greater restriction is in place for eugenol.

Cistus

Botanical name: *Cistus ladanifer* L.
Botanical synonym: *Cistus ladaniferus* Curtis
Family: Cistaceae

Essential oil

Source: Flowering plant
Key constituents:

α-Pinene	3.5–56.0%
Camphene	1.1–10.3%
(3Z)-Hexen-1-ol	0–6.8%
2,2,6-Trimethylcyclohexanone	1.7–5.7%
Bornyl acetate	2.1–4.8%
(2E)-Hexen-1-ol	0–4.5%
Viridiflorol	0–4.5%
p-Cymene	0.7–4.0%
Pinocarveol	1.2–3.4%
p-Menthatriene	0–2.9%
Benzaldehyde	0–2.8%
α-Campholenic aldehyde	0–2.6%
Isopinocamphone	0–2.5%
(+)-Limonene	1.4–2.3%
Eugenol	0–2.3%
Isomenthone	0–2.3%
Acetophenone	0–2.2%
Verbenone	0–2.0%
Geraniol	0–1.7%
γ-Terpinene	1.3–1.6%
α-p-Dimethylstyrene	0–1.6%
(−)-allo-Aromadendrene	0–1.2%
Tricyclene	0–1.2%
Terpinen-4-ol	0.1–1.1%
Dodecanal	0–1.1%
Fenchone	0–1.1%
α-Amorphene	0–1.0%
α-Thujone	0–0.8%

(Lawrence 1989 p. 93–95, 1993 p91–92, 1999d p. 41–50)

Safety summary

Hazards: Skin sensitization if oxidized.
Cautions: Old or oxidized oils should be avoided.

Our safety advice

Because of its potentially high α-pinene content we recommend that oxidation of cistus oil is avoided by storage in a dark, airtight container in a refrigerator. The addition of an antioxidant to preparations containing it is recommended.

Organ-specific effects

Adverse skin reactions: No information found for cistus oil, but autoxidation products of α-pinene can cause skin sensitization (see α-Pinene profile, Chapter 14).

Systemic effects

Acute toxicity: No information found.
Carcinogenic/anticarcinogenic potential: No information found for cistus oil, but it contains no known carcinogens. (+)-Limonene and geraniol display anticarcinogenic activity (see Constituent profiles, Chapter 14).

Comments

Although cistus oil contains small amounts of isopinocamphone and α-thujone, both inhibitors of GABA$_A$ receptor-mediated responses, it also contains higher concentrations of α-pinene, which potentiates these responses. Therefore no restrictions are needed in regard to neurotoxicity. Cistus oil is obtained by direct steam distillation of the whole flowering plant, as distinct from labdanum oil, which is produced from the gum.

Citronella

Botanical names: *Cymbopogon nardus* L. (synonym: *Andropogon nardus* L.) (Sri Lanka type citronella); *Cymbopogon winterianus* Jowitt (Java type citronella)
Family: Poaceae (Gramineae)

Essential oil

Source: Leaves
Key constituents:

Cymbopogon nardus

Citronellal	5.2–46.8%
Geraniol	16.8–29.1%
(−)-Citronellol	3.0–21.8%
(+)-Limonene	2.6–11.3%
(E)-Methyl isoeugenol	0–10.7%
Camphene	0.1–8.0%
Citronellyl acetate	0.9–7.3%
Borneol	0–6.6%
Elemol	1.1–5.0%
α-Pinene	1.9–4.8%
Geranyl formate	0–4.2%
β-Cubebene	0–3.8%
Geranyl acetate	2.1–3.4%
β-Caryophyllene	0.4–3.2%
α-Bergamotene	0–2.3%
(Z)-β-Ocimene	0–2.2%
Isopulegol	0.5–2.1%
Guaiene	0–1.9%
(E)-β-Ocimene	0–1.8%
Methyleugenol	0–1.7%
δ-Cadinene	0.1–1.6%
Linalool	0.5–1.5%
Tricyclene	0–1.5%
Geranyl butyrate	0–1.5%
α-Cadinene	0–1.5%
(Z)-Methyl isoeugenol	0–1.2%

(Wijesekera 1973; Bruns et al 1981; Carlin et al 1988; Lawrence 1989 p. 31; Zhu et al 1993 p. 112)

Cymbopogon winterianus

Citronellal	34.8–42.8%
Geraniol	22.1–25.4%
(−)-Citronellol	9.7–11.5%
Elemol	2.0–5.6%
(+)-Limonene	2.6–5.5%
Geranyl acetate	2.9–5.1%
β-Elemene	1.9–3.2%
β-Cubebene	1.8–2.8%
Eugenol	1.1–2.5%
γ-Cadinene	1.7–2.3%
Citronellyl acetate	1.0–2.0%
T-Amorphol	0.7–1.4%
δ-Cadinene	0.5–1.2%
Linalool	0.5–1.1%
Methyleugenol	0–0.1%

(Carlin et al 1988; Rao et al 1998)

Safety summary

Hazards: Drug interaction; may contain methyleugenol; skin sensitization (low risk).
Cautions (oral): Drugs metabolized by CYP2B6 (Appendix B).
Maximum dermal use level (based on methyleugenol content):

EU	0.01%
IFRA	0.02%
Tisserand & Young	No limit

Maximum dermal use level (based on geraniol content):

EU	No legal limit
IFRA	18.2%
Tisserand & Young	18.2%

Our safety advice

We recommend a dermal maximum of 18.2%, based on 29.1% geraniol with a dermal limit of 5.3% (see Geraniol profile, Chapter 14). Considering its lack of genotoxicity, its chemopreventive activity, and the fact that anticarcinogens constitute over 60% of the oil while methyleugenol is only found at 0–1.7%, we do not consider that citronella oil presents a material risk of carcinogenicity.

Regulatory guidelines

Has GRAS status. IFRA recommends a maximum concentration of 0.0004% methyleugenol in leave-on products such as body lotions (IFRA 2009). The equivalent SCCNFP maximum is 0.0002% (European Commission 2002). Following a re-evaluation of its safety, Canada's Pest Management Regulatory Agency (PMRA) was unable to conclude that insect repellents containing citronella were acceptable for continued use. The PMRA proposes to phase out citronella-based insect repellents unless data to address uncertainties in their human health risk assessment are generated and submitted by manufacturers. The concerns of the PMRA are that citronella oils may contain methyleugenol, and that therefore the carcinogenic hazard posed is unacceptable, and that there are no data on reproductive or developmental toxicity (www.pmra-arla.gc.ca/english/consum/insectrepellents-e.html accessed July 31st 2011). In the EU citronella oil is not restricted in cosmetics, but it is no longer permitted as an ingredient in products making insect repellent claims (http://www.citrefine.com/eudirectives.html accessed July 31st 2011). This ruling was not made on safety grounds, but because no manufacturer registered citronella oil as an insect repellent by the deadline set by the European Biocide Products Directive. (The European chemicals industry was successful in lobbying for registration to be onerous for natural products manufacturers.) In a 1997 report, the EPA concluded: '...based on available data, the use of currently registered products containing oil of citronella in accordance with their approved labeling will not pose unreasonable risks or adverse effects to humans or the environment. Therefore, all currently registered uses of these products are eligible for reregistration.' (www.epa.gov/oppsrrd1/REDs/3105red.pdf accessed July 28th 2012).

Organ-specific effects

Adverse skin reactions: Undiluted citronella oil was irritating to rabbits, the Sri Lankan oil more so than the Javan (Environmental Protection Agency 1997). In a modified Draize procedure on guinea pigs, Sri Lanka type citronella oil was non-sensitizing when used at 40% in the challenge phase, but citronella from Guatemala (Java type) was sensitizing when used at 20% (Sharp 1978). Conversely, in a guinea pig dermal sensitization study, citronella oil Sri Lanka type was was sensitizing, and citronella oil Java type was not (Environmental Protection Agency 1997). In a mouse local lymph node assay, citronella oil Sri Lanka type was only an extremely weak sensitizer (Lalko & Api 2006). Three types of citronella oil (Sri Lanka, Java and 'Formosa') were tested on 25 volunteers at 8%. None were irritating or sensitizing (Opdyke 1973 p. 1067–1068).

There are at least five case reports of contact dermatitis from citronella oil (Lane 1922; Keil 1947; Davies et al 1978). In two instances, patch testing revealed allergy to several constituents of the oil. In three cases, the undiluted oil had been used as an insect repellant, and came in direct contact with the skin, and one case was an occupational accident with the undiluted oil. In the other case, citronella oil was suspected as the cause, but not confirmed.

Of 200 consecutive dermatitis patients, five (2.5%) were sensitive to 2% citronella oil (Rudzki et al 1976). Of 750 consecutive dermatitis patients, 11 (1.5%) were sensitive to 2% citronella oil (Rudzki & Grzywa 1985). In a clinical trial to assess the efficacy of citronella oil as a head lice repellent, a formulation with 3.7% citronella oil was administered daily for four months to the heads of 103 children. One child reported slight itching and burning (Mumcuoglu et al 2004).

Based on literature published in German, citronella oil has been classified as category C, not significantly allergenic, by Schlede et al (2003).

Systemic effects

Acute toxicity, human: A girl of 21 months died after ingesting up to 15 mL of 'Antimate', a product containing citronella oil. Reported signs of poisoning included vomiting, shock, frothing at the mouth, raised body temperature, deep and rapid respiration, cyanosis and mild convulsions. Findings on autopsy included hemorrhages in the white matter of the brain, collapse of the lungs, and congestion of the gastric mucosa. Since the other ingredients of the product were not mentioned in the report, it is not clear whether citronella oil was the sole toxic agent (Mant 1961). Temple et al (1991) pointed out that the child was given a salt water emetic by her grandmother, and the cerebral hemorrhages are consistent with salt intoxication; the girl was also given nikethamide, formerly used as a respiratory stimulant, which could have caused her convulsions, especially since these did not occur until five hours after ingesting the citronella oil. Approximately 25 mL of citronella oil were ingested by a boy of 16 months. Part of his stomach contents were voided 30 minutes later due to medical intervention, but apart from some oral irritation he appeared healthy and was discharged (Temple et al 1991).

Acute toxicity, animal: Citronella oil (type unspecified) acute oral LD_{50} in rats >5 g/kg; acute dermal LD_{50} in rabbits 4.7 mL/kg (Opdyke 1973 p. 1067–1068). Acute oral LD_{50} in rats for Java type citronella oil >4.38 g/kg, and for Sri Lanka type oil >5.0 g/kg; acute rabbit dermal LD_{50} for both types of oil 2.0 g/kg. Rat inhalation toxicity for Java type oil, LC_{50} 3.1 mg/L (Environmental Protection Agency 1997).

Antioxidant/pro-oxidant activity: *Cymbopogon nardus* oil displayed significant scavenging activity against DPPH radicals, with an IC_{50} of 2.0 μL/mL, compared with 31.4 μL/mL for BHT (Lertsatitthanakorn et al 2006).

Carcinogenic/anticarcinogenic potential: Citronella oil (type unspecified) was not mutagenic in an Ames test, using *Salmonella* strains TA98, TA100, TA1537 and TA1535, both with and without S9 activation. The oil was similarly non-genotoxic in CHL fibroblasts (Ishidate et al 1988), Chinese hamster ovary cells (no CA in either), and in a UDS study in rat hepatocytes (Environmental Protection Agency 1997). Citronella oil Sri Lanka type showed significant chemopreventive activity against human mouth epidermal carcinoma (KB) cells and moderate activity against mouse leukemia (P388) cells, with respective IC_{50} values of 0.081 and 1.493 mg/mL (Manosroi et al 2005). Methyleugenol is a rodent carcinogen if exposure is sufficiently high; citronellal, geraniol, (+)-limonene and β-elemene display anticarcinogenic activity (see Constituent profiles, Chapter 14).

Drug interactions: Since geraniol inhibits CYP2B6 (Table 4.11B), there is a theoretical risk of interaction between citronella oil and drugs metabolized by this enzyme (Appendix B).

Comments

The approach of the EPA to citronella oil insect repellents is in contrast to that of the PMRA. The EPA waived the requirement for developmental toxicity, on the basis of the oil's low acute toxicity, its lack of mutagenicity, its GRAS status, and the lack of reports of adverse effects. The EPA report includes this statement: 'Oil of citronella has been in continuous use as an insect repellent with human applications for almost 50 years without any adverse incidents being reported to the EPA. This long use history without adverse incidents, combined with the low acute mammalian toxicity, indicates that oil of citronella is not likely to cause adverse effects resulting from aggregate exposures or cumulative effects.' (Environmental Protection Agency 1997). When the EPA report was written, methyleugenol was not generally regarded as a carcinogen, and this factor was not considered. The PMRA report states: 'Although available data for whole natural citronella oil...did not indicate oncogenic hazard' and then refers to the possible presence of methyleugenol.

Several websites mention that citronella oil has been known to "increase the heart rate of some people", for example: (http://www.cbc.ca/news/background/consumers/citronella. html accessed July 31st 2011). However, this assertion appears to be groundless. In regard to the skin, the available data indicate that the risk to the general population of sensitization from citronella oil is negligible. The extremely low number of reported adverse skin reactions is in spite of widespread dermal application as an insect repellent. *Cymbopogon winterianus* oil is produced in large quantities in Java, Taiwan and China. This type of citronella oil typically has a higher citronellal content than that of *C. nardus*, and is considered to possess a more pleasant odor (Burfield 2000).

Clary sage

Synonym: Muscatel sage
Botanical name: *Salvia sclarea* L.
Family: Lamiaceae (Labiatae)

Absolute

Source: Leaves and flowering tops
Key constituents:

Linalyl acetate	66.5%
Linalool	8.9%
Germacrene D	9.4%
Sclareol	2.4%
β-Caryophyllene	1.9%
α-Copaene	1.1%
Bicyclogermacrene	1.1%

(Fakhry, private communication, 2002)

Safety summary

Hazards: Skin sensitization (moderate risk).
Contraindications: None known.
Maximum dermal use level: 0.25%

Our safety advice

The maximum use level is based on the 0.25% found by Bouhlal et al (1988b) to be the highest concentration producing no adverse skin reactions.

Organ-specific effects

Adverse skin reactions: Tested at 2, 8 and 10% on 25 volunteers with a previous history of reaction to fragrance materials, clary sage absolute produced allergic reactions in five, seven and seven individuals, respectively. In this high-risk group, 0.25% was the concentration at which any observable reaction disappears (Bouhlal et al 1988b).

Systemic effects

Acute toxicity: No information found. Linalyl acetate is non-toxic (see Linalyl acetate profile, Chapter 14).
Carcinogenic/anticarcinogenic potential: No information found for clary sage absolute, but it contains no known carcinogens. Sclareol has demonstrated anticarcinogenic activity (see Sclareol profile, Chapter 14).

Comments

Because sclareol has an extremely low volatility it only shows up as a small percentage when analyzed, as above, by gas chromatography. However, HPLC analysis reveals that clary sage absolute typically consists of 70–75% sclareol and 13-*epi*-sclareol (Burfield, private communication, 2003).

Essential oil

Source: Leaves and flowering tops
Key constituents:

French

Linalyl acetate	49.0–73.6%
Linalool	9.0–16.0%
Germacrene D	1.6–2.0%
β-Caryophyllene	1.4–1.6%

(Lawrence 1993 p. 106–108)

Russian

Linalyl acetate	45.3–61.8%
Linalool	10.4–19.3%
α-Terpineol	1.2–2.5%
Germacrene D	0.7–2.0%
β-Caryophyllene	1.1–1.8%
Geranyl acetate	0.8–1.2%
Geraniol	0.6–1.2%

(Lawrence 1993 p. 106–108)
Quality: Clary sage oil may be adulterated with natural or synthetic mixtures containing linalool and linalyl acetate (Kubeczka 2002).

Safety summary

Hazards: None known.
Contraindications: None known.

Regulatory guidelines

Has GRAS status.

Organ-specific effects

Adverse skin reactions: Undiluted French clary sage oil was moderately irritating to rabbits, but was not irritating to 30 volunteers; tested at 8% on 25 volunteers it was neither irritating nor sensitizing (Opdyke 1974 p. 865–866). Undiluted Russian clary sage oil was not irritating to mice; tested at 8% on two panels of 25 volunteers it was neither irritating nor sensitizing. It is non-phototoxic (Opdyke & Letizia 1982 p. 823–824). In a study of 200 consecutive dermatitis patients, one (0.5%) was sensitive to 2% clary sage oil on patch testing (Rudzki et al 1976).

Systemic effects

Acute toxicity: French clary sage oil acute oral LD_{50} in rats 5.6 g/kg; acute dermal LD_{50} in rabbits >2 g/kg (Opdyke 1974 p. 865–866).

Carcinogenic/anticarcinogenic potential: Clary sage oil was not mutagenic in either the *Bacillus subtilis* rec-assay or the Ames test (Zani et al 1991). French clary sage oil showed strong in vitro activity against four human cancer cell lines: HL60 (leukemia), K562 (myelogenous leukemia), MCF7 (breast) and A2780 (ovarian). The activity was comparable to that of dioxorubicin, used as a positive control (Foray et al 1999).

Comments

Clary sage oil is also produced in China and the USA. American production is primarily for solvent extraction, in order to produce sclareol (see previous profile) which in turn is processed into synthetic ambergris-like compounds. Some clary sage oils are produced from slightly fermented leaves, resulting in a richer, more vegetable-like odor profile (Burfield 2000). According to Franchomme & Pénöel (1990), clary sage oil is estrogen-like due to its content of sclareol. However, clary sage oils typically contain only 0.1 - 0.4% sclareol on GC analysis (Lawrence 1993 p. 106–108). Sclareol is a labdane diterpene derivative which has no known estrogen-like activity (Topçu & Gören 2007), although a sclareol isomer, 13-*epi*-sclareol, inhibits breast and uterine cancer in vitro, possibly by interacting with estrogen receptors (Sashidhara et al 2007). Neither compound, however, bears any obvious structural similarity to endogenous estrogens.

Clementine

Botanical name: *Citrus clementina* Hort. ex Tanaka
Botanical synonym: *Citrus reticulata* Blanco var. *clementina*
Family: Rutaceae

Essential oil

Source: Fruit peel
Key constituents:

(+)-Limonene	94.8–95.0%
β-Myrcene	1.6–1.8%

(Dugo et al 1988, Ruberto et al 1994)

Safety summary

Hazards: Skin sensitization if oxidized.
Cautions: Old or oxidized oils should be avoided.

Our safety advice

Because of its limonene content we recommend that oxidation of clementine oil is avoided by storage in a dark, airtight container in a refrigerator. The addition of an antioxidant to preparations containing it is recommended.

Regulatory guidelines

IFRA recommends that essential oils rich in limonene should only be used when the level of peroxides is kept to the lowest practical level, for instance by adding antioxidants at the time of production (IFRA 2009).

Organ-specific effects

Adverse skin reactions: No information found. Autoxidation products of (+)-limonene can cause skin sensitization (see (+)-Limonene profile, Chapter 14).

Reproductive toxicity: The low developmental toxicity of (+)-limonene in rabbits and mice (Kodama et al 1977a, 1977b) suggests that clementine oil is not hazardous in pregnancy.

Systemic effects

Acute toxicity: No information found. (+)-Limonene is non-toxic (see (+)-Limonene profile, Chapter 14).

Carcinogenic/anticarcinogenic potential: No information found. (+)-Limonene displays anticarcinogenic activity (see (+)-Limonene profile, Chapter 14).

Comments

Clementine oil has not been tested for phototoxicity. Limited availability.

Clove bud

Botanical name: *Syzygium aromaticum* (L.) Merill et L.M. Perry
Botanical synonyms: *Eugenia caryophyllata* Thunb., *Eugenia aromatica* L.
Family: Myrtaceae

Essential oil

Source: Dried flower buds
Key constituents:

Eugenol	73.5–96.9%
β-Caryophyllene	0.6–12.4%
Eugenyl acetate	0.5–10.7%
α-Caryophyllene	0.4–1.4%
Isoeugenol	0.1–0.2%
Methyleugenol	0–0.2%

(Kubeczka 2002, Lawrence 1981 p33–34, 1993 p.36)

Quality: Clove bud oil may be adulterated with clove stem or leaf oils, or with eugenol (Kubeczka 2002, Singhal et al 1997).

Safety summary

Hazards: Drug interaction; may contain methyleugenol; may inhibit blood clotting; embryotoxicity; skin sensitization (moderate risk); mucous membrane irritation (moderate risk).
Cautions (oral): May interact with pethidine, MAOIs or SSRIs. Anticoagulant medication, major surgery, peptic ulcer, hemophilia, other bleeding disorders (Box 7.1).
Cautions (dermal): Hypersensitive, diseased or damaged skin, children under 2 years of age.
Maximum dermal use level (based on methyleugenol content):

EU	0.1%
IFRA	0.2%
Tisserand & Young	10%

Maximum dermal use level (based on eugenol content):

EU	No legal limit
IFRA	0.5%
Tisserand & Young	0.5%

Our safety advice

We recommend a dermal maximum of 0.5% based on 96.9% eugenol content and a limit of 0.5% (see Eugenol profile, Chapter 14).

Regulatory guidelines

IFRA recommends a maximum dermal use level for eugenol of 0.5% for most product types, in order to avoid skin sensitization (IFRA 2009). IFRA recommends a maximum dermal use level for isoeugenol of 0.02% in products that will come into contact with the skin (IFRA 2009). IFRA recommends that the maximum concentration of methyleugenol for leave-on products such as body lotion should be 0.0004% (IFRA 2009). The equivalent SCCNFP maximum is 0.0002% (European Commission 2002).

Organ-specific effects

Adverse skin reactions: In a 48 hour occlusive patch test on 50 Italian volunteers, undiluted clove oil produced no adverse reactions. Similarly tested at 1%, it produced one reaction in 380 eczema patients (Meneghini et al 1971). Undiluted clove bud oil was moderately irritating to rabbits, but was not irritating to mice; tested at 5% on 25 volunteers it was neither irritating nor sensitizing. Both isoeugenol and, to a lesser extent, eugenol are potential sensitizing agents (see Constituent profiles, Chapter 14). Clove bud oil is non-phototoxic (Opdyke 1975 p. 761–763).

Clove oil was cytotoxic to skin cells in vitro, at concentrations as low as 0.03%, suggesting a potential for skin irritancy (Prashar et al 2006). In closed-patch tests, clove oil (type unspecified) caused primary irritation in two out of 25 normal subjects when applied at 20%, but evoked no reaction when tested at 2% on 30 normal subjects, nor when tested at 0.5% on dermatitis patients (Fujii et al 1972). In a study of 200 consecutive dermatitis patients, two (1%) were sensitive to 2% clove oil (type unspecified) on patch testing (Rudzki et al 1976). In a prospective study of adverse skin reactions to cosmetic ingredients identified by patch test (1977–1980) clove oil (type unspecified) was responsible for one case of contact dermatitis of 487 cosmetic-related cases (Eiermann et al 1982).

In a worldwide multicenter study, 42 of 218 fragrance-sensitive dermatitis patients (19.3%) were sensitive to 10% clove bud oil (Larsen et al 2002). Of 713 cosmetic-sensitive dermatitis patients, one reacted to clove oil (type unspecified) (Adams & Maibach 1985). Twelve out of 747 dermatitis patients suspected of fragrance allergy (1.6%) reacted to 2% clove oil (type unspecified) (Wöhrl et al 2001). In a multicenter study, Germany's IVDK reported that 103 of 6,893 dermatitis patients suspected of fragrance allergy (1.49%) tested positive to 2% clove oil (type unspecified) (Uter et al 2010). Spillage of clove oil (type unspecified) on to the skin has caused transient irritation followed by apparent permanent anesthesia and loss of the ability to sweat by the affected area. The skin remained sensitive to deep pressure only (Isaacs 1983).
Cardiovascular effects: Eugenol is a powerful inhibitor of platelet aggregation (Rasheed et al 1984; Janssens et al 1990), an essential step in the blood clotting cascade.
Reproductive toxicity: When clove bud oil (0.25%, 375 mg/kg) was fed to pregnant mice for two weeks it induced a significantly increased rate of embryonic cell death (Domaracky et al 2007). However, since oral administration of 100 mg/kg eugenol to pregnant mice throughout gestation caused no increase in resorption, and no detectable fetal defects (Amini et al 2003), no contraindication is necessary for clove oils.

Systemic effects

Acute toxicity, human: There are three reports of non-fatal oral poisoning from clove oil, all in children. In 1991 a 7-month-old child was given one teaspoon of clove oil (equivalent to 0.5 g/kg of eugenol). Supportive care and gastric lavage were sufficient for total recovery following the resultant severe acidosis, CNS depression and urinary abnormalities (the presence of ketones in the urine) (Lane et al 1991). The second case involves near fatal poisoning of the acetaminophen (paracetamol) type after ingestion of 5–10 mL of clove oil by a 2-year-old boy (equivalent to 0.3–0.7 mL/kg of eugenol). Acidosis, deteriorating liver function, deep coma, generalized seizure and unrecordably low blood glucose were all noted. Heparin (an anticoagulant) was given due to the possible development of disseminated intravascular coagulation. The child was fully conscious by day six and eventually made a full recovery (Hartnoll et al 1993). In the final case, a 15-month-old boy developed fulminant hepatic failure after ingesting 10 mL of clove oil. His ALT (alanine aminotransferase), blood urea and creatinine were all elevated. After intravenous injection of N-acetylcysteine, his liver function and clinical status improved over a period of four days (Janes et al 2005). A 32-year-old woman, who self-injected an unknown quantity of clove oil intravenously, experienced acute respiratory distress due to pulmonary edema which had developed over one hour (Kirsch et al 1990).

Acute toxicity, animal: Clove bud oil acute oral LD_{50} in rats 2.65 g/kg; acute dermal LD_{50} in rabbits ~5 g/kg (Opdyke 1975 p. 761–763).

Antioxidant/pro-oxidant activity: Clove oil displays significant antioxidant activity in lipids (Deans et al 1993, 1995; Recsan et al 1997) and as a radical scavenger (Chaieb et al 2007). In a DPPH assay, an IC_{50} of 0.026 µL/mL was determined for the oil (Tomaino et al 2005). Clove oil protected male rats against free radical damage from aflatoxins, which are potentially mutagenic, carcinogenic, hepatotoxic and teratogenic mycotoxins (Abdel-Wahhab & Aly 2005).

Carcinogenic/anticarcinogenic potential: Clove oil (type unspecified) was not mutagenic in the Ames test, and did not produce CA in Chinese hamster fibroblasts (Ishidate et al 1984). Methyleugenol is a rodent carcinogen if exposure is sufficiently high; anticarcinogenic activity has been reported for eugenol (see Constituent profiles, Chapter 14).

Drug interactions: Anticoagulant medication, because of cardiovascular effects, above. Since eugenol significantly inhibits human MAO-A (Tao et al 2005), oral doses of eugenol-rich essential oils may interact with pethidine, indirect sympathomimetics, MAOIs or SSRIs (Table 4.10B).

Comments

In spite of the chemical similarity between the three types of clove oil, the odor of each is different.

Clove leaf

Botanical name: *Syzygium aromaticum* L.
Botanical synonyms: *Eugenia caryophyllata* Thunb., *Eugenia aromatica* L.
Family: Myrtaceae

Essential oil

Source: Leaves
Key constituents:

Eugenol	77.0–88.0%
β-Caryophyllene	3.5–6.4%
α-Caryophyllene	0.8–1.4%
Eugenyl acetate	tr–1.2%
Isoeugenol	tr

(Lawrence 1995g p178, p. 198)
Quality: May be adulterated with clove stem oil (Singhal et al 1997).

Safety summary

Hazards: Drug interaction may inhibit blood clotting; embryotoxicity; skin sensitization (moderate risk); mucous membrane irritation (moderate risk).
Cautions (oral): May interact with pethidine, MAOIs or SSRIs. Anticoagulant medication, major surgery, peptic ulcer, hemophilia, other bleeding disorders (Box 7.1).
Cautions (dermal): Hypersensitive, diseased or damaged skin, children under 2 years of age.
Maximum dermal use level: 0.6%

Our safety advice

We recommend a dermal maximum of 0.6% based on 88% eugenol content and a limit of 0.5% (see Eugenol profile, Chapter 14). As with the essential oil (see below) no restrictions are required, in our opinion, with regard to carcinogenesis.

Regulatory guidelines

IFRA recommends a maximum dermal use level for eugenol of 0.5% for most product types, in order to avoid skin sensitization (IFRA 2009).

Organ-specific effects

Adverse skin reactions: In a mouse local lymph node assay, which allows comparative measuring of skin sensitizing potency, clove leaf oil was a weak sensitizer, with a similar potency to eugenol (Lalko & Api 2006). Undiluted clove leaf oil was markedly irritating to rabbits, and was irritating to both mice and pigs; tested at 5% on 25 volunteers it was neither irritating nor sensitizing. Clove leaf oil was is non-phototoxic (Opdyke 1978 p. 695). From a total of 11,632 patch tests on eugenol, consumer products containing eugenol, or on clove leaf oil, one instance of induced hypersensitivity at 0.05%, and one instance of pre-existing sensitization at 0.09% were observed (Rothenstein et al 1983). See clove bud profile for data on adverse skin reactions to clove oil (type unspecified).
Cardiovascular effects: Eugenol is a powerful inhibitor of platelet aggregation (Rasheed et al 1984; Janssens et al 1990), an essential step in the blood clotting cascade.

Systemic effects

Acute toxicity, human: See clove bud.
Acute toxicity, animal: Clove leaf oil acute oral LD_{50} in rats 1.37 g/kg; acute dermal LD_{50} in rabbits 1.2 g/kg (Opdyke 1978 p. 695).
Antioxidant/pro-oxidant activity: Clove oils display significant antioxidant activity (Deans et al 1993, 1995; Recsan et al 1997). Clove leaf oil scavenged DPPH radicals at concentrations lower than eugenol, BHA or BHT (Jirovetz et al 2006). Clove oil protected male rats against free radical damage from aflatoxins, which are potentially mutagenic, carcinogenic, hepatotoxic and teratogenic mycotoxins (Abdel-Wahhab & Aly 2005).
Carcinogenic/anticarcinogenic potential: Clove oil (type unspecified) was not mutagenic in the Ames test, and did not produce CA in Chinese hamster fibroblasts (Ishidate et al 1984). Anticarcinogenic activity has been reported for eugenol (see Eugenol profile, Chapter 14).
Drug interactions: Anticoagulant medication, because of cardiovascular effects, above. Since eugenol significantly inhibits human MAO-A (Tao et al 2005), oral doses of eugenol-rich essential oils may interact with pethidine, indirect sympathomimetics, MAOIs or SSRIs (Table 4.10B).

Comments

The most commonly used type of clove oil is clove bud.

Clove stem

Botanical name: *Syzygium aromaticum* L.
Botanical synonyms: *Eugenia caryophyllata* Thunb., *Eugenia aromatica* L.
Family: Myrtaceae

Essential oil

Source: Stems
Key constituents:

Eugenol	76.4–84.8%
β-Caryophyllene	3.5–12.4%
Eugenyl acetate	0.4–8.0%
α-Caryophyllene	1.0–1.5%
Isoeugenol	0.1–0.4%

(Lawrence 1993 p. 36, 1995g p. 178, p.198)

Safety summary

Hazards: Drug interaction; may inhibit blood clotting; embryotoxicity; skin sensitization (moderate risk); mucous membrane irritation (moderate risk).
Cautions (oral): May interact with pethidine, MAOIs or SSRIs. Anticoagulant medication, major surgery, peptic ulcer, hemophilia, other bleeding disorders (Box 7.1).
Cautions (dermal): Hypersensitive, diseased or damaged skin, children under 2 years of age.
Maximum dermal use level: 0.6%

Our safety advice

We recommend a dermal maximum of 0.6%, based on 84.8% eugenol content and a eugenol limit of 0.5% (see Eugenol profile, Chapter 14).

Regulatory guidelines

IFRA recommends maximum dermal use level of 0.5% for eugenol and 0.02% for isoeugenol for most product types, in order to avoid skin sensitization (IFRA 2009).

Organ-specific effects

Adverse skin reactions: Undiluted clove stem oil produced moderate erythema and edema when administered to rabbits, and was severely irritating to mice; tested at 10% on 25 volunteers it was neither irritating nor sensitizing. Eugenol and isoeugenol are potential sensitizing agents, especially in dermatitis patients. Clove stem oil is non-phototoxic (Opdyke 1975 p. 765–767). See clove bud for data on adverse skin reactions to clove oil (type unspecified).
Cardiovascular effects: Eugenol is a powerful inhibitor of platelet aggregation (Rasheed et al 1984; Janssens et al 1990), an essential step in the blood clotting cascade.

Systemic effects

Acute toxicity, human: See Clove bud.
Acute toxicity, animal: Clove stem oil acute oral LD_{50} in rats 2.02 g/kg; acute dermal LD_{50} in rabbits >5 g/kg (Opdyke 1975 p. 765–767).
Antioxidant/pro-oxidant activity: Clove oils display significant antioxidant activity (Deans et al 1993, 1995; Recsan et al 1997). Clove oil protected male rats against free radical damage from aflatoxins, which are potentially mutagenic, carcinogenic, hepatotoxic and teratogenic mycotoxins (Abdel-Wahhab & Aly 2005).
Carcinogenic/anticarcinogenic potential: See Clove stem.
Drug interactions: Anticoagulant medication, because of cardiovascular effects, above. Since eugenol significantly inhibits human MAO-A (Tao et al 2005), oral doses of eugenol-rich essential oils may interact with pethidine, indirect sympathomimetics, MAOIs or SSRIs (Table 4.10B).

Comments

The most commonly used type of clove oil is clove bud.

Coleus

Synonym: Forskohlii
Botanical name: *Plectranthus barbatus* Andrews
Botanical synonyms: *Coleus barbatus* (Andrews) Benth., *Coleus forskohlii* auct., *Plectranthus forskohlii* auct.
Family: Lamiaceae (Labiatae)

Essential oil

Source: Roots
Key constituents:

Bornyl acetate	15.0%
β-Sesquiphellandrene	13.2%
γ-Eudesmol	12.5%
3-Decanone	7.0%
α-Gurjunene	5.0%
α-Selinene	4.4%
Cedran-8-ol	2.8%
γ-Elemene	2.5%
Isolongifolene	2.5%
(Z)-α-Bergamotene	2.4%
Camphene	2.2%
α-Pinene	1.9%
Bicyclogermacrene*	1.5%
(Z)-Calamenene*	1.5%
β-Pinene	1.5%

(Misra et al 1994)

Safety summary

Hazards: None known.
Contraindications: None known.

*Tentative identification

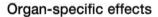

Organ-specific effects

No information found.

Systemic effects

Acute toxicity: No information found. Bornyl acetate is non-toxic (Opdyke 1973 p. 1041–1042).
Carcinogenic/anticarcinogenic potential: No information found. β-Sesquiphellandrene and γ-eudesmol display antitumoral properties (see Constituent profiles, Chapter 14).

Comments

Limited availability. The US Sabinsa corporation has been granted a patent (US Patent #6,607,712) covering CO_2 extraction of this plant, and describing methods to produce antimicrobial compositions which might be used in cutaneous infections such as acne and in preparations to prevent tooth decay. The plant and its extract are widely promoted for certain health benefits. It has been suggested that the sustainability of the wild-grown plant in India is threatened by its collection for medicinal use (Misra et al 1994).

Combava fruit

Synonyms: Colobot oil, kaffir lime, leech-lime, makrut lime, Mauritius papeda, swangi
Botanical name: *Citrus hystrix* DC
Family: Rutaceae

Essential oil

Source: Fruit peel, by steam distillation
Key constituents:

β-Pinene	25.9–31.5%
Sabinene	15.6–20.4%
Citronellal	0.4–16.8%
(+)-Limonene	5.3–13.8%
Terpinen-4-ol	0.4–3.8%
Citronellol	2.9%
α-Pinene	2.0–2.6%
α-Terpineol	1.7–2.1%
Linalool	1.8–1.9%
(E)-Sabinene hydrate	0–1.7%
Citronellyl acetate	0.5–1.5%
β-Myrcene	0–1.3%
Geranyl acetate	1.0%

(Sato et al 1990)

Safety summary

Hazards: None known.
Contraindications: None known.

Organ-specific effects

Reproductive toxicity: The low reproductive toxicity of β-pinene, sabinene and (+)-limonene (see Constituent profiles,

Chapter 14) suggests that combava fruit oil is not hazardous in pregnancy.

Systemic effects

Acute toxicity: No information found.
Carcinogenic/anticarcinogenic potential: Combava fruit oil showed significant chemopreventive activity against human mouth epidermal carcinoma (KB) and mouse leukemia (P388) cell lines, with respective IC_{50} values of 99 and 75 µg/mL. The oil was more effective than three of the four positive control drugs (Manosroi et al 2005). Citronellal and (+)-limonene display antitumoral activity (see Constituent profiles, Chapter 14).

Comments

Because this oil is steam distilled, it is not likely to contain furanocoumarins, or to be phototoxic. The low (+)-limonene content is unusual for a citrus peel oil. Limited availability.

Combava leaf

Synonyms: Kaffir lime, leech-lime, makrut lime, Mauritius papeda, swangi
Botanical name: *Citrus hystrix* DC
Family: Rutaceae

Essential oil

Source: Leaves
Key constituents:

Citronellal	58.9–81.5%
Citronellyl acetate	0.9–5.1%
Isopulegol	0.3–4.9%
Sabinene	1.6–4.8%
Linalool	2.9–4.7%
β-Pinene	0.2–1.5%
β-Myrcene	0.4–1.4%
γ-Terpinene	0.1–1.1%

(Lawrence 1995g p. 122)

Safety summary

Hazards: None known.
Contraindications: None known.

Organ-specific effects

No information found.

Systemic effects

Acute toxicity: No information found.
Carcinogenic/anticarcinogenic potential: Combava leaf oil showed moderate chemopreventive activity against human mouth epidermal carcinoma (KB) and mouse leukemia (P388) cell lines, with respective IC_{50} values of 1.148 and 0.398 mg/mL (Manosroi et al 2005). Citronellal displays anti-carcinogenic activity (see Constituent profiles, Chapter 14).

Comments

The oil is produced to a limited extent in India and Thailand.

Copaiba

Botanical names: *Copaifera langsdorfii* Desf., *Copaifera officinalis* (Jacq.) L.
Family: Fabaceae (Leguminosae)

Essential oil

Source: Balsam from wood
Key constituents:

Copaifera langsdorfii

β-Caryophyllene	53.3%
Germacrene B	8.7%
β-Selinene	6.5%
α-Caryophyllene	6.1%
γ-Elemene	4.8%
α-Selinene	4.5%
β-Elemene	4.4%
γ-Muurolene	2.7%
Cubebene	2.2%
δ-Cadinene	1.7%
α-Guaiene	1.7%
Germacrene D	1.4%

(Gramosa & Silveira 2005)

Copaifera officinalis

β-Caryophyllene	24.7%
α-Copaene	20.7%
δ-Cadinene	7.7%
γ-Cadinene	5.5%
Cedrol	4.8%
α-Selinene	4.1%
α-Ylangene	2.9%
β-Cubebene	2.7%
α-Caryophyllene	2.7%
Germacrene D	2.3%
α-Cubebene	2.0%
(−)-*allo*-Aromadendrene	1.8%
δ-Elemene	1.6%
β-Selinene	1.5%
γ-Muuroolene	1.2%
β-Bisabolol	1.1%
Himachalene	1.1%

(Stashenko et al 1995)

Safety summary

Hazards: None known.
Contraindications: None known.

Organ-specific effects

Adverse skin reactions: Undiluted copaiba oil was irritating to rabbits; tested at 8% on 25 volunteers it was neither irritating nor sensitizing (Opdyke 1973 p. 1075).
Reproductive toxicity: A vaginal cream containing 2.5% oleoresin from *Copaifera duckei* was administered intravaginally to female rats once daily for 30 days before pregnancy and for 20 days following. The dose of 28.6 mg/kg was ten times greater than the relative human intravaginal dose (copaiba creams are used for vaginal infections in Brazil). The cream was considered devoid of reproductive toxicity on the basis of number of implantations and resorptions, pre- and post-implantation loss, number of *corporea lutea*, and skeletal and visceral fetal anomalies. Two other groups of pregnant rats were administered saline or cream base only. β-Caryophyllene was the principal volatile constituent of the oleoresin (Lima et al 2011).

Systemic effects

Acute toxicity: Non-toxic. Copaiba oil acute oral LD_{50} in rats >5 g/kg; acute dermal LD_{50} in rabbits >5 g/kg (Opdyke 1973 p. 1075).
Carcinogenic/anticarcinogenic potential: A copaiba oil with 57.5% β-caryophyllene, 8.3% α-caryophyllene, 2.5% α-copaene, was cytotoxic to B16F10 (mouse) melanoma cells in vitro, and oral administration significantly reduced lung tumors (which had metastasized from injected B16F10 cells) in mice (Lima et al 2003). β-Caryophyllene and α-caryophyllene display antitumoral activity (see Constituent profiles, Chapter 14).

Comments

Copaiba balsam does not carry the same risk of skin reactions as Peru balsam. Both the balsam and essential oil have many traditional medicinal uses. Three patents have been filed relating to cosmetic uses of copaiba (www.amazonlink.org/biopiracy/copaiba.htm accessed August 8th 2011).

Coriander leaf

Synonym: Cilantro
Botanical name: *Coriandrum sativum* L.
Family: Apiaceae (Umbelliferae)

Essential oil

Source: Leaves
Key constituents:

(*E*)-2-Decenal	26.8–46.5%
Decanal	4.4–18.0%
Linalool	4.3–17.5%
Octanal	0.5–11.2%
(*E*)-2-Dodecenal	2.7–10.3%
2-Decen-1-ol	<9.2%
(*E*)-2-Tetradecenal	tr-5.8%
(*E*)-2-Undecenal	1.4–5.6%
Decanol	1.3–4.3%

Nonane	0.2–3.6%
Tridecanal	0.1–2.0%
Dodecanal	1.0–1.7%

(Lawrence 1993 p. 128–130, p. 182–183)

Safety summary

Hazards: None known.
Contraindications: None known.

Regulatory guidelines

Has GRAS status.

Organ-specific effects

Adverse skin reactions: No information found for coriander leaf oil. When applied full strength to rabbits for 24 hours under occlusion, 2-decenal and 2-dodecenal were severely irritating (see Constituent profiles, Chapter 14).

Systemic effects

Acute toxicity: No information found for coriander leaf oil, or most of its constituents.
Carcinogenic/anticarcinogenic potential: No information found for coriander leaf oil, but it contains no known carcinogens.

Comments

Limited availability.

Coriander seed

Botanical name: *Coriandrum sativum* L.
Family: Apiaceae (Umbelliferae)

Essential oil

Source: Seeds
Key constituents:

Linalool	59.0–87.5%
α-Pinene	0.1–10.5%
γ-Terpinene	0.1–9.1%
β-Pinene	0.1–8.6%
p-Cymene	0–8.4%
Camphor	1.6–7.7%
Geraniol	0.3–5.3%
Camphene	tr–4.6%
(+)-Limonene	0.2–3.2%
Geranyl acetate	0–3.1%
Terpinen-4-ol	tr–3.0%
α-Terpineol	0.1–2.2%

(Lawrence 1993 p. 128–130, p. 182–183)
Quality: Coriander seed oil may be adulterated with natural or synthetic linalool (Kubeczka 2002).

Safety summary

Hazards: None known.
Contraindications: None known.

Regulatory guidelines

Has GRAS status. According to IFRA, essential oils rich in linalool should only be used when the level of peroxides is kept to the lowest practical value. The addition of antioxidants such as 0.1% BHT or α-tocopherol at the time of production is recommended (IFRA 2009).

Organ-specific effects

Adverse skin reactions: In a modified Draize procedure on guinea pigs, coriander seed oil was non-sensitizing when used at 40% in the challenge phase (Sharp 1978). Undiluted coriander seed oil was irritating to rabbits; tested at 6% on 25 volunteers it was neither irritating nor sensitizing (Opdyke 1973 p. 1077). A lotion containing 1% coriander seed oil produced no irritation in 40 volunteers on patch testing (Casetti et al 2012). In a study of 200 consecutive dermatitis patients, two (1%) were sensitive to 2% coriander seed oil on patch testing (Rudzki et al 1976). Oxidation products of linalool may be skin sensitizing.
Reproductive toxicity: Coriander seed oil was administered by gavage to pregnant rats at 0, 250, 500 or 1,000 mg/kg/day. The maternal NOAEL was less than 250 mg/kg/day, and the NOAEL of coriander seed oil in the offspring was 500 mg/kg/day. Implantation averages were similar at all doses and neither reproductive performance of female rats nor development of their offspring was affected. The constituents over 1.0% in the coriander seed oil used were 72.9% linalool, 4.6% camphor, 4.0% *p*-cymene, 3.9% α-pinene, 3.6% γ-terpinene, 2.7% (+)-limonene and 1.2% geranyl acetate (RIFM 1989, cited in Letizia et al 2003a).
Immunotoxicity: When female mice were given oral doses of 313, 625 or 1,250 mg/kg coriander seed oil for five days, there were no effects on immune function assessed by plaque-forming cell and host-resistance assays (Gaworski et al 1994).

Systemic effects

Acute toxicity: Coriander seed oil acute oral LD_{50} in rats >5 g/kg; acute dermal LD_{50} in rabbits 4.13 g/kg (Opdyke 1973 p. 1077).
Subacute & subchronic toxicity: In a 28 day study in male and female rats, coriander seed oil with the same composition given above under Reproductive Toxicity, was administered by gavage at 160, 400 or 1,000 mg/kg/day. Increases in kidney and liver weight were observed in the high-dose males and females, and in some mid-dose animals. There were increases in total protein and serum albumin in mid- and high-dose males and high-dose females. Serum calcium was also increased in high-dose males. Histopathological findings included a high incidence of degenerative lesions in the renal cortex of high-dose males, and a high incidence of hepatocellular cytoplasmic vacuolization in the liver of high-dose females. Some stomach lesions were observed in both mid- and high-dose females. No treatment-related effects on survival, clinical observations, body

weight or food consumption were observed and there were no adverse effects in the reproductive organs of either sex at any dose. Based on the findings in this study the NOAEL was 160 mg/kg for male rats and less than 160 mg/kg for female rats (RIFM 1990, cited in Letizia et al 2003a).

Carcinogenic/anticarcinogenic potential: Coriander seed oil was not mutagenic in the *Ames test*, and did not produce CA in Chinese hamster fibroblasts (Ishidate et al 1984). Coriander seed oil dose-dependently inhibited aflatoxin B_1-induced adducts in calf thymus DNA, in the presence of rat liver microsomes (Hashim et al 1994). The oil significantly induced glutathione *S*-transferase in mouse liver (Banerjee et al 1994). (+)-Limonene and geraniol display antitumoral activity (see Constituent profiles, Chapter 14).

Comments

Because of the high content of CNS depressant linalool, it is not thought that the camphor content of coriander seed oil will present a neurotoxic risk. This is borne out by the LD_{50} of the oil.

Cornmint (dementholized)

Synonym: Japanese mint
Botanical names: *Mentha arvensis* L.; *Mentha arvensis* f. *piperascens* Malinv. ex Holmes; *Mentha arvensis* L. var. *glabrata* Benth.; *Mentha arvensis* L. var. *villosa* Benth.; *Mentha canadensis* L.
Family: Lamiaceae (Labiatae)

Essential oil

Source: Leaves
Key constituents:

(−)-Menthol	28.8–34.7%
Menthone	16.3–31.1%
Isomenthone	6.8–12.1%
(+)-Limonene	5.8–9.6%
β-Pinene	2.0–4.5%
α-Pinene	2.0–4.3%
Neomenthol	2.5–4.1%
Piperitone	0.6–3.8%
Menthyl acetate	1.8–3.4%
3-Octanol	0.4–2.4%
β-Myrcene	0.9–2.1%
Sabinene	0.8–1.6%
Isopulegol	0.9–1.4%
β-Caryophyllene	0.6–1.3%
(1*R*)-(+)-β-Pulegone	0.4–1.3%
Iso-isopulegol	0.4–1.2%
Menthofuran	0.4–0.6%

(Kubeczka 2002)

Quality: Cornmint oil is not adulterated, as it is not a commercially attractive proposition (Singhal et al 1997).

Safety summary

Hazards: May be choleretic; mucous membrane irritation (low risk).
Contraindications (all routes): Cardiac fibrillation, G6PD deficiency. Do not apply to or near the face of infants or children.
Contraindications (oral): Cholestasis.
Cautions (oral): Gastroesophageal reflux disease (GERD).

Our safety advice

Cornmint oil should be avoided altogether in cases of cardiac fibrillation and by people with a G6PD deficiency. This is a fairly common inheritable enzyme deficiency, particularly in people of Chinese, West African, Mediterranean or Middle Eastern origin (Olowe & Ransome-Kuti 1980). People with G6PD deficiency will typically have abnormal blood reactions to at least one of the following drugs, or will have been advised to avoid them: antimalarials, sulfonamides, chloramphenicol, streptomycin, aspirin. The pulegone and menthofuran content is not high enough to require restriction in our opinion.

Regulatory guidelines

The Commission E Monograph for cornmint oil allows 5–20% in oil and semisolid preparations, 5–10% in aqueous-alcoholic preparations, 1–5% in nasal ointments and 3–6 drops as an oral dose (Blumenthal et al 1998). The CEFS of the Council of Europe has classed pulegone and menthofuran as hepatotoxic, and has set a group TDI of 0.1 mg/kg bw for the two compounds. Both the UK and EC 'standard permitted proportion' of pulegone in food flavorings is 25 mg/kg of food (Anon 1992b, European Community Council 1988).

Organ-specific effects

Adverse skin reactions: Undiluted cornmint oil was not irritating to rabbit, pig or mouse skin; tested at 8% on 25 volunteers it was neither irritating nor sensitizing. It is non-phototoxic (Opdyke 1975 p. 771–772).
Cardiovascular effects: Cornmint oil inhibits platelet aggregation, but only very weakly (Murayama and Kumaroo 1986). Peppermint confectionery and mentholated cigarettes have been responsible for cardiac fibrillation in patients prone to the condition who are being maintained on quinidine, a stabilizer of heart rhythm (Thomas 1962). Bradycardia has been reported in a person addicted to menthol cigarettes (De Smet et al 1992).
Neonatal toxicity: Menthol can cause neonatal jaundice in babies with a deficiency of the enzyme glucose-6-phosphate dehydrogenase (G6PD). Usually, menthol is detoxified by a metabolic pathway involving G6PD. When babies deficient in this enzyme were given a menthol-containing dressing for their umbilical stumps, menthol accumulated in their bodies (Olowe & Ransome-Kuti 1980).
Gastrointestinal toxicology: Both peppermint oil and menthol are choleretic (Trabace et al 1994) and therefore cornmint oil should not be taken in oral doses by people with cholestasis (obstructed bile flow) (Fujii et al 1994). Since peppermint oil relaxes the lower esophageal sphincter, oral administration of cornmint oil may cause discomfort in cases of GERD.

Hepatotoxicity: Oral doses of menthol or menthone above 200 mg/kg for 28 days produced signs of liver toxicity in rats (Thorup et al 1983b; Madsen et al 1986). Menthofuran is toxic to both liver and lung tissue in mice (Gordon et al 1982). In rats, oral dosing with menthofuran (250 mg/kg/day for three days) caused hepatotoxicity, as demonstrated by changes in blood levels of enzyme markers for liver disease (Madyastha and Raj 1994). Cornmint oil is unlikely to cause liver problems at the doses used in aromatherapy.

Systemic effects

Acute toxicity, human: A proprietary menthol-containing oil was reported to cause incoordination, confusion and delirium when 5 mL of the product (35.5% peppermint oil) was inhaled over a long time period (O'Mullane et al 1982). Nasal preparations containing menthol can cause apnea and collapse in infants following instillation into the nose (Melis et al 1989; Reynolds 1993).
Acute toxicity, animal: Cornmint oil acute oral LD_{50} in rats 1.24 g/kg; acute dermal LD_{50} in rabbits >5 g/kg (Opdyke 1975 p. 771–772).
Carcinogenic/anticarcinogenic potential: The in vitro cell growth of K562 (myelogenous leukemia) cells was inhibited by cornmint oil with an IC_{50} of 40.6 µg/mL (Lampronti et al 2006). Menthone demonstrates some genotoxicity but is not carcinogenic in mice; menthol is neither genotoxic nor carcinogenic, and displays anticarcinogenic activity, as does (+)-limonene (see Constituent profiles, Chapter 14).

Comments

The reports of inhalation toxicity raise the possibility that cornmint might be more acutely toxic, particularly neurotoxic, in humans than rodents. Natural cornmint oil contains 70–90% of menthol, but this oil is rarely seen on the marketplace. The normal article of commerce is 'dementholized' by freezing, a process which removes about 50% of the menthol. Cornmint oil is sometimes used as an adulterant of, or even a substitute for, peppermint oil.

Costus

Botanical name: *Saussurea costus* (Falc.) Lipsch.
Botanical synonyms: *Aplotaxis lappa* Decne., *Aucklandia costus* Falc., *Saussurea lappa* (Decne) C.B. Clarke
Family: Asteraceae (Compositae)

Essential oil

Source: Dried roots
Key constituents:

Aplotaxene	20.0%
Dihydrocostus lactone	15.0%
Costusic acid	14.0%
Costunolide	11.0%
Dehydrocostus lactone	6.0%
Dihydrodehydrocostus lactone	6.0%

(Mahindru 1992 p. 229)

Safety summary

Hazards: Fetotoxicity (based on costunolide and dehydrocostus lactone content); skin sensitization (high risk).
Contraindications: Should not be used on the skin.
Contraindications (all routes): Pregnancy, lactation

Regulatory guidelines

IFRA recommends that costus oil should not be used as a fragrance ingredient due to its sensitizing potential, unless the costus oil being used has been shown not to have sensitizing potential (IFRA 2009). Costus oil is prohibited as a fragrance ingredient in the the EU.

Organ-specific effects

Adverse skin reactions: Undiluted costus oil was mildly irritating to mice; neither of two samples of costus oil tested at 4% on 25 volunteers was irritating. It is non-phototoxic. In a human maximation test at 4%, costus oil produced 25 sensitization reactions in 25 volunteers, and in a similar test at 2%, there were 16 positive reactions in 26 volunteers (62%) (Opdyke 1974 p. 867–868). Costus oil is regarded as a high-risk skin sensitizer in Japan (Nakayama 1998).

Tested on 282 eczema patients, 0.1% costus oil produced only two (0.7%) positive reactions (Mitchell et al 1982). Of 281,100 dermatitis patients, 13,216 had contact dermatitis, and of these 713 were related to cosmetic ingredients. Of this last group, only one reacted to costus oil (Adams & Maibach 1985). In five reports of patch tests using a sesquiterpene lactone mix, consisting of alantolactone, dehydrocostus lactone and costunolide at 0.1%, there were a total of 290 positive reactions in 15,466 dermatitis patients (1.88%), many of which were known or suspected to have sesquiterpene lactone allergy (Ducombs et al 1990; Paulsen et al 1993b; Ross et al 1993; Green & Ferguson 1994; Kanerva et al 2001a).

Dermal sensitization is primarily due to costunolide and dehydrocostus lactone (Benezra & Epstein 1986). Sesquiterpene lactones from Compositae plants are notorious skin sensitizers (Goulden & Wilkinson 1998; Ross et al 1993). A lactone-rich fraction of costus oil produced one positive reaction in 24 volunteers tested (4%) and produced severe reactions in costus-sensitized individuals. A lactone-free fraction of the same oil was not sensitizing in seven subjects, nor did it produce any reactions in costus-sensitized individuals (Opdyke 1974 p. 867–868).
Reproductive toxicity: Since costunolide and dehydrocostus lactone are antiangionenic (Jeong et al 2002; Wang et al 2012), and in view of the probable link between antiangiogenic effects and reproductive toxicity (Chaiworapongsa et al 2010; Zhou et al 2013), we have contraindicated costus oil in pregnancy and lactation.

Systemic effects

Acute toxicity: Costus oil acute oral LD_{50} in rats 3.4 g/kg; acute dermal LD_{50} in rabbits >5 g/kg (Opdyke 1974 p. 867–868).
Subacute & subchronic toxicity: When costus oil was consumed by male rats at 1.77 mg/kg/day, and by female rats at

2.17 mg/kg/day in the diet for 90 days, no adverse effects were observed on growth, food consumption, hematology, blood chemistry, liver weight, kidney weight, or the microscopic or gross appearance of major organs (Oser et al 1965).

Carcinogenic/anticarcinogenic potential: Costus oil inhibited the growth of Meth-A fibrosarcoma cells in mice (Takanami et al 1987). Costunolide displays anticarcinogenic activity (see Costunolide profile, Chapter 14). The oil contains no known carcinogens.

Comments

The data on costus oil and skin sensitization are highly inconsistent. In every study, petrolatum was used as the vehicle. Either sensitivity to this oil is extremely dependent on concentration, or the maximation tests conducted by RIFM produced a large number of false positives. A total of six studies failed to find the degree of sensitization reported by RIFM in 1974, and the consequent IFRA prohibition may be heavy-handed. It seems likely that concentrations up to 0.01%, perhaps even 0.05%, will be safe in almost all circumstances. However, the plant is listed by CITES under their Appendix I: species threatened with extinction, and that are the most endangered.

It has been suggested that the anticarcinogenic activity of costus oil may be due in part to a stimulation of the immune system caused by the delayed hypersensitivity skin response to the lactone content of the oil (Takanami et al 1984, 1985, 1987). It is possible to prepare costus oil so that it is free of skin sensitizing agents by using a polymer, aminoethyl-polystyrene, to which the lactones bind (Cheminat et al 1981), hence the 'unless...' comment by IFRA, above under Regulatory guidelines.

The analysis reported by Mahindru (1992) is far from definitive, but most reports of costus oil constituents do not give amounts. The substance referred to as 'costusic acid' is probably guaia-3,9,11-triene-12 acid, a known constituent of the oil. Other costus oil constituents include: dihydroaplotaxene, α-caryophyllene, β-caryophyllene, caryophyllene oxide, α-ionone, β-elemene, β-selinene and costol (Lawrence 1979 p. 40).

Cubeb

Synonyms: Java pepper, tailed pepper, false pepper
Botanical name: *Piper cubeba* L.
Family: Piperaceae

Essential oil

Source: Fruits
Key constituents:

Sabinene	2.1–28.1%
Cubebol	8.9–15.2%
α-Copaene	4.0–14.3%
β-Cubebene	4.4–11.0%
δ-Cadinene	tr–9.5%
α-Cubebene	1.6–8.5%
α-Pinene	1.3–5.4%
γ-Humulene	4.4–4.9%

(+)-Limonene	0.1–4.4%
(−)-*allo*-Aromadendrene	1.7–4.2%
γ-Muurolene	tr–4.2%
(Z)-Calamenene	tr–3.8%
β-Caryophyllene	1.7–3.7%
α-Asarone	0.9–3.7%
Cesarone	0–3.7%
Nerolidol	1.4–3.5%
epi-Cubenol	0–3.5%
Linalool	tr–3.2%
Germacrene D	0.1–2.9%
(Z)-Sabinene hydrate	tr–2.7%
Terpinen-4-ol	0–2.7%
α-Terpineol	1.9–2.2%
β-Bisabolene	1.5–1.6%
Cubenol	0.6–1.5%
β-Elemene	1.0–1.2%
α-Muurolene	0.6–1.2%
Carvotanacetone	0–1.2%
β-Myrcene	tr–1.1%
γ-Terpinene	tr–1.1%
Safrole	0–0.1%

(Lawrence 1981 p. 43–44, 2001d p. 78–81)
Quality: Cubeb oil may be adulterated with essential oils from other *Piper* species, with Peruvian pepper oil, or with rectified and deodorized clove sesquiterpene fractions (Burfield 2000).

Safety summary

Hazards: Potentially carcinogenic, based on α-asarone content.
Contraindications: None known.
Maximum adult daily oral dose: 243 mg (see Our Safety Advice)
Maximum dermal use level:

EU	10.0%
IFRA	0.26%
Tisserand & Young	7.5%

Our safety advice

We recommend a dermal maximum of 7.5% and an oral maximum of 243 mg, based on 0.1% safrole and 3.7% α-asarone with safrole limits of 0.05% and 0.025 mg/kg and α-asarone limits of 0.33% and 0.15 mg/kg (see Constituent profiles, Chapter 14).

Regulatory guidelines

IFRA recommends that the level of asarone in consumer products should not exceed 0.01% (IFRA 2009). The EU does not restrict asarone. IFRA and the EU recommend a maximum exposure level of 0.01% of safrole from the use of safrole-containing essential oils in cosmetics.

Organ-specific effects

Adverse skin reactions: Undiluted cubeb oil was irritating to rabbits; on mouse and pig skin it produced hyperkeratosis and

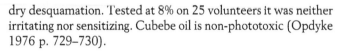

dry desquamation. Tested at 8% on 25 volunteers it was neither irritating nor sensitizing. Cubebe oil is non-phototoxic (Opdyke 1976 p. 729–730).

Systemic effects

Acute toxicity: Cubeb oil acute oral LD_{50} in rats >5 g/kg; acute dermal LD_{50} in rabbits >5 g/kg (Opdyke 1976 p. 729–730). **Carcinogenic/anticarcinogenic potential:** No information found. α-Asarone and safrole are rodent carcinogens; (+)-limonene and β-elemene display anticarcinogenic activity (see Constituent profiles, Chapter 14).

Comments

The safrole content of cubeb oil is not significant. If distillation has been carried through to the highest boiling constituents, the oil may have a slight blue coloring, due to the presence of azulenes.

Cumin

Botanical name: *Cuminum cyminum* L.
Family: Apiaceae (Umbelliferae)

Essential oil

Source: Fruits (seeds)
Key constituents:

Cuminaldehyde	19.8–40.0%
γ-Terpinene	11.2–32.0%
β-Pinene	4.4–17.7%
p-Cymene	5.9–17.5%
p-Mentha-1,3-dien-7-al	7.2–3.2%
p-Mentha-1,4-dien-7-al	2.1–8.6%
β-Myrcene + α-phellandrene	0.5–7.3%
p-Menth-3-en-7-al	0.5–2.5%
Cuminyl alcohol	0.2–2.2%
α-Pinene	0.2–1.2%
Isocaryophyllene	0.1–1.1%

(Lawrence 1995g p. 36–38)
Quality: May be adulterated with additional cuminaldehyde (Burfield 2003).

Safety summary

Hazards: Phototoxic (moderate risk).
Contraindications (dermal): If applied to the skin at over maximum use level, skin must not be exposed to sunlight or sunbed rays for 12 hours.
Maximum dermal use level: 0.4%

Regulatory guidelines

Has GRAS status. To avoid phototoxicity, applications on areas of skin exposed to sunshine, excluding bath preparations, soaps and other wash-off products, cumin oil should be limited to 0.4% (IFRA 2009, SCCNFP 2001a).

Organ-specific effects

Adverse skin reactions: Undiluted cumin oil was moderately irritating to rabbits, but was not irritating to mice; tested at 4% on 25 volunteers it was neither irritating nor sensitizing. Distinct phototoxic effects were reported for cumin oil, but none for cuminaldehyde (Opdyke 1974 p. 869–870). RIFM apparently reported a 5% NOAEL for phototoxicity in human volunteers (IFRA 2009).

Systemic effects

Acute toxicity: Cumin oil acute oral LD_{50} in rats 2.5 mL/kg; acute dermal LD_{50} in rabbits 3.56 mL/kg (Opdyke 1974 p. 869–870).
Carcinogenic/anticarcinogenic potential: Cumin oil was not mutagenic in the *Ames test*, and did not produce CA in Chinese hamster fibroblasts (Ishidate et al 1984). Cumin oil dose-dependently inhibited aflatoxin B_1-induced adducts in calf thymus DNA, in the presence of rat liver microsomes (Hashim et al 1994). It increased glutathione *S*-transferase activity in the stomach, liver and esophagus of mice by more than 78%, and significantly inhibited B[*a*]P-induced squamous cell stomach carcinoma (Aruna and Sivaramakrishnan 1996, Banerjee et al 1994).

Comments

The restriction is poorly worded, since it does not clearly address leave-on products on areas of skin not obviously exposed to sunshine.

Curry leaf

Botanical name: *Murraya koenigii* (L.) Spreng.
Family: Rutaceae

Essential oil

Source: Leaves
Key constituents:

β-Phellandrene	24.4%
α-Pinene	17.5%
β-Caryophyllene	7.3%
Terpinen-4-ol	6.1%
(+)-Limonene	5.1%
γ-Terpinene	4.9%
α-Phellandrene	4.8%
Sabinene	4.1%
β-Pinene	3.7%
α-Terpinene	2.8%
β-Myrcene	2.3%
(*E*)-β-Ocimene	1.8%
α-Terpineol	1.6%
α-Thujene	1.6%
α-Selinene	1.1%
Terpinolene	1.1%
p-Cymene	1.0%

(Wong & Tie 1993)

Safety summary

Hazards: Skin sensitization if oxidized.
Cautions: Old or oxidized oils should be avoided.

Our safety advice

Because of its high combined α-pinene and (+)-limonene content we recommend that oxidation of cypress oil is avoided by storage in a dark, airtight container in a refrigerator. The addition of an antioxidant to preparations containing it is recommended.

Organ-specific effects

Adverse skin reactions: No information found for curry leaf oil or β-phellandrene. Autoxidation products of α-pinene and (+)-limonene can cause skin sensitization (see Constituent profiles, Chapter 14).

Systemic effects

Acute toxicity: No information found for curry leaf oil or β-phellandrene.
Carcinogenic/anticarcinogenic potential: A Malaysian curry leaf oil with 19.5% β-caryophyllene and 15.2% α-caryophyllene showed a dose-dependent antitumoral action against MCF-7 human breast cancer cells in vitro (Nagappan et al 2011).

Comments

Limited availability.

Cypress

Synonyms: Italian cypress, Mediterranean cypress
Botanical name: *Cupressus sempervirens* L.
Family: Cupressaceae

Essential oil

Source: Leaves and terminal branches
Key constituents:

α-Pinene	20.4–52.7%
δ-3-Carene	15.2–21.5%
Cedrol	2.0–7.0%
α-Terpinyl acetate	4.1–6.4%
Terpinolene	2.4–6.3%
(+)-Limonene	2.3–6.0%
β-Pinene	0.8–2.9%
Sabinene	0.7–2.8%
β-Myrcene	<2.7%
δ-Cadinene	1.7–2.6%
Terpinen-4-yl-acetate	1.2–2.1%
α-Terpineol	1.2–1.4%
Sandaracopimaradiene	0.2–1.3%
p-Cymene	0.2–1.2%
γ-Terpinene	0.4–1.1%
Terpinen-4-ol	0.3–1.0%
Borneol	tr–1.0%

(Lawrence 1979 p. 18, 1989 p29–30, 1995d p. 34)
Quality: May be adulterated with additional α-pinene, δ-3-carene and β-myrcene (Burfield 2003).

Safety summary

Hazards: Skin sensitization if oxidized.
Cautions: Old or oxidized oils should be avoided.

Our safety advice

Because of its high α-pinene and δ-3-carene content we recommend that oxidation of cypress oil is avoided by storage in a dark, airtight container in a refrigerator. The addition of an antioxidant to preparations containing it is recommended.

Organ-specific effects

Adverse skin reactions: Undiluted cypress oil was moderately irritating to rabbits, but was not irritating to mice or pigs; tested at 5% on 25 volunteers it was neither irritating nor sensitizing. It is non-phototoxic (Opdyke 1978 p. 699). A 65-year-old aromatherapist with multiple essential oil sensitivities reacted to 5%, and weakly to 1% cypress oil (Selvaag et al 1995). Autoxidation products of α-pinene and δ-3-carene can cause skin sensitization (see Constituent profiles, Chapter 14).
Reproductive toxicity: The low reproductive toxicity of α-pinene, β-myrcene and (+)-limonene (see Constituent profiles, Chapter 14) suggests that cypress oil is not hazardous in pregnancy.

Systemic effects

Acute toxicity: Cypress oil acute oral LD_{50} in rats >5 g/kg; acute dermal LD_{50} in rabbits >5 g/kg (Opdyke 1978 p. 699).
Carcinogenic/anticarcinogenic potential: A leaf essential oil from *Cupressus sempervirens* ssp. *pyramidalis* inhibited the in vitro growth of human melanoma C32 cells with an IC_{50} value of 104.9 µg/mL but was inactive against renal cell adenocarcinoma ACHN cells (Loizzo et al 2008). α-Pinene is not mutagenic (see α-Pinene profile).

Comments

The oil is mainly produced in France and Spain.

Cypress (blue)

Synonym: Northern cypress pine
Botanical name: *Callitris intratropica* R.T. Baker & H.B. Sm.
Family: Cupressaceae

Essential oil

Source: Wood
Key constituents:

β-Eudesmol	14.4%
Dihydrocolumellarin	14.0%
Guaiol	13.7%
γ-Eudesmol	9.1%

α-Eudesmol	7.6%
Guaiazulene	6.2%
Chamazulene	5.6%
Columellarin	2.9%
Callitrin	2.4%
Cadalene	2.3%
β-Selinene	2.2%
α-Selinene	1.5%
Callitrisin	1.4%
Elemol	1.3%

(Doimo 2001)

Safety summary

Hazards: Drug interaction; may be fetotoxic (based on β-eudesmol content).
Contraindications (all routes): Pregnancy and lactation.
Cautions (oral): Low blood pressure, drugs metabolized by CYP2D6 (Appendix B).

Organ-specific effects

Adverse skin reactions: Blue cypress oil was mildly irritating to rabbits at 100% and 75%, but not irritating at 50%. In sensitization testing on guinea pigs, no positive reactions were observed at concentrations up to 75%, but 80% of the guinea pigs (16/20) reacted positively at 100%. In the in vitro Eyetex UMA test the oil was a mild to minimal irritant (McGilvray, private communication, 1999).
Cardiovascular effects: Guaiol and β-eudesmol are hypotensive (Arora et al 1967).
Reproductive toxicity: Since β-eudesmol is antiangionenic (Tsuneki et al 2005), and in view of the probable link between antiangiogenic effects and reproductive toxicity (Chaiworapongsa et al 2010; Zhou et al 2013), we have contraindicated blue cypress oil in pregnancy and lactation.

Systemic effects

Acute toxicity: Blue cypress oil acute oral LD_{50} in rats >2 g/kg, acute dermal LD_{50} in rats >2 g/kg (McGilvray, private communication, 1999).
Antioxidant/pro-oxidant activity: Blue cypress oil exhibited high radical scavenging activity in both ABTS and DPPH assays (Zhao et al 2008).
Carcinogenic/anticarcinogenic potential: Blue cypress oil was not mutagenic in the Ames test (McGilvray, private communication, 1999). The oil contains no known carcinogens. γ-Eudesmol displays anticarcinogenic, and β-eudesmol antiangionenic activity (Hsieh et al 2001, Tsuneki et al 2005).
Drug interactions: Since chamazulene inhibits CYP2D6 (Table 4.11B), there is a theoretical risk of interaction between blue cypress oil and drugs metabolized by this enzyme (see Appendix B).

Comments

The oil is sometimes produced by solvent extraction followed by steam distillation or rectification (Burfield 2000).

Cypress (emerald)

Synonyms: Victorian emerald cypress, green cypress, coastal cypress pine
Botanical name: *Callitris columellaris* F. Muell.
Family: Cupressaceae

Essential oil

Source: Wood
Key constituents:

Citronellic acid	24.3%
Guaiol	20.0%
β-Eudesmol	5.7%
Bulnesol	5.3%
β-Selinene	5.2%
α-Selinene	3.6%
α-Eudesmol	3.5%
γ-Eudesmol	2.4%
γ-Selinene	1.6%
Dihydrocolumellarin	1.0%

(Condon, private communication, 2002)

Safety summary

Hazards: None known.
Cautions: Low blood pressure.

Organ-specific effects

Adverse skin reactions: No information found for emerald cypress oil. Citronellic acid appears to be non-reactive on healthy skin but there are no data on guaiol.
Cardiovascular effects: Guaiol and β-eudesmol are hypotensive (Arora et al 1967).

Systemic effects

Acute toxicity: No information found for emerald cypress oil. Citronellic acid appears to be non-toxic but there are no data on guaiol.
Carcinogenic/anticarcinogenic potential: No information found for emerald cypress oil, but it contains no known carcinogens. γ-Eudesmol displays anticarcinogenic, and β-eudesmol antiangionenic activity (Hsieh et al 2001; Tsuneki et al 2005).

Comments

Limited availability.

Cypress (jade)

Synonyms: Cypress pinewood, white cypress, white cypress pine
Botanical name: *Callitris glaucophylla* Joy Thomps. & L.A.S. Johnson
Family: Cupressaceae

Essential oil

Source: Wood
Key constituents:

α-Guaiene	20.0%
Guaiol	14.7%
α-Eudesmol + β-eudesmol	10.1%
Dihydrocolumellarin	4.6%
δ-Selinene	4.5%
β-Selinene	3.8%
α-Selinene	3.6%
Columellarin	3.3%
Callitrisin	2.9%
Citronellic acid	1.6%
Methyl dehydrogeranate	1.1%

(Condon, private communication, 2002)

Safety summary

Hazards: None known.
Cautions: Low blood pressure.

Organ-specific effects

Adverse skin reactions: No information found for jade cypress oil or any of its major constituents.
Cardiovascular effects: Guaiol and β-eudesmol are hypotensive (Arora et al 1967).

Systemic effects

Acute toxicity: No information found for jade cypress oil or any of its major constituents.
Carcinogenic/anticarcinogenic potential: No information found for jade cypress oil, but it contains no known carcinogens.

Comments

Limited availability. This oil is sometimes mistakenly referred to as deriving from *Callitris columellaris* (see previous profile).

Damiana

Botanical name: *Turnera diffusa* Willd. var. *aphrodisiaca* Urb.
Botanical synonyms: *Turnera aphrodisiaca* L. F. Ward, *Turnera diffusa* Willd. ex Schult. var *diffusa*, *Turnera microphylla* Desv.
Family: Turneraceae

Essential oil

Source: Leaves
Key constituents:

1,8-Cineole	11.4%
β-Opoplenone	10.3%
Cadalene	5.1%
1-*epi*-Cubenol	4.1%
Caryophyllene oxide	2.5%

Thymol	2.3%
Nerolidol	2.2%
γ-Cadinene	1.4%
(E)-Anethole	1.0%
Juniper camphor*	1.0%
Estragole + myrtenol	0.4%

(Bicchi et al 2003)

Safety summary

Hazards: May contain estragole.
Contraindications: None known.
Maximum dermal use level:

EU	No limit
IFRA	2.5%
Tisserand & Young	30%

Our safety advice

We recommend a dermal maximum of 30% for damiana oil, based on 0.4% estragole content with a dermal limit of 0.12% (see Estragole profile, Chapter 14).

Regulatory guidelines

IFRA recommends a maximum dermal use level for estragole of 0.01% in leave-on or wash-off preparations for body and face (IFRA 2009). The EU does not restrict estragole.

Organ-specific effects

No information found for damiana oil, β-opoplenone, cadalene or 1-*epi*-cubenol.

Systemic effects

Acute toxicity: No information found for damiana oil, β-opoplenone, cadalene or 1-*epi*-cubenol.
Carcinogenic/anticarcinogenic potential: No information found for damiana oil. Estragole is a rodent carcinogen when oral exposure is sufficiently high (see Estragole profile, Chapter 14).

Comments

Limited availability.

Davana

Botanical name: *Artemisia pallens* Wall ex DC
Family: Asteraceae (Compositae)

Essential oil

Source: Aerial parts
Key constituents:

(Z)-Davanone	38.0%
Nerol	10.0%

*Tentative identification

Unidentified furans	6.0%
(E)-Davanone	5.0%
Geraniol	5.0%
(Z)-Hydroxy-davanone	3.0%
Isodavanone	3.0%
Davanic acid	2.5%
Cinnamyl cinnamate	2.0%
(E)-Hydroxy-davanone	2.0%
oxo-Nerolidol	2.0%
Artemone	1.5%
Davana ether	1.5%
nor-Davanone	1.5%
(E)-Davanafuran	1.0%

(Lawrence 1995a p. 54)

Quality: The oil tends to become viscous with increasing age (Burfield 2000).

Safety summary

Hazards: None known.
Contraindications: None known.

Organ-specific effects

Adverse skin reactions: Undiluted davana oil was moderately irritating to rabbits, but was not irritating to mice or pigs; tested at 4% on 25 volunteers it was neither irritating nor sensitizing. It is non-phototoxic (Opdyke 1976 p. 737).

Systemic effects

Acute toxicity: Non-toxic. Davana oil acute oral LD_{50} in rats >5 g/kg; acute dermal LD_{50} in rabbits >5 g/kg (Opdyke 1976 p. 737).

Subacute & subchronic toxicity: When davana oil was consumed by male rats at 18.1 mg/kg/day, and by female rats at 21.8 mg/kg/day for 90 days, no adverse effects were observed on growth, food consumption, hematology, blood chemistry, liver weight, kidney weight, or the microscopic or gross appearance of major organs (Oser et al 1965).

Carcinogenic potential. No information found for davana oil, but it contains no known carcinogens.

Comments

The davanone content can be as high as 55%.

Deertongue

Synonyms: Deer's tongue, liatrix
Botanical name: *Trilisa odoratissima* (Walt. ex J. F. Gmel.) Cass.
Botanical synonyms: *Carphephorus odoratissimus* (J. F. Gmel.) H.J.-C. Hebert, *Liatris odoratissima* Willd.
Family: Asteraceae (Compositae)

Absolute

Source: Leaves

Key constituents:

Coumarin	<25.0%

(EFFA 2008)

Safety summary

Hazards: Contains coumarin.
Contraindications: None known.
Maximum adult daily oral dose: 168 mg.

Our safety advice

We recommend a daily oral maximum dose of 168 mg, based on 25.0% coumarin content with a dose limit of 0.6 mg/kg/day (see Coumarin profile, Chapter 14).

Regulatory guidelines

Coumarin was banned by the FDA for food use in 1954.

Organ-specific effects

Adverse skin reactions: Undiluted deertongue absolute was not irritating to rabbits, and tested at 1% it was not irritating to pig or mouse skin. Tested at 5% on 25 volunteers it was neither irritating nor sensitizing. It is non-phototoxic (Opdyke 1979a p. 763). Unlike impure synthetic coumarin, pure, naturally occurring coumarin is not a skin allergen (Floch et al 2002; Vocanson et al 2006).

Reproductive toxicity: Coumarin was not embryotoxic or teratogenic at 25 mg/kg in pigs (Grote et al 1977).

Hepatotoxicity: No information found. High oral doses of coumarin are hepatotoxic in animals and in a very small percentage of humans (see Coumarin profile, Chapter 14).

Systemic effects

Acute toxicity: Deertongue absolute acute oral LD_{50} of a 50% solution in rats >5 g/kg; acute dermal LD_{50} in rabbits >5 g/kg (Opdyke 1979a p763).

Carcinogenic/anticarcinogenic potential: No information found. Coumarin is carcinogenic in rodents, but is anticarcinogenic in humans (Felter et al 2006).

Comments

Dermal application of coumarin is not hazardous (see Coumarin profile, Chapter 14). Deertongue absolute has long been used in tobacco flavoring, and it is also used in fragrances. The leaves contain 2,3-benzofuran, but it is not known whether this is present in the absolute. 2,3-Benzofuran caused DNA fragmentation in human kidney cells from both male and female donors (Robbiano et al 2004).

Dill seed (European)

Botanical name: *Anethum graveolens* L.
Family: Apiaceae (Umbelliferae)

Essential oil

Source: Seeds
Key constituents:

(+)-Limonene	35.9–68.4%
(+)-Carvone	27.3–53.3%
(Z)-Dihydrocarvone	2.9–3.7%
α-Phellandrene	1.0–2.3%
(E)-Dihydrocarvone	1.7–1.8%

(Lawrence 1995g p. 202)
Quality: May be adulterated with terpenes from distilled orange oil (Singhal et al 1997).

Safety summary

Hazards: Drug interaction; skin sensitization if oxidized.
Cautions (oral): Diabetes medication.
Cautions: Old or oxidized oils should be avoided.

Our safety advice

We agree with the IFRA guideline of 1.2% for skin sensitization, but only for (−)-carvone. Our dermal limit for (+)-carvone is 23%, for toxicity. We recommend a human daily oral maximum dose of 12.5 mg/kg for carvone isomers (see Carvone profile, Chapter 14). Therefore, dill seed oil requires no restriction. Because of its limonene content we recommend that oxidation of European dill seed oil is avoided by storage in a dark, airtight container in a refrigerator. The addition of an antioxidant to preparations containing it is recommended.

Regulatory guidelines

The IFRA standard for either isomer of carvone in leave-on products such as body lotions is 1.2%, for skin sensitization. The Council of Europe (1992) has set an ADI of 1 mg/kg for carvone (isomer not specified). This is equivalent to a daily adult dose of 120–240 mg of European dill seed oil (depending on carvone content). IFRA recommends that essential oils rich in limonene should only be used when the level of peroxides is kept to the lowest practical level, for instance by adding antioxidants at the time of production (IFRA 2009).

Organ-specific effects

Adverse skin reactions: Undiluted European dill seed oil was not irritating to rabbit, pig or mouse skin; tested at 4% on 25 volunteers it was neither irritating nor sensitizing. It is non-phototoxic (Opdyke & Letizia 1982 p. 673–674). Autoxidation products of (+)-limonene can cause skin sensitization (see (+)-Limonene profile, Chapter 14).
Cardiovascular effects: Dill oil (type unspecified) reduced blood glucose levels in both normal and alloxan-diabetic rats following sc injection at 27 mg/kg (Essway et al 1995).

Systemic effects

Acute toxicity: European dill seed oil acute oral LD_{50} in rats 4.6 g/kg; acute dermal LD_{50} in rabbits >5 g/kg (Opdyke & Letizia 1982 p. 673–674). Acute subcutaneous LD_{50} in mice 1.35 g/kg (Essway et al 1995).
Carcinogenic/anticarcinogenic potential: European dill seed oil induced chromosome aberrations (mostly chromatid breaks) in human lymphocytes and also was genotoxic in fruit flies (Lazutka et al 2001). (+)-Carvone has been reported as both genotoxic and non-genotoxic, but it is not a rodent carcinogen, and both carvone and (+)-limonene display anticarcinogenic activity (see Constituent profiles, Chapter 14).
Drug interactions: Antidiabetic medication, because of cardiovascular effects, above. See Table 4.10B.

Comments

Unlike Indian dill seed oil, the European type of oil contains no dill apiole, and is similar to caraway seed oil.

Dill seed (Indian)

Synonyms: Sowa, East Indian dill, satapashpi
Botanical name: *Anethum sowa* Roxb. ex Flem.
Family: Apiaceae (Umbelliferae)

Essential oil

Source: Seeds
Key constituents:

Dill apiole	20.7–52.5%
(+)-Limonene	5.9–45.0%
(+)-Carvone	17.4–23.1%
(E)-Dihydrocarvone	4.2–16.6%
α-Phellandrene	tr–6.5%
(Z)-Dihydrocarvone	0.8–5.2%

(Lawrence 1995g p. 202)

Safety summary

Hazards: Hepatotoxicity; nephrotoxicity; may be abortifacient.
Contraindications (all routes): Pregnancy, breastfeeding.
Maximum adult daily oral dose: 53 mg.
Maximum dermal use level: 1.4%.

Our safety advice

We have proposed a daily oral maximum for parsley apiole of 0.4 mg/kg. Because of its structural similarity, dill apiole is likely to present a similar risk. We therefore recommend oral and dermal restrictions of 53 mg and 1.4% for Indian dill seed oil, based on a 52.5% dill apiole with apiole limits of 0.4 mg/kg and 0.76% (see Parsley apiole profile, Chapter 14). Our oral maximum dose of 12.5 mg/kg/day for (+)-carvone can be ignored here since carvone is much less toxic.

Regulatory guidelines

The Council of Europe (1992) has set an ADI of 1 mg/kg for carvone (isomer not specified). This is equivalent to an adult

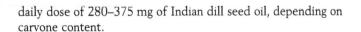

daily dose of 280–375 mg of Indian dill seed oil, depending on carvone content.

Organ-specific effects

Adverse skin reactions: Undiluted Indian dill seed oil was moderately irritating to rabbits, but was not irritating to mice or pigs; tested at 4% on 25 volunteers it was neither irritating nor sensitizing. It is non-phototoxic (Opdyke 1982 p. 673–674).

Reproductive toxicity: Apiole and various preparations of parsley have been used for many years to procure illegal abortion in Italy. Post-abortive vaginal bleeding, sometimes profuse, is a feature of these cases. A cumulative effect is apparent, parsley apiole being taken daily for between two and eight days before either death or abortion ensued. The lowest daily dose of apiole which induced abortion was 0.9 g taken for eight consecutive days (see Parsley apiole profile, Chapter 14).

Systemic effects

Acute toxicity: Indian dill seed oil acute oral LD_{50} in rats 4.6 g/kg, in mice >3 g/kg; acute dermal LD_{50} in rabbits >5 g/kg (Opdyke 1982 p. 673–674). Parsley apiole is toxic in humans; the lowest total dose of apiole causing death is 4.2 g (2.1 g/day for 2 days) the lowest fatal daily dose is 770 mg, which was taken for 14 days; the lowest single fatal dose is 8 g. At least 19 g has been survived (see Parsley apiole profile, Chapter 14).

Carcinogenic/anticarcinogenic potential: No information found for Indian dill seed oil. A very low level of genotoxicity has been reported for dill apiole (Phillips et al 1984; Randerath et al 1984). However, neither dill apiole nor carvone is carcinogenic, and (+)-limonene displays anticarcinogenic activity (see Constituent profiles, Chapter 14). Essential oil of *Piper aduncum*, containing 45.9% dill apiole, was not mutagenic in *S. typhimurium* strains TA98 and TA100, with or without S9 (Guerrini et al 2009).

Comments

Essential oils high in parsley apiole present a high risk of abortion if taken in oral doses, and external use also seems inadvisable in pregnancy. Indian dill seed oil should not be confused with European dill seed oil (*Anethum graveolens*) which contains a maximum of 1% apiole, and is not toxic.

Dill weed

Synonym: Dill herb
Botanical name: *Anethum graveolens* L.
Family: Apiaceae (Umbelliferae)

Essential oil

Source: Aerial parts
Key constituents:

(+)-Carvone	31.6–42.4%
α-Phellandrene	18.2–30.2%
(+)-Limonene	22.5–24.9%
Anethofuran (dill ether)	5.6–6.6%
β-Phellandrene	2.3–3.3%
(*E*)-Dihydrocarvone	0.5–1.9%
(*Z*)-Dihydrocarvone	0.8–1.4%
p-Cymene	1.0–1.1%

(Lawrence 1995g p. 202)

Safety summary

Hazards: Drug interaction.
Cautions (oral): Diabetes medication.

Our safety advice

We agree with the IFRA guideline of 1.2% for skin sensitization, but only for (−)-carvone. Our dermal limit for (+)-carvone is 23%, for toxicity. We recommend a human daily oral maximum dose of 12.5 mg/kg for carvone isomers (see Carvone profile, Chapter 14). Therefore, dill weed oil requires no restriction.

Regulatory guidelines

The IFRA standard for either isomer of carvone in leave-on products such as body lotions is 1.2%, for skin sensitization. The Council of Europe (1992) has set an ADI of 1 mg/kg for carvone (isomer not specified). This is equivalent to a daily adult dose of 150–200 mg of dill weed oil (depending on carvone content).

Organ-specific effects

Adverse skin reactions: Undiluted dill weed oil was not irritating to rabbit, pig or mouse skin; tested at 4% on 25 volunteers it was neither irritating nor sensitizing. It is non-phototoxic (Opdyke 1976 p.747–748).

Cardiovascular effects: Dill oil (type unspecified) reduced blood glucose levels in both normal and alloxan-diabetic rats following sc injection at 27 mg/kg (Essway et al 1995).

Systemic effects

Acute toxicity: Dill weed oil acute oral LD_{50} in rats 4.04 mL/kg; acute dermal LD_{50} in rabbits >5 g/kg (Opdyke 1976 p. 747–748).

Carcinogenic/anticarcinogenic potential: Dill weed oil induced chromosome aberrations (mostly chromatid breaks) in human lymphocytes and also was genotoxic in fruit flies (Lazutka et al 2001). However, it significantly induced glutathione *S*-transferase activity in mouse tissues (Lam & Zheng 1991), as do (+)-carvone, (+)-limonene and anethofuran (Zheng et al 1992d). (+)-Carvone is not a rodent carcinogen; both carvone and (+)-limonene display anticarcinogenic activity (see Constituent profiles, Chapter 14).

Drug interactions: Antidiabetic medication, because of cardiovascular effects, above. See Table 4.10B.

Comments

Dill weed oil is widely used in canned pickles.

Echinacea

Synonym: Purple coneflower
Botanical name: *Echinacea purpurea* (L.) Moench.
Botanical synonyms: *Brauneria purpurea* (L.) Britton, *Echinacea purpurea* (L.) Moench var. *arkansana* Steyerm., *Rudbeckia purpurea* L.
Family: Asteraceae (Compositae)

Essential oil

Source: Whole plant
Key constituents:

Germacrene D	44.6%
β-Caryophyllene	4.5%
δ-Cadinene	3.4%
Caryophyllene oxide	3.0%
β-Myrcene	2.5%
α-Phellandrene	2.3%
Bicyclogermacrene	1.5%
α-Caryophyllene	1.5%
(*E*)-α-Bergamotene	1.4%
γ-Cadinene	1.1%
α-Muurolene	1.1%
Spathulenol	1.0%

(Mainguy, private communication, 2001)

Safety summary

Hazards: None known.
Contraindications: None known.

Organ-specific effects

No information found for echinacea oil or germacrene D.

Systemic effects

Acute toxicity: No information found for echinacea oil or germacrene D.
Carcinogenic/anticarcinogenic potential: No information found for echinacea oil, but it contains no known carcinogens. α-Caryophyllene displays anticarcinogenic activity (see α-Caryophyllene profile, Chapter 14).

Comments

Limited availability.

Elecampane

Synonym: Alantroot
Botanical name: *Inula helenium* L.
Family: Asteraceae (Compositae)

Essential oil

Source: Dried roots
Key constituents:

Alantolactone	52.4%
Isoalantolactone	33.0%
Eudesma-5,7(11)-diene-8 β-12 olide	1.3%
β-Elemene	1.2%

(Bourrel et al 1993b)

Safety summary

Hazards: Skin sensitization (high risk).
Contraindications: Should not be used on the skin.

Regulatory guidelines

IFRA recommends that elecampane oil should not be used as a fragrance ingredient, due to its sensitizing potential (IFRA 2009). Elecampane oil is prohibited as a fragrance ingredient in the EU and Canada (SCCNFP 2001a; Health Canada Cosmetic Ingredient Hotlist, March 2011
http://www.hc-sc.gc.ca/cps-spc/cosmet-person/indust/hotlist-critique/hotlist-liste-eng.php).

Organ-specific effects

Adverse skin reactions: Tested at 4% on 25 volunteers, undiluted elecampane oil was not irritating. A maximation test, using elecampane oil at 4%, elicited "extremely severe allergic reactions" in 23 out of 25 volunteers. Alantolactone elicited positive patch-test responses in sensitized guinea pigs. A 1% concentration of alantolactone produced positive reactions in 4/25 patients (Opdyke 1976 p. 307–308). Sesquiterpene lactones from Compositae plants are notorious skin sensitizers (Ross et al 1993; Goulden & Wilkinson 1998). No phototoxicity data were found.

Systemic effects

Acute toxicity: No information found.
Carcinogenic/anticarcinogenic potential: No information found for elecampane oil, but it contains no known carcinogens. β-Elemene is anticarcinogenic (see β-Elemene profile, Chapter 14).

Comments

Elecampane oil has been frequently employed as an adulterant of costus oil. Elecampane oil should not be confused with *Inula graveolens*; both oils have been referred to as 'inula oil'.

Elemi

Botanical names: *Canarium luzonicum* (Blume) A. Gray, *Canarium vulgare* Leenh. (synonym: *Canarium commune* auct.)
Family: Burseraceae

Essential oil

Source: Gum
Key constituents:

(+)-Limonene	26.9–65.0%
Elemol	2.8–17.3%

α-Phellandrene	4.3–15.1%
Elemicin	1.8–10.6%
p-Cymene	1.4–7.7%
α-Pinene	0.4–5.4%
1,8-Cineole	<2.5%
β-Myrcene	0.6–2.4%
β-Phellandrene	0.8–1.6%
Sabinene	1.3–5.9%
β-Pinene	0.3–1.0%
Methyleugenol	0.2–0.3%

(Lawrence 1981 p. 26–27, 1989 p. 109–110, 2003)
Quality: May be adulterated with additional (+)-limonene and α-phellandrene (Burfield 2003).

Safety summary

Hazards: May contain methyleugenol; skin sensitization if oxidized
Cautions: Old or oxidized oils should be avoided.
Maximum dermal use level:

EU	0.07%
IFRA	0.13%
Tisserand & Young	No limit

Our safety advice

Based purely on 0.3% methyleugenol content, we would recommend a maximum dermal use level of 6.7% for elemi oil, applying a dermal maximum of 0.02% (see Methyleugenol profile, Chapter 14). However, since the antitumoral activity of (+)-limonene is wide-ranging and includes human hepatoma cells (Kim et al 2001), the high level of (+)-limonene in elemi oil is likely to counter any potentially hepatocarcinogenic effect of the very small amount of methyleugenol. We therefore believe that no limit should be applied. We recommend that elemi oil is stored in a dark, airtight container in a refrigerator to minimize oxidation of its (+)-limonene content. The addition of an antioxidant to preparations containing elemi oil is recommended.

Regulatory guidelines

IFRA recommends that the maximum concentration of methyleugenol for leave-on products such as body lotion should be 0.0004% (IFRA 2009). The equivalent SCCNFP maximum is 0.0002% (European Commission 2002). IFRA recommends that essential oils rich in limonene should only be used when the level of peroxides is kept to the lowest practical level, for instance by adding antioxidants at the time of production (IFRA 2009).

Organ-specific effects

Adverse skin reactions: Undiluted elemi oil was slightly irritating to rabbits, but was not irritating to mice or pigs; tested at 4% on 25 volunteers it was neither irritating nor sensitizing. It is non-phototoxic (Opdyke 1976 p. 755). Autoxidation products

of (+)-limonene can cause skin sensitization (see (+)-Limonene profile, Chapter 14).

Systemic effects

Acute toxicity: Elemi oil acute oral LD_{50} in rats 3.37 g/kg; acute dermal LD_{50} in rabbits ~5 g/kg (Opdyke 1976 p. 755).
Carcinogenic/anticarcinogenic potential: No information found for elemi oil. Methyleugenol is a rodent carcinogen if exposure is sufficiently high; (+)-limonene displays anticarcinogenic activity (see Constituent profiles, Chapter 14).

Comments

Elemi oil tends to resinify on ageing. In a report on trees it has been proposed by UNEP-WCMC that CITES add *Canarium luzonicum* to its list of threatened plant species.

Eucalyptus (cineole-rich)

Botanical names: *Eucalyptus camaldulensis* Dehnh. (cineole CT); *Eucalyptus globulus* Labill. (blue gum, Tasmanian blue gum); *Eucalyptus maidenii* F. Muell. (Maiden's gum); *Eucalyptus plenissima* (Gardner) Brooker (synonym: *Eucalyptus kochii* subsp. *plenissima* (Gardner) Brooker); *Eucalyptus polybractea* R. T. Baker (blue-leaved mallee); *Eucalyptus radiata* Sieber ex DC (synonyms: *Eucalyptus Australiana* R. T. Baker, *Eucalyptus phellandra* R. T. Baker) (narrow-leaved peppermint, grey peppermint); *Eucalyptus smithii* R. T. Baker (gully gum, gully peppermint, blackbutt peppermint)
Family: Myrtaceae

Essential oil

Source: Leaves
Key constituents:

Eucalyptus camaldulensis (cineole CT)

1,8-Cineole	46.9–83.7%
α-Pinene	1.3–14.7%
(+)-Limonene	0–11.2%
α-Terpineol	0–8.4%
β-Pinene	tr–7.9%
Globulol	0–5.3%
p-Cymene	0–5.2%
Terpinen-4-ol	0.1–3.3%
α-Phellandrene	tr–2.9%
γ-Terpinene	tr–2.2%
Spathulenol	0–1.8%
(+)-Aromadendrene	0.6–1.4%

(Moudachirou & Gbénou 1999)

Eucalyptus globulus

1,8-Cineole	65.4–83.9%
α-Pinene	3.7–14.7%
(+)-Limonene	1.8–9.0%
Globulol	tr–5.3%

(E)-Pinocarveol 2.3–4.4%
p-Cymene 1.2–3.5%
(+)-Aromadendrene 0.1–2.2%
Pinocarvone tr-1.0%

(Lawrence 1989 p199–200, 1993 p122–125)

Eucalyptus maidenii

1,8-Cineole 76.8%
α-Pinene 13.1%
α-Terpineol 2.1%
(+)-Aromadendrene 1.7%
(E)-Pinocarveol 1.3%

(Zrira et al 1992)

Eucalyptus plenissima

1,8-Cineole 85.0–95.0%
(+)-Limonene 0.5–1.2%

(Day, private communication, 2004)

Eucalyptus polybractea

1,8-Cineole 88.7–91.9%
(+)-Limonene 1.1–2.6%
p-Cymene 2.0–2.5%
α-Pinene 0.9–1.9%

(Lawrence 1993 p122–125, 1997a p49–51)

Eucalyptus radiata

1,8-Cineole 60.4–64.5%
α-Terpineol 0–15.2%
(Z)-Piperitol 0.9–14.9%
(+)-Limonene 5.4–6.3%
Piperitone 0.4–4.7%
Geraniol 0.2–2.8%
α-Pinene 2.0%
β-Caryophyllene 0.1–1.6%
Terpinen-4-ol 0–1.5%
β-Myrcene 1.1%

(Bignell et al 1998)

Eucalyptus smithii

1,8-Cineole 77.5%
β-Eudesmol 6.3%
(E)-Pinocarveol 2.9%
Pinocarvone 1.6%
(Z)-p-Mentha-1(7),8-dien-2-ol 1.4%
(E)-p-Mentha-1(7),8-dien-2-ol 1.3%
(+)-Limonene 1.2%

(Bignell et al 1998)

Quality: Because of their low price, 1,8-cineole type eucalyptus oils are not generally adulterated (Singhal et al 1997; Burfield 2003).

Safety summary

Hazards: Essential oils high in 1,8-cineole can cause CNS and breathing problems in young children.
Contraindications: Do not apply to or near the face of infants or children under ten years of age.
Maximum adult daily oral dose: 600 mg
Maximum dermal use level: 20%

Our safety advice

We agree with the Commission E oral maximum dose of 600 mg and up to 20% for dermal applications.

Regulatory guidelines

Health Canada requires that eucalyptus oil should be used at no more than 25% in cosmetic products (Health Canada Cosmetic Ingredient Hotlist, March 2011). Eucalyptus oil is classed as a 'Schedule 6' poison in Australia. Substances in this category are regarded as having 'a moderate potential for causing harm, the extent of which can be reduced through the use of distinctive packaging with strong warnings and safety directions on the label.' The recommended warnings, to keep out of reach of children and to not take internally, are used by many manufacturers on all their essential oil packaging. However, the recommended use of child-resistant closures on eucalyptus oil is not widely adhered to outside of Australia.

The German Commission E Monograph for eucalyptus oil recommends a daily oral dose of 300–600 mg, and 5–20% for dermal applications. It also contraindicates internal use in cases of inflammatory diseases of the GI tract and bile ducts, and in severe liver disease (Blumenthal et al 1998).

Organ-specific effects

Adverse skin reactions: In an in vitro assay, eucalyptus oil was non-phototoxic (Placzek et al 2007). Undiluted eucalyptus oil was moderately irritating to rabbits, but was not irritating to mice; tested at 10% on 25 volunteers it was neither irritating nor sensitizing (Opdyke 1975 p. 107–108). When injected, E. globulus oil inhibited inflammation induced in rat paw (Silva et al 2003). In a study of 200 consecutive dermatitis patients, three (1.5%) were sensitive to 2% eucalyptus oil (Rudzki et al 1976). Four of 747 dermatitis patients suspected of fragrance allergy (0.54%) reacted to 2% eucalyptus oil (Wöhrl et al 2001). In a multicenter study, Germany's IVDK reported that 17 of 6,680 dermatitis patients suspected of fragrance allergy (0.25%) tested positive to 2% eucalyptus oil (Uter et al 2010). There were only four ++ or +++ reactions, suggesting that eucalyptus oil is virtually non-allergenic. In a worldwide multicenter study, four of 218 dermatitis patients (1.8%) with proven sensitization to fragrance materials were sensitive to 10% eucalyptus oil (Larsen et al 2002). Of 12 workers in a food factory who had developed hand eczema, one tested positive to 2% eucalyptus oil (Peltonen et al 1985). A 65-year-old aromatherapist with multiple essential oil sensitivities reacted to 5%, but not 1% eucalyptus oil (Selvaag et al 1995).
Reproductive toxicity: E. globulus oil was neither embryotoxic nor fetotoxic in pregnant mice when 135 mg was injected sc on

gestational days 6–15 (Pages et al 1990). Eucalyptus oil was not significantly cytotoxic to cultured human umbilical vein endothelial cells (Takarada et al 2004).

Systemic effects

Acute toxicity, human: There are three common signs of eucalyptus poisoning: CNS depression, abnormal respiration and pinpoint pupils. Also likely are epigastric pain, vomiting, weakness in the legs, cold sweats and headache. Cardiovascular collapse is a feature of severe intoxication, and convulsions are notable for their rarity. There is frequently vertigo and lack of coordination, but these are indications of mild poisoning, unless they are rapidly superseded by stupor. Death has occurred from 15 minutes to 15 hours following ingestion, and some cases survive even the most severe stage of intoxication (Gurr & Scroggie 1965). Respiratory effects are variable, with either shallow, or labored breathing (Craig 1953).

Early reports of eucalyptus oil poisoning in children in the UK included fatal cases (Myott 1906; McPherson 1925; Craig 1953), and non-fatal ones (Benjamin 1906; Orr & Edin 1906; Allan 1910; Kirkness 1910; Foggie 1911; Sewell 1925; Gibbon 1927; Hindle 1994). In south-east Queensland, Australia, 41 cases were reported in children aged under 14 years between 1984 and 1991. The authors saw no correlation between the amount ingested and the severity of symptoms, indeed 80% of the children (33/41) were asymptomatic and of these, four had ingested more than 30 mL (Webb & Pitt 1993). There may be great individual variation in sensitivity to eucalyptus poisoning and, at least in Australia, in the content of preparations sold as eucalyptus oil.

During an 11-year period (1981–1992) 109 children were admitted to a Melbourne hospital with eucalyptus oil poisoning. Of these, 31 had some degree of CNS depression, three were unconscious having ingested 5–10 mL, and one was deeply unconscious, having ingested ~75 mL. Vomiting occurred in 37%, ataxia in 15%, and pulmonary dysfunction in 11%. No treatment was given for 12%, ipecac or activated charcoal for 21% and nasogastric activated charcoal for 57%. The authors concluded that eucalyptus oil ingestion usually caused some illness in small children; that significant depression of consciousness was likely after ingesting 5 mL or more, and minor depression after 2–3 mL (Tibballs 1995).

A 3-year-old boy survived the ingestion of ~10 mL eucalyptus oil; severe CNS depression occurred within 30 minutes, followed by equally rapid recovery after gastric lavage (Patel & Wiggins 1980). An 18-month-old child (10–15 mL) and an 11-month-old child (unknown quantity) recovered after ingesting eucalyptus oil. In both cases, severe systemic effects were seen (labored breathing, pallor) and recovery followed gastric lavage and activated charcoal (Hindle 1994). In 1893, a 10-year-old boy died within 15 hours of ingesting about 30 mL of eucalyptus oil. Signs included shortness of breath and vomiting coming on in minutes (Neale 1893).

Under 5 mL of eucalyptus oil has allegedly been fatal in an adult (McPherson 1925) although this is atypical, and seems unlikely. In three early cases, severe symptoms followed adult ingestion of one teaspoon of eucalyptus oil, in each case relieved by induced vomiting (Benham 1905; Taylor 1905). An adult has survived ingestion of 60 mL (Gurr & Scroggie 1965). Death occurs usually after 30 mL, following severe cardiovascular, respiratory and central nervous effects (Myott 1906; Gurr & Scroggie 1965), although 23 mL (untreated) and even 240 mL (treated) have been survived by adults (Mack 1988). Eucalyptus oil appears to be more toxic in humans than would be expected from the animal data on 1,8-cineole.

1,8-Cineole can cause serious poisoning in young children when accidentally instilled into the nose (Melis et al 1989).

Acute toxicity, animal: The acute oral LD_{50} values in mice for *E. camaldulensis* and *E. exserta* (both cineole-rich oils) were 3.67 mL/kg and 3.75 mL/kg (Pho et al 1993). Ingesting 30 mL–60 mL eucalyptus oil is fatal to humans (Gurr & Scroggie 1965), which suggests that it is four times more toxic than would be expected from the rodent data above, or for 1,8-cineole. The rat acute oral LD_{50} for 1,8-cineole is 2.48 g/kg (Jenner et al 1964). This is frequently mis-quoted as an LD_{50} for eucalyptus oil.

Neurotoxicity: A toxic dose of eucalyptus oil usually leads to drowsiness in a few minutes, and the person may be unconscious within 15 minutes. Children may be susceptible even to moderate doses. Over two days, a 6-year-old girl was given repeated topical applications of a home remedy containing eucalyptus oil for pruritic urticaria. She subsequently became drowsy, felt nauseous, vomited, and eventually lost consciousness. Her condition rapidly improved after skin sponging with water (Darben et al 1998). Three hours after the application of a wash-off head lice treatment containing 11% eucalyptus oil, followed by a leave-on conditioner with 2.5% eucalyptus oil, a four-year-old girl felt nauseated and lethargic, became unresponsive, then suffered a grand mal seizure lasting less than one minute (Waldman 2011).

Endocrine toxicity: Eucalyptus oil had no estrogen-like effect in an in vitro assay using MCF-7 cells (Nielsen 2008).

Antioxidant/pro-oxidant activity: Eucalyptus oil has demonstrated scavenging activity against OH radicals (Grassmann et al 2000).

Carcinogenic/anticarcinogenic potential: Eucalyptus oil terpenes significantly induced glutathione *S*-transferase activity in mouse tissues (Lam & Zheng 1991). 1,8-Cineole is neither mutagenic nor carcinogenic (see 1,8-Cineole profile, Chapter 14).

Comments

We have seen no research that would support the Commission E contraindications which are presumably based on the 1,8-cineole content, since they are also applied to cineole-rich niaouli oil. Oral 1,8-cineole was not hepatotoxic in rats at doses of up to 800 mg/kg/day for three days (Kim NH et al 2004), and a single dose of 400 mg/kg significantly protected against chemically induced hepatotoxicity in mice (Santos et al 2001). At 100 mg/kg/day for 60 days, gavage doses of 1,8-cineole protected rat liver from chemically induced oxidative stress (Ciftçi et al 2011). Pre-treatment with 1,8-cineole by rectal instillation at 200 or 400 mg/kg attenuated TNBS-induced colonic damage in rats (Santos et al 2004), and there are many other papers showing an anti-inflammatory action for 1,8-cineole. Most of the research showing anti-hepatotoxic and anti-inflammatory effects for 1,8-cineole has been published since the Commission E contraindications for eucalyptus oil were written. We suggest they now need revision.

There are insufficient data to determine maximum dermal use levels, but for dermatitis patients this may be below 1.0%. Other species from which cineole-rich eucalyptus oils are obtained for commercial use include *E. cneorifolia* (70%), *E. dumosa* (70%), *E. elaeophora* (70–75%), *E. oleosa* (50–80%), *E. sideroxylon* (70–75%) and *E. viridis* (70–80%) (Lawrence 1989 p. 199–200). The European Pharmacopoeia standard for eucalyptus oil requires a minimum 1,8-cineole content of 70% (European Pharmacopoeia Commission 2002). Concentration of 1,8-cineole by fractional distillation is a common practice to ensure that this standard is met. Although there are many different types of eucalyptus oil, the majority of those purchased for household or medical use are chemically similar, being cineole-rich. The main commercial source of cineole-rich eucalyptus is the *E. globulus* produced in the Yunnan province of China. Portugal, Spain, India and South Africa are also major producers, and Australia contributes 5–10% of world production.

Eucalyptus macarthurii

Synonyms: Woolly butt, Camden woollybut, Paddy's river box
Botanical name: *Eucalyptus macarthurii* H. Deane & Maiden
Family: Myrtaceae

Essential oil

Source: Leaves
Key constituents:

1,8-Cineole	28.9–29.0%
Geranyl acetate	18.8–21.8%
(+)-Limonene	9.8–16.2%
Linalool	6.7–7.6%
α-Pinene	4.4–6.7%
p-Cymene	3.1–3.3%
Geraniol	1.9–3.3%
γ-Terpinene	0.5–2.1%
α-Terpineol	1.2–1.6%
Guaiacol	0.8–1.0%

(Lawrence 1981 p. 16–17)

Safety summary

Hazards: May be choleretic.
Contraindications (oral): Cholestasis.

Organ-specific effects

Reproductive toxicity: The low reproductive toxicity of 1,8-cineole, (+)-limonene, linalool and α-pinene (see Constituent profiles, Chapter 14) suggests that eucalyptus macarthurii oil is not hazardous in pregnancy.
Gastrointestinal toxicology: Since geranyl acetate is choleretic (Trabace et al 1994), *Eucalyptus macarthurii* oil should not be taken in oral doses by people with cholestasis (obstructed bile flow) (Fujii et al 1994).

Systemic effects

Acute toxicity: No information found.
Carcinogenic/anticarcinogenic potential: No information found for eucalyptus macarthurii oil, but it contains no known carcinogens. Geranyl acetate is not a rodent carcinogen; (+)-limonene and geraniol are anticarcinogenic (see Constituent profiles, Chapter 14).

Comments

There are three chemotypes, with varying amounts of geranyl acetate, 1,8-cineole, geraniol, (+)-limonene and eudesmol. Geranyl acetate can be as high as 70%. This oil is usually rectified to remove unwanted aldehydes.

Eucalyptus (peppermint)

Synonyms: Broad-leaved peppermint, blue peppermint, peppermint gum
Botanical name: *Eucalyptus dives* Schauer in Walp.
Family: Myrtaceae

Essential oil

Source: Leaves
Key constituents:

Piperitone	54.5%
α-Phellandrene	16.9%
p-Cymene	6.1%
Terpinen-4-ol	4.2%
α-Pinene	2.8%
Terpinolene	1.9%
β-Myrcene	1.4%
α-Terpineol	1.3%
1,8-Cineole	1.2%
(*E*)-*p*-Menth-2-en-1-ol	1.2%
(*Z*)-*p*-Menth-2-en-1-ol	1.0%
(*E*)-Piperitol	1.0%

(Bignell et al 1998)

Safety summary

Hazards: None known.
Contraindications: None known.

Organ-specific effects

No information found.

Systemic effects

Acute toxicity: No information found. Piperitone acute oral LD_{50} in rats 3.55 g/kg, acute dermal LD_{50} in rabbits >5 g/kg, subcutaneous LD_{50} in mice 1.42 g/kg (Wenzel & Ross 1957).
Carcinogenic/anticarcinogenic potential: No information found for peppermint eucalyptus oil, but it contains no known

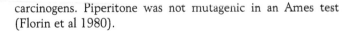

carcinogens. Piperitone was not mutagenic in an Ames test (Florin et al 1980).

Comments

Produced in southeastern Australia. Small quantities of a 1,8-cineole CT may also be produced.

Eucalyptus polybractea (cryptone CT)

Synonym: Blue-leaved mallee
Botanical name: *Eucalyptus polybractea* R. T. Baker
Family: Myrtaceae

Essential oil

Source: Leaves
Key constituents:

p-Cymene	18.3%
1,8-Cineole	16.1%
Spathulenol	14.3%
Cryptone	6.3%
Phellandral	5.7%
α-Phellandrene	3.6%
Terpinen-4-ol	3.5%
Cuminaldehyde	3.3%
(+)-Limonene	2.1%
(–)-*allo*-Aromadendrene	2.0%
α-Pinene	1.7%
γ-Terpinene	1.6%
α-Thujene	1.2%
Carvacrol	1.1%

(Badoux, private communication, 2002)

Safety summary

Hazards: None known.
Contraindications: None known.

Organ-specific effects

No information found.

Systemic effects

Acute toxicity: No information found.
Carcinogenic/anticarcinogenic potential: No information found for *Eucalyptus polybractea* oil cryptone CT, but it contains no known carcinogens.

Comments

Limited availability.

Fennel (bitter)

Botanical name: *Foeniculum vulgare* Mill. subsp. *Capillaceum* Gilib.
Family: Apiaceae (Umbelliferae)

Essential oil

Source: Seeds
Key constituents:

(*E*)-Anethole	52.5–84.3%
Fenchone	4.0–24.0%
α-Pinene	tr–10.4%
(+)-Limonene	0.5–9.4%
Estragole	2.8–6.5%
α-Phellandrene	0.3–1.2%
(*Z*)-Anethole	tr–0.2%

(Lawrence 1995g p. 199)

Safety summary

Hazards: Drug interaction; reproductive hormone modulation; potentially carcinogenic, based on estragole content; may inhibit blood clotting; skin sensitization if oxidized.
Contraindications (all routes): Pregnancy, breastfeeding, endometriosis, estrogen-dependent cancers, children under five years of age.
Cautions (oral): Diabetes medication, anticoagulant medication, major surgery, peptic ulcer, hemophilia, other bleeding disorders (Box 7.1).
Maximum adult daily oral dose: 54 mg
Maximum dermal use level:

EU	No limit
IFRA	0.15%
Tisserand & Young	1.8%

Our safety advice

We recommend a maximum adult oral dose of 54 mg and a dermal maximum of 1.8%, based on 6.5% estragole content with oral and dermal limits of 0.05 mg/kg and 0.12% (see Estragole profile, Chapter 14).

Regulatory guidelines

The Comission E Monograph for fennel oil (type unspecified) recommends that it is not used in pregnancy, or "for infants and toddlers" (Blumenthal et al 1998). IFRA recommends a maximum dermal use level for estragole of 0.01% in leave-on or wash-off preparations for body and face (IFRA 2009). The EU does not restrict estragole.

Organ-specific effects

Adverse skin reactions: Undiluted bitter fennel oil was non-phototoxic in hairless mice and swine. The undiluted oil was irritating to rabbits, but was not irritating to mice or pigs; tested at 4% on two panels of 25 volunteers it was not irritating

(Opdyke 1976 p. 309; Opdyke & Letizia 1983 p. 529). A maximation test using bitter fennel oil at 4% produced sensitization reactions in three out of 25 test subjects (Opdyke 1976 p. 309). It was later shown that the fennel oil used in this test had oxidized, and subsequent testing with a non-oxidized sample on 29 subjects produced no sensitization reactions (Opdyke & Letizia 1983 p. 529).

Cardiovascular effects: (*E*)-anethole inhibits platelet aggregation (Yoshioka & Tamada 2005), an essential step in the blood clotting cascade. Sweet fennel oil (which is very similar to bitter fennel in composition) reduced blood glucose levels in both normal and alloxan-diabetic rats following sc injection at 21.5 mg/kg (Essway et al 1995).

Hepatotoxicity: (*E*)-Anethole has a dose-dependent hepatotoxicity which is due to a metabolite, anethole 1′,2′-epoxide (AE) and different amounts of AE are produced in different species. High doses of (*E*)-anethole or AE deplete glutathione (Marshall & Caldwell 1992, 1993) but sweet fennel oil, which has a very similar composition to bitter fennel, significantly induced glutathione *S*-transferase activity in mouse tissues (Lam & Zheng 1991). The amounts of (*E*)-anethole-rich essential oils used in aromatherapy pose no risk to humans (see (*E*)-Anethole profile).

Systemic effects

Acute toxicity: Bitter fennel acute oral LD_{50} in rats 4.52 mL/kg; acute dermal LD_{50} in rabbits >5 g/kg (Opdyke 1976 p. 309).

Carcinogenic/anticarcinogenic potential: No information found for bitter fennel oil. Estragole is a rodent carcinogen when exposure is sufficiently high; (*E*)-anethole is not a rodent carcinogen; (+)-limonene is anticarcinogenic (see Constituent profiles, Chapter 14).

Drug interactions: Antidiabetic or anticoagulant medication, because of cardiovascular effects, above. See Table 4.10B.

Comments

The Expanded Commission E Monographs list bitter fennel oil as an oil that should not be used in pregnancy, or for infants and toddlers (Blumenthal et al 2000 p. 126). No explanation is given. Bitter fennel is the official fennel oil of the European Pharmacopoeia, and should contain >60% (*E*)-anethole, >15% fenchone, and <5% estragole (European Pharmacopoeia Commission 2002). It is clearly important to ensure that bitter fennel oil has not oxidized before employing it for therapeutic purposes, although this raises the issue of what oxidized in the oil, and whether anise and sweet fennel oils, which are similar to bitter fennel in composition, might be similarly prone to oxidation. (*E*)-Anethole is susceptible to oxidation, and its oxidation products, (*Z*)-anethole, anisaldehyde and anisic ketone, may be skin sensitizing (see (*E*)-Anethole profile, Chapter 14).

Fennel (sweet)

Botanical name: *Foeniculum vulgare* Mill.
Family: Apiaceae (Umbelliferae)

Essential oil

Source: Seeds
Key constituents:

(*E*)-Anethole	58.1–92.5%
(+)-Limonene	0.2–21.0%
Fenchone	0.2–8.0%
Estragole	1.1–4.8%
α-Pinene	0.1–3.4%
α-Phellandrene	0.1–2.0%
(*Z*)-Anethole	tr–0.7%

(Lawrence 1995g p. 199; Kubeczka 2002)

Quality: Sweet fennel oil may be adulterated with monoterpene hydrocarbons such as limonene, and with synthetic anethole, which usually contains the more toxic (*Z*)- isomer. (Kubeczka 2002). Bitter fennel oil may be passed off as sweet fennel oil (Burfield 2000).

Safety summary

Hazards: Drug interaction; reproductive hormone modulation; potentially carcinogenic, based on estragole content; may inhibit blood clotting; skin sensitization if oxidized.

Contraindications (all routes): Pregnancy, breastfeeding, endometriosis, estrogen-dependent cancers, children under five years of age.

Cautions (oral): Diabetes medication, anticoagulant medication, major surgery, peptic ulcer, hemophilia, other bleeding disorders (Box 7.1).

Maximum adult daily oral dose: 73 mg
Maximum dermal use level:

EU	No limit
IFRA	0.2%
Tisserand & Young	2.5%

Our safety advice

We recommend an oral maximum of 73 mg and a dermal maximum of 2.5%, based on 4.8% estragole content with oral and dermal limits of 0.05 mg/kg and 0.12% (see Estragole profile, Chapter 14).

Regulatory guidelines

The Commission E Monograph for fennel oil (type unspecified) recommends that it is not used in pregnancy, or "for infants and toddlers" (Blumenthal et al 1998). IFRA recommends a maximum dermal use level for estragole of 0.01% in leave-on or wash-off preparations for body and face (IFRA 2009). The EU does not restrict estragole.

Organ-specific effects

Adverse skin reactions: Undiluted sweet fennel oil was moderately irritating to rabbits and was severely irritating to mice; tested at 4% on 25 volunteers it was neither irritating nor sensitizing. It is non-phototoxic (Opdyke 1974 p. 879–880). (*E*)-Anethole is prone to oxidation, and its oxidation products may be skin sensitizing (see (*E*)-Anethole profile). Oxidation of sweet fennel oil progressed rapidly during storage in the light, but progressed only slowly in dark conditions (Misharina & Polshkov 2005). Sweet fennel oil has demonstrated antioxidant activity in relation to two lipid peroxidation models (Ruberto et al 2000).

Cardiovascular effects: Sweet fennel oil inhibits platelet aggregation (Tognolini et al 2006), an essential step in the blood clotting cascade. Sweet fennel oil reduced blood glucose levels in both normal and alloxan-diabetic rats following sc injection at 21.5 mg/kg (Essway et al 1995).

Reproductive toxicity: Sweet fennel oil, containing 72% (E)-anethole, 12.0% fenchone and 5% estragole, was tested at various concentrations on a rat embryo limb bud culture. Compounds that inhibit differentiation of these cells by more than 50% have a high correlation with teratogenicity. At a concentration as low as 0.93 mg/mL, the oil produced a significant reduction (approximately 50%) in differentiated limb bud foci. However, this was due to cytotoxicity, resulting from exposing the cells directly to the essential oil. It was concluded that fennel oil, at certain concentrations, is toxic to fetal cells, but does not impact normal development (Ostad et al 2004).

When orally administered to male mice at 1 or 2 mL/kg/day for three days, sweet fennel oil had no adverse effect on sperm, and it significantly inhibited sperm abnormalities caused by cyclophosphamide (Tripathi et al 2013).

In an ex vivo study, sweet fennel oil showed a dose-dependent reduction in the intensity of uterine contractions induced by either oxytocin or prostaglandin E_2 (PGE$_2$). Some effect was seen at 25 μg/mL for oxytocin and 10 μg/mL for PGE$_2$; more significant effects were seen at 50 μg/mL for oxytocin and 20 μg/mL for PGE$_2$ (Ostad et al 2001). Consequently, sweet fennel oil might not be advisable to use during labor, especially if it is progressing very slowly. However, we know nothing about the clinical relevance of these findings to human childbirth.

Four girls, all between 5 months and 5 years of age, presented with premature breast development, and their serum estradiol levels were 15–20 times higher than normal. All had been taking fennel seed tea for colic, daily for several months (fennel tea contains 1.3–10.0% of fennel oil [Bilia et al 2002]). On stopping the fennel tea, the premature thelarche resolved in 3–6 months, and estradiol levels decreased to within the normal range (Türkyilmaz et al 2008). Since in vitro estrogenic effects have been seen for both (E)-anethole (Tabanca et al 2004) and for fennel oil (Melzig et al 2003), the essential oil is the most likely suspect in these cases. In a clinical trial for infantile colic, daily amounts of up to 12 mg/kg/day of fennel seed oil were taken by 62 infants for 7 days, and no side effects were noted (Alexandrovich et al 2003). However, one week is probably not long enough for estrogenic effects to show.

Hepatotoxicity: (E)-Anethole is dose-dependently hepatotoxic which is due to a metabolite, anethole 1′,2′-epoxide (AE) and different amounts of AE are produced in different animal species. However, the amounts of (E)-anethole-rich essential oils used in aromatherapy pose no risk to humans (see (E)-Anethole profile). Sweet fennel oil demonstrated a potent hepatoprotective action against carbon tetrachloride-induced liver injury in rats, almost normalizing liver function tests (Özbek et al 2003). High doses of (E)-anethole or AE deplete glutathione

(Marshall & Caldwell 1992, 1993) but sweet fennel oil significantly induced glutathione S-transferase activity in mouse tissues (Lam & Zheng 1991).

Systemic effects

Acute toxicity: Sweet fennel oil acute oral LD$_{50}$ in rats reported as 1.33 g/kg (Ostad et al 2001) and 3.8 g/kg; acute dermal LD$_{50}$ in rabbits >5 g/kg (Opdyke 1974 p. 879–880). Given subcutaneously to mice, the LD$_{50}$ was 1.08 g/kg (Essway et al 1995).

Antioxidant/pro-oxidant activity: Sweet fennel oil is an effective antioxidant and free radical scavenger (Parejo et al 2002; Shahat et al 2011).

Carcinogenic/anticarcinogenic potential: Sweet fennel oil was not mutagenic in the Ames test, and did not produce CA in Chinese hamster fibroblasts (Ishidate et al 1984). When orally administered to mice at 1 or 2 mL/kg/day for three days, sweet fennel oil was not genotoxic, and it significantly inhibited both the genotoxicity and reduction of antioxidant enzymes caused by cyclophosphamide (Tripathi et al 2013). (E)-Anethole is not a rodent carcinogen. Estragole is a rodent carcinogen when exposure is sufficiently high; (+)-limonene is anticarcinogenic (see Constituent profiles, Chapter 14).

Drug interactions: Antidiabetic or anticoagulant medication, because of cardiovascular effects, above. See Table 4.10B.

Comments

Both (+)-limonene and fennel oil induce glutathione synthesis, and (+)-limonene is anticarcinogenic while estragole is carcinogenic. In the absence of any further information, sweet fennel oil should be treated as a potential carcinogen, because of its estragole content. There are four chemotypes of fennel, an anethole, a (+)-limonene, an estragole and an estragole/fenchone, although only the anethole chemotype is used for commercial essential oil production. In an analysis of 30 anethole chemotype oils, the estragole content ranged from 2.0–4.3% (Krüger & Hammer 1999). Anisaldehyde, an oxidation product of anethole, increases if the oil is improperly stored.

Fenugreek

Botanical name: *Trigonella foenum-graecum* L.
Family: Fabaceae (Leguminoseae)

Essential oil

Source: Seeds
Key constituents:

Neryl acetate	17.3%
Camphor	16.3%
β-Pinene	15.1%
β-Caryophyllene	14.6%
2,5-Dimethylpyrazine	6.1%
Geranial	4.8%
6-Methyl-5-hepten-2-one	4.5%
3-Octen-2-one	4.3%
α-Selinene	4.0%

α-Terpineol	2.8%
α-Campholenal	2.6%
α-Pinene	2.6%
γ-Terpinene	2.1%

(Hamden et al 2011)

Absolute

Source: Seeds
Key constituents:

Hexanol	5–10%
Heptanoic acid	5–10%
Phenol	<5%
1,8-Cineole	<5%
Dihydrobenzofuran	<5%

(Lawrence 1989 p. 237)

Safety summary

Hazards: Drug interaction.
Cautions (oral): Diabetes medication.

Regulatory guidelines

Has GRAS status.

Organ-specific effects

Adverse skin reactions: No information found for fenugreek oil. Undiluted fenugreek absolute was moderately irritating to rabbits, but was not irritating to mice or pigs; tested at 2% on 25 volunteers it was neither irritating nor sensitizing. It is non-phototoxic (Opdyke 1978 p755–756).
Cardiovascular effects: Dietary fenugreek oil (composition as above) fed to male alloxan-diabetic rats at 5%, significantly inhibited α-amylase and maltase activity in the pancreas and plasma, and improved glucose tolerance (Hamden et al 2011).

Systemic effects

Acute toxicity: Fenugreek absolute acute oral LD_{50} in rats >5 g/kg; acute dermal LD_{50} in rabbits >2 g/kg (Opdyke 1978 p. 755–756). No information was found for fenugreek oil.
Carcinogenic/anticarcinogenic potential: No information found for fenugreek oil or absolute, but neither contains any known carcinogens. α-Cadinol is active against the human colon cancer cell line HT-29 (He et al 1997a).
Drug interactions: Antidiabetic medication, because of cardiovascular effects, above. See Table 4.10B.

Comments

Limited availability. The absolute is more correctly described as a resinoid, and is usually extracted with either alcohol or aqueous alcohol (Burfield 2000). CO_2 extracts are also produced from the seeds.

Fern (sweet)

Botanical name: *Comptonia peregrina* (L.) J. M. Coult.
Family: Pteridophytae

Essential oil

Source: Leaves
Key constituents:

β-Caryophyllene	24.5%
1,8-Cineole	6.0%
β-Myrcene	5.1%
δ-Cadinene	4.2%
(E)-Nerolidol	3.7%
α-Caryophyllene	3.0%
Linalool	2.6%
γ-Terpinene	2.5%
γ-Cadinene	2.2%
α-Pinene	2.2%
β-Selinene	2.1%
β-Chamigrene	1.7%
(E)-β-Ocimene	1.7%
1(10)-Aromadendrene	1.7%
Caryophyllene oxide	1.5%
(Z)-β-Ocimene	1.5%
p-Cymene	1.2%
Bornyl acetate	1.0%
α-Selinene	1.0%

(Mainguy, private communication, 2003)

Safety summary

Hazards: None known.
Contraindications: None known.

Organ-specific effects

Adverse skin reactions: No information found for sweet fern oil, but judging from its composition the risk of skin reactions is likely to be low.

Systemic effects

Acute toxicity: No information found for sweet fern oil, but its composition does not raise any red flags.
Carcinogenic/anticarcinogenic potential: A fraction of sweet fern oil collected at 30–60 minutes during distillation, and containing 15.6% β-caryophyllene and 7.4% β-caryophyllene, was cytotoxic to human cell lines for both lung cancer (A-549) and colon cancer (DLD-1) (Sylvestre et al 2007). β-Caryophyllene, nerolidol and α-caryophyllene display anticarcinogenic activity (see Constituent profiles, Chapter 14).

Comments

Limited availability.

Ferula

Botanical name: *Ferula jaeschkeana* Vatke
Family: Apiaceae (Umbelliferae)

Essential oil

Source: Rhizomes
Key constituents:

α-Pinene	79.5%
β-Pinene	12.7%
Camphene	1.0%

(Lawrence 2012)

Safety summary

Hazards: Skin sensitization if oxidized.
Cautions: Old or oxidized oils should be avoided.

Our safety advice

Because of its high α-pinene content we recommend that oxidation of ferula oil is avoided by storage in a dark, airtight container in a refrigerator. The addition of an antioxidant to preparations containing it is recommended.

Organ-specific effects

Adverse skin reactions: Autoxidation products of α-pinene can cause skin sensitization (see α-Pinene profile, Chapter 14).
Reproductive toxicity: The low reproductive toxicity for α-pinene, β-pinene and camphene (see Constituent profiles, Chapter 14) suggests that no ferula oil is not hazardous in pregnancy.

Systemic effects

Acute toxicity: The α-pinene acute oral LD$_{50}$ in rats has been reported as 2.1, 3.2 and 3.7 g/kg; acute dermal LD$_{50}$ in rabbits <5 g/kg (Opdyke 1978 p. 853–857).
Carcinogenic/anticarcinogenic potential: No information found for ferula oil, but it contains no known carcinogens. α-Pinene is antimutagenic, and is not carcinogenic in rats (see α-Pinene profile, Chapter 14).

Comments

Limited availability.

Feverfew

Synonyms: Nosebleed, midsummer daisy
Botanical name: *Tanacetum parthenium* (L.) Sch. Bip.
Botanical synonym: *Chrysanthemum parthenium* (L.) Bernh.
Family: Asteraceae (Compositae)

Essential oil

Source: Leaves
Key constituents:

Camphor	28.0–44.2%
(*E*)-Chrysanthenyl acetate	22.9–30.2%
Camphene	5.4–7.7%
Germacrene D	0.7–4.6%
α-Terpinene	2.2–3.8%
p-Cymene	0.6–3.1%
β-Farnesene	0.8–3.0%
Terpinen-4-ol	0.3–2.8%
γ-Terpinene	1.0–2.7%
α-Pinene	1.0–2.4%
Caryophyllene oxide	1.0–2.1%
(*E*)-Chrysanthenol	1.3–2.0%
Bornyl acetate	0.7–1.9%
Linalool	0–1.3%
Borneol	0.6–1.1%

(Lawrence 1999e p. 56-59)

Safety summary

Hazards: Moderate neurotoxicity, based on camphor content.
Contraindications (all routes): Pregnancy, breastfeeding.
Maximum adult daily oral dose: 318 mg
Maximum dermal use level: 10%

Our safety advice

Our oral and dermal restrictions are based on 44.2% camphor content with camphor limits of 2 mg/kg and 4.5% (see Estragole profile, Chapter 14). The high concentration of camphor suggests that this oil may be unsafe in pregnancy and breastfeeding.

Organ-specific effects

No information found.

Systemic effects

Acute toxicity: No information found for feverfew oil. Camphor is potentially neurotoxic (see Camphor profile, Chapter 14).
Carcinogenic/anticarcinogenic potential: No information found for feverfew oil, but it contains no known carcinogens.

Comments

Limited availability.

Fig leaf

Botanical name: *Ficus carica* L.
Family: Moraceae

Absolute

Source: Leaves
Key constituents: No useful data was found.

Safety summary

Hazards: Skin sensitization (high risk); skin irritation (low risk); phototoxic (high risk).
Contraindications: Should not be used, either internally or externally.

Regulatory guidelines

IFRA recommends that fig leaf absolute should not be used as a fragrance ingredient because of its sensitizing and extreme phototoxic potential (IFRA 2009). Fig leaf absolute is prohibited as a fragrance ingredient in the EU and Canada (SCCNFP 2001a, Health Canada Cosmetic Ingredient Hotlist, March 2011).

Organ-specific effects

Adverse skin reactions: Undiluted fig leaf absolute was irritating to mice. Tested at 5% on two panels of 25 volunteers it produced one irritation reaction. In maximation tests at 5% on two panels of 25 volunteers, the absolute produced 2/28 and 2/25 positive reactions (Opdyke & Letizia 1982 p. 691–692). Fig leaf absolute produced strong phototoxic effects on hairless mice at a 12.5% dilution; a 0.001% dilution still resulted in phototoxic reactions in three out of six mice. In two maximation tests, using fig leaf absolute at a 5% dilution on 25 and 28 volunteers, there were two sensitization reactions in each group. Fig leaves contain furanocoumarins, although their presence in fig leaf absolute has not been established (Opdyke & Letizia 1982 p. 691–692).

Systemic effects

Acute toxicity: No information found.
Carcinogenic/anticarcinogenic potential: No information found.

Comments

Fig leaf absolute is typical of materials which are produced for the fragrance industry, but are unlikely to be used in aromatherapy.

Finger root

Synonyms: Fingerroot, Chinese ginger, Thai ginger, lesser ginger
Botanical name: *Boesenbergia pandurata* (Roxb.) Schlecht
Botanical synonyms: *Kaempferia pandurata, Boesenbergia rotunda*
Family: Zingiberaceae

Essential oil

Source: Rhizomes
Key constituents:

Thailand

(*E*)-β-Ocimene	22.8%
Geraniol	20.8%
Camphor	16.9%
1,8-Cineole	7.8%
Camphene	5.4%
(*Z*)-β-Ocimene	3.2%

Methyl cinnamate	3.0%
δ-3-Carene	2.0%
Geranial	1.5%
Terpinolene	1.2%
β-Pinene	1.1%
β-Elemene	1.0%

(Jantan et al 2001)

Safety summary

Hazards: Drug interaction.
Cautions (oral): Drugs metabolized by CYP2B6 (Appendix B).

Organ-specific effects

No information found.

Systemic effects

Carcinogenic/anticarcinogenic potential: No information found for finger root oil, but it contains no known carcinogens.
Drug interactions: Since geraniol inhibits CYP2B6 (Table 4.11B), there is a theoretical risk of interaction between finger root oil and drugs metabolized by this enzyme (Appendix B).

Comments

Limited availability.

Fir (Douglas)

Botanical name: *Pseudotsuga menziesii* (Mirbel) Franco
Family: Pinaceae

Essential oil

Source: Wood
Key constituents:

Camphene	16.7%
α-Pinene	13.0%
β-Pinene	11.6%
Bornyl acetate	10.0%
Terpinolene	9.1%
Sabinene	7.4%
Terpinen-4-ol	4.6%
Santene	3.5%
(+)-Limonene	3.4%
γ-Terpinene	3.2%
Tricyclene	2.3%
Citronellol	2.1%
δ-3-Carene	2.0%
α-Terpinene	2.0%
β-Myrcene	1.5%
Citronellyl acetate	1.1%

(Kubeczka & Schultze 1987)

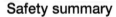

Safety summary

Hazards: Skin sensitization if oxidized.
Cautions: Old or oxidized oils should be avoided.

Regulatory guidelines

Essential oils derived from the *Pinaceae* family, including *Pinus* and *Abies* genera, should only be used when the level of peroxides is kept to the lowest practicable level, for example by the addition of antioxidants at the time of production (SCCNFP 2001a; IFRA 2009).

Organ-specific effects

Adverse skin reactions: Douglas fir oil was neither irritant nor sensitizing when patch tested on a panel of 25 volunteers at 8% (Opdyke 1979b p. 369). Autoxidation products of (+)-limonene, α-pinene and δ-3-carene can cause skin sensitization (see Constituent profiles, Chapter 14). Douglas fir oil is not phototoxic (Opdyke 1979b p. 369).

Systemic effects

Acute toxicity: Acute oral LD_{50} in rats >5 g/kg; acute dermal LD_{50} in rabbits 2.82 >5 g/kg (Opdyke 1979b p. 369).
Carcinogenic/anticarcinogenic potential: No information found for Douglas fir oil, but it contains no known carcinogens.

Comments

Douglas firs can grow as tall as 80–100 m, and their wood is used for timber. The oil is steam distilled from the oleoresin collected from felled wood (Burfield 2000).

Fir cones (silver)

Synonyms: White fir, silver spruce, templin
Botanical name: *Abies alba* Mill.
Family: Pinaceae

Essential oil

Source: Cones
Key constituents:

(+)-Limonene	28.5–34.1%
α-Pinene	18.0–31.7%
β-Pinene	3.0–22.5%
Bornyl acetate	1.3–12.5%
Camphene	5.8–8.0%
p-Cymene	0.1–7.5%
β-Caryophyllene	0.1–4.2%
β-Himachalene	0–2.6%
α-Caryophyllene	0–2.0%
Borneol	0.2–1.5%
β-Myrcene	0–1.0%

(Tsankova & Ognyanov 1968; Kubeczka & Schultze 1987)

Quality: Silver fir cone oil may be adulterated with pinenes, bornyl acetate, isobornyl acetate and similar materials (Burfield 2000).

Safety summary

Hazards: Skin sensitization if oxidized.
Cautions: Old or oxidized oils should be avoided.

Our safety advice

Because of its (+)-limonene and α-pinene content we recommend that oxidation of silver fir cone oil is avoided by storage in a dark, airtight container in a refrigerator. The addition of an antioxidant to preparations containing it is recommended.

Regulatory guidelines

Essential oils derived from the *Pinaceae* family, including *Pinus* and *Abies* genera, should only be used when the level of peroxides is kept to the lowest practicable level, for example by the addition of antioxidants at the time of production (SCCNFP 2001a; IFRA 2009).

Organ-specific effects

Adverse skin reactions: Undiluted silver fir cone oil was moderately irritating to rabbits, but was not irritating to the backs of hairless mice; tested at 20% on 25 volunteers it was neither irritating nor sensitizing (Opdyke 1974 p. 809–810). In a study of 200 consecutive dermatitis patients, two were sensitive to 2% silver fir oil (type unspecified) on patch testing (Rudzki et al 1976). Autoxidation products of (+)-limonene and α-pinene can cause skin sensitization (see Constituent profiles, Chapter 14). Silver fir cone oil is non-phototoxic (Opdyke 1974 p. 809–810).
Reproductive toxicity: The low reproductive toxicity of (+)-limonene, α-pinene, β-pinene and camphene (see Constituent profiles, Chapter 14) suggest that silver fir cone oils are not hazardous in pregnancy.

Systemic effects

Acute toxicity: Templin oil acute oral LD_{50} in rats >5 g/kg; acute dermal LD_{50} in rabbits >5 g/kg (Opdyke 1974 p. 809–810).
Carcinogenic/anticarcinogenic potential: No information found for silver fir cone oil, but it contains no known carcinogens. (+)-Limonene and α-caryophyllene display antitumoral activity (see Constituent profiles, Chapter 14).

Comments

Limited availability.

Fir needle (Canadian)

Synonym: Balsam fir, fir balsam
Botanical name: *Abies balsamea* L.
Family: Pinaceae

Essential oil

Source: Needles (leaves) and twigs
Key constituents:

β-Pinene	28.1–56.1%
δ-3-Carene	0–27.3%
Bornyl acetate	4.9–16.2%
α-Pinene	6.2–14.3%
(+)-Limonene	1.8–15.6%
β-Phellandrene	4.4–12.6%
Camphene	3.5–9.7%
α + β-Terpineol	0.6–4.5%
Thymol	0–2.9%
β-Myrcene	0.6–2.3%
Borneol	0.3–2.1%
Tricyclene	0.6–1.7%
Terpinolene	0.2–1.7%
Santene	0.3–1.4%

(Régimbal & Collin 1994)

Quality: Fir needle oils may be adulterated with turpentine oil fractions, mixtures of camphene, (−)-bornyl acetate and so on (Burfield 2003).

Safety summary

Hazards: Skin sensitization if oxidized.
Cautions: Old or oxidized oils should be avoided.

Our safety advice

Because of its (+)-limonene, α-pinene and δ-3-carene content we recommend that oxidation of Canadian fir needle oil is avoided by storage in a dark, airtight container in a refrigerator. The addition of an antioxidant to preparations containing it is recommended.

Regulatory guidelines

Essential oils derived from the *Pinaceae* family, including *Pinus* and *Abies* genera, should only be used when the level of peroxides is kept to the lowest practicable level, for example by the addition of antioxidants at the time of production (SCCNFP 2001a; IFRA 2009).

Organ-specific effects

Adverse skin reactions: Undiluted Canadian fir needle oil was not irritating to rabbit or mouse skin; tested at 10% on 25 volunteers it was neither irritating nor sensitizing. It is non-phototoxic (Opdyke 1975 p. 449–450). Autoxidation products of (+)-limonene, α-pinene and δ-3-carene can cause skin sensitization (see Constituent profiles, Chapter 14).
Reproductive toxicity: The low reproductive toxicity of (+)-limonene, β-pinene and α-pinene (see Constituent profiles, Chapter 14) and the structural similarity of δ-3-carene to

α-pinene suggest that Canadian fir needle oil is not hazardous in pregnancy.

Systemic effects

Acute toxicity: Canadian fir needle oil acute oral LD_{50} in rats >5 g/kg; acute dermal LD_{50} in rabbits >5 g/kg (Opdyke 1975 p. 449–450).
Carcinognenic potential: Canadian fir needle oil was active against the human solid tumor cell lines MCF-7 (breast), PC-3 (prostate), A-549 (lung), DLD-1 (colon), M4BEU (melanoma) and CT-26 (colon). This activity seemed to be due to α-caryophyllene, since no other constituent was active. Both α-caryophyllene and Canadian fir needle oil induced dose- and time-dependent glutathione depletion and an increase of reactive oxygen species in the tumor cells (Legault et al 2003). α-Caryophyllene constitutes only 0.06–0.6% of the essential oil (Régimbal & Collin 1994).

Comments

The tree produces thick resin blisters, which contain a clear, yellow fluid known as Canada balsam. A separate essential oil (Canada balsam oil) is distilled from this. Canada balsam oil is also produced from *Abies alba, Abies fraseri* and *Tsuga canadensis* (Burfield 2000).

Fir needle (Himalayan)

Synonyms: East Himalayan fir, Himalayan silver fir
Botanical name: *Abies spectabilis* (D. Don) Spach
Botanical synonyms: *Abies webbiana* (Wall ex D. Don) Lindl., *Pinus spectabilis* D. Don, *Pinus webbiana* Wall ex D. Don
Family: Pinaceae

Essential oil

Source: Needles (leaves) and twigs
Key constituents:

(+)-Limonene	29.6%
α-Pinene	19.1%
β-Pinene	9.1%
β-Caryophyllene	5.3%
Bornyl acetate	4.7%
Calarene*	4.2%
Camphene	3.7%
β-Bourbonene	3.3%
β-Maaliene	3.3%
γ-Selinene	3.3%
β-Myrcene	2.5%
α-Caryophyllene	2.4%
δ-Cadinene	2.1%

(Vossen, private communication, 2004)

*Tentative identification

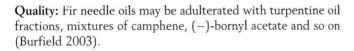

Quality: Fir needle oils may be adulterated with turpentine oil fractions, mixtures of camphene, (−)-bornyl acetate and so on (Burfield 2003).

Safety summary

Hazards: Skin sensitization if oxidized.
Cautions: Old or oxidized oils should be avoided.

Our safety advice

Because of its (+)-limonene and α-pinene content we recommend that oxidation of Himalayan fir needle oil is avoided by storage in a dark, airtight container in a refrigerator. The addition of an antioxidant to preparations containing it is recommended.

Regulatory guidelines

Essential oils derived from the *Pinaceae* family, including *Pinus* and *Abies* genera, should only be used when the level of peroxides is kept to the lowest practicable level, for example by the addition of antioxidants at the time of production (SCCNFP 2001a; IFRA 2009).

Organ-specific effects

Reproductive toxicity: The low reproductive toxicity of (+)-limonene, α-pinene and β-pinene (see Constituent profiles, Chapter 14) suggests that Himalayan fir needle oil is not hazardous in pregnancy.

Systemic effects

Carcinogenic/anticarcinogenic potential: No information found for Himalayan fir needle oil, but it contains no known carcinogens. (+)-Limonene exhibits anticarcinogenic activity (see (+)-Limonene profile, Chapter 14).

Comments

Limited availability.

Fir needle (Japanese)

Synonyms: Japanese pine needle, sachalin fir
Botanical name: *Abies sachalinensis* F. W. Schmidt
Family: Pinaceae

Essential oil

Source: Needles (leaves) and twigs
Key constituents:

Bornyl acetate	27.9%
Camphene	18.5%
α-Pinene	12.2%
β-Phellandrene	7.5%
β-Pinene	7.0%
(+)-Limonene	6.5%
Sesquiterpene alcohols (unknown)	4.6%
Santene	2.1%
Tricyclene	2.0%
β-Caryophyllene	1.5%
β-Myrcene	1.3%

(Holm et al 1994)

Quality: Fir needle oils may be adulterated with turpentine oil fractions, mixtures of camphene, (−)-bornyl acetate and so on (Burfield 2003).

Safety summary

Hazards: Skin sensitization if oxidized.
Cautions: Old or oxidized oils should be avoided.

Our safety advice

Because of its (+)-limonene and α-pinene content we recommend that oxidation of Japanese fir needle oil is avoided by storage in a dark, airtight container in a refrigerator. The addition of an antioxidant to preparations containing it is recommended.

Regulatory guidelines

Essential oils derived from the *Pinaceae* family, including *Pinus* and *Abies* genera, should only be used when the level of peroxides is kept to the lowest practicable level, for example by the addition of antioxidants at the time of production (SCCNFP 2001a; IFRA 2009).

Organ-specific effects

Adverse skin reactions: Undiluted Japanese fir needle oil was mildly to moderately irritating to rabbits. Tested at 20% on two panels of 25 and 28 volunteers it was not irritating. In an initial test for skin sensitization with 20% Japanese fir needle oil, there were two positive reactions out of the 25 volunteers tested. A second test was carried out on a new panel of 28 volunteers using a sample of Japanese fir needle oil which had been collected under nitrogen, and had had BHA (an antioxidant) added to it. There were no positive reactions. Autoxidation products of (+)-limonene and α-pinene can cause skin sensitization (see Constituent profiles, Chapter 14). Japanese fir needle oil is non-phototoxic (Letizia et al 2000 p. S1–S2).

Systemic effects

Acute toxicity: Acute oral LD_{50} in rats >5 g/kg; acute dermal LD_{50} in rabbits >5 g/kg (Letizia et al 2000 p. S1–S2).
Carcinogenic/anticarcinogenic potential: No information was found for Japanese fir needle oil, but it contains no known carcinogens. (+)-Limonene is anticarcinogenic (see (+)-Limonene profile, Chapter 14).

Comments

Limited availability.

Fir needle (Siberian)

Synonyms: Russian fir, Siberian silver fir, Siberian pine needle
Botanical name: *Abies sibirica* Ledeb.
Family: Pinaceae

Essential oil

Source: Needles (leaves) and twigs
Key constituents:

Bornyl acetate	31.0%
Camphene	24.2%
α-Pinene	13.7%
δ-3-Carene	12.2%
(+)-Limonene	4.0%
Santene	2.5%
Tricyclene	2.4%
β-Phellandrene	2.4%
β-Pinene	1.6%
Borneol	1.6%
Terpinolene	1.1%

(Orav et al 1995)

Quality: Fir needle oil may be adulterated with turpentine oil, with mixtures of camphene, pinene and bornyl acetate, or with other chemicals. The oil may contain up to 40% bornyl acetate (Kubeczka 2002).

Safety summary

Hazards: Skin irritation (low risk); skin sensitization if oxidized.
Cautions: Old or oxidized oils should be avoided.

Our safety advice

Because of its (+)-limonene, α-pinene and δ-3-carene content we recommend that oxidation of Siberian fir needle oil is avoided by storage in a dark, airtight container in a refrigerator. The addition of an antioxidant to preparations containing it is recommended.

Regulatory guidelines

Essential oils derived from the *Pinaceae* family, including *Pinus* and *Abies* genera, should only be used when the level of peroxides is kept to the lowest practicable level, for example by the addition of antioxidants at the time of production (IFRA 2009, SCCNFP 2001a).

Organ-specific effects

Adverse skin reactions: Undiluted Siberian fir needle oil was moderately irritating to rabbits; tested at 2.5% on 25 volunteers it produced a mild irritation, but no sensitization reactions (Opdyke 1975 p. 450). Autoxidation products of (+)-limonene, α-pinene and δ-3-carene can cause skin sensitization (see Constituent profiles, Chapter 14).

Systemic effects

Acute toxicity: Acute oral LD_{50} in rats 10.2 g/kg; acute dermal LD_{50} in rabbits >3 g/kg (Opdyke 1975 p. 450).
Carcinogenic/anticarcinogenic potential: No information was found for Siberian fir needle oil, but it contains no known carcinogens. (+)-Limonene is anticarcinogenic (see Constituent profiles, Chapter 14).

Comments

The oil is produced in large quantities, and is widely used in wash products and air fresheners.

Fir needle (silver)

Synonyms: White fir, silver spruce, templin
Botanical name: *Abies alba* Mill.
Family: Pinaceae

Essential oil

Source: Needles (leaves)
Key constituents:

(+)-Limonene	54.7%
Camphene	14.8%
α-Pinene	7.4%
Santene	5.0%
β-Caryophyllene	2.3%
Tricyclene	2.1%
β-Myrcene	1.9%
Bornyl acetate	1.0%

(Kubeczka & Schultze 1987)

Quality: May be adulterated with pinenes, bornyl acetate, isobornyl acetate and similar materials (Burfield 2000).

Safety summary

Hazards: Skin sensitization if oxidized.
Cautions: Old or oxidized oils should be avoided.

Our safety advice

Because of its (+)-limonene and α-pinene content we recommend that oxidation of silver fir needle oil is avoided by storage in a dark, airtight container in a refrigerator. The addition of an antioxidant to preparations containing it is recommended.

Regulatory guidelines

Essential oils derived from the *Pinaceae* family, including *Pinus* and *Abies* genera, should only be used when the level of peroxides is kept to the lowest practicable level, for example by the addition of antioxidants at the time of production (SCCNFP 2001a; IFRA 2009).

Organ-specific effects

Adverse skin reactions: Undiluted silver fir needle oil was not irritating to rabbits or to the backs of hairless mice; tested at 20% on 25 volunteers it was neither irritating nor sensitizing (Opdyke 1974 p. 811). In a study of 200 consecutive dermatitis patients, two were sensitive to 2% silver fir oil (type unspecified) on patch testing (Rudzki et al 1976). Autoxidation products of (+)-limonene and α-pinene can cause skin sensitization (see Constituent profiles, Chapter 14). Silver fir needle oil is non-phototoxic (Opdyke 1974 p. 811).

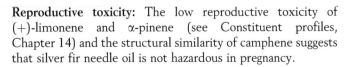

Reproductive toxicity: The low reproductive toxicity of (+)-limonene and α-pinene (see Constituent profiles, Chapter 14) and the structural similarity of camphene suggests that silver fir needle oil is not hazardous in pregnancy.

Systemic effects

Acute toxicity: Silver fir needle oil acute oral LD_{50} in rats >5 g/kg; acute dermal LD_{50} in rabbits >5 g/kg (Opdyke 1974 p. 811).
Carcinogenic/anticarcinogenic potential: No information was found for silver fir needle oil, but it contains no known carcinogens. (+)-Limonene displays anticarcinogenic activity (see (+)-Limonene profile, Chapter 14).

Comments

The oil is produced in Eastern Europe and Siberia.

Fleabane

Synonyms: Canadian fleabane, horseweed, fleawort
Botanical name: *Conyza canadensis* (L.) Cronquist
Botanical synonym: *Erigeron Canadensis* L.
Family: Asteraceae (Compositae)

Essential oil

Source: Flowering herb
Key constituents:

(+)-Limonene	56.4%
(Z,Z)-Matricaria methyl ester	11.5%
(E)-α-Bergamotene	8.2%
Germacrene D	5.5%
γ-Curcumene	2.9%
(E)-β-Ocimene	2.8%
β-Myrcene	2.1%
(Z,E)-Matricaria methyl ester	1.8%
α-Amorphene*	1.4%
α-Zingiberene	1.4%
(E)-β-Farnesene	1.3%

(Mainguy, private communication, 2003)

Safety summary

Hazards: Skin sensitization if oxidized.
Cautions: Old or oxidized oils should be avoided.

Our safety advice

Because of its limonene content we recommend that oxidation of fleabane oil is avoided by storage in a dark, airtight container in a refrigerator. The addition of an antioxidant to preparations containing it is recommended.

Regulatory guidelines

IFRA recommends that essential oils rich in limonene should only be used when the level of peroxides is kept to the lowest practical level, for instance by adding antioxidants at the time of production (IFRA 2009).

Organ-specific effects

Adverse skin reactions: Autoxidation products of (+)-limonene can cause skin sensitization (see (+)-Limonene profile, Chapter 14).
Reproductive toxicity: The low developmental toxicity of (+)-limonene in rabbits and mice (Kodama et al 1977a, 1977b) suggests that fleabane oil is not hazardous in pregnancy.

Systemic effects

Carcinogenic/anticarcinogenic potential: No information was found for fleabane oil, but it contains no known carcinogens. (+)-Limonene displays anticarcinogenic activity (see (+)-Limonene profile, Chapter 14).

Comments

Limited availability. The oil is a water-white, or pale yellow liquid, which becomes darker and more viscous on ageing (Arctander 1960).

Fragonia

Synomym: Fragrant agonis
Botanical name: *Agonis fragrans* J.R.Wheeler & N.G.Marchant
Family: Myrtaceae

Essential oil

Source: Leaves
Key constituents:

1,8-Cineole	31.0–33.0%
α-Pinene	21.0–27.0%
Linalool	11.7–12.4%
α-Terpineol	5.6–5.7%
Terpinen-4-ol	3.7–4.0%
Myrtenol	3.1–3.8%
γ-Terpinene	1.8–3.6%
p-Cymene	2.0–2.9%
(+)-Limonene	2.5%
β-Myrcene	1.6–2.4%
β-Pinene	1.5–1.7%

(Day, private communication, 2004)

Safety summary

Hazards: Skin sensitization if oxidized.
Cautions: Old or oxidized oils should be avoided.

*Tentative identification

Our safety advice

Because of its high α-pinene content we recommend that oxidation of fragonia oil is avoided by storage in a dark, airtight container in a refrigerator. The addition of an antioxidant to preparations containing it is recommended.

Organ-specific effects

Adverse skin reactions: No information found for fragonia oil. Autoxidation products of α-pinene can cause skin sensitization; 1,8-cineole presents only a low risk of both skin irritation and sensitization, and it has antioxidant properties (see 1,8-Cineole profile, Chapter 14).

Reproductive toxicity: The low reproductive toxicity of 1,8-cineole, α-pinene, linalool and (+)-limonene (see Constituent profiles, Chapter 14) suggests that fragonia oil is not hazardous in pregnancy.

Systemic effects

Acute toxicity: No information found for fragonia oil. None of its key constituents is significantly toxic (see Constituent profiles, Chapter 14).

Carcinogenic/anticarcinogenic potential: No information found for fragonia oil, but it contains no known carcinogens. (+)-Limonene displays anticarcinogenic activity (see (+)-Limonene profile, Chapter 14).

Comments

The name 'fragonia' has been trademarked by the sole producer of this oil in Australia.

Frankincense

Synonym: Olibanum
Botanical names: *Boswellia frereana* Birdwood (synonym: *Boswellia hildebrandtii* Engl.) (African elemi, elemi frankincense); *Boswellia papyrifera* (Del.) Hochst (synonyms: *Amyris papyrifera, Boswellia chariensis, Boswellia occidentalis, Boswellia odorata, Ploesslea floribunda*) Sudanese frankincense; *Boswellia sacra* Flueck. (synonyms: *Boswellia carteri* Birdwood, *Boswellia bhau-dajiana* Birdwood, *Boswellia undulato-crenata*) Saudi frankincense; *Boswellia serrata* Roxb. (synonyms: *Boswellia glabra* Roxb., *Boswellia thurifera* Roxb., *Chloroxylon dupada*) Indian frankicnese; *Boswellia neglecta* S. Moore ('Borena' type frankincense); *Boswellia rivae* Engl. ('Ogaden' type frankincense)
Family: Burseraceae

Essential oil

Source: Gum resin
Key constituents:

Boswellia frereana

α-Pinene	41.7–80.0%
Sabinene	0.5–21.0%
α-Thujene	0–19.3%
(+)-Limonene	0–17.0%
Viridiflorol	0–15.2%
p-Cymene	0.7–11.7%
β-Pinene	0–6.9%
Verbenone	0–6.5%
β-Myrcene	0–6.0%
α-Phellandrene	0–5.9%
Bornyl acetate	0–5.6%
Carvone	0–4.4%
δ-3-Carene	0–3.4%
Linalool	0–3.0%
1,8-Cineole	0–2.9%
γ-Terpinene	0–2.5%
Camphene	0–2.1%
Thujol	0–1.8%
α-Pinocarveol	0–1.7%
Campholenic aldehyde	0–1.5%
Octyl acetate	0–1.5%
α-Terpinene	0–1.5%
β-Elemene	0–1.3%
β-Caryophyllene	0–1.2%
α-Thujone	0–1.2%
(Z)-β-Ocimene	0–1.0%
β-Phellandrene	0–1.0%
β-Selinene	0–1.0%

(Tucker 1986; Lawrence 1995g p. 20–23; Hall 2000)

Boswellia papyrifera

Octyl acetate	50.0–60.0%
1-Octanol	3.5–12.7%
Terpinen-4-ol	0–8.0%
(+)-Limonene	1.7–5.0%
α-Pinene	1.0–4.6%
Incensyl acetate	3.0–4.1%
Cadinol	0–3.0%
Incensol	2.1–2.7%
Thymol	0–2.6%
Linalool	0.2–2.5%
Cembrene A	1.4–2.3%
Isocembrene	0–1.8%
1,8-Cineole	0–1.6%
(E)-β-Ocimene	1.3–5%
α-Thujene	0–1.4%
Bornyl acetate	1.0–.1%
Camphene	0–1.1%

(Tucker 1986; Lawrence 1995g p. 20–23; Hall 2000)

Boswellia sacra (α-pinene CT)

α-Pinene	10.3–51.3%
α-Phellandrene	0–41.8%
(+)-Limonene	6.0–21.9%
β-Myrcene	0–20.7%

β-Pinene	0–9.1%
β-Caryophyllene	1.9–7.5%
p-Cymene	0–7.5%
Terpinen-4-ol	0–6.9%
Verbenone	0–6.5%
Sabinene	0–5.5%
Linalool	0–5.4%
α-Thujene	0–4.5%
Bornyl acetate	0–2.9%
δ-3-Carene	0–2.6%
δ-Cadinene	0–2.3%
Camphene	0–2.0%
α-Caryophyllene	0–1.8%
Campholenic aldehyde	0–1.5%
Octyl acetate	0–1.5%
Caryophyllene oxide	0–1.4%
α-Copaene	0–1.4%
Calamenene	0–1.3%
Thujol	0–1.2%
1,8-Cineole	0–1.0%
(E)-Cinnamyl acetate	0–1.0%

(Hall 2000)

Boswellia serrata (Indian)

α-Thujene	26.2–47.4%
α-Pinene	0–11.2%
Tetrahydro-linalool	7.0–10.6%
δ-3-Carene	3.6–9.6%
epi-Cubenol	3.4–9.1%
(+)-Limonene	0.7–8.5%
α-Terpineol	1.5–5.8%
Benzyl tiglate	1.9–5.5%
10-epi-γ-Eudesmol	0–5.3%
Terpinyl isobutyrate	0–3.9%
Eudesmol	0.9–3.4%
Methyl isoeugenol	1.3–3.1%
p-Cymene	1.6–2.8%
α-Terpinene	0.3–2.7%
Geraniol	0–2.4%
Nerolidol	0–2.1%
β-Phellandrene	0–1.2%
Sabinene	0.4–1.0%
Estragole	0–0.4%

(Singh et al 2007a)

Boswellia neglecta

α-Thujene	19.2%
α-Pinene	16.7%
Terpinen-4-ol	12.5%
p-Cymene	9.5%
δ-3-Carene	3.7%
Sabinene	2.9%
(E)-Verbenol	2.6%

(+)-Limonene	2.2%
β-Thujone	1.8%
α-Terpineol	1.4%
p-Cymen-8-ol	1.2%
(Z)-Sabinol	1.1%
β-Pinene	1.1%
Verbenone	1.0%

(Baser et al 2003)

Boswellia rivae

(+)-Limonene	28.0%
δ-3-Carene	15.7%
α-Pinene	13.3%
p-Cymene	7.1%
(E)-Verbenol	5.8%
γ-Terpinene	2.3%
Terpinen-4-ol	1.9%
α-Terpineol	1.7%
α-Thujene	1.7%
(E)-Pinocarveol	1.6%
α-Terpinene	1.6%
p-Cymen-8-ol	1.4%
Thymol	1.4%
(E)-Carveol	1.2%
α-Phellandrene	1.2%
α-Phellandren-8-ol	1.0%

(Camarda et al 2007)

Safety summary

Hazards: Skin sensitization if oxidized.
Cautions: Old or oxidized oils should be avoided.

Our safety advice

Because of their high content of α-pinene, (+)-limonene and/or δ-3-carene we recommend that oxidation of *B. frereana*, *B. sacra* and *B. rivae* oils is avoided by storage in a dark, airtight container in a refrigerator. The addition of an antioxidant to preparations containing these oils is recommended. *B. Serrata* oil may contain a small amount of estragole, but this is unlikely to present a problem, since it contains larger amounts of anticarcinogens. No maximum is given for *B. frereana* or *B. neglecta* which, in addition to small amounts of thujone (an inhibitor of GABA$_A$ receptor-mediated responses), contain higher concentrations of pinenes (which potentiate these responses).

Organ-specific effects

Adverse skin reactions: A 65-year-old aromatherapist with multiple essential oil sensitivities reacted to 5%, and weakly to 1% frankincense oil (Selvaag et al 1995). *B. frereana*, *B. sacra* and *B. rivae* are rich in α-pinene, (+)-limonene and/or δ-3-carene. Autoxidation products of these compounds can cause skin sensitization (see Constituent profiles, Chapter 14).

Reproductive toxicity: The low reproductive toxicity of sabinene, α-pinene, (+)-limonene and octyl acetate (see Constituent profiles, Chapter 14) suggests that frankincense oils are not hazardous in pregnancy.

Systemic effects

Acute toxicity: No information found for any frankincense oil. For α-pinene, the acute oral LD_{50} in rats has been reported as 2.1, 3.2 and 3.7 g/kg; acute dermal LD_{50} in rabbits <5 g.kg (Opdyke 1978 p. 853–857). *B. serrata* can contain low concentrations of α-thujone and β-thujone. The thujones are potentially neurotoxic, but these levels are not significant.
Subacute & subchronic toxicity: No information found for any frankincense oil. Oral octyl acetate is not subchronically toxic in rats at 500 mg/kg (Daughtrey et al 1989a).
Carcinogenic potential: A commercially purchased essential oil said to be from *B. carteri* was cytotoxic to J82 human bladder cancer cells, but not to normal urothelial UROtsa cells, within a range of concentration. IC_{50} values were 1:600 and 1:1,250, respectively (Frank et al 2009). *B. serrata* can contain low concentrations of estragole, which is a rodent carcinogen when oral exposure is sufficiently high (see Estragole profile, Chapter 14). (+)-Limonene, geraniol and nerolidol display antitumoral activity (see Constituent profiles, Chapter 14).

Comments

For many years there has been little clarity about the various types of frankincense and their essential oils. The current consensus is that *B. carteri* and *B. sacra* are the same plant, though this is still disputed by some. *B. thurifera* has sometimes been given as a synonym for these. *B. bhau-dajiana* is a synonym for *B. sacra*, but has often been given as a separate taxon in the past. Amid the confusion over nomenclature, some frankincense oils may have been ascribed to incorrect origins. A complicating factor has been that some reports were based on materials obtained from markets rather than from properly identified trees. Some of the compositional data used here for *B. papyrifera* were originally ascribed to *B. carteri*, but there now seems little doubt that frankincense oils rich in octyl acetate originate from *B. papyrifera* (Hall 2000). High α-pinene levels (50–80%) probably indicates *B. frereana*, and lower concentrations (10–50%) probably point to *B. sacra*, but more work needs to be done to confirm these findings. There may also be an α-thujene CT for *B. sacra*. There is a (+)-limonene/(E)-β-ocimene CT of *B. sacra* (Al-Harrasi & Al-Saidi 2008) though this is probably not used for commercial essential oil production. Some sources give α-pinene as the major constituent of *B. rivae*.

B. frereana originates almost exclusively from Somalia, with small amounts coming from Oman; *B. papyrifera* is found in Eritrea, Ethiopia and Sudan; *B. sacra* is found in Saudi Arabia, Somalia, Eritrea, Oman and Yemen; *B. neglecta* and *B. rivae* are both found in Ethiopia and Somalia; *B. serrata* grows in India. Most commercial frankincense oil comes from Somalia (with most of the rest coming from Yemen and India) and most of that is from *B. frereana*, but *B. sacra* is also an important source. The resin of *B. papyrifera* is produced in abundance but the oil is not, as the yield is low relative to other species. In a report on trees, it has been proposed by UNEP-WCMC that CITES add *Boswellia sacra* to its list of threatened plant species.

Galangal (greater)

Synonym: Siamese ginger
Botanical name: *Alpinia galanga* L.
Botanical synonyms: *Amomum galanga* L., *Languas vulgare* Koenig., *Languas galanga* L.
Family: Zingiberaceae

Essential oil

Source: Rhizomes
Key constituents:

1,8-Cineole	30.2–33.6%
Camphor	5.0–14.0%
β-Pinene	0.9–12.9%
α-Fenchyl acetate	1.1–12.7%
α-Terpineol	2.3–9.3%
(Z)-β-Ocimene	0–6.4%
(E)-Methyl cinnamate	2.6–5.3%
(+)-Limonene	3.5–3.7%
Camphene	0.5–3.1%
Farnesol	0–3.1%
α-Pinene	0.5–3.0%
Bornyl acetate	0.6–1.5%
β-Patchoulene	0.3–1.5%
Terpinen-4-ol	0.9–1.3%
β-Eudesmol	0.4–1.1%
Geraniol	0.3–1.1%
Pentadecane	0.6–1.0%

(Mallavarapu et al 2002)

Safety summary

Hazards: None known.
Contraindications: None known.

Organ-specific effects

Adverse skin reactions: No information found.
Reproductive toxicity: The low reproductive toxicity of 1,8-cineole, camphor, β-pinene (+)-limonene, camphene and α-pinene (see Constituent profiles, Chapter 14) suggests that greater galangal oil is not hazardous in pregnancy.

Systemic effects

Acute toxicity: No information found.
Carcinogenic/anticarcinogenic potential: Galangal rhizome oil (type unspecified) significantly induces glutathione S-transferase activity in mouse tissues (Lam & Zheng 1991). The oil contains no known carcinogens. 1,8-Cineole is non-mutagenic and shows no evidence of carcinogenesis in rodents; (+)-limonene is anticarcinogenic (see Constituent profiles, Chapter 14).

Comments

There appear to be at least two chemotypes, a 1,8-cineole, and a (E)-β-farnesene. Methyl cinnamate has also been reported as a major component.

Galangal (lesser)

Synonym: Chinese ginger
Botanical name: *Alpinia officinarum* Hance
Botanical synonym: *Languas officinarum* Hance
Family: Zingiberaceae

Essential oil

Source: Rhizomes
Key constituents:

1,8-Cineole	49.6%
β-Pinene	6.6%
α-Pinene	5.8%
α-Terpineol	5.0%
Camphene	4.6%
(+)-Limonene	4.0%
δ-Cadinene	2.5%
γ-Cadinene	2.1%
Terpinen-4-ol	1.9%
p-Cymene	1.6%
(E)-α-Bergamotene	1.6%
Camphor	1.0%

(Lawrence 1989 p. 171–172)

Safety summary

Hazards: Essential oils high in 1,8-cineole can cause CNS and breathing problems in young children.
Contraindications: Do not apply to or near the face of infants or children.

Regulatory guidelines

Has GRAS status.

Organ-specific effects

Adverse skin reactions: No information found.
Reproductive toxicity: The low reproductive toxicity of 1,8-cineole, and monoterpenes such as α-pinene and (+)-limonene (see Constituent profiles, Chapter 14) suggest that lesser galangal oil is not hazardous in pregnancy.

Systemic effects

Acute toxicity: No information found for lesser galangal oil. 1,8-Cineole has been reported to cause serious poisoning in young children when accidentally instilled into the nose (Melis et al 1989).

Carcinogenic/anticarcinogenic potential: Lesser galangal oil showed moderate chemopreventive activity against human mouth epidermal carcinoma (KB) cells and significant activity against mouse leukemia (P388) cells, with respective IC_{50} values of 0.722 and 0.083 mg/mL (Manosroi et al 2005). Galangal rhizome oil (type unspecified) significantly induces glutathione S-transferase activity in mouse tissues (Lam & Zheng 1991). The oil contains no known carcinogens. 1,8-Cineole is non-mutagenic and shows no evidence of carcinogenesis in rodents; (+)-limonene is anticarcinogenic (see Constituent profiles, Chapter 14).

Comments

The plant is widely cultivated in Southeast Asia. Also see Maraba oil.

Galbanum

Botanical name: *Ferula galbaniflua* Boiss. & Buhse
Botanical synonyms: *Ferula gummosa* Boiss., *Ferula erubescens* Boiss.
Family: Apiaceae (Umbelliferae)

Essential oil

Source: Resin
Key constituents:

β-Pinene	45.1–58.8%
δ-3-Carene	2.0–12.1%
α-Pinene	5.7–12.0%
Sabinene	0–6.4%
β-Myrcene	0–4.6%
(+)-Limonene	2.7–4.0%
γ-Elemene	0–2.4%
1,3,5-Undecatriene	1.6–1.8%
(Z)-β-Ocimene	0–1.2%

(Lawrence 1993 p. 82–83; Ghannadi & Amree 2002)

Safety summary

Hazards: Skin sensitization if oxidized.
Cautions: Old or oxidized oils should be avoided.

Our safety advice

Because of its combined α-pinene, δ-3-carene and (+)-limonene content we recommend that oxidation of galbanum oil is avoided by storage in a dark, airtight container in a refrigerator. The addition of an antioxidant to preparations containing it is recommended.

Organ-specific effects

Adverse skin reactions: In a modified Draize procedure on guinea pigs, galbanum oil was non-sensitizing when used at 20% in the challenge phase (Sharp 1978). Undiluted galbanum oil was slightly irritating to rabbits; tested at 4% on 25 volunteers it was neither irritating nor sensitizing (Opdyke 1978 p. 765–766). Autoxidation products of α-pinene, δ-3-carene and (+)-limonene can cause skin sensitization (see Constituent profiles, Chapter 14).

Reproductive toxicity: The low reproductive toxicity of α-pinene, β-pinene, β-myrcene and (+)-limonene (see Constituent profiles, Chapter 14) suggests that galbanum oil is not hazardous in pregnancy.

Systemic effects

Acute toxicity: Galbanum oil acute oral LD_{50} in rats >5 g/kg; acute dermal LD_{50} in rabbits >5 g/kg (Opdyke 1978 p. 765–766).
Carcinogenic/anticarcinogenic potential: No information found for galbanum oil, but it contains no known carcinogens. (+)-Limonene is anticarcinogenic (see (+)-Limonene profile, Chapter 14).

Comments

The oil does not age very rapidly, but when it does it tends to polymerize. The main producers are Iran and Turkey. Galbanum oil may also derive from *Ferula rubicaulis* Boiss.

Garlic

Botanical name: *Allium sativum* L.
Family: Liliaceae

Essential oil

Source: Bulbs
Key constituents:

Diallyl trisulfide	18.0–48.8%
Diallyl disulfide	25.2–46.8%
Methyl allyl trisulfide	8.3–18.2%
Methyl allyl disulfide	3.9–12.2%
Propyl allyl disulfide	0.26–7.2%
Methyl allyl tetrasulfide	0.04–5.9%
Dimethyl trisulfide	0.5–3.3%
Diallyl sulfide	1.1–2.4%
Diallyl pentasulfide	2.1%
2-Vinyl-4*H*-1,3-dithiin	0–1.7%
Methyl allyl pentasulfide	1.6%
Dimethyl tetrasulfide	1.3%
Propyl methyl disulfide	0.06–1.3%
Dimethyl disulfide	0.4–1.2%
Diallyl tetrasulfide	0.5–1.1%

(Yu et al 1989; Lawson et al 1991; Rao PGP et al 1999)
Quality: May be adulterated with synthetic sulfur compounds such as propenyl disulfides (Burfield 2003).

Safety summary

Hazards: Moderately toxic; inhibits blood clotting; skin irritation (moderate risk); skin sensitization (moderate risk).
Contraindications (oral): Anticoagulant medication, major surgery, peptic ulcer, hemophilia, other bleeding disorders (Box 7.1).
Cautions (dermal): Hypersensitive, diseased or damaged skin, children under 2 years of age.

Organ-specific effects

Adverse skin reactions: Garlic has frequently been cited as causing ACD (Delaney & Donnelly 1996; Jappe et al 1999). Fresh garlic paste has been the cause of irritant dermatitis in children (Parish et al 1987; Garty 1993); garlic oil has caused similar problems, also in children (Mayerhofer 1934, cited in De Smet et al 1992). Diallyl disulfide is the most common cause of skin sensitization, including one case of systemic contact dermatitis (Delaney & Donnelly 1996; Fernandez-Vozmediano et al 2000; Pereira et al 2002). Propyl allyl disulfide and other allergens, not present in the essential oil, have also been identified (Papageorgiou et al 1983). There are two reports of photoallergic contact dermatitis to diallyl disulfide, so garlic oil may be photoallergic (Scheman & Gupta 2001; Alvarez et al 2003).
Cardiovascular effects: Garlic oil (18 mg per day for four weeks) was hypotensive in humans after oral administration (Barrie et al 1987). Garlic oil demonstrates antiplatelet activity. In six healthy adults it dose-dependently inhibited in vitro platelet aggregation induced by ADP, epinephrine (adrenaline) or collagen (Bordia 1978). Given orally to cardiovascular patients at a daily dose of 120 mg for up to 30 days, garlic oil similarly inhibited platelet aggregation promoted by the same substances (Co-operative Group for Essential Oil of Garlic 1986). Garlic oil inhibits platelet thromboxane formation in vitro, and at a daily dose of 18 mg for four weeks, it significantly reduced platelet aggregation in 20 healthy volunteers (Barrie et al 1987; Bordia et al 1998). Several constituents of garlic oil have been associated with this action. Methyl allyl trisulfide was active at a very low concentration (10 μmol/L; 1.52 mg/L) in human platelet-rich plasma, while in whole blood the most potent activity was attributed to diallyl trisulfide (Boullin 1981; Fenwick & Hanley 1985; Lawson et al 1992).

Systemic effects

Acute toxicity: Garlic oil mouse LD_{100} 10 mg (Belman 1983).
Chronic toxicity: In a clinical trial, 3,411 male and female Chinese volunteers were divided into three groups, a vitamin/mineral supplement group, a garlic group, and a placebo group. The garlic preparation consisted of 400 mg of aged garlic extract and 2 mg of garlic oil, and this was taken twice daily for 39 months. Compliance was monitored, and was 92.9% in the garlic group. No treatment-related toxicity was observed, and there were no differences in side effects between the garlic group and the placebo group (Gail et al 1998; You et al 2001).
Carcinogenic/anticarcinogenic potential: Garlic oil did not produce chromosomal aberrations in CHL cells (Ishidate et al 1988). Given orally to mice, it reduced the genotoxicity of stavudine, an anti-HIV drug (Kaur & Singh 2007). It inhibited the proliferation of human leukemia HL-60 cells (Seki et al 2000).

Garlic oil demonstrated an inhibitory effect on PMA-mediated mouse skin tumor promotion both in vitro and in vivo (Belman 1983; Zelikoff & Belman 1985) and inhibited B[a]P-induced mouse skin carcinogenesis at the initiation stage (Sadhana et al 1988). Garlic oil significantly reduced 3-methylcholan-threne-induced cervical cancer in mice (Rai & Ahujarai 1990). In mouse epidermal cells, garlic oil increased glutathione peroxidase activity, and abolished the inhibitory effect of a tumor promoter on the enzyme (Perchellet et al 1986). In rats, garlic oil protected against nicotine-induced lipid peroxidation, increasing activities of antioxidant enzymes and concentrations of glutathione (Helen et al 1999). Garlic oil significantly increased the glutathione content of red blood cells and the activity of glutathione *S*-transferase and PROD in rats when given orally at 80 or 200 mg/kg (Wu et al 2001, 2002).

Diallyl sulfide, diallyl disulfide, diallyl trisulfide and methyl allyl disulfide display anticarcinogenic activity (see Constituent profiles, Chapter 14). The first three of these compounds also protect erythrocytes against glucose-induced oxidation (Chan et al 2002). The same three compounds markedly inhibited the growth of cultured canine mammary tumor cells, while three water-soluble constituents of garlic did not. This inhibition was closely correlated with a reduction of intracellular glutathione (Sundaram & Milner 1993).

Drug interactions: Anticoagulant medication, because of cardiovascular effects, above. See Table 4.10B. Garlic oil protects the liver from toxic doses of acetaminophen (paracetamol) (Kalantari & Salehi 2001).

Comments

Safe levels for application of garlic oil to the skin are not known, but there is a potential for allergic reaction, and some irritancy is strongly suspected. A maximum concentration of 0.1% is recommended for initial application. Other *Allium* oils rich in sulfur compounds, such as leek, may present similar problems to garlic oil. Sulfur-rich oils such as garlic are not used in fragrances, hence the lack of RIFM data; they are more commonly administered internally than externally in aromatherapy. The protective action of garlic oil against cancer is due in part to the induction of phase II detoxifying enzymes.

Genipi

Synonym: Genepi
Botanical name: *Artemisia genepi* Weber syn.
Botanical synonyms: *Artemisia spicata* Wulfen, *Artemisia mutellina* Vill.
Family: Asteraceae (Compositae)

Essential oil

Source: Aerial parts
Key constituents:

α-Thujone	79.8%
β-Thujone	10.4%
β-Pinene	1.3%
Terpinen-4-ol	1.0%

(Mucciarelli et al 1995)

Safety summary

Hazards: Expected to be neurotoxic, based on thujone content.
Contraindications (all routes): Pregnancy, breastfeeding.
Contraindications: Should not be taken in oral doses.
Maximum dermal use level: 0.3%

Our safety advice

Our dermal maximum is based on 90.2% total thujone content with a limit of 0.25% (see Thujone profile, Chapter 14).

Organ-specific effects

Neurotoxicity: No information found. There is a risk of convulsions with moderately high doses of thujone. The thujone NOAEL for convulsions was reported to be 10 mg/kg in male rats and 5 mg/kg in females (Margaria 1963).

Systemic effects

Acute toxicity: No information found. Both α- and β-thujone are moderately toxic, with reported oral LD_{50} values ranging from 190–500 mg/kg for different species (see Thujone profile, Chapter 14). There is a risk of convulsions with moderately high doses of thujone.
Carcinogenic/anticarcinogenic potential: No information found for genipi oil, but it contains no known carcinogens.

Comments

In the EU SCF report on thujone it was concluded that the available data were inadequate to establish a TDI/ADI (SCF 2003b).

Geranium

Botanical name: *Pelargonium x asperum* Ehrh. ex Willd.
Family: Geraniaceae

Essential oil

Source: Leaves
Key constituents:

Chinese

Citronellol	36.5–39.1%
Citronellyl formate	9.2–10.1%
Geraniol	8.7–8.9%
Guaia-6,9-diene	6.5–6.8%
Isomenthone	5.4–5.7%
Linalool	3.6–3.9%
Menthone	1.4–2.4%
Geranyl formate	1.9–2.1%
(Z)-+(E)-Rose oxide	1.8–2.0%
Germacrene D	0.4–1.5%
Geranyl tiglate	1.2–1.3%
Citronellyl propionate	0.9–1.2%
β-Caryophyllene	0.7–1.2%
Citronellyl tiglate	0.9–1.0%

Geranyl butyrate   0.6–1.0%
β-Bourbonene   0–1.0%

(Benveniste & Azzo 1992a; Southwell & Stiff 1995)

Egyptian

Citronellol	24.8–27.7%
Geraniol	15.7–18.0%
Linalool	0.5–8.6%
Citronellyl formate	6.5–6.7%
Isomenthone	5.7–6.1%
10-*epi*-γ-Eudesmol	5.5–5.7%
Geranyl formate	3.6–3.7%
Geranyl butyrate	1.5–1.9%
Geranyl tiglate	1.5–1.9%
β-Caryophyllene	1.2–1.3%
Guaia-6,9-diene	0.3–1.2%
Germacrene D	0.3–1.2%
Geranyl propionate	1.0–1.1%
(Z)-Rose oxide	0.9–1.0%
2-Phenylethyl butyrate	0–1.0%

(Benveniste & Azzo 1992a; Southwell & Stiff 1995)

Moroccan

Citronellol	18.6–37.8%
Geraniol	15.1–20.6%
Linalool	5.6–10.0%
Citronellyl formate	5.5–8.1%
Geranyl formate	2.8–6.6%
Isomenthone	3.8–5.6%
10-*epi*-γ-Eudesmol	0–5.2%
Citronellyl propionate	0–2.5%
Geranyl tiglate	1.1–2.4%
Geranyl butyrate	0.4–2.4%
Menthone	0.8–2.1%
Geranyl propionate	0.7–1.6%
(Z)-Rose oxide	0.8–1.3%
Citronellyl actetate	0.9–1.2%
Nerol	0.6–1.2%
Citronellyl butyrate	0.4–1.1%
α-Terpineol	0.9–1.0%
2-Phenylethyl tiglate	0.4–1.0%

(Lawrence 1989 p. 119–121, 1996f p. 58–62, 1999a p. 56–61)

Reunion

Citronellol	20.3–47.7%
Geraniol	7.3–30.3%
Linalool	3.1–13.8%
Citronellyl formate	4.8–12.4%
Isomenthone	3.4–9.8%
10-*epi*-γ-Eudesmol	tr–8.9%
Geranyl formate	1.6–7.6%
Guaia-6,9-diene	0.1–6.8%

α-Caryophyllene	0.4–6.0%
Geranyl acetate	0.2–4.4%
Geranyl tiglate	0.2–3.0%
β-Myrcene	0.2–2.3%
Menthone	0.1–2.1%
β-Bourbonene	0.3–2.0%
Citronellyl tiglate	1.4–1.8%
Geranyl butyrate	0.6–1.7%
Geranyl propionate	0.1–1.7%
Citronellyl propionate	0–1.7%
β-Caryophyllene	0.4–1.6%
(Z)-Rose oxide	0.3–1.4%
Citronellyl butyrate	0.3-1.3%
2-Phenylethyl tiglate	0.2–1.2%
Nerol	0–1.2%
Neral	0–1.1%

(Lawrence 1989 p. 119–121, 1996f p. 58–62, 1999a p. 56–61)

Safety summary

Hazards: Drug interaction; skin sensitization (low risk).
Cautions (oral): Diabetes medication, drugs metabolized by CYP2B6 (Appendix B).
Maximum dermal use level: 17.5%

Our safety advice

We recommend a dermal maximum of 17.5% based on 30.3% geraniol content with a dermal limit of 5.3% (see Constituent profiles, Chapter 14).

Regulatory guidelines

Has GRAS status.

Organ-specific effects

Adverse skin reactions: In a mouse local lymph node assay, geranium oil was an extremely weak sensitizer (Lalko & Api 2006). Undiluted Moroccan geranium oil was slightly irritating to rabbit and guinea pig skin, but was not irritating to mouse skin; tested at 10% on 25 healthy volunteers it was neither irritating nor sensitizing. It is non-phototoxic (Opdyke 1975 p. 451). Undiluted Reunion geranium oil was moderately irritating to rabbit skin, but was not irritating to mouse skin; tested at 10% on 25 healthy volunteers it was neither irritating nor sensitizing. It is non-phototoxic (Opdyke 1974 p. 883–884).

In a group of 100 consecutive dermatitis patients tested with 5% Bourbon geranium oil there were two irritant reactions and no allergic reactions (Frosch et al 1995a). From 1990 to 1998 the average patch test positivity rate to 20% geranium oil in a total of 1,483 Japanese dermatitis patients (99% female) suspected of cosmetic sensitivity was 1.93% (Sugiura et al 2000). In a study of 200 consecutive dermatitis patients, three (1.5%) were sensitive to 2% geranium oil on patch testing (Rudzki et al 1976). A 65-year-old aromatherapist with multiple essential oil sensitivities reacted to 5%, but not 1% geranium oil (Selvaag et al 1995). In 178 dermatitis patients who were

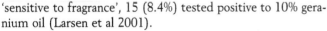

'sensitive to fragrance', 15 (8.4%) tested positive to 10% geranium oil (Larsen et al 2001).

Cardiovascular effects: When a laboratory-distilled Tunisian geranium oil (citronellol 16.2%, geraniol 15.3%) was given to alloxan-induced diabetic male rats at 75 and 150 mg/kg/day po for 30 days, blood glucose was reduced by an amount comparable with that elicited by glibenclamide (600 μg/kg), while hepatic glycogen concentration increased (Boukhris et al 2012).

Systemic effects

Acute toxicity: Bourbon geranium oil acute oral LD_{50} in rats >5 g/kg; acute dermal LD_{50} in rabbits 2.5 g/kg (Opdyke 1974 p. 883–884). Algerian geranium oil acute dermal LD_{50} in rabbits >5 g/kg (Opdyke 1976 p. 781–782). Moroccan geranium oil acute dermal LD_{50} in rabbits >5 g/kg (Opdyke 1975 p. 451).

Antioxidant/pro-oxidant activity: Moderate antioxidant activity has been reported for *Pelargonium graveolens* oil, against the free radical DPPH, and against lipid peroxidation in chicken liver, muscle and egg yolk (Dorman et al 1995; Sun et al 2005).

Carcinogenic/anticarcinogenic potential: A South African geranium oil (32.7% citronellol, 19.6% geraniol) was not mutagenic in *S. typhimurium* strains TA98 or TA100, with or without metabolic activation, and inhibited the mutagenic activity of 2-aminoanthracene (Guerrini et al 2011). Geraniol and α-caryophyllene display anticarcinogenic activity (see Constituent profiles, Chapter 14).

Drug interactions: Antidiabetic medication, because of cardiovascular effects, above. See Table 4.10.b. Since geraniol inhibits CYP2B6 (Table 4.11B), there is a theoretical risk of interaction between geranium oil and drugs metabolized by this enzyme (Appendix B).

Comments

In addition to China, Egypt and Morocco, geranium oil is produced on a large scale in Crimea, Ukraine, Georgia, India, Madagascar and South Africa. The name 'rose geranium' was originally reserved for geranium oil from Reunion, which derived from a particular cultivar known as geranium Bourbon. However, the Bourbon oil from Reunion is now only produced in very small quantities, and is no longer sold on the open market. 'Rose geranium' oils are now offered from other sources. There is some confusion concerning the precise botanical species from which geranium oils are derived. The binomials *P. capitatum* and *P. roseum* are sometimes seen, and *P. graveolens* is frequently cited in aromatherapy literature. According to Tucker & Debaggio (2000, p. 433) *Pelargonium x asperum* is a cross between *P. capitatum* and *P. radens*, while *P. graveolens*, the oil from which contains 30–83% isomenthone, is not in fact the source of commercial geranium oil.

Ghandi root

Synonyms: Sugandhmantri
Botanical name: *Homalomena aromatica* Schott.
Family: Araceae

Essential oil

Source: Rhizomes
Key constituents:

Linalool	62.1%
Terpinen-4-ol	17.2%
α-Terpineol	2.4%
γ-Terpinene	1.9%
α-Cadinol	1.5%
Geraniol	1.4%
Nerol	1.4%
α-Terpinene	1.0%
Spathulenol	1.0%
T-Cadinol	1.0%

(Singh G et al 2000)

Safety summary

Hazards: None known.
Contraindications: None known.

Regulatory guidelines

According to IFRA, essential oils rich in linalool should only be used when the level of peroxides is kept to the lowest practical value. The addition of antioxidants such as 0.1% BHT or α-tocopherol at the time of production is recommended (IFRA 2009).

Organ-specific effects

Adverse skin reactions: No information found for Ghandi root oil, but judging from its composition the risk of skin reactions is likely to be low.

Reproductive toxicity: The virtual absence of reproductive toxicity for linalool (Politano et al 2008) suggests that Ghandi root oil is not hazardous in pregnancy.

Systemic effects

Acute toxicity: No information found.

Carcinogenic/anticarcinogenic potential: No information found for Ghandi root oil. Geraniol displays anticarcinogenic activity (see Geraniol profile, Chapter 14), and α-cadinol is active against the human colon cancer cell line HT-29 (He et al 1997a).

Comments

Limited availability in the West, but produced in quantity in India.

Ginger

Botanical name: *Zingiber officinale* Roscoe
Family: Zingiberaceae

Essential oil

Source: Dried rhizomes
Key constituents:

Chinese

Zingiberene	38.1%
ar-Curcumene	17.1%
β-Sesquiphellandrene	7.2%
Camphene	4.7%
β-Bisabolene	5.2%
β-Phellandrene	2.5%
Borneol	2.2%
1,8-Cineole	2.1%
α-Pinene	1.3%
β-Elemene	1.2%

(Lawrence 1995b p. 55)

Indian

Zingiberene	40.2%
ar-Curcumene	17.1%
β-Sesquiphellandrene	7.3%
β-Bisabolene	6.0%
Camphene	4.5%
β-Phellandrene	3.4%
Borneol	2.8%
1,8-Cineole	1.7%
α-Pinene	1.4%
2-Undecanone	1.4%

(Lawrence 1995b p. 55)
Quality: Ginger oil is not commonly adulterated (Singhal et al 1997).

Safety summary

Hazards: None known.
Contraindications: None known.

Regulatory guidelines

Has GRAS status.

Organ-specific effects

Adverse skin reactions: Undiluted ginger oil was moderately irritating to rabbits, but was not irritating to mice; tested at 4% on 25 volunteers it was neither irritating nor sensitizing. Low-level phototoxic effects reported for ginger oil are not considered significant (Opdyke 1974 p. 901–902). Oral administration of ginger oil dose-dependently weakened the delayed hypersensitivity response, so any allergic reaction from the oil is likely to be minimal (Zhou et al 2006).

Systemic effects

Acute toxicity: Ginger oil acute oral LD_{50} in rats >5 g/kg; acute dermal LD_{50} in rabbits >5 g/kg (Opdyke 1974 p. 901–902).

Subacute & subchronic toxicity: In a 13 week oral toxicity study, ginger oil (31.1% zingiberene) was administered to male and female rats at 100, 250 or 500 mg/kg/day. No adverse effects were seen, including mortality, decreased food consumption, changes in body weight or organ weights, hematological parameters, hepatic or renal function. No histopathological changes were noted in selected organs (Jeena et al 2011).
Antioxidant/pro-oxidant activity: Ginger oil showed moderate antioxidant activity in lipid peroxidation tests, and high activity as a DPPH radical scavenger (Sacchetti et al 2005; Singh et al 2008).
Carcinogenic/anticarcinogenic potential: Ginger oil did not produce CA in CHL cells (Ishidate et al 1988). Ginger oil dose-dependently inhibited aflatoxin B_1-induced adducts in calf thymus DNA, in the presence of rat liver microsomes (Hashim et al 1994). Lam & Zheng (1991) reported that ginger oil induced glutathione *S*-transferase activity to more than 2.5 times control level in mouse tissues, and Banerjee et al (1994) that it significantly induced both glutathione *S*-transferase and aryl hydrocarbon hydroxylase in mouse liver, all of these being indicative of anticarcinogenic activity. Ginger oil was cytotoxic to human prostate and lung cancer cells with IC_{50} values of 0.08%, 0.11% respectively, but it was not cytotoxic to breast cancer cells (Zu et al 2010). (+)-Limonene, β-sesquiphellandrene, and β-elemene display anticarcinogenic activity (see Constituent profiles, Chapter 14).

Comments

In addition to China and India, major ginger oil producers include England (from Nigerian ginger) and Jamaica. CO_2 extracts are also available.

Gingergrass

Synonym: Russa grass, sofia
Botanical name: *Cymbopogon martinii* Roxb. var. *sofia* Gupta
Botanical synonym: *Andropogon martinii* Roxb. var. *sofia* Gupta
Family: Poaceae (Gramineae)

Essential oil

Source: Leaves
Key constituents:

(+)-Limonene	30.1%
(*Z*)-*p*-Mentha-1(7), 8-dien-2-ol	13.0%
(*E*)-*p*-Mentha-1(7), 8-dien-2-ol	12.1%
(*Z*)-*p*-Mentha-2,8-dien-1-ol	11.1%
(*E*)-*p*-Mentha-2,8-dien-1-ol	6.8%
p-Menthadienol	5.3%
Carvone	3.2%
(*E*)-Carveol	3.0%
p-Menthadienol	2.6%
p-Menthatrienol	1.7%
p-Mentha-1(7),2,8-triene	1.6%
p-Mentha-1,5,8-triene	1.1%

(Boelens 1994)

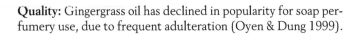

Quality: Gingergrass oil has declined in popularity for soap perfumery use, due to frequent adulteration (Oyen & Dung 1999).

Safety summary

Hazards: Skin sensitization if oxidized.
Cautions: Old or oxidized oils should be avoided.

Our safety advice

Because of its (+)-limonene content we recommend that oxidation of gingergrass oil is avoided by storage in a dark, airtight container in a refrigerator. The addition of an antioxidant to preparations containing it is recommended.

Regulatory guidelines

IFRA recommends that essential oils rich in limonene should only be used when the level of peroxides is kept to the lowest practical level, for instance by adding antioxidants at the time of production (IFRA 2009).

Organ-specific effects

Adverse skin reactions: No information found for gingergrass oil. Autoxidation products of (+)-limonene can cause skin sensitization (see (+)-Limonene profile, Chapter 14).

Systemic effects

Acute toxicity: No information found.
Carcinogenic/anticarcinogenic potential: No information found for gingergrass oil, but it contains no known carcinogens. (+)-Limonene displays anticarcinogenic activity (see (+)-Limonene profile, Chapter 14).

Comments

Limited availability. Menthadienols are not found in abundance in any other commercially available essential oil.

Ginger lily

Synonyms: White ginger lily, butterfly lily
Botanical name: *Hedychium coronarium* Koenig
Family: Zingiberaceae

Absolute

Source: Flowers
Key constituents:

Linalool	29.3%
(*E*)-Isoeugenol	18.4%
Indole	7.0%
Methyl benzoate	5.7%
Valeric acid	4.0%
Jasmine lactone	3.5%
Benzyl benzoate	2.9%
Methyl jasmonate	1.8%
β-Caryophyllene	1.6%
Methyl *epi*-jasmonate	1.6%
Eugenol	1.4%
Benzyl cyanide	1.3%
1,8-Cineole	1.3%
(*Z*)-Jasmone	1.2%
β-Ocimene	1.2%
Phenylacetaldehyde	1.1%
(*E,E*)-2,6,10-trimethyl-2,6,10,12-tridecatetraene	1.1%

(Matsumoto et al 1993)

Safety summary

Hazards: Skin sensitization (moderate risk).
Cautions (dermal): Hypersensitive, diseased or damaged skin, children under 2 years of age.
Maximum dermal use level: 1.0%

Our safety advice

Our dermal maximum is based on 18.4% isoeugenol content with a dermal limit of 0.2% (see Isoeugenol profile, Chapter 14). We believe the IFRA guideline of 0.02% for isoeugenol to be over-restrictive.

Regulatory guidelines

Essential oils containing isoeugenol should not be used such that the level of isoeugenol exceeds 0.02% for most product types (SCCNFP 2001a; IFRA 2009). IFRA recommends that benzyl cyanide is not used as a fragrance ingredient, but that exposure from oils and extracts is not significant and their use is authorized so long as the level of benzyl cyanide in the finished product does not exceed 100 ppm (0.01%) (IFRA 2009). According to IFRA, essential oils rich in linalool should only be used when the level of peroxides is kept to the lowest practical value. The addition of antioxidants such as 0.1% BHT or α-tocopherol at the time of production is recommended (IFRA 2009). Phenylacetaldehyde is restricted by IFRA, but this would not apply, since it would allow ginger lily absolute to be used at 27.3%.

Organ-specific effects

Adverse skin reactions: No information found for ginger lily absolute. Isoeugenol is a potential skin sensitizer (see Isoeugenol profile, Chapter 14). Oxidation products of linalool may be skin sensitizing.

Systemic effects

Acute toxicity: No information found for ginger lily absolute. Karo karoundé absolute, which contains 4.8% benzyl cyanide, has a rat acute oral LD$_{50}$ of 1.4 g/kg and an acute dermal LD$_{50}$ of >5 g/kg in rabbits (Ford et al 1988a p. 61S).
Carcinogenic/anticarcinogenic potential: No information found for ginger lily absolute but it contains no known carcinogens. Methyl jasmonate and (*Z*)-jasmone display anticarcinogenic activity (see Constituent profiles, Chapter 14).

Comments

The maximum level for benzyl cyanide does not apply to ginger lily absolute, as it is higher than the maximum for isoeugenol. Although benzyl cyanide is moderately toxic, with a rat acute oral LD_{50} of 270 mg/kg, as an organic cyanide it is much less toxic than inorganic cyanides like hydrogen cyanide. Its presence as a constituent of ginger lily absolute is not a cause for concern. The material used for the compositional analysis was simultaneously steam distilled and solvent extracted with diethyl ether from a concrete. Ginger lily absolute comes from the flowers of the same plant as longoza oil.

Goldenrod

Synonym: Canada goldenrod
Botanical name: *Solidago canadensis* L.
Family: Asteraceae (Compositae)

Essential oil

Source: Flowering herb
Key constituents:

Bornyl acetate	19.5%
Sabinene	18.8%
(+)-Limonene	17.8%
α-Phellandrene	11.9%
β-Myrcene	9.4%
γ-Terpinene	4.2%
Terpinolene	4.2%
β-Pinene	2.8%
Borneol	2.0%
Linalool	1.9%
p-Cymene	1.2%
Bornyl benzoate	1.1%
Terpinen-4-ol	1.1%

(Rondeau, private communication, 1999)

Safety summary

Hazards: None known.
Contraindications: None known.

Organ-specific effects

No information found.

Systemic effects

Acute toxicity: No information found for goldenrod oil, but bornyl acetate is non-toxic (Opdyke 1973 p. 1041–1042).
Carcinogenic/anticarcinogenic potential: No information found for goldenrod oil, but it contains no known carcinogens; (+)-limonene is anticarcinogenic (see (+)-Limonene profile, Chapter 14).

Comments

Limited availability.

Grapefruit

Botanical name: *Citrus* x *paradisi* Macfady
Family: Rutaceae

Essential oil

Source: Fruit peel, by expression
Key constituents:

(+)-Limonene	84.8–95.4%
β-Myrcene	1.4–3.6%
α-Pinene	0.2–1.6%
Sabinene	0.4–1.0%
Nootkatone	0.1–0.8%

Non-volatile compounds

Bergapten	0.012–0.19%
Epoxy-bergamottin	0.1126%
Bergamottin	<0.11%

(Dugo et al 1999a, Lawrence 1989 p. 91–92, 1993 p167–168, SCCP 2005b)
Quality: Grapefruit oil may be adulterated with orange terpenes, or with purified limonene (Burfield 2000).

Safety summary

Hazards: Phototoxic (low risk); skin sensitization if oxidized.
Contraindications (dermal): If applied to the skin at over maximum use level skin must not be exposed to sunlight or sunbed rays for 12 hours.
Cautions: Old or oxidized oils should be avoided.
Maximum dermal use level: 4% (see IFRA regulatory guidelines below).

Our safety advice

Because of its (+)-limonene content we recommend that oxidation of grapefruit oil is avoided by storage in a dark, airtight container in a refrigerator. The addition of an antioxidant to preparations containing it is recommended.

Regulatory guidelines

Has GRAS status. In Europe, essential oils containing furanocoumarins must be used so that the total level of bergapten will not exceed: (a) 15 ppm in finished cosmetic products intended for application to skin areas likely to be exposed to sunshine, excluding rinse-off products; or (b) 1 ppm in sun protection and in bronzing products. In the presence of other phototoxic ingredients, the sum of their concentrations (expressed as % of the respective maximum levels) shall not exceed 100% (SCCNFP 2000).

IFRA recommends that, for application to areas of skin exposed to sunshine, expressed grapefruit oil be limited to a maximum of 4% in products applied to the skin except for bath

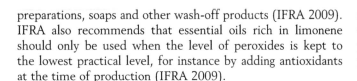

preparations, soaps and other wash-off products (IFRA 2009). IFRA also recommends that essential oils rich in limonene should only be used when the level of peroxides is kept to the lowest practical level, for instance by adding antioxidants at the time of production (IFRA 2009).

Organ-specific effects

Adverse skin reactions: Undiluted grapefruit oil was slightly irritating to rabbits, but was not irritating to mice or pigs. Tested at 10% or 100% on two panels of 25 volunteers it was not irritating. Tested at 10% on 25 volunteers it was not sensitizing. It is non-phototoxic (Opdyke 1974 p. 723–724). Autoxidation products of (+)-limonene can cause skin sensitization (see (+)-Limonene profile).

Reproductive toxicity: The low developmental toxicity of (+)-limonene in rabbits and mice (Kodama et al 1977a, 1977b) suggests grapefruit oil is not hazardous in pregnancy.

Systemic effects

Acute toxicity: Grapefruit oil acute oral LD_{50} in rats >5 g/kg; acute dermal LD_{50} in rabbits >5 g/kg (Opdyke 1974 p. 723–724).

Carcinogenic/anticarcinogenic potential: Grapefruit oil was not mutagenic in the *Ames test*, and did not produce CA in Chinese hamster fibroblasts (Ishidate et al 1984). It significantly induced glutathione *S*-transferase in mouse liver and small bowel mucosa, and inhibited B[*a*]P-induced neoplasia of both forestomach and lungs (Wattenberg et al 1985). Grapefruit oil was cytotoxic to human prostate and lung cancer cells with IC_{50} values of 0.09% and 0.10% respectively, but it was not cytotoxic to human breast cancer cells (Zu et al 2010). Grapefruit oil induced apoptosis in human leukemia (HL-60) cells, as did three minor constituents of the oil: citral, decanal and octanal (Hata et al 2003). (+)-Limonene displays anticarcinogenic activity (see (+)-Limonene profile, Chapter 14).

Drug interactions: Grapefruit juice inhibits the metabolism of many medications (Fuhr 1998). The constituent primarily responsible is 6,7-dihydroxybergamottin (DHB), a furanocoumarin not present in grapefruit oil, which inhibits CYP3A4 (Paine et al 2005). DHB probably hydrolyses from epoxybergamottin, which is in the peel and the essential oil, during juice extraction (Wangensteen et al 2003). Bergamottin and bergapten also inhibit CYP3A4, and they are present in grapefruit oil and other citrus oils (Ho et al 2001; Dresser & Bailey 2003). Bergamottin has weaker inhibitory action than DHB, and is not primarily responsible for CYP3A4 inhibition (Schmiedlin-Ren et al 1997; Bailey et al 2003; Greenblatt et al 2003). Grapefruit flavonoids (not present in the essential oil) also contribute to the enzyme inhibition of grapefruit juice (Li et al 2007). Based on the IC_{50} values for CYP3A4 inhibition (Table 4.11B) and the concentrations of bergamottin and bergapten in grapefruit oil, it is not at all likely to cause drug interactions.

Comments

Phototoxicity is due to bergapten, and other furanocoumarins found in the oil.

Grindelia

Botanical name: *Grindelia oregana* A. Grey
Family: Asteraceae (Compositae)

Essential oil

Source: Aerial parts
Key constituents:

β-Myrcene	14.0–26.0%
α-Pinene	17.0–24.0%
Citronellol	1.0–5.0%
Longifolene	1.0–2.5%
Nonadecane	0.4–1.0%

(Apostolova, private communication, 1999)

Safety summary

Hazards: Skin sensitization if oxidized.
Cautions: Old or oxidized oils should be avoided.

Our safety advice

Because of its α-pinene content we recommend that oxidation of grindelia oil is avoided by storage in a dark, airtight container in a refrigerator. Grindelia oil also has a tendency to polymerize, and so does not keep well. The addition of an antioxidant to preparations containing it is recommended.

Organ-specific effects

Adverse skin reactions: No information found for grindelia oil. Autoxidation products of α-pinene can cause skin sensitization (see α-Pinene profile, Chapter 14). Little is known about the action of β-myrcene on the skin.

Reproductive toxicity: Oral β-myrcene was reproductively toxic in pregnant rats at 500 mg/kg, but not at 250 mg/kg (Delgado et al 1993a, 1993b, Paumgartten et al 1998). This does not suggest any dose limitation for grindelia oil.

Systemic effects

Acute toxicity: No information found.
Carcinogenic/anticarcinogenic potential: No information found for grindelia oil. β-Myrcene is not genotoxic and demonstrates antigenotoxic activity; it is a male mouse-specific hepatocarcinogen (see β-Myrcene profile, Chapter 14).

Comments

Limited availability; produced in Bulgaria.

Guaiacwood

Botanical name: *Bulnesia sarmientoi* Lorentz ex Griseb.
Family: Zygophyllaceae

Essential oil

Source: Wood
Key constituents:

Bulnesol	40.5%
Guaiol	26.8%
10-*epi*-γ-Eudesmol	2.2%
Guaiol isomer	1.4%
Elemol	1.2%

(Prudent et al 1991)

Safety summary

Hazards: None known.
Contraindications: None known.

Organ-specific effects

Adverse skin reactions: Undiluted guaiacwood oil was moderately irritating to rabbits, but was not irritating to mice; tested at 8% on 25 volunteers it was neither irritating nor sensitizing. It is non-phototoxic (Opdyke 1974 p. 905). In a study of 200 consecutive dermatitis patients, none were sensitive to 2% guaiacwood oil on patch testing (Rudzki et al 1976).

Systemic effects

Acute toxicity: Non-toxic. Guaiacwood oil acute oral LD_{50} in rats >5 g/kg; acute dermal LD_{50} in rabbits >5 g/kg (Opdyke 1974 p. 905).
Subacute & subchronic toxicity: When guaiacwood oil was consumed by male rats at 30.7 mg/kg/day, and by female rats at 36.0 mg/kg/day for 90 days, no adverse effects were observed on growth, food consumption, hematology, blood chemistry, liver weight, kidney weight, or the microscopic or gross appearance of major organs (Oser et al 1965). In a second 90 day feeding study in rats, the NOAEL for guaiacwood oil was 31.8 mg/kg (Bär & Griepentrog 1967).
Carcinogenic/anticarcinogenic potential: No information found for guaiacwood oil, but it contains no known carcinogens.

Comments

Bulnesia sarmientoi (both wood and 'extracts', which presumably includes the essential oil) is listed by CITES under their Appendix II: 'species that are not necessarily now threatened with extinction but that may become so unless trade is closely controlled.' This has legal implications for trade of bulk essential oil, although these limitations specifically do not apply to 'finished products packaged and ready for retail sale.'

Gurjun

Botanical names: *Dipterocarpus tuberculatus* Roxb.; *Dipterocarpus turbinatus* C. F. Gaertn.; *Dipterocarpus jourdainii* Pierre ex Laness.; *Dipterocarpus alatus* Roxb.
Family: Dipterocarpaceae

Essential oil

Source: Balsamic resin
Key constituents:

Dipterocarpus tuberculatus

α-Gurjunene	90.0%
(−)-*allo*-Aromadendrene	4.0–6.0%
β-Caryophyllene	2.0–4.0%

(Lawrence 1981 p. 34–35)

Dipterocarpus turbinatus

α-Gurjunene	20.0–75.0%
Calarene	15.0%
(−)-*allo*-Aromadendrene	4.0–6.0%
Copaene	5.0%

(Lawrence 1981 p. 34–35)

Safety summary

Hazards: None known.
Contraindications: None known.

Organ-specific effects

Adverse skin reactions: Undiluted gurjun balsam oil was not irritating to rabbit, pig or mouse skin; tested at 8% on 25 volunteers it was neither irritating nor sensitizing. It is non-phototoxic (Opdyke 1976 p. 791).

Systemic effects

Acute toxicity: Non-toxic. Gurjun balsam oil acute oral LD_{50} in rats >5 g/kg acute dermal LD_{50} in rabbits >5 g/kg (Opdyke 1976 p. 791).
Carcinogenic/anticarcinogenic potential: No information found for gurjun balsam oil, but it contains no known carcinogens.

Comments

Other chemotypes apparently exist, with either α-copaene or calarene as the major constituent. Gurjun balsam oil is a common adulterant of patchouli oil.

Hay

Synonym: Foin
Botanical names: *Anthoxylum odoratum* L.; *Cynosurus cristatus* L.; *Lolium italicum* L.; *Lolium perenne* L.; *Phleum pratense* L.; *Poa pratense* L.
Family: Poaceae (Gramineae)

Absolute

Source: Leaves
Key constituents:

Coumarin	<8.0%

(EFFA 2008)

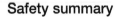

Safety summary

Hazards: Contains coumarin.
Contraindications: None known.
Maximum adult daily oral dose: 525 mg

Our safety advice

Our oral maximum is based on 8.0% coumarin content with a dose limit of 0.6 mg/kg/day (see Coumarin profile, Chapter 14).

Regulatory guidelines

Coumarin was banned by the FDA for food use in 1954.

Organ-specific effects

Adverse skin reactions: Undiluted hay absolute was slightly irritating to rabbits, but was not irritating to mice or pigs; tested at 4% on 25 volunteers it was neither irritating nor sensitizing. It is non-phototoxic (Opdyke 1976 p. 777). Unlike impure synthetic coumarin, pure or naturally-occurring coumarin is not a skin allergen (Floch et al 2002, Vocanson et al 2006).
Hepatotoxicity: No information found for hay absolute. High oral doses of coumarin are hepatotoxic in animals and in a very small percentage of humans (see Coumarin profile, Chapter 14).

Systemic effects

Acute toxicity: Hay absolute acute oral LD_{50} in rats >5 g/kg; acute dermal LD_{50} in rabbits >5 g/kg (Opdyke 1976 p. 777).
Carcinogenic/anticarcinogenic potential: No information found for hay absolute. Coumarin is carcinogenic in rodents, but is anticarcinogenic in humans (Felter et al 2006).

Comments

Dermal application of coumarin is not hazardous.

Hemp

Synonym: Cannabis
Botanical name: *Cannabis sativa* L.
Botanical synonym: *Cannabis indica* L.
Family: Cannabaceae

Essential oil

Source: Flowering tops
Key constituents:

French

β-Myrcene	31.1%
β-Caryophyllene	13.7%
(*E*)-β-Ocimene	10.2%
Terpinolene	8.9%
α-Pinene	7.6%
α-Caryophyllene	4.5%
β-Pinene	3.0%
β-Caryophyllene oxide	2.2%
(−)-β-Farnesene	1.7%
(*E*)-α-Bergamotene	1.3%
(*Z*)-β-Ocimene	1.1%
(+)-Limonene	1.0%

(Meier & Mediavilla 1998, Sonnay, private communication, 2011)

Swiss

β-Myrcene	21.2–31.1%
β-Caryophyllene	14.3–19.4%
(*E*)-β-Ocimene	2.1–6.7%
Terpinolene	1.6–9.1%
α-Pinene	14.3–19.4%
α-Caryophyllene	5.0–7.4%
β-Pinene	6.0–7.2%
β-Caryophyllene oxide	2.0–5.8%
(−)-β-Farnesene	tr-1.7%
(*E*)-α-Bergamotene	0.9–1.5%
(+)-Limonene	3.7–4.4%
β-Phellandrene	tr-1.5%

(Meier & Mediavilla 1998, Sonnay, private communication, 2011)

Safety summary

Hazards: Skin sensitization if oxidized.
Cautions: Old or oxidized oils should be avoided.

Our safety advice

Because of its combined (+)-limonene, α-pinene and δ-3-carene content we recommend that oxidation of hemp oil is avoided by storage in a dark, airtight container in a refrigerator. The addition of an antioxidant to preparations containing it is recommended.

Regulatory guidelines

The Canadian Industrial Hemp Regulations allow up to 10 μg/g of THC in cosmetics (Health Canada Cosmetic Ingredient Hotlist, March 2011).

Organ-specific effects

Adverse skin reactions: No information found for hemp oil, but autoxidation products of (+)-limonene, α-pinene and δ-3-carene can cause skin sensitization (see Constituent profiles, Chapter 14).
Reproductive toxicity: Oral β-myrcene was reproductively toxic in pregnant rats at 500 mg/kg, but not at 250 mg/kg (Delgado et al 1993a, 1993b; Paumgartten et al 1998). This does not suggest any dose limitation for hemp oil.

Systemic effects

Acute toxicity: No information found for hemp oil. β-Myrcene is non-toxic (see β-Myrcene profile, Chapter 14).
Carcinogenic/anticarcinogenic potential: No information found for hemp oil. β-Myrcene is not genotoxic and demonstrates anti-genotoxic activity; it is a male mouse-specific hepatocarcinogen (see β-Myrcene profile, Chapter 14). β-Caryophyllene and

α-caryophyllene display anticarcinogenic activity (see Constituent profiles, Chapter 14).

Comments

The analyses above are for commercially produced oils in France and Switzerland, and hemp essential oil is also produced in Canada. Analyses of non-commercial hemp oils show much greater ranges (β-myrcene 12.5–65.8%, β-caryophyllene 10.6–37.5%, α-pinene 3.4–31.0%, and so on (Mediavilla & Steinmann 1997; Nissen et al 2010). The psychotropic compounds in hemp, the cannabinols (mainly δ-9-tetrahydrocannabinol, or THC), are present in varying amounts in different cultivars of this plant, and many are now cultivated which contain none at all, or only trace amounts. Only essential oils with extremely low TCH are being produced commercially. The fixed oil from hemp seeds is also known as 'hemp oil'.

Hibawood

Synonyms: Hiba, false arborvitae
Botanical name: *Thujopsis dolobrata* (L. fil.) Siebold & Zucc. var. *hondai* Makino
Family: Cupressaceae

Essential oil

Source: Wood
Key constituents:

β-Thujaplicin	Major constituent
β-Dolabrin	Major constituent
α-Thujaplicin	Minor constituent
γ-Thujaplicin	Minor constituent
4-Acetyltropolone	Minor constituent

(Morita et al 2004)

Safety summary

Hazards: May be reproductively toxic.
Contraindications (all routes): Pregnancy, breastfeeding.

Organ-specific effects

Adverse skin reactions: Undiluted hibawood oil was moderately irritating to rabbits, but was not irritating to mice or pigs; tested at 12% on 25 volunteers it was neither irritating nor sensitizing. It is non-phototoxic (Opdyke 1979a p. 817).
Reproductive toxicity: In rats, oral doses of β-thujaplicin were reproductively toxic at 135 mg/kg (fetal malformations) and 45 mg/kg (decrease in fetal weight), but not at 15 mg/kg (Ema et al 2004). β-Thujaplicin was not estrogenic in a yeast screen (Nishihara et al 2000).

Systemic effects

Acute toxicity: Hibawood oil acute oral LD_{50} in rats >5 g/kg; acute dermal LD_{50} in rabbits >5 g/kg (Opdyke 1979a p. 817).
Carcinogenic/anticarcinogenic potential: No information found for hibawood oil, but it contains no known carcinogens.

β-Thujaplicin is not carcinogenic (Imai et al 2006). α-Thujaplicin, β-thujaplicin, γ-thujaplicin, β-dolabrin and 4-acetyltropolone display antitumoral activity (Matsumura et al 2001; Morita et al 2001, 2002, 2004).
Drug interactions: Hibawood oil induced CYP2B1 in male rat hepatic microsomes (Hiroi et al 1995), but not at a level suggestive of drug interaction.

Comments

If we assume the whole essential oil is as reproductively toxic as β-thujaplicin, this would imply a maximum oral dose of 1,050 mg, and a maximum dermal use level of 30%. No quantitative data was found for the constituents of hibawood oil.

Hinoki leaf

Botanical name: *Chamaecyparis obtusa* (Siebold & Zucc.) Endl. var. *obtusa*
Botanical synonym: *Cupressus obtusa* K. Koch
Family: Cupressaceae

Essential oil

Source: Leaves and terminal branches
Key constituents:

Elemol	14.8%
α-Terpinyl acetate	9.1%
γ-Eudesmol	8.3%
Bornyl acetate	7.2%
β-Eudesmol	6.5%
γ-Muurolene	5.7%
α-Eudesmol	5.4%
β-Cedrene	4.7%
α-Muurolene	3.8%
(+)-Limonene	3.1%
δ-Cadinene	2.8%
β-Pinene	2.8%
α-Fenchol	2.1%
γ-Terpinene	1.8%
Cadin-10(15)-en-4-ol	1.7%
(Z)-Caryophyllene	1.7%
Sabinene	1.6%
α-Elemene	1.5%
Borneol	1.2%
α-Terpinene	1.1%
α-Terpineol	1.1%
α-Pinene	1.0%
Terpinolene	1.0%

(Shieh et al 1981)

Safety summary

Hazards: None known.
Contraindications: None known.

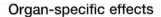

Organ-specific effects

Adverse skin reactions: No information found.

Systemic effects

Acute toxicity: No information found.
Carcinogenic/anticarcinogenic potential: No information found for hinoki leaf oil, but it contains no known carcinogens. (+)-Limonene and γ-eudesmol display anticarcinogenic activity (see Constituent profiles, Chapter 14).
Drug interactions: Hinoki leaf oil induced CYP2B1 in male rat hepatic microsomes (Hiroi et al 1995), but not at a level suggestive of drug interaction.

Comments

Two varieties exist, var. *obtusa* (Hinoki false cypress), and var. *formosana* (Formosan hinoki). In a report on trees it has been proposed by UNEP-WCMC that CITES add *Chamaecyparis obtusa* var. *formosana* to its list of threatened plant species. Major constituents from various different hinoki leaf oils include α-pinene, longifolene, sabinene, thujopsene, as well as elemol.

Hinoki root

Botanical name: *Chamaecyparis obtusa* (Siebold & Zucc.) Endl. var. *obtusa*
Botanical synonym: *Cupressus obtusa* K. Koch
Family: Cupressaceae

Essential oil

Source: Roots
Key constituents:

Longi-α-nojigiku alcohol	19.7%
α-Terpinyl acetate	9.1%
Longi-β-camphenilan aldehyde	8.4%
T-Cadinol	5.9%
α-Cadinol	5.3%
Cadin-1(10)-en-4, β-ol	5.0%
Longicyclenyl alcohol	4.8%
T-Muurolol	4.5%
δ-Cadinene	3.8%
α-Terpineol	3.5%
β-Caryophyllene alcohol	2.6%
Verbenone	2.4%
Longiisohomocamphenilone	2.2%
γ-Cadinene	2.1%
α-Muurolene	1.7%
Calamenene	1.6%
Longiverbenol	1.3%
Caryophylla-3,8(13)-dien-5,α-ol	1.3%
Cadin-1(10)-en-4,α-ol	1.2%

(Shieh et al 1981)

Safety summary

Hazards: None known.
Contraindications: None known.

Organ-specific effects

Adverse skin reactions: No information found for hinoki root oil or most of its constituents.

Systemic effects

Acute toxicity: No information found for hinoki root oil or most of its constituents.
Carcinogenic/anticarcinogenic potential: No information found for hinoki root oil, but it contains no known carcinogens. α-Cadinol is active against the human colon cancer cell line HT-29 (He et al 1997a).

Comments

Two varieties exist, var. *obtusa* (Hinoki false cypress), and var. *formosana* (Formosan hinoki). In a report on trees it has been proposed by UNEP-WCMC that CITES add *Chamaecyparis obtusa* var. *formosana* to its list of threatened plant species.

Hinoki wood

Botanical name: *Chamaecyparis obtusa* (Siebold & Zucc.) Endl. var. *obtusa*
Botanical synonym: *Cupressus obtusa* K. Koch
Family: Cupressaceae

Essential oil

Source: Wood
Key constituents:

α-Cadinol	20.5%
T-Muurolol	18.4%
γ-Cadinene	12.5%
δ-Cadinene	10.8%
T-Cadinol	10.6%
Cadin-1(10)-en-4,β-ol	6.8%
α-Muurolene	5.8%
β-Caryophyllene alcohol	1.5%
Cadin-1(10)-en-4,α-ol	1.0%

(Shieh et al 1981)

Safety summary

Hazards: None known.
Contraindications: None known.

Organ-specific effects

Adverse skin reactions: No information found for hinoki wood oil, α-cadinol or T-muurolol.

Systemic effects

Acute toxicity: No information found.
Carcinogenic/anticarcinogenic potential: No information found for hinoki wood oil, but it contains no known carcinogens. α-Cadinol is active against the human colon cancer cell line HT-29 (He et al 1997a).
Drug interactions: Hinoki wood oil induced CYP2B1 in male rat hepatic microsomes (Hiroi et al 1995), but not at a level suggestive of drug interaction.

Comments

Limited availability. The Japanese government has protected the trees since 1982, but some wood is still available from trees that die naturally, from large stocks felled before 1982, and from wood recycled from old buildings (Burfield 2000). In a report on trees it has been proposed by UNEP-WCMC that CITES add *Chamaecyparis obtusa* var. *formosana* to its list of threatened plant species.

Ho leaf (camphor CT)

Synonym: Hon-sho (true camphor tree)
Botanical name: *Cinnamomum camphora* L.
Family: Lauraceae

Essential oil

Source: Leaves
Key constituents:

Camphor	42.0–84.1%
Linalool	0.5–15.0%
Safrole	0.1–5.0%
Bicyclogermacrene	0–5.0%
α-Caryophyllene	0.1–4.0%
β-Caryophyllene	0.2–3.4%
Spathulenol	0–2.6%
(+)-Limonene	0–2.1%
α-Terpineol	1.3–2.0%
1,8-Cineole	1.0–1.7%
α-Pinene	0.1–1.7%
β-Myrcene	0.1–1.5%
Camphene	0–1.5%
Terpinen-4-ol	0–1.2%
Borneol	0.8–1.1%
β-Pinene	0–1.0%
Methyleugenol	0–0.5%

(Zhu et al 1993, 1994; Pélissier et al 1995)

Safety summary

Hazards: Drug interaction; may contain safrole and methyleugenol; expected to be neurotoxic, based on camphor content.
Contraindications (all routes): Pregnancy, breastfeeding.
Cautions (oral): Drugs metabolized by CYP2E1 (Appendix B).
Maximum adult daily oral dose: 28 mg

Maximum dermal use level:

EU	0.03%
IFRA	0.06%
Tisserand & Young	0.8%

Our safety advice

We recommend a dermal maximum of 0.8% and a daily oral maximum dose of 28 mg, based on 5.0% safrole and 0.5% methyleugenol content, with dermal and oral limits of 0.05% (0.025 mg/kg) for safrole and 0.02% (0.01 mg/kg) for methyleugenol (see Constituent profiles, Chapter 14). (Limits based on camphor would be much higher.)

Regulatory guidelines

IFRA and the EU recommend a maximum exposure level of 0.01% of safrole from the use of safrole-containing essential oils in cosmetics. IFRA recommends that the maximum concentration of methyleugenol for leave-on products such as body lotion should be 0.0004% (IFRA 2009). The equivalent SCCNFP maximum is 0.0002% (European Commission 2002).

Organ-specific effects

Adverse skin reactions: No information found.

Systemic effects

Acute toxicity: No information found. Camphor is potentially neurotoxic and is thought to be more toxic in humans than in rodents. Camphor minimum LD_{50} is 1.7 g/kg in rats (Christensen & Lynch 1937).
Carcinogenic/anticarcinogenic potential: No information found. Safrole and methyleugenol are rodent carcinogens; (+)-limonene and α-caryophyllene display anticarcinogenic activity (see Constituent profiles, Chapter 14).
Drug interactions: Since safrole inhibits CYP2E1 (Table 4.11B), there is a theoretical risk of interaction between ho leaf oil (camphor CT) and drugs metabolized by this enzyme (Appendix B).

Comments

This plant is the main source of natural camphor.

Ho leaf (cineole CT)

Synonyms (Chinese): Yu-sho (camphor oil tree)
Synonym (Madagascan): Ravintsara
Botanical name: *Cinnamomum camphora* L.
Family: Lauraceae

Essential oil

Source: Leaves

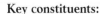

Key constituents:

Chinese

1,8-Cineole	50.0 %
α-Terpineol	14.3%
β-Pinene	6.9%
Bornyl acetate	3.1%
Linalool	2.0%
β-Bisabolene	1.7%
α-Pinene	1.6%
p-Cymene	1.1%
Safrole	0.2%
Methyleugenol	0.1%

(Zhu et al 1993)

Madagascan

1,8-Cineole	56.7–63.7%
Sabinene	11.4–14.0%
α-Terpineol	6.9–8.3%
α-Pinene	3.7–4.6%
β-Pinene	2.7–3.3%
Terpinen-4-ol	1.6–2.4%
p-Cymene	0.9–1.8%
α-Caryophyllene	0.4–1.7%
β-Caryophyllene	0.1–1.3%
β-Myrcene	0.6–1.2%

(Chalchat & Valade 2000)

Safety summary

Hazards: May contain methyleugenol; essential oils high in 1,8-cineole can cause CNS and breathing problems in young children.
Contraindications: Do not apply to or near the face of infants or children.
Maximum dermal use level (Chinese ho leaf (cineole CT) oil):

EU	0.2%
IFRA	0.4%
Tisserand & Young	11%

Our safety advice

We recommend a dermal maximum of 11%, based on 0.2% safrole and 0.1% methyleugenol content, and dermal limits of 0.05% for safrole and 0.02% for methyleugenol (see Constituent profiles, Chapter 14). No restriction is required for the Madagascan oil.

Regulatory guidelines

IFRA and the EU recommend a maximum exposure level of 0.01% of safrole from the use of safrole-containing essential oils in cosmetics. IFRA recommends that the maximum concentration of methyleugenol for leave-on products such as body lotion should be 0.0004% (IFRA 2009). The equivalent SCCNFP maximum is 0.0002% (European Commission 2002).

Organ-specific effects

Adverse skin reactions: No information found.

Systemic effects

Acute toxicity: No information found. 1,8-Cineole has been reported to cause serious poisoning in young children when accidentally instilled into the nose (Melis et al 1989).
Carcinogenic potential: Madagascan *Cinnamomum camphora* oil has demonstrated antigenotoxic effects (Bakkali et al 2006). Safrole and methyleugenol are rodent carcinogens (see Constituent profiles, Chapter 14).

Comments

The Madagascan oil is known as ravintsara oil, which can lead to confusion with ravensara oil, also from Madagascar. Unlike the Chinese oil, ravintsara oil does not contain the carcinogens safrole and methyleugenol.

Ho leaf (linalool CT)

Synonyms: Ho-sho (fragrant camphor tree), shiu, shiu-sho (bad-smelling camphor tree)
Botanical name: *Cinnamomum camphora* Sieb. var. *glavescens* Hayata
Family: Lauraceae

Essential oil

Source: Leaves
Key constituents:

Linalool	66.7–90.6%
1,8-Cineole	0.2–13.3%
Nerolidol	0.5–3.2%
Sabinene	0.1–3.2%
(*E*)-Linalool oxide	0–2.8%
β-Caryophyllene	0–2.0%
α-Pinene	0.1–1.1%
δ-Elemene	1.1%
Safrole	0.01–0.9%
Methyleugenol	0.1–0.4%

(Zhu et al 1993; Lawrence 1995d p30–33)

Safety summary

Hazards: May contain methyleugenol
Contraindications: None known
Maximum dermal use level:

EU	0.05%
IFRA	0.1%
Tisserand & Young	No limit

Our safety advice

Although ho leaf oil (linalool CT) can contain up to ~1% of potentially carcinogenic constituents; it also contains an average of 80% linalool and nerolidol, which are anticarcinogenic. Consequently we see no need for any dose limitation.

Regulatory guidelines

IFRA and the EU recommend a maximum exposure level of 0.01% of safrole from the use of safrole-containing essential oils in cosmetics. IFRA recommends that the maximum concentration of methyleugenol for leave-on products such as body lotion should be 0.0004% (IFRA 2009). The equivalent SCCNFP maximum is 0.0002% (European Commission 2002). According to IFRA, essential oils rich in linalool should only be used when the level of peroxides is kept to the lowest practical value. The addition of antioxidants such as 0.1% BHT or α-tocopherol at the time of production is recommended (IFRA 2009).

Organ-specific effects

Adverse skin reactions: Undiluted ho leaf oil was moderately irritating to rabbits; tested at 10% on 25 volunteers it was neither irritating nor sensitizing (Opdyke 1974 p. 917). Oxidation products of linalool may be skin sensitizing, but 1,8-cineole has antioxidant properties.

Systemic effects

Acute toxicity: Acute oral LD_{50} in rats 3.27 g/kg; acute dermal LD_{50} in rabbits >5 g/kg (Jenner et al 1964).
Carcinogenic/anticarcinogenic potential: No information found. Safrole and methyleugenol are rodent carcinogens; linalool and nerolidol display anticarcinogenic activity (see Constituent profiles, Chapter 14).

Comments

This oil is produced in much larger quantities than the other types of ho leaf oil, and is generally referred to simply as 'ho leaf oil'. Curiously, it is sometimes referred to as 'ho wood oil'.

Honeysuckle

Botanical names: *Lonicera periclymenum* L and other *Lonicera* species such as *L. caprifolium* L. and *L. etrusca* Santi
Family: Caprifoliaceae

Absolute

Source: Flowers
Key constituents:

Linalool	75.0%
Germacrene D	5.8%
Indole	3.3%
α-Farnesene	3.0%
Nerolidol	2.2%
Jasmine lactone	1.4%

(Joulain 1986)
Note: this is a headspace analysis of *L. caprifolium* flowers

Safety summary

Hazards: None known.
Contraindications: None known.

Regulatory guidelines

According to IFRA, essential oils rich in linalool should only be used when the level of peroxides is kept to the lowest practical value. The addition of antioxidants such as 0.1% BHT or α-tocopherol at the time of production is recommended (IFRA 2009).

Organ-specific effects

Adverse skin reactions: Tested at 3% on 25 volunteers honeysuckle absolute was neither irritating nor sensitizing. Minimal phototoxic effects were observed when honeysuckle absolute was used at 100%; in concentrations of 50% in benzene or 12.5, 50 or 70% in methanol it did not produce phototoxic effects (Ford et al 1988a p. 357). Oxidation products of linalool may be skin sensitizing.
Reproductive toxicity: The virtual absence of reproductive toxicity for linalool (Politano et al 2008) suggests that honeysuckle absolute oil is not hazardous in pregnancy.

Systemic effects

Carcinogenic/anticarcinogenic potential: Honeysuckle absolute was mutagenic to *S. typhimurium* at 100 mg/mL in water, but was not mutagenic when in dimethyl sulfoxide; it was not mutagenic in a *Bacillus subtilis* rec-assay (Ford et al 1988a p. 357). Honeysuckle absolute contains no known carcinogens; linalool and nerolidol display anticarcinogenic activity (see Constituent profiles, Chapter 14).

Comments

Limited availability.

Hop

Synonym: Common hop
Botanical name: *Humulus lupulus* L.
Family: Moraceae

Essential oil

Source: Inflorescence
Key constituents:

α-Caryophyllene	36.7%
β-Myrcene	25.4%
β-Caryophyllene	9.8%
γ-Cadinene	5.5%
δ-Cadinene	4.1%
α-Muurolene	3.0%
α-Copaene	1.5%
Geraniol	1.5%
Sabinene	1.4%

β-Selinene	1.2%
Linalool	1.1%
α-Selinene	1.0%
(E)-β-Ocimene	1.0%

(Malizia et al 1999)

Safety summary

Hazards: None known.
Contraindications: None known.

Regulatory guidelines

Has GRAS status.

Organ-specific effects

Adverse skin reactions: No information found for hop oil or α-caryophyllene.
Reproductive toxicity: Oral β-myrcene was reproductively toxic in pregnant rats at 500 mg/kg, but not at 250 mg/kg (Delgado et al 1993a, 1993b; Paumgartten et al 1998). This does not suggest any dose limitation for hop oil.

Systemic effects

Acute toxicity: No information found for hop oil or α-caryophyllene. β-Myrcene is not acutely toxic.
Carcinogenic/anticarcinogenic potential: Hop oil did not produce CA in CHL cells (Ishidate et al 1988) and it significantly induced glutathione S-transferase activity in mouse tissues (Lam & Zheng 1991). β-Myrcene is not genotoxic and demonstrates antigenotoxic activity; it is a male mouse-specific hepatocarcinogen (see β-Myrcene profile, Chapter 14). Geraniol, α-caryophyllene and β-caryophyllene display anticarcinogenic activity (see Constituent profiles, Chapter 14).

Comments

It has been stated that hop oil has estrogen-like properties (Franchomme & Pénöel 1990). However, although the plant contains estrogenic substances (Bradley 1992), no evidence could be found either for their presence in the essential oil, or for a hormone-like activity in the oil.

Horseradish

Botanical name: *Armoracia rusticana* P. Gaertn. et al.
Botanical synonyms: *Cochlearia armoracia* L., *Armoracia lapathifolia* Gilib.
Family: Brassicaceae (Cruciferae)

Essential oil

Source: Roots
Key constituents:

Allyl isothiocyanate	44.3–55.7%
2-Phenylethyl isothiocyanate	38.4–51.3%
4-Pentenyl isothiocyanate	0.6–4.0%

| 2-Butyl isothiocyanate | 0–2.7% |
| Allyl thiocyanate | 1.6–2.5% |

(Lawrence 1989 p. 5)

Safety summary

Hazards: Toxicity; skin irritation (high risk); mucous membrane irritation (high risk).
Contraindications: Should not be used, either internally or externally.

Our safety advice

Due to the toxicity and irritancy of allyl isothiocyanate, and the lack of information on safe use levels, we recommend that horseradish oil is not used in therapy.

Regulatory guidelines

Allyl isothiocyanate is prohibited in fragrances by IFRA, and as a cosmetic ingredient in the EU, which effectively means that horseradish oil is similarly prohibited.

Organ-specific effects

Adverse skin reactions: According to King's American Dispensatory (1898), horseradish oil possesses 'the pungent properties of the plant in a high degree, causing irritation and even blistering when in contact with the skin' (http://www.henriettesherbal.com/eclectic/kings/armoracia.html accessed August 8th 2011). Allyl isothiocyanate is a severe irritant to skin and mucous membranes (Evans & Schmidt 1980; Budavari 1989).
Reproductive toxicity: No information found. Allyl isothiocyanate caused embryonic death and decreased fetal weight in pregnant rats when given at 50 mg/kg sc on two consecutive days (Nishie & Daxenbichler 1980).

Systemic effects

Acute toxicity: No information found. Allyl isothiocyanate acute oral LD_{50} is 340 mg/kg in rats, producing jaundice (Jenner et al 1964). In oral doses, it is toxic to rat liver, thymus, kidney and blood at 40 mg/kg (Lewerenz et al 1988) and goitrogenic in rats at 2–4 mg (Langer & Stolc 1965).
Subacute & subchronic toxicity: No information found. Given to rats at 50 mg/kg in the diet for 20 days, allyl isothiocyanate caused acute to subacute stomach ulceration in all animals. At 20 mg/kg for 20 days the ulceration occurred in 50% of the animals. At 50 mg/kg for 14 days, it caused thickening of the mucosal surface of the stomach in both rats and mice, and thickening of the urinary bladder wall in male mice. No gross or microscopic lesions were seen after feeding allyl isothiocyanate to rats and mice for 13 weeks at 25 mg/kg (National Toxicology Program 1982). Given to rats in the diet for 26 weeks at 1,000, 2,500 or 10,000 ppm there were no apparent adverse effects (Hagan et al 1967).
Carcinogenic/anticarcinogenic potential: No information found. Allyl isothiocyanate was genotoxic in tests on Chinese hamster cells in vitro (Kasamaki et al 1982). It can cause hyperplasia and transitional cell papillomas in male rats

(Dunnick et al 1982). Phenylethyl isothiocyanate has demonstrated both mutagenicity and antimutagenicity. It is carcinogenic to male rat bladder, but anticarcinogenic in prostate, colon and lung cancers (see Phenylethyl isothiocyanate profile).

Comments

One of the most hazardous essential oils. The composition of horseradish oil is similar to that of mustard oil.

Hyacinth

Botanical name: *Hyacinthus orientalis* L.
Family: Liliaceae

Absolute

Source: Flowers
Key constituents:

Benzyl alcohol	40.0%
(*E*)-Cinnamyl alcohol	11.0%
Benzyl acetate	8.1%
Benzyl benzoate	6.0%
2-Phenylethanol	3.7%
1,2,4-Trimethoxybenzene	3.0%
Methyleugenol	1.5%
Phenylethyl benzoate	1.2%
p-Methoxyphenylethanol	1.2%

(Lawrence 1979 p. 5)

Safety summary

Hazards: Potentially carcinogenic, based on methyleugenol content.
Contraindications: None known.
Maximum dermal use level:

EU	0.01%
IFRA	0.03%
Tisserand & Young	1.3%

Our safety advice

We recommend a dermal maximum of 1.3%, based on 1.5% methyleugenol content with a dermal limit of 0.02% (see Methyleugenol profile, Chapter 14).

Regulatory guidelines

IFRA recommends that the maximum concentration of methyleugenol for leave-on products such as body lotion should be 0.0004% (IFRA 2009). The equivalent SCCNFP maximum is 0.0002% (European Commission 2002).

Organ-specific effects

Adverse skin reactions: Undiluted hyacinth absolute was moderately irritating to rabbits, but was not irritating to mice or pigs;

tested at 8% on 25 volunteers it was neither irritating nor sensitizing. It is non-phototoxic (Opdyke 1976 p. 795).

Systemic effects

Acute toxicity: Hyacinth absolute acute oral LD_{50} in rats 4.2 g/kg; acute dermal LD_{50} in rabbits >1.25 g/kg (Opdyke 1976 p. 795).
Carcinogenic/anticarcinogenic potential: No information found for hyacinth absolute. Methyleugenol is a rodent carcinogen if exposure is sufficiently high (see Methyleugenol profile, Chapter 14).

Comments

There are doubts about whether any genuine hyacinth absolute is produced.

Hyssop (linalool CT)

Botanical name: *Hyssopus officinalis* L. var. *decumbens* Briq.
Family: Lamiaceae (Labiatae)

Essential oil

Source: Aerial parts
Key constituents:

Linalool	48.0–51.7%
1,8-Cineole	12.3–14.9%
(+)-Limonene	5.0–6.0%
γ-Pinene	2.9–3.3%
Caryophyllene oxide	1.7–3.2%
α-Pinene	2.2–2.5%
Camphene	1.7–2.0%
β-Myrcene	1.3–1.7%
Isopinocamphone	1.0–1.5%
β-Bourbonene	1.0–1.2%
Sabinene	0.8–1.0%
Pinocamphone	0.5–1.0%

(Salvatore et al 1998)

Safety summary

Hazards: None known.
Contraindications: None known.

Regulatory guidelines

According to IFRA, essential oils rich in linalool should only be used when the level of peroxides is kept to the lowest practical value. The addition of antioxidants such as 0.1% BHT or α-tocopherol at the time of production is recommended (IFRA 2009).

Organ-specific effects

Adverse skin reactions: No information found. Oxidation products of linalool may be skin sensitizing, but 1,8-cineole has antioxidant properties.

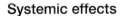

Systemic effects

Acute toxicity: No information found. Neither linalool nor 1,8-cineole is toxic (see Constituent profiles, Chapter 14).
Carcinogenic/anticarcinogenic potential: No information found. Neither linalool nor 1,8-cineole is carcinogenic; (+)-limonene is antitumoral (see Constituent profiles, Chapter 14).

Comments

The very low content of pinocamphones means that this chemotype of hyssop oil will not possess the kind of GABA$_A$ receptor inhibitory neurotoxicity normally associated with hyssop oils (see Hyssop (pinocamphone CT) profile) especially since linalool, α-pinene and β-pinene potentiate GABA$_A$ receptor-mediated responses, and so would counter pinocamphone toxicity.

Hyssop (pinocamphone CT)

Botanical name: *Hyssopus officinalis* L.
Family: Lamiaceae (Labiatae)

Essential oil

Source: Leaves and flowering tops
Key constituents:

Pinocamphone	31.2–42.7%
Isopinocamphone	30.9–39.2%
β-Pinene	4.0–8.8%
Myrtenyl methyl ether	0–3.9%
Myrtenol	0.4–2.1%
Sabinene	1.3–1.7%
β-Myrcene	0.7–1.2%
α-Terpineol	0–1.0%
Methyleugenol	0–0.5%
β-Thujone	0–0.3%
α-Thujone	0–0.1%

(Lawrence 1989 p. 110, 1999c p. 58–60)

Safety summary

Hazards: Neurotoxicity; may contain the carcinogen methyleugenol.
Contraindications (all routes): Pregnancy, breastfeeding, children under 2 years of age.
Contraindications: Should not be taken in oral doses.
Maximum dermal use level:

EU	0.04%
IFRA	0.08%
Tisserand & Young	0.3%

Our safety advice

We recommend a dermal maximum of 0.3%, based on 82.3% total pinocamphone, isopinocamphone and thujone content, with a dermal limit of 0.25% (see Constituent profiles, Chapter 14).

Regulatory guidelines

IFRA recommends that the maximum concentration of methyleugenol for leave-on products such as body lotion should be 0.0004% (IFRA 2009). The equivalent SCCNFP maximum is 0.0002% (European Commission 2002).

Organ-specific effects

Adverse skin reactions: Undiluted hyssop oil (pinocamphone CT) was not irritating to rabbit, pig or mouse skin; tested at 4% on 25 volunteers it was neither irritating nor sensitizing. It is non-phototoxic (Opdyke 1978 p. 783–784).
Neurotoxicity: The amounts of hyssop oil used in the animal tests (see below) were generally high. However, there are three reported cases of low-dose hyssop oil ingestion resulting in epileptiform convulsions (O'Mullane et al 1982). The first case was a 6-year-old whose mother frequently gave him 2–3 drops of hyssop oil for his asthma. During one severe attack, he was given 'half a coffee spoon' (15–20 drops?) shortly after which he suffered a convulsion. He fully recovered after three days in hospital. The second case, an 18-year-old girl, drank 30 drops of hyssop oil to treat a cold. One hour later she lost consciousness for 10 minutes, during which she suffered generalized contractions and bit her tongue. In the third case a 26-year-old woman took 10 drops of hyssop oil on each of two consecutive days, and suffered a seizure on the second day (Millet et al 1981).

Systemic effects

Acute toxicity: Hyssop oil (pinocamphone CT) acute oral LD$_{50}$ in mice 1.4 mL/kg; acute dermal LD$_{50}$ in rabbits 5 mL/kg (Opdyke 1978 p. 783–784). Intraperitoneal pinocamphone was convulsant and lethal to rats above 0.05 mL/kg and convulsions appeared for hyssop oil at doses over 130 mg/kg. The ip LD$_{50}$ was 1.25 g/kg (Millet et al 1979, 1981). In mice, protection against the convulsant actions of ip hyssop oil was afforded by diazepam (Höld et al 2002). The convulsant effects of hyssop oil were first researched more than a century ago. Doses of 2.5 mg/kg were injected into dogs, producing almost immediate seizures (Cadéac & Meunier 1891). In 1945, similar tests, injecting hyssop oil at 1–2 mL, revealed a two-phase response. During the first phase, blood pressure went down, breathing became rapid, and random clonic movements appeared. The second phase was characterized by hypertension, rapid heartbeat and numerous clonic contractions. The rapid onset of both phases was noted (Caujolle & Franck 1945b).
Carcinogenic/anticarcinogenic potential: A hyssop oil (pinocamphone CT) with 0.67% methyleugenol was not mutagenic in *S. typhimurium* strains T98 and T100, with or without metabolic activation (De Martino et al 2009a). Methyleugenol is a rodent carcinogen if exposure is sufficiently high (see Methyleugenol profile, Chapter 14).

Comments

This chemotype is so common it is normally referred to simply as 'hyssop oil'. Hyssop oil should be regarded as hazardous oil because of its potential to cause convulsions, especially if taken orally.

Immortelle

Synonyms: Everlasting, helichrysum, curry plant
Botanical names: *Helichrysum italicum* (Roth) G. Don (synonym: *Helichrysum angustifolium* (Lam.) DC; *Helichrysum stoechas* L. subsp. *stoechas*
Family: Asteraceae (Compositae)

Absolute

Source: Flowering plant
Key constituents: No useful data could be found.

Safety summary

Hazards: Skin irritation (moderate risk).
Contraindications: None known.
Maximum dermal use level: 0.5%

Our safety advice

The 0.5% maximum dermal use level is based on the Bouhlal et al (1988b) data, to avoid skin irritation.

Organ-specific effects

Adverse skin reactions: Undiluted immortelle absolute was mildly to moderately irritating to rabbits, but was not irritating to mice or pigs; tested at 2% on 25 volunteers it was neither irritating nor sensitizing. It is non-phototoxic (Opdyke 1979a p. 821). Immortelle absolutes from two different sources were moderately irritating in fragrance-sensitive volunteers, with concentration-dependent irritation being seen in dilutions ranging from 1.0% to 100%, but none at 0.5% (Bouhlal et al 1988b).

Systemic effects

Acute toxicity: Immortelle absolute acute oral LD_{50} in rats 4.4 g/kg; acute dermal LD_{50} in rabbits >5 g/kg (Opdyke 1979a p. 821).
Carcinogenic/anticarcinogenic potential: No information found.

Comments

The two types of helichrysum are commonly harvested and processed together.

Essential oil

Source: Flowering plant
Key constituents:

Helichrysum italicum

α-Pinene	21.7%
γ-Curcumene	10.4%
Neryl acetate	6.1%
β-Selinene	6.0%
Italidione I	5.1%
β-Caryophyllene	5.0%
ar-Curcumene	4.0%
Italicene	4.0%
α-Selinene	3.6%
Caryophyllene oxide	2.6%
(+)-Limonene	2.4%
Selina-4,11-diene	2.0%
Italidione III	2.0%
α-Copaene	1.6%
Isoitalicene	1.5%
(Z)-α-Bergamotene	1.3%
(E)-α-Bergamotene	1.2%

(Weyerstahl et al 1986)

Helichrysum italicum subsp. italicum

Neryl acetate	34.5–39.9%
γ-Curcumene	5.1–12.9%
(+)-Limonene	5.1–7.3%
Neryl propionate	4.8–6.7%
ar-Curcumene	2.3–4.6%
Italidione I	3.5–4.5%
Nerol	2.6–3.4%
Italicene	2.4–3.4%
α-Pinene	1.5–2.9%
Linalool	1.5–2.8%
Italidione II	0.6–2.6%
Eudesm-5-en-11-ol	0–2.3%
Italidione II isomer	0.6–2.0%
4,6-Dimethyloctan-3,5-dione	1.0–1.3%
4-Methylhexan-3-one	0–1.1%
Isoitalicene	0.7–1.0%
1,8-Cineole	0–1.0%

(Bianchini et al 2001)

Helichrysum italicum subsp. microphyllum

Neryl acetate	38.6%
Linalool	17.3%
Nerol	14.6%
(+)-Limonene	10.7%
Neryl propionate	1.8%
δ-Cadinene	1.1%
Italicene	1.1%

(Tucker et al 1997)

Safety summary

Hazards: None known.
Contraindications: None known.

Regulatory guidelines

Has GRAS status.

Organ-specific effects

Adverse skin reactions: Undiluted immortelle oil (type unspecified) was slightly irritating to guinea pigs, but was not irritating

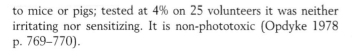

to mice or pigs; tested at 4% on 25 volunteers it was neither irritating nor sensitizing. It is non-phototoxic (Opdyke 1978 p. 769–770).

Systemic effects

Acute toxicity: Non-toxic. Immortelle oil acute oral LD_{50} in rats >5 g/kg; acute dermal LD_{50} in rabbits >5 g/kg (Opdyke 1978 p. 769–770).
Subacute & subchronic toxicity: Guinea pigs, given a 2% solution of helichrysum oil in oil at 5 mL/kg/day (so 0.1 mL/kg/day of helichrysum oil) over 14 days, showed occasional gastric ulceration (Opdyke 1978 p. 769–770).
Carcinogenic/anticarcinogenic potential: A *H. italicum* oil with 28.7% α-pinene and 21.3% γ-curcumene was not genotoxic in fruit flies, and showed significant antigenotoxic activity (Idaomar et al 2002). Immortelle oils contain no known carcinogens. (+)-Limonene displays anticarcinogenic activity (see (+)-Limonene profile, Chapter 14).

Comments

Distinguishing species of *Helichrysum* and their essential oils is problematic. Sometimes more than one species is harvested and processed together, and very small quantities of subspecies are sometimes produced by small distillers. Some regard *H. angustifolium* as synonymous only with *H. italicum* subsp. *italicum*.

Inula

Synonyms: Sweet inula, camphor inula
Botanical name: *Dittrichia graveolens* (L.) Greuter
Botanical synonym: *Inula graveolens* (L.) Desf.
Family: Asteraceae (Compositae)

Essential oil

Source: Flowering tops
Key constituents:

Bornyl acetate	46.1%
Borneol	15.3%
T-Cadinol	7.5%
Camphene	4.5%
2,3-Dehydro-1,8-cineole	2.5%
β-Caryophyllene	2.4%
Caryophyllene oxide	2.2%
γ-Cadinene	1.5%
α-Terpineol	1.4%
p-Menthadienol	1.2%
p-Menthadienol isomer	1.2%
Dimethyl-dimethylenebicycloundecan-β-ol	1.2%

(Badoux, private communication, 2002)

Safety summary

Hazards: None known.
Contraindications: None known.

Organ-specific effects

Adverse skin reactions: No information found. Bornyl acetate and borneol are relatively non-reactive in relation to the skin (see Constituent profiles, Chapter 14).

Systemic effects

Acute toxicity: No information found. Neither bornyl acetate nor borneol appear to present any toxicity (see Constituent profiles, Chapter 14).
Carcinogenic/anticarcinogenic potential: No information found for inula oil, but it contains no known carcinogens.

Comments

Limited availability. Should not be confused with elecampane oil, *Inula helenium*.

Jaborandi

Botanical names: *Pilocarpus jaborandi* Holmes, *Pilocarpus microphyllus* Stapf.
Family: Rutaceae

Essential oil

Source: Leaves
Key constituents:

Pilocarpus jaborandi

(+)-Limonene	0–67.1%
2-Tridecanone	18.6–60.7%
2-Pentadecanone	0–18.8%
Sandaracopimara-8(14),15-diene	0–13.1%
Spathulenol	0–7.6%
γ-Muurolene	0–4.9%
β-Caryophyllene	0–3.5%
α-Cadinol	0–1.6%
β-Elemene	0–1.5%
α-Pinene	0–1.3%
2-Tridecanol	0–1.3%
2-Undecanone	0–1.2%
Caryophyllene oxide	0–1.0%

(Andrade-Neto et al 2000)

Pilocarpus microphyllus

β-Caryophyllene	23.9–40.6%
2-Pentadecanone	14.2–28.1%
2-Tridecanone	2.4–20.4%
Caryophyllene oxide	2.7–15.4%
Germacrene D	6.6–10.5%
α-Caryophyllene	1.7–5.4%
α-Copaene	1.8–4.7%
β-Bourbonene	0.9–3.4%
β-Sesquiphellandrene	0.5–3.4%
β-Cubebene	1.4–2.8%

Spathulenol	0–2.7%
Humulene epoxide II	0–1.7%
2-Tetradecanone	0–1.5%

(Taveira et al 2003)

Safety summary

Hazards: May be toxic.
Cautions (all routes): Use with caution due to uncertain toxicity.

Regulatory guidelines

Jaborandi extracts and oils are prohibited as cosmetic ingredients in the EU and Canada. In the UK, jaborandi preparations can only be sold in a pharmacy under the supervision of a pharmacist.

Organ-specific effects

Adverse skin reactions: No information found.

Systemic effects

Acute toxicity: No information found for jaborandi oil, 2-pentadecanone or 2-tridecanone.
Carcinogenic/anticarcinogenic potential: No information found for jaborandi oil, but it contains no known carcinogens. (+)-Limonene, β-caryophyllene and α-caryophyllene display anticarcinogenic activity (see Constituent profiles, Chapter 14).

Comments

The UK regulation, which has been in force since 1968, is presumably based on the fact that the jaborandi plant contains some very powerful and potentially toxic alkaloids such as pilocarpine. Alkaloids are not generally found in essential oils, although Burfield maintains that jaborandi oil contains 0.8% of toxic alkaloids (www.cropwatch.org/Banned%20essential%20oils%20v1.07a.pdf, accessed August 8th 2011). None were reported in the above analyses. It appears from the Andrade-Neto et al (2000) data that there are (+)-limonene and tridecanone CTs for *Pilocarpus jaborandi*. However, Craveiro et al (1979) reported (+)-limonene and 2-undecanone as the main constituents of *P. jaborandi*, and Guenther (1949, vol. 3, p. 375) cited 2-undecanone as the main consitituent. Jaborandi oil is produced in South America and is used commercially on a very limited scale.

Jamrosa

Botanical name: *Cymbopogon nardus* L. var. *confertiflorus* Steud. x *Cymbopogon jawarancusa*
Family: Poaceae (Gramineae)

Essential oil

Source: Leaves
Key constituents:

Geraniol	54.0–85.0%
Geranyl acetate	18.0–25.0%

β-Ocimene isomers	7.8%
Linalool	3.4%
Piperitone	3.4%
Isopulegol	1.0%

(Mahindru 1992)

Safety summary

Hazards: Drug interaction; may be choleretic; skin sensitization (low risk).
Contraindications (oral): Cholestasis.
Cautions (oral): Drugs metabolized by CYP2B6 (Appendix B).
Maximum dermal use level: 6.2%

Our safety advice

Our dermal maximum is based on 85% geraniol content with a dermal limit of 5.3% (see Constituent profiles, Chapter 14).

Organ-specific effects

Adverse skin reactions: No information found. Geraniol is a low-risk skin allergen (see Geraniol profile, Chapter 14).
Gastrointestinal toxicology: Since geranyl acetate is choleretic (Trabace et al 1994), jamrosa oil should not be taken in oral doses by people with cholestasis (obstructed bile flow) (Fujii et al 1994).

Systemic effects

Acute toxicity: No information found. Geraniol acute toxicity is in the 3–5 g/kg range (see Geraniol profile, Chapter 14).
Carcinogenic/anticarcinogenic potential: No information was found for jamrosa oil, but it contains no known carcinogens, and geraniol displays anticarcinogenic activity (see Geraniol profile, Chapter 14).
Drug interactions: Since geraniol inhibits CYP2B6 (Table 4.11B), there is a theoretical risk of interaction between jamrosa oil and drugs metabolized by this enzyme (Appendix B).

Comments

Produced in India.

Jasmine

Synonyms: Royal jasmine, Spanish jasmine
Botanical name: *Jasminum grandiflorum* L.
Botanical synonyms: *Jasminum officinale* L. var. *grandiflorum* L., *Jasminum officinale* L. f. *grandiflorum* L.
Family: Oleaceae

Absolute

Source: Flowers
Key constituents:

Benzyl acetate	15.0–24.5%
Benzyl benzoate	8.0–20.0%

Phytol	7.0–12.5%
Squalene 2,3-oxide	5.8–12.0%
Isophytol	5.0–8.0%
Phytyl acetate	3.5–7.0%
Linalool	3.0–6.5%
Squalene	2.5–6.0%
Geranyl linalool	2.5–5.0%
Indole	0.7–3.5%
(Z)-Jasmone	1.5–3.3%
Eugenol	1.1–3.0%
(Z)-Methyl jasmonate	0.2–1.3%
Jasmolactone	0.3–1.2%
Methyl benzoate	0.2–1.0%

(Bassett 1994)

Quality: Jasmine absolute is frequently adulterated with materials such as indole, α-amyl cinnamic aldehyde, ylang-ylang fractions, artificial jasmine bases, synthetic jasmones and so on (Arctander 1960). α-Amyl cinnamic aldehyde is a low–moderate skin allergen. Coniferyl benzoate, a more potent skin allergen, may be present in jasmine absolute, as it is a constituent of Sumatra benzoin, which is sometimes added to jasmine concrete as an adulterant (http://www.cropwatch.org/nwsletters.htm Newsletter 14 January 2009 accessed August 8th 2011).

Safety summary

Hazards: Skin sensitization (moderate risk).
Contraindications: None known.
Maximum dermal use level: 0.7% (see Regulatory Guidelines).

Regulatory guidelines

Has GRAS status. IFRA recommends a dermal limit of 0.7% for jasmine absolute.

Organ-specific effects

Adverse skin reactions: See Table 13.1. Undiluted jasmine absolute was not irritating to rabbit, pig or mouse skin; tested at 3% on 25 volunteers it was not irritating. Tested at 3% on a second panel of 25 volunteers jasmine absolute produced two false positive sensitization reactions. These were said to be due to a spillover effect from tests of costus oil on the same subjects. When jamine absolute was tested at 3% on a separate panel of 25 volunteers, there were no positive reactions. Jasmine absolute is non-phototoxic (Opdyke 1976 p. 331). When tested at 10% on 20 dermatitis patients who were sensitive to fragrance, jasmine absolute induced seven positive reactions (Larsen 1977). Similarly, tested at 2% and 3% on 25 human volunteers with a history of reaction to fragrance materials, jasmine absolute produced allergic reactions in eight individuals at both concentrations. In this high-risk group of 25, 0.25% was the concentration at which any observable reaction disappears (Bouhlal et al 1988b).

When jasmine absolute was tested at 10% on 50 dermatitis patients who were not thought to be sensitive to fragrance there

Table 13.1 Allergic reactions to jasmine absolute

A. Dermatitis patients

Concentration	Percentage who reacted	Number of reactors	Reference
2%	0.4%	7/1,603	Belsito et al 2006
2%	1.1%	13/1,200	Santucci et al 1987
2%	1.1%	34/4,900	Pratt et al 2004
5%	0%	0/100	Frosch et al 1995a
5%	0.3%	1/318	Paulsen and Andersen 2005
5%	1.2%	20/1,606	Frosch et al 2002b
5%	1.7%	62/3,668	Uter et al 2010
10%	0%	0/50	Larsen 1977
Various	0.4%	2/487	Eiermann et al 1982

B. Dermatitis patients suspected of cosmetic or fragrance sensitivity

Concentration	Percentage who reacted	Number of reactors	Reference
5%	0.92%	13/1,483	Sugiura et al 2000
5%	1.2%	12/982	Uter et al 2010
Unspecified	0.4%	22/5,202	Broeckx et al 1987

C. Fragrance-sensitive dermatitis patients

Concentration	Percentage who reacted	Number of reactors	Reference
0.25%	0%	0/25	Bouhlal et al 1988b
2%	32%	8/25	Bouhlal et al 1988b
10%	16.9%	30/178	Larsen et al 2001
10%	35%	7/20	Larsen 1977

were no positive reactions (Larsen 1977). There were no irritant or allergic reactions in a group of 100 consecutive dermatitis patients tested with 5% Egyptian jasmine absolute (Frosch et al 1995a). Tested at 5%, jasmine absolute induced allergic responses in 20 (1.2%) of 1,606, and one of 318 (0.3%) consecutive dermatitis patients (Frosch et al 2002b; Paulsen & Andersen 2005). Of 1,200 dermatitis patients patch tested, 13 (1.1%) were sensitive to 2% jasmine absolute (Santucci et al 1987). In a multicenter study, 0.7% of 4,900 dermatitis patients tested positive to 2% jasmine absolute (Pratt et al 2004). In a North American multicenter study,

0.4% (7/1,603) patients reacted to 2% Egyptian jasmine absolute (Belsito et al 2006). An unspecified concentration of jasmine absolute produced reactions in 22 of 5,202 dermatitis patients (0.4%) suspected of contact dermatitis, and in four of 156 of the same group (2.6%) identified as being allergic to cosmetics (Broeckx et al 1987). In a multicenter study, Germany's IVDK reported that 62 of 3,668 consecutive dermatitis patients (1.69%) and 12 of 982 patients suspected of fragrance allergy (1.2%) tested positive to 5% jasmine absolute (Uter et al 2010).

In a prospective study of adverse skin reactions to cosmetic ingredients identified by patch test (1977–1980) jasmine absolute elicited contact dermatitis in two (0.4%) of 487 cosmetic-related cases (Eiermann et al 1982). Of 281,100 dermatitis patients, 13,216 had contact dermatitis, and of these 713 were related to cosmetic ingredients. Of this last group, three reacted to jasmine absolute (Adams & Maibach 1985). From 1990 to 1998 the average patch test positivity rate to 5% jasmine absolute in a total of 1,483 Japanese eczema patients (99% female) suspected of cosmetic sensitivity was 0.92% (Sugiura et al 2000).

Systemic effects

Acute toxicity: Non-toxic. Jasmine absolute acute oral LD_{50} in rats >5 g/kg; acute dermal LD_{50} in rabbits >5 g/kg (Opdyke 1976 p. 331).
Antioxidant/pro-oxidant activity: Jasmine absolute showed high activity as a DPPH radical scavenger (~90%) and in the aldehyde/carboxylic acid assay (100%) (Wei & Shibamoto 2007a).
Carcinogenic/anticarcinogenic potential: Jasmine absolute was cytotoxic to human prostate, lung and breast cancer cells with IC_{50} values of 0.02%, 0.01% and 0.08%, respectively (Zu et al 2010). (Z)-Jasmone and methyl jasmonate display anticarcinogenic activity (see Constituent profiles, Chapter 14).

Comments

Jasmine absolute appears to be a moderate-risk skin sensitizer that has caused problems in 0–1.2% of people with dermatitis when patch tested at 2 or 3%. There may be a slightly higher risk from jasmine absolutes to people of Asian origin, compared to those with black or caucasian skins. However, considering the issue of adulteration in jasmine absolute (see Quality, above), it is possible that adulterants might have played a part in some of the allergic reactions reported. It is to be regretted that the provenance and purity of the essential oils and fragrance materials used in dermatological testing is frequently not recorded in any detail. Without such attention to purity, the data cannot be relied upon for establishing safety concentrations. Egyptian jasmine absolute may contain traces of benzyl cyanide. Benzyl cyanide should not be present in products at more than 0.01% (IFRA 2009). However, at the level it is found in Egyptian jasmine absolute, no restriction is necessary. People with Refsum's disease cannot metabolize phytanic acid, a metabolite of phytol (see Phytol profile, Chapter 14), but jasmine absolute is used in such small quantities that no contraindication is needed.

Jasmine sambac

Synonym: Arabian jasmine
Botanical name: *Jasminum sambac* L.
Family: Oleaceae

Absolute

Source: Flowers
Key constituents:

Chinese

α-Farnesene	18.4%
Indole	14.1%
Linalool	13.9%
Methyl anthranilate	5.5%
Benzyl acetate	4.3%
Methyl benzoate	2.6%
2-Phenylethanol	2.4%
(3Z)-Hexen-1-yl benzoate	2.3%
Methyl palmitate	2.3%
Benzyl alcohol	1.3%

(Kaiser 1988)

Safety summary

Hazards: Drug interaction; skin sensitization (low risk).
Cautions (oral): Drugs metabolized by CYP2D6 (Appendix B).
Maximum dermal use level: 4.0% (see Regulatory Guidelines).

Regulatory guidelines

Has GRAS status. The maximum dermal use level of 4.0% is the IFRA guideline for category 4 (body creams, oils, lotions) (IFRA 2009).

Organ-specific effects

No information found.

Systemic effects

Carcinogenic/anticarcinogenic potential: No information was found for jasmine sambac absolute, but it contains no known carcinogens.
Drug interactions: Since farnesene inhibits CYP2D6 (Table 4.11B), there is a theoretical risk of interaction between jasmine sambac absolute and drugs metabolized by this enzyme (see Appendix B).

Comments

People with Refsum's disease cannot metabolize phytanic acid, a metabolite of phytol (see Phytol profile, Chapter 14), but jasmine absolute is used in such small quantities that no contraindication seems appropriate. Principal production in India and China. The major constituents of Indian hydrodistilled jasmine sambac oil are benzyl acetate, (3Z)-hexen-1-yl benzoate and linalool (Rao & Rout 2003).

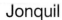

Jonquil

Botanical name: *Narcissus jonquilla* L.
Family: Amaryllidaceae

Absolute

Source: Flowers
Key constituents:

(*E*)-β-Ocimene	35.3%
Methyl benzoate	23.4%
Linalool	17.8%
(*E*)-Methyl cinnamate	7.8%
Benzyl benzoate	4.4%
Prenyl benzoate	1.8%
Indole	1.7%
Benzyl acetate	1.0%

(Lawrence 1995f p. 45)
Note: this is a headspace analysis of jonquil concrete

Safety summary

Hazards: None known.
Contraindications: None known.

Organ-specific effects

Adverse skin reactions: Undiluted jonquil absolute was not irritating to mice; tested at 2% on 25 volunteers it was neither irritating nor sensitizing. It is non-phototoxic (Opdyke & Letizia 1983 p. 861).

Systemic effects

Acute toxicity: No information was found for jonquil absolute, but none of the major constituents present any degree of toxicity.
Carcinogenic/anticarcinogenic potential: No information was found for jonquil absolute, but it contains no known carcinogens.

Comments

Limited availability.

Juniperberry

Synonym: Juniper
Botanical name: *Juniperus communis* L.
Family: Cupressaceae (Coniferae)

Essential oil

Source: Berries
Key constituents:

15 Lab-distilled oils

α-Pinene	24.1–55.4%
Sabinene	0–28.8%
β-Myrcene	0–22.0%
Terpinen-4-ol	1.5–17.0%
(+)-Limonene	0–10.9%
β-Pinene	2.1–6.0%
γ-Terpinene	0–5.8%
δ-3-Carene	0–3.0%
α-Terpinene	0–2.6%
β-Caryophyllene	1.3–2.2%
p-Cymene	0–2.0%
Terpinolene	0–1.9%
α-Thujene	0–1.8%
α-Terpineol	0–1.6%

(Schilcher et al 1993)

Single lab-distilled oil

α-Pinene	41.1%
β-Myrcene	15.2%
Sabinene	9.8%
Germacrene D	6.3%
(+)-Limonene	3.1%
β-Pinene	2.8%
δ-Cadinene	2.7%
Terpinen-4-ol	1.9%
Germacrene B	1.8%
β-Caryophyllene	1.7%
α-Caryophyllene	1.4%
β-Elemene	1.0%

(Kubeczka 2002)

Quality: Common adulterants of juniperberry oil include the oil from fermented fruits, juniper wood and twig oil, turpentine oil and terpene hydrocarbon fractions. In one comparative analysis, 15 minor constituents, present in a lab-distilled oil at between 0.1 and 1.0%, were not detected in a commercial oil (Kubeczka 2002).

Safety summary

Hazards: Skin sensitization if oxidized.
Cautions: Old or oxidized oils should be avoided.

Our safety advice

Because of its high α-pinene content we recommend that oxidation of juniperberry oil is avoided by storage in a dark, airtight container in a refrigerator. The addition of an antioxidant to preparations containing it is recommended.

Regulatory guidelines

Has GRAS status. A warning about kidney irritation appears in the Expanded Commission E Monographs: 'excessive use [of juniperberry oil] may cause kidney irritation and damage because terpinen-4-ol has demonstrated irritant activities' (Blumenthal et al 2000).

Organ-specific effects

Adverse skin reactions: Undiluted juniperberry oil was moderately irritating to rabbits, but was not irritating to mice or pigs (Opdyke 1976 p. 333). A patch test using undiluted juniperberry oil for 24 hours produced positive reactions in 2/20 volunteers tested (Katz 1946). When tested at 8% on 25 volunteers it was neither irritating nor sensitizing. It is non-phototoxic (Opdyke 1976 p. 333). In a study of 200 consecutive dermatitis patients, one was sensitive to 2% juniperberry oil on patch testing (Rudzki et al 1976). Since autoxidation products of α-pinene can cause skin sensitization (see α-Pinene profile), oxidation of α-pinene and other monoterpenes in the oil may be responsible for the skin reactions reported above.

Nephrotoxicity: We found no evidence to support the Commission E Monographs statement about kidney irritation. Blumenthal et al (2000) references two other books, which in turn reference other books, but we could find no definitive source for this warning. However, we did find evidence of a lack of nephrotoxicity. Two different batches of juniperberry oil were tested for 28 days in male rats with 100, 333 or 1,000 mg/kg, and 100, 300 or 900 mg/kg orally. Additionally, terpinen-4-ol was tested at 400 mg/kg. In spite of the high doses used, none of the tested substances induced changes in kidney function or morphology (Schilcher & Leuschner 1997). Juniperberry oil has demonstrated renoprotective activity, completely reversing the decrease in inulin clearance caused by tacrolimus (a drug used to prevent the rejection of transplanted tissue) in rats (Butani et al 2003).

Reproductive toxicity: Several sources have flagged juniperberry as being contraindicated in both pregnancy and kidney disease (Anon 1934; List & Hörhammer 1976; BHMA Scientific Committee 1983; Duke 1985; Chandler 1986; Czygan 1987; De Smet et al 1993). A vigorous attempt was made to trace the source of these contraindications. Most of the above referenced sources refer to 'juniper' generically, without specifying a preparation. None of theses refer to the probable scientific basis for the abortifacient activity of juniper. Ethanolic and acetone extracts of juniper berries have a significant antifertility effect in rats (Agrawal et al 1980; Prakash et al 1985). An ethanolic extract of juniper berries demonstrated both an early and a late abortifacient activity in rats (Agrawal et al 1980). An ethanolic extract would contain some essential oil, but there is no evidence that the essential oil is responsible for these effects. Since the oil constitutes only 1.5% of the raw material, and since all the major constituents of the essential oil are apparently non-toxic (see Constituent profiles, Chapter 14), it seems inconceivable that juniperberry oil could be responsible for the reproductive toxicity noted above. Isocupressic acid, a constituent of *Juniperus communis* needles, is abortifacient in cattle (Gardner et al 1998).

Nutmeg oil contains 10–25% α-pinene, 2–3% β-myrcene, 12% β-pinene, 5–6% terpinen-4-ol, 15-35% sabinene and 3–4% (+)-limonene. These same constituents account for some 75% of juniperberry oil. The administration of up to 560 mg/kg of nutmeg oil to pregnant rodents for 10 consecutive days had no effect on implantation or on maternal or fetal survival; no teratogenic effect was observed (NTIS 1972, cited in Opdyke 1976). The low reproductive toxicity of α-pinene, β-pinene, sabinene, β-myrcene and (+)-limonene (see Constituent profiles, Chapter 14) suggests that juniperberry oil is not hazardous in pregnancy.

Systemic effects

Acute toxicity: Juniperberry oil acute oral LD_{50} in rats reported as 8.0 g/kg (Jenner et al 1964) and as >5 g/kg; acute dermal LD_{50} in rabbits >5 g/kg (Opdyke 1976 p. 333).

Antioxidant/pro-oxidant activity: Juniperberry oil showed moderate antioxidant activity as a DPPH radical scavenger and in the aldehyde/carboxylic acid assay (Wei & Shibamoto 2007a).

Carcinogenic/anticarcinogenic potential: No information found. (+)-Limonene displays anticarcinogenic activity (see Constituent profiles, Chapter 14).

Comments

We believe that there is no reason to regard (unoxidized) juniperberry oil as being hazardous. There are two likely reasons why juniperberry oil acquired a 'tainted' reputation, which has since been quoted and re-quoted. Firstly, there has been some confusion between juniper (*Juniperus communis*) and savin (*Juniperus sabina*). One research paper, published in 1928, has the sub-heading: 'Emmenagogue Oils (Pennyroyal, Tansy and *Juniper*)'. In the body of the text it later states: 'The popular idea has always been that pennyroyal, tansy, *savin* and other oils produce abortion' (Datnow 1928). It is obvious that savin (*Juniperus sabina*) and juniper (*Juniperus communis*) have been confused. This could explain why juniperberry oil was considered dangerous in pregnancy, since savin oil certainly is so (see Ch.13, p. 237). Secondly, if juniper berries are abortifacient, and if the component responsible for this is unknown, then suspicion could naturally fall on the essential oil. Gin has a reputation as an abortifacient, but again juniperberry oil is very unlikely to be responsible for any such effects, since the average maximum concentration of juniperberry oil in alcoholic beverages is only 0.006% (Leung & Foster 2003). Most commercial juniperberry oil is a by-product of gin manufacture, and is derived from fermented fruits; this oil is not very aromatic.

Juniper (Phoenician)

Synonym: Phoenician savin
Botanical name: *Juniperus phoenicea* L.
Family: Cupressaceae

Essential oil

Source: Leaves and branches
Key constituents:

α-Pinene	41.8–53.5%
Manoyl oxide	tr–14.4%
β-Phellandrene	3.5–5.9%
(+)-Limonene	tr–4.7%
α-Terpinyl acetate	0–4.6%
β-Myrcene	4.0–4.5%
Isopulegyl acetate	0–3.3%
β-Pinene	1.3–2.5%
α-Terpineol	0.8–2.5%
1-*epi*-Cubenol	0–2.3%

Linalyl acetate	0–2.0%
δ-3-Carene	0–1.7%
Isopulegol	tr–1.6%
Terpinolene	0.6–1.3%
Linalool	0.7–1.3%
δ-Cadinene	tr–1.3%
Terpinen-4-ol	tr–1.3%
Elemol	0–1.2%
β-Caryophyllene	0.5–1.0%

(Adams et al 1996)

Safety summary

Hazards: Skin sensitization if oxidized.
Cautions: Old or oxidized oils should be avoided.

Our safety advice

Because of its high α-pinene content we recommend that oxidation of Phoenician juniper oil is avoided by storage in a dark, airtight container in a refrigerator. The addition of an antioxidant to preparations containing it is recommended.

Organ-specific effects

Adverse skin reactions: Undiluted Phoenician juniper oil was moderately irritating to rabbits; tested at 1% on 25 volunteers it was neither irritating nor sensitizing. No phototoxic effects were produced in mice or swine (Ford et al 1992 p. 59S). Autoxidation products of α-pinene can cause skin sensitization (see α-Pinene profile).

Systemic effects

Acute toxicity: Phoenician juniper oil acute oral LD_{50} in rats >5 g/kg; acute dermal LD_{50} in rabbits >5 g/kg (Ford et al 1992 p. 59S).
Carcinogenic/anticarcinogenic potential: No information was found for Phoenician juniper oil, but it contains no known carcinogens.

Comments

Phoenician juniper oil is sometimes confused with savin oil.

Kanuka

Synonyms: White tea tree, burgan
Botanical name: *Kunzea ericoides* (A. Rich.) Joy Thomp.
Botanical synonym: *Kunzea peduncularis* F. Muell., *Leptospermum ericoides* A. Rich
Family: Myrtaceae

Essential oil

Source: Leaves and terminal branches
Key constituents:

α-Pinene	55.5%
Viridiflorol	7.2%
1,8-Cineole	3.9%
(+)-Limonene	3.9%
p-Cymene	3.4%
Calamenene	3.0%
γ-Terpinene	2.5%
α-Selinene	2.4%
Ledol	1.9%
β-Nerolidol	1.8%
Linalool	1.5%
Cadina-1,4-diene	1.3%
Spathulenol	1.3%

(Porter & Wilkins 1998)

Safety summary

Hazards: Skin sensitization if oxidized.
Cautions: Old or oxidized oils should be avoided.

Our safety advice

Because of its high α-pinene content we recommend that oxidation of kanuka oil is avoided by storage in a dark, airtight container in a refrigerator. The addition of an antioxidant to preparations containing it is recommended.

Organ-specific effects

Adverse skin reactions: No information was found for kanuka oil, but autoxidation products of α-pinene can cause skin sensitization (see α-Pinene profile, Chapter 14).
Reproductive toxicity: The low reproductive toxicity of α-pinene, 1,8-cineole and (+)-limonene (see Constituent profiles, Chapter 14) suggests that kanuka oil is not hazardous in pregnancy.

Systemic effects

Acute toxicity: No information found. α-Pinene oral toxicity in rodents reported as 2.1–3.7 g/kg (Opdyke 1978 p. 853–857).
Carcinogenic/anticarcinogenic potential: Kanuka oil was moderately cytotoxic to mouse P388 leukemia cells, but showed greater toxicity to normal rat hepatocytes (Wyatt et al 2005). The oil contains no known carcinogens.

Comments

The oil is produced in New Zealand. It is botanically related to manuka, but the two oils are quite different in composition.

Karo karoundé

Botanical name: *Leptactina senegambica* Hook. f.
Family: Rubiaceae

Absolute

Source: Flowers
Key constituents:

Benzyl cyanide	4.8%
2-Phenylnitroethane	1.1%
Isoeugenol	0.5%

(Joulain & Laurent 1986)

Safety summary

Hazards: Contains benzyl cyanide.
Contraindications: None known.
Maximum dermal use level: 0.2%

Our safety advice

Our dermal maximum is based on on 4.8% benzyl cyanide content and its IFRA dermal limit of 0.01% (see below).

Regulatory guidelines

The occurrence of benzyl cyanide in fragranced products is prohibited in the EU (Anon 2003a). IFRA recommends that benzyl cyanide is not used as a fragrance ingredient, but that exposure from oils and extracts is not significant and their use is authorized so long as the level of benzyl cyanide in the finished product does not exceed 100 ppm (0.01%) (IFRA 2009). The IFRA maximum for isoeugenol, to avoid skin sensitization, is 0.02% for most product types.

Organ-specific effects

Adverse skin reactions: Undiluted karo karoundé absolute was slightly irritating to rabbits; tested at 1% on 25 volunteers it was neither irritating nor sensitizing. It is non-phototoxic (Ford et al 1988a p. 61S).

Systemic effects

Acute toxicity: Karo karoundé absolute acute oral LD_{50} in rats 1.4 g/kg; acute dermal LD_{50} in rabbits >5 g/kg (Ford et al 1988a p. 61S).
Carcinogenic/anticarcinogenic potential: No information was found for karo karoundé absolute, but it contains no known carcinogens.

Comments

Although benzyl cyanide is moderately toxic, with a rat acute oral LD_{50} of 270 mg/kg, as an organic cyanide it is much less toxic than inorganic cyanides like hydrogen cyanide (see Benzyl cyanide and Hydrocyanic acid profiles). Joulain & Laurent (1986) reported some 230 constituents in karo karoundé absolute, and benzyl cyanide is the major component. Limited availability.

Katrafay

Botanical name: *Cedrelopsis grevei* Baill.
Family: Ptaeroxylaceae

Essential oil

Source: Bark
Key constituents:

α-Himachalene	11.0–15.0%
Calamenene	4.0–6.0%
β-Caryophyllene	3.0–6.0%
β-Elemene	3.0–6.0%
β-Pinene	2.0–6.0%
α-Copaene	3.0–5.0%
ar-Curcumene	3.0–5.0%
γ-Cadinene	1.0–5.0%
β-Bisabolene	1.0–3.0%
Cyclosativene	1.0–3.0%
Linalool	1.0–3.0%
δ-3-Carene	0.5–2.0%
α-Pinene	0.5–2.0%
β-Bourbonene	0.5–1.0%
(Z)-β-Farnesene	0.5–1.0%
(+)-Limonene	0.3–1.0%
(–)-*allo*-Aromadendrene	0.2–1.0%
γ-Muurolene	tr–1.0%

(Behra, private communication, 2003)

Safety summary

Hazards: None known.
Contraindications: None known.

Organ-specific effects

Adverse skin reactions: No information was found for katrafay oil or α-himachalene.

Systemic effects

Acute toxicity: No information was found for katrafay oil or α-himachalene.
Carcinogenic/anticarcinogenic potential: No information was found for katrafay oil, but it contains no known carcinogens. β-Elemene displays anticarcinogenic activity (see β-Elemene profile, Chapter 14).

Comments

Produced in Madagascar. Limited availability.

Kesom

Botanical name: *Polygonum minus* Huds.
Family: Polygonaceae

Essential oil

Source: Aerial parts
Key constituents:

Dodecanal	44.1%
Decanal	27.7%
Decanol	10.9%
β-Caryophyllene	3.8%
Dodecanol	2.6%
α-Caryophyllene	1.5%
Undecane	1.1%

(Hunter et al 1997)

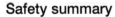

Safety summary

Hazards: None known.
Cautions (dermal): May be a skin irritant.

Organ-specific effects

Adverse skin reactions: No information found. When applied full strength to rabbits for 24 hours under occlusion, dodecanal was severely irritating (see Dodecanal profile, Chapter 14).

Systemic effects

Acute toxicity: No information found. Dodecanal does not appear to be toxic (see Dodecanal profile, Chapter 14).
Carcinogenic/anticarcinogenic potential: No information was found for kesom oil, but it contains no known carcinogens. α- and β-caryophyllene display anticarcinogenic activity (see Constituent profiles, Chapter 14).

Comments

Limited availability. The source of kesom in Malaysia (where the oil is produced) is said to be *P. minus* but the culinary herb, in Vietnam and the USA, is said to be *P. odoratum* Loureiro. It is very likely that they are one and the same species (Tucker, private communication, 2003).

Kewda

Synonyms: Keora, padang, pandanus
Botanical name: *Pandanus fascicularis* Lam.
Botanical synonym: *Pandanus odoratissimus* L. fil.
Family: Pandanaceae

Essential oil

Source: Flowers
Key constituents:

Phenylethyl methyl ether	65.6–75.4%
Terpinen-4-ol	0–21.0%
2-Phenylethyl acetate	2.8–3.5%
p-Cymene	0.3–3.1%
α-Terpineol	0–2.9%
γ-Terpinene	tr–2.4%
β-Pinene	0.1–1.2%

(Maheshwari 1995, Misra et al 2000)

Safety summary

Hazards: None known.
Contraindications: None known.

Organ-specific effects

Adverse skin reactions: No information found. Phenylethyl methyl ether was mildly irritating when applied undiluted to rabbits for 24 hours under occlusion; the material was neither irritating nor sensitizing when tested at 8% on 25 volunteers (Opdyke 1982 p. 807).

Systemic effects

Acute toxicity: No information found. Phenylethyl methyl ether acute oral LD_{50} in rats 4.1 g/kg; acute dermal LD_{50} in rabbits 3.97 g/kg (Opdyke 1982 p. 807).
Carcinogenic/anticarcinogenic potential: No information was found for kewda oil, but it contains no known carcinogens.

Comments

Limited availability.

Khella

Synonym: Toothpick ammi, chellah
Botanical name: *Ammi visnaga* L.
Family: Apiaceae (Umbelliferae)

Essential oil

Source: Seeds
Key constituents:

Linalool	28.8%
Isoamyl 2-methylbutyrate	18.2%
Amyl isobutyrate	10.6%
Amyl valerate	9.6%
Geranyl linalool	4.1%
Isoamyl isovalerate	3.1%
2-Methylbutyl isovalerate	2.8%
Pulegone	1.8%
Isoamyl isobutyrate	1.7%
Decyl isobutyrate	1.4%
Isobutyl isovalerate	1.3%
Citronellyl propionate	1.2%
(+)-Limonene	1.1%
Isopropyl isovalerate	1.0%

(Badoux, private communication, 2003)

Safety summary

Hazards: None known.
Cautions (dermal): May be phototoxic.

Our safety advice

Our dermal and oral limits of 1% and 0.5 mg/kg for pulegone do not translate to any meaningful restriction in the use of khella oil.

Regulatory guidelines

The CEFS of the Council of Europe has classed pulegone and menthofuran as hepatotoxic, and has set a group TDI of 0.1 mg/kg bw for the two compounds. According to IFRA, essential oils rich in linalool should only be used when the level of peroxides is kept to the lowest practical value. The addition of antioxidants such as 0.1% BHT or α-tocopherol at the time of production is recommended (IFRA 2009). In Australia, khella oil is classed as a poison, due to its khellin content (see Acute toxicity, below).

Organ-specific effects

Adverse skin reactions: No information found. Khella oil has been reported to contain the furanocoumarins marmesine and 8-hydroxybergapten, but of unknown quantity (Franchomme & Pénöel 1990). The oil has not been tested for phototoxicity. Oxidation products of linalool may be skin sensitizing.

Systemic effects

Acute toxicity: No information found. Khella oil has been reported to contain 1.0% of the furanochromone khellin (Franchomme and Pénöel 1990) although the analysis reported above found no khellin, and another source states that he has never detected khellin in a commercial khella oil (Burfield, private communication, 2003). Khellin is a toxic material, with an oral LD_{50} in rats of 80 mg/kg (Budavari 1989).

Carcinogenic/anticarcinogenic potential: No information was found for khella oil, but it contains no known carcinogens.

Comments

It is unlikely that a 1% khellin content would impart any significant toxicity to the essential oil.

Labdanum

Botanical name: *Cistus ladanifer* L.
Botanical synonym: *Cistus ladaniferus* Curtis
Family: Cistaceae

Essential oil

Source: Gum from leaves and terminal branches
Key constituents:

α-Pinene	4.9–44.0%
3-Phenylproprionic acid	0–22.2%
Camphene	1.4–7.0%
α-Selinene	0–6.4%
p-Cymene	2.1–6.3%
Caryophyllene oxide	0–4.4%
Viridiflorol	1.4–3.7%
Heptyl vinyl ketone	0–2.9%
α-Terpineol	0–2.4%
Fenchone	1.4–2.3%
Bornyl acetate	1.2–2.1%
2,2,6-Trimethylcyclohexanone	1.7–2.0%
α-*p*-Dimethylstyrene	0–1.9%
Pinocarveol	0–1.8%
(*Z*)-Tagetenone	0–1.8%
Terpinen-4-ol	0–1.8%
Benzyl 3-phenylpropionate	0–1.7%
(*E*)-Cinnamic acid	0–1.4%

Borneol	1.1–1.3%
Pinocamphone	0–1.3%
Verbenone	0–1.2%
Ledol	0–1.1%
Germacrene D	0–1.0%

(Lawrence 1989 p. 24–25, 1999d p. 41–44)

Safety summary

Hazards: None known.
Contraindications: None known.

Organ-specific effects

Adverse skin reactions: Undiluted labdanum oil was moderately irritating to rabbits; tested at 8% on 25 volunteers it was neither irritating nor sensitizing. It is non-phototoxic (Opdyke 1976 p. 335).

Systemic effects

Acute toxicity: Non-toxic. Labdanum oil acute oral LD_{50} in rats 8.98 g/kg; acute dermal LD_{50} in rabbits >5 g/kg (Opdyke 1976 p. 335). 3-Phenylproprionic acid acute oral LD_{50} in mice 1.6 g/kg (Schafer & Bowles 1985).

Carcinogenic/anticarcinogenic potential: No information was found for labdanum oil, but it contains no known carcinogens.

Comments

The very low content of pinocamphone does not require any restriction for the $GABA_A$ receptor inhibitory neurotoxicity normally associated with pinocamphone, especially since α-pinene potentiates $GABA_A$ receptor-mediated responses. Labdanum oil is distilled from the gum, obtained by immersing the harvested plant material in boiling water. Also see cistus oil. Labdanum gum, and possibly absolute, contains labdane diterpenes such as labdane and sclareol.

Labrador tea

Synonym: Greenland moss
Botanical name: *Ledum groenlandicum* Oeder
Botanical synonyms: *Ledum palustre* L. ssp. *groenlandicum* (Oeder) Hulten, *Ledum palustre* L. var. *latifolium* (Jacq.) Michx., *Rhododendron groenlandicum* (Oeder) Kron & Judd
Family: Ericaceae

Essential oil

Source: Leaves
Key constituents:

Sabinene	15.7%
Terpinen-4-ol	7.6%
β-Selinene	5.7%
Myrtenal	3.5%

Bornyl acetate	3.3%
γ-Elemene	3.1%
γ-Terpinene	2.9%
β-Pinene	2.3%
Pinocarvone	2.3%
α-Caryophyllene	2.2%
α-Pinene	1.9%
α-Selinene	1.9%
Cuminaldehyde	1.6%
Camphene	1.5%
(Z)-Carveol	1.5%
α-Terpinene	1.5%
p-Cymene	1.3%
(+)-Limonene	1.1%

(Rondeau, private communication, 1999)

Safety summary

Hazards: None known.
Contraindications: None known.

Organ-specific effects

Adverse skin reactions: No information was found for Labrador tea oil or sabinene.

Systemic effects

Acute toxicity: No information was found for Labrador tea oil or sabinene.
Carcinogenic/anticarcinogenic potential: A labrador tea oil with 36.6% (+)-limonene and 8.7% terpinen-4-ol was not genotoxic in fruit flies, and showed significant antigenotoxic activity (Idaomar et al 2002). However, oils with this profile are not commercially available. Labrador tea oil contains no known carcinogens.

Comments

Limited availability.

Lantana

Botanical name: *Lantana camara* L.
Family: Verbenaceae

Essential oil

Source: Flowering tops
Key constituents:

Madagascan

Davanone	15.9%
β-Caryophyllene	12.0%
Sabinene	9.0%
α-Caryophyllene	6.2%
α-Pinene	3.7%

Linalool	3.4%
β-Bisabolene	3.0%
1,8-Cineole	2.8%
Bicyclogermacrene	2.6%
β-Pinene	2.6%
δ-3-Carene	2.3%
Nerolidol	2.3%
Camphene	2.0%
Humulene epoxide	1.9%
Cubebol	1.6%
(+)-Limonene	1.6%
Germacrene D	1.4%
Caryophyllene epoxide II	1.2%
α-Muurolene	1.2%
(E)-β-Ocimene	1.1%
β-Cubebene	1.0%
(E)-β-Farnesene	1.0%
γ-Terpinene	1.0%

(Ngassoum et al 1999)

Safety summary

Hazards: None known.
Contraindications: None known.

Organ-specific effects

Adverse skin reactions: No information was found for lantana oil or davanone.
Hepatotoxicity: Consumption of *Lantana camara* by grazing animals causes acute hepatotoxicity. This is due to the presence of triterpenoids called lantadenes, which are not present in the essential oil (Sharma et al 2007). Davanone is not hepatotoxic since davana oil, which contains 38.0% davanone, showed no signs of either acute or subacute toxicity in a 90 day feeding study in rats (Oser et al 1965; Opdyke 1976 p. 737).

Systemic effects

Acute toxicity: No information was found for lantana oil or for davanone, but see Hepatotoxicity above.
Carcinogenic/anticarcinogenic potential: No information was found for lantana oil, but it contains no known carcinogens. β-Caryophyllene and α-caryophyllene display anticarcinogenic activity (see Constituent profiles, Chapter 14).

Comments

Lantana camara grows in many parts of the world and oils are also produced in the Comoro islands and South Africa.

Lanyana

Synonym: African wormwood
Botanical name: *Artemisia afra* von Jacquin
Family: Asteraceae (Compositae)

Essential oil

Source: Leaves and stems
Key constituents:

α-Thujone	22.5%
(E)-Chrysanthenyl acetate	19.2%
1,8-Cineole	19.1%
Camphor	11.0%
β-Thujone	8.9%
β-Myrcene	2.4%
Camphene	1.8%
β-Pinene	1.3%
α-Pinene	1.2%
Germacrene D	1.2%

(Graven, private communication, 1999)

Safety summary

Hazards: Expected to be neurotoxic, based on thujone content.
Contraindications (all routes): Pregnancy, breastfeeding.
Maximum adult daily oral dose: 22 mg
Maximum dermal use level: 0.8%

Our safety advice

Our oral and dermal restrictions are based on 31.4% total thujone content and thujone limits of 0.1 mg/kg and 0.25% (see Thujone profile, Chapter 14).

Organ-specific effects

Adverse skin reactions: No information found.
Neurotoxicity: No information found. There is a risk of convulsions with moderately high doses of thujone. The thujone NOAEL for convulsions was reported to be 10 mg/kg in male rats and 5 mg/kg in females (Margaria 1963).

Systemic effects

Acute toxicity: No information found. Both α- and β-thujone are moderately toxic, with reported oral LD_{50} values ranging from 190–500 mg/kg for different species (see Thujone profile, Chapter 14).
Antioxidant/pro-oxidant activity: Lanyana oil demonstrated radical scavenging activity in relation to both DPPH and hydroxyl radicals (Burits et al 2001).
Carcinogenic/anticarcinogenic potential: No information was found for lanyana oil, but it contains no known carcinogens.

Comments

There are *Artemisia afra* chemotypes which may not contain significant amounts of toxic constituents, but none of these are commercially available.

*Tentative identification

Larch needle

Synonyms: American larch, larch tamarack, hackmatack
Botanical name: *Larix laricina* Du Roi
Family: Pinaceae

Essential oil

Source: Needles (leaves)
Key constituents:

α-Pinene	38.5%
δ-3-Carene	14.0%
β-Pinene	10.2%
Bornyl acetate	7.9%
β-Phellandrene*	4.0%
Camphene	3.6%
(+)-Limonene	2.7%
β-Myrcene	2.5%
δ-Cadinene	2.1%
β-Caryophyllene	1.4%
Terpinolene	1.3%

(Mainguy, private communication 2001)

Safety summary

Hazards: Skin sensitization if oxidized.
Cautions: Old or oxidized oils should be avoided.

Our safety advice

Because of its α-pinene and δ-3-carene content we recommend that oxidation of larch needle oil is avoided by storage in a dark, airtight container in a refrigerator. The addition of an antioxidant to preparations containing it is recommended.

Regulatory guidelines

Essential oils derived from the *Pinaceae* family, including *Pinus* and *Abies* genera, should only be used when the level of peroxides is kept to the lowest practicable level, for example by the addition of antioxidants at the time of production (SCCNFP 2001a; IFRA 2009).

Organ-specific effects

Adverse skin reactions: No information was found for larch needle oil, but autoxidation products of α-pinene and δ-3-carene can cause skin sensitization (see Constituent profiles, Chapter 14).
Reproductive toxicity: The low reproductive toxicity of α-pinene and (+)-limonene (see Constituent profiles, Chapter 14) and the structural similarity of monoterpenes such as β-pinene and δ-3-carene suggest that larch needle oil is not hazardous in pregnancy.

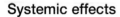

Systemic effects

Acute toxicity: No information found.
Carcinogenic/anticarcinogenic potential: No information was found for larch needle oil, but it contains no known carcinogens.

Comments

Limited availability.

Laurel berry

Botanical names: *Laurus nobilis* L., *Laurus novocanariensis* (previously *Laurus azorica*)
Family: Lauraceae

Essential oil/fixed oil

Source: Berries
Key constituents:

Volatile constituents (hydrodistilled Laurus nobilis *essential oil from Tunisia)*

(*E*)-β-Ocimene	23.7%
α-Pinene	10.3%
1,8-Cineole	8.1%
β-Longipinene	6.8%
β-Pinene	5.8%
Linalool	4.2%
δ-Cadinene	3.9%
Camphene	3.8%
(*Z*)-β-Ocimene	3.0%
α-Terpinyl acetate	3.0%
α-Bulnesene	2.7%
Sabinene	2.6%
Bornyl acetate	2.1%
trans-Cadinene*	2.1%
β-Cubebene	1.9%
(*E*)-Caryophyllene	1.9%
Germacrene D	1.8%
p-Mentha-1,5-dien-8-ol	1.5%
Spathulenol	1.4%
Linalyl acetate	1.3%
α-Cadinol	1.1%
5-Isocedranol	1.1%
Methyleugenol	1.0%

(Marzouki et al 2008)

Non-volatile constituents (cold-pressed Laurus novocanariensis *fixed oil from Madeira)*

Lauric acid	30.0%
Linoleic acid	25.6%
Oleic acid	22.1%
Palmitic acid	14.7%
Capric acid	1.3%
Linolenic acid	1.1%

(Castilho et al 2005)

Note: Laurel oil from *L. nobilis* is produced in Syria and Turkey; oil from *L. novocanariensis* is produced in Madeira. As made in Madeira, laurel berry oil is a combination of approximately 90% fixed oil, 10% essential oil (Castilho et al 2005). There may be less than 10% essential oil with different methods of preparation. The expressed oil of *Laurus novocanariensis* fruits contains 3.4–3.9% costunolide and 1.3–1.7% dehydrocostus lactone (Ferrari et al 2005).

Safety summary

Hazards: Skin sensitization.
Contraindications: Should not be used on the skin.

Regulatory guidelines

Laurus nobilis seed (i.e. berry) oil is prohibited as a cosmetic ingredient in the EU and Canada.

Organ-specific effects

Adverse skin reactions: Laurel berry oil (either cold-pressed, or produced as described below) was such a widely used and well-known item in Europe in the early 20th century, that it was simply known as 'laurel oil', but only a small percentage consisted of essential oil. It was used in popular skin preparations in France and Germany. Along with Switzerland, these were the countries reporting most cases of ACD to laurel oil. Of several thousand dermatitis patients tested in Germany between 1953 and 1962, 3.1%, 3.55%, 3.9% and 6.9% were allergic to 'laurel oil' in four reports cited by Foussereau et al (1967a). These, and similar reports, may have contributed to the current classification in Germany of laurel *leaf* essential oil as a high-risk skin allergen.

Systemic effects

Acute toxicity: No information found.
Carcinogenic/anticarcinogenic potential: Laurel berry oil contains 0.1% methyleugenol (1.0% methyleugenol is listed above, but the volatile constituents are only 10% of the total oil). Methyleugenol is a rodent carcinogen if exposure is sufficiently high.

Comments

Laurel oil skin allergy reached almost epidemic proportions in the mid-20th century and its use has declined considerably since then. A complete ban on use in cosmetics is understandable, though there may be a level that could be safely used. No dermatological testing has been carried out in recent times. Technically speaking, the EU ban only applies to oils produced from *L. nobilis*, and not to oils made from *L. novocanariensis*. The sesquiterpene lactones costunolide and dehydrocostus lactone are assumed to be responsible for skin reactions, and

---

*We are not familiar with this isomer of cadinene

paradoxically, these have only been identified in the oil from *L. novocanariensis*.

Laurel berries contain both fixed oil and essential oil, and the 'laurel oil' referred to in most pre-1960 literature was a combination of the two. It was widely used, and a common cause of skin allergy. Foussereau et al (1967a) reports that the dried and powdered berries were treated with steam and expressed to yield 30% of a "strong smelling thick oil" containing 1–3% of essential oil and resin. This was used both medicinally and non-medicinally. Occupational dermatitis was reported in "hatters, cooks, housewives, grocers, drysalters etc." The oil was used to condition felt hats and other felt garments, and most cases of allergy were to felt or laurel-based ointments. From about 1860 to 1960, most Westerners wore felt hats. In 1962, the use of laurel oil for conditioning felt ceased.

This is probably the same type of laurel oil referred to by Culpeper in 1652: 'The oil made of the berries is very comfortable in all cold griefs of the joints…by anointing the parts affected therewith…The oil takes away the marks of the skin and flesh by bruises, falls, &c.' It seems to have been in common use for several centuries in many European countries.

Laurel berry oil is still produced by traditional methods in Syria, with some production in Turkey and Madeira. It is used in soaps and cosmetics, and very little reaches the open market. 'In Syrian mountain communities, villagers collect laurel berries and manually extract the oil using traditional, multi-staged methods. The whole berries are boiled in water for six to eight hours in a metal container over a wood fire. As the oil rises to the surface, it is skimmed off with a wooden spoon then filtered and bottled. Sixteen kilograms of laurel berries produce about one liter of laurel oil…The extracted oil is sold to local soap makers and herbal traders, who then re-sell the oil at the city markets in Aleppo and Damascus.' (http://www.underutilized-species.org/species/brochures/Laurel.pdf accessed July 31st 2011).

For 50–100 years, laurel berry essential oil was steam distilled for perfumery use. In 1960, Arctander described it as 'Almost obsolete, but undoubtedly still imprinted in the minds of older perfumers.' Laurel berry concretes and absolutes have also been produced by French perfume manufacturers for in-house use. A laurel berry essential oil is sold by several internet-based suppliers, but this oil is from the berries of *Cinnamomum glaucescens* (see Sugandha profile). The words 'laurel' and 'bay' are among the most potentially confusing of all aromatic descriptors. 'Bay leaf oil' can refer to: *Laurus nobilis* leaves, *Pimenta dioica* leaves or *Pimenta racemosa* leaves. 'Laurel oil' *can refer to: Laurus nobilis* leaves, *Cinnamomum cecidodaphne* fruits or *Pimenta racemosa* fruits. 'Laurel' can also refer to: *Umbellularia californica*, *Prunus caroliniana*, *Prunus laurocerasus* or *Prunus lusitanica*.

Laurel leaf

Synonyms: Bay leaf, bay laurel, sweet bay
Botanical name: *Laurus nobilis* L.
Family: Lauraceae

Essential oil

Source: freshly picked leaves

Key constituents:

1,8-Cineole	38.1–43.5%
α-Pinene	7.1–15.9%
α-Terpinyl acetate	4.5–7.0%
Linalool	6.2–6.5%
β-Pinene	4.9–6.5%
Sabinene	4.5–6.5%
Methyleugenol	1.4–3.8%
Eugenol	1.2–3.0%
Camphene	0.7–2.9%
Linalyl acetate	0.4–2.7%
Bornyl acetate	0.4–2.3%
Terpinen-4-ol	2.1–2.2%
α-Terpineol	0.9–1.9%
β-Myrcene	0.7–1.5%
Borneol	0.1–1.5%
β-Caryophyllene	0.1–1.5%
Terpinolene	0.1–1.1%
γ-Terpinene	0–1.0%

(Lawrence 1995a p. 51–52)

Safety summary

Hazards: Potentially carcinogenic, based on methyleugenol content; essential oils high in 1,8-cineole can cause CNS and breathing problems in young children; skin sensitization (low risk); mucous membrane irritation (low risk).
Cautions (dermal): Hypersensitive, diseased or damaged skin, children under 2 years of age. Some laurel leaf oils may cause skin sensitization.
Maximum adult daily oral dose: 18 mg
Maximum dermal use level:

EU	0.005%
IFRA	0.01%
Tisserand & Young	0.5%

Our safety advice

We recommend a dermal maximum of 0.5% and an oral maximum of 18 mg, based on 3.8% methyleugenol content with dermal and oral limits of 0.02% and 0.01 mg/kg (see Methyleugenol profile, Chapter 14).

Regulatory guidelines

IFRA recommends that the maximum concentration of methyleugenol for leave-on products such as body lotion should be 0.0004% (IFRA 2009). The equivalent SCCNFP maximum is 0.0002% (European Commission 2002).

Organ-specific effects

Adverse skin reactions: In a 48 hour occlusive patch test on 50 Italian volunteers, undiluted laurel leaf oil produced no adverse reactions. Similarly tested at 1%, it produced no reactions in 380 eczema patients (Meneghini et al 1971). Undiluted laurel leaf oil was moderately irritating to rabbits, but was not irritating to mice or pigs. Tested at 2% on 25 volunteers it was not irritating, nor was it irritating when re-tested at 10%. A second sample of laurel leaf oil was not irritating when tested at 10% on two separate panels of volunteers. Laurel leaf oil was non-phototoxic in hairless mice and swine (Opdyke 1976 p. 337–338). Laurel leaf *absolute* was phototoxic at 10% or over, but not at 2% (Bouhlal et al 1988b).

Neither of two different laurel leaf oils were sensitizing when tested on separate panels of 25 volunteers, one at 2% and one at 10%. A third sample was not sensitizing in either of two further panels of volunteers when tested at 10%. When laurel leaf oil was tested at 10% on six costus-sensitized individuals, there were positive reactions in all six (Opdyke 1976 p. 337–338). Four of 747 dermatitis patients suspected of fragrance allergy (0.54%) reacted to 2% laurel leaf oil (Wöhrl et al 2001). In a multicenter study, Germany's IVDK reported that 62 of 6,297 dermatitis patients suspected of fragrance allergy (0.98%) tested positive to 2% laurel leaf oil (Uter et al 2010).

There are many case reports of contact dermatitis from laurel leaf oil (Adisen & Onder 2007; Athanasiadis et al 2007, Foussereau 1963; Foussereau et al 1967a, 1967b, 1975; Özden et al 2001). Some laurel leaf oils are thought to contain small amounts of costunolide (De Smet et al 1992). However, it is likely that costunolide is not the allergen responsible for most reactions to this essential oil (Foussereau et al 1975). An individual known to be allergic to oakmoss had a +++ reaction to 10% laurel leaf oil in acetone (Benezra et al 1978).

Systemic effects

Acute toxicity: Laurel leaf oil acute oral LD_{50} in rats 3.95 g/kg; acute dermal LD_{50} in rabbits >5 g/kg (Opdyke 1976 p. 337–338). 1,8-Cineole has been reported to cause serious poisoning in young children when accidentally instilled into the nose (Melis et al 1989).

Antioxidant/pro-oxidant activity: A laurel leaf oil showed moderate antioxidant activity in scavenging DPPH radicals and inhibiting lipid peroxidation (Ferreira et al 2006).

Carcinogenic/anticarcinogenic potential: Laurel leaf oil containing 2.5% methyleugenol was active against human melanoma, renal cell adenocarcinoma, and human chronic myelogenous leukemia cell lines in vitro (Loizzo et al 2007, Saab et al 2012b). Methyleugenol is a rodent carcinogen if exposure is sufficiently high (see Methyleugenol profile, Chapter 14).

Comments

Laurel leaves contain various sesquiterpene lactones, some of them known skin sensitizers. These include costunolide and deacetyl laurenobiolide; dehydrocostuslactone was indentified in a laurel leaf concrete (Tada & Takeda 1976; Cheminat et al 1984). It is not clear from the literature whether or not laurel leaf oil is likely to cause sensitization problems. This may be because some laurel leaf oils contain sensitizing agents and others do not. Some fragrance houses internally restrict the use of laurel leaf oil because of customer sensitization issues (Burfield 2004). Based on literature published in German, laurel leaf oil has been classified as category A, a significant contact allergen (Schlede et al 2003).

The species is known in three forms: *nobilis*, *angustifolius* and *crispa*. Laurel leaf oil should not be confused with the leaf oil of *Pimenta racemosa*, West Indian bay oil, used in 'bay rum', and also known as bay leaf oil. There is potential for confusion between 'laurel oil' (produced by solvent extraction of the leaves) and 'laurel essential oil' (produced by steam distillation of the leaves) (Foussereau et al 1975). A laurel leaf absolute is also produced. No information was found about either its composition or its safety. There is also a cold-pressed laurel *berry* oil (see previous profile).

Lavandin

Botanical name: *Lavandula x intermedia* Emeric ex Loisel.
Botanical synonyms: *Lavandula hybrida* Reverchon, *Lavandula hortensis* Hy
Family: Lamiaceae (Labiatae)

Absolute

Source: Flowering tops
Key constituents:

Linalool	42.0%
Coumarin	5.0%
Geraniol	1.5%
(+)-Limonene	1.0%

(EFFA 2008)

Safety summary

Hazards: Skin sensitization (moderate risk).
Contraindications: None known.
Maximum dermal use level: 0.03%

Our safety advice

The dermal maximum is based on the 0.03% found by Bouhlal et al (1988b) to be the highest concentration producing no adverse skin reactions.

Organ-specific effects

Adverse skin reactions: Undiluted lavandin absolute produced slight erythema and edema in guinea pig skin; moderate erythema and edema were seen in one rabbit during a dermal LD_{50} study; it was not irritating to mice or pigs. Tested at 10% on 25 volunteers it was neither irritating nor sensitizing. It is non-phototoxic (Ford et al 1992 p. 65S). Tested at 2, 5 and 10% on 25 volunteers with a previous history of reaction to fragrance materials, lavandin absolute produced allergic reactions in 9, 10 and 11 individuals, respectively. In this high-risk group, 0.03% was the concentration at which any observable reaction disappeared (Bouhlal et al 1988b).

Systemic effects

Acute toxicity: Non-toxic. Lavandin absolute acute oral LD_{50} in rats >5 g/kg; acute dermal LD_{50} in rabbits >5 g/kg (Ford et al 1992 p. 65S).

Carcinogenic/anticarcinogenic potential: No information found.

Comments

This species is the natural and artificial hybrid of *Lavandula angustifolia* x *Lavandula latifolia*.

Essential oil

Source: Flowering tops
Key constituents:

Lavandin Abrialis

Linalool	30.0–38.0%
Linalyl acetate	20.0–30.0%
Camphor	7.0–11.0%
1,8-Cineole	6.0–11.0%
(E)-β-Ocimene	3.0–7.0%
Borneol	2.0–4.0%
(Z)-β-Ocimene	1.5–4.0%
Lavandulyl acetate	1.0–2.0%
Lavandulol	0.5–1.5%
Terpinen-4-ol	<1.0%

(Lawrence 1989 p. 241–243)

Lavandin Grosso

Linalyl acetate	26.2–37.5%
Linalool	22.5–28.0%
Camphor	6.6–12.2%
1,8-Cineole	5.2–10.2%
Terpinen-4-ol	0–3.3%
Borneol	2.4–2.9%
β-Caryophyllene	1.9–2.7%
Lavandulyl acetate	2.3–2.4%
(Z)-β-Farnesene	1.1–1.6%
β-Myrcene	0–1.5%
Geranyl acetate	0–1.2%
α-Terpineol	0–1.2%
(Z)-β-Ocimene	0.9–1.1%
Germacrene D	0–1.1%

(Naef & Morris 1992; Milchard et al 2004)

Lavandin Super

Linalyl acetate	38.6–44.3%
Linalool	29.4–32.7%
Camphor	4.5–5.3%
1,8-Cineole	3.0–3.6%
Borneol	1.7–2.9%
Lavandulyl acetate	1.5–1.7%
(Z)-β-Ocimene	1.5%
β-Caryophyllene	1.4%
(E)-β-Ocimene	1.3%

(Lawrence 2001a p. 45; Milchard et al 2004)

Safety summary

Hazards: Drug interaction; may inhibit blood clotting.

Cautions (oral): Anticoagulant medication, major surgery, peptic ulcer, hemophilia, other bleeding disorders (Box 7.1).

Regulatory guidelines

Has GRAS status. According to IFRA, essential oils rich in linalool should only be used when the level of peroxides is kept to the lowest practical value. The addition of antioxidants such as 0.1% BHT or α-tocopherol at the time of production is recommended (IFRA 2009).

Organ-specific effects

Adverse skin reactions: Undiluted lavandin oil (type unspecified) was slightly irritating to rabbits, but was not irritating to mice or pigs; tested at 5% on 25 volunteers it was neither irritating nor sensitizing. It is non-phototoxic (Opdyke 1976 p. 447). In a study of 200 consecutive dermatitis patients, one (0.5%) was sensitive to 2% lavandin oil on patch testing (Rudzki et al 1976). In a group of 100 consecutive dermatitis patients there were no irritant or allergic reactions to 1% lavandin oil. In a second similar group there was one irritant reaction and no allergic reactions to 5% lavandin oil (Frosch et al 1995a). Oxidation products of linalool may be skin sensitizing. 1,8-Cineole has antioxidant properties.
Cardiovascular effects: Lavandin Grosso oil inhibited platelet aggregation induced by arachidonic acid, U46619, collagen and ADP, with IC_{50} values of 51, 84, 191 and 640 µg/mL, respectively (Ballabeni et al 2004).

Systemic effects

Acute toxicity: Lavandin oil acute oral LD_{50} in rats >5 g/kg; acute dermal LD_{50} in rabbits >5 g/kg (Opdyke 1976 p. 447).
Carcinogenic/anticarcinogenic potential: No information was found for lavandin oil, but it contains no known carcinogens.
Drug interactions: Anticoagulant medication, because of cardiovascular effects, above. See Table 4.10B.

Comments

Abrialis and Grosso are the two principal cultivars of lavandin grown for essential oil production. Lavandin Abrialis has the highest 1,8-cineole content, lavandin Super is the sweetest and most similar to the oil from *Lavandula angustifolia*, and Grosso has the highest essential oil yield. Lavandin is the natural and artificial hybrid of *Lavandula angustifolia* and *Lavandula latifolia*.

Lavender

Synonyms: Common lavender, English lavender
Botanical name: *Lavandula angustifolia* Mill.
Botanical synonyms: *Lavandula officinalis* Chaix in Villars, *Lavandula vera* DC
Family: Lamiaceae (Labiatae)

Absolute

Source: Flowering tops
Key constituents:

Linalyl actetate	44.7%
Linalool	28.0%
Coumarin	4.3%
β-Caryophyllene	3.2%
Geranyl acetate	2.7%
Terpinen-4-ol	2.7%
Herniarin (7-methoxycoumarin)	2.3%
(E)-β-Farnesene	1.2%
Camphor	1.2%
1-Octen-3-yl acetate	1.1%

(Jones, private communication, 2002)

Safety summary

Hazards: Skin sensitization (moderate risk).
Contraindications: None known.
Maximum dermal use level: 0.1%

Our safety advice

The dermal maximum of 0.1% is based on the 0.12% found by Bouhlal et al (1988b) to be the highest concentration producing no adverse skin reactions.

Organ-specific effects

Adverse skin reactions: Undiluted lavender absolute was slightly irritating to rabbits; tested at 10% on 25 volunteers it was neither irritating nor sensitizing (Opdyke 1976 p. 449). Tested at 2, 5 and 10% on 25 volunteers with a previous history of reaction to fragrance materials, lavender absolute produced allergic reactions in 7, 11 and 13 individuals, respectively. In this high-risk group, 0.12% was the concentration at which any observable reaction disappears (Bouhlal et al 1988b). The cause of facial dermatitis in a physiotherapist was due to a pharmaceutical gel she often used on patients. She also reacted to 2% lavender absolute, which was present in the gel (Rademaker 1995). Two cases of facial dermatitis are reported following the nightly application of a few drops of undiluted lavender oil to the bed pillow as a sedative; both tested positive to 2% lavender absolute (Coulson and Khan 1999). An eczema patient using an aromatherapy lavender gel tested positive to 10% lavender absolute, but not to 2% (Varma et al 2000).
Carcinogenic/anticarcinogenic potential: No information found. Coumarin is carcinogenic in rodents, but is anticarcinogenic in humans (Felter et al 2006).

Systemic effects

Acute toxicity: Lavender absolute acute oral LD_{50} in rats 4.25 g/kg; acute dermal LD_{50} in guinea pigs >5 g/kg (Opdyke 1976 p. 449).

Comments

Lavender absolute causes more skin reactions than lavender oil, but it is not known which constituent(s) may be responsible for this. Dermal application of coumarin is not hazardous (see Coumarin profile, Chapter 14).

Essential oil

Source: Flowering tops
Key constituents:

Australian

Linalool	39.1% (25–38%)
Linalyl acetate	36.2% (25–45%)
(Z)-β-Ocimene	4.3% (3–9%)
Terpinen-4-ol	3.0% (1.5–6%)
3-Octanone	2.9% (2–5%)
β-Caryophyllene	2.6%
Lavandulyl acetate	2.5% (>1.0%)
3-Octanyl acetate	1.8%

(Schmidt 2003)

Bulgarian

Linalyl acetate	46.6% (30–42%)
Linalool	27.1% (22–34%)
(Z)-β-Ocimene	5.5% (3–9%)
Lavandulyl acetate	4.7% (2–5%)
Terpinen-4-ol	4.6% (2–5%)
β-Caryophyllene	4.1%
(E)-β-Farnesene	2.4%
(E)-β-Ocimene	2.2% (2–5%)
3-Octanyl acetate	1.1%

(Schmidt 2003)

French

Linalool	44.4% (30–45%)
Linalyl acetate	41.6% (33–46%)
Lavandulyl acetate	3.7% (<1.3%)
β-Caryophyllene	1.8%
Terpinen-4-ol	1.5% (<1.5%)
Borneol	1.0%
α-Terpineol	0.7% (<1.5%)
(Z)-β-Ocimene	0.3% (<2.5%)
3-Octanone	0.2% (1–2.5%)
(E)-β-Ocimene	0.1% (<2%)

(Schmidt 2003)

Moldovan

Linalyl acetate	38.6% (29–44%)
Linalool	34.0% (20–35%)
(Z)-β-Ocimene	5.5% (3–8%)
β-Caryophyllene	3.9%
Lavandulyl acetate	2.5% (1–3.5%
Terpinen-4-ol	2.0% (1.2–5%)

1,8-Cineole	1.6% (<2.5%)
(E)-β-Farnesene	1.6%
(E)-β-Ocimene	1.3% (2–5%)
α-Terpineol	1.1% (0.5–2%)
3-Octanyl acetate	1.1%

(Schmidt 2003)

Ukranian

Linalyl acetate	43.3% (29–44%)
Linalool	27.5% (20–35%)
β-Caryophyllene	5.9%
(Z)-β-Ocimene	4.2% (3–8%)
(E)-β-Ocimene	2.4% (2–5%)
Lavandulyl acetate	2.1% (1–3.5%
Terpinen-4-ol	2.1% (1.2–5%)
(E)-β-Farnesene	2.0%
1,8-Cineole	1.5%
3-Octanyl acetate	1.1%
Borneol	1.0%
α-Terpineol	0.6% (0.5–2%)

(Schmidt 2003)

Note: The figures in parentheses are the ISO standards for lavender oil (© ISO 2002). For French lavender the ISO standard for clonal lavender is given here, there is a different standard for 'population' lavender. ISO have a single standard for 'Russian Federation'.

Quality: Lavender oil is often adulterated with lavandin oil. Other possible adulterants include spike lavender oil, Spanish sage oil, white camphor oil fractions, rectified or acetylated ho oil, acetylated lavandin oil, synthetic linalool and linalyl acetate (Kubeczka 2002; Burfield 2003). The linalool content of lavender oil should comprise at least 85% of the (R)-(–)- enantiomer, and the linalyl acetate content should comprise at least 98% of the (R)-(–)- enantiomer (http://www.users.globalnet.co.uk/~nodice/new/magazine/october/october.htm, accessed 5th August 2012).

Safety summary

Hazards: None known.
Contraindications: None known.

Regulatory guidelines

Has GRAS status. According to IFRA, essential oils rich in linalool should only be used when the level of peroxides is kept to the lowest practical value. The addition of antioxidants such as 0.1% BHT or α-tocopherol at the time of production is recommended (IFRA 2009).

Organ-specific effects

Adverse skin reactions: In a 48 hour occlusive patch test on 50 Italian volunteers, undiluted lavender oil produced no adverse reactions. Similarly tested at 1%, it produced no reactions in 273 eczema patients (Meneghini et al 1971). The undiluted oil was slightly irritating to rabbits, but was not irritating to mice

or pigs; tested at 10% on 25 volunteers it was neither irritating nor sensitizing (Opdyke 1976 p. 451). In a modified Draize procedure on guinea pigs, lavender oil was non-sensitizing when used at 30% in the challenge phase (Sharp 1978). Oxidation products of linalool may be skin sensitizing (see Linalool profile, Chapter 14). There is one confirmed report of photoallergy to lavender oil, tested at 2% (Goiriz et al 2007). However, lavender oil is not phototoxic (Opdyke 1976 p. 451).

In a study of 200 consecutive dermatitis patients, none were sensitive to 2% lavender oil on patch testing (Rudzki et al 1976). In a Danish study, two of 217 consecutive dermatitis patients (0.9%) tested positive to 2% lavender oil (Veien et al 2004). In a worldwide multicenter study, of 218 dermatitis patients with proven sensitization to fragrance materials, six (2.8%) were sensitive to 10% lavender oil (Larsen et al 2002). Lavender oil is regarded as a high-risk skin sensitizer in Japan (Nakayama 1998), possibly due to a rise in the incidence of positive patch test results. From 1990 to 1996 the average patch test positivity rate to 20% lavender oil in a total of 1,483 Japanese eczema patients (99% female) suspected of cosmetic sensitivity was 1.4%, but in 1997 it was 8.7%, and by 1998 had risen to 13.9% (Sugiura et al 2000). This dramatic increase has been attributed to a fashion for introducing dried lavender flowers into the home. A much more likely explanation is that it was due to oxidation of the test material being used (Matura et al 2005).

An 18-year-old female hairdresser with hand dermatitis had a ++ reaction when patch tested with 1% lavender oil in ethanol. She had been using a shampoo containing lavender oil several times a day (Brandão 1986). An aromatherapist who developed hand eczema tested positive to 2% lavender oil (Keane et al 2000). Dermatitis of the face and chest in a 39-year-old woman resolved after she stopped using essential oil based personal care products, including a spray perfume said to include lavender oil. No causative substance was identified (Weiss & James 1997).

In cases of multiple sensitivity, a 65-year-old aromatherapist with widespread dermatitis showed marked sensitivity to thirteen essential oils including a ++ reaction to 1% lavender oil (Selvaag et al 1995); a dermatitis patient was sensitive to five essential oils including lavender (De Groot 1996); another tested positive to six essential oils, including 1% lavender oil (Schaller & Korting 1995). There is evidence of an antiallergic action in lavender oil. Topically applied, the oil concentration-dependently inhibited immediate-type allergic reactions in rats and mice by inhibiting the release of histamine and TNF-α by mast cells (Kim & Cho 1999).

Reproductive toxicity: Lavender oil is estrogenic in vitro (Henley et al 2007) but is not estrogenic in vivo (Politano et al 2013). See discussion in Chapter 11, p. 151. Inhaled lavender oil (1 mL/hour) attenuated the damage caused by inhaled formaldehyde (10 ppm/hour) to male rat sperm count and motility (Köse et al 2011).

Systemic effects

Acute toxicity: Non-toxic. Lavender oil acute oral LD_{50} 6.5 g/kg in mice (Altaei 2012), >5 g/kg in rats; acute dermal LD_{50} in rabbits >5 g/kg (Opdyke 1976 p. 451). Lavender oil was not

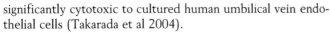
significantly cytotoxic to cultured human umbilical vein endothelial cells (Takarada et al 2004).

Antioxidant/pro-oxidant activity: Lavender oil showed moderate antioxidant activity as a DPPH radical scavenger and low activity in the aldehyde/carboxylic acid assay (Wei & Shibamoto 2007a).

Carcinogenic/anticarcinogenic potential: Lavender oil was not mutagenic in *S. typhimurium* strains TA98 and TA100, or on *E. coli* WP2 uvrA strain, either with or without metabolic activation. The oil was dose-dependently antimutagenic, reducing mutant colonies in the TA98 strain exposed to 2-nitrofuorene, and was moderately antimutagenic when the same strain was exposed to 1-nitropyrene (Evandri et al 2005). De Martino et al (2009a) also found lavender oil non-mutagenic in T98 and T100 with or without S9. Lavender oil showed moderate chemopreventive activity against human mouth epidermal carcinoma (KB) and mouse leukemia (P388) cell lines, with respective IC_{50} values of 0.445 and 0.206 mg/mL (Manosroi et al 2005). Lavender oil was cytotoxic to human prostate, lung and breast cancer cells with IC_{50} values of 0.05%, 0.13% and 0.14%, respectively (Zu et al 2010). Lavender oil contains no known carcinogens.

Comments

Considering the high usage of lavender oil on the skin in aromatherapy, the reported incidence of skin reactions is low. All the cultivars of *Lavandula angustifolia* are selections of subsp. *angustifolia* (Craker & Simon 1986 p. 54). The values given by Schmidt (2003) are for the mean composition of 46 oils over five years (Australia), 30 oils over two years (Bulgaria), 200 oils over 15 years (France), six oils (Moldova) and 22 oils (Ukraine). All are from clonal lavenders. The Australian lavender oil industry has only developed seriously since the mid-1990s, and the oil is chemically and odoriferously distinct from European lavender oils. Lavender oil is also commercially produced on a small scale in several other countries, including Croatia, England, India and Italy. Moldovan and Ukranian lavender used to be known as 'Russian'.

Lavender cotton

Synonyms: Cotton lavender, santolina
Botanical name: *Santolina chamaecyparissus* L.
Family: Asteraceae (Compositae)

Essential oil

Source: Seeds
Key constituents:

Artemisia ketone	30.6–45.0%
β-Phellandrene	5.0–17.9%
β-Myrcene	3.6–15.0%
Longiverbenone	9.1–10.2%
Sabinene	3.9–5.5%
β-Pinene	2.9–5.2%
Camphene	0.6–3.0%
Camphor	1.5–2.6%

Terpinolene	0.8–2.3%
1,8-Cineole	tr–2.0%
γ-Curcumene	0–1.9%
Longipinene	1.3–1.8%
ar-Curcumene	0.1–1.7%
Artemisia alcohol	1.1–1.5%
Borneol	0.8–1.5%
(+)-Limonene	0.8–1.5%
Yomogi alcohol	0–1.3%
Germacrene D	0.4–1.1%
α-Thujene	0–1.0%

(Vernin 1991; Lawrence 1995g p. 57–59)

Safety summary

Hazards: None known.
Contraindications: None known.

Regulatory guidelines

In 2006 lavender cotton oil was placed on the IFRA list of prohibited materials, due to insufficient safety information (IFRA 2009).

Organ-specific effects

Adverse skin reactions: No information found.

Systemic effects

Acute toxicity: No information found. An annual wormwood oil containing 35.7% artemisia ketone had a mouse i.p. LD50 of 1,832 mg/kg. Doses higher than 1,500 mg/kg were neurototic, but lower doses were not (Radulovic et al 2013).
Carcinogenic/anticarcinogenic potential: No information was found for lavender cotton oil, but it contains no known carcinogens.

Comments

Limited availability. IFRA placed santolina oil on its list of prohibited materials, not because of any information about toxicity, but because of a lack of information about toxicity. However, the new data on annual wormwood oil suggests that any concerns about artemisia ketone or lavender cotton oil toxicity are probably misplaced.

Lavender (Spanish)

Synonyms: French lavender, maritime lavender
Botanical name: *Lavandula stoechas* L. ssp. *stoechas*
Family: Lamiaceae (Labiatae)

Essential oil

Source: Flowering tops
Key constituents:

Camphor	16.4–56.2%
(+)-Fenchone	14.9–49.1%

1,8-Cineole	3.6–14.5%
α-Pinene	3.4–4.5%
Camphene	2.8–5.5%
Myrtenyl acetate	2.0–4.3%
Bornyl acetate	1.8–3.1%
Linalool	0.8–2.2%
Myrtenol	0.6–2.4%
δ-3-Carene	tr–1.9%
(+)-Limonene	1.0–1.4%
Ledol	0.5–1.2%

(Ristorcelli et al 1998)

Safety summary

Hazards: May be neurotoxic, based on camphor content.
Contraindications (all routes): Pregnancy, breastfeeding.
Maximum adult daily oral dose: 250 mg
Maximum dermal use level: 8%

Our safety advice

Our oral and dermal restrictions are based on 56.2% camphor content and camphor limits of 2 mg/kg/day and 4.5% (see Camphor profile, Chapter 14).

Organ-specific effects

Adverse skin reactions: No information found. Fenchone is relatively non-irritant and non-sensitizing (Opdyke 1976 p. 769–771).

Systemic effects

Acute toxicity: No information found. The rat acute oral LD_{50} for fenchone is 6.16 g/kg (Jenner et al 1964). Camphor minimum LD_{50} is 1.7 g/kg in rats (Christensen & Lynch 1937). Camphor is potentially neurotoxic and is thought to be more toxic in humans than in rodents (see Camphor profile, Chapter 14).
Carcinogenic/anticarcinogenic potential: No information was found for Spanish lavender oil, but it contains no known carcinogens.

Comments

The camphor content is significantly higher than that of true lavender oil (<1%). Mainly produced in Portugal, though the analysis above is from Corsican oils. Six subspecies are known, *stoechas* being the most important (Craker & Simon 1986 p. 55).

Lavender (spike)

Synonym: Spike
Botanical name: *Lavandula latifolia* Medic.
Botanical synonym: *Lavandula spica* DC
Family: Lamiaceae (Labiatae)

Essential oil

Source: Flowering tops
Key constituents:

Linalool	27.2–43.1%
1,8-Cineole	28.0–34.9%
Camphor	10.8–23.2%
Borneol	0.9–3.6%
β-Pinene	0.8–2.6%
(E)-α-Bisabolene	0.5–2.3%
α-Pinene	0.6–1.9%
β-Caryophyllene	0.5–1.9%
α-Terpineol	0.8–1.6%
Germacrene D	0.3–1.0%

(Salido et al 2004)
Quality: Spike lavender oil may be adulterated with Spanish sage oil, eucalyptus oil, lavandin oil, and fractions of these and other cheap oils (Kubeczka 2002).

Safety summary

Hazards: May be mildly neurotoxic, based on camphor content.
Contraindications: None known.
Maximum daily oral dose: 603 mg
Maximum dermal use level: 19%

Our safety advice

Our oral and dermal restrictions are based on 23.2% camphor content with camphor limits of 2.0 mg/kg/day and 4.5% (see Camphor profile, Chapter 14).

Regulatory guidelines

Has GRAS status. According to IFRA, essential oils rich in linalool should only be used when the level of peroxides is kept to the lowest practical value. The addition of antioxidants such as 0.1% BHT or α-tocopherol at the time of production is recommended (IFRA 2009).

Organ-specific effects

Adverse skin reactions: Undiluted spike lavender oil was moderately irritating to rabbits; tested at 8% on 25 volunteers it was neither irritating nor sensitizing (Opdyke 1976 p. 453). In a study of 200 consecutive dermatitis patients, one (0.5%) was sensitive to 2% spike lavender oil on patch testing (Rudzki et al 1976). Oxidation products of linalool may be skin sensitizing, but 1,8-cineole has antioxidant properties (see Constituent profiles, Chapter 14).
Reproductive toxicity: The low reproductive toxicity of linalool, 1,8-cineole and camphor (see Constituent profiles, Chapter 14) suggests that spike lavender oil is not hazardous in pregnancy.

Systemic effects

Acute toxicity: Spike lavender oil acute oral LD_{50} in rats 3.8 g/kg; acute dermal LD_{50} in rabbits >2 g/kg

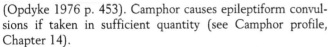

(Opdyke 1976 p. 453). Camphor causes epileptiform convulsions if taken in sufficient quantity (see Camphor profile, Chapter 14).

Carcinogenic/anticarcinogenic potential: No information was found for spike lavender oil, but it contains no known carcinogens.

Comments

Camphor content is significantly higher than that of true lavender oil. Spike lavender is slightly more toxic and more irritant. Since linalool is anticonvulsant, it may mitigate the neurotoxicity of camphor in spike lavender oil.

Leek

Botanical name: *Allium porrum* L.
Family: Liliaceae

Essential oil

Source: Aerial parts
Key constituents:

Dipropyl disulfide	34.0%
Dipropyl trisulfide	19.5%
Propyl allyl disulfide	8.1%
Methyl propyl trisulfide	3.9%
Methyl propyl disulfide	3.1%
Dipropyl tetrasulfide	3.0%
Methyl allyl sulfide	2.5%
Octadecanoic acid	2.2%
Dipropenyl trisulfide	2.1%
Dipropenyl tetrasulfide	1.9%

(Abisset, private communication, 2004)

Safety summary

Hazards: Drug interaction; may inhibit blood clotting; skin sensitization.
Cautions (oral): Anticoagulant medication, major surgery, peptic ulcer, hemophilia, other bleeding disorders (Box 7.1).
Cautions (dermal): Use with caution on skin, especially if hypersensitive, diseased or damaged.

Organ-specific effects

Adverse skin reactions: No information found for leek oil or its two major constituents. Since garlic oil is moderately skin sensitizing, there is a suspicion that other essential oils rich in sulfur compounds might present a similar risk.
Cardiovascular effects: Onion oil possesses significant antiplatelet activity (see Onion profile). Since onion and leek oils share over 60% of their constituents, it seems likely that leek oil will possess a similar action.

Systemic effects

Acute toxicity: No information found for leek oil or its two major constituents.

Carcinogenic/anticarcinogenic potential: No information found for leek oil, but it contains no known carcinogens.
Drug interactions: Anticoagulant medication, because of cardiovascular effects, above. See Table 4.10B.

Comments

Safe levels for dermal application of leek oil are not known, but essential oils of the *Allium* genus are rarely used on the skin.

Lemon (distilled)

Botanical name: *Citrus x limon* L.
Botanical synonym: *Citrus limonum* Risso
Family: Rutaceae

Essential oil

Source: Fruit peel, by distillation
Key constituents:

(+)-Limonene	64.0–70.5%
β-Pinene	8.2–14.0%
γ-Terpinene	8.4–10.7%
Geranial	0.7–2.2%
α-Pinene	1.1–2.1%
Sabinene	0.8–1.7%
β-Myrcene + methyl heptenone	1.4–1.6%
Neral	0.5–1.5%

(Lawrence 1993 p. 62)

Safety summary

Hazards: Skin sensitization if oxidized.
Cautions: Old or oxidized oils should be avoided.
Maximum dermal use level: 20%

Our safety advice

Our dermal maximum is based on 3% citral content with a citral limit of 0.6% (see Citral profile, Chapter 14). Because of its (+)-limonene content we recommend that oxidation of distilled lemon oil is avoided by storage in a dark, airtight container in a refrigerator. The addition of an antioxidant to preparations containing it is recommended.

Regulatory guidelines

IFRA recommends that essential oils rich in limonene should only be used when the level of peroxides is kept to the lowest practical level, for instance by adding antioxidants at the time of production (IFRA 2009).

Organ-specific effects

Adverse skin reactions: Undiluted distilled lemon oil was moderately irritating to rabbits, and was slightly irritating to mice; tested at 10% on 25 volunteers it was neither irritating nor sensitizing. It is non-phototoxic (Opdyke 1974 p. 727).

Autoxidation products of (+)-limonene can cause skin sensitization (see (+)-Limonene profile, Chapter 14).

Reproductive toxicity: The low developmental toxicity of (+)-limonene, β-pinene, α-pinene and sabinene (see Constituent profiles, Chapter 14) suggests that distilled lemon oil is not hazardous in pregnancy.

Systemic effects

Acute toxicity: Distilled lemon oil acute oral LD_{50} in rats >5 g/kg; acute dermal LD_{50} in rabbits >5 g/kg (Opdyke 1974 p. 727).

Carcinogenic/anticarcinogenic potential: No information was found for distilled lemon oil, but see lemon (expressed) below. The oil contains no known carcinogens. Citral (geranial + neral) and (+)-limonene display anticarcinogenic activity (see Constituent profiles, Chapter 14).

Comments

Distilled lemon oil is generally used in flavoring, rather than fragrances. It is regarded as having an inferior odor to the expressed oil.

Lemon (expressed)

Botanical name: *Citrus x limon* L.
Botanical synonym: *Citrus limonum* Risso
Family: Rutaceae

Essential oil

Source: Fruit peel, by expression
Key constituents:

(+)-Limonene	56.6–76.0%
β-Pinene	6.0–17.0%
γ-Terpinene	3.0–13.3%
α-Terpineol	0.1–8.0%
α-Pinene	1.3–4.4%
Geranial	0.5–4.3%
Sabinene	0.5–2.4%
p-Cymene	tr–2.3%
β-Myrcene	tr–2.2%
Neral	0.4–2.0%
Terpinen-4-ol	tr–1.9%
Neryl acetate	0.1–1.5%

(Lawrence 1993 p. 61–69, 1995g p1–4, p158–162, 1996a p41–45, 2002b p62–88)

Non-volatile compounds

Oxypeucedanin	0.09–0.82%
Bergamottin	0.16–0.54%
5-Geranoxy-7-methoxycoumarin	0.18–0.28%
Citropten	0.05–0.17%
Byakangelicol	0.006–0.16%
8-Geranyloxypsoralen	0.01–0.045%
Bergapten	0.0001–0.035%
Isopimpinellin	0–0.011%

(Lawrence 2002b p62–88; SCCP 2005b)

Quality: Lemon oil may be adulterated with natural or synthetic limonene, natural or synthetic citral, and numerous other cheap products (Kubeczka 2002). These may include orange terpenes, lemon terpenes or by-products (Burfield 2003).

Safety summary

Hazards: Skin sensitization if oxidized; phototoxic (low risk).
Contraindications (dermal): If applied to the skin at over maximum use level, skin must not be exposed to sunlight or sunbed rays for 12 hours.
Cautions: Old or oxidized oils should be avoided.
Maximum dermal use level: 2.0% (see Regulatory Guidelines).

Our safety advice

Because of its (+)-limonene content we recommend that oxidation of lemon oil is avoided by storage in a dark, airtight container in a refrigerator. The addition of an antioxidant to preparations containing it is recommended.

Regulatory guidelines

Has GRAS status. In Europe, essential oils containing furanocoumarins must be used so that the total level of bergapten will not exceed: (a) 15 ppm in finished cosmetic products intended for application to skin areas likely to be exposed to sunshine, excluding rinse-off products; or (b) 1 ppm in sun protection and in bronzing products. In the presence of other phototoxic ingredients, the sum of their concentrations (expressed as % of the respective maximum levels) shall not exceed 100% (SCCNFP 2000).

IFRA recommends that, for application to areas of skin exposed to sunshine, expressed lemon oil be limited to a maximum of 2% in products applied to the skin except for bath preparations, soaps and other wash-off products (IFRA 2009). IFRA also recommends that essential oils rich in limonene should only be used when the level of peroxides is kept to the lowest practical level, for instance by adding antioxidants at the time of production (IFRA 2009).

Organ-specific effects

Adverse skin reactions: Undiluted expressed lemon oil was moderately irritating to rabbits and three different lemon oils were mildly irritating to mice but three further samples were not. Tested at 10% or 100% on two panels of 25 volunteers expressed lemon oil was not irritating. In a modified Draize procedure on guinea pigs, lemon oil was non-sensitizing when used at 20% in the challenge phase (Sharp 1978). Tested at 10% on 25 volunteers it was not sensitizing (Opdyke 1974 p725–726).

In a study of 200 consecutive dermatitis patients, one was sensitive to 2% lemon oil on patch testing (Rudzki et al 1976). Two of 747 dermatitis patients suspected of fragrance allergy (0.27%) reacted to 2% lemon oil (Wöhrl et al 2001). In a multicenter study, Germany's IVDK reported that 19 of 6,467 dermatitis patients (0.29%) suspected of fragrance allergy tested positive to 2% lemon oil. There were only 4 or 5 ++ or +++ reactions (Uter et al 2010). This suggests that (presumably unoxidized) lemon oil is virtually non-allergenic. A 65-year-old aromatherapist with multiple essential oil sensitivities reacted to 5%, but not 1% lemon oil (Selvaag et al 1995). A 47-year-old man who handled lemons as a barman developed hand eczema. Patch testing revealed allergies to lemon oil, lemongrass oil and geraniol (Audicana & Bernaola 1994). Autoxidation products of (+)-limonene can cause skin sensitization (see (+)-Limonene profile, Chapter 14).

Distinct phototoxic effects were found for five samples of expressed lemon oil, three Italian, one Greek and one Ivory Coast; low-level phototoxic effects were found in a Californian expressed lemon oil (Opdyke 1974 p. 725–726). The phototoxicity of expressed lemon oil is almost entirely accounted for by bergapten and oxypeucedanin, the content of which varies by a factor of up to 20 depending on country of origin (Naganuma et al 1985). Bergapten is photocarcinogenic (Young et al 1990). A woman was treated for minor burns after a 20-minute session on a sunbed, taken immediately after a sauna bath with expressed lemon oil. A few drops of the oil were placed in a pot in the sauna room, not on the woman's skin. The burns were to one arm and leg (Anon 1992a).

Reproductive toxicity: The low developmental toxicity of (+)-limonene, β-pinene, α-pinene, sabinene and β-myrcene (see Constituent profiles, Chapter 14) suggests that expressed lemon oil is not hazardous in pregnancy.

Systemic effects

Acute toxicity: Expressed lemon oil acute oral LD_{50} in rats >5 g/kg; acute dermal LD_{50} in rabbits >5 g/kg (Opdyke 1974 p. 725–726).

Antioxidant/pro-oxidant activity: Lemon oil has demonstrated marked DPPH radical scavenging activity (Choi et al 2000).

Carcinogenic/anticarcinogenic potential: Lemon oil was not mutagenic in the *Ames test*, and did not produce CA in Chinese hamster fibroblasts (Ishidate et al 1984). Lemon oil significantly induced glutathione *S*-transferase in mouse liver and small bowel mucosa and inhibited B[*a*]P-induced neoplasia of both forestomach and lungs (Wattenberg et al 1985). It also inhibited NNK-induced pulmonary adenoma formation and the occurrence of forestomach tumors in mice (Wattenberg & Coccia 1991). Apoptosis in human leukemia (HL-60) cells was induced by lemon oil and by citral (geranial + neral), octanal and decanal, all minor constituents of the oil (Hata et al 2003). Lemon oil was cytotoxic to human prostate, lung and breast cancer cells with IC_{50} values of 0.08%, 0.06% and 0.14% respectively (Zu et al 2010). Citral (geranial + neral) and (+)-limonene display anticarcinogenic activity (see Constituent profiles, Chapter 14).

Comments

Expressed lemon oil has not been studied for long-term photogenotoxic or photocarcinogenic effects. Lemon oil is also produced by distillation, notably for particular flavor applications, such as soluble essences for lemon drinks. Distilled lemon oil is non-phototoxic but has an inferior odor to that of expressed lemon oil.

Lemon balm (Australian)

Synonym: Lemon-scented ironbark
Botanical name: *Eucalyptus staigeriana* F. v. Muell. ex F. M. Bailey
Family: Myrtaceae

Essential oil

Source: Leaves
Key constituents:

(+)-Limonene + β-phellandrene	30.5%
Geranial	9.9%
Neral	7.7%
α-Phellandrene	7.1%
Terpinolene	6.6%
Geranyl acetate	4.0%
Geraniol	3.7%
1,8-Cineole	3.5%
Methyl geranate	3.4%
α-Pinene	2.5%
P-Cymene	2.1%
β-Pinene	1.9%
Nerol	1.9%
Terpinen-4-ol	1.8%
Linalool	1.6%
Neryl acetate	1.6%
α-Terpineol	1.1%

(Cornwell, private communication, 2004)

Safety summary

Hazards: Drug interaction; teratogenicity; skin sensitization (low risk).
Cautions (oral): Drugs metabolized by CYP2B6 (Appendix B).
Cautions: Old or oxidized oils should be avoided.
Maximum daily oral dose in pregnancy: 238 mg
Maximum dermal use level: 3.4%

Our safety advice

We recommend a dermal maximum of 3.4% to avoid skin sensitization, and a daily oral maximum in pregnancy of 238 mg. This is based on 17.6% citral content, with dermal and oral citral limits of 0.6% and 0.6 mg/kg (see Citral profile, Chapter 14). Because of its (+)-limonene content we recommend that oxidation of Australian lemon balm oil is avoided by storage in a dark, airtight container in a refrigerator. The addition of an antioxidant to preparations containing it is recommended.

Regulatory guidelines

IFRA recommends a maximum dermal use level for citral of 0.6% for body oils and lotions, in order to avoid skin sensitization (IFRA 2009). IFRA recommends that essential oils rich in limonene should only be used when the level of peroxides is kept to the lowest practical level, for instance by adding antioxidants at the time of production (IFRA 2009).

Organ-specific effects

Adverse skin reactions: No information found. Autoxidation products of (+)-limonene can cause skin sensitization (see (+)-Limonene profile, Chapter 14). Citral (geranial + neral) is a potential skin sensitizer (see Citral profile, Chapter 14).
Reproductive toxicity: Citral is dose-dependently teratogenic because it inhibits retinoic acid synthesis, and this can affect fetal development (see Citral profile, Chapter 14).
Drug interactions: Since citral and geraniol inhibit CYP2B6 (Table 4.11B), there is a theoretical risk of interaction between lemon balm (Australian) oil and drugs metabolized by this enzyme (Appendix B).

Systemic effects

Acute toxicity: No information found.
Antioxidant/pro-oxidant activity: Australian lemon balm oil exhibited high radical scavenging activity in both ABTS and DPPH assays (Zhao et al 2010).
Carcinogenic/anticarcinogenic potential: No information was found for Australian lemon balm oil, but it contains no known carcinogens. Citral (geranial + neral) and (+)-limonene display anticarcinogenic activity (see Constituent profiles, Chapter 14).

Comments

The compositional data here are averages.

Lemon leaf

Synonym: Lemon petitgrain
Botanical name: *Citrus x limon* L.
Botanical synonym: *Citrus limonum* Risso
Family: Rutaceae

Essential oil

Source: Leaves
Key constituents:

Geranial	10.9–39.0%
(+)-Limonene	8.1–30.7%
Neral	6.5–25.3%
Geraniol	0.5–15.0%
β-Pinene	3.5–13.6%
Neryl acetate	3.7–7.4%
Nerol	1.3–7.4%
α-Terpinyl acetate	tr–7.3%
Linalyl acetate	tr–6.5%
Geranyl acetate	tr–4.0%
Citronellal	1.5–2.9%
γ-Terpinene	0.4–2.3%
α-Pinene	0.1–2.2%
β-Caryophyllene	0.6–2.0%
Linalool	1.2–1.8%
β-Myrcene	0.4–1.5%
α-Terpineol	0.4–1.1%

(Lawrence 1995a p. 114–117)

Safety summary

Hazards: Drug interaction; teratogenicity; skin sensitization (low risk).
Cautions (oral): Diabetes medication, drugs metabolized by CYP2B6 (Appendix B), pregnancy.
Cautions (dermal): Hypersensitive, diseased or damaged skin, children under 2 years of age.
Maximum daily oral dose in pregnancy: 84 mg
Maximum dermal use level: 1.2%

Our safety advice

We recommend a dermal maximum of 1.2% to avoid skin sensitization, and a daily oral maximum in pregnancy of 84 mg. This is based on 50% citral content, with dermal and oral citral limits of 0.6% and 0.6 mg/kg (see Citral profile, Chapter 14). Because of its (+)-limonene content we recommend that oxidation of lemon leaf oil is avoided by storage in a dark, airtight container in a refrigerator. The addition of an antioxidant to preparations containing it is recommended.

Regulatory guidelines

IFRA recommends a maximum dermal use level for citral of 0.6% for body oils and lotions, in order to avoid skin sensitization (IFRA 2009). IFRA recommends that essential oils rich in limonene should only be used when the level of peroxides is kept to the lowest practical level, for instance by adding antioxidants at the time of production (IFRA 2009).

Organ-specific effects

Adverse skin reactions: Undiluted lemon leaf oil was not irritating to rabbits, but was slightly irritating to mice and pigs; tested at 10% on 25 volunteers it was neither irritating nor sensitizing. It is non-phototoxic (Opdyke 1978 p. 807). Citral (geranial + neral) is a potential skin sensitizer, and autoxidation products of (+)-limonene can cause skin sensitization (see Constituent profiles, Chapter 14).
Cardiovascular effects: Gavage doses of 10, 15 or 20 mg/kg/day citral for 28 days, dose-dependently lowered plasma insulin levels and increased glucose tolerance in obese rats (Modak & Mukhopadhaya 2011).
Reproductive toxicity: Citral is dose-dependently teratogenic because it inhibits retinoic acid synthesis, and this can affect fetal development (see Citral profile, Chapter 14).

Systemic effects

Acute toxicity: Lemon leaf oil acute oral LD_{50} in rats >5 g/kg; acute dermal LD_{50} in rabbits >5 g/kg (Opdyke 1978 p. 807).
Carcinogenic/anticarcinogenic potential: No information was found for lemon leaf oil, but it contains no known carcinogens. Citral, (+)-limonene, geraniol and citronellal display anticarcinogenic activity (see Constituent profiles, Chapter 14).

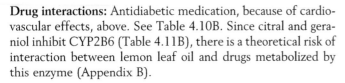

Drug interactions: Antidiabetic medication, because of cardiovascular effects, above. See Table 4.10B. Since citral and geraniol inhibit CYP2B6 (Table 4.11B), there is a theoretical risk of interaction between lemon leaf oil and drugs metabolized by this enzyme (Appendix B).

Comments

The main producer of this oil is Italy, and compositional data is for Italian lemon leaf oils.

Lemongrass

Botanical names: *Cymbopogon flexuosus* Nees ex Steud. (synonym: *Andropogon flexuosus* Nees ex Steud.) (East Indian); *Cymbopogon citratus* DC (synonym: *Andropogon citratus* DC) (West Indian)
Family: Poaceae (Gramineae)

Essential oil

Source: Leaves
Key constituents:

East Indian

Geranial	45.1–54.5%
Neral	30.1–36.1%
Geranyl acetate	0.1–4.0%
Geraniol	0.2–3.8%
(+)-Limonene	0.1–3.8%
Caryophyllene oxide	0–1.6%
6-Methyl-5-hepten-2-one	0.3–1.4%
Linalool	0.4–1.3%

(Lawrence 1989 p. 111, 2002f p. 58)

West Indian

Geranial	36.7–55.9%
Neral	25.0–35.2%
β-Myrcene	5.6–19.2%
Geraniol	0–6.7%
Limonene oxide	0–6.4%
1,8-Cineole	0–2.9%
6-Methylhept-5-en-2-one	0.1–2.6 %
Geranyl acetate	0.4–1.9%
Linalool	0.2–2.0%

(Lawrence 1989 p. 111; Zhu et al 1993 p200; Chagonda & Makanda 2000)
Quality: May be adulterated with synthetic citral (Singhal et al 1997).

Safety summary

Hazards: Drug interaction; teratogenicity; skin sensitization.
Cautions (all routes): Drugs metabolized by CYP2B6 (Appendix B).
Cautions (oral): Diabetes medication, pregnancy.

Cautions (dermal): Hypersensitive, diseased or damaged skin, children under 2 years of age.
Maximum daily oral dose in pregnancy: 46 mg
Maximum dermal use level: 0.7%

Our safety advice

We recommend a dermal maximum of 0.7% to avoid skin sensitization, and a daily oral maximum in pregnancy of 46 mg. This is based on 90% citral content, with dermal and oral citral limits of 0.6% and 0.6 mg/kg (see Citral profile, Chapter 14).

Regulatory guidelines

Has GRAS status. IFRA recommends a maximum dermal use level for citral of 0.6% for body oils and lotions, in order to avoid skin sensitization (IFRA 2009).

Organ-specific effects

Adverse skin reactions: Undiluted East or West Indian lemongrass oil was moderately irritating to rabbits, and was mildly irritating to mice and pigs; tested at 4% on 25 volunteers it was neither irritating nor sensitizing. It is non-phototoxic (Opdyke 1976 p. 455, p. 457). Lemongrass oil (type unspecified) tested at 2%, induced allergic responses in 25 (1.6%) of 1,606 consecutive dermatitis patients (Frosch et al 2002b). In 318 such patients, there were four reactions (1.3%) to 2% East Indian lemongrass oil (Paulsen & Andersen 2005). There were no irritant or allergic reactions to 1% lemongrass oil (type unspecified) in a group of 100 such patients (Frosch et al 1995a). Six of 747 dermatitis patients suspected of fragrance allergy (0.8%) reacted to 2% lemongrass oil (type unspecified) (Wöhrl et al 2001). In a multicenter study, Germany's IVDK reported that 15 of 2,435 consecutive dermatitis patients (0.61%), and 210 of 8,445 patients suspected of fragrance allergy (2.49%) tested positive to 2% lemongrass oil (type unspecified) (Uter et al 2010).

Citral (geranial + neral) can induce sensitization reactions on patch testing at concentrations above 0.5% and this effect can allegedly be reduced by the co-presence of (+)-limonene or α-pinene (see Constituent profiles, Chapter 14). In a mouse local lymph node assay, which allows comparative measuring of skin sensitizing potency, East Indian lemongrass oil was a weak sensitizer, with a similar potency to citral (Lalko & Api 2006). There is strong circumstantial evidence linking exposure to the undiluted oil with dermatitis in eight men who had worked on a boat carrying lemongrass oil from India. Some of the oil had spilled (Mendelsohn 1944).
Cardiovascular effects: Gavage doses of 10, 15 or 20 mg/kg/day citral for 28 days, dose-dependently lowered plasma insulin levels and increased glucose tolerance in obese rats (Modak & Mukhopadhaya 2011).
Reproductive toxicity: Citral is dose-dependently teratogenic because it inhibits retinoic acid synthesis, and this can affect fetal development (see Citral profile, Chapter 14).

Systemic effects

Acute & subacute toxicity: East Indian lemongrass oil acute oral LD_{50} in rats 5.6 g/kg; acute dermal LD_{50} in rabbits >2 g/kg

(Opdyke 1976 p. 455). West Indian lemongrass oil acute oral LD$_{50}$ in rats >5 g/kg; acute dermal LD$_{50}$ in rabbits >5 g/kg (Opdyke 1976 p. 457). When West Indian lemongrass oil was administered orally to mice for 21 days at 1, 10 or 100 mg/kg, there were no significant changes in gross pathology, body weight, absolute or relative organ weights, histology (brain, heart, kidneys, liver, lungs, stomach, spleen and urinary bladder), urinalysis or clinical biochemistry in the treated mice relative to the control groups (Costa et al 2011). In rats, West Indian lemongrass oil in the diet at 1,500 ppm for 60 days had no effect on levels of leukocytes, hemoglobin, urea, protein, cholesterol, blood glucose, ALP (alkaline phosphatase), ALT or AST (Mishra et al 1991).

Antioxidant/pro-oxidant activity: In both egg yolk and rat liver assays, West Indian lemongrass oil showed a strong pro-oxidant activity at all the concentrations tested (Baratta et al 1998). West Indian lemongrass oil (composition unstated) scavenged DPPH radicals, with an IC$_{50}$ of 27.0 µL/mL, compared with 31.4 µL/mL for BHT (Lertsatitthanakorn et al 2006). Lemongrass oil (type unspecified) significantly induced glutathione S-transferase activity in mouse tissues (Lam & Zheng 1991).

Carcinogenic/anticarcinogenic potential: When given to mice at 500 mg/kg for six weeks, West Indian lemongrass oil was antigenotoxic, mitigating leukocyte DNA damage induced by MNU (Bidinotto et al 2010). Doses of 100 mg/kg for 3 weeks had no such antigenotoxic effect, but were not genotoxic (Costa et al 2011). East Indian lemongrass oil showed good in vitro cytotoxic activity against 12 human cancer cell lines, representing cancers of the cervix, lung, liver, colon, prostate, mouth and nerves (neuroblastoma), with IC$_{50}$ values ranging from 4.2–79.0 µg/mL. Administration of the oil at 200 mg/kg ip in mice, inhibited Ehrlich and Sarcoma-180 tumors from 37–97%, primarily due to apoptosis (Sharma et al 2009). Treatment of mice with gavage doses of West Indian lemongrass oil (500 mg/kg/day five days/week for up to five weeks) significantly reduced pre-cancerous changes in breast tissue (alveolar/ductal hyperplasia) induced by MNU, but increased apoptosis. This suggests a protective action in the early stages of breast cancer (Bidinotto et al 2012). West Indian lemongrass oil showed significant chemopreventive activity against human mouth epidermal carcinoma (KB) and mouse leukemia (P388) cell lines, with respective IC$_{50}$ values of 115 and 75 µg/mL. The oil was more effective than three of the four positive control drugs (Manosroi et al 2005). West Indian lemongrass oil was lethal to 50–81% of various leukemic cells in vitro after four hours, but was not toxic to normal thymocytes (Dudai et al 2005). Citral, geraniol and (+)-limonene all exhibit anticarcinogenic activity (see Constituent profiles, Chapter 14).

Drug interactions: Antidiabetic medication, because of cardiovascular effects, above. See Table 4.10B. Since citral and geraniol inhibit CYP2B6 (Table 4.11B), there is a theoretical risk of interaction between lemongrass oil and drugs metabolized by this enzyme (see Appendix B).

Comments

The validity of the quenching phenomenon is disputed, and sensitization reactions from lemongrass oil are certainly possible. Uter et al (2010) reported a good correlation between sensitivity to lemongrass and citral among 1,777 patients tested with both substances. Their data also show four times as many reactions to lemongrass oil in patients suspected of fragrance sensitivity as in consecutive dermatitis patients. There are insufficient data to determine maximum dermal use levels, but for dermatitis patients this will be below 1.0%, possibly in the region of 0.5%. Lemongrass oils are sometimes rectified to produce an oil with up to 95% citral. A novel chemotype of C. citratus is now being cultivated in Uttarakhand, India, containing 40% geraniol, 24% citronellol, 7% geranial and 5% neral (Singh, private communication, 2009).

Lemon-scented gum

Synonyms: Eucalyptus citriodora, lemon-scented iron gum, spotted gum, lemon eucalyptus
Botanical name: *Corymbia citriodora* Hook.
Botanical synonyms: *Eucalyptus citriodora* Hook., *Eucalyptus maculata* Hook. var. *citriodora* Hook., *Eucalyptus melissiodora* Lindley
Family: Myrtaceae

Essential oil

Source: Leaves and terminal branchlets
Key constituents:

Australian

Citronellal	81.7%
Citronellol	4.9%
Isopulegol	1.3%

(Condon, private communication, 2003)

Chinese

Citronellal	86.2%
Citronellol	4.2%
α-Pinene	2.4%
Isopulegol	2.2%
Citronellyl acetate	1.1%

(Zhu et al 1993)

Indian

Citronellal	79.8%
Citronellol	5.4%
Isopulegol	4.0%
β-Caryophyllene	1.8%

(Lawrence 2001d p. 75–78)

Madagascan

Citronellal	66.9%
Citronellyl acetate	9.7%
Linalyl acetate	4.5%
β-Caryophyllene	1.5%
Chavicol	1.4%
β-Pinene	1.0%

(De Medici et al 1992)

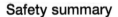
Safety summary

Hazards: None known.
Contraindications: None known.

Organ-specific effects

Adverse skin reactions: Undiluted lemon-scented gum oil was irritating to rabbits, producing scab formation and sloughing; tested at 10% on 25 volunteers it was neither irritating nor sensitizing. It is non-phototoxic (Ford et al 1988a p. 323). When injected, lemon-scented gum oil inhibited inflammation induced in rat paw (Silva et al 2003).

Systemic effects

Acute toxicity: Lemon-scented gum oil acute oral LD_{50} in rats >5 g/kg; acute dermal LD_{50} in rabbits 2.48 g/kg (Ford et al 1988a p. 323).
Antioxidant/pro-oxidant activity: Lemon-scented gum oil exhibited high radical scavenging activity in both ABTS and DPPH assays (Zhao et al 2008).
Carcinogenic/anticarcinogenic potential: No information was found for lemon-scented gum oil, but it contains no known carcinogens. Citronellal displays anticarcinogenic activity (see Constituent profiles, Chapter 14).

Comments

Lemon-scented gum oil is also produced in Brazil, Ethiopia and several other countries.

Lime (distilled)

Family: Rutaceae

Essential oil

Source: Ripe (yellow) fruit peel, by distillation

Mexican type

Synonyms: West Indian lime, Key lime
Botanical name: *Citrus x aurantifolia* Christm.
Key constituents:

(+)-Limonene + 1,8-cineole	40.4–49.4%
α-Terpineol	5.4–12.7%
γ-Terpinene	9.5–10.7%
Terpinolene	8.1–8.7%
1,4-Cineole	2.0–3.0%
β-Pinene	2.0–2.9%
p-Cymene	1.6–2.5%
Terpinen-1-ol	1.0–2.3%
(Z)-β-Terpineol	0.5–2.2%
β-Myrcene	1.3–2.1%
α-Pinene	1.2–2.1%
α-Terpinene	tr–2.1%
Terpinen-4-ol	0.7–1.9%
β-Bisabolene	1.6–1.8%

γ-Terpineol	0.8–1.6%
α-Fenchol	0.6–1.4%
Borneol	0.5–1.4%
Camphene	0.5–1.3%

(Pino & Rosado 2001; Kubeczka 2002)

Persian type

Synonym: Lime Tahiti
Botanical name: *Citrus x latifolia* Tanaka
Key constituents:

(+)-Limonene + 1,8-cineole	55.6%
γ-Terpinene	11.8%
α-Terpineol	6.6%
Terpinolene	5.2%
β-Myrcene	2.6%
(Z)-β-Terpineol	2.2%
Terpinen-1-ol	1.9%
α-Pinene	1.8%
β-Pinene	1.8%
1,4-Cineole	1.8%
p-Cymene	1.5%
Terpinen-4-ol	1.3%
α-Fenchol	1.1%

(Pino & Rosado 2001)

Quality: Distilled lime oil may be adulterated with added α-terpineol, terpinolene and other lime terpenes (Singhal et al 1997).

Safety summary

Hazards: Skin sensitization if oxidized.
Cautions: Old or oxidized oils should be avoided.

Our safety advice

Because of its (+)-limonene content we recommend that oxidation of distilled lime oil is avoided by storage in a dark, airtight container in a refrigerator. The addition of an antioxidant to preparations containing it is recommended.

Regulatory guidelines

Has GRAS status. IFRA recommends that essential oils rich in limonene should only be used when the level of peroxides is kept to the lowest practical level, for instance by adding antioxidants at the time of production (IFRA 2009).

Organ-specific effects

Adverse skin reactions: Undiluted distilled lime oil was slightly irritating to rabbits; tested at 15% or 100% on two panels of 25 volunteers it was not irritating. Tested at 15% on 25 volunteers it was not sensitizing. It is non-phototoxic (Opdyke 1974 p. 729). Autoxidation products of (+)-limonene can cause skin sensitization (see (+)-Limonene profile, Chapter 14).

Reproductive toxicity: The low developmental toxicity of (+)-limonene in rabbits and mice (Kodama et al 1977a, 1977b) suggests that lime oil is not hazardous in pregnancy.

Systemic effects

Acute toxicity: Distilled lime oil acute oral LD_{50} in rats >5 g/kg; acute dermal LD_{50} in rabbits >5 g/kg (Opdyke 1974 p. 729).
Carcinogenic/anticarcinogenic potential: Lime oil (type unspecified) has been reported as a promoter of tumors in the forestomach and in the skin of rats pre-treated with DMBA; most of these papillomas were benign, but a few were malignant (Roe & Field 1965). Lime oil (type unspecified) was not mutagenic in the Ames test, and did not produce CA in Chinese hamster fibroblasts (Ishidate et al 1984). Lime terpenes induced glutathione S-transferase activity to more than 2.5 times control level in mouse tissues (Lam & Zheng 1991).

Comments

The terms 'Mexican', 'Persian', etc. refer to the type of lime, and not necessarily the country of origin. Distilled lime oil is produced on a much larger scale than the expressed oil, and most of the production is used in food flavoring. Although distilled lime oils are not regarded as phototoxic, citropten (0.9%) and bergapten (0.3%) have been reported as constituents of a distilled Mexican lime oil (Lawrence 1989 p. 43). Distilled lime oil contains some relatively rare constituents such as 1,4-cineole, β-terpineol and terpinen-1-ol, because of the acidic conditions present during processing (Kubeczka 2002). The research in the 1960s that identified limonene in several citrus oils as a promotor of malignant tumors was probably flawed, since we now know that limonene, and its metabolite perillyl alcohol, are both anticarcinogenic (see Constituent profiles, Chapter 14). Oxidation products of (+)-limonene may have caused these early results.

Lime (expressed)

Family: Rutaceae

Essential oil

Source: Unripe (green) fruit peel, by expression

Mexican type

Synonyms: West Indian lime, Key lime
Botanical name: *Citrus x aurantifolia* Christm.
Key constituents:

(+)-Limonene	48.2%
β-Pinene	21.1%
γ-Terpinene	8.1%
Sabinene	3.1%
α-Pinene	2.5%
Geranial	2.4%
β-Bisabolene	1.8%
Neral	1.4%
β-Myrcene	1.3%

(E)-α-Bergamotene	1.1%
β-Caryophyllene	1.0%
(2E,6E)-α-Farnesene	1.0%

(Kubeczka 2002)

Persian type

Synonym: Lime Tahiti
Botanical name: *Citrus x latifolia* Tanaka
Key constituents:

(+)-Limonene	51.5–59.6%
β-Pinene	12.2–16.0%
γ-Terpinene	1.3–14.4%
p-Cymene	0.4–10.4%
α-Pinene	2.0–5.0%
Geranial	2.2–3.9%
Sabinene	0.9–2.1%
β-Myrcene	0.9–1.8%
β-Bisabolene	0.2–1.7%
Neryl acetate	0.4–1.5%
α-Bergamotene	1.0–1.4%
Neral	0.5–1.2%

(Lawrence 1989 p. 176, 1993 p. 137)

Non-volatile compounds

7-Methoxy-5-geranoxycoumarin	1.7–5.2%
5-Geranoxy-7-methoxycoumarin	1.7–3.2%
Bergamottin	1.7–3.0%
Citropten	0.4–2.2%
Isopimpinellin	0.1–1.3%
5-Geranoxy-8-methoxypsoralen	0.2–0.9%
Bergapten	0.17–0.33%
Oxypeucedanin	0.02–0.3%
8-Geranoxypsoralen	0.10–0.14%

(Lawrence 1989 p. 42–43; Dugo et al 1999a; SCCP 2005b)

Safety summary

Hazards: Skin sensitization if oxidized; phototoxic (moderate risk); may be photocarcinogenic.
Contraindications (dermal): If applied to the skin at over maximum use level, skin must not be exposed to sunlight or sunbed rays for 12 hours.
Cautions: Old or oxidized oils should be avoided.
Maximum dermal use level: 0.7% (see Regulatory Guidelines)

Our safety advice

Because of its (+)-limonene content we recommend that oxidation of expressed lime oil is avoided by storage in a dark, airtight container in a refrigerator. The addition of an antioxidant to preparations containing it is recommended.

Regulatory guidelines

Has GRAS status. In Europe, essential oils containing furanocoumarins must be used so that the total level of bergapten will not exceed: (a) 15 ppm in finished cosmetic products intended for application to skin areas likely to be exposed to sunshine, excluding rinse-off products; or (b) 1 ppm in sun protection and in bronzing products. In the presence of other phototoxic ingredients, the sum of their concentrations (expressed as % of the respective maximum levels) shall not exceed 100% (SCCNFP 2000). In order to avoid phototoxicity, IFRA recommends that, for application to areas of skin exposed to sunshine, expressed lime oil be limited to a maximum of 0.7% in products applied to the skin except for bath preparations, soaps and other wash-off products (IFRA 2009). IFRA also recommends that essential oils rich in limonene should only be used when the level of peroxides is kept to the lowest practical level, for instance by adding antioxidants at the time of production (IFRA 2009).

Organ-specific effects

Adverse skin reactions: No irritation or sensitization data could be found. Expressed lime oil was phototoxic when applied to human skin (Opdyke 1974 p. 731). Phototoxicity is due to bergapten and other furanocoumarins. Bergapten is photocarcinogenic (Young et al 1990) (see Ch. 14, p. 507). Eleven cases of photodermatitis from expressed lime oil have been reported, and photodynamic reaction was experimentally produced by expressed lime oil on the skin and subsequent solar irradiation (Opdyke 1974 p. 731). Autoxidation products of (+)-limonene can cause skin sensitization (see (+)-Limonene profile, Chapter 14).

Reproductive toxicity: The low reproductive toxicity of (+)-limonene and β-pinene (see Constituent profiles, Chapter 14) suggests that expressed lime oil is not hazardous in pregnancy.

Systemic effects

Acute toxicity: No information found.

Antioxidant/pro-oxidant activity: Persian lime oil has demonstrated marked DPPH radical scavenging activity (Choi et al 2000). Lime terpenes induced glutathione S-transferase activity to more than 2.5 times control level in mouse tissues (Lam & Zheng 1991).

Carcinogenic/anticarcinogenic potential: Lime oil (type unspecified) has been reported as a promotor of tumors in the forestomach and in the skin of rats pre-treated with DMBA; most of these papillomas were benign, but a few were malignant (Roe & Field 1965). Lime oil (type unspecified) was not mutagenic in the Ames test, and did not produce CA in Chinese hamster fibroblasts (Ishidate et al 1984). Citral (geranial + neral) and (+)-limonene display anticarcinogenic activity (see Constituent profiles, Chapter 14).

Comments

Lime oil is not regarded as a carcinogen by any agency. The non-volatile residue of cold-pressed lime oil is thought to be higher than for any other citrus oil, and has been reported as 6.7–15.4% (Lawrence 1989 p. 43). The terms 'Mexican', 'Persian', etc. are employed to describe the type of lime, and do not necessarily denote country of origin.

Linaloe wood

Botanical names: *Bursera glabrifolia* Humb. (synonym: *Bursera delpechiana* Poisson) and other *Bursera* species such as *B. aloexylon* Schiede, *B. fagaroides* Humb., *B. penicillata* Sesse & Moc. and *B. simaruba* L)
Family: Burseraceae

Essential oil

Source: Wood
Key constituents:

Linalyl acetate	47.0%
Linalool	30.0%
α-Terpineol	8.5%
Geranyl acetate	3.5%
Neryl acetate	2.5%
(Z)-Linalool oxide	2.0%
Methyl heptenol	1.5%
Geraniol	1.0%
(E)-Linalool oxide	1.0%

(Lawrence 1979 p.3)

Safety summary

Hazards: None known.
Contraindications: None known.

Regulatory guidelines

According to IFRA, essential oils rich in linalool should only be used when the level of peroxides is kept to the lowest practical value. The addition of antioxidants such as 0.1% BHT or α-tocopherol at the time of production is recommended (IFRA 2009).

Organ-specific effects

Adverse skin reactions: Undiluted linaloe wood oil was moderately irritating to rabbits, but was not irritating to mice or pigs; tested at 8% on 25 volunteers it was neither irritating nor sensitizing. It is non-phototoxic (Opdyke 1979a p. 849). Oxidation products of linalool may be skin sensitizing.

Systemic effects

Acute toxicity: Linaloe wood acute oral LD_{50} in rats >5 g/kg; acute dermal LD_{50} in rabbits >5 g/kg (Opdyke 1979a p. 849).

Carcinogenic/anticarcinogenic potential: No information was found for linaloe wood oil, but it contains no known carcinogens.

Comments

According to Arctander (1960) the essential oil can be considered partly a pathological product, since the oil content in undamaged trees is too low for economical exploitation. The felling of entire, old and damaged trees is less practical and less environmentally sound that harvesting the leaves or fruits for distillation.

Longoza

Synonym: Longozo
Botanical name: *Hedychium coronarium* J. Koenig
Family: Zingiberaceae

Essential oil

Source: Rhizomes
Key constituents:

β-Pinene	30.0–52.0%
α-Pinene	18.0–24.0%
β-Caryophyllene	0.8–8.0%
β-Phellandrene	2.0–6.0%
β-Myrcene	1.0–5.0%
p-Cymene	1.0–4.0%
γ-Terpinene	1.0–4.0%
(+)-Limonene	1.5–3.0%
Sabinene	1.5–3.0%
α-Ylangene	0.2–1.0%

(Behra, private communication, 2003)

Safety summary

Hazards: Skin sensitization if oxidized.
Cautions: Old or oxidized oils should be avoided.

Our safety advice

Because of its α-pinene and generally high monoterpene content we recommend that oxidation of longoza oil is avoided by storage in a dark, airtight container in a refrigerator. The addition of an antioxidant to preparations containing it is recommended.

Organ-specific effects

Adverse skin reactions: No information was found for longoza oil. Autoxidation products of α-pinene can cause skin sensitization (see α-Pinene profile, Chapter 14).
Reproductive toxicity: The low reproductive toxicity of β-pinene, α-pinene, β-myrcene and (+)-limonene (see Constituent profiles, Chapter 14) suggest that longoza oil is not hazardous in pregnancy.

Systemic effects

Acute toxicity: No information found.
Carcinogenic/anticarcinogenic potential: No information was found for longoza oil, but it contains no known carcinogens.

Comments

Limited availability.

Lovage leaf

Botanical name: *Levisticum officinale* W.S. Koch
Family: Apiaceae (Umbelliferae)

Essential oil

Source: Leaves
Key constituents:

α-Terpinyl actetate	43.4–47.3%
(*Z*)-Ligustilide	15.5–22.4%
β-Phellandrene	15.0–20.0%
β-Myrcene	1.8–4.6%
(+)-Limonene	1.2–3.0%
(*E*)-Ligustilide	0.5–2.7%
α-Terpineol	0.4–2.2%
α-Pinene	0.5–1.4%

(Lawrence 1999b p. 35–39)

Safety summary

Hazards: May be phototoxic.
Cautions (dermal): Has not been tested for phototoxicity.

Organ-specific effects

Adverse skin reactions: No information was found for lovage leaf oil, but terpinyl acetate is notably non-allergenic (see Terpinyl acetate profile, Chapter 14). Although there are no data on (*Z*)-ligustilide, it is the main component of lovage root oil (see below) which seems to be well tolerated. Lovage leaves contain furanocoumarins, and the essential oil has not been tested for phototoxicity.

Systemic effects

Acute toxicity: No information found. Terpinyl acetate is non-toxic (see Terpinyl acetate profile, Chapter 14). Although there are no data on (*Z*)-ligustilide, it is the main component of lovage root oil (see below) which appears to be non-toxic.
Carcinogenic/anticarcinogenic potential: Lovage leaf oil was cytotoxic to human head and neck squamous carcinoma cells, with an IC_{50} of 292.6 µg/mL (Sertel et al 2011b). (*Z*)-Ligustilide was cytotoxic to human colon cancer (HT-29) cells with an IC_{50} of 11.52 µg/mL (Kan et al 2008).

Comments

Produced in Europe.

Lovage root

Botanical name: *Levisticum officinale* Koch
Family: Apiaceae (Umbelliferae)

Essential oil

Source: Roots
Key constituents:

(*Z*)-Ligustilide	67.5%
Pentylcyclohexadiene	7.5%
β-Phellandrene	3.8%
β-Pinene	2.9%

α-Pinene	2.1%
(Z)-3-Butylidenephthalide	1.5%
(Z)-3-n-Validene-3,4-dihydrophthalide	1.5%
(E)-3-Butylidene-4,5-dihydrophthalide	1.3%

(Toulemonde & Noleau 1988)

Safety summary

Hazards: None known.
Contraindications: None known.

Organ-specific effects

Adverse skin reactions: Undiluted lovage root oil was moderately irritating to rabbits, slightly irritating to guinea pigs, but was not irritating to mice or pigs; tested at 2% on 25 volunteers it was neither irritating nor sensitizing. It is non-phototoxic (Opdyke 1978 p. 813–814).

Systemic effects

Acute toxicity: Lovage root oil acute oral LD_{50} in rats 3.4 g/kg; acute dermal LD_{50} in rabbits >5 g/kg (Opdyke 1978 p. 813–814).
Carcinogenic/anticarcinogenic potential: No information was found for lovage root oil, but it contains no known carcinogens. (Z)-Ligustilide is cytotoxic to human colon cancer cells with an IC_{50} of 11.52 μg/mL (Kan et al 2008).

Comments

The major constituent is also known as (Z)-3-butylidene-4,5-dihydrophthalide.

Lovage seed

Botanical name: *Levisticum officinale* Koch
Family: Apiaceae (Umbelliferae)

Essential oil

Source: Seeds
Key constituents:

β-Phellandrene	63.2%
(Z)-β-Ocimene	9.2%
(Z)-Ligustilide	5.6%
(+)-Limonene	3.1%
α-Terpinyl acetate	3.1%
α-Phellandrene	2.9%
β-Myrcene	2.0%
α-Pinene	1.9%

(Toulemonde & Noleau 1988)

Safety summary

Hazards: None known.
Contraindications: None known.

Organ-specific effects

Adverse skin reactions: No information was found for lovage seed oil or β-phellandrene.

Systemic effects

Acute toxicity: No information was found for lovage seed oil or β-phellandrene.
Carcinogenic/anticarcinogenic potential: No information was found for lovage seed oil, but it contains no known carcinogens.

Comments

Lovage oils are among the most pungent.

Mace

Botanical name: *Myristica fragrans* Houtt.
Botanical synonyms: *Myristica officinalis* L. fil., *Myristica moschata* Thunb., *Myristica aromatica* O. Schwartz, *Myristica amboinensis* Gand.
Family: Myristicaceae

Essential oil

Source: Aril (pericarp) which surrounds the ripe seed
Key constituents:

East Indian

α-Pinene	16.3–26.7%
β-Pinene	10.6–20.0%
Sabinene	12.5–14.5%
Terpinen-4-ol	4.4–14.0%
γ-Terpinene	4.9–11.6%
β-Phellandrene + 1,8-cineole	4.9–11.6%
(+)-Limonene	4.2–9.4%
α-Terpinene	4.8–7.5%
Myristicin	1.3–3.8%
Elemicin	0.2–2.0%
Safrole	0.2–1.9%
α-Terpineol	0.7–1.2%
Methyleugenol	0.1–0.2%
Isoeugenol	0–0.1%

(Forrest et al 1972; Lawrence 1995g p. 202)

Indian

β-Pinene + sabinene	45.5%
α-Pinene	15.2%
1,8-Cineole + (+)-limonene	7.0%
Myristicin	5.9%
Terpinen-4-ol	4.5%
α-Terpinene + p-cymene	3.5%
α-Phellandrene	3.2%
Elemicin	3.1%

β-Phellandrene	2.8%
γ-Terpinene	1.8%
Safrole + p-cymen-8-ol	0.7%
Methyleugenol	0.2%

(Lawrence 2000c p. 6–68)

Safety summary

Hazards: Potentially carcinogenic, based on safrole and methyleugenol content; may be psychotropic.
Contraindications: None known.
Maximum adult daily oral dose (East Indian mace oil): 73 mg
Maximum adult daily oral dose (Indian mace oil): 146 mg
Maximum dermal use level (East Indian mace oil):

EU	0.08%
IFRA	0.2%
Tisserand & Young	2%

Maximum dermal use level (Indian mace oil):

EU	0.1%
IFRA	0.18%
Tisserand & Young	4.1%

Our safety advice

We recommend a dermal maximum of 2% for the East Indian oil and a maximum oral dose of 73 mg based on 1.9% safrole and 0.2% methyleugenol content, and a dermal maximum of 4.1% and a maximum oral dose of 146 mg for the Indian oil based on 0.7% safrole and 0.2% methyleugenol. These are based on dermal limits of 0.05% and 0.02%, and oral dose limits of 0.025 and 0.01 mg/kg for safrole and methyleugenol, respectively (see Constituent profiles, Chapter 14).

Regulatory guidelines

IFRA and the EU recommend a maximum exposure level of 0.01% of safrole from the use of safrole-containing essential oils in cosmetics. IFRA recommends a maximum concentration of 0.0004% methyleugenol in leave-on products such as body lotions (IFRA 2009). The equivalent SCCNFP maximum is 0.0002% (European Commission 2002).

Organ-specific effects

Adverse skin reactions: Undiluted mace oil was moderately irritating to rabbits, but was not irritating to mice or pigs; tested at 8% on 25 volunteers it was neither irritating nor sensitizing. It is non-phototoxic (Opdyke 1979a p. 851–852).
Neurotoxicity: Psychotropic effects have been reported for nutmeg in high doses. Myristicin and elemicin are thought to be responsible, but other synergistic elements may need to be present for a psychotropic effect to take place (see Ch. 10, p. 144/145).

Systemic effects

Acute toxicity: Mace oil acute oral LD_{50} in rats 3.64 g/kg; acute dermal LD_{50} in rabbits >5 g/kg (Opdyke 1979a p. 851–852).

Carcinogenic/anticarcinogenic potential: No information was found for mace oil. Safrole and methyleugenol are carcinogenic if the dose is sufficiently high; (+)-limonene and myristicin display anticarcinogenic activity (see Constituent profiles, Chapter 14).

Comments

No compositional data was found for West Indian mace oil, but a CO_2 extract contained 0.2% safrole and 0.1% methyleugenol (Lawrence 2000c p. 66–68). It is feasible that the myristicin in mace oil might counter the potentially carcinogenic effect of methyleugenol and safrole.

Magnolia flower

Synonyms: White champaca, white jade orchid
Botanical name: *Michelia alba* DC
Botanical synonyms: *Michelia longifolia* Blume, *Sampacca longifolia* (Blume) Kuntze
Family: Magnoliaceae

Essential oil

Source: Flowers
Key constituents:

Linalool	69.9%
β-Caryophyllene	4.2%
Butanoic acid, 2-methyl methyl ester	3.7%
Selinene	3.1%
(E)-β-Ocimene	2.7%
β-Elemene	2.3%
(Z)-β-Ocimene	2.1%

(Maire, private communication, 2004)
Quality: May be co-distilled with (cheaper) ylang-ylang flowers (Oyen & Dung 1999).

Safety summary

Hazards: None known.
Contraindications: None known.

Regulatory guidelines

According to IFRA, essential oils rich in linalool should only be used when the level of peroxides is kept to the lowest practical value. The addition of antioxidants such as 0.1% BHT or α-tocopherol at the time of production is recommended (IFRA 2009).

Organ-specific effects

Adverse skin reactions: No information found. Oxidation products of linalool may be skin sensitizing.
Reproductive toxicity: The virtual absence of reproductive toxicity for linalool (Politano et al 2008) suggests that magnolia flower oil is not hazardous in pregnancy.

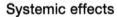

Systemic effects

Acute toxicity: No information found. Linalool is not toxic, but does possess enzyme inducing and sedative properties (see Linalool profile, Chapter 14).

Carcinogenic/anticarcinogenic potential: No information was found magnolia flower oil, but it contains no known carcinogens. β-Elemene displays anticarcinogenic activity (see β-Elemene profile, Chapter 14).

Comments

Limited availability. This is a steam distilled oil. See champaca (white) for the absolute made from this plant.

Magnolia leaf

Synonym: White champaca, white jade orchid
Botanical name: *Michelia alba* DC
Botanical synonyms: *Michelia longifolia* Blume, *Sampacca longifolia* (Blume) Kuntze
Family: Magnoliaceae

Essential oil

Source: Flowers
Key constituents:

Linalool	78.9%
β-Caryophyllene	4.4%
β-Elemene	2.4%
(*E*)-β-Ocimene	2.3%
α-Caryophyllene	1.4%
(*Z*)-β-Ocimene	1.3%
Methyleugenol	0.1%

(Maire, private communication, 2004)

Safety summary

Hazards: May contain methyleugenol.
Contraindications: None known.
Maximum dermal use level:

EU	0.2%
IFRA	0.4%
Tisserand & Young	No limit

Our safety advice

Considering that 87% of magnolia leaf oil consists of anticarcinogenic constituents, we do not consider that the 0.1% of methyleugenol requires a use restriction of the essential oil.

Regulatory guidelines

IFRA recommends a maximum concentration of 0.0004% methyleugenol in leave-on products such as body lotions (IFRA 2009). The equivalent SCCNFP maximum is 0.0002% (European Commission 2002). According to IFRA, essential oils rich in linalool should only be used when the level of peroxides is kept to the lowest practical value. The addition of antioxidants such as 0.1% BHT or α-tocopherol at the time of production is recommended (IFRA 2009).

Organ-specific effects

Adverse skin reactions: No information found. Oxidation products of linalool may be skin sensitizing.
Reproductive toxicity: The virtual absence of reproductive toxicity for linalool (Politano et al 2008) suggests that magnolia leaf oil is not hazardous in pregnancy.

Systemic effects

Acute toxicity: No information found. Linalool is not toxic, but does possess enzyme inducing and sedative properties (see Linalool profile, Chapter 14).
Carcinogenic/anticarcinogenic potential: No information found. Methyleugenol is a rodent carcinogen if exposure is sufficiently high; linalool, β-caryophyllene, α-caryophyllene and β-elemene display anticarcinogenic activity (see Constituent profiles, Chapter 14).

Comments

Limited availability.

Mandarin

Synonym: Common mandarin
Botanical name: *Citrus reticulata* Blanco
Botanical synonym: *Citrus nobilis* Andrews
Family: Rutaceae

Essential oil

Source: Fruit peel, by expression
Key constituents:

(+)-Limonene	65.3–74.2%
γ-Terpinene	16.4–22.7%
α-Pinene	2.0–2.7%
β-Pinene	1.4–2.1%
β-Myrcene	1.5–1.8%
p-Cymene	0.1–1.4%
α-Thujene	0.7–1.0%
Terpinolene	0.7–1.0%

(Lawrence 1996b p. 25–28)

Non-volatile compounds

Bergamottin	0–0.001%
Bergapten	0–0.0003%

(SCCP 2005b)

Safety summary

Hazards: Skin sensitization if oxidized.
Cautions: Old or oxidized oils should be avoided.

Our safety advice

Because of its (+)-limonene content we recommend that oxidation of mandarin oil is minimized by storage in a dark, airtight container in a refrigerator. The addition of an antioxidant to preparations containing it is also recommended.

Regulatory guidelines

Has GRAS status. In Europe, essential oils containing furanocoumarins must be used so that the total level of bergapten will not exceed: (a) 15 ppm in finished cosmetic products intended for application to skin areas likely to be exposed to sunshine, excluding rinse-off products; or (b) 1 ppm in sun protection and in bronzing products. In the presence of other phototoxic ingredients, the sum of their concentrations (expressed as % of the respective maximum levels) shall not exceed 100% (SCCNFP 2000). IFRA recommends that essential oils rich in limonene should only be used when the level of peroxides is kept to the lowest practical level, for instance by adding antioxidants at the time of production (IFRA 2009).

Organ-specific effects

Adverse skin reactions: Undiluted mandarin oil produced slight edema and erythema in rabbits; two of three samples of mandarin oil were irritating to mice and pigs. Tested at 8% on 25 volunteers mandarin oil was neither irritating nor sensitizing. Three different samples of mandarin oil were non-phototoxic (Ford et al 1992 p. 69S–70S). Autoxidation products of (+)-limonene can cause skin sensitization (see (+)-Limonene profile, Chapter 14).

Reproductive toxicity: The low developmental toxicity of (+)-limonene in rabbits and mice (Kodama et al 1977a, 1977b) suggests that mandarin oil is not hazardous in pregnancy.

Systemic effects

Acute toxicity: Mandarin oil acute oral LD_{50} in rats >5 g/kg, acute dermal LD_{50} in rabbits >5 g/kg (Ford et al 1992 p. 69S–70S). (+)-Limonene displays anticarcinogenic activity (see Constituent profiles, Chapter 14).

Carcinogenic/anticarcinogenic potential: No information was found for mandarin oil but it contains no known carcinogens. (+)-Limonene displays anticarcinogenic activity (see (+)-Limonene profile, Chapter 14).

Comments

The furanocoumarin content of mandarin fruit oil is not sufficient to cause a phototoxic reaction, but it may contribute to the total psoralen content of a mixture.

Mandarin leaf

Synonyms: Mandarin petitgrain, petitgrain mandarin
Botanical name: *Citrus reticulata* Blanco
Botanical synonym: *Citrus nobilis* Andrews
Family: Rutaceae

Essential oil

Source: Leaves
Key constituents:

Dimethyl anthranilate	43.2–51.9%
γ-Terpinene	23.9–28.5%
(+)-Limonene	7.2–11.7%
p-Cymene	3.0–4.8%
β-Pinene	1.9–2.5%
α-Pinene	1.8–2.3%
β-Caryophyllene	1.2–1.4%
α-Thujene	0.8–1.0%

(Dugo et al 1996)

Safety summary

Hazards: Phototoxic (moderate risk).
Contraindications (dermal): If applied to the skin at over maximum use level, skin must not be exposed to sunlight or sunbed rays for 12 hours.
Maximum dermal use level: 0.17% (see Regulatory Guidelines, IFRA).

Regulatory guidelines

Has GRAS status. IFRA recommends that, for application to areas of skin exposed to sunshine, mandarin leaf oil be limited to a maximum of 0.17% except for bath preparations, soaps and other wash-off products (IFRA 2009). This recommendation is based on the phototoxicity of dimethyl anthranilate and its assumed presence in mandarin leaf oil at <60%. EU regulations require that dimethyl anthranilate, as a constituent of mandarin leaf oil, should not be used in leave-on cosmetics, and its use in rinse-off products should be limited to 0.1% (SCCP 2006). In Canada, mandarin leaf oil is permitted in leave-on products at up to 0.1% (Health Canada Cosmetic Ingredient Hotlist, March 2011). In Europe, essential oils containing furanocoumarins must be used so that the total level of bergapten will not exceed: (a) 15 ppm in finished cosmetic products intended for application to skin areas likely to be exposed to sunshine, excluding rinse-off products; or (b) 1 ppm in sun protection and in bronzing products. In the presence of other phototoxic ingredients, the sum of their concentrations (expressed as % of the respective maximum levels) shall not exceed 100% (SCCNFP 2000).

Organ-specific effects

Adverse skin reactions: No information found. Mandarin leaf oil typically contains 50 ppm (0.005%) bergapten which is not sufficient to cause a phototoxic reaction (IFRA 2009). However, dimethyl anthranilate was phototoxic to mice at 5%, with an NOAEL of 0.5% in humans (Opdyke 1979a p. 273).

Systemic effects

Acute toxicity: No information found. Dimethyl anthranilate and γ-terpinene are slightly toxic orally, and non-toxic dermally (see Constituent profiles, Chapter 14).
Carcinogenic/anticarcinogenic potential: No information was found for mandarin leaf oil, but it contains no known

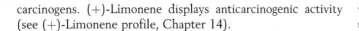

carcinogens. (+)-Limonene displays anticarcinogenic activity (see (+)-Limonene profile, Chapter 14).

Comments

A bergapten content of 50 ppm would not be sufficient to impart phototoxicity to mandarin leaf oil. Assuming a bergapten content of 50 ppm, and to comply with the 15 ppm SCCNFP guideline for bergapten, mandarin leaf oil should not be used at more than 30%. Major constituents vary considerably between different cultivars, and also according to the time of year. If the dimethyl anthranilate concentration is lower than 60% the maximum use level could be proportionately increased.

Mango ginger

Botanical name: *Curcuma amada* Roxb.
Family: Zingiberaceae

Essential oil

Source: Rhizomes
Key constituents:

ar-Curcumene	28.1%
β-Curcumene	11.2%
Camphor	11.2%
Curzerenone	7.1%
1,8-Cineole	6.0%
Isoborneol	4.5%
β-Elemene	2.8%
Camphene	1.7%
Zingiberene	1.4%
Borneol	1.3%

(Srivastava et al 2001)

Safety summary

Hazards: None known.
Contraindications: None known.

Organ-specific effects

Adverse skin reactions: No information was found for mango ginger oil or the curcumenes.

Systemic effects

Acute toxicity: No information was found for mango ginger oil or the curcumenes.
Carcinogenic/anticarcinogenic potential: No information was found for mango ginger oil, but it contains no known carcinogens. β-Elemene displays anticarcinogenic activity (see β-Elemene profile, Chapter 14); curzerenone has been used as an anticancer agent in China (Hsu 1980).

Comments

This oil was previously reported as containing 9.3% of safrole (Mahindru 1992, citing a 1941 report) but safrole has not been found in recent investigations. Mustafa et al (2005) reported a totally different composition for *Curcuma amada* rhizome oil,

with 21.9% (Z)-β-farnesene, 19.8% guaia-6,9-diene, 14.8% α-longipinene, and 14.5% α-guaiene as the major constituents.

Manuka

Botanical name: *Leptospermum scoparium* J. R. Forster & G. Forster
Family: Myrtaceae

Essential oil

Source: Leaves
Key constituents:

Leptospermone	8.7–19.4%
(*E*)-Calamenene	0.6–18.5%
α-Pinene	1.3–11.0%
Cadina-3,5-diene	3.0–10.0%
δ-Cadinene	4.8–7.2%
α-Copaene	4.7–6.5%
Flavesone	1.3–5.8%
Cadina-1,4-diene	4.0–5.3%
β-Selinene	2.8–5.1%
α-Selinene	2.7–5.0%
Isoleptospermone	1.4–4.7%
α-Cubebene	3.0–4.4%
δ-Amorphene	2.0–4.2%
β-Caryophyllene	2.0–3.2%
(+)-Aromadendrene	1.6–2.2%
β-Elemene	0.6–1.6%
(*E,E*)-α-Farnesene	0.7–1.5%
Cubenol	0.1–1.5%
Globulol	tr–1.5%
γ-Muurolene	0.9–1.4%
α-Gurjunene	0.8–1.2%
1(10)-Aromadendrene	0.6–1.1%
1,8-Cineole	0.2–1.0%
Bicyclogermacrene	tr–1.0%

(Lawrence 2001b p. 22–25)

Safety summary

Hazards: None known.
Contraindications: None known.

Organ-specific effects

Adverse skin reactions: No information was found for manuka oil, leptospermone, (*E*)-calamenene, or cadina-3,5-diene.

Systemic effects

Acute toxicity: Manuka oil was not significantly cytotoxic to cultured human umbilical vein endothelial cells (Takarada et al 2004).
Antioxidant/pro-oxidant activity: Antioxidant activity has been reported for makuka oil (Lis-Balchin et al 2000).

Carcinogenic/anticarcinogenic potential: Manuka oil contains no known carcinogens. β-Elemene displays anticarcinogenic activity (see β-Elemene profile, Chapter 14).

Comments

There are no obvious reasons to suspect any kind of toxicity.

Maraba

Synonyms: False galangal, false ginger, small galangal, resurrection lily
Botanical name: *Kaempferia galanga* L.
Family: Zingiberaceae

Essential oil

Source: Rhizomes
Key constituents:

Ethyl (*E*)-*p*-methoxycinnamate	49.5–51.6%
Pentadecane	9.0–21.6%
(*E*)-Ethyl cinnamate	13.2–16.5%
1,8-Cineole	0.9–5.7%
Ethyl (*Z*)-*p*-methoxycinnamate	0–3.6%
δ-3-Carene	0.6–3.3%
Borneol	1.0–2.7%
Anethole*	0–2.6%

(Wong et al 1992; Zhu et al 1993)

Safety summary

Hazards: None known.
Contraindications: None known.

Organ-specific effects

Adverse skin reactions: No information was found for maraba oil, pentadecane or ethyl (*E*)-*p*-methoxycinnamate.

Systemic effects

Acute toxicity: No information was found for maraba oil, pentadecane or ethyl (*E*)-*p*-methoxycinnamate.
Carcinogenic/anticarcinogenic potential: No information was found for maraba oil, but it contains no known carcinogens.

Comments

On standing, the oil deposits crystals of ethyl (*E*)-*p*-methoxycinnamate (Burfield 2000 p283).

Marigold (Mexican)

Synonyms: Spanish tarragon, Mexican tarragon, Texas tarragon, winter tarragon, Mexican mint marigold, sweet dragon, pericon, sweet mace, sweet-scented marigold

Botanical name: *Tagetes lucida* Cav.
Family: Asteraceae (Compositae)

Essential oil

Source: Flowering tops
Key constituents:

Estragole	84.7%
β-Myrcene	1.4%

(Jones, private communication, 2003, from a commercially purchased oil)

Safety summary

Hazards: Potentially carcinogenic; may inhibit blood clotting.
Contraindications: Should not be taken in oral doses.
Maximum dermal use level:

EU	No limit
IFRA	0.01%
Tisserand & Young	0.1%

Our safety advice

We recommend a dermal maximum of 0.1%, based on 84.7% estragole content with a dermal limit of 0.12% (see Estragole profile, Chapter 14).

Regulatory guidelines

IFRA recommends a maximum dermal use level for estragole of 0.01% in leave-on or wash-off preparations for body and face (IFRA 2009). The EU does not restrict estragole.

Organ-specific effects

Adverse skin reactions: No information found.
Cardiovascular effects: Estragole inhibits platelet aggregation (Yoshioka & Tamada 2005), an essential step in the blood clotting cascade.

Systemic effects

Acute toxicity: No information found. Estragole acute oral LD_{50} in mice 1.25 g/kg, in rats 1.82 g/kg (Opdyke 1976 p. 603).
Carcinogenic/anticarcinogenic potential: No information found. Estragole is a rodent carcinogen when oral exposure is sufficiently high (see Estragole profile, Chapter 14).

Comments

Limited availability. There are several chemotypes, including one with 33.9% estragole, 24.3% methyleugenol and 23.8% (*E*)-anethole, reported by Bicchi et al (1997). As far as we are aware, the estragole chemotype is the only one commercially available. The herb is cultivated commercially in Costa Rica, and an analysis of the essential oil showed an estragole content of 95–97% (Cicció 2004). The plant is frequently described as

*Isomer not specified

smelling like tarragon (from which it derives several common names), suggesting a high estragole content. An analysis from experimentally grown *Tagetes lucida* leaves in Italy, found 78.2% estragole, 3.6% methyleugenol, and 9.4% β-caryophyllene. The oil from the flowers contained 93.8% estragole, 0.1% methyleugenol, and 2.1% β-caryophyllene (Marotti et al 2004).

The name 'lucida' derives from a psychotropic action dating back to the Aztecs, who threw the powdered leaves in the faces of captives about to be sacrificed, presumably to deaden their senses. There are anecdotal reports of narcotic effects; the dried herb is smoked and is said to be mildly psychoactive. However, no active ingredient has been identified (Emboden 1979).

Marjoram (Spanish)

Synonyms: Mastic thyme, Spanish wild marjoram
Botanical name: *Thymus mastichina* L. ssp. *mastichina*
Family: Lamiaceae (Labiatae)

Essential oil

Source: Aerial parts of flowering plant
Key constituents:

1,8-Cineole	45.1–58.6%
Camphor	5.5–8.9%
α-Pinene	4.6–6.8%
Camphene	4.3–6.0%
Borneol	3.8–5.9%
β-Pinene	2.3–5.1%
α-Terpineol	2.8–4.5%
Linalool	0.4–4.0%
Sabinene	1.9–3.4%
Terpinen-4-ol	1.1–3.1%
(E)-Sabinene hydrate	0.1–3.0%
Elemol	0.4–2.2%
(E)-β-Ocimene	0.5–2.1%
δ-Terpineol	1.0–2.0%
β-Myrcene	0.7–1.6%
(+)-Limonene	1.3–1.5%
γ-Terpinene	0.4–1.3%
Intermedeol	0.2–1.3%

(Miguel et al 2003a)

Safety summary

Hazards: Essential oils high in 1,8-cineole can cause CNS and breathing problems in young children.
Contraindications: Do not apply to or near the face of infants or children.

Organ-specific effects

Adverse skin reactions: Undiluted Spanish marjoram oil was mildly irritating to rabbits, but was not irritating to mice or pigs;

tested at 6% on 25 volunteers it was neither irritating nor sensitizing. It is non-phototoxic (Opdyke 1976 p. 467).
Reproductive toxicity: The low reproductive toxicity of 1,8-cineole, camphor and α-pinene (see Constituent profiles, Chapter 14) suggests that Spanish marjoram oil is not hazardous in pregnancy.

Systemic effects

Acute toxicity: Spanish marjoram oil acute oral LD$_{50}$ in rats >5 g/kg; acute dermal LD$_{50}$ in rabbits >5 g/kg (Opdyke 1976 p. 467). 1,8-Cineole has been reported to cause serious poisoning in young children when accidentally instilled into the nose (Melis et al 1989).
Antioxidant/pro-oxidant activity: Antioxidant activity has been reported for Spanish marjoram oil (Miguel et al 2003b).
Carcinogenic/anticarcinogenic potential: No information was found for Spanish marjoram oil, but it contains no known carcinogens.

Comments

Considering that the oil is mostly distilled from wild-growing plants there is probably more variation in composition than the constituents listed above suggest. The plant is oddly named, as it has little in common with sweet marjoram (see Marjoram (sweet) profile) either chemically or botanically.

Marjoram (sweet)

Botanical name: *Origanum majorana* L.
Botanical synonyms: *Majorana hortensis* Moench, *Origanum dubium* Boiss.
Family: Lamiaceae (Labiatae)

Essential oil

Source: Freshly dried flowering plant
Key constituents:

Terpinen-4-ol	16.4–31.6%
(Z)-Sabinene hydrate	7.1–13.8%
Linalyl acetate	7.4–10.5%
γ-Terpinene	7.3–9.8%
α-Terpineol	3.8–8.3%
(E)-Sabinene hydrate	2.4–6.7%
α-Terpinene	3.0–5.9%
Terpinen-4-yl acetate	2.3–5.7%
Sabinene	3.0–5.3%
p-Cymene	2.2–5.3%
Linalool	1.7–3.3%
Terpinolene	2.0–2.8%

(Lawrence 1989 p. 96–97)

Safety summary

Hazards: None known.
Contraindications: None known.

Regulatory guidelines

Organ-specific effects

Adverse skin reactions: Undiluted sweet marjoram oil was not irritating to rabbits; tested at 6% on 25 volunteers it was neither irritating nor sensitizing (Opdyke 1976 p. 469). Terpinen-4-ol is not regarded as a skin sensitizer (see Terpinen-4-ol profile, Chapter 14). A 65-year-old aromatherapist with multiple essential oil sensitivities reacted to 1% and 5% marjoram oil (Selvaag et al 1995).

Systemic effects

Acute toxicity: Sweet marjoram oil acute oral LD_{50} in rats 2.24 g/kg; acute dermal LD_{50} in rabbits >5 g/kg (Opdyke 1976 p. 469). Terpinen-4-ol is not nephrotoxic, or generally toxic on chronic administration (see Terpinen-4-ol profile, Chapter 14).

Carcinogenic/anticarcinogenic potential: No information was found for sweet marjoram oil, but it contains no known carcinogens. Terpinen-4-ol appears to be non-carcinogenic (see Terpinen-4-ol profile, Chapter 14).

Antioxidant/pro-oxidant activity: An Egyptian marjoram oil inhibited DPPH radicals, hydroxyl radicals, hydrogen peroxide and lipid peroxidation, with IC_{50} values of 58.7, 67.1 91.3 and 68.8 μg/mL, respectively (Mossa & Nawwar 2011). A marjoram oil with 20.8% terpinen-4-ol and 14.1% γ-terpinene showed significant antioxidant activity in egg yolk and rat liver assays, both with and without the presence of a radical inducer. It was more effective than α-tocopherol in both egg yolk assays (Baratta et al 1998).

Comments

Oils are produced from other chemotypes of sweet marjoram, often sold as 'wild oregano' and labeled as being from *Origanum dubium*. These are generally rich in either carvacrol or linalool.

Marjoram wild (carvacrol CT)

Synonym: Wild oregano
Botanical name: *Origanum majorana* L.
Botanical synonyms: *Majorana hortensis* Moench, *Origanum dubium* Boiss.
Family: Lamiaceae (Labiatae)

Essential oil

Source: Leaves
Key constituents:

Carvacrol	76.4–81.0%
p-Cymene	5.2–6.0%
γ-Terpinene	3.0–3.6%
α-Phellandrene	0–1.8%
α-Terpineol	0.9–1.6%
β-Myrcene	0.1–1.4%

Terpinen-4-ol	1.0–1.2%
α-Terpinene	1.2%
α-Pinene	0.9–1.0%

(Arnold et al 1993)

Safety summary

Hazards: Drug interaction; may inhibit blood clotting; skin irritation (low risk).
Cautions (oral): Diabetic medication, anticoagulant medication, major surgery, peptic ulcer, hemophilia, other bleeding disorders (Box 7.1).
Maximum dermal use level: 1.2%

Our safety advice

Our dermal maximum is based on 81% carvacrol content and a dermal limit of 1% for carvacrol to avoid skin irritation (see Carvacrol profile, Chapter 14).

Organ-specific effects

Adverse skin reactions: No information found. Other carvacrol-rich essential oils, such as oregano and savory, are irritant to animals when applied undiluted, as is carvacrol, but when applied to humans at dilutions in the 2–6% range these are non-irritant (see Constituent profiles, Chapter 14).
Cardiovascular effects: Carvacrol inhibits platelet aggregation (Enomoto et al 2001), an essential step in the blood clotting cascade. An essential oil high in carvacrol *(Satureja khuzestanica,* 93.9% carvacrol) significantly reduced plasma glucose concentrations in diabetic rats when given orally at 100 mg/kg/day for 21 days (Shahsavari et al 2009).
Reproductive toxicity: No information was found for wild marjoram oil carvacrol CT, however see comments for this section under Oregano oil.

Systemic effects

Acute toxicity: No information found. For oregano oil, which has a very similar composition, the acute oral LD_{50} in rats was 1.85 g/kg and the acute dermal LD_{50} in rabbits was 480 mg/kg (Opdyke 1974 p. 945–946).
Carcinogenic/anticarcinogenic potential: No information was found for wild marjoram oil carvacrol CT, but it contains no known carcinogens. Carvacrol is reported to be genotoxic, very weakly genotoxic, non-genotoxic and antigenotoxic. This may be dose-related, with only high concentrations presenting a risk. Some in vitro anticarcinogenic activity has been observed (see Carvacrol profile, Chapter 14).
Drug interactions: Antidiabetic or anticoagulant medication, because of cardiovascular effects, above. See Table 4.10B.

Comments

This essential oil is extremely similar to oregano oil in composition. Limited availability.

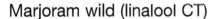

Marjoram wild (linalool CT)

Synonym: Wild oregano
Botanical name: *Origanum majorana* L.
Botanical synonyms: *Majorana hortensis* Moench, *Origanum dubium* Boiss.
Family: Lamiaceae (Labiatae)

Essential oil

Source: Leaves
Key constituents:

Linalool	67.7%
Carvacrol	23.3%
γ-Terpinene	2.1%
p-Cymene	2.0%
β-Caryophyllene	1.8%

(Owen, private communication, 2004)

Safety summary

Hazards: Dermal irritation.
Contraindications: None known.
Maximum dermal use level: 4.3%.

Our safety advice

Our dermal maximum is based on 23.3% carvacrol content and a dermal limit of 1% for carvacrol to avoid skin irritation (see Carvacrol profile, Chapter 14).

Regulatory guidelines

According to IFRA, essential oils rich in linalool should only be used when the level of peroxides is kept to the lowest practical value. The addition of antioxidants such as 0.1% BHT or α-tocopherol at the time of production is recommended (IFRA 2009).

Organ-specific effects

Adverse skin reactions: No information found.
Reproductive toxicity: The low reproductive toxicity of linalool and carvacrol (see Constituent profiles, Chapter 14) suggests that wild marjoram oil linalool CT is not hazardous in pregnancy.

Systemic effects

Acute toxicity: No information found. For linalool, the acute oral LD_{50} has been reported as 2.79 g/kg in rats (Jenner et al 1964) and 2.2, 3.5 and 3.92 g/kg in mice (Letizia et al 2003a). Acute dermal LD_{50} in rabbits 5.61 g/kg (Opdyke 1975 p. 827–832).
Carcinogenic/anticarcinogenic potential: No information was found for wild marjoram oil linalool CT, but it contains no known carcinogens. Carvacrol is reported to be genotoxic, very weakly genotoxic, non-genotoxic and antigenotoxic. This may be dose-related, with only high concentrations presenting a risk. Some in vitro anticarcinogenic activity has been observed (see Carvacrol profile, Chapter 14).

Comments

Limited availability.

Massoia

Botanical name: *Cryptocarya massoy* (Oken) Kosterm.
Botanical synonyms: *Cryptocaria massoia* (Becc.) Kosterm., *Massoia aromatica* Becc.
Family: Lauraceae

Essential oil

Source: Bark
Key constituents:

C-10 Massoia lactone	64.8–68.2%
C-12 Massoia lactone	14.6–17.4%
Benzyl benzoate	8.1–13.4%
β-Bisabolene	0–1.4%

(Garnero and Joulain 1983; Rali et al 2007)

Safety summary

Hazards: Skin irritation/sensitization (high risk); mucous membrane irritation (high risk).
Contraindications: Hypersensitive, diseased or damaged skin, children under 2 years of age. Do not use on mucous membranes.
Maximum dermal use level: 0.01%

Our safety advice

A producer of massoia CO_2 extract recommends a maximum use level of 0.01% for products applied to the skin. In the absence of any published maximum dermal use level for massoia lactones, we have adopted this recommendation.

Regulatory guidelines

IFRA prohibits the use of massoia bark oil as a fragrance ingredient (IFRA 2009).

Organ-specific effects

Adverse skin reactions: There is no RIFM monograph for massoia, which has been suspected of irritation, sensitization and phototoxicity. In a private communication from RIFM, we were informed that, in private tests, 'massoia lactone was so irritating that the standard tests for sensitization and phototoxicity could not be conducted.'

Systemic effects

Acute toxicity: No information found.
Carcinogenic/anticarcinogenic potential: No information was found for massoia bark oil, but it contains no known carcinogens.

Comments

It is unfortunate that no published data can be referenced, either for massoia lactone or massoia oil. Since the oil has not been tested it would seem premature to totally restrict its use, and we are recommending a low maximum use level. If massoia lactone is a strong skin irritant, the essential oil is likely to cause similar problems, but at what concentration is not known. Of two massoia CO_2 extracts sold, one contains 78% and the other 98% massoia lactone.

Mastic

Botanical name: *Pistacia lentiscus* L.
Family: Anacardiaceae

Essential oil

Source: Gum resin
Key constituents:

α-Pinene	58.8–78.6%
β-Myrcene	0.2–12.3%
Linalool	0.1–3.7%
β-Pinene	1.2–3.3%
Verbenone	0–2.9%
Pinocarveol	tr–2.1%
β-Caryophyllene	0.2–2.0%
(+)-Limonene	0.4–1.6%
Methyl-*o*-cresol	0.4–1.2%
Camphoraldehyde II	tr–1.1%
Caryophyllene oxide	tr–1.1%
Methyleugenol	tr–0.1%

(Lawrence 1995g p. 19, p. 69; Magiatis et al 1999)

Safety summary

Hazards: May contain methyleugenol.
Contraindications: None known.
Maximum dermal use level:

EU	0.2%
IFRA	0.4%
Tisserand & Young	20%

Our safety advice

We recommend a dermal maximum of 20%, based on 0.1% methyleugenol content with a dermal limit of 0.02% (see Methyleugenol profile, Chapter 14). Because of its high α-pinene content we recommend that oxidation of mastic oil is avoided by storage in a dark, airtight container in a refrigerator. The addition of an antioxidant to preparations containing it is recommended.

Regulatory guidelines

IFRA recommends a maximum concentration of 0.0004% for methyleugenol in leave-on products such as body lotion (IFRA 2009). The equivalent SCCNFP maximum is 0.0002% (European Commission 2002).

Organ-specific effects

Adverse skin reactions: No information was found for the essential oil, but autoxidation products of α-pinene can cause skin sensitization (see α-Pinene profile, Chapter 14).
Reproductive toxicity: The low reproductive toxicity of α-pinene, β-myrcene and linalool (see Constituent profiles, Chapter 14) suggests that mastic oil is not hazardous in pregnancy.

Systemic effects

Acute toxicity: No information was found for mastic oil. The α-pinene acute oral LD_{50} in rats has been reported as 2.1, 3.2 and 3.7 g/kg; acute dermal LD_{50} in rabbits <5 g.kg (Opdyke 1978 p. 853–857).
Carcinogenic/anticarcinogenic potential: An oil from *Pistacia lentiscus* L. var. *chia* inhibited the proliferation and angiogenesis of human leukemia K562 cells (Loutrari et al 2006). (+)-Limonene displays anticarcinogenic activity; methyleugenol is a rodent carcinogen if exposure is sufficiently high (see Constituent profiles, Chapter 14).

Comments

Limited availability.

May chang

Synonym: Pheasant pepper tree
Botanical name: *Litsea cubeba* (Lour.) Pers.
Botanical synonyms: *Litsea citrata* Blume, *Laurus cubeba* Lour.
Family: Lauraceae

Essential oil

Source: Fruits
Key constituents:

Geranial	37.9–40.6%
Neral	25.5–33.8%
(+)-Limonene	8.4–22.6%
Methyl heptenone	0.5–4.4%
β-Myrcene	0.5–3.0%
Linalool	1.2–1.7%
Geraniol	0.5–1.6%
Sabinene	0.1–1.6%
Linalyl acetate	0–1.6%
α-Pinene	0.8–1.4%
β-Pinene	0.4–1.2%
Nerol	0.2–1.1%

(Lawrence 1989 p. 11, 1996e p. 62; Zhu et al 1993)
Quality: May be adulterated with synthetic citral (Oyen & Dung 1999).

Safety summary

Hazards: Drug interaction; teratogenicity; skin allergy.
Cautions (all routes): Drugs metabolized by CYP2B6 (Appendix B).
Cautions (oral): Diabetes medication, pregnancy.

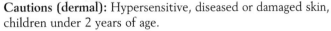

Cautions (dermal): Hypersensitive, diseased or damaged skin, children under 2 years of age.
Maximum daily oral dose in pregnancy: 56 mg
Maximum dermal use level: 0.8%

Our safety advice

We recommend a dermal maximum of 0.8% to avoid skin sensitization. This is based on the IFRA maximum for citral of 0.6% for body oils and lotions (IFRA 2009) and 75% citral content. We recommend a daily oral maximum in pregnancy of 56 mg. This is based on 74% citral content, with dermal and oral citral limits of 0.6% and 0.6 mg/kg (see Citral profile, Chapter 14).

Organ-specific effects

Adverse skin reactions: Undiluted may chang oil was moderately to markedly irritating to rabbits, and was strongly irritating to both mice and pigs; tested at 8% on 25 volunteers it was neither irritating nor sensitizing. It is non-phototoxic (Opdyke 1982 p.731–732). In a study of 200 consecutive dermatitis patients, three were sensitive to 2% may chang oil on patch testing (Rudzki et al 1976). Citral can induce sensitization reactions, and this effect can allegedly be reduced by the co-presence of (+)-limonene (Hanau et al 1983). In a mouse local lymph node assay, which allows comparative measuring of skin sensitizing potency, may chang oil was a weak sensitizer, with a similar potency to citral (Lalko & Api 2006).
Cardiovascular effects: Gavage doses of 10, 15 or 20 mg/kg/day citral for 28 days, dose-dependently lowered plasma insulin levels and increased glucose tolerance in obese rats (Modak & Mukhopadhaya 2011).
Reproductive toxicity: Citral is dose-dependently teratogenic because it inhibits retinoic acid synthesis, and this can affect fetal development (see Citral profile, Chapter 14).

Systemic effects

Acute toxicity: May chang oil acute oral LD_{50} in rats >5 g/kg; acute dermal LD_{50} in rabbits 4.8 g/kg (Opdyke 1982 p. 731–732). Tests using both rats and mice resulted in the following approximate values for may chang oil: acute oral LD_{50} 4.0 g/kg, acute dermal LD_{50} >5.0 g/kg, inhalation LC_{50} 12,500 ppm (Luo et al 2005).
Carcinogenic/anticarcinogenic potential: May chang oil was not genotoxic to *Salmonella tymphimurium*, and did not induce micronuclei in bone marrow cells or chromosome aberrations in mouse spermatocyte cells (Luo et al 2005). Citral, (+)-limonene, and geraniol display anticarcinogenic activity (see Constituent profiles, Chapter 14).
Drug interactions: Antidiabetic medication, because of cardiovascular effects, above. See Table 4.10B. Since citral and geraniol inhibit CYP2B6 (Table 4.11B), there is a theoretical risk of interaction between may chang oil and drugs metabolized by this enzyme (see Appendix B).

Comments

As with lemongrass, the majority of people do not react allergically to may chang oil, but occasional reactions are possible. May chang oil is produced in very high volumes, and is used in the manufacture of citral, ionone, methyl ionone, and vitamins A, E and K (Luo et al 2005). In Java, essential oils from *Litsea cubeba* leaves are produced for local consumption. (May chang oils of commerce are produced from the fruit.) There are two types, one from central Java with 50% 1,8-cineole, 10% citral, the other from West Java with 25% 1,8-cineole, 25% citronellal (Oyen & Dung 1999).

Melissa

Synonyms: Balm, lemon balm
Botanical name: *Melissa officinalis* L.
Family: Lamiaceae (Labiatae)

Essential oil

Source: Fresh aerial parts of plant
Key constituents:

Geranial	12.5–38.3%
Neral	9.7–26.1%
β-Caryophyllene	0.3–19.1%
Citronellal	4.5–13.3%
Germacrene D	0–13.0%
Caryophyllene oxide	0.8–10.0%
Geraniol	1.0–8.1%
(E)-β-Ocimene	0–4.9%
Neryl acetate	1.5–4.0%
6-Methyl-5-hepten-2-ol	0–3.8%
Geranyl acetate	0.7–3.3%
Citronellol + δ-cadinene	0–3.1%
6-Methyl-5-hepten-2-one	0–2.5%
α-Copaene	0–1.7%
Methyl citronellate	0–1.6%
α-Terpineol	0.1–1.4%
α-Caryophyllene	0–1.4%
Nerol	0.6–1.3%
1-Octen-3-ol	0–1.3%

(Lawrence 1996d p. 59–60, 1999c p. 47)
Quality: Shalaby et al (1995) reported that melissa oil degraded readily, even when kept at 4°C. Melissa oil is frequently imitated by mixing oils of citronella, may chang and lemon, plus various isolates and synthetics (Burfield 2003). Such mixtures are sold at prices considerably less than the market value of genuine melissa oil. Synthetic citral and citronellal may be used as adulterants.

Safety summary

Hazards: Drug interaction; teratogenicity; skin sensitization.
Cautions (oral): Diabetes medication, drugs metabolized by CYP2B6 (Appendix B), pregnancy.
Cautions (dermal): Hypersensitive, diseased or damaged skin, children under 2 years of age.
Maximum daily oral dose in pregnancy: 65 mg
Maximum dermal use level: 0.9%

Our safety advice

We recommend a dermal maximum of 0.9% to avoid skin sensitization, and a daily oral maximum in pregnancy of 65 mg. This is based on 64% citral content, with dermal and oral citral limits of 0.6% and 0.6 mg/kg (see Citral profile, Chapter 14). We recommend that an antioxidant is added to melissa oil to guard against oxidation.

Regulatory guidelines

IFRA previously recommended that melissa oil should not be used as a fragrance ingredient (IFRA 2009). In 2009, IFRA introduced a dermal limit of 0.63%.

Organ-specific effects

Adverse skin reactions: No information found. Citral (geranial + neral) may induce sensitization reactions on patch testing at concentrations above 0.5% (see Citral profile, Chapter 14).
Cardiovascular effects: When fed to male mice at 0.015 mg/day for six weeks, melissa oil caused a 65% reduction in blood glucose, a significant increase in serum insulin levels, and an improvement in glucose tolerance (Chung et al 2010).
Reproductive toxicity: Citral is dose-dependently teratogenic because it inhibits retinoic acid synthesis, and this can affect fetal development (see Citral profile, Chapter 14).

Systemic effects

Acute toxicity: No information found.
Antioxidant/pro-oxidant activity: A melissa oil from Serbia and Montenegro, containing 23.4% geranial, 16.5% neral, 13.7% citronellal and 4.6% β-caryophyllene, exhibited very strong, dose-dependent radical scavenging activity. The oil scavenged DPPH radicals with an IC_{50} of 7.6 µg/mL, compared to 5.4 µg/mL for BHT. The most powerful scavenging constituents included the ones cited above for this oil (Mimica-Dukic et al 2004). A Brazilian melissa oil, containing 47.3% geranial, 39.3% neral, 2.9% isomenthol and 1.8% chrysanthenol, demonstrated antioxidant activity (measured using a reduction assay) with an EC_{50} of 2 µL (De Sousa et al 2004).
Carcinogenic/anticarcinogenic potential: The same Brazilian melissa oil was tested for cytotoxicty against human cell lines for lung cancer (A549), breast cancer (MCF-7), colon cancer (CaCo-2), leukemia (HL60 and K562), and a mouse melanoma cell line (B16F10). It was dose-dependently cytotoxic to all cell lines, at concentrations ranging from 1:2,000 to 1:50,000 (De Sousa et al 2004). Melissa oil inhibited proliferation of HEP-2 cells derived from human laryngeal cancer (Allahverdiyev et al 2001). A melissa oil with 39.6% citronellal and no neral or geranial was non-mutagenic in both T98 and T100 *S. typhimurium* strains, with or without metabolic activation (De Martino et al 2009a). Melissa oil contains no known carcinogens. Citral (geranial + neral), β-caryophyllene, citronellal and geraniol display anticarcinogenic activity (see Constituent profiles, Chapter 14).
Drug interactions: Antidiabetic medication, because of cardiovascular effects, above. See Table 4.10B. Since citral and geraniol inhibit CYP2B6 (Table 4.11B), there is a theoretical risk of interaction between melissa oil and drugs metabolized by this enzyme (Appendix B).

Comments

Melissa oil was previously banned by IFRA for use in fragrances. According to RIFM, 'animal sensitization tests were done and found that melissa oil was a sensitizer', but because no member company was willing to fund further testing, the oil was prohibited, due to 'insufficient data' (Api, private communication, 2006). IFRA changed its ruling in 2009, largely due to lobbying by Tony Burfield of Cropwatch, who showed why original ban by IFRA could not be justified (www.cropwatch.org/Melissa%20oil;%20the%20Cropwatch%20articles%202006-9.pdf, accessed August 11th 2011). Melissa oils, both steam distilled and solvent extracted, became commercially available during the early 1990s. (Previously the only melissa oils on the market were fabricated ones, and many are still offered.) These represent several chemotypes.

Mimosa

Botanical name: *Acacia dealbata* Link
Botanical synonyms: *Acacia decurrens* Willd. var. *dealbata* (Link) Muller, *Racosperma dealbatum* (Link) Pedley
Family: Mimosaceae

Absolute

Source: Flowers
Key constituents:

Lupenone	20%
Lupeol	7.8%
(Z)-Heptadec-8-ene	6.0%

(Perriot et al 2010)

Safety summary

Hazards: None known.
Contraindications: None known.

Organ-specific effects

Adverse skin reactions: Undiluted mimosa absolute was slightly irritating to guinea pigs, but was not irritating to mice; tested at 1% on 25 volunteers it was neither irritating nor sensitizing. It is non-phototoxic (Opdyke 1975 p. 874–874).

Systemic effects

Acute toxicity: Non-toxic. Mimosa absolute acute oral LD_{50} in rats >5 g/kg; acute dermal LD_{50} in rabbits >5 g/kg (Opdyke 1975 p. 874–874).
Carcinogenic/anticarcinogenic potential: No information found.

Comments

The constituents of mimosa absolute comprise 50% semivolatile, 30% non-volatile and 20% volatile compounds. Many constituents are triterpene ketones, alcohols and esters (Perriot et al 2010). The concrete is extracted with hexane. The plant

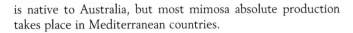

is native to Australia, but most mimosa absolute production takes place in Mediterranean countries.

Mint (bergamot)

Botanical name: *Mentha aquatica* L. var. *citrata* (Her.) Fresen
Botanical synonym: *Mentha citrata* Ehrh.
Family: Lamiaceae (Labiatae)

Essential oil

Source: Aerial parts
Key constituents:

Linalyl acetate	34.0–57.3%
Linalool	24.9–55.2%
β-Terpineol	1.0–2.8%
1,8-Cineole	0.5–2.3%
Geranyl acetate	0.7–1.8%
(*E*)-Linalool oxide	1.3–1.7%
(*Z*)-Linalool oxide	1.2–1.6%
3-Octyl acetate	0.7–1.2%

(Lawrence 1979 p. 20)
Quality: May be adulterated with added linalyl acetate and linalool (Burfield 2003).

Safety summary

Hazards: None known.
Contraindications: None known.

Regulatory guidelines

According to IFRA, essential oils rich in linalool should only be used when the level of peroxides is kept to the lowest practical value. The addition of antioxidants such as 0.1% BHT or α-tocopherol at the time of production is recommended (IFRA 2009).

Organ-specific effects

Adverse skin reactions: Undiluted bergamot mint oil produced slight to moderate edema and erythema on guinea pigs; tested at 8% on 25 volunteers it was neither irritating nor sensitizing. No phototoxic effects were produced in mice (Ford et al 1992 p. 73S). Oxidation products of linalool may be skin sensitizing, but 1,8-cineole has antioxidant properties (see Constituent profiles, Chapter 14).

Systemic effects

Acute toxicity: Bergamot mint oil acute oral LD$_{50}$ in rats ~5 g/kg; acute dermal LD$_{50}$ in rabbits >5 g/kg (Ford et al 1992 p. 73S).
Carcinogenic/anticarcinogenic potential: No information was found for bergamot mint oil, but it contains no known carcinogens.

Comments

The plant has been designated as a variety of peppermint (*Mentha x piperita* L. var. *citrata* Ehrh.) but seems more likely to be a selection of *Mentha aquatica*, the correct infraspecific taxon of which is not known (Craker and Simon 1986 p. 55).

Mint (wild forest)

Synonym: Common horsemint common
Botanical name: *Mentha longifolia* L.
Family: Lamiaceae (Labiatae)

Essential oil

Source: Leaves
Key constituents:

Piperitone oxide	50.8%
Germacrene D	12.7%
Piperitenone oxide	10.3%
Carvone	4.1%
β-Caryophyllene	4.1%
1,8-Cineole	4.0%
(+)-Limonene	2.1%
(*Z*)-β-Ocimene	1.6%
Viridiflorol	1.4%
β-Pinene	1.1%
β-Myrcene	1.0%

(Badoux, private communication, 2003)

Safety summary

Hazards: None known.
Contraindications: None known.

Organ-specific effects

Adverse skin reactions: No information was found for either wild forest mint oil or piperitone oxide.

Systemic effects

Acute toxicity: No information found.
Antioxidant/pro-oxidant activity: Wild forest mint oil significantly scavenged DPPH and OH radicals (Mimica-Dukic et al 2003).
Carcinogenic/anticarcinogenic potential: No information was found for wild forest mint oil or piperitone oxide. The oil contains no known carcinogens.

Comments

Limited availability. The plant exists in several chemotypes, including a pulegone, a rotundifolone, a carvone and a linalool.

Mugwort (common, camphor/thujone CT)

Synonyms: Mugwort, Indian wormwood
Botanical name: *Artemisia vulgaris* L.
Family: Asteraceae (Compositae)

Essential oil

Source: Aerial parts of flowering plant
Key constituents:

Camphor	20.8%
Artemisia alcohol	15.3%
α-Thujone	11.4%
β-Caryophyllene	10.6%
Isoborneol	9.3%
1,8-Cineole	9.0%
Sabinene	6.1%
α-Terpineol	3.9%
δ-Guaiene	1.2%
α-Pinene	1.2%
Germacrene D	1.0%

(Haider et al 2003)

Safety summary

Hazards: Expected to be mildly neurotoxic, based on thujone content.
Contraindications (all routes): Pregnancy, breastfeeding.
Maximum adult daily oral dose: 56 mg
Maximum dermal use level: 2%

Our safety advice

Our oral and dermal restrictions are based on 20.8% camphor and 11.4% α-thujone content with limits of 2.0 mg/kg and 4.5% for camphor and 0.1 mg/kg and 0.25% for thujone (see Constituent profiles, Chapter 14).

Organ-specific effects

Adverse skin reactions: No information found.
Neurotoxicity: There is a risk of convulsions with high doses of thujone. The thujone NOAEL for convulsions was reported to be 10 mg/kg in male rats and 5 mg/kg in females (Margaria 1963).

Systemic effects

Acute toxicity: No information found. Both α- and β-thujone are moderately toxic, with reported oral LD$_{50}$ values ranging from 190–500 mg/kg for different species (see Thujone profile, Chapter 14).
Antioxidant/pro-oxidant activity: Essential oil of *Artemisia vulgaris* var. *indica* strongly scavenged DPPH radicals (Xiufen et al 2004).
Carcinogenic/anticarcinogenic potential: *Artemisia vulgaris* var. *indica* oil was antimutagenic in an assay with *S. typhimurium* TA98 (Hiramatsu et al 2004).

Comments

This analysis is for an oil from a small plantation in Lucknow, India. *Artemisia vulgaris* is sometimes erroneously given as the source of white wormwood oil.

Mugwort (common, chrysanthenyl acetate CT)

Synonyms: Mugwort, Indian wormwood
Botanical name: *Artemisia vulgaris* L.
Family: Asteraceae (Compositae)

Essential oil

Source: Aerial parts
Key constituents:

Chrysanthenyl acetate	31.7–32.8%
Germacrene D	12.1–15.9%
β-Caryophyllene	3.8–3.9%
Artemisia ketone	0–3.1%
β-Selinene	2.8–2.9%
1,8-Cineole	2.2–2.9%
β-Thujone	2.1–2.3%
α-Selinene	1.5–2.2%
Sabinene	1.8–1.9%
Santolina triene	0–1.9%
Terpinen-4-ol	1.7–1.8%
Borneol	1.6–1.7%
α-Caryophyllene	1.5–1.6%
Caryophyllene oxide	1.2–1.5%
p-Cymene	0.9–1.5%
β-Myrcene	1.2–1.3%
Phytol	0.9–1.2%
Spathulenol	~1.2%
α-Copaene	1.0–1.1%
α-Thujone	0.2–0.3%

(Fakhry, private communication, 2003)

Safety summary

Hazards: Slight neurotoxicity.
Contraindications (all routes): Pregnancy, breastfeeding.
Maximum adult daily oral dose: 269 mg
Maximum dermal use level: 9.6%

Our safety advice

Our oral and dermal restrictions are based on 2.6% total thujone content with thujone limits of 0.1 mg/kg and 0.25% (see Thujone profile, Chapter 14).

Organ-specific effects

Adverse skin reactions: No information found.
Neurotoxicity: There is a risk of convulsions with moderately high doses of thujone. The thujone NOAEL for convulsions

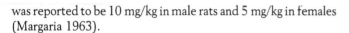

was reported to be 10 mg/kg in male rats and 5 mg/kg in females (Margaria 1963).

Systemic effects

Acute toxicity: No information was found for the essential oil or its two major constituents. Both α- and β-thujone are moderately toxic, with reported oral LD$_{50}$ values ranging from 190–500 mg/kg for different species (see Thujone profile, Chapter 14).
Antioxidant/pro-oxidant activity: Essential oil of *Artemisia vulgaris* var. *indica* strongly scavenged DPPH radicals (Xiufen et al 2004).
Carcinogenic/anticarcinogenic potential: *Artemisia vulgaris* var. *indica* oil was antimutagenic in an assay with *S. typhimurium* TA98 (Hiramatsu et al 2004).

Comments

We could not establish for certain whether the chrysanthenyl acetate-rich essential oil sold as deriving from *Artemisia vulgaris* might actually be the chrysanthenyl acetate chemotype of *Artemisia herba-alba* (see White wormwood, below). *Artemisia vulgaris* is sometimes erroneously given as the source of white wormwood oil.

Mugwort (Douglas)

Synonyms: Douglas sagewort, California mugwort
Botanical name: *Artemisia douglasiana* Bess.
Family: Asteraceae (Compositae)

Essential oil

Source: Leaves
Key constituents:

Artemisia ketone	55.8%
1,8-Cineole	6.4%
Artemisia alcohol	5.6%
Yomogi alcohol	1.8%
p-Cymene	1.7%
β-Caryophyllene + terpinen-4-ol	1.5%
Sabinene	1.4%

(http://libertynatural.com/coa/179.htm accessed 6th August 2012)

Safety summary

Hazards: None known.
Contraindications: None known.

Organ-specific effects

Adverse skin reactions: No information found.

Systemic effects

Acute toxicity: No information found. An annual wormwood oil containing 35.7% artemisia ketone had a mouse i.p. LD50 of

1,832 mg/kg. Doses higher than 1,500 mg/kg were neurototic, but lower doses were not (Radulovic et al 2013).
Carcinogenic/anticarcinogenic potential: No information was found for Douglas mugwort oil, but it contains no known carcinogens.

Comments

Limited availability. The data on annual wormwood oil suggest that neither artemisia ketone nor Douglas mugwort oil are particularly toxic.

Mugwort (great)

Botanical name: *Artemisia arborescens* L.
Family: Asteraceae (Compositae)

Essential oil

Source: Aerial parts
Key constituents:

β-Thujone	34.0%
Chamazulene	22.4%
Camphor	11.8%

(Tucker et al 1993)

Safety summary

Hazards: Drug interaction; expected to be neurotoxic, based on thujone content.
Contraindications (all routes): Pregnancy, breastfeeding.
Cautions (all routes): Drugs metabolized by CYP2D6 (Appendix B).
Cautions (oral): Drugs metabolized by CYP1A2 or CYP3A4 (Appendix B).
Maximum adult daily oral dose: 20 mg
Maximum dermal use level: 0.7%

Our safety advice

Our oral and dermal restrictions are based on 34.0% {τσ}-thujone content with thujone limits of 0.1 mg/kg and 0.25% (see Thujone profile, Chapter 14).

Organ-specific effects

Adverse skin reactions: No information found.
Neurotoxicity: There is a risk of convulsions with moderately high doses of thujone. The thujone NOAEL for convulsions was reported to be 10 mg/kg in male rats and 5 mg/kg in females (Margaria 1963).

Systemic effects

Acute toxicity: No information was found for great mugwort oil, but toxicity is likely to be comparable to that of white mugwort (see below) as the composition of the two oils is so similar.

Carcinogenic/anticarcinogenic potential: No information was found for great mugwort oil but it contains no known carcinogens.

Drug interactions: Since chamazulene inhibits CYP1A2, CYP3A4 and CYP2D6 (Table 4.11B), there is a theoretical risk of interaction between great mugwort oil and drugs metabolized by these enzymes (Appendix B).

Comments

Great mugwort oil is occasionally available.

Muhuhu

Botanical name: *Brachylaena huillensis* O. Hoffm.
Botanical synonym: *Brachylaena hutchinsii* Hutch.
Family: Asteraceae (Compositae)

Essential oil

Source: Wood
Key constituents:

α-Amorphene	16.5%
Brachyl oxide	10.0%
Copaenol	7.5%
Copaenal + unknown	7.5%
δ-Cadinene	6.5%
α-Calacorene	5.0%
Ylangenal	4.0%
Cubebol	3.5%
Cadalene	3.0%
α-Muurolene	3.0%
α-Copaene	2.0%
Ylangenol	1.5%
γ-Amorphene	1.0%
α-Ylangene	1.0%

(Lawrence 1981 p. 30)

Safety summary

Hazards: None known.
Contraindications: None known.

Organ-specific effects

Adverse skin reactions: No information was found for muhuhu oil, and little is known about its major constituents.

Systemic effects

Acute toxicity: No information was found for muhuhu oil, and little is known about its major constituents.
Carcinogenic/anticarcinogenic potential: No information was found for muhuhu oil, but it contains no known carcinogens.

Comments

Limited availability. This slow-growing, hardwood tree is indigenous to Angola, Kenya, Mozambique, Tanzania and Uganda. It is rare for Asteraceae species to be classed as trees.

Mullilam

Synonym: Salai
Botanical name: *Zanthoxylum rhetsa* (Roxb.) DC
Botanical synonym: *Zanthoxylum limonella* (Dennst.) Alston
Family: Rutaceae

Essential oil

Source: Dried fruit pods
Key constituents:

Sabinene	66.3%
α-Pinene	6.6%
β-Pinene	6.4%
Terpinen-4-ol	3.5%
Decanal	2.3%
β-Myrcene	1.4%
β-Phellandrene	1.4%
α-Terpineol	1.3%
Linalool	1.2%
γ-Terpinene	1.0%

(Shafi et al 2000)

Safety summary

Hazards: None known.
Contraindications: None known.

Organ-specific effects

Adverse skin reactions: No information found for mullilam oil or sabinene.
Reproductive toxicity: The low reproductive toxicity of sabinene, α-pinene and β-pinene (see Constituent profiles, Chapter 14) suggests that no mullilam oil is not hazardous in pregnancy.

Systemic effects

Acute toxicity: No information found for mullilam oil or sabinene.
Carcinogenic/anticarcinogenic potential: No information was found for mullilam oil, but it contains no known carcinogens.

Comments

Limited availability.

Mustard

Botanical names: *Brassica nigra* L. (black mustard); *Brassica juncea* (L.) Czern.
Family: Brassicaceae (Cruciferae)

Essential oil

Source: Black or brown mustard seeds

Key constituents:

Brassica nigra

Allyl isothiocyanate	23.2%
Dimethyl trisulfide	15.6%
Methyl linoleate	9.5%
3-Butenonitrile	6.0%
2-Phenylethyl isothiocyanate	5.0%
Methyl linolenate	4.5%
Ethyl acetate	3.8%
Methyl palmitate	3.5%
(3Z)-Hexen-1-ol	3.3%
3-Phenylpropionitrile	2.3%
Ethyl pentadecanoate	1.4%
Furfural	1.3%
2-Methylpent-2-enal	1.0%

(Zheng-kui & Ying-fang 1986)

Brassica juncea

Allyl isothiocyanate	54.8–68.8%
Diallyl trisulfide	7.8–9.7%
3-Butenyl isothiocyanate	4.8–5.9%
Diallyl sulfide	3.2–5.5%
Diallyl disulfide	2.7–4.1%
Butyl isothiocyanate	0–3.6%
Phenylethyl isothiocyanate	2.4–3.4%
Diallyl tetrasulfide	0.7–3.3%

(Yu et al 2003)

Quality: Allyl isothiocyanate may be passed off as mustard oil (Burfield 2003).

Safety summary

Hazards: Toxicity; skin irritation (high risk); mucous membrane irritant (high risk).
Contraindications: Should not be used, either internally or externally.

Our safety advice

There is little doubt that the toxicity of mustard oil is largely due to its content of allyl isothiocyanate. Due to the toxicity of this constituent, and to the severe lachrymatory and irritant nature of the essential oil, we recommend that mustard oil is not used in therapy. It is possible that there are safe levels for therapeutic use, but there are no data which indicate what these levels might be.

Regulatory guidelines

Allyl isothiocyanate is prohibited in fragrances by IFRA, and as a cosmetic ingredient in the EU, which effectively means that mustard oil is similarly prohibited.

Organ-specific effects

Adverse skin and mucous membrane reactions: Mustard oil is said to be a severe skin irritant, producing almost instant blistering (Leung & Foster 2003). Allyl isothiocyanate is similarly described as a severe irritant to skin and mucous membranes (Evans & Schmidt 1980; Budavari 1989). At 0.125%, mustard oil was slightly irritating to human oral mucous membrane. Successive application of this concentration at one minute intervals resulted in a perceived reduction in irritation, indicating desensitization (Simons et al 2003). Inhalation of mustard oil produces unpleasant sensations in the head and greatly irritates the eyes and mucous membranes of the nose and respiratory system (Von Skramlik 1959).

Reproductive toxicity: No information found. Allyl isothiocyanate caused embryonic death and decreased fetal weight in pregnant rats when given at 50 mg/kg sc on two consecutive days (Nishie & Daxenbichler 1980). Ethyl acetate is widely considered to be neurotoxic.

Systemic effects

Acute toxicity: No information found. Allyl isothiocyanate acute oral LD_{50} is 340 mg/kg in rats, producing jaundice (Jenner et al 1964). It is orally toxic to rat liver, thymus, kidney and blood at 40 mg/kg (Lewerenz et al 1988). Goitrogenic in rats at 2–4 mg po (Langer & Stolc 1965).

Subacute & subchronic toxicity: No information found. Given to rats at 50 mg/kg in the diet for 20 days, allyl isothiocyanate caused stomach ulceration in all animals, while at 20 mg/kg the ulceration occurred in 50% of animals. At 50 mg/kg for 14 days, it caused thickening of the mucosal surface of the stomach in both rats and mice, and thickening of the urinary bladder wall in male mice. No gross or microscopic lesions were seen after feeding allyl isothiocyanate to rats and mice for 13 weeks at 25 mg/kg (National Toxicology Program 1982). Given to rats in the diet for 26 weeks at 1,000, 2,500 or 10,000 ppm there were no apparent adverse effects (Hagan et al 1967).

Carcinogenic/anticarcinogenic potential: Mustard oil was not mutagenic in the Ames test but produced CA in Chinese hamster fibroblasts (Ishidate et al 1984). Mustard oil had a significant chemopreventive effect in DMBA-induced transplacental and translactational carcinogenesis in mice. It is believed that this effect is due to the induction of detoxifying enzymes (Hashim et al 1998). Allyl isothiocyanate was genotoxic in tests on Chinese hamster cells (Kasamaki et al 1982). It can cause hyperplasia and transitional cell papillomas in male rats (Dunnick et al 1982). Diallyl trisulfide, diallyl disulfide and diallyl sulfide display anticarcinogenic activity (see Constituent profiles, Chapter 14).

Comments

Zhu et al (1995) reports a *Brassica juncea* oil consisting of 92.3% allyl isothiocyanate, and Burfield (2000) states that mustard oils can contain up to 97% of this compound. Mustard is one of the most hazardous essential oils. The oil is not present in the free state in the seed or powdered seed, but in the form of glycosides, so preparations made from these by mechanical means (i.e. pressing) do not contain allyl isothiocyanate. The essential oil is only formed after fermentation, then distillation. When the mustard comes into contact with water, this hydrolyses sinigrin, a glycoside contained within the seeds' cells under the influence of myrosinase, an enzyme which is also present. White mustard seeds do not produce any allyl isothiocyanate under these conditions (Arctander 1960). The fixed oil from the seeds is also known as mustard oil.

Myrrh

Synonym: Somalian myrrh
Botanical name: *Commiphora myrrha* (Nees) Engl.
Botanical synonym: *Commiphora molmol* Engl.
Family: Burseraceae

Essential oil

Source: Dried gum oleoresin
Key constituents:

Furanoeudesma-1,3-diene	34.0%
Furanodiene	19.7%
Lindestrene	12.0%
β-Elemene	8.7%
Germacrene B	4.3%
Germacrene D	3.2%
δ-Elemene	2.1%
2-Methoxyfuranodiene	2.1%
Isofuranogermacrene (curzerene)	2.0%
T-Cadinol	1.6%
β-Caryophyllene	1.3%
β-Bourbonene	1.2%
γ-Cadinene	1.2%
Furanoeudesma-1,4-diene	1.2%
γ-Elemene	1.1%

(Dekebo et al 2002)

Safety summary

Hazards: May be fetotoxic, due to β-elemene and furanodiene content.
Contraindications (all routes): Pregnancy, lactation.

Organ-specific effects

Adverse skin reactions: Undiluted myrrh oil was not irritating to mice or pigs; tested at 8% on 25 volunteers it was neither irritating nor sensitizing. Myrrh oil is not phototoxic (Opdyke 1976 p. 621). Myrrh oil was concentration-dependently irritating to the ear of albino mice, causing irritation in 12/12 animals at 0.1 mg/μL (~10%) and 4/12 animals at ~0.15% (Saeed & Sabir 2004). A 65-year-old aromatherapist with multiple essential oil sensitivities reacted to both 1% and 5% myrrh oil (Selvaag et al 1995).
Reproductive toxicity: The administration of a combination of myrrh resin and essential oil to pregnant rats at 50–200 mg/kg/day on gestational days 6–15 did not increase abnormalities of the fetal skeleton (Massoud et al 2000, cited in Mills & Bone 2005). Both furanodiene and β-elemene are antiangiogenic (Chen et al 2011; Zhong et al 2012). In view of the probable link between antiangiogenic effects and reproductive toxicity (Chaiworapongsa et al 2010; Zhou et al 2013), we have contraindicated myrrh oil in pregnancy and lactation.
Hepatotoxicity: A single oral dose of 12.5, 25 or 50 mg/kg of furanodiene dose-dependently protected mice against liver injury induced by D-galactosamine/lipopolysaccharide or TNF-α (Morikawa et al 2002).

Systemic effects

Acute toxicity: Myrrh oil acute oral LD_{50} in rats: 1.65 g/kg (Opdyke 1976 p. 621).
Antioxidant/pro-oxidant activity: The essential oil from Somalian *Commiphora myrrha* displayed an antioxidant activity against singlet oxygen greater than that of (±)-α-tocopherol (Racine & Auffray 2005; Auffray 2007). Singlet oxygen is a major player in lipid peroxidation, phototoxicity and DNA degradation.
Carcinogenic/anticarcinogenic potential: No information was found for myrrh oil, but it contains no known carcinogens. Furanodiene demonstrated an in vitro anticarcinogenic action against human liver cancer cells by preventing tumor cell growth and inducing apoptosis (Xiao et al 2007). Furanodiene inhibited proliferation of six cancer cell lines with IC_{50} values of 0.6–4.8 μg/mL, and of uterine cervical and sarcoma tumors in mice (Sun et al 2009). β-Elemene displays anticarcinogenic activity (see β-Elemene profile).

Comments

There appears to be a considerable discrepancy in the mouse skin irritation data reported by Opdyke (1976 p. 621) and Saeed & Sabir (2004). The general perception is that myrrh oil should only derive from C. *myrrha*. However, there are over 150 species of *Commiphora*, and myrrh oil may wholly or partly come from species such as C. *Africana*, C. *erythraea*, C. *holtziana*, C. *kataf*, C. *madagascariensis*, C. *mukul*, C. *schimperi* and C. *sphaerocarpa*. Essential oils from other species have significantly different chemical compositions to that of true myrrh (Hanus et al 2005). Curzerene is the major constituent of C. *myrrha* var. *molmol* oil (Morteza-Semnani & Saeedi 2003). Many early reports of myrrh oil composition include constituents that are not present in true myrrh oil, such as curzerenone and dihydropyrocurzerenone; a careful analysis of the oil will reveal such adulteration (Dekebo et al 2002).

Myrtle

Botanical name: *Myrtus communis* L.
Family: Myrtaceae

Essential oil

Source: Leaves
Key constituents:

α-Pinene	18.5–56.7%
1,8-Cineole	18.9–37.5%
Myrtenyl acetate	0.1–21.1%
(+)-Limonene	5.1–12.7%

Linalool	1.7–9.5%
α-Terpinyl acetate	0–4.4%
α-Terpineol	0–3.3%
Geranyl acetate	1.4–2.9%
Linalyl acetate	tr–2.5%
p-Cymene	0.4–1.8%
Estragole	0–1.4%
Isobutyl isobutyrate	0.3–1.1%
Methyleugenol	0.3–0.8%

(Lawrence 1995g p. 80–82)

Myrtle (red)

1,8-Cineole	34.3%
α-Pinene	24.8%
Myrtenyl acetate	13.7%
(+)-Limonene	10.7%
α-Terpineol	4.0%
Geranyl acetate	2.8%
Linalool	2.3%
Methyleugenol	1.0%
Estragole	0.2%

(Berger, private communication, 1998)

Safety summary

Hazards: Drug interaction; potentially carcinogenic, based on estragole and methyleugenol content.
Cautions (oral): Diabetes medication.
Maximum adult daily oral dose: 65 mg
Maximum dermal use level:

EU	0.02%
IFRA	0.04%
Tisserand & Young	1.9%

Our safety advice

We recommend a maximum adult daily oral dose of 65 mg for each myrtle oil, based on limits of 0.05 mg/kg/day for estragole, and 0.01 mg/kg/day for methyleugenol. We also recommend a dermal maximum of 1.9% for myrtle oils based on either 1.4% estragole and 0.8% methyleugenol content or 0.2% estragole and 1.0% methyleugenol content, and dermal limits of 0.12% and 0.02% for estragole and methyleugenol, respectively (see Constituent profiles, Chapter 14).

Regulatory guidelines

IFRA recommends a maximum dermal use level for estragole of 0.01% in leave-on or wash-off preparations for body and face (IFRA 2009). IFRA recommends a maximum concentration of 0.0004% methyleugenol in leave-on products such as body lotions (IFRA 2009). The equivalent SCCNFP maximum is 0.0002% (European Commission 2002).

Organ-specific effects

Adverse skin reactions: Undiluted myrtle oil was moderately irritating to rabbits, but was not irritating to mice; tested at 4% on 25 volunteers it was neither irritating nor sensitizing. Myrtle oil produced no sensitization reactions in 100 subjects when tested at concentrations ranging from 0.28–0.9% in two perfume compositions in a repeat insult patch test. Myrtle oil was non-phototoxic in hairless mice. (Opdyke 1983 p. 869).
Cardiovascular effects: Myrtle oil reduced blood glucose by 51% in alloxan-diabetic rabbits four hours after an oral dose of 50 mg/kg, but had no affect serum insulin concentrations (Sepici et al 2004).

Systemic effects

Acute toxicity: Acute oral LD_{50} in rats reported as >5 g/kg; acute dermal LD_{50} in rabbits >5 g/kg (Opdyke 1983 p. 869) and 3.68 mL/kg (Uehleke & Brinkschulte-Freitas 1979). Acute oral LD_{50} in mice 2.23 mL/kg (Uehleke & Brinkschulte-Freitas 1979).
Antioxidant/pro-oxidant activity: Two myrtle oils exhibited moderate DPPH scavenging activity with IC_{50} values of 5.99 and 6.24 mg/mL (Mimica-Dukic et al 2010).
Carcinogenic/anticarcinogenic potential: Myrtle oil has demonstrated weak-to-moderate antimutagenic activity (Hayder et al 2003, 2004; Mimica-Dukic et al 2010). Estragole and methyleugenol are rodent carcinogens; (+)-limonene has demonstrated anticarcinogenic activity (see (+)-Limonene profile, Chapter 14).
Drug interactions: Antidiabetic medication, because of cardiovascular effects, above. See Table 4.10B.

Comments

In addition to regular myrtle oil, 'green' and 'red' myrtle oils are available. Green myrtle oil is high in myrtenyl acetate/linalool, and is produced in Corsica, and red myrtle refers to the cineole-rich type available from Morocco (Burfield 2000). At least two subspecies of *Myrtus communis* exist, with subsp. *communis* being the most often encountered (Craker & Simon 1987).

Myrtle (aniseed)

Synonyms: Anise-scented myrtle
Botanical name: *Backhousia anisata* Vickery
Family: Myrtaceae

Essential oil

Source: Leaves
Key constituents:

(E)-Anethole	95.0%
Estragole	4.4%

(Brophy et al 1995)

Safety summary

Hazards: Drug interaction; potentially carcinogenic, based on estragole content; reproductive hormone modulation; may inhibit blood clotting.
Contraindications (all routes): Pregnancy, breastfeeding, endometriosis, estrogen-dependent cancers, children under 5 years of age.
Cautions (oral): Diabetes medication, anticoagulant medication, major surgery, peptic ulcer, hemophilia, other bleeding disorders (Box 7.1)
Maximum adult daily oral dose: 80 mg
Maximum dermal use level:

EU	No limit
IFRA	0.2%
Tisserand & Young	2.7%

Our safety advice

We recommend an oral maximum of 80 mg/day, and a dermal maximum of 2.7%, based on 4.4% estragole with oral and dermal limits of 0.05 mg/kg/day and 0.12% (see Estragole profile, Chapter 14).

Regulatory guidelines

IFRA recommends a maximum dermal use level for estragole of 0.01% in leave-on or wash-off preparations for body and face (IFRA 2009). Estragole is not restricted in the EU.

Organ-specific effects

Adverse skin reactions: No information found. (E)-Anethole is prone to oxidation, and its oxidation products may be skin sensitizing (see (E)-Anethole profile, Chapter 14).
Cardiovascular effects: (E)-anethole inhibits platelet aggregation (Yoshioka & Tamada 2005), an essential step in the blood clotting cascade. Sweet fennel oil (which is similar to aniseed myrtle oil in composition) reduced blood glucose levels in both normal and alloxan-diabetic rats following sc injection at 21.5 mg/kg (Essway et al 1995).
Reproductive toxicity: (E)-Anethole is estrogenic in in vitro yeast assays (Albert-Puleo 1980, Howes et al 2002) and sweet fennel tea (containing (E)-anethole) has shown in vivo estrogenic effects in humans (Türkyilmaz et al 2008).
Hepatotoxicity: No information found. (E)-Anethole shows a dose-dependent hepatotoxicity which is due to a metabolite, anethole 1',2'-epoxide (AE) and different amounts of AE are produced in different species. However, the amounts of (E)-anethole-rich essential oils used in aromatherapy pose no risk to humans (see (E)-Anethole profile). High doses of (E)-anethole or AE deplete glutathione (Marshall & Caldwell 1992, 1993) but sweet fennel oil, which has a similar composition to aniseed myrtle, significantly induced glutathione S-transferase activity in mouse tissues (Lam & Zheng 1991).

Systemic effects

Acute toxicity: No information found.

Carcinogenic/anticarcinogenic potential: No information found. Estragole is a rodent carcinogen when oral exposure is sufficiently high; (E)-anethole is not a rodent carcinogen (see (E)-Anethole profile, Chapter 14).
Drug interactions: Antidiabetic or anticoagulant medication, because of cardiovascular effects, above. See Table 4.10B.

Comments

There is also an estragole chemotype, with 77.5% of estragole, which is not commercially available.

Myrtle (bog)

Synonym: Sweet gale
Botanical name: *Myrica gale* L.
Family: Myrtaceae

Essential oil

Source: Leaves
Key constituents:

β-Caryophyllene	11.0%
β-Myrcene	9.5%
(+)-Limonene	7.2%
δ-Cadinene	4.7%
α-Caryophyllene	4.4%
α-Phellandrene	4.2%
Germacrone	3.7%
γ-Elemene	3.3%
α-Cadinol + unidentified	2.9%
α-Selinene	2.6%
p-Cymene	2.5%
(E)-β-Ocimene	2.3%
α-Longipinene	1.7%
(Z)-β-Ocimene	1.7%
Selin-11-en-4-ol	1.7%
(E)-Nerolidol	1.5%
Caryophyllene oxide	1.2%
1,8-Cineole	1.1%
α-Bisabolol	1.0%

(Mainguy, private communication 2001)

Safety summary

Hazards: None known.
Contraindications: None known.

Organ-specific effects

Adverse skin reactions: No information found.

Systemic effects

Acute toxicity: No information found.
Carcinogenic/anticarcinogenic potential: A bog myrtle oil hydrodistilled in Canada and containing 12.1–23.2% myrcene,

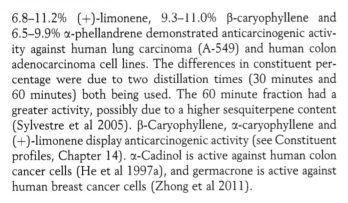

6.8–11.2% (+)-limonene, 9.3–11.0% β-caryophyllene and 6.5–9.9% α-phellandrene demonstrated anticarcinogenic activity against human lung carcinoma (A-549) and human colon adenocarcinoma cell lines. The differences in constituent percentage were due to two distillation times (30 minutes and 60 minutes) both being used. The 60 minute fraction had a greater activity, possibly due to a higher sesquiterpene content (Sylvestre et al 2005). β-Caryophyllene, α-caryophyllene and (+)-limonene display anticarcinogenic activity (see Constituent profiles, Chapter 14). α-Cadinol is active against human colon cancer cells (He et al 1997a), and germacrone is active against human breast cancer cells (Zhong et al 2011).

Comments

The plant, which has a reputation for repelling small flying insects, grows in many parts of the world, but the oil is only distilled in Canada. Limited availability.

Myrtle (honey)

Synonym: Marsh honey myrtle
Botanical name: *Melaleuca teretifolia* Endl.
Family: Myrtaceae

Essential oil

Source: Leaves
Key constituents:

Geranial	37.5%
Neral	29.0%
β-Myrcene	10.9%
Geraniol	3.4%
Nerol	2.8%
(*E*)-Isocitral	2.3%
1,8-Cineole	2.0%
(*Z*)-Isocitral	1.5%
α-Pinene	1.2%
Geranyl acetate	1.0%

(Day, private communication, 2004)

Safety summary

Hazards: Drug interaction; teratogenicity; skin sensitization.
Cautions (all routes): Drugs metabolized by CYP2B6 (Appendix B).
Cautions (oral): Diabetes medication, pregnancy.
Cautions (dermal): Hypersensitive, diseased or damaged skin, children under 2 years of age.
Maximum daily oral dose in pregnancy: 63 mg
Maximum dermal use level: 0.9%

Our safety advice

We recommend a dermal maximum of 0.9% to avoid skin sensitization, and a daily oral maximum in pregnancy of 63 mg. This is based on 66.5% citral content, with dermal and oral citral limits of 0.6% and 0.6 mg/kg (see Citral profile, Chapter 14).

Regulatory guidelines

IFRA recommends a maximum dermal use level for citral of 0.6% for body oils and lotions, in order to avoid skin sensitization (IFRA 2009).

Organ-specific effects

Adverse skin reactions: No information found. Citral (geranial + neral) is a potential skin sensitizer (see Citral profile, Chapter 14).
Cardiovascular effects: Gavage doses of 10, 15 or 20 mg/kg/day citral for 28 days, dose-dependently lowered plasma insulin levels and increased glucose tolerance in obese rats (Modak & Mukhopadhaya 2011).
Reproductive toxicity: Citral is dose-dependently teratogenic because it inhibits retinoic acid synthesis, and this can affect fetal development (see Citral profile. Chapter 14).
Drug interactions: Antidiabetic medication, because of cardiovascular effects, above. See Table 4.10B. Since citral and geraniol inhibit CYP2B6 (Table 4.11B), there is a theoretical risk of interaction between honey myrtle oil and drugs metabolized by this enzyme (Appendix B).

Systemic effects

Acute toxicity: No information found.
Carcinogenic/anticarcinogenic potential: No information was found for honey myrtle oil but it contains no known carcinogens. Citral (geranial + neral) and geraniol display anticarcinogenic activity (see Constituent profiles, Chapter 14).

Comments

Limited availability. There is also a 1,8-cineole chemotype, which is not produced commercially.

Myrtle (lemon)

Synonyms: Lemon-scented myrtle, lemon ironwood, sweet verbena tree
Botanical name: *Backhousia citriodora* F. Muell.
Family: Myrtaceae

Essential oil

Source: Leaves
Key constituents:

Geranial	46.1–60.7%
Neral	32.0–40.9%
Isogeranial	1.0–4.2%
Isoneral	0.6–2.7%
6-Methyl-5-hepten-2-one	0.1–2.5%
Linalool	0.3–1.0%

(Southwell et al 2000)
Quality: May be adulterated with synthetic citral.

Safety summary

Hazards: Drug interaction; teratogenicity; skin sensitization.
Cautions (all routes): Drugs metabolized by CYP2B6 (Appendix B).
Cautions (oral): Diabetes medication, pregnancy.
Cautions (dermal): Hypersensitive, diseased or damaged skin, children under 2 years of age.
Maximum daily oral dose in pregnancy: 46 mg
Maximum dermal use level: 0.7%

Our safety advice

We recommend a dermal maximum of 0.7% to avoid skin sensitization, and a daily oral maximum in pregnancy of 46 mg. This is based on 90% citral content, with dermal and oral citral limits of 0.6% and 0.6 mg/kg (see Citral profile, Chapter 14).

Regulatory guidelines

IFRA recommends a maximum dermal use level for citral of 0.6% for body oils and lotions, in order to avoid skin sensitization (IFRA 2009).

Organ-specific effects

Adverse skin reactions: In a Danish study, none of 217 consecutive dermatitis patients tested positive to 2% lemon myrtle oil (Veien et al 2004). In a clinical trial, 31 children (mean age 4.6 years) were treated for molluscum contagiosum with a 10% solution of lemon myrtle oil in olive oil daily for 21 days. There were no significant adverse effects (Burke et al 2004). After exposing human abdominal skin to 100 µL (one-tenth of 1 mL) of the undiluted essential oil for 12 hours, the only constituents detected in the skin were neral and geranial. It was estimated that the final amounts absorbed by a 70 kg adult would be 0.02 mg/kg, and by a 10 kg child would be 0.14 mg/kg, both of which are less than the NOAEL of 0.5 mg/L. However, histopathological skin changes suggested mild skin irritation and corrosion (Hayes & Markovic 2003). Citral (geranial + neral) can induce sensitization reactions on patch testing at concentrations above 0.5% and this can allegedly be inhibited by the co-presence of (+)-limonene or α-pinene (see Constituent profiles, Chapter 14).
Cardiovascular effects: Gavage doses of 10, 15 or 20 mg/kg/day citral for 28 days, dose-dependently lowered plasma insulin levels and increased glucose tolerance in obese rats (Modak & Mukhopadhaya 2011).
Reproductive toxicity: Citral is dose-dependently teratogenic because it inhibits retinoic acid synthesis, and this can affect fetal development (see Citral profile. Chapter 14).

Systemic effects

Acute toxicity: No information found.
Carcinogenic/anticarcinogenic potential: Lemon myrtle oil was strongly cytotoxic against various human cancer cell lines including HepG2 (liver), F1-73 (epithelial cells) and skin fibroblasts (Hayes & Markovic 2002). Its NOAEL was calculated as 0.5 mg/L at 24 hours exposure. Citral displays anticarcinogenic activity (see Citral profile, Chapter 14).

Drug interactions: Antidiabetic medication, because of cardiovascular effects, above. See Table 4.10B. Since citral inhibits CYP2B6 (Table 4.11B), there is a theoretical risk of interaction between lemon myrtle oil and drugs metabolized by this enzyme (Appendix B).

Comments

If 10 mL of lemon myrtle oil was to come into contact with the skin accidentally, concentrations of neral and geranial in the body could be as high as 2.0 mg/kg in an adult and 14.0 mg/kg in a child. This would exceded the NOAEL (Hayes & Markovic 2003). Lemon myrtle oil became commercially available in 1997.

Nagarmotha

Synonyms: Cypriol, cyperus
Botanical name: *Cyperus mitis* Seud.
Botanical synonym: *Cyperus scariosus* R. Br.
Family: Cupressaceae

Essential oil

Source: Dried rhizomes
Key constituents:

Cyperene	15.8–24.4%
Isopatchoulenone	2.3–16.5%
Corymbolone	3.2–11.9%
Patchoulenone	0.8–7.6%
Isopatchoul-3-ene	2.3–7.5%
Rotundone	3.5–5.1%
Rotundene	0–4.8%
Patchouli alcohol	<3.5%
α-Copaene	<3.2%
β-Selinene	2.2–3.0%
Agarol	1.2–2.5%
Patchoulanol	0–2.2%
Calamenol	<2.1%
Isopatchouli-3,5-diene	0–2.0%
Rotundenol	0.9–1.9%
ar-Himachalene	<1.9%
3,4,5-Trimethoxybenzaldehyde	0–1.9%
Cyperolone	<1.6%
Myrtenol	0–1.5%
Valencene	<1.4%
δ-Cadinene	<1.3%
α-Selinene	<1.3%
(Z)-Pinocarveol	0–1.0%

(Garg et al 1989; Vaze 2003)

Safety summary

Hazards: None known.
Contraindications: None known.

Organ-specific effects

No information found for nagarmotha oil or most of its constituents.

Systemic effects

Acute toxicity: No information found for nagarmotha oil or most of its constituents.

Carcinogenic/anticarcinogenic potential: No information found for nagarmotha oil, but it contains no known carcinogens.

Comments

Limited availability.

Narcissus

Synonym: Poet's narcissus
Botanical name: *Narcissus poeticus* L.
Family: Amaryllidaceae

Absolute

Source: Flowers
Key constituents:

γ-Terpinene	10.3–27.2%
(E)-Methyl cinnamate	1.1–15.8%
Linalool	0.6–11.7%
Benzyl acetate	9.5–9.6%
Benzyl benzoate	0.7–8.9%
p-Cymene	1.3–8.5%
δ-3-Carene	6.6–8.4%
α-Terpineol	0.3–7.0%
α-Pinene	2.4–6.1%
(E)-Ethyl cinnamate	0.5–5.6%
Benzyl alcohol	1.7–4.8%
(+)-Limonene	2.1–3.3%
1,8-Cineole	1.5–3.0%
Cinnamyl alcohol	0.8–2.9%
(E)-β-Ocimene	0–2.2%
2-Phenylethanol	0–1.6%
(E)-Methyl isoeugenol	0–0.6%
Indole	0–1.5%
Coumarin	0–1.2%
(Z)-β-Ocimene	0–1.1%

(Lawrence 1995g p. 33–36, 1997b p. 63–65)

Safety summary

Hazards: Skin sensitization (moderate risk).
Contraindications: None known.
Maximum dermal use level: 0.8%

Our safety advice

There are no regulatory guidelines for narcissus absolute. Our maximum dermal use level is based on the fact that allergenic incidence for narcissus absolute is very similar to that of ylang-ylang oil and lemongrass oil (Table 4.10B) and these both have maximum use levels of 0.8%. To a degree the matter is academic, since the cost of naricisus absolute is so great that concentrations greater than a fraction of a percent are unlikely.

Organ-specific effects

Adverse skin reactions: Undiluted narcissus absolute was slightly irritating to guinea pigs, but was not irritating to mice or pigs. Tested at 2% on 25 volunteers it was neither irritating nor sensitizing. It is non-phototoxic (Opdyke 1978 p. 827). Tested at 2%, narcissus absolute induced allergic responses in 21 (1.3%) of 1,606 consecutive dermatitis patients (Frosch et al 2002b). Similarly, four of 318 consecutive dermatitis patients (1.3%) were sensitive to 2% narcissus absolute (Paulsen & Andersen 2005). Tested at concentrations ranging from 0.06% to 2.0% on human volunteers with a previous history of reaction to fragrance materials, narcissus absolute was non-irritant and non-sensitizing (Bouhlal et al 1988b). However, Larsen et al (1996b) found that, of 167 fragrance-sensitive dermatitis patients, 11 (6.6%) were allergic to 2% narcissus absolute. In a multicenter study, Germany's IVDK reported that 15 of 2,445 consecutive dermatitis patients, and 5 of 809 patients suspected of fragrance allergy (0.61% in both cases) tested positive to 2% narcissus absolute. Only three of the total of 3,254 patients had ++ or +++ reactions (Uter et al 2010).

Systemic effects

Acute toxicity: Narcissus absolute acute oral LD_{50} in rats >5 g/kg; acute dermal LD_{50} in rabbits >5 g/kg (Opdyke 1978 p. 827).
Carcinogenic/anticarcinogenic potential: No information was found for narcissus absolute, but it contains no known carcinogens.

Comments

Absolutes are highly subject to adulteration, and no detailed compositional data were given in any of the papers cited above. The divergence in allergenicity data may therefore be due to differences in the purity of the absolutes used.

Nasturtium

Synonym: Indian cress
Botanical name: *Tropaeolum majus* L.
Family: Tropaeolaceae

Absolute

Source: Flowers
Key constituents:

Benzyl isothiocyanate	72.3%
Unidentified nitrogen compound	16.0%
Benzyl cyanide	2.0%
Linalool	1.0%

(Fakhry, private communication, 2002)

Safety summary

Hazards: Moderate toxicity assumed from benzyl cyanide content.
Contraindications: None known.
Maximum daily oral dose in pregnancy and breastfeeding: 8.7 mg
Maximum dermal use level in pregnancy and breastfeeding: 0.26%
Maximum dermal use level: 0.5% (see Regulatory Guidelines)

Our safety advice

We recommend dermal and oral limits of 0.26% and 8.7 mg, respectively, in pregnancy and breastfeeding, based on 72.3% benzyl isothiocyanate, with a NOAEL of 12.5 mg/kg/day and an uncertainty factor of $100 \times$, assuming 3 mL maximum dermal absorption.

Regulatory guidelines

IFRA recommends that benzyl cyanide is not used as a fragrance ingredient. However, exposure from oils and extracts is permitted so long as the level of benzyl cyanide in the finished product does not exceed 100 ppm (0.01%) (IFRA 2009).

Organ-specific effects

Adverse skin reactions: No information found.
Reproductive toxicity: Benzyl isothiocyanate shows minor signs of fetal toxicity at 25 mg/kg, in rats, and the reproductive toxicity NOAEL was 12.5 mg/kg (Adebiyi et al 2004).

Systemic effects

Acute toxicity: No information found. Karo karoundé absolute, which contains 4.8% of benzyl cyanide, has a rat acute oral LD_{50} of 1.4 g/kg and an acute dermal LD_{50} of >5 g/kg in rabbits (Ford et al 1988a p. 61S).
Carcinogenic/anticarcinogenic potential: No information found. Benzyl isothiocyanate is anticarcinogenic (see Benzyl isothiocyanate profile, Chapter 14).

Comments

Although benzyl cyanide is moderately toxic, with a rat acute oral LD_{50} of 270 mg/kg, as an organic cyanide it is much less toxic than inorganic cyanides like hydrogen cyanide. The reproductive toxicity NOAEL of 12.5 mg/kg for benzyl isothiocyanate suggests a dermal limit of 42% for nasturtium absolute, so no restriction on this basis is required. Limited availability.

Neroli

Synonym: Orange blossom
Botanical name: *Citrus x aurantium* L.
Family: Rutaceae

Essential oil

Source: Flowers
Key constituents:

Egyptian

Linalool	43.7–54.3%
(+)-Limonene	6.0–10.2%
Linalyl acetate	3.5–8.6%
(*E*)-β-Ocimene	4.6–5.8%
α-Terpineol	3.9–5.8%
β-Pinene	3.5–5.3%
Geranyl acetate	3.4–4.1%
(*E*)-Nerolidol	1.3–4.0%
Geraniol	2.8–3.6%
(*E,E*)-Farnesol	1.6–3.2%
Neryl acetate	1.7–2.1%
β-Myrcene	1.4–2.1%
Sabinene	0.4–1.6%
Nerol	1.1–1.3%
(*Z*)-β-Ocimene	0.7–1.0%

(Fakhry, private communication, 2002)

Spanish

Linalool	31.4–47.1%
(+)-Limonene	12.9–17.9%
β-Pinene	10.5–13.0%
Linalyl acetate	0.6–10.0%
(*E*)-β-Ocimene	5.6–7.0%
α-Terpineol	1.1–3.5%
(*E*)-Nerolidol	2.2–3.4%
β-Myrcene	1.4–3.1%
Geranyl acetate	0.7–3.0%
Sabinene	1.4–2.8%
Geraniol	0.8–2.3%
(*E,Z*)-Farnesol	0.7–1.6%
Neryl acetate	0.3–1.6%
Terpinen-4-ol	0.3–1.3%
α-Pinene	0.8–1.1%

(Boelens & Boelens 1997)
Quality: Neroli oils are expensive and are subject to frequent adulteration. Reconstituted oils may be added, or passed off as neroli oil (Burfield 2003). Considerable quantities of leaf and twig material may be distilled along with the blossoms.

Safety summary

Hazards: None known.
Contraindications: None known.

Regulatory guidelines

Has GRAS status. According to IFRA, essential oils rich in linalool should only be used when the level of peroxides is kept to the lowest practical value. The addition of antioxidants such as 0.1% BHT or α-tocopherol at the time of production is recommended (IFRA 2009).

Organ-specific effects

Adverse skin reactions: Undiluted neroli oil was not irritating to rabbit, pig or mouse skin; tested at 4% on 25 volunteers it was neither irritating nor sensitizing. It is non-phototoxic (Opdyke 1976 p. 813–814). In a multicenter study, Germany's IVDK reported that 49 of 6,220 dermatitis patients suspected of fragrance allergy (0.79%) tested positive to 2% neroli oil. Only nine patients had ++ or +++ reactions (Uter et al 2010). Two cases of alleged ACD to neroli oil have been reported, but in neither case was clinical relevance established, and patch testing only elicited + reactions (Newsham et al 2011). Oxidation products of linalool may be skin sensitizing.

Reproductive toxicity: The low reproductive toxicity of linalool, (+)-limonene and β-pinene (see Constituent profiles, Chapter 14) suggests that neroli oil is not hazardous in pregnancy.

Systemic effects

Acute toxicity: Neroli oil acute oral LD_{50} in rats 4.55 g/kg; acute dermal LD_{50} in rabbits >5 g/kg (Opdyke 1976 p. 813–814).

Carcinogenic/anticarcinogenic potential: No information was found for neroli oil, but it contains no known carcinogens. (+)-Limonene, nerolidol and geraniol display anticarcinogenic activity (see Constituent profiles, Chapter 14).

Comments

Boelens & Boelens (1997) also analyzed a Tunisian neroli oil, and found no significant differences between this and the ranges given above for Spanish neroli. See Orange flower for the equivalent absolute of this flower oil.

Niaouli (cineole CT)

Botanical name: *Melaleuca quinquenervia* Cav.
Family: Myrtaceae

Essential oil

Source: Leaves
Key constituents:

1,8-Cineole	55.0–65.0%
α-Pinene	7.0–12.0%
(+)-Limonene	6.0–12.0%
α-Terpineol	4.0–10.0%
β-Pinene	1.5–4.5%
Viridiflorol	1.0–3.5%
β-Caryophyllene	tr–2.0%
β-Myrcene	tr–2.0%

(McGilvray, private communication, 1999)

Quality: A very high 1,8-cineole content may indicate adulteration with eucalyptus oil. 'Modified' eucalyptus oil is commonly used as a substitute for niaouli oil. Kerosene or fatty acids are occasionally used as adulterants (Oyen & Dung 1999).

Safety summary

Hazards: Essential oils high in 1,8-cineole can cause CNS and breathing problems in young children.

Contraindications: Do not apply to or near the face of infants or children.

Regulatory guidelines

The German Commission E Monograph for niaouli oil recommends a daily oral dose of 300–600 mg, and 50–20% for dermal applications. It also contraindicates internal use in cases of inflammatory diseases of the GI tract and bile ducts, and in severe liver disease (Blumenthal et al 1998).

Organ-specific effects

Adverse skin reactions: No information found. 1,8-Cineole is not a high-risk skin irritant or allergen (see 1,8-Cineole profile, Chapter 14).

Reproductive toxicity: Niaouli oil (50.6% 1,8-cineole) was both maternally toxic and fetotoxic when injected ip to pregnant rats for 18 days at 1,350 mg/kg/day. Signs of maternal toxicity included: low relative weight, higher mortality, and increased weight of both liver and kidneys. Signs of fetotoxicity included: low number of surviving fetuses, high rate of fetal resorption, low birth weight and low placental weight (Laleye et al 2004). Since the dose used is equivalent to injecting 94.5 g of essential oil into the abdomen of a pregnant woman every day for 18 days, this information has no bearing on the real world use of essential oils. The low reproductive toxicity of eucalyptus oil, α-pinene and (+)-limonene (see Constituent profiles, Chapter 14) suggests that niaouli oil cineole CT is not hazardous in pregnancy.

Systemic effects

Acute toxicity: No information found. 1,8-Cineole has been reported to cause serious poisoning in young children when accidentally instilled into the nose (Melis et al 1989).

Carcinogenic/anticarcinogenic potential: No information was found for niaouli oil (cineole CT). It contains no known carcinogens.

Comments

We are not aware of any research that would support the Commission E contraindications which are presumably based on the 1,8-cineole content, since they are also applied to some eucalyptus oils. Oral 1,8-cineole was not hepatotoxic in rats at doses of up to 800 mg/kg/day for three days (Kim NH et al 2004), and a single dose of 400 mg/kg significantly protected against chemically induced hepatotoxicity in mice (Santos et al 2001). At 100 mg/kg/day for 60 days, gavage doses of 1,8-cineole protected rat liver from chemically induced oxidative stress (Ciftçi et al 2011). Pre-treatment with 1,8-cineole by rectal instillation at 200 or 400 mg/kg attenuated TNBS-induced colonic damage in rats (Santos et al 2004), and there are many other papers showing an anti-inflammatory action for 1,8-cineole. Most of the research showing anti-hepatotoxic and anti-inflammatory effects for 1,8-cineole has been published since the Commission E contraindications for niaouli oil were written. We suggest they now need revision.

The only dose used in the fetotoxic study is equivalent to 85 mL being injected into a human adult; over 18 days the total dose would be over 1.5 kg. Nothing useful can be extrapolated from the outcomes of such massive dosing. The German Commission E Monograph for niaouli recommends a daily oral dose of 200–2,000 mg for niaouli oil (Blumenthal et al 1998). However, the higher range may be unsafe, considering the toxicity of eucalyptus oil in humans. This chemotype of *M. quinquenervia* is the one normally referred to as 'niaouli oil', though the other three (below) are also commercially available.

Niaouli (linalool CT)

Synonym: Nerolina
Botanical name: *Melaleuca quinquenervia* Cav.
Family: Myrtaceae

Essential oil

Source: Leaves
Key constituents:

(*E*)-Nerolidol	61.1%
Linalool	23.9%
1,8-Cineole	2.6%
α-Pinene	1.9%
Terpinen-4-ol	1.8%
Viridiflorol	1.6%
β-Caryophyllene	1.1%

(Cornwell, private communication, 2004)

Safety summary

Hazards: None known.
Contraindications: None known.

Organ-specific effects

Adverse skin reactions: No information found.

Systemic effects

Acute toxicity: No information found.
Carcinogenic/anticarcinogenic potential: No information was found for the essential oil but it contains no known carcinogens. Nerolidol displays anticarcinogenic activity (see Nerolidol profile, Chapter 14).

Comments

The distinction between this chemotype and the nerolidol chemotype is not well established. Although it is a mixed chemotype, oils with this profile are generally referred to as linalool chemotype. The compositional values given here are averages. A further 77 constituents have been identified (Cornwell, private communication, 2004).

Niaouli (nerolidol CT)

Botanical name: *Melaleuca quinquenervia* Cav.
Family: Myrtaceae

Essential oil

Source: Leaves
Key constituents:

(*E*)-Nerolidol	75.7–92.5%
β-Caryophyllene	0.5–8.7%
1,8-Cineole	tr–6.6%
Caryophyllene oxide	0.1–6.1%
α-Pinene + α-thujene	0–4.5%
δ-Cadinol	0–2.5%
Viridiflorol	0.1–1.7%
α-Terpineol + viridiflorene	0–1.5%

(Ramanoelina et al 1994a)

Safety summary

Hazards: None known.
Contraindications: None known.

Organ-specific effects

Adverse skin reactions: No information was found for niaouli oil nerolidol CT. None of its major constituents show any tendency to skin reactivity.

Systemic effects

Acute toxicity: No information found. Nerolidol acute oral LD_{50} in rats >5 g/kg; acute dermal LD_{50} in rabbits >5 g/kg (Opdyke 1975 p. 887).
Carcinogenic/anticarcinogenic potential: No information was found for niaouli oil (nerolidol CT), but it contains no known carcinogens. Nerolidol exhibits anticarcinogenic activity (see Nerolidol profile, Chapter 14).

Comments

Even though there are no published data for this essential oil, its constituents are mostly well known, and it is unlikely to present any significant safety issues.

Niaouli (viridiflorol CT)

Botanical name: *Melaleuca quinquenervia* Cav.
Family: Myrtaceae

Essential oil

Source: Leaves
Key constituents:

Viridiflorol	40.0–45.0%
1,8-Cineole	30.0–35.0%
(*E*)-Nerolidol	3.0–6.0%
Ledol	tr–4.0%

(Behra, private communication, 2003)

Safety summary

Hazards: None known.
Contraindications: None known.

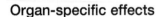
Organ-specific effects

Adverse skin reactions: No information found for niaouli oil (viridiflorol CT) or viridiflorol.

Systemic effects

Acute toxicity: No information found for niaouli oil (viridiflorol CT) or viridiflorol.

Carcinogenic/anticarcinogenic potential: No information found for niaouli oil (viridiflorol CT), but it contains no known carcinogens. Nerolidol exhibits anticarcinogenic activity (see Nerolidol profile, Chapter 14).

Comments

The oil is produced in South Africa.

Nut grass

Synonyms: Coco grass, motha
Botanical name: *Cyperus rotundus* L.
Family: Cyperaceae

Essential oil

Source: Rhizomes
Key constituents:

Cyperene	30.9%
Cyperotundene	8.8%
Rotundene	7.6%
α-Cyperone	4.5%
Cyperol	4.0%
β-Pinene	3.9%
Muskatone	3.8%
Isorotundene	3.6%
α-Cubebene	3.4%
Isocyperol	2.7%
α-Cadinol	2.5%
Cypera-2,4-diene	2.4%
T-Muurolol	2.2%
(E)-Calamenene	2.0%
α-Muurolol	1.9%
β-Selinene	1.5%
T-Cadinol	1.4%
α-Calacorene	1.4%
α-Pinene	1.4%
α-Muurolene	1.1%
(E,E)-Farnesol	1.0%

(Kilani et al 2005)

Safety summary

Hazards: None known.
Contraindications: None known.

Organ-specific effects

Adverse skin reactions: No information found for nut grass oil or any of its major constituents.

Systemic effects

Acute toxicity: No information found for nut grass oil or any of its major constituents.

Antioxidant/pro-oxidant activity: Nut grass oil exhibits antioxidant activity in DPPH and other assays (Kilani et al 2008).

Carcinogenic/anticarcinogenic potential: Nut grass oil was not mutagenic in the SOS chromotest (a bacterial assay) nor in *Salmonella* strains TA98 or T100 in the Ames test, and showed significant antimutagenic activity (Kilani et al 2005). Nut grass oil was highly cytotoxic to L1210 (mouse) leukemia cells in vitro, this activity correlating with apoptosis (Kilani et al 2008). Nut grass oil contains no known carcinogens.

Comments

The analysis of the oil given above is for an oil distilled in Tunisia, where the plant grows wild. The commercial oil is produced in India, but the composition of the oil is similar. In a recent dissertation Sonwa (2000) reported many sesquiterpenes in *Cyperus rotundus*. No quantitative data were given but in descending order, the major constituents were: (−)-cyperene, rotundene, cyperotundone, (−)-α-copaene, cyperenol, caryophyllene oxide and muskatone.

Nutmeg

Botanical name: *Myristica fragrans* Houtt.
Botanical synonyms: *Myristica officinalis* L. fil., *Myristica moschata* Thunb., *Myristica aromatica* O. Schwartz, *Myristica amboinensis* Gand.
Family: Myristicaceae

Essential oil

Source: Kernels
Note: There are two types of nutmeg oil, with important chemotype differences.
Key constituents:

East Indian

Sabinene	14.0–44.1%
α-Pinene	18.0–26.5%
β-Pinene	8.7–17.7%
Myristicin	3.3–13.5%
Terpinen-4-ol	1.0–10.9%
γ-Terpinene	1.3–7.7%
Linalool	0.2–7.4%
(+)-Limonene	2.0–7.0%
α-Phellandrene	0.4–5.8%
α-Terpinene	0.1–5.2%
Elemicin	0.1–4.6%
β-Myrcene	0.3–4.0%

Safrole	0.3–3.3%
α-Thujene	0.9–2.7%
p-Cymene	0.3–2.7%
Terpinolene	0.6–2.6%
β-Phellandrene	0.1–2.4%
δ-3-Carene	0.5–1.5%
α-Terpineol	0.1–1.4%
Methyleugenol	0.1–1.2%
(Z)-p-Menth-2-en-1-ol	0.1–1.2%

(Lawrence 1995 g p. 202; Simpson & Jackson 2002)

West Indian

Sabinene	42.0–57.0%
α-Pinene	1.6–12.6%
β-Pinene	7.8–12.1%
Terpinen-4-ol	3.0–6.4%
γ-Terpinene	1.7–4.7%
(+)-Limonene	2.9–4.4%
α-Terpinene	0.8–4.2%
β-Myrcene	2.2–3.4%
p-Cymene	0.7–3.2%
(E)-Sabinene hydrate	0.3–2.4%
Terpinolene	1.4–1.7%
Elemicin	1.2–1.4%
α-Thujene	1.2%
(Z)-p-Piperitol	0.4–.2%
Myristicin	0.5–0.9%
Safrole	0.1–0.5%
Methyleugenol	0.1–0.2%

(Lawrence 1995 g p. 202; Simpson & Jackson 2002)

Quality: Nutmeg oil may be adulterated by the addition of nutmeg terpenes, (+)-limonene α-pinene or turpentine fractions (Burfield 2003).

Safety summary

Hazards: Potentially carcinogenic, based on safrole and methyleugenol content; psychotropic in high doses.
Contraindications: None known.
Maximum adult daily oral dose (East Indian nutmeg oil): 28 mg
Maximum adult daily oral dose (West Indian nutmeg oil): 175 mg
Maximum dermal use level (East Indian nutmeg oil):

EU	0.016%
IFRA	0.03%
Tisserand & Young	0.8%

Maximum dermal use level (West Indian nutmeg oil):

EU	0.1%
IFRA	0.2%
Tisserand & Young	5%

Our safety advice

We recommend a dermal maximum of 0.8% for the East Indian oil based on 3.3% safrole and 1.2% methyleugenol content, and 5% for the Indian oil based on 0.5% safrole and 0.2% methyleugenol content, applying dermal limits of 0.05% and 0.02% for safrole and methyleugenol, respectively. The maximum daily oral doses are based on 0.025 mg/kg for safrole and 0.01 mg/kg for methyleugenol (see Constituent profiles, Chapter 14).

Regulatory guidelines

IFRA recommends a maximum concentration of 0.0004% methyleugenol in leave-on products such as body lotions (IFRA 2009). The equivalent SCCNFP maximum is 0.0002% (European Commission 2002). IFRA and the EU recommend a maximum exposure level of 0.01% of safrole from the use of safrole-containing essential oils in cosmetics.

Organ-specific effects

Adverse skin reactions: Undiluted nutmeg oil was moderately irritating to rabbits; tested at 2% on 25 volunteers it was neither irritating nor sensitizing (Opdyke 1976 p. 631–633).
Neurotoxicity: Whole nutmeg has been known for its narcotic, intoxicating properties since the sixteenth century (Weil 1965). Psychotropic effects have been reported for whole nutmeg in high doses. Myristicin and elemicin are thought to be responsible, but other synergistic elements may need to be present for a psychotropic effect to take place (see Ch. 10, p. 144/145). There is little information concerning psychotropic effects for the essential oil. One of us (R.T.) has ingested 1 mL of nutmeg oil with no noticeable effect, and 1.5 mL which resulted in a moderately strong psychotropic effect. Three other individuals each ingested 1.5 mL of nutmeg oil, and two experienced psychotropic effects. See Ch. 10, p. 145 for cases of nutmeg intoxication.
Reproductive toxicity: The administration of nutmeg oil at up to 260 mg/kg to pregnant rats for 10 consecutive days, up to 560 mg/kg to pregnant mice for 10 consecutive days, and up to 600 mg/kg to pregnant hamsters for five consecutive days had no effect on implantation or on maternal or fetal survival; no teratogenic effect was observed in comparison with controls (NTIS 1976). Sabinene is not reproductively toxic (see Sabinene profile, Chapter 14). A 30-year-old woman, at 30 weeks of gestation, ingested several cookies made with 7 g of ground nutmeg, instead of the recommended one-eighth of a teaspoon (Lavy 1987). Four hours later she experienced a sudden onset of palpitations, blurred vision, agitation and a sense of impending doom. The fetal heartbeat was 160–170 bpm, and returned to a baseline of 120–140 within 12 hours. The fetal response was attributed to the myristicin content of nutmeg oil, and its anticholinergic (i.e., stimulant) effect. It is thought that myristicin readily crosses the placenta. This case, with its assumed conclusions, is not a sufficient basis to contraindicate nutmeg oil in pregnancy.

High oral doses of East Indian nutmeg oil reduced fertility in male mice (Pecevski et al 1981). The effect was dose-dependent, between 60 and 400 mg/kg/day given 5 days per

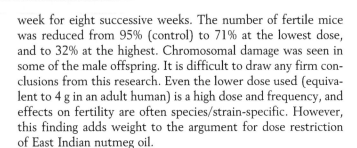

week for eight successive weeks. The number of fertile mice was reduced from 95% (control) to 71% at the lowest dose, and to 32% at the highest. Chromosomal damage was seen in some of the male offspring. It is difficult to draw any firm conclusions from this research. Even the lower dose used (equivalent to 4 g in an adult human) is a high dose and frequency, and effects on fertility are often species/strain-specific. However, this finding adds weight to the argument for dose restriction of East Indian nutmeg oil.

Systemic effects

Acute toxicity: Nutmeg oil acute oral LD_{50} has been reported as 2.62 g/kg (Jenner et al 1964) and 2.6 g/kg in rats, 5.6 g/kg in mice and 6 g/kg in hamsters; acute dermal LD_{50} in rabbits >10 mL/kg (Opdyke 1976 p. 631–633).
Antioxidant/pro-oxidant activity: Nutmeg oil has demonstrated significant antioxidant activity in vitro and in vivo (Deans et al 1993; Dorman et al 1995; Recsan et al 1997). It showed potent DPPH radical scavenging activity, with an IC_{50} of 0.13 μL/mL (Tomaino et al 2005).
Carcinogenic/anticarcinogenic potential: Nutmeg oil contains both rodent carcinogens and anticarcinogens. Methyleugenol and safrole are carcinogenic and (+)-limonene and myristicin display anticarcinogenic activity (see Constituent profiles, Chapter 14). Nutmeg oil was not mutagenic in the Ames test, and did not produce CA in Chinese hamster fibroblasts (Ishidate et al 1984). Nutmeg oil dose-dependently inhibited aflatoxin B_1-induced adducts in calf thymus DNA, in the presence of rat liver microsomes (Hashim et al 1994). Nutmeg oil significantly induced glutathione *S*-transferase in mouse liver (Banerjee et al 1994).
Drug interactions: Nutmeg oil is a weak inhibitor of MAO (Truitt et al 1963), not at a level suggestive of drug interaction. (Essential oils with higher concentrations of myristicin pose a greater risk.)

Comments

While nutmeg oil contains both carcinogens and anticarcinogens, the anticarcinogens are present in higher concentrations, and the existing data suggest either that the oil is not carcinogenic or that it is anticarcinogenic. If myristicin is important in any of the therapeutic actions of nutmeg oil, the East Indian oil might be more useful than the West Indian oil. Camphene has been cited as the major constituent of nutmeg oil, but this is a historical error. The 1989 edition of the Merck Index cites camphene as constituting 60–80% of nutmeg oil. Guenther (1949–1952 vol. 5 p. 77) cites a 1907 reference from Power and Salway, in which '*d*-pinene' and '*d*-camphene' were identified as constituting 80% of nutmeg oil. However, any analysis published since about 1970 shows sabinene as the major constituent, with camphene occurring at 0–0.6%.

Oakmoss

Botanical name: *Evernia prunastri* L.
Family: Usneaceae

Absolute

Source: Dried moss
Key constituents:

Methyl β-orcinolcarboxylate	18.6–25.5%
Ethyl everninate	0.2–3.7%
Ethyl hematommate	1.4–3.0%
Ethyl chlorohematommate	1.0–1.3%

(Terajima et al 1988; Joulain & Tabacchi 2009b)

Safety summary

Hazards: Skin sensitization (high risk).
Contraindications (dermal): Hypersensitive, diseased or damaged skin, children under 2 years of age.
Maximum dermal use level: 0.1% (see Regulatory Guidelines).

Regulatory guidelines

Dermal maximum based on IFRA guidelines for category five (women's facial creams, hand creams) and category four (body creams, oils, lotions) (IFRA 2009). The maximum concentration of combined oakmoss and treemoss extracts should not exceed 0.1% (SCCNFP 2001a; IFRA 2009).

Organ-specific effects

Adverse skin reactions: In a multicenter project, 6,701 of 59,298 dermatitis patients (11.3%) tested positive to the fragrance mix over a seven year period (1996–2002). Of the 6,701, 1,680 were patch tested with oakmoss absolute, and 502 had positive reations. This represents 0.84% of the original cohort (Schnuch et al 2004a). Of 1,200 patients patch tested, there were no irritant reactions and 17 allergic reactions (1.4%) to 3% oakmoss absolute. In a second group of 1,500 patients, there were no irritant reactions and 19 allergic reactions (1.26%) to 1% oakmoss absolute (Santucci et al 1987). The results of other reports of oakmoss testing are shown in Table 13.2.

There were 21 reactions to 10% oakmoss (presumably absolute) in 179 dermatitis patients (11.7%) suspected of cosmetic allergy (De Groot et al 1985). Of 167 fragrance-sensitive patients, 22 (13.2%) were allergic to 5% oakmoss absolute on

Table 13.2 Allergic reactions to oakmoss absolute in dermatitis patients

Concentration used	Percentage who reacted	Number of reactors	Reference
1%	1.26%	19/1,500	Santucci et al 1987
1%	1.85%	13/702	Frosch et al 1995b
1%	2.23%	46/2,063	Schnuch et al 2007a
1%	2.27%	81/3,566	Heisterberg et al 2011
2%	0.5%	1/200	Rudzki et al 1976
3%	1.42%	17/1,200	Santucci et al 1987

patch testing (Larsen et al 1996b). A survey of 59 household products found oakmoss in only one (Rastogi et al 2001). An unpublished survey conducted by RIFM and IFRA found oakmoss absolute in 0.4% of household products tested (cited in Schnuch et al 2004a). However, it has been widely used in perfumes. There are several reports of contact dermatitis being caused by oakmoss in fragranced products (Calnan 1979; Held et al 1988; Kanerva et al 1999). Oakmoss is the most prevalent sensitizer in people sensitive to the fragrance mix.

Following suspicions that allergy to oakmoss absolute was partly or entirely due to contamination with resin acids of the type found in oakmoss, treemoss and colophony, two investigations concluded that allergic reactions to oakmoss are primarily due to constituents of the absolute, and not to resin acid contamination (Buckley et al 2002; Johansen et al 2002). However, resin acids have been found in oakmoss absolute samples, and they are highly allergenic (Lepoittevin & Meschkat 2000). IFRA warns that oakmoss absolute should not contain more than traces of resin acids, and that oxidation products of resin acids are sensitizing.

Atranol, chloroatranol and methyl-β-orcinol carboxylate have been identified as strong elicitants in most patients sensitized to oakmoss absolute (Bernard et al 2003). In further work, 12 of 13 oakmoss-sensitive individuals (92%) reacted positively to a 5 ppm solution of chloroatranol, the other reacting to 25 ppm. At 0.2 ppm, six of the test subjects reacted. None of the controls reacted to concentrations of up to 200 ppm. The researchers commented that chloroatranol was probably the most potent allergen present in consumer products (Johansen et al 2003a). Further work on atranol and chloroatranol found both, at significant concentrations, in 87% of perfumes and eaux de toilette analyzed. One sample of oakmoss absolute contained ~2.1% atranol and ~0.9% chloroatranol (Rastogi et al 2004). (Note that a high incidence of oakmoss in perfume, and a low incidence in perfumed household products, is not contradictory.)

An early RIFM monograph on oakmoss *concrete* concluded that it was non-phototoxic (Opdyke 1975 p. 891–892). In an in vitro assay using human erythrocytes, oakmoss (presumably absolute) was phototoxic in the presence of both UVA and UVB radiation (Placzek et al 2007). There are several reports of oakmoss photosensitivity (Fernández de Corres et al 1983; Fernández de Corres 1986; Guin & Jackson 1988). Of seven dermatitis patients allergic to oakmoss absolute, three reacted positively to photopatch testing. It was concluded that photoallergy following ACD, rather than phototoxicity, was much more likely (Thune et al 1982).

Systemic effects

Acute toxicity: No information found for oakmoss absolute or any of its known constituents. For oakmoss *concrete*, the rat acute oral LD_{50} is reported as 2.9 g/kg, and the rabbit acute dermal LD_{50} as >5 g/kg (Opdyke 1975 p. 891–892).
Carcinogenic/anticarcinogenic potential: No information found.

Comments

The SCCP (2004b) published an Opinion that concluded that 'As chloroatranol and atranol are such potent allergens (and

chloroatranol particularly so), they should not be present in cosmetic products.' We do not agree that prohibiting oakmoss altogether on the basis of constituent data is sensible, nor do we view it as necessary. Oakmoss concretes and resinoids are also produced. Over 40 constituents of oakmoss extracts have been identified, but most have not been quantified (Joulain & Tabacchi 2009a).

Onion

Botanical name: *Allium cepa* L.
Family: Liliaceae

Essential oil

Source: Seeds
Key constituents:

Dipropyl disulfide	26.0%
Methyl propyl trisulfide	16.0%
Methyl propyl disulfide	12.5%
Propyl (*E*)-1-propenyl disulfide	9.5%
Dipropyl trisulfide	8.0%
Propyl (*Z*)-1-propenyl disulfide	6.0%
Methyl (*E*)-1-propenyl disulfide	4.0%
Dimethyl trisulfide	3.6%
Methyl (*Z*)-1-propenyl disulfide	2.1%
(*E*)-1-Propenyl propyl trisulfide	1.3%
Dimethyl sulfide	1.1%
2-Methylpent-2-enal	1.0%
(*Z*)-1-Propenyl propyl trisulfide	1.0%
Di(1-propenyl) trisulfide	1.0%

(Boelens et al 1971)
Quality: May be adulterated with aliphatic sulfide mixtures (Burfield 2003).

Safety summary

Hazards: Drug interaction; inhibits blood clotting; may be skin sensitizing.
Caution (oral): Anticoagulant medication, major surgery, peptic ulcer, hemophilia, other bleeding disorders (Box 7.1).
Cautions (dermal): Use with caution on skin or mucous membranes, especially if hypersensitive, diseased or damaged.

Regulatory guidelines

Has GRAS status.

Organ-specific effects

Adverse skin reactions: Since onion and garlic oils have a great deal in common, there is a suspicion that onion oil might, like garlic oil, present some risk of sensitization.
Cardiovascular effects: Onion oil demonstrates antiplatelet activity (Fenwick & Hanley 1985; Barrie et al 1987; Co-operative Group for Essential Oil of Garlic 1986; Nutrition International 1990). Platelet activity is essential for blood clotting. Onion oil is more potent than garlic oil (Fenwick & Hanley 1985).

Systemic effects

Acute toxicity: No information found.

Antioxidant/pro-oxidant activity: In rats, onion oil protected against nicotine-induced lipid peroxidation, increasing activities of antioxidant enzymes and concentrations of glutathione (Helen et al 1999).

Carcinogenic/anticarcinogenic potential: Onion oil was not mutagenic in the Ames test, but was marginally mutagenic in a chromosomal aberration test (Ishidate et al 1984). In mouse micronucleus tests, onion oil showed no genotoxicity (Hayashi et al 1988). The proliferation of human leukemia HL-60 cells was inhibited by onion oil (Seki et al 2000). It also demonstrated an inhibitory effect on PMA-mediated mouse skin tumor promotion both in vitro and in vivo (Belman 1983; Zelikoff & Belman 1985). In mouse epidermal cells, onion oil increased glutathione peroxidase activity, and abolished the inhibitory effect of a tumor promoter on the enzyme (Perchellet et al 1986). Onion oil contains no known carcinogens.

Drug interactions: Anticoagulant medication, because of cardiovascular effects, above. See Table 4.10B.

Comments

Safe levels for dermal application of onion oil are not known. Sulfur-rich oils such as onion are more commonly administered internally than externally in aromatherapy. Shallot oil, *Allium cepa* var. *aggregatum*, is occasionally available.

Opopanax

Synonyms: Opoponax, scented myrrh, sweet myrrh, bisabol myrrh
Botanical name: *Commiphora guidottii* Chiov.
Family: Burseraceae

Essential oil

Source: Gum
Key constituents:

(E)-β-Ocimene	33.0%
(Z)-α-Bisabolene	22.2%
α-Santalene	15.8%
(E)-β-Bergamotene	6.6%
α-Bergamotene	3.0%
Germacrene D	1.6%
Decanol	1.2%

(Baser et al 2003)

Safety summary

Hazards: Skin sensitization (moderate risk).
Cautions (dermal): Hypersensitive, diseased or damaged skin, children under 2 years of age.
Maximum dermal use level: 0.6% (see Regulatory Guidelines).

Regulatory guidelines

IFRA recommends that opopanax preparations, whether steam distilled oils or solvent extracted products, should not be used at levels over 0.6% for products applied to the skin. This is based on unpublished tests referred to below, and is apparently in relation to sensitization, and not to phototoxicity.

Organ-specific effects

Adverse skin reactions: A 1977 RIFM report on phototoxicity testing for 160 fragrance raw materials concluded that opopanax oil was phototoxic (Forbes et al 1977). An SCCP Opinion cites 11 unpublished RIFM reports on human maximation tests using nine different opopanax oils (two samples were tested twice) at 8%. In 8 of the 11 tests there were no reactions, and the other three elicited 1/25, 2/25 and 4/25 positive reactions. The collective tally was 7/298 reactions, or 2.35%. In tests of two absolutes and one concrete, there were 0/89 reactions; in tests of five resinoids there were, collectively, 2/125 reactions (1.6%). The botanical origin of the samples used is not known. It is concluded that opopanax oil has an allergenic potential, but that the quality of the data is poor (SCCP 2005c).

Systemic effects

Acute toxicity: No information found. Mixed isomer ocimene acute oral LD_{50} in rats >5 g/kg; acute dermal LD_{50} in rabbits >5 g/kg (Opdyke 1978 p. 829).

Carcinogenic/anticarcinogenic potential: No information was found for opopanax oil, but it contains no known carcinogens.

Comments

Since opopanax oil appeared in a list of substances found by RIFM to be phototoxic in 1977, IFRA has never specifically referred to opopanax as phototoxic, even though the IFRA restriction of 0.6% for the oil originated in 1978. RIFM has never published a full monograph on opopanax oil. The current IFRA statement for opopanax includes: 'This recommendation is based on test results of RIFM with samples of resinoids, concretes, absolutes and oil of opoponax. Earlier samples showed limited sensitization reactions when tested at 8% whereas tests on a larger number of more recent samples showed no sensitization at 8%.' Apparently, some time between 1977 and the present, IFRA dropped the idea of opopanax being phototoxic. The IFRA comment that recent samples produced no reactions does not explain their maximum use level of 0.6%. Anyway, the "recent" samples dated from 1979–1980, and it is difficult to understand how the RIFM data could be interpreted as suggesting any specific maximum use level. No allergens have ever been identified in opopanax oil. The 0.6% remains an arbitrary level, based on poor data.

There is confusion about botanical sources. According to Guenther (1949–1952, vol 4, p. 349), opopanax originally derived from *Opopanax chironium* Koch., but by the early 1950s the origin of commerical opopanax gum had been replaced by *Commiphora erythraea* Engl. var. *glabrescens* Engl., synonym: *Commiphora erythraea* Ehrenb. This has been regarded as the principal source by most authorities since, for example Craker & Simon (1987 p. 215). However, the current principal source is in fact *Commiphora guidottii* (Thulin & Claeson 1991). According to Burfield (2000, vol I p. 212) opopanax oil is also derived from other *Commiphora* species, including *C. kataf* (Forssk.) Engl., *C. pseudopaoli* JB Gillet, and *C. holtziana* Engl. ssp. *holtziana* Kenya.

Orange (bitter)

Synonym: Seville orange
Botanical name: *Citrus x aurantium* L.
Botanical synonyms: *Citrus aurantium* L. subsp. *amara* L., *Citrus aurantium* L. subsp. *aurantium*
Family: Rutaceae

Essential oil

Source: Fruit peel, by expression
Key constituents:

(+)-Limonene	89.7–94.7%
β-Myrcene	1.6–2.4%
Linalool	0.1–2.0%

(Lawrence 1989 p. 41, 2000b p. 46–49)

Non-volatile compounds

Bergapten	0.035–0.073%
Epoxy-bergamottin	0.082%
Psoralen	0.007%

(Dugo et al 1999a; Lawrence 2000b p. 46–49; SCCP 2005b)
Quality: May be adulterated with sweet orange oil, orange terpenes, and traces of character compounds (Burfield 2003).

Safety summary

Hazards: Skin sensitization if oxidized; phototoxic (low risk).
Contraindications (dermal): If applied to the skin at over maximum use level, skin must not be exposed to sunlight or sunbed rays for 12 hours.
Cautions: Old or oxidized oils should be avoided.
Maximum dermal use level: 1.25% (for phototoxicity).

Our safety advice

Because of its (+)-limonene content we recommend that oxidation of bitter orange oil is avoided by storage in a dark, airtight container in a refrigerator. The addition of an antioxidant to preparations containing it is recommended.

Regulatory guidelines

Has GRAS status. To avoid phototoxicity, IFRA recommends that, for application to areas of skin exposed to sunshine, bitter orange oil be limited to a maximum of 1.25% in products applied to the skin, except for bath preparations, soaps and other products which are washed off. This NOAEL was based on studies conducted with pooled samples of bitter orange oil in miniature swine and hairless mice, which showed a NOEL of 6.25% (IFRA 2009). IFRA also recommends that essential oils rich in limonene should only be used when the level of peroxides is kept to the lowest practical level, for instance by adding antioxidants at the time of production (IFRA 2009).

In Europe, essential oils containing furanocoumarins must be used so that the total level of bergapten will not exceed: (a) 15 ppm in finished cosmetic products intended for application to skin areas likely to be exposed to sunshine, excluding rinse-off products; or (b) 1 ppm in sun protection and in bronzing products. In the presence of other phototoxic ingredients, the sum of their concentrations (expressed as % of the respective maximum levels) shall not exceed 100% (SCCNFP 2000).

Organ-specific effects

Adverse skin reactions: Undiluted bitter orange oil was moderately irritating to rabbits and was very mildly irritating to mice; tested at 10% on 25 volunteers it was neither irritating nor sensitizing (Opdyke 1974 p. 735–736). In a study of 200 consecutive dermatitis patients, three (1.5%) were sensitive to 2% bitter orange oil on patch testing (Rudzki et al 1976). In a clinical trial, bitter orange oil was applied to three groups of 20 patients each, at 20% in alcohol three times daily (group 1), at 25% in an emulsion three times daily (group 2), or 100% once daily (group 3) for 1–3 weeks. The patients were being treated for superficial dermatophyte infections, one of the most common types of fungal skin conditions. There were no side effects, except for "mild irritation" in group three (Ramadan et al 1996). A 65-year-old aromatherapist with multiple essential oil sensitivities reacted to 5%, but not 1% orange oil (Selvaag et al 1995). Autoxidation products of (+)-limonene can cause skin sensitization (see (+)-Limonene profile). Distinct phototoxic effects were found for bitter orange oil (Opdyke 1974 p. 735–736; Kaidbey & Kligman 1980).
Reproductive toxicity: The low reproductive toxicity of (+)-limonene (see Constituent profile, Chapter 14) suggests that bitter orange oil is not hazardous in pregnancy. Also, see sweet orange oil, below.

Systemic effects

Acute toxicity: Non-toxic. Bitter orange oil acute oral LD_{50} in rats >5 g/kg; acute dermal LD_{50} in rabbits >10 g/kg (Opdyke 1974 p. 735–736).
Carcinogenic/anticarcinogenic potential: Orange oil (type unspecified) was not mutagenic in the Ames test, and did not produce CA in Chinese hamster fibroblasts (Ishidate et al 1984). Orange oil (type unspecified) significantly induced glutathione *S*-transferase in mouse liver and small bowel mucosa and inhibited B[*a*]P-induced neoplasia of both forestomach and lungs (Wattenberg et al 1985). Orange oil (type unspecified) demonstrated a chemopreventive action in both nitrosomethylurea-induced rat mammary carcinomas and *N*-nitrosodiethylamine-induced preneoplastic hepatic lesions in rats (Bodake et al 2002, Maltzman et al 1989). Orange oil (type unspecified) also inhibited NNK-induced pulmonary adenoma formation and the occurrence of forestomach tumors in mice (Wattenberg & Coccia 1991). (+)-Limonene displays anticarcinogenic activity (see (+)-Limonene profile).

Comments

Expressed *sweet* orange oil is not phototoxic. It might, therefore, be preferable for use in some instances. Some authorities believe that the bitter orange is a hybrid of C. *reticulata* and C. *maxima* (Oyen & Dung 1999 p. 81).

Orange (sweet)

Botanical name: *Citrus sinensis* L.
Botanical synonym: *Citrus aurantium* L. var. *sinensis*
Family: Rutaceae

Essential oil

Source: Fruit peel, by expression
Key constituents:

American

(+)-Limonene	93.2–94.9%
β-Myrcene	2.6–3.1%
α-Pinene	0.6–1.0%

(Lawrence 1995g p. 48–49)

Brazilian

(+)-Limonene	86.1–93.4%
β-Myrcene	1.3–3.3%
β-Bisabolene	0–1.5%
α-Pinene	0.8–1.0%

(Lawrence 1995g p. 48–49)

Chinese

(+)-Limonene	83.9%
Linalool	5.6%
Geranial	1.8%
Neral	1.3%
β-Myrcene	0.9%

(Zhu et al 1993)

Italian

(+)-Limonene	93.7–95.9%
β-Myrcene	1.7–2.5%
Sabinene	0.2–1.0%

(Dugo 1994)

Spanish

(+)-Limonene	95.6%
β-Myrcene	1.8%

(Lawrence 1993 p. 119)

Quality: Sweet orange oil may be adulterated with natural or synthetic limonene, or with mixtures of terpene hydrocarbons, though adulteration of this inexpensive oil is not common (Kubeczka 2002).

Safety summary

Hazards: Skin sensitization if oxidized.
Cautions: Old or oxidized oils should be avoided.

Our safety advice

Because of its (+)-limonene content we recommend that oxidation of sweet orange oil is avoided by storage in a dark, airtight container in a refrigerator. The addition of an antioxidant to preparations containing it is recommended.

Regulatory guidelines

Has GRAS status. IFRA recommends that essential oils rich in limonene should only be used when the level of peroxides is kept to the lowest practical level, for instance by adding antioxidants at the time of production (IFRA 2009).

Organ-specific effects

Adverse skin reactions: Undiluted expressed sweet orange oil was moderately irritating to rabbits, but was not irritating to mice. Tested at 8% or 100% on two panels of 25 volunteers it was not irritating. Tested at 8% on 25 volunteers it was not sensitizing. Sweet orange oil is non-phototoxic (Opdyke 1974 p. 733–734) and no bergapten was detected in five samples from different types of C. *sinensis* (Sawamura et al 2009). There were no irritant or allergic reactions in a group of 100 consecutive dermatitis patients tested with 5% Brazilian orange oil (Frosch et al 1995a). In a study of 200 consecutive dermatitis patients, one (0.5%) was sensitive to 2% sweet orange oil on patch testing (Rudzki et al 1976). One out of 747 dermatitis patients suspected of fragrance allergy (0.13%) reacted to 2% orange oil (type unspecified) (Wöhrl et al 2001). In a multicenter study, Germany's IVDK reported that 13 of 6,246 dermatitis patients (0.2%) suspected of fragrance allergy tested positive to 2% sweet orange oil. There were no ++ or +++ reactions (Uter et al 2010). This suggests that (presumably unoxidized) orange oil is non-allergenic. Autoxidation products of (+)-limonene can cause skin sensitization (see (+)-Limonene profile). A 65-year-old aromatherapist with multiple essential oil sensitivities reacted to 5%, but not 1% orange oil (Selvaag et al 1995).

Reproductive toxicity: Female rats were given gavage doses of 375, 750 or 1,500 mg/kg/day sweet orange oil in corn oil, for one week before cohabitation, all through gestation, and for four days post-delivery. Adverse effects consisted of reduced food consumption and reduced weight gain in the 750 and 1,500 mg/kg groups during the pre-mating period, and a significant increase in stillbirths and pup deaths in the high-dose group. No adverse effects on mating performance or fertility were seen in any group. The NOAEL values for maternal and fetal toxicity were 375 and 750 mg/kg, respectively (Hoberman et al 1989). Therefore, sweet orange oil is not hazardous in pregnancy.

Systemic effects

Acute toxicity: Non-toxic. Sweet orange acute oral LD_{50} in rats >5 g/kg; acute dermal LD_{50} in rabbits >5 g/kg (Opdyke 1974 p. 733–734).

Carcinogenic/anticarcinogenic potential: Apoptosis in human leukemia (HL-60) cells was induced by sweet orange oil and by citral (geranial+neral), octanal and decanal, all minor constituents of the oil (Hata et al 2003). Also see bitter orange (above). (+)-Limonene displays anticarcinogenic activity (see (+)-Limonene profile).

Comments

The blood orange, *Citrus sinensis* L. cv. *Sanguinelli* and *Citrus sinensis* L. cv. *Moro*, is a variety of sweet orange. Orange is produced in greater quantity than any other essential oil, and most of this production is used in foods and beverages.

Orange flower

Botanical name: *Citrus x aurantium* L.
Family: Rutaceae

Essential oil

See Neroli

Absolute

Source: Flowers
Key constituents:

2-Phenylethanol	4.5–35.0%
Linalool	30.0–32.0%
Linalyl acetate	7.0–16.8%
Methyl anthranilate	3.0–15.0%
Farnesol	tr–7.7%
Nerolidol	0–7.6%
(+)-Limonene+(Z)-β-ocimene	0–5.1%
Nerol	0.9–4.0%
Neryl acetate	0.8–4.0%
α-Terpineol	2.0–2.4%
Geraniol	<1.5%
Benzyl cyanide	1.0%
Indole	0.1–1.0%

(Anonis 1993; IFRA 2009)

Safety summary

Hazards: May contain benzyl cyanide.
Contraindications: None known.
Maximum dermal use level: 1.0%

Our safety advice

Our dermal maximum is based on 1.0% benzyl cyanide content and the IFRA maximum of 0.01% for benzyl cyanide.

Regulatory guidelines

IFRA recommends that benzyl cyanide is not used as a fragrance ingredient, but that exposure from oils and extracts is not significant and their use is authorized so long as the level of benzyl

cyanide in the finished product does not exceed 100 ppm (0.01%) (IFRA 2009). According to IFRA, essential oils rich in linalool should only be used when the level of peroxides is kept to the lowest practical value. The addition of antioxidants such as 0.1% BHT or α-tocopherol at the time of production is recommended (IFRA 2009).

Organ-specific effects

Adverse skin reactions: Undiluted orange flower absolute was slightly irritating to rabbits; tested at 20% on 25 volunteers it was neither irritating nor sensitizing (Opdyke & Letizia 1982 p. 785). Oxidation products of linalool may be skin sensitizing. Orange flower absolute, tested on 14 human volunteers, was detemined to be "weakly phototoxic" (Bouhlal et al 1988b).
Reproductive toxicity: The low reproductive toxicity of 2-phenylethanol and linalool (see Constituent profiles, Chapter 14) suggests that orange flower absolute is not hazardous in pregnancy.

Systemic effects

Acute toxicity: Non-toxic. Orange flower absolute acute oral LD_{50} in rats >5 g/kg; acute dermal LD_{50} in rabbits >5 g/kg (Opdyke & Letizia 1982 p. 785).
Carcinogenic/anticarcinogenic potential: No information was found for orange flower absolute, but it contains no known carcinogens. Farnesol, geraniol nerolidol and (+)-limonene display anticarcinogenic activity (see Constituent profiles, Chapter 14).

Comments

Neroli is the equivalent essential oil.

Orange flower water

Botanical name: *Citrus x aurantium* L.
Family: Rutaceae

Absolute

Source: Orange flower water
Key constituents:

Linalool+2-phenylethanol	67.5%
α-Terpineol	20.0%
Methyl anthranilate	3.0%
Nerol	3.0%
(Z)-Linalool oxide	1.9%
(E)-Linalool oxide	1.1%

(Fakhry, private communication, 2003)

Safety summary

Hazards: None known.
Contraindications: None known.

Organ-specific effects

Adverse skin reactions: Orange flower water absolute, tested on 14 human volunteers, was detemined to be 'weakly phototoxic' (Bouhlal et al 1988b). Linalool, 2-phenylethanol and α-terpineol

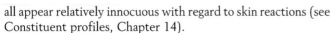

all appear relatively innocuous with regard to skin reactions (see Constituent profiles, Chapter 14).

Reproductive toxicity: The low reproductive toxicity of 2-phenylethanol and linalool (see Constituent profiles, Chapter 14) suggests that orange flower water absolute is not hazardous in pregnancy.

Systemic effects

Acute toxicity: No information found. Linalool, 2-phenylethanol and α-terpineol all appear to be non-toxic (see Constituent profiles, Chapter 14).

Carcinogenic/anticarcinogenic potential: No information was found for orange flower water absolute, but it contains no known carcinogens.

Comments

Unusually, the absolute is not prepared from a concrete that has been made with the botanical raw material, but is produced directly from distillation water.

Orange flower & leaf water

Synonym: Eau de brouts
Botanical name: *Citrus x aurantium* L.
Family: Rutaceae

Absolute

Source: A mixture of orange flower water and orange leaf water
Key constituents:

Linalool	51.6%
α-Terpineol	23.5 %
Geraniol	10.0%
Linalyl acetate	4.1%
Nerol	3.7%
Geranyl acetate	1.8%

(Fakhry, private communication, 2003)

Safety summary

Hazards: None known.
Contraindications: None known.

Organ-specific effects

Adverse skin reactions: Undiluted eau de brouts absolute was moderately irritating to rabbits, but was not irritating to mice or pigs; tested at 4% on 25 volunteers it was neither irritating nor sensitizing. It is non-phototoxic (Opdyke 1976 p. 753). Oxidation products of linalool may be skin sensitizing.

Systemic effects

Acute toxicity: Eau de Brouts absolute acute oral LD$_{50}$ in rats >5 g/kg; acute dermal LD$_{50}$ in rabbits >5 g/kg (Opdyke 1976 p. 753).

Carcinogenic/anticarcinogenic potential: No information was found for eau de brouts absolute, but it contains no known carcinogens. Linalool is neither mutagenic nor carcinogenic; geraniol displays anticarcinogenic activity (see Constituent profiles, Chapter 14).

Regulatory guidelines

According to IFRA, essential oils rich in linalool should only be used when the level of peroxides is kept to the lowest practical value. The addition of antioxidants such as 0.1% BHT or α-tocopherol at the time of production is recommended (IFRA 2009).

Comments

Like the previous profile, the absolute is not prepared from a concrete that has been made with the botanical raw material, but is produced directly from a mixture of distillation waters.

Orange leaf

Synonyms: Petitgrain, orange petitgrain, bitter orange leaf, sour orange leaf, Seville orange leaf
Botanical name: *Citrus x aurantium* L.
Family: Rutaceae

Absolute

Source: Leaves
Key constituents:

Linalyl acetate	48.9%
Linalool	42.5%
β-Myrcene	2.5%
Geranyl acetate	1.6%
(*E*)-β-Ocimene	1.2%
Neryl acetate	1.0%

(Fakhry, private communication, 2002)

Essential oil

Source: Flowering leaves and terminal branches
Key constituents:

Bigarade

Linalyl acetate	51.0–71.0%
Linalool	12.3–24.2%
(+)-Limonene	0.4–8.0%
α-Terpineol	2.1–5.2%
Geranyl acetate	1.9–3.4%
β-Pinene	0.3–2.7%
Neryl acetate	0–2.6%
Geraniol	1.4–2.3%
(*E*)-β-Ocimene	0.2–2.2%
β-Myrcene	0–2.0%
Nerol	0.4–1.1%

(Lawrence 1995g p. 107–110)

Paraguayan

Linalyl acetate	47.4–58.0%
Linalool	20.8–25.2%
α-Terpineol	4.4–6.8%
Geranyl acetate	2.9–4.5%
Geraniol	2.1–3.0%
Neryl acetate	2.1–3.0%
β-Myrcene	0–2.0%
(E)-β-Ocimene	0–2.0%
β-Pinene	0.3–1.2%
(+)-Limonene	0.3–1.1%

(Lawrence 1995g p. 107–110)

Quality: Orange leaf bigarade may be adulterated with the cheaper Paraguayan oil, which itself is frequently adulterated (Kubeczka 2002). The Paraguayan oil may be adulterated with a mixture of linalyl acetate, α-terpineol, geranyl acetate, neryl acetate and trace amounts of pyrazines (Burfield 2003).

Safety summary

Hazards: None known.
Contraindications: None known.

Regulatory guidelines

Has GRAS status. According to IFRA, essential oils rich in linalool should only be used when the level of peroxides is kept to the lowest practical value. The addition of antioxidants such as 0.1% BHT or α-tocopherol at the time of production is recommended (IFRA 2009).

Organ-specific effects

Adverse skin reactions: Undiluted orange leaf bigarade oil was slightly irritating to rabbits; tested at 0.1%, 2%, 5% or 8% on different panels of 25 volunteers it was not irritating; an 8% concentration of orange leaf bigarade oil was not sensitizing in 25 volunteers (Ford et al 1992 p. 101S). In a study of 200 consecutive dermatitis patients, one (0.5%) was sensitive to 2% orange leaf bigarade oil on patch testing (Rudzki et al 1976). No phototoxic effects were produced in mice or swine (Ford et al 1992 p. 101S). Oxidation products of linalool may be skin sensitizing.

Undiluted orange leaf Paraguayan oil was slightly irritating to rabbits, but not to mice or pigs. Tested at 2%, 5%, 7% or 8% on four panels of 25 volunteers it was not irritating, nor was it to subjects with dermatoses at 0.1%. In sensitization tests orange leaf Paraguayan oil produced three false positive reactions at 7%, and no positive reactions on a second panel when tested at 8% (Opdyke & Letizia 1982 p. 801–802). In a study of 200 consecutive dermatitis patients, one (0.5%) was sensitive to 2% orange leaf Paraguayan oil on patch testing (Rudzki et al 1976). No phototoxic effects were produced in mice or swine (Opdyke & Letizia 1982 p. 801–802). No information was found for orange leaf absolute.

Systemic effects

Acute toxicity: For both types of orange leaf oil, the acute oral LD$_{50}$ in rats was >5 g/kg, and the acute dermal LD$_{50}$ in rabbits was <2 g/kg (Opdyke & Letizia 1982 p. 801–802; Ford et al 1992 p. 101S). No information was found for orange leaf absolute.

Carcinogenic/anticarcinogenic potential: No information was found for orange leaf oil or absolute but neither contains any known carcinogens. Geraniol and (+)-limonene display anticarcinogenic ativity (see Constituent profiles, Chapter 14).

Comments

Orange leaf oil Paraguay is produced in the greatest quantity. The 'bigarade' oil is produced from a different variety of tree, and is produced in several countries, including Haiti, Italy, Spain, France and North Africa. There are important differences in the minor constituents of the two types of oil.

Oregano

Synonym: Origanum
Botanical names: *Origanum onites* L. (synonym: *Origanum smyrnaeum* L.); *Origanum vulgare* L. subsp. *hirtum* (Link) Ietswaart (synonyms: *Origanum compactum*, *Origanum hirtum* Link); *Thymbra capitata* (L.) Cav. (synonyms: *Thymus capitatus* L., *Coridothymus capitatus* L., *Satureja capitata* L.); and occasionally other *Origanum* species
Family: Lamiaceae (Labiatae)

Essential oil

Source: Dried aerial parts of flowering plant
Key constituents:

Origanum onites (Turkish)

Carvacrol	66.5–80.4%
p-Cymene	3.0–10.9%
γ-Terpinene	1.6–8.7%
Thymol	0.3–1.9%
Linalool	0.04–1.9%

(Baser et al 1993)

Origanum vulgare subsp. hirtum *(Greek/Turkish)*

Carvacrol	61.6–83.4%
p-Cymene	4.9–9.7%
γ-Terpinene	3.8–8.2%
Thymol	0–4.4%
β-Caryophyllene	1.4–2.5%
α-Pinene	0.5–2.2%
β-Myrcene	0–1.9%
α-Terpinene	0.8–1.4%

(Sezik et al 1993; Baser et al 1994; Karpouhtsis et al 1998; Owen, private communication, 2004)

Thymbra capitata (Greek)

Carvacrol	81.5–82.3%
p-Cymene	5.8–6.4%
γ-Terpinene	2.3–2.7%
β-Caryophyllene	0.9–1.9%
Thymol	0.3–1.5%

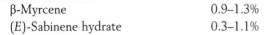

| β-Myrcene | 0.9–1.3% |
| (E)-Sabinene hydrate | 0.3–1.1% |

(Lagouri et al 1993; Karpouhtsis et al 1998)

Quality: Oregano oil may be adulterated by the addition of carvacrol and p-cymene (Burfield 2003).

Safety summary

Hazards: Drug interaction; inhibits blood clotting; embryotoxicity; skin irritation (low risk); mucous membrane irritation (moderate risk).

Contraindications (all routes): Pregnancy, breastfeeding.

Cautions (dermal): Hypersensitive, diseased or damaged skin, children under two years of age.

Cautions (oral): Diabetic medication, anticoagulant medication, major surgery, peptic ulcer, hemophilia, other bleeding disorders (Box 7.1).

Maximum dermal use level: 1.1%

Our safety advice

Our dermal maximum is based on 87.8% total thymol and carvacrol content and a dermal limit of 1% for carvacrol and thymol to avoid skin irritation (see Carvacrol and Thymol profiles, Chapter 14).

Regulatory guidelines

Has GRAS status.

Organ-specific effects

Adverse skin reactions: Undiluted oregano oil was severely irritating to mice, and moderately irritating to rabbits. Tested at 2% on 25 volunteers it was neither irritating nor sensitizing. Oregano oil is non-phototoxic (Opdyke 1974 p945–946). In a CAM (chorioallantoic membrane of the fertile chicken egg) assay, a model for detecting irritants, *Origanum onites* oil with 57.4% carvacrol and 11.6% thymol was strongly irritating. This irritation was due to thymol and not to carvacrol (Demirci et al 2004).

Cardiovascular effects: *Origanum vulgare* oil inhibits platelet aggregation (Tognolini et al 2006), an essential step in the blood clotting cascade. An essential oil high in carvacrol *(Satureja khuzestanica,* 93.9% carvacrol) significantly reduced plasma glucose concentrations in diabetic rats when given orally at 100 mg/kg/day for 21 days (Shahsavari et al 2009).

Reproductive toxicity: When *Origanum vulgare* oil was fed to pregnant mice for two weeks at 1,000 ppm (equivalent to ~150 mg/kg), there was a related increase in the rate of embryonic cell death (Domaracky et al 2007). *Satureja khuzestanica,* an essential oil consisting of 93.9% carvacrol, was given orally to pregnant rats during gestational days 0–15 at doses of 100, 500 or 1,000 ppm. There were no signs of maternal toxicity or teratogenicity at any dose, and in the two higher dose groups there was a significant increase in the number of implantation and live fetuses, a positive outcome (Abdollahi et al 2003; Abdollahi, private communication, 2004).

Systemic effects

Acute toxicity: Oregano oil acute oral LD_{50} in rats 1.85 g/kg; acute dermal LD_{50} in rabbits 480 mg/kg (Opdyke 1974 p. 945–946).

Antioxidant/pro-oxidant activity: *Origanum vulgare* L. subsp. *hirtum* oil displayed antioxidant activity in chicken liver, muscle tissue and egg yolk (Dorman et al 1995) and was significantly antioxidant (comparable with α-tocopherol or BHT) in three different assays (Kusilic et al 2004).

The oil scavenged DPPH radicals with an IC_{50} of 0.17 μg/mL (Bozin et al 2006). *Thymbra capitata* oil had more than double the antioxidant potency of BHT in sunflower oil (Miguel et al 2003b).

Carcinogenic/anticarcinogenic potential: Oregano oil significantly induced glutathione *S*-transferase activity in mouse tissues (Lam & Zheng 1991). *Origanum onites* oil (74.0% carvacrol, 7.2% linalool, 4.4% thymol) was not mutagenic in *S. tymphimurium* strains TA98 and TA100 with or without S9, and strongly inhibited induced mutagenicity in the same strains (Ipek et al 2005). *Thymbra capitata* oil was not mutagenic in either the *Bacillus subtilis rec*-assay or the *Salmonella*/microsome reversion assay (Zani et al 1991). *Origanum vulgare* L. subsp. *hirtum* oil is reported to be non-genotoxic and antigenotoxic (Bakkali et al 2006; Mezzoug et al 2007). An *Origanum vulgare* L. subsp. *hirtum* oil with 79.6% carvacrol caused complete cell death in two human cancer cell lines, Hep-2 and HeLa, at 0.01% (Sivropoulou et al 1996). Carvacrol displays anticarcinogenic activity (see Carvacrol profile, Chapter 14).

Drug interactions: Antidiabetic or anticoagulant medication, because of cardiovascular effects, above. See Table 4.10B.

Comments

Oils from many origins may be offered as 'oregano' or 'origanum' oils. Wild marjoram oil (carvacrol CT) is chemically similar to oregano oil. While most commercial oils are high in carvacrol, thymol chemotypes or thymol/carvacrol chemotypes are also found, though this is unlikely to significantly affect the safety profile of the oil. There is a (non-commercial) chemotype of *Origanum onites,* with 80–92% linalool.

Oregano (Mexican)

Botanical name: *Lippia graveolens* HBK
Botanical synonyms: *Lippia berlandieri* Schauer, *Lippia amentacea* M. E. Jones, *Lippia tomentosa* Sessé & Moc.
Family: Verbenaceae

Essential oil

Source: Dried aerial parts of flowering plant
Key constituents:

Thymol	0.2–60.6%
p-Cymene	7.7–28.0%
Carvacrol	0.5–24.8%
1,8-Cineole	1.8–14.0%

β-Phellandrene	4.5–4.8%
γ-Terpinene	0.5–3.9%
Methyl thymol	2.4–3.8%
Terpinen-4-ol	0.3–3.8%
β-Caryophyllene	0.8–3.4%
α-Terpineol	0.4–2.8%
β-Myrcene	0.9–2.5%
Linalool	0.4–2.4%
α-Caryophyllene	1.3–2.1%
Terpinen-4-yl acetate	1.6–1.9%
δ-3-Carene	0.9–1.5%
α-Terpinene	0.2–1.4%
Borneol	0.1–1.4%
α-Pinene	0.2–1.3%
α-Thujene	0.1–1.3%
Piperitone	0.9–1.2%
(E)-p-Menth-2-en-1-ol	0.8–1.2%
β-Bisabolene	0.2–1.2%

(Terblanché & Kornelius 1996)

Safety summary

Hazards: Drug interaction; may inhibit blood clotting; skin irritation (low risk); mucous membrane irritation (moderate risk).
Cautions (dermal): Hypersensitive, diseased or damaged skin, children under 2 years of age.
Cautions (oral): Anticoagulant medication, major surgery, peptic ulcer, hemophilia, other bleeding disorders (Box 7.1).
Maximum dermal use level: 1.2%

Our safety advice

Our dermal maximum is based on 85.4% total thymol and carvacrol content and a dermal limit of 1% for carvacrol and thymol to avoid skin irritation (see Carvacrol and Thymol profiles, Chapter 14).

Organ-specific effects

Adverse skin reactions: No information found.
Cardiovascular effects: Thymol and carvacrol inhibit platelet aggregation (Enomoto et al 2001), an essential step in the blood clotting cascade.

Systemic effects

Acute toxicity: No information found.
Carcinogenic/anticarcinogenic potential: No information was found for Mexican oregano oil, but it contains no known carcinogens.
Drug interactions: Anticoagulant medication, because of cardiovascular effects, above. See Table 4.10B.

Comments

Limited availability.

Orris

Synonym: Iris
Botanical names: *Iris pallida* Lam., *Iris* x *germanica* L.
Family: Iridaceae

Absolute

Source: Rhizomes
Key constituents:

Iris pallida

(Z)-γ-Irone	54–59.4%
(Z)-α-Irone	34.9–39.8%
(E)-α-Irone	4.7–5.0%
(Z)-β-Irone	0.9–2.2%

(Galfré et al 1993)

Iris × *germanica*

(Z)-γ-Irone	32.3–36.9%
(Z)-α-Irone	58.4–62.7%
(E)-α-Irone	1.7–3.9%
(Z)-β-Irone	0.4–2.3%

(Galfré et al 1993)

Safety summary

Hazards: None known.
Contraindications: None known.

Organ-specific effects

Adverse skin reactions: Undiluted orris absolute was not irritating either to pigs or mice; tested at 3% on 25 volunteers it was neither irritating nor sensitizing. It is non-phototoxic (Opdyke 1975 p. 895–896).

Systemic effects

Acute toxicity: Non-toxic. Orris absolute acute oral LD_{50} in rats >5 g/kg acute dermal LD_{50} in rabbits >5 g/kg (Opdyke 1975 p. 895–896).
Carcinogenic/anticarcinogenic potential: No information was found for orris absolute. In male and female mice given 24 ip injections of α-irone in impure tricaprylin in a total dose of 1.95 or 9.6 g/kg over 24 weeks the incidence of primary lung tumors was no higher than in the control group (Stoner et al 1973).

Comments

While orris is often referred to as originating from *Iris florentina* auct. (*Iris* × *germanica* var. *florentina* Dykes) it would be more correctly described as a cultivar, 'Florentina' (Craker & Simon 1987 p.199).

Essential oil

Source: Rhizomes

Key constituents:

Iris pallida

(Z)-γ-Irone	55.4–69.2%
(Z)-α-Irone	26.0–40.6%
(E)-α-Irone	3.7–4.8%
(Z)- β-Irone	0–0.5%

(Galfré et al 1993)

Iris × germanica

(Z)-α-Irone	57.6–66.2%
(Z)- γ-Irone	33.8–39.4%
(E)-α-Irone	0.5–2.7%
(Z)-β-Irone	0–2.2%

(Galfré et al 1993)

Safety Summary

Hazards: None known.
Contraindications: None known.

Organ-specific effects

Adverse skin reactions: No information found.

Systemic effects

Acute toxicity: No information was found for orris oil. Orris absolute is non-toxic (see above) as is α-irone (Lalko et al 2007c). **Carcinogenic/anticarcinogenic potential:** No information was found for orris oil. In male and female mice given 24 ip injections of α-irone in impure tricaprylin in a total dose of 1.95 or 9.6 g/kg over 24 weeks the incidence of primary lung tumors was no higher than in the control group (Stoner et al 1973).

Comments

Considering the chemical similarity between orris oil and absolute, the known safety of the absolute (see above) and the known safety of α-irone, orris oil is unlikely to present any toxicity concerns. Orris essential oil is a cream-colored solid, and is often referred to as orris butter, or sometimes (incorrectly) as orris concrete. A concrete does exist, but is a dark viscous material, and is perhaps more correctly described as a resinoid. While orris is often referred to as originating from *Iris florentina* auct. (*Iris x germanica* var. *florentina* Dykes) it would be more correctly described as a cultivar, 'Florentina' (Craker & Simon 1987 p. 199).

Osmanthus

Synonyms: Fragrant olive, sweet olive, tea olive
Botanical name: *Osmanthus fragrans* Lour.
Botanical synonym: *Olea fragrans* Thunb.
Family: Oleaceae

Absolute

Source: Flowers

Key constituents:

β-Ionone	7.6–33.8%
Dihydro-β-ionone	6.4–15.7%
γ-Decalactone	4.7–12.7%
Linalool	0.8–8.7%
Geraniol	1.2–7.1%
(E)-Linalool oxide	0.6–7.0%
(Z)-Linalool oxide	0.7–5.6%
Decan-4-olide	0–4.0%
Dihydro-β-ionol	0–3.0%
α-Ionone	tr–2.3%
2-Phenylethanol	tr–2.2%

(Lawrence 1989 p. 188–190; Anonis 1993)

Safety summary

Hazards: None known.
Contraindications: None known.

Organ-specific effects

Adverse skin reactions: No information was found for osmanthus absolute, but ionones tend to be non-reactive on the skin (see Constituent profiles, Chapter 14).

Systemic effects

Acute toxicity: No information found. Ionones are not acutely toxic (see Constituent profiles, Chapter 14). **Carcinogenic/anticarcinogenic potential:** No information was found for osmanthus absolute. β-Ionone is not mutagenic and demonstrates anticarcinogenic activity (see Constituent profiles, Chapter 14).

Comments

The absolute is produced in China, and is mostly used in fine perfumery.

Palmarosa

Synonyms: Motia, rosha grass
Botanical name: *Cymbopogon martinii* Roxb. var. *martinii*
Botanical synonyms: *Andropogon martinii* Roxb. *var martinii*, *Cymbopogon martinii* Roxb. var. *motia*
Family: Poaceae (Gramineae)

Essential oil

Source: Leaves
Key constituents:

Indian

Geraniol	74.5–81.0%
Geranyl acetate	0.5–10.7%
(E,Z)-Farnesol	0.5–6.1%
Linalool	2.6–4.5%
(E)-β-Ocimene	1.3–3.1%

β-Caryophyllene	0.9–2.6%
Geranial	0.5–1.9%
Caryophyllene oxide	0.1–1.8%
β-Myrcene	0.6–1.3%
Elemol	0.2–1.0%
(Z,Z)-Farnesol	0.1–1.0%

(Lawrence 2002a p. 56–57)
Quality: Palmarosa oil may be adulterated by the addition of geraniol (Burfield 2003).

Safety summary

Hazards: Drug interaction; skin sensitization (low risk).
Cautions (oral): Drugs metabolized by CYP2B6 (Appendix B).
Maximum dermal use level: 6.5%

Our safety advice

We recommend a dermal maximum of 6.5%, based on 81% geraniol content with a dermal limit of 5.3% (see Geraniol profile, Chapter 14).

Regulatory guidelines

Has GRAS status.

Organ-specific effects

Adverse skin reactions: In a mouse local lymph node assay, palmarosa oil was a weak sensitizer, with a similar potency to geraniol (Lalko & Api 2006). Undiluted palmarosa oil was moderately irritating to rabbits, but was not irritating to mice; tested at 8% on 25 volunteers it was neither irritating nor sensitizing. It is non-phototoxic (Opdyke 1974 p. 947).

Systemic effects

Acute toxicity: Non-toxic. Palmarosa oil acute oral LD$_{50}$ in rats >5 g/kg; acute dermal LD$_{50}$ in rabbits >5 g/kg (Opdyke 1974 p. 947).
Carcinogenic/anticarcinogenic potential: No information was found for palmarosa oil, but it contains no known carcinogens. Geraniol, farnesol, β-caryophyllene and geranial display anticarcinogenic activity (see Constituent profiles, Chapter 14). Considering these constitute 85% of palmarosa oil, it is very likely to possess anticarcinogenic activity.
Drug interactions: Since citral and geraniol inhibit CYP2B6 (Table 4.11B), there is a theoretical risk of interaction between palmarosa oil and drugs metabolized by this enzyme (Appendix B).

Comments

In spite of European legislation listing geraniol as an allergen, the risk of geraniol allergy is relatively low (see Geraniol profile, Chapter 14).

Palo santo

Botanical name: *Bursera graveolens* (Kunth) Triana et Planch
Family: Burseraceae

Essential oil

Source: Wood
Key constituents:

(+)-Limonene	58.6–63.3%
(+)-Menthofuran	6.6–11.8%
α-Terpineol	7.1–10.9%
Carvone	1.6–2.0%
Germacrene D	1.7%
β-Pulegone	1.1–1.2%
γ-Muurolene	0.7–1.2%
(E)-Carveol	0.4–1.1%

(Young et al 2007; Aromatics International website)

Safety summary

Hazards: Skin sensitization if oxidized; hepatotoxicity.
Cautions: Old or oxidized oils should be avoided.
Maximum adult daily oral dose: 94 mg
Maximum dermal use level: 3.4%

Our safety advice

Our oral and dermal restrictions are based on 11.8% menthofuran and 1.2% pulegone content, with limits of 0.2 mg/kg/day and 0.5% for menthofuran, and of 0.5 mg/kg/day and 1.2% for pulegone (see Constituent profiles, Chapter 14). Because of its (+)-limonene content, we recommend that oxidation of palo santo oil is avoided by storage in a dark, airtight container in a refrigerator. The addition of an antioxidant to preparations containing it is recommended.

Regulatory guidelines

IFRA recommends that essential oils rich in limonene should only be used when the level of peroxides is kept to the lowest practical level, for instance by adding antioxidants at the time of production (IFRA 2009).

Organ-specific effects

Adverse skin reactions: No information found.
Hepatotoxicity: Menthofuran is toxic to both liver and lung tissue in mice (Gordon et al 1982). In rats, high oral doses of menthofuran (250 mg/kg/day for 3 days) caused hepatotoxicity, detected as changes in blood levels of liver enzyme markers for liver disease (Madyastha & Raj 1994). β-Pulegone is also hepatotoxic (see β-Pulegone profile, Chapter 14).

Systemic effects

Acute toxicity: No information found.
Carcinogenic potential: No information found. (+)-Limonene displays anticarcinogenic activity (see (+)-Limonene profile, Chapter 14).

Comments

Bursera graveolens is a wild-growing small tree. It is regarded as a critically endangered species in Peru. The essential oil is mainly produced in Ecuador, where the plant is unofficially also endangered.

Parsley leaf

Synonym: Parsley herb
Botanical name: *Petroselinum crispum* Mill.
Botanical synonyms: *Petroselinum sativum* Hoffm., *Petroselinum hortense* auct.
Family: Apiaceae (Umbelliferae)

Essential oil

Source: Leaves
Key constituents:

Egyptian

p-Mentha-1,3,8-triene	6.2–45.2%
β-Myrcene	7.8–23.8%
β-Phellandrene	6.7–19.5%
Myristicin	1.9–8.8%
α-Pinene	6.9–7.6%
Terpinolene	2.8–6.6%
(+)-Limonene	3.3–5.4%
α-*p*-Dimethylstyrene	2.7–5.4%
Dill apiole	0.2–5.2%
β-Pinene	4.6–4.9%
α-Phellandrene	1.0–1.5%
p-Mentha-1,4,8-triene	0–1.2%

(Lawrence 2001b p38; Fakhry, private communication, 2002)

Safety summary

Hazards: Toxicity; may be abortifacient.
Contraindications (all routes): Pregnancy, breastfeeding.
Maximum adult daily oral dose: 538 mg
Maximum dermal use level: 14.6%

Our safety advice

We have proposed limits for parsley apiole of 0.4 mg/kg/day (oral) and 0.76% (dermal) for general toxicity, and because of its structural similarity, we have made the assumption that dill apiole presents a similar risk. On this basis, we recommend a dermal maximum of 14.6% and a daily oral maximum of 538 mg for an oil containing 5.2% dill apiole. Parsley herb is routinely contraindicated in pregnancy in herbal medicine texts (including the Commission E Monographs), and since the the safety of *p*-mentha-1,3,8-triene is unknown, a similar restriction for the essential oil seems prudent.

Organ-specific effects

Adverse skin reactions: Undiluted parsley leaf oil was severely irritating to rabbits, but was not irritating to mice or pigs; tested at 2% on 25 volunteers it was neither irritating nor sensitizing.

It is non-phototoxic (Opdyke & Letizia 1983 p. 871–872). Parsley leaf oil typically contains 20 ppm (0.002%) bergapten (www.ifraorg.org/view_document.aspx?docId=22594 accessed November 12th 2012). This is not sufficient to cause a phototoxic reaction, although it may contribute to the total psoralen content of a mixture.

Reproductive toxicity: Parsley is a commonly used abortifacient in South America (Ciganda & Laborde 2003). Apiole and various preparations of parsley have been used for many years to procure illegal abortion in Italy. Post-abortive vaginal bleeding, sometimes profuse, is a feature of these cases.

Systemic effects

Acute toxicity: Acute oral LD_{50} in rats 3.3 g/kg; acute dermal LD_{50} in rabbits >5 g/kg (Opdyke & Letizia 1983 p. 871–872).
Carcinogenic/anticarcinogenic potential: Parsley leaf oil significantly induced glutathione *S*-transferase activity in mouse tissues (Lam & Zheng 1991). It contains no known carcinogens. Myristicin and (+)-limonene display anticarcinogenic activity (see Constituent profiles, Chapter 14).

Comments

Essential oils high in parsley apiole present a high risk of abortion if taken in oral doses, and external use also seems inadvisable in pregnancy. Myristicin is suspected of being psychotropic, and is a moderate MAO inhibitor. However the amount present in parsley leaf oil is very unlikely to have any adverse effect in either scenario.

Parsleyseed

Botanical name: *Petroselinum crispum* Mill.
Botanical synonyms: *Petroselinum sativum* Hoffm., *Petroselinum hortense* auct.
Family: Apiaceae (Umbelliferae)

Essential oil

Source: Seeds
Key constituents:

Parsley apiole	11.3–67.5%
Myristicin	0.7–37.9%
Allyltetramethoxybenzene	0.6–29.0%
α-Pinene	8.3–16.9%
β-Pinene	5.4–10.7%
Elemicin	0–8.8%
(+)-Limonene	1.3–3.0%

(Lamarti et al 1991)

Safety summary

Hazards: Drug interaction; hepatotoxicity; nephrotoxicity; potentially abortifacient; skin irritation (low risk).
Contraindications (all routes): Pregnancy, breastfeeding.
Cautions (oral): May interact with pethidine, MAOIs or SSRIs.
Maximum adult daily oral dose: 42 mg
Maximum dermal use level: 1.1%

Our safety advice

Our oral and dermal restrictions are based on 67.5% parsley apiole and limits of 0.76% and 0.4 mg/kg/day (see Parsley apiole profile, Chapter 14).

Regulatory guidelines

The Commission E Monograph for parsleyseed oil concludes that 'a therapeutic application cannot be justified because of high risks.' (Blumenthal et al 1998)

Organ-specific effects

Adverse skin reactions: Undiluted parsleyseed oil was slightly irritating to rabbits, but was not irritating to mice or pigs; tested at 2% on 25 volunteers it was mildly irritating, but was not sensitizing. It is non-phototoxic (Opdyke 1975 p. 897–898).
Neurotoxicity: Psychotropic effects have been reported for whole nutmeg, and myristicin and elemicin are thought to be responsible. However, other synergistic constituents may need to be present for a psychotropic effect to take place (see Ch. 10, p. 144/145). One of us (R.T.) ingested 1.0 mL of parsleyseed oil with no apparent psychotropic effect.
Reproductive toxicity: Parsley is a commonly used abortifacient in South America (Ciganda & Laborde 2003). Apiole and various preparations of parsley have been used for many years to procure illegal abortion in Italy. Post-abortive vaginal bleeding, sometimes profuse, is a feature of these cases. A cumulative effect is apparent, parsley apiole being taken daily for between two and eight days before either death or abortion ensued. The lowest daily dose of parsley apiole which induced abortion was 900 mg taken for eight consecutive days (see Parsley apiole profile, Chapter 14).

Systemic effects

Acute toxicity, human: Parsley apiole is toxic to humans; the lowest total dose of parsley apiole causing death is 4.2 g (2.1 g/day for two days) the lowest fatal daily dose is 770 mg, which was taken for 14 days; the lowest single fatal dose is 8 g. At least 19 g has been survived. Parsley apiole is hepatotoxic and nephrotoxic (see Parsley apiole profile, Chapter 14).
Acute toxicity, animal: Parsleyseed oil acute oral LD_{50} in rats 3.96 g/kg, in mice 1.52 g/kg; acute dermal LD_{50} in rabbits >5 g/kg (Opdyke 1975 p. 897–898).
Antioxidant/pro-oxidant activity: Antioxidant activity has been reported for parsleyseed oil (Fejes et al 1998). Parsleyseed oil showed moderate DPPH radical scavenging activity, and high activity in the aldehyde/carboxylic acid assay (Wei & Shibamoto 2007a).
Carcinogenic/anticarcinogenic potential: No information found. Parsley apiole, myristicin and (+)-limonene display anti-tumoral activity (see Constituent profiles, Chapter 14).
Drug interactions: Myristicin is an inhibitor of MAO in rodents; nutmeg oil was less potent an inhibitor of MAO than myristicin (Truitt et al 1963). MAO inhibitors should not be taken in conjunction with pethidine (Reynolds 1993) or with MAO inhibiting drugs (Table 4.10B).

Comments

Essential oils high in parsley apiole present a risk of abortion if taken in substantial oral doses, and external use also seems inadvisable in pregnancy. There are three chemotypes of parsleyseed oil, with either parsley apiole, allyltetramethoxybenzene or myristicin as the major constituent (Lawrence 1989 p. 27). The majority of commercial oils contain high concentrations of parsley apiole.

Parsnip

Botanical name: *Pastinaca sativa* L.
Family: Apiaceae (Umbelliferae)

Essential oil

Source: Roots
Key constituents:

Terpinolene	40.3–69.0%
Myristicin	17.2–40.1%
β-Pinene	2.4–8.6%
(Z)-β-Ocimene	0.7–3.7%
(+)-Limonene	1.7–3.2%
(E)-β-Ocimene + γ-terpinene	0.5–1.3%
β-Myrcene	0.7–1.2%

(Kubeczka & Stahl 1975)

Safety summary

Hazards: Drug interaction; may be phototoxic.
Cautions (dermal): Has not been tested for phototoxicity.
Cautions (oral): May interact with pethidine, MAOIs or SSRIs.

Organ-specific effects

Adverse skin reactions: No information found. Parsnip roots are phototoxic (Bang Pedersen & Pla Arles 1998) and both the flowers and fruits contain methoxsalen, bergapten, psoralen, imperatorin and isopimpinellin (Berenbaum et al 1984; Zangerl et al 1997).

Systemic effects

Acute toxicity: No information found.
Carcinogenic/anticarcinogenic potential: No information was found for parsnip oil, but it contains no known carcinogens. Myristicin and (+)-limonene display anticarcinogenic activity (see Constituent profiles, Chapter 14).
Drug interactions: Myristicin is an inhibitor of MAO in rodents; nutmeg oil was less potent an inhibitor of MAO than myristicin (Truitt et al 1963). MAO inhibitors should not be taken in conjunction with pethidine (Reynolds 1993) or with MAO inhibiting drugs (Table 4.10B).

Comments

The fruiting or flowering tops may be distilled in addition to the roots.

Patchouli

Botanical name: *Pogostemon cablin* (Blanco) Benth.
Botanical synonym: *Pogostemon patchouly* Pellet
Family: Lamiaceae (Labiatae)

Essential oil

Source: Leaves
Key constituents:

Chinese

Patchouli alcohol	17.5–32.3%
α-Bulnesene (δ-guaiene)	8.7–20.7%
α-Guaiene	8.8–15.3%
Seychellene	0–9.6%
β-Patchoulene	4.8–9.3%
α-Patchoulene	4.8–8.5%
γ-Patchoulene	0–6.7%
(−)-*allo*-Aromadendrene	0–5.0%
1(10)-Aromadendrene	0–3.9%
Pogostone	0–3.8%
β-Caryophyllene	2.1–3.2%
Pogostol	0–2.4%
β-Elemene	0–1.3%

(Lawrence 1989 p. 15, 1995c p. 73; Milchard et al 2004)

Indonesian

Patchouli alcohol	28.2–32.7%
α-Bulnesene (δ-guaiene)	15.8–18.8%
α-Guaiene	13.5–14.6%
Seychellene	0–9.0%
γ-Patchoulene	0–6.7%
α-Patchoulene	4.5–5.7%
β-Caryophyllene	3.1–4.2%
1(10)-Aromadendrene	0–3.7%
β-Patchoulene	2.0–3.4%
Pogostol	tr–2.4%
(−)-*allo*-Aromadendrene	0–2.4%
δ-Cadinene	0–2.4%

(Bruns 1978; Lawrence 1989 p. 15, 1993 p. 91; Milchard et al 2004)

Quality: May be adulterated with gurjun balsam oil, in which case α-gurjunene will appear as a constituent. Other possible adulterants include copaiba balsam oil, cedarwood oil, patchouli, vetiver and camphor distillate residues, hercolyn D, benzyl benzoate, propylene glycol and vegetable oils. The superior Indonesian oil may be blended with the cheaper Chinese oil (Oyen & Dung 1999; Kubeczka 2002; Burfield 2003).

Safety summary

Hazards: Drug interaction; may inhibit blood clotting.
Cautions (oral): Anticoagulant medication, major surgery, peptic ulcer, hemophilia, other bleeding disorders (Box 7.1).

Organ-specific effects

Adverse skin reactions: In a modified Draize procedure on guinea pigs, patchouli oil was non-sensitizing when used at 20% in the challenge phase (Sharp 1978). Undiluted patchouli oil was slightly irritating to rabbits, but was not irritating to mice or pigs; tested at 10% on 25 volunteers it was neither irritating nor sensitizing. In one study patchouli oil was mildly phototoxic, in another there were no phototoxic effects (Opdyke & Letizia 1982 p. 791–792). Patchouli oil, tested at 10% in consecutive dermatitis patients, induced allergic responses in 13 of 1,606 (0.8%) (Frosch et al 2002b), and three of 318 (0.95%) (Paulsen & Andersen 2005). Of 167 fragrance-sensitive dermatitis patients, five (3%) were allergic to 10% patchouli oil on patch testing (Larsen et al 1996b). In a multicenter study, Germany's IVDK reported that 15 of 2,446 consecutive dermatitis patients (0.61%), and 11 of 828 dermatitis patients suspected of fragrance allergy (1.32%) tested positive to 10% patchouli oil. Only one of the 2,446 had a ++ or +++ reaction (Uter et al 2010).
Cardiovascular effects: Patchouli oil displays antiplatelet activity, and this is due to its α-bulnesene content (Hsu et al 2006; Tsai et al 2007).

Systemic effects

Acute toxicity: Patchouli oil acute oral LD_{50} in rats >5 g/kg; acute dermal LD_{50} in rabbits >5 g/kg (Opdyke & Letizia 1982 p. 791–792).
Subacute & subchronic toxicity: When patchouli oil was consumed by male rats at 11.9 mg/kg/day, and by female rats at 14.5 mg/kg/day for 90 days, no adverse effects were seen on growth, food consumption, hematology, blood chemistry, liver weight, kidney weight, or the microscopic or gross appearance of major organs (Oser et al 1965).
Antioxidant/pro-oxidant activity: Patchouli oil showed moderate antioxidant activity as a DPPH radical scavenger and in the aldehyde/carboxylic acid assay (Wei & Shibamoto 2007a).
Carcinogenic/anticarcinogenic potential: No information was found for patchouli oil, but it contains no known carcinogens. β-Elemene displays anticarcinogenic activity (see β-Elemene profile, Chapter 14).
Drug interactions: Anticoagulant medication, because of cardiovascular effects, above. See Table 4.10B.

Comments

Patchouli oil is a low-risk allergen and does not require a dermal use restriction. Indonesia is the main producer of patchouli oil, followed by China. Brazil and Malaysia also produce small quantities (Burfield 2000).

Pennyroyal (N. American, European and Turkish)

Botanical names: *Hedeoma pulegioides* L. (N. American); *Mentha pulegium* L. (European); *Micromeria fruticosa* L. (Turkish)
Family: Lamiaceae (Labiatae)

Essential oil

Source: Fresh aerial parts
Note: Due to their compositional similarity these three essential oils are treated here in one profile.
Key constituents:

Hedeoma pulegioides

(1R)-(+)-β-Pulegone	61.3–82.3%
Isomenthone	0.8–31.0%
Piperitenone	0.2–4.7%
(+)-Limonene	0.6–1.9%
Menthone	0.6–1.4%

(Lawrence 1979 p. 21)

Mentha pulegium

(1R)-(+)-β-Pulegone	67.6–86.7%
Menthone	1.5–16.0%
Isomenthone	0.8–8.6%
Piperitenone	0.5–2.5%
Neoisomenthol	tr–2.4%
3-Octanol	0.6–2.0%
(−)-(E)-α-Pulegone	0.2–1.6%
α-Caryophyllene	0.1–1.1%
(+)-Limonene	0.1–1.0%
3-Octyl acetate	tr–1.0%
Menthofuran	tr–0.3%

(Lawrence 1993 p. 56, 1998c p. 63–68)

Micromeria fruticosa

(1R)-(+)-β-Pulegone	66.7%
Isomenthone	11.1%
Piperitenone	3.6%
Menthone	3.5%
Isomenthol	1.8%
(−)-(E)-α-Pulegone	1.5%
(Z)-Piperitenone oxide	1.2%

(Owen, private communication, 2003)

Safety summary

Hazards: Hepatotoxicity; neurotoxicity.
Contraindications (all routes): Pregnancy, breastfeeding.
Contraindications: Should not be taken in oral doses.
Maximum dermal use level: 1.3%

Our safety advice

We recommend a dermal maximum of 1.3% for all pennyroyal oils, based on 86.7% (1R)-(+)-β-pulegone content and a limit of 1.0% (see β-Pulegone profile, Chapter 14).

Regulatory guidelines

The CEFS of the Council of Europe has classed pulegone and menthofuran as hepatotoxic, and has set a group TDI of 0.1 mg/kg bw for the two compounds. Both the UK and EC 'standard permitted proportion' of pulegone in food flavorings is 25 mg/kg of food (European Community Council 1988; Anon 1992b).

Organ-specific effects

Adverse skin reactions: Undiluted pennyroyal oil was moderately irritating to mice, but was not irritating to rabbits; tested at 6% on 25 volunteers it was neither irritating nor sensitizing. It is non-phototoxic (Opdyke 1974 p. 949–950).
Pumonary toxicity: There was moderate necrosis of epithelial cells in the lungs in mice given ip doses of 400–600 mg/kg pennyroyal oil (Gordon et al 1982).
Neurotoxicity: Neurological symptoms of varying severity have occurred in some cases of pennyroyal overdose (Braithwaite 1906; Jones 1913; Anon 1978; Bakerink et al 1996). Pennyroyal oil has been an occasional cause of seizures when taken in an attempt to produce abortion (Wingate 1889; Holland 1902; Early 1961; Kimball 1898). In these four cases the amounts ingested were all substantial, including one teaspoon in one case, and 30 mL in another.
Reproductive toxicity: The plant has enjoyed folk status as an emmenagogue and an abortifacient since ancient times (Girling 1887; Flynn 1893; Stephen & Rishton 1894; Gunby 1979). Pennyroyal oil, however, is not abortifacient unless taken in such massive quantities that it causes acute hepatotoxicity in the mother. She miscarries only because she is so poisoned that the pregnancy cannot be maintained (Macht 1921). In fact both *Mentha pulegium* oil and pulegone inhibit the contractile activity of rat uterine muscle (Soares PM et al 2005). Although not abortifacient *per se*, pennyroyal and other pulegone-rich oils should not be used in pregnancy, due to their hepatotoxicity.
Hepatotoxicity: Severe liver damage has been reported in several cases of pennyroyal poisoning (Sullivan et al 1979; Anderson et al 1996). In the case of an infant who survived, hepatic dysfunction is cited, and in the case of an infant who died, liver failure (Bakerink et al 1996). When male mice were injected with ip doses of 400, 500 or 600 mg/kg pennyroyal oil, there was dose-dependent hepatic necrosis, and 50% of mice died in the high-dose group (Gordon et al 1982). In rats, (1R)-(+)-β-pulegone depletes hepatic glutathione (Thomassen et al 1990), and in doses of >200 mg/kg, it destroys hepatic CYP (Moorthy et al 1989a).

Systemic effects

Acute toxicity, human: The clinical pathology of pennyroyal intoxication is characterized by massive centrilobular necrosis (death of liver cells), pulmonary edema and internal hemorrhage (Anderson et al 1996). These effects are similar to those produced by ip administration of both pennyroyal oil and pulegone in mice (Gordon et al 1982). A review of 18 cases of pennyroyal ingestion, all in adult women, noted moderate to severe toxicity in patients who had ingested a single dose of 10 mL or more of the essential oil (Anderson et al 1996). The cases cited below suggest that 5–7 mL of pennyroyal oil will elicit symptoms of toxicity in an adult.

We found 14 reported cases of poisoning from pennyroyal overdoses, nine non-fatal, and five fatal; three of these from the essential oil, and two from the tea. In Britain, a 23-year-old woman ingested one tablespoon (~15 mL) of pennyroyal oil, and soon proceeded to vomit. She was admitted to hospital four days later with symptoms of acute gastritis, and died later that day. Post-mortem examination showed congestion of the abdominal organs (Allen 1897). She had taken the oil to stimulate menstruation. At the inquest, the pharmacist who sold her the oil stated that, in 30 years, he had never heard of a case of pennyroyal oil poisoning. It would seem that pennyroyal oil was readily available over the counter at that time, and was regarded as a safe menstrual stimulant and abortifacient. This belief almost certainly contributed to further accidents.

Three non-fatal cases are reported where the oil was ingested as a menstrual stimulant. In 1906, a woman took half an ounce (about 15 mL) of pennyroyal oil. She became extremely ill within 10 minutes, and experienced tingling and numbness of the extremities. Within two hours she was unconscious but had recovered the next day (Braithwaite 1906). In the second case, the woman concerned vomited, became febrile, delirious, and experienced involuntary twitching. She had recovered by the next day (Jones 1913). In the third case a woman ingested 15 mL of American pennyroyal oil. She experienced minor symptoms of acute poisoning, vomited many times, and survived (Buechel et al 1983).

A more serious case was reported in *The Lancet* in 1955. It is not known how much oil was taken, but the effects were abortion, vaginal bleeding, hemolytic anemia (destruction of red blood cells) and rapid destruction of the kidney tubules, with death following massive urea leakage into the blood (Vallance 1955).

Four cases of pennyroyal oil poisoning from attempts to self-induce abortion were reported in Colorado in 1978/79. In the first, a 21-year-old woman, who was less than one month pregnant, took a quarter-ounce of pennyroyal oil. She presented with nausea, numbness and tingling of the extremities and dizziness. Her pregnancy did not abort and she recovered the same day. She later had a legal abortion (Anon 1978). In the second case, a 24-year-old woman also ingested a quarter-ounce of pennyroyal oil. She was dizzy and nauseated, but her pregnancy survived. She was discharged the following day (Anon 1978). In the third case a 22-year-old pregnant woman ingested 10 mL of pennyroyal oil. She experienced no symptoms other than dizziness, and did not miscarry (Sullivan et al 1979).

The fourth case was of an 18-year-old, frightened of being pregnant but actually not, depressed and with a tendency to irregular menses. She took one ounce of pennyroyal oil and presented with rash, abdominal pain and frequent vomiting of blood. These effects persisted over the following 12 hours and she began to bleed from the vagina as well as from injection sites. 24 hours after ingestion, liver function tests had become abnormal, she lapsed into coma, developed fluid on the lungs and died on the sixth day in hospital. The cause was brain stem dysfunction due to liver damage (Anon 1978; Sullivan et al 1979).

A 24-year-old woman died after repeated ingestion of pennyroyal tea over a two week period in an unsuccessful attempt to induce abortion. Post-mortem serum examination revealed 18 ng/mL of pulegone and 1 ng/mL of menthofuran (Anderson et al 1996). One infant died and another survived after ingesting pennyroyal tea. In both cases there was severe hepatic and neurological injury (Bakerink et al 1996). A 22-month-old girl ingested < 20 mL of pennyroyal oil, and was given gastric lavage, followed by activated charcoal and sorbitol 30 minutes later. N-acetylcysteine was also administered. 10 hours following ingestion 40 ng/mL serum of menthofuran was detected, and there was no laboratory evidence of abnormal liver function (Mullen et al 1994). Ingestion by an adult of almost 30 g pennyroyal oil was survived with little to report other than vomiting, following treatment with N-acetylcysteine (McCormick & Manoguerra 1988). N-acetylcysteine replenishes hepatic glutathione and probably contributed to the positive outcome in the last two cases.

Acute toxicity, animal: Pennyroyal (*Mentha pulegium*) oil acute oral LD_{50} in rats 400 mg/kg; acute dermal LD_{50} in rabbits 4.2 g/kg (Opdyke 1974 p. 949–950). A 7-year-old, 30 kg female dog was treated topically for fleas by its owner with 60 mL of undiluted pennyroyal oil. Less than one hour later the dog became listless, and the owner attempted to remove the oil by shampooing, but within 30 hours the dog had diarrhea and vomiting, and was bleeding from the nose and mouth. She was admitted to a veterinary hospital where, in spite of supportive therapy, she developed seizures and died. On autopsy, multiple sites of internal hemorrhage were found, including the heart, lungs, stomach and small intestine. There were large areas of gross necrotic lesions in the liver, which was the organ most obviously affected, and the spleen and kidneys were congested. Tissue from the liver was tested for xenobiotics, and pulegone was identified (Sudekum et al 1992).

Carcinogenic/anticarcinogenic potential: Pennyroyal oil was not mutagenic in fruit flies (Franzios et al 1997). β-Pulegone is not mutagenic (see β-Pulegone profile, Chapter 14).

Comments

The rat oral LD_{50} is equivalent to about 30 g or 35 mL in an adult, which correlates with human toxicity. Many of the toxic signs seen in a dog that died from pennyroyal toxicity are similar to those seen in humans, but dogs may be more susceptible to pennyroyal toxicity. Pennyroyal oil is only abortifacient in almost fatal doses, but the oil is too toxic to be safely used during pregnancy, especially since there is no information on reproductive toxicity. Our oral maximum for pulegone is 0.5 mg/kg/day, which would extrapolate to an adult oral dose of 40 mg. However, since there is no significant benefit from using pennyroyal oil medicinally, on a risk/benefit basis, it is best avoided.

Pepper (black)

Botanical name: *Piper nigrum* L.
Family: Piperaceae

Essential oil

Source: Fruits
Key constituents:

β-Caryophyllene	9.4–30.9%
(+)-Limonene	16.4–24.4%
α-Pinene	1.1–16.2%
δ-3-Carene	tr–15.5%

β-Pinene	4.9–14.3%
Sabinene	0.1–13.8%
β-Bisabolene	0.1–5.2%
α-Copaene	0.1–3.9%
(E)-β-Farnesene	tr–3.3%
α-Cubebene	0.2–1.6%

(Lawrence 1995g p. 199)

Safety summary

Hazards: Skin sensitization if oxidized.
Cautions: Old or oxidized oils should be avoided.

Our safety advice

Because of its combined (+)-limonene, α-pinene and δ-3-carene content we recommend that oxidation of black pepper oil is avoided by storage in a dark, airtight container in a refrigerator. The addition of an antioxidant to preparations containing it is recommended.

Regulatory guidelines

Has GRAS status. IFRA recommends that essential oils rich in limonene should only be used when the level of peroxides is kept to the lowest practical level, for instance by adding antioxidants at the time of production (IFRA 2009).

Organ-specific effects

Adverse skin reactions: Undiluted black pepper oil was moderately irritating to rabbits, but was not irritating to mice or pigs; tested at 4% on 25 volunteers it was neither irritating nor sensitizing. Autoxidation products of (+)-limonene, α-pinene and δ-3-carene can cause skin sensitization (see Constituent profiles, Chapter 14). Antioxidant properties have been reported for black pepper oil (Deans et al 1993; Recsan et al 1997). Low-level phototoxic effects reported for black pepper oil are not considered significant (Opdyke 1978 p. 651–652).

Systemic effects

Acute toxicity: Non-toxic. Black pepper oil acute oral LD_{50} in rats >5 g/kg; acute dermal LD_{50} in rabbits >5 g/kg (Opdyke 1978 p. 651–652).
Carcinogenic/anticarcinogenic potential: Black pepper oil dose-dependently inhibited aflatoxin B_1-induced adducts in calf thymus DNA, in the presence of rat liver microsomes (Hashim et al 1994). Black pepper oil showed moderate chemopreventive activity against human mouth epidermal carcinoma (KB) cells and mouse leukemia (P388) cells, with respective IC_{50} values of 0.215 and 0.201 mg/mL (Manosroi et al 2005). The oil contains no known carcinogens. β-Caryophyllene and (+)-limonene display anticarcinogenic activity (see Constituent profiles, Chapter 14).

Comments

Because of the pungency of fresh pepper, it is often incorrectly assumed that the oil must be a strong skin irritant. It is not

unusual for a substance to have both antioxidant and pro-oxidant properties.

Pepper (pink)

Synonyms: California pepper, Peruvian pepper, Peruvian mastic
Botanical name: *Schinus molle* L.
Family: Anacardiaceae

Essential oil

Source: Fruits
Key constituents:

β-Myrcene	5.0–20.4%
α-Phellandrene	5.3–17.3%
p-Cymene	2.9–11.5%
δ-Cadinene	4.7–9.1%
(+)-Limonene	7.2–9.0%
β-Phellandrene	4.8–7.2%
α-Cadinol	0.2–6.6%
Viridiflorol	0–6.5%
α-Cadinene	0–3.8%
Spathulenol	0–3.6%
α-Pinene	1.4–3.1%
α-Caryophyllene	0.6–3.0%
T-Cadinol	0.7–2.5%
Germacrene D	tr–2.4%
T-Muurulol	0.2–2.3%
β-Caryophyllene	0.3–2.0%
α-Muurolene	tr–1.5%
Elemol	0.2–1.3%
Terpinen-4-ol	0–1.3%

(Lawrence 1997e p. 76–78)

Safety summary

Hazards: None known.
Contraindications: None known.

Organ-specific effects

Adverse skin reactions: Undiluted pink pepper oil was moderately irritating to rabbits, but was not irritating to mice or pigs; tested at 4% on 25 volunteers it was neither irritating nor sensitizing. It is non-phototoxic (Opdyke 1976 p. 861).
Reproductive toxicity: The low reproductive toxicity of β-myrcene and (+)-limonene (see Constituent profiles, Chapter 14) suggests that pink pepper oil is not hazardous in pregnancy.

Systemic effects

Acute toxicity: Pink pepper oil acute oral LD_{50} in rats >5 g/kg; acute dermal LD_{50} in rabbits >5 g/kg (Opdyke 1976 p. 861).
Carcinogenic/anticarcinogenic potential: Pink pepper oil inhibited the growth of human MCF-7 breast cancer cells in vitro, with an IC_{50} of 54 mg/L (Bendaoud et al 2010). (+)-Limonene and α-caryophyllene display anticarcinogenic

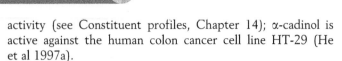

activity (see Constituent profiles, Chapter 14); α-cadinol is active against the human colon cancer cell line HT-29 (He et al 1997a).

Regulatory guidelines

Has GRAS status.

Comments

The tree is commonly found in parts of Southern Europe, Southern USA and S. America.

Pepper (Sichuan)

Synonyms: Japanese pepper, fagara, prickly ash, hua jiao
Botanical name: *Zanthoxylum piperitum* DC
Family: Rutaceae

Essential oil

Source: Fruits
Key constituents:

(+)-Limonene	44.4%
β-Myrcene	16.4%
3,7-Dimethyl-1,6-octadien-3-ol	13.6%
3,7-Dimethyl-1,6-octadien-3-yl acetate	12.2%
(*E*)-3,7-Dimethyl-1,3,6-octatriene	4.3%
C$_{15}$ Alkenes	2.0%
(*E*)-3,7-Dimethyl-2,6-octadien-1-yl acetate	1.3%

(Wang, private communication, 1999)

Safety summary

Hazards: Skin sensitization if oxidized.
Cautions: Old or oxidized oils should be avoided.

Our safety advice

Because of its (+)-limonene content we recommend that oxidation of Sichuan pepper oil is avoided by storage in a dark, airtight container in a refrigerator. The addition of an antioxidant to preparations containing it is recommended.

Regulatory guidelines

IFRA recommends that essential oils rich in limonene should only be used when the level of peroxides is kept to the lowest practical level, for instance by adding antioxidants at the time of production (IFRA 2009).

Organ-specific effects

Adverse skin reactions: Undiluted Sichuan pepper oil was mildly irritating to rabbits (Wang, private communication, 1999). Autoxidation products of (+)-limonene can cause skin sensitization (see (+)-Limonene profile, Chapter 14).
Reproductive toxicity: The low reproductive toxicity of β-myrcene and (+)-limonene (see Constituent profiles,

Chapter 14) suggests that pink pepper oil is not hazardous in pregnancy.

Systemic effects

Acute toxicity: Sichuan pepper oil acute oral LD$_{50}$ in male mice >5.0 g/kg, acute oral LD$_{50}$ in female mice 4.32 g/kg; acute inhaled LD$_{50}$ in rabbits >8.3 g/m^3 (Wang, private communication, 1999).
Carcinogenic/anticarcinogenic potential: No information was found for Sichuan pepper oil but it contains no known carcinogens. (+)-Limonene displays anticarcinogenic activity (see (+)-Limonene profile, Chapter 14).

Comments

Limited availability.

Pepper (white)

Botanical name: *Piper nigrum* L.
Family: Piperaceae

Essential oil

Source: Fruits
Key constituents:

δ-3-Carene	25.2%
β-Caryophyllene	23.4%
(+)-Limonene	22.6%
β-Pinene	9.3%
α-Phellandrene	4.5%
α-Pinene	4.0%
β-Myrcene	2.7%
δ-Elemene	2.1%
m-Cymene	1.0%
α-Caryophyllene	1.0%

(Lawrence 2002c p. 48)

Safety summary

Hazards: Skin sensitization if oxidized.
Cautions: Old or oxidized oils should be avoided.

Our safety advice

Because of its content of δ-3-carene and (+)-limonene we recommend that oxidation of white pepper oil is avoided by storage in a dark, airtight container in a refrigerator. The addition of an antioxidant to preparations containing it is recommended.

Regulatory guidelines

Has GRAS status. IFRA recommends that essential oils rich in limonene should only be used when the level of peroxides is kept to the lowest practical level, for instance by adding antioxidants at the time of production (IFRA 2009).

Organ-specific effects

Adverse skin reactions: No information found. Autoxidation products of δ-3-carene and (+)-limonene can cause skin sensitization (see Constituent profiles, Chapter 14).

Systemic effects

Acute toxicity: No information found.
Carcinogenic/anticarcinogenic potential: No information was found for white pepper oil, but it contains no known carcinogens. β-Caryophyllene, (+)-limonene and α-caryophyllene display anticarcinogenic activity (see Constituent profiles, Chapter 14).

Comments

White pepper oil is not likely to be very different to black pepper oil in toxicity, due to compositional similarity. Both are from the same plant, but white peppercorns have had the outer skin of the fruit removed. Limited availability.

Peppermint

Botanical name: *Mentha × piperita* L.
Family: Lamiaceae (Labiatae)

Essential oil

Source: Leaves
Key constituents:

(−)-Menthol	19.0–54.2%
Menthone	8.0–31.6%
(−)-Menthyl acetate	2.1–10.6%
Neomenthol	2.6–10.0%
1,8-Cineole	2.9–9.7%
(6R)-(+)-Menthofuran	tr–9.4%
Isomenthone	2.0–8.7%
Terpinen-4-ol	0–5.0%
(1R)-(+)-β-Pulegone	0.3–4.7%
(+)-Limonene	0.8–4.5%
Germacrene D	tr–4.4%
β-Caryophyllene	0.1–2.8%
(E)-Sabinene hydrate	0.2–2.4%
β-Pinene	0.6–2.0%
Piperitone	0–1.3%
Isomenthol	0.2–1.2

(Lawrence 1993 p. 31–35, 1995g p. 94–105, 1997d p. 57–66)

ISO standards: US oil

(−)-Menthol	36.0–46.0%
Menthone	15.0–25.0%
(−)-Menthyl acetate	3.0–6.5%
Neomenthol	2.5–4.5%
1,8-Cineole	4.0–6.0%
(6R)-(+)-Menthofuran	1.5–6.0%
Isomenthone	2.0–4.5%
(1R)-(+)-β-Pulegone	0.5–2.5%
(+)-Limonene	1.0–2.5%
β-Caryophyllene	1.0–2.5%
(E)-Sabinene hydrate	0.5–2.3%

(© ISO 2006)

ISO standards: non-US oil

(−)-Menthol	32.0–49.0%
Menthone	13.0–28.0%
(−)-Menthyl acetate	2.0–8.0%
Neomenthol	2.0–6.0%
1,8-Cineole	3.0–8.0%
(6R)-(+)-Menthofuran	1.0–8.0%
Isomenthone	2.0–8.0%
(1R)-(+)-β-Pulegone	0.5–3.0%
(+)-Limonene	1.0–3.0%
β-Caryophyllene	1.0–3.5%
(E)-Sabinene hydrate	0.5–2.0%

(© ISO 2006)
Quality: Peppermint oil is frequently adulterated with cornmint oil (Kubeczka 2002).

Safety summary

Hazards: Choleretic; neurotoxicity; mucous membrane irritation (low risk).
Contraindications (all routes): Cardiac fibrillation, G6PD deficiency. Do not apply to or near the face of infants or children.
Contraindications (oral): Cholestasis.
Cautions (oral): Gastroesophageal reflux disease (GERD).
Maximum adult daily oral dose: 152 mg
Maximum dermal use level: 5.4%

Our safety advice

Our oral and dermal restrictions are based on 8.0% menthofuran and 3.0% pulegone content, with limits of 0.2 mg/kg/day and 0.5% for menthofuran, and of 0.5 mg/kg/day and 1.2% for pulegone (see Constituent profiles, Chapter 14). Peppermint oil should be avoided altogether in cases of cardiac fibrillation, and by people with a G6PD deficiency. This is a fairly common inherited enzyme deficiency, particularly in people of Chinese, West African, Mediterranean or Middle Eastern origin (Olowe & Ransome-Kuti 1980). People with G6PD deficiency will typically have abnormal blood reactions to at least one of the following drugs, or will have been advised to avoid them: antimalarials; sulfonamides (antimicrobial); chloramphenicol (antibiotic); streptomycin (antibiotic); aspirin.

Regulatory guidelines

Has GRAS status. The Commission E Monograph for peppermint oil allows 5–20% in oily and semisolid preparations, 5–10% in aqueous-alcoholic preparations, 1–5% in nasal ointments and 6–12 drops (or 0.6 mL in enterically coated capsules) as an average daily oral dose (Blumenthal et al 1998). The Cosmetic Ingredient Review Expert Panel has concluded that peppermint oil is safe as used in cosmetic formulations, so long as the pulegone content of the essential oil does not exceed

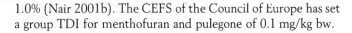

1.0% (Nair 2001b). The CEFS of the Council of Europe has set a group TDI for menthofuran and pulegone of 0.1 mg/kg bw.

Organ-specific effects

Adverse skin reactions: In a 48 hour occlusive patch test on 380 eczema patients, 1% peppermint oil produced no adverse reactions (Meneghini et al 1971). Urticarial hypersensitivity has been reported for pharmaceutical products containing peppermint oil (Wilkinson & Beck 1994; Lewis et al 1995). Such reactions are rare and generally occur where there is a history of skin sensitivity. When tested at 2% on consecutive dermatitis patients, peppermint oil produced reactions in three (0.25%) of 1,200 (Santucci et al 1987), one of 200 (0.5%) (Rudzki et al 1976), nine of 1,606 (0.6%) (Frosch et al 2002b) and two of 318 (0.6%) (Paulsen & Andersen 2005). One out of 747 dermatitis patients suspected of fragrance allergy (0.13%) reacted to 2% peppermint oil (Wöhrl et al 2001). In a multicenter study, Germany's IVDK reported 42 of 6,546 dermatitis patients suspected of fragrance allergy (0.64%) testing positive to 2% peppermint oil (Uter et al 2010).

In a retrospective multicenter study in Finland, there were no irritant or allergic reactions to peppermint oil in 73 dermatitis patients (Kanerva et al 2001a). Of 18,747 dermatitis patients, 1,781 had contact dermatitis and one (0.005% of dermatitis patients and 0.06% of contact dermatitis patients) was allergic to peppermint oil. Of the 1,781 patients 75 were allergic to cosmetic products, so the one reaction constituted 1.4% of this group (De Groot 1987). Of 12 workers in a food factory who had developed hand eczema, one tested positive to 2% peppermint oil (Peltonen et al 1985). A 65-year-old aromatherapist with multiple essential oil sensitivities reacted weakly to 5%, but not 1% peppermint oil (Selvaag et al 1995). A man handling undiluted peppermint oil at work spilled some on the back of one hand. Five years previously he had spilled acid on the same hand, and needed skin grafts. The peppermint oil caused substantial necrosis, and fresh skin grafting was successful (Parys 1983). In an in vitro assay, peppermint oil was non-phototoxic (Placzek et al 2007).

Mucous membrane sensitivity: There have been occasional reports of oral mucous membrane sensitivity to peppermint oil and menthol either on contact (Morton et al 1995) or after excessive prolonged use (Rogers & Pahor 1995; Fleming & Forsyth 1998). In each case, a burning sensation, ulceration and inflammation were the result. These reactions are excessively rare given peppermint's widespread use in dental hygiene products.

Cardiovascular effects: Menthol and menthone inhibit platelet aggregation, but only very weakly (Murayama & Kumaroo 1986). Peppermint confectionery and mentholated cigarettes have been responsible for cardiac fibrillation in patients prone to the condition who are being maintained on quinidine, a stabilizer of heart rhythm (Thomas 1962). Bradycardia was reported in a person addicted to menthol cigarettes (De Smet et al 1992). Menthol blocks cardiovascular calcium channels, which could lead to a depressant effect on the heart (Teuscher et al 1989). Peppermint oil may interfere both with calcium influx into myocardial cells and with the release of intracellular calcium stores. There is no direct evidence that

the oil presents any health risk, nor of what dose might present a risk (Schafer et al 1986; Hills & Aaronson 1991). Menthol appears to be peppermint's active pharmacological ingredient (Sidell et al 1990).

Neonatal toxicity: Menthol has caused neonatal jaundice in babies with a deficiency of the enzyme glucose-6-phosphate dehydrogenase (G6PD). Usually, menthol is detoxified by a metabolic pathway involving G6PD. When babies deficient in this enzyme were given a menthol-containing dressing for their umbilical stumps, menthol accumulated in their bodies (Olowe & Ransome-Kuti 1980).

Neurotoxicity: Peppermint oil was reported to produce microscopic dose-related lesions in rat cerebellum when given for 28 days at 40 or 100 mg/kg/day, though no effect was seen at 10 mg/kg/day (Thorup et al 1983a; Olsen & Thorup 1984). Mengs & Stotzem (1989) failed to find similar lesions at 500 mg/kg, despite looking specifically for them, but Spindler & Madsen (1992) observed cerebellar lesions at 100 mg/kg/day, and not 40 mg/kg/day. Gavage dosing and Wistar rats were used in all these studies, and the last two are described under Subacute & subchronic toxicity, below. Massive doses of peppermint oil produce signs of neurotoxicity (see Acute toxicity, animal, below).

Immunotoxicity: At the massively high oral dose of 2.5 g/kg for five consecutive days, peppermint oil reduced the resistance of mice to infection with *L. monocytogenes* (Gaworski et al 1994).

Gastrointestinal toxicology: Peppermint oil is choleretic (Trabace et al 1994) and therefore should not be taken in oral doses by people with cholestasis (obstructed bile flow) (Fujii et al 1994). Since peppermint oil relaxes the lower esophageal sphincter, oral administration may exacerbate gastroesophageal reflux disease (GERD).

Hepatotoxicity: Large doses of menthol or menthone (above 200 mg/kg po for 28 days) can produce signs of liver toxicity in rats (Thorup et al 1983a; Madsen et al 1986). Menthofuran is toxic to both liver and lung tissue in mice (Gordon et al 1982). In rats, high oral doses of menthofuran (250 mg/kg/day for 3 days) caused hepatotoxicity, detected as changes in blood levels of liver enzyme markers for liver disease (Madyastha & Raj 1994). β-Pulegone is also hepatotoxic (see β-pulegone profile).

Although several constituents of peppermint oil show varying degrees of hepatotoxicity, this does not carry over to the essential oil in the doses used in therapy. Rats were given a single gavage dose of 8.3, 83 or 830 µL/kg (approximately 10, 100 and 1,000 times the maximum recommended human oral dose) of peppermint oil, or doses of 83 µL/kg for 28 days. The acute dose had no effect on liver enzyme activities, and chronic dosing had no effect on bilirubin or γ-glutamyltranspeptidase. No change in histology was observed from either acute or chronic dosing. The only significant effects were an increase in bile flow from the acute dose (hepatotoxicity is often correlated with a decrease in bile flow) and an increase in ALP activity after chronic dosing at the two higher levels (Vo et al 2003). ALP is commonly used as a non-specific indicator of hepatic injury. Oral dosing with menthone resulted in dose-dependent increases in plasma activity of ALP in rats (Madsen et al 1986). At 160 mg/kg/day (but not at 80 mg/kg/day) there was an increase in rat plasma ALP following oral dosing with pulegone for 28 days (Mølck et al 1998).

The lack of histological change contrasts with findings for the constituents cited above, but this may be due to dosage differences since, for example, 83 µL/kg of peppermint oil is a lower dose than either 200 mg/kg of menthol (by approximately 5–10 times) or 200 mg of menthone (by approximately 10–20 times). Vo et al (2003) gave no compositional data for the peppermint oil used in their study.

Systemic effects

Acute toxicity, human: A proprietary menthol-containing oil was reported to produce incoordination, confusion and delirium when 5 mL of the product (35.5% peppermint oil) was inhaled over a long time period (O'Mullane et al 1982). There are reports of nasal preparations containing menthol causing apnea and instant collapse in infants following instillation into the nose (Melis et al 1989; Reynolds 1993).

Acute toxicity, animal: The acute ip LD_{50} in rats for peppermint oil was 819 mg/kg; the acute oral LD_{50} has been reported as 4.44 g/kg in rats (Eickholt & Box 1965) and >4 g/kg in both rats and mice (Mengs & Stotzem 1989). In the latter study signs of toxicity were observed in both the liver and stomach of rats, but none were seen in mice. Both studies reported clinical signs of ataxia and convulsions, suggesting a central nervous target site. Elevated doses of peppermint oil (0.5–2 mL/kg, ip) produce convulsions and ataxia, with paralysis, loss of reflexes and very slowed breathing in rats (Eickholt & Box 1965).

Subacute & subchronic toxicity: Rats were given gavage doses of 20, 150, or 500 mg/kg/day peppermint oil for 35 days. The highest dose increased the relative mean weight of liver and kidneys, reduced plasma triglyceride levels (probably due to lower food consumption) and increased water consumption; all doses caused slightly raised plasma ALP, although this effect was not dose-dependent. There were no changes at any dose in general condition, behavior, body weight development, hematological or urinary parameters. No toxic lesions were found in the liver, kidneys or cerebellum. In a subacute toxicity study in dogs, neither 25 nor 125 g/kg/day given orally for 35 days resulted in any observable effect, with the exception of slightly raised ALP and urea levels in the higher dose males during week five. The urea levels in dogs, and the ALP levels in rats and dogs were within normal limits (Mengs & Stotzem 1989).

In a 90 day study, peppermint oil (1.1% pulegone) was administered by gavage to groups of rats at 0, 10, 40 and 100 mg/kg/day. No effects were observed in either the low or intermediate dose groups, but at the high-dose nephropathy was noted in males. This was interpreted as an early manifestation of sex- and species-specific toxicity due to α2$_u$-globulin. Also at the high dose, cyst-like spaces in the cerebellum were seen. A NOAEL of 40 mg/kg/day was determined (Spindler & Madsen 1992)

Antioxidant/pro-oxidant activity: Peppermint oil significantly savenged DPPH radicals, with an IC_{50} of 2.53 µg/mL (Mimica-Dukic et al 2003). The essential oil was moderately antioxidant in human liver microsomes, producing reversible inhibition of nifedipine oxidation (Dresser et al 2002).

Carcinogenic/anticarcinogenic potential: Peppermint oil was not mutagenic in the Ames test (Andersen & Jensen 1984).

Ishidate et al (1984) came to the same conclusion, but found the oil to be marginally mutagenic in a chromosomal aberration test using Chinese hamster fibroblasts. Lazutka et al (2001) reported that peppermint oil induced CA (mostly chromatid breaks) in human lymphocytes and also was genotoxic in fruit flies. Menthone demonstrates similar genotoxicity (Franzios et al 1997) and may be responsible for that of peppermint oil. However, menthone was not carcinogenic in mice (Stoner et al 1973). Peppermint oil was not mutagenic in a MLA, and was not genotoxic in rat hepatocytes (Heck et al 1989). Peppermint tail fractions induced glutathione S-transferase activity to more than 2.5 times control level in mouse tissues (Lam & Zheng 1991). Incubation of human hepatoma cells with 0.5 µL/mL (but not 0.05 µL/mL) peppermint oil resulted in increased cell death (Vo et al 2003). At a concentration of 0.02 µL/mL, peppermint oil was cytotoxic to 98.5% of HeLa cervical cancer cells (Sharafi et al 2010). Menthol is not genotoxic or carcinogenic, and has demonstrated antitumoral activity (see Menthol profile, Chapter 14).

Drug interactions: Peppermint oil is a moderately potent reversible inhibitor of CYP3A4 activity in vitro and, possibly through this mechanism, increased the bioavailability of felodipine (a calcium antagonist used to control hypertension) in 12 volunteers when given orally at 600 mg (Dresser et al 2002). It is not clear from this small study whether there is a potential for clinically relevant interaction, but since this dose of peppermint oil is four times greater than our recommended maximum we have not flagged an interaction. In rats, 100 mg/kg of peppermint oil tripled the bioavailability of cyclosporin, an immune-suppressant drug (Wacher et al 2002). The implication of this finding for humans is uncertain, but this is a massive dose of essential oil. Samojlik et al (2012) reported variable effects on the actions of pentobarbitone, codeine and midazolam from oral peppermint oil at 0.1 or 0.2 mL/kg, in either single or prepeated doses. The results strongly suggest that a human therapeutic dose of peppermint oil (even at up to 1.2 mL/day) would be insufficient to interact with these drugs. Peppermint oil increased the permeability of rat skin to 5-fluorouracil (Abdullah et al 1996), but it decreased the permeability of benzoic acid across human skin (Nielsen 2006).

Comments

Peppermint oil is a low-risk skin allergen, and no use restriction for skin reactivity is needed. It is clear from both acute and subchronic data that peppermint oil is neurotoxic in high doses. The difference in findings between Spindler & Madsen (1992) and Olsen & Thorup (1984) could be due to variations in the menthone and pulegone content of the peppermint oils used. NOAELs of 10 and 40 mg/kg is the difference between a daily oral dose 0.7 g and 2.8 g in an adult human. Even after allowing for possible interspecies differences, these levels do not indicate a need for contraindication. However, if peppermint oil is instilled into the noses of young children, a neurotoxic dose could be attained.

In calculating the maximum safe doses (for pulegone and menthofuran content), we have used the ISO standards, since these are a good representation of commercially available peppermint oils. As with all our safety guidelines, they assume a maximum of toxic constituents – in this case menthofuran and pulegone. Consequently, peppermint oil preparations may be found that exceed our guidelines, but the essential oil used in these may contain less than the maximum assumed for the toxic constituents. Some reports give pulegone contents for commercial peppermint oils of up to 8 or 9%, but these do not represent the type of peppermint oil traded today, at least in the Western world. A 1996 report by the Joint Food Safety and Standards Group in the UK found that peppermint oils traded in the UK contain 0.2–2.9% pulegone (http://archive.food.gov.uk/maff/archive/food/infsheet/1996/no79/79pmint.htm, accessed August 12th 2011). There are many commercial sources of peppermint oil containing less than 1% pulegone. The pulegone content of peppermint oil depends on the type of soil in which the plant is grown and the time of picking, as well as on other, more elusive factors (Farley & Howland 1980).

Perilla

Synonyms: Beefsteak plant, shiso
Botanical name: *Perilla frutescens* (L.) Britt.
Family: Lamiaceae (Labiatae)

Essential oil

Source: Leaves and flowering tops
Key constituents:

(−)-Perillaldehyde	86.8%
Perillyl alcohol	5.4%
Linalool	1.6%

(Zhu et al 1995)

Safety summary

Hazards: Skin sensitization (low risk).
Cautions (all routes): Some chemotypes of perilla oil may be toxic to the lungs.

Organ-specific effects

Adverse skin reactions: Undiluted perilla oil produced skin irritant effects in both rabbits and guinea pigs patch tested for 24 hours under occlusion at 5.0 g/kg as part of a dermal LD_{50} study. Tested at 4% on 25 volunteers perilla oil was not irritating, and produced one questionably positive sensitization reaction in 26 people in a maximation test. Out of 152 perilla workers, dermal effects were observed in about 50%; perilla oil produced allergic reactions in all of 17 perilla workers with dermatitis. The oil is non-phototoxic (Ford et al 1988a p. 397–398).
Pulmonary toxicity: Perilla ketone (found in some perilla chemotypes) is a potent pulmonary toxin in mice, rats, heifers and sheep (Ford et al 1988a p. 397–398). Perilla ketone is a potent lung toxin to laboratory animals, and it often poisons grazing cattle that eat perilla leaves (Wilson et al 1977; Wilson 1979). Some chemotypes of perilla oil contain egomaketone or isoegomaketone, both of which are similar pulmonary toxins in animals to perilla ketone (Wilson et al 1977; Wilson 1979).

Systemic effects

Acute toxicity: Perilla oil acute oral LD_{50} 2.77 g/kg (mouse); 5.0 g/kg (rat); acute dermal LD_{50} in both rabbits and guinea pigs >5 g/kg (Ford et al 1988a p. 397–398).
Carcinogenic/anticarcinogenic potential: Perilla oil was not mutagenic in the Ames test, and was marginally mutagenic in a chromosomal aberration test (Ishidate et al 1984). The oil contains no known carcinogens, and perillyl alcohol is anticarcinogenic (see Perillyl alcohol profile, Chapter 14).

Comments

Some perilla chemotypes contain substantial amounts of perilla ketone or egomaketone, which can cause pulmonary toxicity in mammals. Other chemotypes also exist. However, the perillaldehyde chemotype is the only one that is currently produced, and it is used in food flavorings in Asia. (−)-Perillaldehyde is 2,000 times sweeter than sucrose, and is used as a sweetening agent in Japan. There is a fixed oil pressed from the seeds, and also known as 'perilla oil.'

Peru balsam

Botanical name: *Myroxylon balsamum* (L.) Harms var. *pereirae* (Royle) Harms
Botanical synonyms: *Myroxylon pereirae* Royle; *Myroxylon peruiferum* L.F. *Myrospermum pereirae* Royle; *Toluifera pereirae* Royle
Family: Fabaceae (Leguminosae)

Essential oil

Source: Gum resin
Key constituents:

Benzyl benzoate	59.0–86.2%
(E)-Benzyl cinnamate	0.4–30.1%
Benzoic acid	1.4–6.3%
(E)-Cinnamic acid	0–5.8%
(E)-Nerolidol	2.0–3.1%
(E)-Methyl cinnamate	tr–1.7%
Benzyl alcohol	1.3–1.6%

(Akisue 1977; Moyler 1998; Cornwell, private communication, 2004)

Safety summary

Hazards: Skin sensitization (moderate risk).
Cautions (dermal): Hypersensitive, diseased or damaged skin, children under 2 years of age.
Maximum adult daily oral dose: 372 mg (see Our Safety Advice).
Maximum dermal use level: 0.4% (see Regulatory Guidelines).

Our safety advice

We recommend a daily oral maximum of 372 mg, based on an oral limit of 5 mg/kg for benzyl alcohol, benzyl benzoate and benzoic acid, which constitute up to 94% of the oil.

Regulatory guidelines

The maximum dermal use level of 0.4% is the IFRA guideline for Peru balsam oil for category 5 (women's facial creams, hand creams) and category 4 (body creams, oils, lotions) (IFRA 2009). (Crude Peru balsam, not the essential oil, is prohibited as a cosmetic ingredient in the EU.) A group ADI of 0–5 mg/kg body weight for benzoic acid, the benzoate salts (calcium, potassium and sodium), benzaldehyde, benzyl acetate, benzyl alcohol and benzyl benzoate, expressed as benzoic acid equivalents, was established by JECFA in 1996.

Organ-specific effects

Adverse skin reactions: One sample of undiluted Peru balsam oil was not irritating to rabbits, a second sample was slightly irritating; neither sample was irritating to mice when applied undiluted. Tested at 8% on panels of 25 volunteers, none of five different samples of Peru balsam oil was either irritating or sensitizing. Neither of two samples of Peru balsam oil was phototoxic (Opdyke 1974 p. 953–954).

Crude Peru balsam, not the essential oil, is notorious as a skin sensitizer and, although it was prohibited by IFRA in 1974, positive reactions to it increased significantly in the period 1975–1983 (Brun 1982; Gollhausen et al 1988). In three large scale studies (totalling 13,558 subjects) Peru balsam produced a positive reaction in 6.9–27% of those tested. The RIFM monograph on Peru balsam states that seven of 25 subjects (28%) were sensitive to it (Opdyke 1974 p. 951). When patch tested at 25% on 20 dermatitis patients who were sensitive to fragrance, Peru balsam induced nine positive reactions. However, when tested at 5% on 50 dermatitis patients not thought to be sensitive to fragrance there were no positive reactions (Larsen 1977).

Of 2,273 dermatitis patients, 445 (19.6%) were sensitive to Peru balsam, and 102 of these agreed to participate in further testing. Of the 102, 38 tested positive to cinnamyl alcohol, 33 to cinnamic acid, 20 to benzoic acid, 20 to cinnamyl cinnamate, eight to benzyl alcohol four to benzyl benzoate three to benzyl cinnamate, three to methyl cinnamate and three to nerolidol (Hausen 2001). These results are not inconsistent with those from an earlier report, in which 47% of patients sensitive to Peru balsam were not sensitive to any of benzyl benzoate, benzyl cinnamate, cinnamic acid, benzoic acid and vanillin (Hjorth 1961). In this same report it is suggested that coniferyl alcohol esters are the most important allergens in Peru balsam, since 70 of 82 Peru balsam-sensitive patients (85.4%) reacted to them.

Reproductive toxicity: The reproductive toxicity data for benzyl benzoate, benzyl alcohol benzoic acid and cinnamic acid (Table 11.3) do not suggest any restriction in the use of Peru balsam oil in pregnancy.

Systemic effects

Acute toxicity: Peru balsam oil acute oral LD_{50} in rats reported as 3.5 mL/kg and 2.36 mL/kg; acute dermal LD_{50} in rabbits reported as >2.0 g/kg and >5.0 g/kg (Opdyke 1974 p. 953–954).

Carcinogenic/anticarcinogenic potential: No information was found for Peru balsam oil, but it contains no known carcinogens.

Comments

There are several sensitizing compounds in Peru balsam that are not generally found in the essential oil. These include: coniferyl benzoate, coniferyl alcohol, benzyl isoferulate and resorcinol monobenzoate (Hausen et al 1992; Hausen 2001). The coniferyl benzoate content of Peru balsam oil depends on the exact conditions of its manufacture. Ultra high vacuum distillation will strip most of the coniferyl benzoate, which can also be removed chemically (Burfield, private communication, 2003). The proportion of constituents found in the balsam is different to that found in the essential oil.

The published data do not support the conclusion that Peru balsam oil is a strong sensitizer. It is possible that, in spite of the lack of any positive reactions cited in the published RIFM report, some commercial Peru balsam oils could contain levels of sensitizing chemicals significantly higher than those of the tested oils. However, there seems little doubt that Peru balsam oils in general are markedly less sensitizing than crude Peru balsam.

Peru balsam derives from El Salvador, not Peru.

Peta

Botanical name: *Helichrysum splendidum* Less.
Family: Asteraceae (Compositae)

Essential oil

Source: Leaves and flowers
Key constituents:

α-Terpinene	14.9%
β-Pinene	10.2%
1,8-Cineole	8.6%
Bicyclogermacrene	7.9%
δ-Cadinene	7.4%
Cubebol	7.3%
α-Phellandrene	5.5%
p-Cymene	3.0%
Germacrene D-4-ol	2.5%
Sabinene	2.4%
α-Cadinol	1.6%
Camphor	1.2%

(Teubes, private communication, 2003)

Safety summary

Hazards: None known.
Contraindications: None known.

Organ-specific effects

No information found.

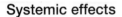
Systemic effects

Acute toxicity: No information found.
Carcinogenic/anticarcinogenic potential: No information was found for peta oil, but it contains no known carcinogens. α-Cadinol is active against the human colon cancer cell line HT-29 (He et al 1997a).

Comments

The oil is produced on a small scale in South Africa.

Phoebe

Botanical name: *Phoebe porosa* Mez.
Botanical synonym: *Oreodaphne porosa* Nees ex Mart
Family: Lauraceae

Essential oil

Source: Wood
Key constituents:

Eremoligneol	8.4–8.8%
β-Eudesmol	6.8–8.4%
Valerianol	5.0–7.6%
α-Copaene	5.6–6.2%
α-Bisabolol	3.3–3.6%
γ-Cadinene	1.2–3.6%
δ-Cadinene	3.1–3.3%
Hinesol	1.9–3.2%
β-Bisabolol	2.5–2.9%
(−)-*allo*-Aromadendrene	2.4–2.6%
Eremophil-9,10-en-11-ol	1.6–2.5%
(*E*)-α-Bergamotene	1.5–2.5%
β-Curcumene	0–2.5%
α-Eudesmol	0–2.3%
7-*epi*-δ-Eudesmol	0–2.3%
Agarospirol	0–2.2%
10-*epi*-γ-Eudesmol	1.2–2.1%
Carquejyl acetate	0–2.1%
Sesquithujene	0.5–2.0%
Viridiflorol	1.2–1.8%
α-Calacorene	1.0–1.7%
epi-Sesquithujene	0–1.7%
γ-Muurolene	0.2–1.6%
α-Pinene	1.3–1.5%
Calamenene	1.3–1.4%
α-Caryophyllene	1.2–1.3%
(*E*)-β-Farnesene	0–1.3%
7-*epi*-α-Eudesmol	0–1.2%
β-Selinene	0–1.1%
β-Caryophyllene	1.0–1.1%
Caryophyllene oxide	1.0–1.1%
Ledol	0.7–1.1%

1,10-Aristolene	0.6–1.0%
β-Bisabolene	0–1.0%
α-Cadinol	0–1.0%
Humulene oxide I	0–1.0%
α-Selinene	0–1.0%
Safrole	0.5–0.7%

(Lawrence 1995f p. 47–48)

Safety summary

Hazards: May contain safrole
Contraindications: None known
Maximum dermal use level:

EU	1.4%
IFRA	1.4%
Tisserand & Young	7%

Our safety advice

We recommend a dermal maximum of 7%, based on 0.7% safrole content with a dermal limit of 0.05% (see Safrole profile, Chapter 14).

Regulatory guidelines

IFRA and the EU recommend a maximum exposure level of 0.01% of safrole from the use of safrole-containing essential oils in cosmetics.

Organ-specific effects

Adverse skin reactions: No information was found for phoebe oil or its four major constituents.

Systemic effects

Acute toxicity: No information was found for phoebe oil or its four major constituents.
Carcinogenic/anticarcinogenic potential: No information found. Safrole is a rodent carcinogen when oral exposure is sufficiently high (see Safrole profile, Chapter 14). δ-Cadinene and β-caryophyllene display moderate anticarcinogenic activity (see Constituent profiles, Chapter 14); α-cadinol is active against the human colon cancer cell line HT-29 (He et al 1997a).

Comments

Limited availability.

Pimento berry

Synonyms: Allspice, Jamaica pepper
Botanical name: *Pimenta dioica* L.
Botanical synonym: *Pimenta officinalis* Lindl.
Family: Myrtaceae

Essential oil

Source: Berries

Key constituents:

Eugenol	67.0–80.0%
Methyleugenol	2.9–13.1%
β-Caryophyllene	4.0–6.6%
(+)-Limonene	tr–4.2%
1,8-Cineole	0.2–3.0%
α-Phellandrene	0–1.8%
Terpinolene	0.1–1.5%
α-Caryophyllene	0–1.5%
α-Selinene	0–1.0%
β-Selinene	0–1.0%

(Lawrence 1979 p. 72, 1993 p. 86–87, 1995 g p. 184; Analytical Methods Committee 1988, Green & Espinosa 1988)

Safety summary

Hazards: Potentially carcinogenic, based on methyleugenol content; may inhibit blood clotting; skin sensitization (moderate risk); mucous membrane irritation (moderate risk).
Contraindications: Should not be taken in oral doses.
Maximum dermal use level:

EU	0.0015%
IFRA	0.003%
Tisserand & Young	0.15%

Our safety advice

We recommend a dermal maximum of 0.15%, based on 13.1% methyleugenol content with a dermal limit of 0.02% (see Methyleugenol profile, Chapter 14).

Regulatory guidelines

IFRA recommends a dermal limit for eugenol of 0.5% for both leave-on and rinse-off products, in order to avoid skin sensitization (IFRA 2009). IFRA recommends a maximum concentration of 0.0004% methyleugenol in leave-on products such as body lotions (IFRA 2009). The equivalent SCCNFP maximum is 0.0002% (European Commission 2002).

Organ-specific effects

Adverse skin reactions: Pimento berry oil was neither irritant nor sensitizing when patch tested on a panel of 32 volunteers at 8% (Opdyke 1979b p. 381). Eugenol is a potential cause of skin sensitization in dermatitis patients. Pimento berry oil is not phototoxic (Opdyke 1979b p. 381).
Cardiovascular effects: Eugenol is a powerful inhibitor of platelet aggregation (Janssens et al 1990), an essential step in the blood clotting cascade.

Systemic effects

Acute toxicity: No information found.
Antioxidant/pro-oxidant activity: Two pimento berry oils, containing 74.7% and 73.4% eugenol and 4.1% and 9.5% methyleugenol, scavenged DPPH radicals (IC_{50} values 4.8 and 5.1 µg/mL) and ABTS radicals (IC_{50} values 2.3 and 2.9 µg/mL) showing excellent antioxidant activity (Padmakumari et al 2011).
Carcinogenic/anticarcinogenic potential: In mouse micronucleus tests, pimento berry oil showed no genotoxicity (Hayashi et al 1988). Methyleugenol is a rodent carcinogen when exposure is sufficiently high; eugenol, (+)-limonene and α-caryophyllene display anticarcinogenic activity (see Constituent profiles, Chapter 14).

Comments

The berries of this plant are known as allspice, and yield pimento berry oil, which has a superior odor and taste to the leaf oil. This should not be confused with the berries of *Pimenta racemosa*, or West Indian bay oil, which in turn is sometimes confused with *Laurus nobilis* ('laurel leaf', or 'bay leaf') oil.

Pimento leaf

Synonym: Pimenta leaf
Botanical name: *Pimenta dioica* L.
Botanical synonym: *Pimenta officinalis* Lindl.
Family: Myrtaceae

Essential oil

Source: Leaves
Key constituents:

Eugenol	66.0–84.0%
1,8-Cineole	1.8–3.2%
β-Caryophyllene	4.1–5.0%
α-Caryophyllene	1.4–2.2%
Methyleugenol	tr–1.9%
γ-Cadinenel	0–1.3%
Caryophyllene oxide	0.2–1.0%

(Lawrence 1979 p. 72, 1993 p. 86–87, 1995 g p. 184; Green & Espinosa 1988; Tucker et al 1991b)

Safety summary

Hazards: Drug interaction; potentially carcinogenic, based on methyleugenol content; may inhibit blood clotting; skin sensitization (moderate risk); mucous membrane irritation (moderate risk).
Cautions (oral): May interact with pethidine, MAOIs or SSRIs. Anticoagulant medication, major surgery, peptic ulcer, hemophilia, other bleeding disorders (Box 7.1).
Maximum adult daily oral dose: 37 mg
Maximum dermal use level (based on methyleugenol content):

EU	0.01%
IFRA	0.02%
Tisserand & Young	1.0%

Maximum dermal use level (based on eugenol content):

EU	No legal limit
IFRA	0.6%
Tisserand & Young	0.6%

Our safety advice

We recommend a dermal maximum of 0.6%, based on 84.0% eugenol content, and a dermal limit of 0.5% (see Eugenol profile, Chapter 14). The maximum oral dose of 37 mg is based on a limit of 0.01 mg/kg for methyleugenol (see Constituent profiles, Chapter 14).

Regulatory guidelines

IFRA recommends a dermal limit for eugenol of 0.5% for most product types, in order to avoid skin sensitization (IFRA 2009). IFRA recommends a maximum concentration of 0.0004% methyleugenol in leave-on products such as body lotions (IFRA 2009). The equivalent SCCNFP maximum is 0.0002% (European Commission 2002).

Organ-specific effects

Adverse skin reactions: Undiluted pimento leaf oil was severely irritating to rabbits, but was not irritating to mice; tested at 12% on 25 volunteers it was neither irritating nor sensitizing. Eugenol is a potential cause of skin sensitization in dermatitis patients. Pimento leaf oil is non-phototoxic (Opdyke 1974 p. 971–972).
Cardiovascular effects: Eugenol is a powerful inhibitor of platelet aggregation (Janssens et al 1990; Rasheed et al 1984), an essential step in the blood clotting cascade.

Systemic effects

Acute toxicity: Acute oral LD_{50} in rats 3.6 mL/kg; acute dermal LD_{50} in rabbits 2.82 mL/kg (Opdyke 1974 p. 971–972).
Antioxidant/pro-oxidant activity: A hydroalcoholic extract of *Pimenta dioica* leaves displayed DPPH radical scavenging activity, with an IC_{50} of 21 µg/mL (Ramos et al 2003).
Carcinogenic/anticarcinogenic potential: No information found. A hydroalcoholic extract of *Pimenta dioica* leaves was antimutagenic, as was eugenol, against *t*-butyl hydroperoxide-induced mutagenesis in *E. coli* (Ramos et al 2003). Methyleugenol is a rodent carcinogen when exposure is sufficiently high; α-caryophyllene and eugenol display anticarcinogenic activity (see Constituent profiles, Chapter 14).
Drug interactions: Anticoagulant medication, because of cardiovascular effects, above. Since eugenol significantly inhibits human MAO-A (Tao et al 2005), oral doses of eugenol-rich essential oils may interact with pethidine, indirect sympathomimetics, MAOIs or SSRIs (Table 4.10B).

Comments

The berries of this plant are known as allspice, and yield pimento berry oil, which has a superior odor and taste to the leaf oil. This should not be confused with the berries of *Pimenta racemosa*, or West Indian bay oil which in turn is sometimes confused with *Laurus nobilis* ('laurel leaf', or 'bay leaf') oil.

Pine (black)

Botanical name: *Pinus nigra* J. F. X Arnold
Family: Pinaceae

Essential oil

Source: Needles (leaves)
Key constituents:

1-Epibicyclosesquiphellandrene	23.4–36.8%
α-Pinene	11.5–35.1%
β-Caryophyllene	5.3–11.8%
β-Pinene	2.4–4.4%
δ-Cadinene	1.9–3.2%
p-Menth-1-en-8-yl acetate	1.7–2.9%
α-Caryophyllene	0.8–1.7%
Tricyclene	0.5–1.5%
(+)-Limonene	0.7–1.4%
(*E*) 3,7-Dimethylocta-1,3,6-triene	0.4–1.1%

(Vidrich et al 1996)
Quality: Pine needle oils may be adulterated with turpentine oil, mixtures of terpenes such as α-pinene, camphene and (+)-limonene, and esters such as (−)-bornyl acetate and isobornyl acetate (Kubeczka 2002; Burfield 2003).

Safety summary

Hazards: Skin sensitization if oxidized.
Cautions: Old or oxidized oils should be avoided.

Our safety advice

Because of its high α-pinene content we recommend that oxidation of black pine oil is avoided by storage in a dark, airtight container in a refrigerator. The addition of an antioxidant to preparations containing it is recommended.

Regulatory guidelines

Essential oils derived from the *Pinaceae* family, including *Pinus* and *Abies* genera, should only be used when the level of peroxides is kept to the lowest practicable level, for example by the addition of antioxidants at the time of production (SCCNFP 2001a; IFRA 2009).

Organ-specific effects

Adverse skin reactions: Undiluted black pine oil was slightly to moderately irritating to rabbits when applied for 24 hours under occlusion. Tested at 12% on 25 volunteers it was neither irritating nor sensitizing; phototoxicity testing produced no positive reactions in hairless mice (Letizia et al 2000 p. S177–S179). Autoxidation products of α-pinene can cause skin sensitization (see α-Pinene profile, Chapter 14).

Systemic effects

Acute toxicity: Black pine oil acute oral LD_{50} in rats >5.0 g/kg; acute dermal LD_{50} in rabbits >5 g/kg (Letizia et al 2000 p. S177–S179).
Carcinogenic/anticarcinogenic potential: No information was found for black pine oil, but it contains no known carcinogens. β-Caryophyllene, (+)-limonene and α-caryophyllene display anticarcinogenic activity (see Constituent profiles, Chapter 14).

Comments

Limited availability.

Pine (dwarf)

Synonyms: Mountain pine, dwarf mountain pine, mugo pine, pumilio pine
Botanical names: *Pinus mugo* Turra (synonym: *Pinus Montana* Mill.); *Pinus mugo* Turra var. *pumilio* Haenke (synonym: *Pinus pumilio* Haenke); *Pinus mugo* Turra var. *mugo* Zenari (synonym: *Pinus mugus* Scop.)
Family: Pinaceae

Essential oil

Source: Needles (leaves) and terminal branches
Key constituents:

Terpinolene	1.0–29.2%
β-Pinene	1.3–20.7%
β-Phellandrene	0.5–16.5%
Bornyl acetate	1.0–7.9%
β-Myrcene	0.5–7.0%
p-Cymene	0.4–6.9%
Camphene	1.3–6.7%
γ-Terpinene	0.1–5.0%
α-Terpineol	0.3–4.5%
α-Terpinene	0.2–4.5%
β-Caryophyllene	tr–2.5%
Sabinene	tr–1.7%
Terpinen-4-ol	0.2–1.5%
Tricyclene	0.2–1.5%
α-Phellandrene	0.1–1.3%
δ-Cadinene	tr–1.0%

(Lawrence 1999c p. 62–64)
Quality: Dwarf pine oil may be adulterated with cheaper pine needle or turpentine oils.

Safety summary

Hazards: Skin sensitization if oxidized; skin irritation (low risk).
Cautions: Old or oxidized oils should be avoided.

Our safety advice

Because of its (+)-limonene, α-pinene and δ-3-carene content we recommend that oxidation of dwarf pine oil is avoided by storage in a dark, airtight container in a refrigerator. The addition of an antioxidant to preparations containing it is recommended.

Regulatory guidelines

Essential oils derived from the *Pinaceae* family, including *Pinus* and *Abies* genera, should only be used when the level of peroxides is kept to the lowest practicable level, for example by the addition of antioxidants at the time of production (SCCNFP 2001a; IFRA 2009).

Organ-specific effects

Adverse skin reactions: Tested at 12% dwarf pine oil produced irritation in three out of 22 volunteers, but produced no sensitization reactions (Opdyke 1976 p. 843–844). Autoxidation products of (+)-limonene, α-pinene and δ-3-carene can cause skin sensitization (see Constituent profiles, Chapter 14). Dwarf pine needle oil, tested at 2% in consecutive dermatitis patients, induced allergic responses in 12 of 1,606 (0.7%) (Frosch et al 2002b), and two of 318 (0.6%) (Paulsen & Andersen 2005).

Systemic effects

Acute toxicity: Dwarf pine needle oil acute oral LD$_{50}$ in rats reported as >5 g/kg (Opdyke 1976 p. 843–844) and 10.64 g/kg (von Skramlik 1959). Ingestion of 400–500 mL of (unspecified) pine oil with suicidal intent has been survived following hemodialysis and hemoperfusion. Pine seems to possess low toxicity with a human lethal dose reported as 60–120 mL (Köppel et al 1981). Several cases of pine oil cleaner ingestion have been reported. This product contains 20–35% pine oil and various ingredients described as 'inert'. The main toxic manifestations were mucous membrane and gastrointestinal irritation, CNS depression, ataxia and pneumonitis. Recovery was typically rapid and ingesting the cleaner was not considered to be life-threatening (Brock et al 1989).
Carcinogenic/anticarcinogenic potential: No information was found for dwarf pine oil but it contains no known carcinogens. (+)-Limonene displays anticarcinogenic activity (see (+)-Limonene profile, Chapter 14).

Comments

Dwarf pine oil is a frequent cause of contact dermatitis, although it is almost certainly only oxidized oils which cause problems, due to monoterpene oxidation.

Pine (grey)

Synonym: Jack pine
Botanical name: *Pinus divaricata* Aiton
Botanical synonym: *Pinus banksiana* Lamb.
Family: Pinaceae

Essential oil

Source: Needles (leaves) and terminal branches
Key constituents:

α-Pinene	23.1–32.1%
β-Pinene	11.1–15.4%
δ-3-Carene	7.3–12.7%
Bornyl acetate	12.5–12.6%
Camphene	2.8–12.1%
(+)-Limonene	7.1–10.9%
β-Myrcene	4.1–6.1%
β-Phellandrene	40–4.8%
α-Terpineol	40–4.0%

Terpinolene	1.5–2.0%
Tricyclene	0.5–1.7%

(Rondeau, private communication 1999; Mainguy, private communication 2001)

Quality: Pine needle oils may be adulterated with turpentine oil, mixtures of terpenes such as α-pinene, camphene and (+)-limonene, and esters such as (–)-bornyl acetate and isobornyl acetate (Kubeczka 2002; Burfield 2003).

Safety summary

Hazards: Skin sensitization if oxidized.
Cautions: Old or oxidized oils should be avoided.

Our safety advice

Because of its α-pinene, (+)-limonene and δ-3-carene content we recommend that oxidation of grey pine oil is avoided by storage in a dark, airtight container in a refrigerator. The addition of an antioxidant to preparations containing it is recommended.

Regulatory guidelines

Essential oils derived from the *Pinaceae* family, including *Pinus* and *Abies* genera, should only be used when the level of peroxides is kept to the lowest practicable level, for example by the addition of antioxidants at the time of production (SCCNFP 2001a; IFRA 2009).

Organ-specific effects

Adverse skin reactions: No information was found for grey pine oil, but autoxidation products of α-pinene, (+)-limonene and δ-3-carene can cause skin sensitization (see Constituent profiles, Chapter 14).
Reproductive toxicity: The low reproductive toxicity of α-pinene, β-pinene, camphene, (+)-limonene and β-myrcene (see Constituent profiles, Chapter 14) suggests that grey pine oil is not hazardous in pregnancy.

Systemic effects

Acute toxicity: No information found.
Carcinogenic/anticarcinogenic potential: No information was found for grey pine oil but it contains no known carcinogens. (+)-Limonene displays anticarcinogenic activity (see (+)-Limonene profile, Chapter 14).

Comments

Limited availability.

Pine (huon)

Botanical name: *Dacrydium franklinii* J. D. Hook.
Botanical synonym: *Lagarostrobos franklinii* Hook.
Family: Podocarpaceae

Essential oil

Source: Wood
Key constituents:

Methyleugenol	95.0–97%
Eugenol	0.5–1.0%

(Guenther 1949–1952 Vol. 6 p. 196)

Safety summary

Hazards: Potentially carcinogenic, based on methyleugenol content.
Contraindications: Should not be used, either internally or externally.

Our safety advice

Due to its high methyleugenol content, we recommend that huon pine oil is not used in therapy.

Regulatory guidelines

IFRA recommends a maximum concentration of 0.0004% methyleugenol in leave-on products such as body lotions (IFRA 2009). The equivalent SCCNFP maximum is 0.0002% (European Commission 2002).

Organ-specific effects

Adverse skin reactions: No information found.

Systemic effects

Acute toxicity: No information found.
Carcinogenic/anticarcinogenic potential: No information found. Methyleugenol is potentially carcinogenic, depending on dosage (see Methyleugenol profile, Chapter 14).

Comments

Distillation takes place in Tasmania, on an irregular basis, from the shavings and sawdust. The wood is used for very insect-resistant furniture, floorboards and in ship building (Arctander 1960).

Pine (ponderosa)

Synonym: Western yellow pine
Botanical name: *Pinus ponderosa* Douglas ex P. Lawson & C. Lawson
Family: Pinaceae

Essential oil

Source: Needles (leaves)
Key constituents:

β-Pinene	28.9%
Estragole	22.0%
δ-3-Carene	17.2%

α-Pinene	8.8%
(+)-Limonene	3.0%
Terpinolene	2.0%
β-Myrcene	1.6%
α-Terpineol	1.4%
β-Phellandrene	1.2%
Geranyl acetate	1.1%
Linalool	1.0%

(Abisset, private communication, 2004)
Quality: Pine needle oils may be adulterated with turpentine oil, mixtures of terpenes such as α-pinene, camphene and (+)-limonene, and esters such as (−)-bornyl acetate and isobornyl acetate (Kubeczka 2002; Burfield 2003).

Safety summary

Hazards: Potentially carcinogenic, based on estragole content.
Contraindications: None known.
Maximum adult daily oral dose: 16 mg
Maximum dermal use level:

EU	No limit
IFRA	0.05%
Tisserand & Young	0.5%

Our safety advice

We recommend a maximum adult oral dose of 16 mg and a dermal maximum of 0.5%, based on 22.0% estragole content with a maximum oral dose of 0.05 mg/kg and a dermal limit of 0.12% (see Estragole profile, Chapter 14). We recommend that oxidation of ponderosa pine oil is avoided by storage in a dark, airtight container in a refrigerator. The addition of an antioxidant to preparations containing it is recommended.

Regulatory guidelines

IFRA recommends a dermal limit for estragole of 0.01% in leave-on or wash-off preparations for body and face (IFRA 2009). Estragole is not restricted in the EU. Essential oils derived from the *Pinaceae* family, including *Pinus* and *Abies* genera, should only be used when the level of peroxides is kept to the lowest practicable level, for example by the addition of antioxidants at the time of production (SCCNFP 2001a; IFRA 2009).

Organ-specific effects

Adverse skin reactions: No information found.

Systemic effects

Acute toxicity: No information found.
Carcinogenic/anticarcinogenic potential: No information found. Estragole is a rodent carcinogen when oral exposure is sufficiently high (see Estragole profile, Chapter 14).

Comments

The high estragole content is very unusual for a pine oil.

Pine (red)

Synonym: Norway pine
Botanical name: *Pinus resinosa* Ait.
Family: Pinaceae

Essential oil

Source: Needles (leaves) and terminal branches
Key constituents:

α-Pinene	47.7–52.8%
β-Pinene	29.4–29.9%
δ-3-Carene	4.2–7.3%
β-Myrcene	4.3–5.0%
(+)-Limonene	1.1–2.0%
β-Phellandrene	1.1–1.8%
α-Terpineol	1.0–1.8%
Camphene	1.5–1.6%
β-Caryophyllene	0.4–1.1%

(Rondeau, private communication, 1999; Mainguy, private communication 2001)
Quality: Pine needle oils may be adulterated with turpentine oil, mixtures of terpenes such as α-pinene, camphene and (+)-limonene, and esters such as (−)-bornyl acetate and isobornyl acetate (Kubeczka 2002; Burfield 2003).

Safety summary

Hazards: Skin sensitization if oxidized.
Cautions: Old or oxidized oils should be avoided.

Our safety advice

Because of its α-pinene and δ-3-carene content we recommend that oxidation of red pine oil is avoided by storage in a dark, airtight container in a refrigerator. The addition of an antioxidant to preparations containing it is recommended.

Regulatory guidelines

Essential oils derived from the *Pinaceae* family, including *Pinus* and *Abies* genera, should only be used when the level of peroxides is kept to the lowest practicable level, for example by the addition of antioxidants at the time of production (SCCNFP 2001a; IFRA 2009).

Organ-specific effects

Adverse skin reactions: No information was found for red pine oil, but autoxidation products of α-pinene and δ-3-carene can cause skin sensitization (see Constituent profiles, Chapter 14).
Reproductive toxicity: The low reproductive toxicity of α-pinene, β-pinene, β-myrcene and (+)-limonene (see Constituent profiles, Chapter 14) suggests that red pine oil is not hazardous in pregnancy.

Systemic effects

Acute toxicity: No information found.

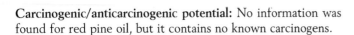

Carcinogenic/anticarcinogenic potential: No information was found for red pine oil, but it contains no known carcinogens.

Comments

Limited availability.

Pine (Scots)

Synonym: Scotch pine
Botanical name: *Pinus sylvestris* L.
Family: Pinaceae

Essential oil

Source: Needles (leaves)
Key constituents:

α-Pinene	20.3–45.8%
β-Pinene	1.9–33.3%
δ-3-Carene	0.4–31.8%
β-Phellandrene	0.3–10.9%
δ-Cadinene	tr–9.5%
Camphene	1.6–9.4%
α-Muurolene	tr–7.8%
β-Bisabolene	0–6.3%
γ-Cadinene	tr–5.4%
(+)-Limonene	0.7–5.2%
Caryophyllene oxide	0–4.9%
Bornyl acetate	0–4.2%
β-Myrcene	2.1–3.8%
β-Caryophyllene	0.7–3.8%
Longifolene	0–3.5%
α-Terpinene	0.1–3.2%
Terpinolene	tr–3.0%
1,8-Cineole	0–2.9%
α-Cadinol	0–2.7%
Fenchone	0–2.1%
γ-Muurolene	0–2.0%
α-Terpineol	0–1.9%
Tricyclene	0.4–1.8%
α-Caryophyllene	tr–1.8%
(Z)-β-Ocimene	0–1.8%
Chamazulene	0–1.7%
(E)-β-Ocimene	0–1.5%
Germacrene D	0–.4%
T-Muurolol	0–1.0%
Sabinene	0–1.0%

(Lawrence 1993 p. 140–143; Orav et al 1996)
Quality: Pine needle oils may be adulterated with turpentine oil, mixtures of terpenes such as α-pinene, camphene and (+)-limonene, and esters such as (−)-bornyl acetate and isobornyl acetate (Kubeczka 2002; Burfield 2003).

Safety summary

Hazards: Skin sensitization if oxidized.
Cautions: Old or oxidized oils should be avoided.

Our safety advice

Because of its α-pinene and δ-3-carene content we recommend that oxidation of Scots pine oil is avoided by storage in a dark, airtight container in a refrigerator. The addition of an antioxidant to preparations containing it is recommended.

Regulatory guidelines

The Expanded Commission E Monographs lists Scots pine oil as being contraindicated in bronchial asthma and whooping cough (Blumenthal et al 2000 p. 305). Essential oils derived from the *Pinaceae* family, including *Pinus* and *Abies* genera, should only be used when the level of peroxides is kept to the lowest practicable level, for example by the addition of antioxidants at the time of production (SCCNFP 2001a; IFRA 2009).

Organ-specific effects

Adverse skin reactions: Undiluted Scots pine oil was not irritating to rabbit, pig or mouse skin; tested at 12% on 25 volunteers it was neither irritating nor sensitizing. It is non-phototoxic (Opdyke 1976 p. 845–846). In a study of 200 consecutive dermatitis patients, four were sensitive to 2% 'pine needle oil' on patch testing (Rudzki et al 1976). Autoxidation products of α-pinene and δ-3-carene can cause skin sensitization (see Constituent profiles, Chapter 14).
Reproductive toxicity: The low reproductive toxicity of α-pinene, β-pinene, β-myrcene and (+)-limonene (see Constituent profiles, Chapter 14) suggests that Scots pine oil is not hazardous in pregnancy.

Systemic effects

Acute toxicity, human: Ingestion of 400–500 mL of pine oil with suicidal intent has been survived following hemodialysis and hemoperfusion. Pine seems to possess very low toxicity with a human lethal dose reported as 60–120 mL. The unidentified pine oil comprised 57% α-pinene, 26% δ-3-carene, 8% β-pinene, 6% (+)-limonene and 3% other hydrocarbons (Köppel et al 1981). Several cases of pine oil cleaner ingestion are known. This product contains 20–35% pine oil and various ingredients described as 'inert'. The main toxic manifestations were mucous membrane and gastrointestinal irritation, CNS depression, ataxia and pneumonitis. Recovery was typically rapid and ingesting the cleaner was not considered to be life-threatening (Brock et al 1989).
Acute toxicity, animal: Scots pine needle oil acute oral LD_{50} in rats >5 g/kg; acute dermal LD_{50} in rabbits >5 g/kg (Opdyke 1976 p. 845–846).
Carcinogenic/anticarcinogenic potential: Scots pine needle oil was genotoxic to fruit flies and weakly induced chromosome aberrations in human lymphocytes (Lazutka et al 2001). The oil contains no known carcinogens. (+)-Limonene and α-caryophyllene display anticarcinogenic activity (see Constituent

profiles, Chapter 14); α-cadinol is active against the human colon cancer cell line HT-29 (He et al 1997a).

Comments

There is considerable variation between different Scots pine needle oils. There are possibly two chemotypes, a β-pinene and a δ-3-carene. Pine needle oils may be adulterated with turpentine oil, with mixtures of camphene, pinene and bornyl acetate, or with other chemicals (Kubeczka 2002).

Pine (white)

Botanical name: *Pinus strobus* L.
Family: Pinaceae

Essential oil

Source: Needles (leaves) and terminal branches
Key constituents:

α-Pinene	30.8–36.8%
β-Pinene	31.1–33.3%
β-Myrcene	4.7–13.1%
β-Phellandrene	5.4–6.0%
Camphene	5.2%
(+)-Limonene	4.0–5.1%
δ-3-Carene	0–3.7%
Bornyl acetate	0.9–1.9%
Terpinolene	0.9–1.0%
α-Terpineol	0.4–1.0%

(Rondeau, private communication 1999; Mainguy, private communication 2001)
Quality: Pine needle oils may be adulterated with turpentine oil, mixtures of terpenes such as α-pinene, camphene and (+)-limonene, and esters such as (−)-bornyl acetate and isobornyl acetate (Kubeczka 2002; Burfield 2003).

Safety summary

Hazards: Skin sensitization if oxidized.
Cautions: Old or oxidized oils should be avoided.

Our safety advice

Because of its high α-pinene content we recommend that oxidation of white pine oil is avoided by storage in a dark, airtight container in a refrigerator. The addition of an antioxidant to preparations containing it is recommended.

Regulatory guidelines

Essential oils derived from the *Pinaceae* family, including *Pinus* and *Abies* genera, should only be used when the level of peroxides is kept to the lowest practicable level, for example by the addition of antioxidants at the time of production (SCCNFP 2001a; IFRA 2009).

Organ-specific effects

Adverse skin reactions: No information was found for white pine oil, but autoxidation products of α-pinene can cause skin sensitization (see α-Pinene profile, Chapter 14).
Reproductive toxicity: The low reproductive toxicity of α-pinene, β-pinene, β-myrcene and (+)-limonene (see Constituent profiles, Chapter 14) suggests that white pine oil is not hazardous in pregnancy.

Systemic effects

Acute toxicity: No information found.
Carcinogenic/anticarcinogenic potential: No information was found for white pine oil, but it contains no known carcinogens. (+)-Limonene displays anticarcinogenic activity (see (+)-Limonene profile, Chapter 14).

Comments

Limited availability.

Piri-piri

Synonyms: Jointed flat sedge, priprioca, adrue
Botanical name: *Cyperus articulatus* L.
Family: Cyperaceae

Essential oil

Source: Rhizomes
Key constituents:

β-Caryophyllene oxide	4.6–13.7%
α-Pinene	5.7–12.9%
Humulene epoxide II	1.3–11.2%
Myrtenal+myrtenol	4.1–7.7%
(E)-Pinocarveol	3.8–7.5%
β-Pinene	4.2–7.4%
α-Cyperone	1.4–5.9%
Cyperotundone	2.1–5.4%
Ledol	3.2–4.6%
Cyperene	1.1–4.3%
Verbenone	1.1–3.9%
p-Mentha-1,5-dien-8-ol	0.8–3.0%
(E)-Verbenol	1.4–2.7%
β-Selinene	0.3–2.7%
α-Copaene	2.0–2.3%
Pinocarvone	1.4–2.1%
α-Bulnesene	0.6–2.1%
α-Selinene	0–1.7%
Patchoulenone	0.4–1.6%
Eudesma-3,11-dien-5-ol	0–.6%
α-Caryophyllene	0–1.5%
α-Calacorene	0.7–1.4%
Dill apiole	0–1.4%
(+)-Limonene	0.6–1.3%
Thuja-2,4(10)-diene	0.4–1.2%

(Z)-Verbenol	0.3–1.2%
δ-Cadinene	0.4–1.0%
Terpinen-4-ol	0.2–1.0%

(Zoghbi et al 2006)

Safety summary

Hazards: None known.
Cautions: None known.

Organ-specific effects

Adverse skin reactions: No information found. The dermal allergenic potency of β-caryophyllene oxide is negligible.

Systemic effects

Acute toxicity: No information found. β-Caryophyllene oxide and β-pinene are non-toxic.
Carcinogenic potential: No information found. The oil contains no known carcinogens. β-Caryophyllene oxide, α-pinene and β-pinene are non-mutagenic, as is nut grass oil, which contains similar unusual constituents.

Comments

The oil is produced in Brazil and is used in local cosmetics. Some of its unusual constituents are also found in nut grass (C. rotundus) or nagarmotha (C. mitis) essential oils.

Plai

Botanical name: Zingiber montanum (J. König) Theilade
Botanical synonyms: Amomum montanum J. König, Zingiber cassumunar Roxb.; Zingiber purpureum Roscoe
Family: Zingiberaceae

Essential oil

Source: Rhizomes
Key constituents:

Terpinen-4-ol	41.7%
Sabinene	27.0%
γ-Terpinene	6.5%
(E)-1-(3,4-Dimethoxyphenyl)butadiene	4.6%
α-Terpinene	3.5%
β-Pinene	2.7%
p-Cymene	1.6%
β-Myrcene	1.3%
α-Pinene	1.3%
Terpinolene	1.1%
β-Phellandrene	1.0%

(Pappas, private communication, 2003)

Safety summary

Hazards: None known.
Contraindications: None known.

Organ-specific effects

Adverse skin reactions: No information found. Terpinen-4-ol is not likely to cause skin reactions (see Terpinen-4-ol profile, Chapter 14).

Systemic effects

Acute toxicity: One supplier cites an LD_{50} for plai oil of 2.15 g/kg, but no further details are given, and the source of this information could not be traced. Terpinen-4-ol appears to be non-toxic (see Terpinen-4-ol profile, Chapter 14).
Antioxidant/pro-oxidant activity: Plai oil demonstrates moderate radical scavenging activity against DPPH radicals, with an IC_{50} of 6.9 μL/mL, compared with 31.4 μL/mL for BHT (Lertsatitthanakorn et al 2006).
Carcinogenic/anticarcinogenic potential: Plai oil demonstrated significant chemopreventive activity against human mouth epidermal carcinoma (KB) and mouse leukemia (P388) cell lines, with respective IC_{50} values of 94 and 99 μg/mL. The oil was more effective than three of the four positive control drugs (Manosroi et al 2005).

Comments

Limited availability.

Plectranthus

Botanical name: Plectranthus fruticosus L'Hérit.
Family: Lamiaceae (Labiatae)

Essential oil

Source: Leaves
Key constituents:

Sabinyl acetate	> 60.0%

(Fournier et al 1986)

Safety summary

Hazards: Embryo-fetotoxicity; may be abortifacient.
Contraindications (all routes): Pregnancy, breastfeeding.

Our safety advice

Sabinyl acetate is thought to be responsible for all of the effects described below under Reproductive toxicity. It is present in higher concentrations in plectranthus than in any other essential oil. These data are most probably applicable to humans and suggest that plectranthus oil should be avoided altogether by pregnant women.

Organ-specific effects

Adverse skin reactions: No information found.
Reproductive toxicity: Plectranthus oil is embryotoxic, fetotoxic, teratogenic and abortifacient in rodents. Plectranthus oil dramatically increased the rate of resorption in pregnant rats after oral administration of 0.5, 2.5 or 5.0 mg/kg on gestational days 6–15. Fetal toxicity, which increased with dose, included

cerebral hemorrhage, hydrocephalus, microphthalmia and anophthalmia. There was no evidence of maternal toxicity at any dose (Pages et al 1988).

Plectranthus oil is embryotoxic and fetotoxic in mice, producing malformed embryos and an increased frequency of resorption. Its effects on mouse fetal development include kidney and heart defects, skeletal alterations and anophthalmia. Pregnant mice were injected sc with 15, 45 or 135 mg/kg of plectranthus oil on gestational days 6–15. Toxicity increased with dose, and included a reduction in weight gain attributed to the number of fetal resorptions in the treated groups. A slight maternal toxicity was observed (Pages et al 1991).

A fraction of Spanish sage oil containing 50% sabinyl acetate, caused dose-dependent maternal toxicity in rodents, and was dose-dependently abortifacient, but was not fetotoxic. The abortifacient effect was apparent even at 15 mg/kg, and was probably due to sabinyl acetate (Pages et al 1992). Subcutaneously administered savin oil, containing 50% sabinyl acetate, prevented implantation in mice at 45 and 135 mg/kg, but not at 15 mg/kg when given on gestational days 0–4. The same pattern was observed with sabinyl acetate given at 70 mg/kg. However, no antifertility effect was found when savin oil was given on gestational days 8–11, indicating that the abortifacient action of sabinyl acetate is due to inhibition of implantation (Pages et al 1996).

Systemic effects

No information found.

Comments

Plectranthus oil has never been commercially available, although the leaves are used in traditional Romanian medicine. The profile is included here because of its implications for other essential oils rich in sabinyl acetate.

Pteronia

Synonyms: Blue dog, blue bush
Botanical name: *Pteronia incana* DC
Family: Asteraceae (Compositae)

Essential oil

Source: Aerial parts
Key constituents:

β-Pinene	32.5%
α-Pinene	18.6%
p-Cymene	11.3%
β-Myrcene	10.3%
1,8-Cineole	9.0%
Sabinene	7.4%
Methyleugenol	7.2%
(+)-Limonene	7.0%
Terpinen-4-ol	5.3%

β-Caryophyllene	3.2%
1(10)-Aromadendrene	3.1%
δ-Cadinene	2.3%
ar-Curcumene	2.1%
epi-Globulol	1.5%
Isospathulenol*	1.4%
(*E*)-Pinocarveol	1.3%
α-Terpineol	1.3%
Bicyclogermacrene	1.2%
α-Caryophyllene	1.2%
α-Muurolene	1.1%

(Bruns & Meiertoberens 1987)

Safety summary

Hazards: Potentially carcinogenic, based on methyleugenol content; skin sensitization if oxidized.
Contraindications: Should not be taken in oral doses.
Maximum dermal use level:

EU	0.003%
IFRA	0.006%
Tisserand & Young	0.3%

Our safety advice

We recommend a dermal maximum of 0.3%, based on 7.2% methyleugenol content with a dermal limit of 0.02% (see Methyleugenol profile, Chapter 14).

Regulatory guidelines

IFRA recommends a maximum concentration of 0.0004% methyleugenol in leave-on products such as body lotions (IFRA 2009). The equivalent SCCNFP maximum is 0.0002% (European Commission 2002).

Organ-specific effects

Adverse skin reactions: No information found. Autoxidation products of (+)-limonene and α-pinene can cause skin sensitization (see Constituent profiles, Chapter 14).

Systemic effects

Acute toxicity: No information found.
Carcinogenic/anticarcinogenic potential: No information found. Methyleugenol is a rodent carcinogen when oral exposure is sufficiently high; (+)-limonene and α-caryophyllene display anticarcinogenic activity (see Constituent profiles, Chapter 14).

Comments

Pteronia oil does not keep well, and may polymerize as well as oxidize. Limited availability.

*Tentative identification

Rambiazana

Synonym: Rambiazinza vavy
Botanical name: *Helichrysum gymnocephalum* Humbert
Family: Asteraceae (Compositae)

Essential oil

Source: Leaves
Key constituents:

1,8-Cineole	47.4%
Bicyclosesquiphellandrene	5.6%
γ-Curcumene	5.6%
α-Amorphene	5.1%
Bicyclogermacrene	5.0%
p-Cymene	4.3%
δ-Cadinene	3.6%
β-Selinene	3.3%
Terpinen-4-ol	2.7%
(*E*)- β-Ocimene	2.4%
2,3-Dihydro-1,8-cineole	2.1%
Aromadendrene	2.0%
Calamenene	1.8%
α-Terpineol	1.8%
α-Terpinene	1.3%
α-Terpinolene	1.3%
β-Pinene	1.1%
α-Thujene	1.0%

(Afoulous et al 2011)

Safety summary

Hazards: Essential oils high in 1,8-cineole can cause CNS and breathing problems in young children.
Contraindications: Do not apply to or near the face of infants or children.

Organ-specific effects

Adverse skin reactions: No information was found for rambiazana oil, but judging from its composition the risk of skin reactions is likely to be low.

Systemic effects

Acute toxicity: No information found. 1,8-Cineole has been reported to cause serious poisoning in young children when accidentally instilled into the nose (Melis et al 1989).
Carcinogenic/anticarcinogenic potential: Rambiazana oil showed weak in vitro activity against MCF-7 human breast cancer cells, with an IC_{50} of 16 mg/L (Afoulous et al 2011).

Comments

Produced in Madagascar. Limited availability.

Ravensara bark

Synonym: Havozo
Botanical name: *Ravensara aromatica* Sonnerat
Botanical synonym: *Ravensara anisata* Danguy et Choux
Family: Lauraceae

Essential oil

Source: Bark
Key constituents:

Estragole	90.0–95.0%
Linalool	2.0–6.8%

(Behra et al 2001)

Safety summary

Hazards: Potentially carcinogenic; may inhibit blood clotting.
Contraindications: Should not be taken in oral doses.
Maximum dermal use level:

EU	No limit
IFRA	0.01%
Tisserand & Young	0.1%

Our safety advice

We recommend a dermal maximum of 0.1% based on 95.0% estragole with a dermal limit of 0.12% (see Estragole profile, Chapter 14). Estragole is not restricted in the EU.

Regulatory guidelines

IFRA recommends a maximum dermal use level for estragole of 0.01% in leave-on or wash-off preparations for body and face (IFRA 2009).

Organ-specific effects

Adverse skin reactions: No information found.
Cardiovascular effects: Estragole inhibits platelet aggregation (Yoshioka & Tamada 2005), an essential step in the blood clotting cascade.

Systemic effects

Acute toxicity: No information found.
Carcinogenic/anticarcinogenic potential: No information found. Estragole is a rodent carcinogen when oral exposure is sufficiently high (see Estragole profile, Chapter 14).

Comments

Tucker & Maciarello (1995) report 61.6% estragole, 20.1% (*E*)-anethole and 0.9% methyleugenol (in addition to other constituents) for ravensara bark oil. The production of ravensara bark oil is not currently sustainable (Behra et al 2001). Also see comments under ravensara leaf, below.

Ravensara leaf

Synonym: Aromatic ravensare
Botanical name: *Ravensara aromatica* Sonnerat
Botanical synonym: *Ravensara anisata* Danguy et Choux
Family: Lauraceae

Essential oil

Source: Leaves
Key constituents:

(+)-Limonene	13.9–22.5%
Sabinene	10.2–16.4%
Isoledene	0.9–14.2%
Estragole	2.4–11.9%
β-Caryophyllene	1.5–8.4%
β-Myrcene	5.0–7.3%
α-Terpinene	1.8–7.1%
α-Pinene	3.0–6.4%
Linalool	3.0–5.7%
δ-3-Carene	4.9–5.0%
Terpinen-4-ol	1.7–4.8%
γ-Terpinene	1.8–4.1%
1,8-Cineole	1.8–3.3%
β-Pinene	2.2–2.9%
β-Phellandrene	1.0–2.9%
α-Thujene	0.4–2.1%
Camphene	0.9–1.8%
γ-Cadinene	tr–1.8%
α-Copaene	0.2–1.7%
p-Cymene	0.5–1.6%
β-Elemene	tr–1.1%
(Z)-β-Ocimene	0.3–1.0%

(Behra et al 2001)

Safety summary

Hazards: Potentially carcinogenic, based on estragole content.
Contraindications: None known.
Maximum adult daily oral dose: 29 mg
Maximum dermal use level:

EU	No limit
IFRA	0.08%
Tisserand & Young	1%

Our safety advice

We recommend a maximum oral dose of 29 mg and a dermal maximum of 1%, based on 11.9% estragole with a maximum oral dose of 0.05 mg/kg and a dermal limit of 0.12% (see Estragole profile, Chapter 14). Because of its limonene content, oxidation of ravensara leaf oil should be avoided by storage in a dark, airtight container in a refrigerator. The addition of an antioxidant to preparations containing it is recommended.

Regulatory guidelines

IFRA recommends a dermal limit for estragole of 0.01% in leave-on or wash-off preparations for body and face (IFRA 2009). Estragole is not restricted in the EU. IFRA recommends that essential oils rich in limonene should only be used when the level of peroxides is kept to the lowest practical level, for instance by adding antioxidants at the time of production (IFRA 2009).

Organ-specific effects

Adverse skin reactions: No information found.

Systemic effects

Acute toxicity: No information found.
Carcinogenic/anticarcinogenic potential: A ravensara leaf oil with 56.5% 1,8-cineole, 13.0% sabinene, 7.6% α-terpineol (and no estragole) was not genotoxic in fruit flies, and showed significant antigenotoxic activity (Idaomar et al 2002). Estragole is a rodent carcinogen when oral exposure is sufficiently high (see Estragole profile, Chapter 14).

Comments

The leaf oil is the one generally sold for aromatherapy use. Various reports show ravensara leaf oil to be rich in 1,8-cineole (Théron et al 1994; Tucker & Maciarello 1995; Möllenbeck et al 1997). According to Behra et al (2001) this is due to confusion between 'ravensara' and 'ravintsara', a Malagasy word meaning 'fragrant leaf'. Ravintsara is the local Malagasy name for *Cinnamomum camphora*, and such reports are said to relate to the leaf oil of *C. camphora*. *C. camphora* oil from Madagascar is still being sold under the name 'ravensara oil' due to this confusion. This does not, however, explain all the anomalies in analysis of ravensara bark and leaf oils, and the existence of chemotypes cannot be excluded. Estragole has been reported as the major constituent (76.6–83.4%) of the leaf oil (Ramanoelina & Rasoarahona 2006). According to professor Chantal Menut, University of Montpellier, there are four leaf chemotypes (sabinene, estragole, methyleugenol and α-terpinene) but all bark or root oils are estragole-rich. *Ravensara anisata*, once thought to be a different species, is now considered a synonym of *R. aromatica* (Rasoanaivo & De La Gorce 1998).

Rhododendron

Synonyms: Anthopogon, sunpati
Botanical name: *Rhododendron anthopogon* D. Don.
Family: Ericaceae

Essential oil

Source: Leaves and branchlets
Key constituents:

α-Pinene	37.4%
β-Pinene	16.0%
(+)-Limonene	13.3%

δ-Cadinene	9.1%
(3Z)-β-Ocimene	5.3%
α-Amorphene	3.2%
α-Muurolene	2.7%
p-Cymene	2.6%
β-Caryophyllene	2.3%
Germacrene D	1.8%
γ-Terpinene	1.5%
β-Myrcene	1.1%

(Innocenti et al 2010)

Safety summary

Hazards: Skin sensitization if oxidized.
Cautions: Old or oxidized oils should be avoided.

Our safety advice

Because of its high α-pinene content we recommend that oxidation of rhododendron oil is avoided by storage in a dark, airtight container in a refrigerator. The addition of an antioxidant to preparations containing it is recommended.

Organ-specific effects

Adverse skin reactions: Autoxidation products of α-pinene can cause skin sensitization (see α-Pinene profile, Chapter 14).
Reproductive toxicity: The low reproductive toxicity of α-pinene, β-pinene and (+)-limonene (see Constituent profiles, Chapter 14) suggests that rhododendron oil is not hazardous in pregnancy.

Systemic effects

Acute toxicity: No information was found for rhododendron oil or any of its major constituents.
Carcinogenic/anticarcinogenic potential: Rhododendron oil was cytotoxic to human cell lines for cancers of the ovary (2008 cells, IC_{50} 224.0 µg/mL), cervix (A-431 cells, IC_{50} 218.6 µg/mL) and colon (LoVo cells, IC_{50} 217.6 µg/mL) (Innocenti et al 2010).

Comments

The commercial essential oil is produced in Nepal, and has the composition given above. Zhu et al (1993) describe a *Rhododendron anthopogon* oil with 35.6% 3-phenyl-2-butanone, 8.1% γ-elemene and 6.1% selin-3,7(11)-diene.

Rosalina

Synonyms: Lavender tea tree, Swamp paperbark tree
Botanical name: *Melaleuca ericifolia* Smith
Family: Myrtaceae

Essential oil

Source: Leaves

Key constituents:

Linalool	35.0–55.0%
1,8-Cineole	18.0–26.0%
α-Pinene	5.0–10.0%
Terpinolene	2.0–5.0%
(+)-Limonene	1.5–5.0%
(+)-Aromadendrene	1.5–4.0%
γ-Terpinene	1.5–4.0%
α-Terpineol	1.5–4.0%
p-Cymene	1.0–4.0%
Terpinen-4-ol	0.5–3.5%
1(10)-Aromadendrene	0.5–3.0%

(McGilvray, private communication, 1999)

Safety summary

Hazards: None known.
Contraindications: None known.

Regulatory guidelines

According to IFRA, essential oils rich in linalool should only be used when the level of peroxides is kept to the lowest practical value. The addition of antioxidants such as 0.1% BHT or α-tocopherol at the time of production is recommended (IFRA 2009).

Organ-specific effects

Adverse skin reactions: No information found. Oxidation products of linalool may be skin sensitizing, but 1,8-cineole has antioxidant properties.
Reproductive toxicity: The low reproductive toxicity of linalool, 1,8-cineole, α-pinene and (+)-limonene (see Constituent profiles, Chapter 14) suggests that rosalina oil is not hazardous in pregnancy.

Systemic effects

Acute toxicity: No information was found for rosalina oil, but its composition does not raise any red flags.
Carcinogenic/anticarcinogenic potential: No information was found for rosalina oil, but it contains no known carcinogens. (+)-Limonene displays anticarcinogenic activity (see (+)-Limonene profile, Chapter 14).

Comments

Limited availability. There is a methyleugenol-rich chemotype, but this is not produced commercially.

Rose (Damask)

Synonym: Rose otto
Botanical name: *Rosa × damascena* Mill.
Botanical synonyms: *Rosa damascena* Mill. var. *trigintipetala* (Dieck) Koehne; *Rosa gallica* f. *trigintipetala* Dieck
Family: Rosaceae

Essential oil

Source: Flowers
Key constituents:

Bulgarian

(−)-Citronellol	16.0–35.9%
Geraniol	15.7–25.7%
Alkenes & alkanes	19.0–24.5%
Nerol	3.7–8.7%
Methyleugenol	0.5–3.3%
Linalool	0.4–3.1%
Citronellyl acetate	0.4–2.2%
Ethanol	0.01–2.2%
2-Phenylethanol	1.0–1.9%
(E,E)-Farnesol	0–1.5%
β-Caryophyllene	0.5–1.2%
Eugenol	0.5–1.2%
Geranyl acetate	0.2–1.0%

(Kovats 1987; Tucker & Maciarello 1988; Boelens & Boelens 1997; Jirovetz et al 2002)

Turkish

(−)-Citronellol	24.5–43.5%
Nonadecane	6.4–20.6%
Geraniol	2.1–18.0%
Heneicosane	2.0–8.9%
Nerol	0.8–7.6%
1-Nonadecene	1.8–6.0%
Ethanol	0–5.2%
Methyleugenol	0.6–3.3%
γ-Muurolene	tr–3.0%
α-Guaiaene	tr–2.9%
Heptadecane	0.4–2.4%
Geranyl acetate	0.4–2.3%
Eicosane	0.6–2.2%
α-Pinene	0.1–2.2%
2-Phenylethanol	0.3–2.0%
Tricosane	0.3–1.9%
Linalool	0.2–1.6%
α-Caryophyllene	tr–1.5%
Octadecane	0–1.4%
Eugenol	0.3–1.3%
(E,E)-Farnesol	0.3–1.3%
δ-Guaiaene	0.1–1.3%

(Lawrence 1997c p. 57-66)

Quality: Damask rose oil may be adulterated with ethanol, 2-phenylethanol, fractions of geranium oil or of rhodinol. Reconstructions with damascones, β-ionone, alkenes, alkanes, (−)-citronellol and other rose alcohols may be added or passed off as rose oil (Kubeczka 2002; Burfield 2003).

Safety summary

Hazards: May contain methyleugenol.

Contraindications: None known.
Maximum adult daily oral dose: 21 mg
Maximum dermal use level:

EU	0.006%
IFRA	0.012%
Tisserand & Young	0.6%

Our safety advice

We recommend a dermal maximum of 0.6% and a maximum oral dose of 21 mg, based on 3.3% methyleugenol content, with dermal and oral limits of 0.02% and 0.01 mg/kg for methyleugenol (see Methyleugenol profile, Chapter 14).

Regulatory guidelines

Has GRAS status. IFRA recommends a maximum concentration of 0.0004% methyleugenol in leave-on products such as body lotions (IFRA 2009). The equivalent SCCNFP maximum is 0.0002% (European Commission 2002).

Organ-specific effects

Adverse skin reactions: Undiluted Bulgarian and Turkish rose oils were slightly or moderately irritating to rabbits, but were not irritating to mice. Tested at 2% on panels of 25 volunteers, these oils were neither irritating nor sensitizing. They were non-phototoxic (Opdyke 1974 p. 979–980, 1975 p. 913). From 1990 to 1998 the average patch test positivity rate to 2% Bulgarian rose oil in a total of 1,483 Japanese dermatitis patients (99% female) suspected of cosmetic sensitivity was 0.4% (Sugiura et al 2000). A 48-year-old female developed contact dermatitis which was traced to Bulgarian rose oil (positive at 2%) and geraniol (also positive at 2%). The authors commented that this was the only one of 326 dermatitis patients with suspected contact dermatitis from perfumes (0.31%) to test positive to rose oil, and that they could find no previous case of rose sensitivity. The rose oil consisted of 18.5% geraniol (Vilaplana et al 1991). **Reproductive toxicity:** Inhaled Turkish rose oil (1 mL/hour) attenuated the damage to male rat sperm count and motility caused by inhaled formaldehyde at 10 ppm/hour (Köse et al 2012). **Hepatotoxicity:** Bulgarian rose oil, orally administered to two groups of 20 male rats at 0.01 or 0.05 mL/kg daily for six months, dose-dependently reduced ethanol-induced liver damage. Two further groups of 20 rats were given ethanol only, or just food and water. Dystrophy and lipid infiltration were notably reduced in the rose oil groups, cellular necrosis was prevented, lowered glycogen levels tended to complete recovery, and perturbation of various enzymes was normalized (Kirov et al 1988b).

Systemic effects

Acute toxicity: Turkish rose oil acute oral LD_{50} in rats >5 g/kg; acute dermal LD_{50} in rabbits 2.5 g/kg (Opdyke 1975 p. 913). Bulgarian rose oil acute oral LD_{50} in rats >5 g/kg; acute dermal LD_{50} in rabbits 2.5 g/kg (Opdyke 1974 p. 979–980). In subsequent work, both age and sex differences were seen in rats given Bulgarian rose oil. Acute oral LD_{50} values varied between 5,525 mg/kg for males, 2,975 mg/kg for mature females, and

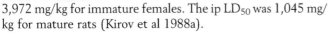

3,972 mg/kg for immature females. The ip LD_{50} was 1,045 mg/kg for mature rats (Kirov et al 1988a).

Subacute toxicity: Bulgarian rose oil was administered daily to male and female rats 5 days a week for 30 days, at 85 or 425 mg/kg. The high dose caused CNS depression, reduced body weight, anemia, functional hepatic changes, and altered weight ratios of liver, kidneys and testes. Toxic effects were more pronounced in female rats. The low dose had no toxic effects in either sex, and is suggested as the NOAEL (Kirov et al 1988a).

Antioxidant/pro-oxidant activity: Rose oil showed high antioxidant activity, both as a DPPH radical scavenger and in the aldehyde/carboxylic acid assay (Wei & Shibamoto 2007a).

Carcinogenic/anticarcinogenic potential: Damask rose oil was cytotoxic to human prostate, lung and breast cancer cells with IC_{50} values of 0.04%, 0.05% and 0.07%, respectively (Zu et al 2010). Methyleugenol causes liver cancer in rodents if exposure is sufficiently high (see Methyleugenol profile, Chapter 14). During the initial phases of induced liver carcinogenesis in rats, geraniol reduced both DNA damage and pre-cancerous cell proliferation, increasing apoptosis (Ong et al 2006). Geraniol significantly suppressed the growth of hepatomas transplanted to rats (Yu et al 1995a).

Comments

The geraniol content of rose otto may counteract the carcinogenicity of the methyleugenol. It is significant that rats given oral Bulgarian rose otto at 0.05 mL/kg/day for six months developed no signs of hepatotoxicity. This dose is equivalent to <1.5 mg/kg/day of methyleugenol, which is 150 times more than our maximum for methyleugenol. As a percentage of dermatitis patients suspected of fragrance or cosmetic sensitivity, the single case of contact dermatitis reported in Spain (0.31%) is consistent with the Japanese data (0.4%) and these are very low prevalence rates for a high-risk group. Rose otto is another term for the essential oil from *Rosa Damascena*. The main producing countries are Bulgaria and Turkey. Small quantities are produced in Iran and Morocco, but are not exported.

Rose (Japanese)

Synonyms: Ramanas rose, rugosa rose
Botanical name: *Rosa rugosa* Thunb.
Family: Rosaceae

Essential oil

Source: Flowers
Key constituents:

Citronellol	44.5%
Geraniol	12.8%
Farnesol	3.8%
2-Tridecanone	3.3%
(+)-Aromadendrene	2.5%
2-Dodecanone	2.5%
2-Pentadecanone	1.2%
Linalool	1.1%
2-Tridecanol	1.1%

β-Cubebene	1.0%
Eugenol	1.0%
Methyleugenol	0.1%

(Zhu et al 1993)

Safety summary

Hazards: May contain methyleugenol.
Contraindications: None known.
Maximum dermal use level:

EU	0.2%
IFRA	0.4%
Tisserand & Young	No limit

Our safety advice

Considering that Japanese rose oil contains 128 times more anticarcinogenic geraniol than methyleugenol, available evidence suggests that there is no need for restriction in the use of this oil.

Regulatory guidelines

Has GRAS status. IFRA recommends a maximum concentration of 0.0004% methyleugenol in leave-on products such as body lotions (IFRA 2009). The equivalent SCCNFP maximum is 0.0002% (European Commission 2002).

Organ-specific effects

Adverse skin reactions: No information found.

Systemic effects

Acute toxicity: No information found. Citronellol acute oral LD_{50} in rats 3.45 g/kg, acute dermal LD_{50} in rabbits 2.65 g/kg (Opdyke 1975 p. 757–758).

Carcinogenic/anticarcinogenic potential: No information found. Methyleugenol causes liver cancer in rodents if exposure is sufficiently high (see Methyleugenol profile, Chapter 14). During the initial phases of induced liver carcinogenesis in rats, geraniol reduced both DNA damage and pre-cancerous cell proliferation, increasing apoptosis (Ong et al 2006). Geraniol significantly suppressed the growth of hepatomas transplanted to rats (Yu et al 1995a).

Comments

Although citronellol, geraniol and farnesol are all listed as high-risk allergens by the EU, the patch test data for these constituents do not justify this classification. Damask rose oil, similarly rich in citronellol and geraniol, is not a high-risk allergen. *Rosa rugosa* oil is produced commercially in China, but the plant is traditionally known as Japanese rose.

Rose (Provence)

Synonyms: Cabbage rose, rose de Mai, French rose, hundred-leaved rose
Botanical name: *Rosa x centifolia* L.
Botanical synonyms: *Rosa gallica* L. var. *centifolia* (Regel.)
Family: Rosaceae

Absolute

Source: Flowers
Key constituents:

2-Phenylethanol	64.8–73.0%
(−)-Citronellol	8.8–12.0%
Alkanes & alkenes	1.1–8.5%
Geraniol	4.9–6.4%
Nerol	0–3.0%
Eugenol	0.7–2.8%
(E,E)-Farnesol	0.5–1.3%
Terpinen-4-ol	0–1.0%
Methyleugenol	0–0.8%

(Buccellato 1980; Jones, private communication, 2002; Chana & Harkiss, private communication, 2004)

Safety summary

Hazards: May contain methyleugenol.
Contraindications: None known.
Maximum dermal use level:

EU	0.025%
IFRA	0.05%
Tisserand & Young	2.5%

Our safety advice

We recommend a dermal maximum of 2.5% based on 0.8% methyleugenol content with a dermal limit of 0.02% (see Methyleugenol profile, Chapter 14).

Regulatory guidelines

Has GRAS status. IFRA recommends a maximum concentration of 0.0004% methyleugenol in leave-on products such as body lotions (IFRA 2009). The equivalent SCCNFP maximum is 0.0002% (European Commission 2002).

Organ-specific effects

Adverse skin reactions: Undiluted rose absolute was moderately irritating to rabbits, but was not irritating to mice or pigs; tested at 2% on 25 healthy human volunteers (three different samples) it was not irritating. There was one reaction from 25 subjects in a maximation test, but it was determined that this was a false positive. Rose absolute is non-phototoxic (Opdyke 1975 p. 911–912).

Systemic effects

Acute toxicity: Acute oral LD_{50} in rats >5 g/kg; acute dermal LD_{50} in rabbits 800 mg/kg (Opdyke 1975 p. 911–912). The dermal LD_{50} seems a little low, and the RIFM report states that it was 'determined on an inadequate sample'. The acute oral LD_{50} for 2-phenylethanol is ~1 g/kg (0.4–0.79) so the dermal LD_{50} may not be an anomaly.
Carcinogenic/anticarcinogenic potential: No information found. Methyleugenol is a rodent carcinogen if exposure is sufficiently high; geraniol displays anticarcinogenic activity (see Constituent profiles, Chapter 14).

Comments

The potential toxicity of rose absolute is not likely to cause any problems in terms of aromatherapy use. *Rosa x centifolia* is cultivated on a small scale in France and Morocco. The origins of this hybrid are uncertain, but it is generally believed that Dutch rose breeders developed it, possibly from crossing *R. gallica, R. moschata, R. canina,* and *R. damascena.*

Rosemary

Botanical name: *Rosmarinus officinalis* L.
Family: Lamiaceae (Labiatae)

Essential oil

Source: Aerial parts
Key constituents:

Borneol CT

1,8-Cineole	20.0%
Borneol	15.6%
Camphor	15.3%
Verbenone	8.4%
α-Pinene	8.3%
Bornyl acetate	4.9%
Linalool	3.5%
Camphene	3.1%
β-Caryophyllene	2.2%
α-Terpineol	2.0%
p-Cymene	1.8%
ar-Curcumene	1.3%
1-Nonanol	1.2%
Terpinen-4-ol	1.0%

(Reverchon & Senatore 1992)

Bornyl acetate CT

α-Pinene	24.0–28.5%
Bornyl acetate	11.5–14.3%
1,8-Cineole	6.8–13.6%
Camphor	9.9–10.4%
Borneol	5.0–8.4%
Camphene	5.9–7.0%
Verbenone	4.3–5.7%
(+)-Limonene	4.1–4.6%
β-Pinene	2.2–2.9%
β-Myrcene	1.7–2.4%
p-Cymene	1.1–2.4%
Linalool	1.4–2.1%
Terpinen-4-ol	0.7–1.4%
α-Terpineol	0.8–1.2%
1-Octen-3-ol	0–1.1%

(Jones, private communication, 2002; Badoux, private communication, 2003)

Camphor CT

Camphor	17.0–27.3%
1,8-Cineole	17.0–22.5%
α-Pinene	4.4–22.0%
γ-Terpinene	0.5–10.8%
Camphene	2.8–10.0%
Borneol	2.0–9.0%
Verbenone	0–6.3%
(+)-Limonene	0–5.8%
β-Pinene	0.3–5.0%
β-Myrcene	0–4.6%
α-Terpineol	0–3.8%
α-Phellandrene	0–3.2%
β-Caryophyllene	0–2.5%
p-Cymene	0.5–2.4%
Terpinen-4-ol	0.6–1.7%
Bornyl acetate	1.0–1.5%
Linalool	0.9–1.5%
Sabinene	0.1–1.0%
Methyleugenol	0–0.02%

(Formacek and Kubeczka 1982; Boelens 1985; Bourrel et al 1995; Chalchat et al 1993)

1,8-Cineole CT

1,8-Cineole	39.0–57.7%
Camphor	7.4–14.9%
α-Pinene	9.6–12.7%
β-Pinene	5.5–7.8%
β-Caryophyllene	0.5–6.3%
α-Caryophyllene	0.1–5.4%
Borneol	3.0–4.5%
Camphene	3.2–4.0%
α-Terpineol	0–3.1%
p-Cymene	0.9–2.5%
(+)-Limonene	1.5–2.1%
Linalool	0.7–1.7%
β-Myrcene	0.7–1.6%
Terpinen-4-ol	0.5–1.2%
γ-Terpinene	0–1.2%

(Chalchat et al 1993; Badoux, private communication, 2003)

β-Myrcene CT

β-Myrcene	19.5–52.1%
α-Pinene	12.0–25.0%
(+)-Limonene	2.4–10.6%
Terpinen-4-ol	1.8–6.8%
p-Cymene	2.4–6.0%
1,8-Cineole	4.2–5.6%
Camphor	2.1–4.4%
α-Terpineol+borneol	1.3–4.1%
β-Pinene	1.5–3.4%
Bornyl acetate	0.5–2.0%
Linalool	0.4–2.0%
Camphene	1.3–1.9%
Verbenone	tr–1.8%

(Lawrence 1995a p. 51)

α-Pinene CT

α-Pinene	19.1–35.8%
1,8-Cineole	15.0–25.1%
Camphor	6.6–20.7%
Camphene	7.0–10.0%
β-Pinene	3.0–7.7%
β-Myrcene	1.1–6.0%
Verbenone	0.5–6.0%
(+)-Limonene	2.9–5.0%
α-Terpineol+borneol	2.0–5.0%
β-Caryophyllene	1.8–4.3%
Bornyl acetate	0.4–4.2%
p-Cymene	0.4–2.4%
Terpinen-4-ol	0.7–2.0%
Linalool	0.5–2.0%

(Lawrence 1995a p. 51)

Verbenone CT (Egyptian)

Camphor	11.3–14.9%
Verbenone	7.6–12.3%
α-Pinene	2.5–9.3%
1,8-Cineole	0–9.0%
Bornyl acetate	2.0–7.6%
(+)-Limonene	0–7.1%
Linalool	5.4–6.6%
p-Cymene	1.8–6.3%
β-Myrcene	0.5–5.4%
α-Terpineol	3.3–4.9%
Camphene	1.6–3.7%
Terpinen-4-ol	2.2–2.9%
Isopinocamphone	1.2–2.9%
β-Caryophyllene	1.5–2.8%
Terpinen-4-yl-acetate	0.9–2.8%
(E)-Pinocarveol	1.0–2.3%
(E)-Myrtanol	0.8–2.3%
α-Phellandrene	0.5–2.2%
β-Pinene	1.2–1.8%
Carvone*	0.4–1.7%
Borneol*	0.3–1.7%
Caryophyllene oxide	0.3–1.3%
(Z)-Myrtanol	0.3–1.2%

(Soliman et al 1994)

Quality: Rosemary oil may be adulterated with eucalyptus oil, white camphor oil, turpentine oil and fractions thereof (Kubeczka 2002).

*Isomer not specified

Safety summary

Hazards: May be neurotoxic, based on camphor content
Contraindications (1,8-cineole CT): Do not apply to or near the face of infants or children.
Maximum use levels:

Camphor CT   16.5% (dermal maximum); 513 mg (daily adult oral maximum)

α-Pinene CT   22% (dermal maximum); 676 mg (daily adult oral maximum)

Verbenone CT   6.5% (dermal maximum); 192 mg (daily adult oral maximum)

Our safety advice

The maximum doses recommended above for the camphor and α-pinene CT oils are based on camphor contents of 27.3% and 20.7%, respectively, and dermal and oral limits of 4.5% and 2 mg/kg/day (see Camphor profile, Chapter 14). The verbenone chemotype limits are based on 14.9% camphor and 2.9% isopinocamphone, with limits of 0.24% and 0.1 mg/kg/day for isopinocamphone.

Regulatory guidelines

Has GRAS status.

Organ-specific effects

Adverse skin reactions: Undiluted rosemary oil was moderately irritating to rabbits; tested at 10% on 25 volunteers it was neither irritating nor sensitizing; it is non-phototoxic (Opdyke 1974 p. 977–978). In a study of 200 consecutive dermatitis patients, none were sensitive to 2% rosemary oil on patch testing (Rudzki et al 1976).
Cardiovascular effects: In normal rabbits, 25 mg/kg im rosemary oil produced 20–55% increases in plasma glucose levels after 60–120 minutes, and a 30% decrease in serum insulin levels (Al-Hader et al 1994). In spite of being contraindicated for people with high blood pressure in several aromatherapy books (see Table 7.1) there is no evidence that rosemary oil is hypertensive.
Reproductive toxicity: The low reproductive toxicity of camphor, 1,8-cineole, α-pinene, β-myrcene and (+)-limonene (see Constituent profiles, Chapter 14) suggest that most rosemary oils are not hazardous in pregnancy. However, bornyl acetate and verbenone have not been studied.

Systemic effects

Acute toxicity: Rosemary oil acute oral LD_{50} in rats ~5 mL/kg; acute dermal LD_{50} in rabbits >10 mL/kg (Opdyke 1974 p. 977–978). Rosemary oil was not significantly cytotoxic to cultured human umbilical vein endothelial cells (Takarada et al 2004). Camphor is potentially neurotoxic and may be more toxic in humans than in rodents. Camphor minimum LD_{50} is 1.7 g/kg in rats (Christensen & Lynch 1937). 1,8-Cineole has been reported to cause serious poisoning in young children when accidentally instilled into the nose (Melis et al 1989).

Antioxidant/pro-oxidant activity: Rosemary oil showed high antioxidant activity as a DPPH radical scavenger (IC_{50} 3.82 µg/mL) and against lipid peroxidation (Bozin et al 2007). A rosemary oil (verbenone CT) showed high antioxidant activity in the same two assays (Sacchetti et al 2005).
Carcinogenic/anticarcinogenic potential: Orally administered rosemary oil (bornyl acetate CT) was hepatoprotective in rats and antimutagenic in Swiss mice. The antimutagenic dose of 1,100 mg/kg/day for seven days prevented the formation of micronuclei (Fahim et al 1999). In a similar study, there was a significant *increase* in micronuclei in Swiss mice given a single dose of 1,000 or 2,000 mg/kg, but there was no genotoxicity in a group on 300 mg/kg. However, a comet assay found all three doses to be genotoxic (Maistro et al 2010). Rosemary oil induced apoptosis in human liver cancer (HepG2) cells (Wei et al 2008).
Drug interactions: Given to male rats in their diet at 0.5% for two weeks, rosemary oil selectively induced CYP2B1 and CYP2B2 in rat liver (Debersac et al 2001). This high-dose regimen does not suggest a significant risk of drug interaction.

Comments

Many of the above studies do not specify which chemotype was used. Rosemary oil is produced in many parts of the world, and this summary of chemotypes may not represent every type of commercial oil. 1,8-Cineole chemotypes tend to be Moroccan or Tunisian, α-pinene chemotypes are often from Spain (the main producer of rosemary oil) bornyl acetate chemotypes may be French, myrcene chemotypes are probably Portuguese and verbenone chemotypes are generally Egyptian. Rosemary oils are also produced in England, Russia, Germany, Romania and the Balkans. Most research papers do not identify the type of rosemary oil used.

Rosewood

Synonyms: Bois de rose, Pau-rosa
Botanical names: *Aniba rosaeodora* Ducke, *Aniba amazonica* Ducke, *Aniba parviflora* Meissner Mez.
Family: Lauraceae

Essential oil

Source: Wood
Key constituents:

Linalool	82.3–90.3%
α-Terpineol	0.5–5.4%
(Z)-Linalool oxide	~1.5%
(E)-Linalool oxide	~1.3%
1,8-Cineole	0.2–2.3%

(Lawrence 1989 p. 118–119)
Quality: Rosewood oil may be adulterated with synthetic linalool, along with trace amounts of methyl heptenone, methyl heptenol, 3-octanol, *p*-methyl acetophenone and others (Burfield 2003).

Safety summary

Hazards: None known.
Contraindications: None known.

Regulatory guidelines

According to IFRA, essential oils rich in linalool should only be used when the level of peroxides is kept to the lowest practical value. The addition of antioxidants such as 0.1% BHT or α-tocopherol at the time of production is recommended (IFRA 2009).

Organ-specific effects

Adverse skin reactions: Undiluted rosewood oil was not irritating to rabbit, pig or mouse skin; tested at 5% on 25 volunteers it was neither irritating nor sensitizing. It is non-phototoxic (Opdyke 1978 p. 653–654). A 65-year-old aromatherapist with multiple essential oil sensitivities reacted to 5%, and weakly to 1% rosewood oil (Selvaag et al 1995). Oxidation products of linalool may be skin sensitizing.
Reproductive toxicity: The virtual absence of reproductive toxicity for linalool (Politano et al 2008) suggests that rosewood oil is not hazardous in pregnancy.

Systemic effects

Acute toxicity: Rosewood oil acute oral LD_{50} in rats 4.3 g/kg; acute dermal LD_{50} in rabbits >5 g/kg (Opdyke 1978 p. 653–654).
Carcinogenic/anticarcinogenic potential: Rosewood oil selectively killed human epithelial carcinoma A431 cells while only having a minor cytotoxic effect on normal keratinocytes (Sœur et al 2011). Linalool is neither genotoxic nor carcinogenic, and displays in vitro antitumoral effects (see Linalool profile, Chapter 14).

Comments

Aniba rosaeodora (both wood and essential oil) is listed by CITES under their Appendix II: 'species that are not necessarily now threatened with extinction but that may become so unless trade is closely controlled.' This has legal implications for trade of bulk essential oil, although these limitations specifically do not apply to 'finished products packaged and ready for retail sale.'

Rue

Botanical names: *Ruta graveolens* L., *Ruta Montana* Mill.
Family: Rutaceae

Essential oil

Source: Aerial parts
Key constituents:

R. graveolens (Egyptian)

2-Undecanone	49.2%
2-Nonanone	24.7%
2-Nonyl acetate	6.2%
2-Decanone	2.8%
Pregeijerene	2.1%
2-Dodecanone	1.1%
2-Tridecanone	1.0%

(Aboutabl et al 1988)

R. graveolens (Italian)

2-Undecanone	46.8%
2-Nonanone	18.8%
Methyl salicylate	3.9%
Octanoic acid	3.4%
(+)-Limonene	3.0%
1,8-Cineole	2.9%
2-Tridecanone	2.5%
2-Decanone	2.2%
Valeric acid	1.6%
Linalool	1.5%
2-Nonanol	1.5%
α-Pinene	1.3%

(De Feo et al 2002)

Non-volatile compounds

Angelicin	0.043%
Methoxsalen	0.032%
Isopimpinellin	0.02%
Bergapten	0.018%
Psoralen	0.015%

(SCCP 2005b)

Safety summary

Hazards: May be abortifacient; phototoxic (moderate risk); may be photocarcinogenic.
Contraindications (dermal): If applied to the skin at over maximum use level, skin must not be exposed to sunlight or sunbed rays for 12 hours.
Contraindications (all routes): Pregnancy, breastfeeding.
Maximum dermal use level: 0.15% (see Regulatory Guidelines, IFRA).

Regulatory guidelines

To avoid phototoxicity, IFRA recommends that, for application to areas of skin exposed to sunshine, rue oil is limited to a maximum of 0.15% except for bath preparations, soaps and other wash-off products. This is based on the no-effect level of 0.8% found in hairless mice (IFRA 2009). In Europe, essential oils containing furanocoumarins must be used so that the total level of bergapten will not exceed: (a) 15 ppm in finished cosmetic products intended for application to skin areas likely to be exposed to sunshine, excluding rinse-off products; or (b) 1 ppm in sun protection and in bronzing products. In the presence of other phototoxic ingredients, the sum of their concentrations (expressed as % of the respective maximum levels) should not exceed 100% (SCCNFP 2000).

The FDA considers that rue oil is safe for human consumption as it is currently used in food flavorings, 'but not necessarily under different conditions of use'; in particular, further teratological research is recommended (Anon 1974). In the EU, rue oil is permitted in foods and beverages at up to 9,000 µg/kg (Committee for Veterinary Medicinal Products 1999).

Organ-specific effects

Adverse skin reactions: Undiluted rue oil was slightly irritating to rabbits, but was not irritating to mice; tested at 1% on 25 volunteers it was neither irritating nor sensitizing. In phototoxicity tests, distinct positive results were obtained with concentrations of 100%, 50%, 25%, 12.5%, 6.25% and 3.125%. Borderline results were obtained with 1.56%, and 0.78% was not phototoxic (Opdyke 1975 p. 455–456). In human testing, rue *absolute* was phototoxic at 1.0% or over, and non-phototoxic at 0.5% (Bouhlal et al 1988b). Bergapten, methoxsalen and psoralen all possess similar phototumorigenic properties (Grube 1977) (see Ch. 5, p. 88). There are anecdotal reports of rue oil being an irritant to both skin and mucous membranes (Arctander 1960). Our own tests found it to be non-irritant to mucous membranes. Martindale cites rue oil as a 'powerful local irritant' (Reynolds 1993).

Neurotoxicity: In aromatherapy literature, rue oil is often referred to as neurotoxic and/or convulsant, purely on the basis that it is ketone-rich, and that all ketones are assumed to be neurotoxic. However, in King's American Dispensatory (1898), oral rue oil is said to be beneficial for convulsions, and the plant is a traditional anticonvulsant remedy (Aguilar-Santamaría & Tortoriello 1998). A convulsant effect for rue oil seems unlikely, since both methanol and ethanol extracts of *Ruta chalapensis* counteracted PTZ-induced convulsions, and were sedative in mice (Aguilar-Santamaría & Tortoriello 1998; Gonzalez-Trujano et al 2006).

Reproductive toxicity: There seems little doubt that the plant is abortifacient in humans, although this only occurs at close to maternally toxic doses, is probably due to constituents not found in the essential oil. There are several documented cases of abortion from *Ruta chalapensis* or *Ruta graveolens* ingestion in Uruguay, many of which involved multiple organ failure and there have been four fatalities (Ciganda & Laborde 2003). The constituents in the plant thought to be responsible for its abortifacient effects are rutin and philocarpine (do not confuse with pilocarpine, found in jaborandi) (Farnsworth et al 1975). However, a later study in rats and hamsters found rutin to be inactive (Gandhi et al 1991). Neither of these compounds are present in the essential oil. A hot water extract of rue was reportedly abortifacient after ingestion, and administration of this extract at 1 mL/kg showed significant anti-implantation effects in rats. The chloroform extract of rue had an antifertility effect and chalepensin, a coumarin acting in the early stages of pregnancy, was the active component (Kong et al 1989). Similarly, aqueous extracts of *R. graveolens* reduced fertility both in female mice and rats, as did an alcoholic extract in rats (Guerra & Andrade 1978; Gandhi et al 1991; Alkofahi et al 1996). However, a hydroalcoholic extract of *R. graveolens* had no antifertility effect on female mice (de Freitas et al 2005). An aqueous extract of *R. graveolens* was embryotoxic in mice, significantly altering pre-implantation development. Alkaloids are suggested as the toxic agents (Gutiérrez-Pajares & Lidia Zúñiga 2003).

There is one early report that rue oil has a direct action on the uterus, but the details of the research on which this is based are obscure (Papavassiliou & Eliakis 1937). Rue oil showed no stimulant action on the isolated uteri of pregnant and non-pregnant cats (Macht 1913) nor on isolated non-pregnant fallopian tubes (Gunn 1921). A freshly prepared infusion of rue, ingested shortly after childbirth by three women, had no stimulant effect on the uterus, while six of the total of nine herbs tested were uterine stimulants (Kapur 1948).

Used in massive amounts on pregnant rabbits (12 mL/kg) and guinea pigs (50 mL/kg) rue oil, not surprisingly, was equally toxic to mother and fetus, causing widespread tissue damage (especially in the liver and kidneys), diarrhea, dyspnea and some fatalities (Patoir et al 1938b). These doses are equivalent to adult human ingestion of approximately 800 mL and 3.2 liters. Two pregnant guinea pigs, each fed 12 drops of rue oil, aborted; rue oil was found in the fetal tissue, and was considered toxic to it (Anon 1974). This is still a high dose (approximately 3 mL/kg, or 195 mL in an adult human) and the abortifacient activity seen here may be due to maternal toxicity. In teratology studies on rats and mice, at doses of rue oil up to 820 and 970 mg/kg, respectively, no significant maternotoxic, embryotoxic or teratogenic effects were observed (cited in Committee for Veterinary Medicinal Products 1999).

Systemic effects

Acute toxicity, human: According to the Merck Index 'Ingestion of large quantities [of rue oil] causes epigastric pain, nausea, vomiting, confusion, convulsions, death; may cause abortion' (Budavari 1989). No further details are given, but it seems that the toxic effects of the plant have been assumed to also apply to the essential oil, since we could find no reports of human overdose, nor any of these toxic effects, involving rue oil.

Acute toxicity, animal: Rue oil acute oral LD_{50} reported as >5 g/kg in rats and 2.54 g/kg in mice; acute dermal LD_{50} in rabbits >5 g/kg (Opdyke 1975 p. 455–456). A single oral dose at 400 mg/kg has been reported as causing death in guinea pigs due to liver, kidney and adrenal gland damage (Leung & Foster 2003).

Carcinogenic/anticarcinogenic potential: According to an EMEA review of *Ruta graveolens*, rue oil is not mutagenic in *S. typhimurium* nor in *S. cerevisiae* (Committee for Veterinary Medicinal Products 1999).

Comments

The acute toxicity data suggest that rue oil is more toxic to guinea pigs than rats or mice, and the only evidence of an abortifacient effect is in guinea pigs. The oil had no effect on isolated cat uterus; it caused abortion in guinea pigs at doses only about three times higher than the dose which was non-teratogenic in mice and rats. Guinea pigs, therefore, may be particularly sensitive to rue oil toxicity. The plant is abortifacient in humans at maternally toxic doses, due at least in part to constituents not found in the essential oil. It is not known whether rue oil, in therapeutic doses, presents any risk in human pregnancy. In the absence of any further information, we must assume that it does.

Data on the composition of rue oil are scarce but bergapten and methoxsalen are well-known constituents of the plant, responsible for cases of phototoxic contact dermatitis caused by touching the leaves (Schempp et al 1999). An analysis of

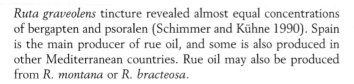

Ruta graveolens tincture revealed almost equal concentrations of bergapten and psoralen (Schimmer and Kühne 1990). Spain is the main producer of rue oil, and some is also produced in other Mediterranean countries. Rue oil may also be produced from *R. montana* or *R. bracteosa*.

Saffron

Botanical name: *Crocus sativus* L.
Family: Iridaceae

Essential oil

Source: Stigmas
Key constituents:

Safranal	47.0–60.3%
4-Hydroxy-2,6,6-trimethyl-1-cyclohexenecarbaldehyde	0.1–13.8%
Isophorone	1.9–8.8%
4-Hydroxy-2,6,6-trimethyl-3-oxo-1,4-cyclohexadienecarbaldehyde	2.3–6.0%
4-Hydroxy-3,3,5-trimethyl-2-cyclohexen-1-one	0.2–6.0%
3,5,5-Trimethyl-2-cyclohexene-1,4-dione	1.1–4.1%
3-(But-1-enyl)-2,4,4-trimethylcyclohex-2-en-1-ol	0–3.6%
2-Hydroxy-4,4,6-trimethylcyclohexa-2,5-dien-1-one	0–3.6%
3,5,5-Trimethyl-1,4-cyclohexanedione	1.5–1.8%
6,6-Dimethyl-2-methylene-3-cyclohexenecarbaldehyde	0.1–1.4%
2,2-Dimethyl-4-oxocyclohexane-1-carboxaldehyde	0–1.4%
2,6,6-Trimethyl-3-oxo-1,4-cyclohexadienecarbaldehyde	0.1–1.3%
2-Hydroxy-3,5,5-trimethyl-2-cyclohexene-1,4-dione	1.1–1.2%
2,3-Epoxy-4-(hydroxymethylene)-3,3,5-rimethylcyclohexanone	0–1.0%
2,6,6-Trimethyl-3-oxocyclohex-1-ene-1-carboxaldehyde	0–1.0%

(Zarghami & Heinz 1971; Roedel & Petrzika 1991)

Safety summary

Hazards: May be skin sensitizing.
Cautions (dermal): Hypersensitive, diseased or damaged skin, children under 2 years of age.
Maximum dermal use level: 0.02%

Our safety advice

If the IFRA guideline for safranal is extrapolated to an oil containing 60.3% safranal, we calculate a maximum concentration of 0.02% for any application to the body. However, the compositional data shown above are for the 'volatile constituents' of

saffron. Essential oils, absolutes and resinoids are offered, and these should be used at maximum levels depending on their safranal content.

Regulatory guidelines

Has GRAS status. IFRA recommends that safranal should not be used in skin-contact products such that the concentration exceeds 0.005%. The maximum for products not intended for use on the body (air fresheners, etc.) is 0.05%. These guidelines are based on test results showing skin sensitization when tested at 0.1%, and none at 0.05% (IFRA 2009).

Organ-specific effects

Adverse skin reactions: No information was found for saffron oil, absolute or resinoid, but safranal is a skin sensitizer (see Regulatory Guidelines).

Systemic effects

Acute toxicity: No information was found for saffron oil, absolute or resinoid. An ethanol extract of saffron had an LD_{50} of 600 mg/kg in mice. Hematological and biochemical studies showed an absence of toxicity to the liver, kidneys and bladder, and the extract was not cytotoxic to normal spleen cells, but a significant decrease in hemoglobin levels was observed (Nair et al 1991).

Carcinogenic/anticarcinogenic potential: An ethanol extract of saffron was cytotoxic to intraperitoneally transplanted sarcoma 180 cells, P388 leukemia cells, Ehrlich ascites carcinoma cells and Dalton's lymphoma ascites cells in mice (Nair et al 1991). Safranal completely inhibited the growth of ascites sarcoma BP8 cells (a rat cell line) at concentrations of 1.0 and 0.1 mM (Pilotti et al 1975).The antigenotoxic and antitumoral properties of various extracts of saffron have been reviewed by Abdullaev & Espinosa-Aguirre (2004). Safranal is one of the active constituents, and induced 50% growth inhibition on HeLa cells at 0.8 mM (Escribano et al 1996). However, the antitumoral action of safranal is less potent than that of many other constituents of saffron, which are not found in the essential oil or absolute (Abdullaev et al 2002). Safranal is suspected of a co-mutagenic effect in 2-amino-anthracene-induced mutagenicity (Abdullaev et al 2003).

Comments

Saffron is reputed to be toxic and abortifacient, but no information was found to support these notions. The aldehyde safranal is a decomposition product of picrocrocin, and very little is present in fresh saffron. Limited availability.

Sage (African wild)

Synonyms: Leleshwa, camphor bush, wild camphor tree, Hottentot tobacco
Botanical name: *Tarchonanthus camphoratus* L.
Family: Asteraceae

Essential oil

Source: Leaves and flowers
Key constituents:

1,8-Cineole	15.5%
α-Fenchol	12.4%
α-Pinene	11.5%
γ-Curcumene	6.7%
Camphene	6.5%
α-Terpineol	5.7%
(E)-Pinene hydrate	3.4%
β-Pinene	3.4%
α-Terpinene	3.4%
p-Cymene	3.3%
Terpinen-4-ol	3.3%
ar-Curcumene	2.6%
γ-Terpinene	1.6%
Terpinolene	1.6%
Fenchone	1.4%
α-Phellandrene	1.4%
Borneol	1.2%

(Pappas, private communication, 2003)

Safety summary

Hazards: None known.
Contraindications: None known.

Organ-specific effects

Adverse skin reactions: No information found for African wild sage oil or α-fenchol.

Systemic effects

Acute toxicity: No information found for African wild sage oil or α fenchol.
Carcinogenic/anticarcinogenic potential: No information found for African wild sage oil, but it contains no known carcinogens.

Comments

This oil is reputed to possess impressive antimicrobial properties. It is unusual to find α-fenchol as a major constituent. The cineole/fenchol chemotype is commercially available, and there may also be a camphor-rich chemotype. Much of the literature about the plant refers to its strong camphoraceous odor, and one student report at Zimbabwe University refers to extracting camphor from *Tarchonanthis camphoratus* (http://uzweb.uz.ac.zw/medicine/pharmacy/pubs/19983.html accessed August 12th 2011).

Sage (blue mountain)

Synonym: Stenophylla
Botanical name: *Salvia stenophylla* Burch. ex Benth.
Family: Lamiaceae (Labiatae)

Essential oil

Source: Leaves and stem
Key constituents:

δ-3-Carene	38.1%
epi-α-Bisabolol	27.1%
(+)-Limonene + 1,8-cineole	8.8%
β-Myrcene	6.2%
Manool	5.2%
Camphene	3.8%
α-Pinene	3.0%
Camphor	2.7%
α-Phellandrene	1.2%
Borneol	1.1%

(Graven, private communication, 1999)

Safety summary

Hazards: Skin sensitization if oxidized.
Cautions: Old or oxidized oils should be avoided.

Our safety advice

Because of its δ-3-carene content we recommend that oxidation of blue mountain sage oil is avoided by storage in a dark, airtight container in a refrigerator. The addition of an antioxidant to preparations containing it is recommended.

Organ-specific effects

Adverse skin reactions: No information found. Autoxidation products of δ-3-carene can cause skin sensitization (see δ-3-Carene profile, Chapter 14).

Systemic effects

Acute toxicity: No information found.
Carcinogenic/anticarcinogenic potential: No information was found for blue mountain sage oil, but it contains no known carcinogens. (+)-Limonene displays anticarcinogenic activity (see (+)-Limonene profile, Chapter 14).

Comments

Limited availability.

Sage (Dalmatian)

Botanical name: *Salvia officinalis* L.
Family: Lamiaceae (Labiatae)

Essential oil

Source: Leaves
Key constituents:

Camphor	7.3–50.2%
α-Thujone	13.1–48.5%
Borneol	1.5–23.9%
1,8-Cineole	1.8–21.7%

β-Thujone	3.9–19.1%
β-Caryophyllene	0.2–9.7%
Camphene	0–8.6%
α-Pinene	0–8.0%
Bornyl acetate	0.3–5.7%
β-Pinene	0–1.2%

(Lawrence 1998b p50)

Safety summary

Hazards: Neurotoxicity.
Contraindications: Should not be taken in oral doses.
Contraindications (all routes): Pregnancy, breastfeeding.
Maximum dermal use level: 0.4%

Our safety advice

Our dermal maximum is based on 60% total thujone content with a dermal thujone limit of 0.25% (see Thujone profile, Chapter 14).

Regulatory guidelines

The Commission E Monograph for Dalmatian sage oil gives a contraindication for oral dosing in pregnancy, and a warning that prolonged ingestion may cause seizures, but otherwise a daily dose range of 100–300 mg (Blumenthal et al 1998). In 2009, the European Medicines Agency concluded that 'the benefits of sage oil do not outweigh its risks.' (www.ema.europa.eu/ema/pages/includes/document/open_document.jsp?webContentId=WC500098002 accessed May 27th 2012).

Organ-specific effects

Adverse skin reactions: Undiluted Dalmatian sage oil was moderately irritating to rabbits; tested at 8% on 25 volunteers it was neither irritating nor sensitizing. A 24-hour patch test using undiluted sage oil produced one irritation reaction in 20 volunteers (Opdyke 1974 p. 987–988). A 65-year-old aromatherapist with multiple essential oil sensitivities reacted to both 1% and 5% sage oil (Selvaag et al 1995).
Cardiovascular effects: A subcutaneous injection of 39 mg/kg of sage oil (type not specified) caused hypoglycemia in both normal and alloxan-diabetic rats after one hour (Essway et al 1995). In contrast, Eidi et al (2005) found no significant change in serum glucose levels in streptozotocin-diabetic rats for up to five hours after ip administration of 0.042, 0.125, 0.2 or 0.4 mL/kg of Dalmatian sage oil.
Neurotoxicity: Convulsions appeared for sage oil at over 500 mg/kg ip in rats (Millet et al 1981). A 44-year-old woman who weighed 133 lb (~60 kg) died hours after ingesting two teaspoons of sage oil as a treatment for asthma (a friend had suggested she take 1–5 drops in two teaspoons of brandy). Before dying she suffered epileptiform convulsions. Doctors reported cardiac failure and dyspnea, and estimated that she had drunk 0.25 oz (7 mL). Post-mortem examination showed only slight damage to the stomach and small intestine. The lungs smelled strongly of sage, and were 'emphysematous'. No other organ showed any sign of damage (Whitling 1908). In a second case, convulsions occurred in an adult who accidentally ingested one 'swallow' of sage oil (Arditti et al 1978). In a third case, a 54-year-old woman ingested at least one 'swallow' of sage oil. After 30 minutes she suffered a tonic-clonic seizure and remained unconscious for one hour. In a fourth case, a 53-year-old man ingested 12 drops of sage oil. He rapidly developed a tonic-clonic seizure followed by a 15 minute coma. Neurological tests were normal (Burkhard et al 1999). In three further non-fatal cases, all in Turkey, accidental ingestion of sage oil by a newborn, a 1-month-old boy and a 5 1/2-year-old girl (who ingested an estimated 5 mL) was followed by seizures (Sarici et al 2004; Halicioglu et al 2011).
Reproductive toxicity: When Dalmatian sage oil (0.25%, 375 mg/kg) was fed to pregnant mice for two weeks, it negatively influenced the distribution of embryos according to nucleus number (Domaracky et al 2007).
Hepatotoxicity: An essential oil of *Salvia officinalis* with 17.4% α-thujone, 13.3% α-caryophyllene, 12.7% 1,8-cineole, 8.3% borneol 3.9% β-thujone, 3.3% camphor (and other constituents) was tested for toxicity to rat hepatocytes. The oil was not toxic when present at concentrations of 200 nL/mL or less. However at 2,000 nL/mL significant LDH leakage and glutathione decrease occurred, indicating cell damage (Lima et al 2004).

Systemic effects

Acute toxicity: Dalmatian sage oil acute oral LD_{50} in rats reported as 2.6 g/kg both by Opdyke (1974 p. 987–988) and Von Skramlik (1959); acute subcutaneous LD_{50} in mice 1.95 g/kg (Essway et al 1995); acute dermal LD_{50} in rabbits >5 g/kg (Opdyke 1974 p. 987–988).
Antioxidant/pro-oxidant activity: Dalmatian sage oil showed high antioxidant activity as a DPPH radical scavenger (IC_{50} 1.78 µg/mL) and against lipid peroxidation (Bozin et al 2007).
Carcinogenic/anticarcinogenic potential: Dalmatian sage oil was not mutagenic in a chromosomal aberration test, a *Bacillus subtilis rec*-assay or the Ames test (Ishidate et al 1984; Zani et al 1991). It was similarly non-mutagenic in *S. typhimurium* strains T98 and T100, with or without S9 (De Martino et al 2009a). Sage oil was not mutagenic in *S. typhimurium* TA100, and inhibited UV-induced mutations (Vuković-Gačić et al 2006). Dalmatian sage oil (37.5% α-thujone, 14.4% 1,8-cineole, 13.8% camphor) was antimutagenic in *Salmonella*/microsome, *E. coli* K12, and *S. cerevisiae* D7 reversion assays (Knežević-Vukčević et al 2005). Given orally to mice at 25, 50 or 100 µL/kg, Dalmatian sage oil was not mutagenic at the low dose, but was slightly mutagenic at 50 µL/kg. At 100 µL/kg the oil was cytotoxic. Both of the lower doses inhibited CA induced by mitomycin C (Vujosevic & Blagojevic 2004). Dalmatian sage oil was active against human melanoma and renal cell adenocarcinoma cell lines in vitro (Loizzo et al 2007). It was cytotoxic to human oral squamous cell carcinoma cells, with an IC_{50} of 135 µg/mL (Sertel et al 2011a).

Comments

In an analysis of thujones in *Salvia officinalis*, three chemotypes were determined with total thujone contents of 9%, 22–28% and 39–44% (Perry et al 1999). However, a total thujone content of 30–50% is not unusual in Dalmatian sage oils

(Lawrence 1998b p. 47–52). More than 50% is very uncommon, but we have allowed for 60% in the above safety calculations. The Commission E Monograph daily oral dose of 100–300 mg seems unsafe.

Sage (Greek)

Synonym: Turkish sage
Botanical name: *Salvia fruticosa* Mill.
Botanical synonym: *Salvia triloba* L.
Family: Lamiaceae (Labiatae)

Essential oil

Source: Leaves
Key constituents:

1,8-Cineole	59.0%
β-Pinene	6.7%
α-Pinene	5.9%
β-Caryophyllene	5.5%
Camphor	2.8%
β-Myrcene	2.3%
α-Terpineol	1.8%
α-Caryophyllene	1.6%
β-Thujone	1.6%
Camphene	1.3%
(+)-Limonene	1.3%

(Owen, private communication, 2003)

Safety summary

Hazards: Essential oils high in 1,8-cineole can cause CNS and breathing problems in young children.
Contraindications: Do not apply to or near the face of infants or children.

Organ-specific effects

Adverse skin reactions: No information found.
Reproductive toxicity: The low reproductive toxicity of 1,8-cineole and α-pinene (see Constituent profiles, Chapter 14) suggests that Greek sage oil is not hazardous in pregnancy.

Systemic effects

Acute toxicity: No information found. 1,8-Cineole has been reported to cause serious poisoning in young children when accidentally instilled into the nose (Melis et al 1989).
Carcinogenic/anticarcinogenic potential: Greek sage oil was not genotoxic in the wing somatic mutation and recombination test (SMART) of *Drosophila melanogaster* (Pavlidou et al 2004). Greek sage oil contains no known carcinogens, and both α-caryophyllene and (+)-limonene display anticarcinogenic activity (see Constituent profiles, Chapter 14).

Comments

Although Greek sage oil contains a small amount of thujone (an inhibitor of GABA$_A$ receptor-mediated responses), it also contains higher concentrations of pinenes (which potentiate these responses). Therefore no assumptions have been made regarding thujone neurotoxicity. The oil is produced in both Greece and Turkey, and is similar in composition to white sage oil.

Sage (Spanish)

Synonym: Lavender sage
Botanical name: *Salvia lavandulifolia* Vahl.
Botanical synonym: *Salvia hispanorum* Lag.
Family: Lamiaceae (Labiatae)

Essential oil

Source: Flowering tops
Key constituents:

1,8-Cineole	12.0–40.3% (10.0–30.0%)*
Camphor	12.9–36.1% (11.0–36.0%)
α-Terpinyl acetate	0–15.5% (0.5–9.0%)
Linalool	0.2–11.2% (0.3–4.0%)
α-Pinene	4.7–10.9% (4.0–11.0%
Camphene	4.6–10.6%
β-Pinene	3.3–7.3%
(Z)-Sabinyl acetate	0–.6% (0.5–9.0%)
Borneol	1.5–6.4% (1.0–7.0%)
Linalyl acetate	0.1–5.8% (0.1–5.0%)
(+)-Limonene	2.4–5.0% (2.0–6.0%)
β-Myrcene	1.0–4.9%
Bornyl acetate	0.8–4.9%
β-Caryophyllene	0.2–3.7%
Sabinene	0.6–2.2% (0.1–3.5%)
(Z)-β-Ocimene	0–2.2%
p-Cymene	0.4–2.1%
Isoborneol	0.2–1.9%
α-Terpineol	0.1–1.9%
α-Caryophyllene	0–1.0%
Terpinen-4-ol	0.2–0.8% (0–2.0%)

(Cordoba Rodriguez, cited in: Lawrence 1993 p84–86)

Safety summary

Hazards: Abortifacient.
Contraindications (all routes): Pregnancy, breastfeeding.
Maximum adult daily oral dose: 388 mg
Maximum dermal use level: 12.5%

Our safety advice

Our oral and dermal restrictions are based on 36.1% camphor content with limits of 2 mg/kg/day and 4.5% (see Camphor profile, Chapter 14).

---

*The values in parentheses are the ISO standards for Spanish sage oil (© ISO 2005)

Organ-specific effects

Adverse skin reactions: Undiluted Spanish sage oil was not irritating to rabbit, pig or mouse skin; tested at 8% on 25 volunteers it was neither irritating nor sensitizing. It is non-phototoxic (Opdyke 1976 p. 857–858).

Reproductive toxicity: A fraction of Spanish sage oil, containing 50% sabinyl acetate, 41% 1,8-cineole, and 5% camphor, was injected sc into pregnant mice on gestational days 6–15 at 15, 45 and 135 mg/kg. It was dose-dependently abortifacient and maternally toxic, but was not fetotoxic (Pages et al 1992). Plectranthus oil, containing 60% sabinyl acetate, is teratogenic to pregnant mice (Pages et al 1991), but 1,8-Cineole is not (Pages et al 1990).

Systemic effects

Acute toxicity: Spanish sage oil acute oral LD_{50} in rats >5 g/kg; acute dermal LD_{50} in rabbits >5 g/kg (Opdyke 1976 p. 857–858). Possible estrogenic activity (via induction of β-galactosidase in yeast cells) has been reported for Spanish sage oil (Perry et al 2001).

Carcinogenic/anticarcinogenic potential: Spanish sage oil was not mutagenic in either the *Bacillus subtilis rec*-assay or the *Salmonella*/microsome reversion assay (Zani et al 1991). The oil contains no known carcinogens, and showed moderate in vitro activity against four human cancer cell lines: HL60 (leukemia), K562 (myelogenous leukemia), MCF7 (breast) and A2780 (ovarian) (Foray et al 1999).

Comments

The abortifacient action of sabinyl acetate is due to inhibition of implantation (Pages et al 1996). Since sabinyl acetate presents a risk of abortion, maternal toxicity and teratogenicity in mice, and since an NOAEL has not been established, Spanish sage oil should be avoided in pregnancy, and is likely to present a greater risk during the first trimester. Small amounts of thujones have been reported in Spanish sage oils.

Sage (white)

Botanical name: *Salvia apiana* Jeps.
Family: Lamiaceae (Labiatae)

Essential oil

Source: Leaves
Key constituents:

1,8-Cineole	68.4%
β-Pinene	8.0%
α-Pinene	5.7%
β-Myrcene	2.3%
(+)-Limonene	1.7%
β-Caryophyllene	1.6%
Camphor	1.3%

(Mainguy, private communication 2001)

Safety summary

Hazards: Essential oils high in 1,8-cineole can cause CNS and breathing problems in young children.
Contraindications: Do not apply to or near the face of infants or children.

Organ-specific effects

Adverse skin reactions: No information found.
Reproductive toxicity: The low reproductive toxicity of 1,8-cineole and α-pinene (see Constituent profiles, Chapter 14) suggests that white sage oil is not hazardous in pregnancy.

Systemic effects

Acute toxicity: No information found. 1,8-Cineole has been reported to cause serious poisoning in young children when accidentally instilled into the nose (Melis et al 1989).
Carcinogenic/anticarcinogenic potential: No information was found for white sage oil, but it contains no known carcinogens. (+)-Limonene displays anticarcinogenic activity (see (+)-Limonene profile, Chapter 14).

Comments

Limited availability. Although there are no data for white sage oil it seems unlikely that it would present any significant degree of toxicity.

Sage (wild mountain)

Synonym: Mountain salvia
Botanical name: *Hemizygia petiolata* Ashby
Family: Lamiaceae (Labiatae)

Essential oil

Source: Aerial parts
Constituents:

(*E*)-β-Farnesene	69.6%
Linalool	15.0%
Germacrene B	4.8%
Germacrene D	2.6%
Massoia lactone	1.4%

(Teubes, private communication, 2003)
Quality: Wild mountain sage oil is subject to resinification.

Safety summary

Hazards: Drug interaction; skin irritation/sensitization (moderate risk).
Cautions (all routes): Drugs metabolized by CYP2D6 (Appendix B).
Cautions (dermal): Hypersensitive, diseased or damaged skin, children under 2 years of age.
Maximum dermal use level: 0.7%

Our safety advice

Our dermal maximum is based on a 1.4% massoia lactone content with a dermal limit of 0.01%.

Regulatory guidelines

IFRA recommends that massoia lactone is not used as a fragrance ingredient (IFRA 2009).

Organ-specific effects

Adverse skin reactions: No information was found for either wild mountain sage oil or farnesene, but massoia lactone is regarded as a powerful irritant and sensitizer (see Massoia lactone profile, Chapter 14).

Systemic effects

Acute toxicity: No information was found for wild mountain sage oil or farnesene.
Carcinogenic/anticarcinogenic potential: No information was found for wild mountain sage oil but it contains no known carcinogens.
Drug interactions: Since farnesene inhibits CYP2D6 (Table 4.11B), there is a theoretical risk of interaction between wild mountain sage oil and drugs metabolized by this enzyme (Appendix B).

Comments

It is unfortunate that no published data can be referenced for massoia lactone. Since wild mountain sage oil has not been dermatologically tested it would seem premature to totally restrict its use, and we are recommending a maximum use level in line with the level for massoia oil and its concentration of massoia lactone.

St. John's wort

Botanical name: *Hypericum perforatum* L.
Family: Hypericaceae

Essential oil

Source: Aerial parts
Key constituents:

2-Methyloctane	37.1%
α-Pinene	31.4%
β-Pinene	10.7%
Sabinene	2.1%
β-Myrcene	1.7%
β-Caryophyllene	1.5%
Methyl nonane	1.2%

(Badoux, private communication, 2004)

Safety summary

Hazards: Skin sensitization if oxidized.
Cautions: Old or oxidized oils should be avoided.

Our safety advice

Because of its high α-pinene content we recommend that oxidation of St. John's Wort oil is avoided by storage in a dark, airtight container in a refrigerator. The addition of an antioxidant to preparations containing it is recommended.

Organ-specific effects

Adverse skin reactions: No information found. Autoxidation products of α-pinene and can cause skin sensitization (see α-Pinene profile, Chapter 14).

Systemic effects

Acute toxicity: No information found.
Carcinogenic/anticarcinogenic potential: No information was found for St. John's wort oil but it contains no known carcinogens.

Comments

The plant contains hypericin, which can be powerfully photoactive when ingested (Traynor et al 2005). However, this large molecule is not present in the distilled oil. Limited availability. Indian and Canadian oils may be different in composition.

Sandalwood (East African)

Botanical names: *Osyris lanceolata* Hochst. & Steud.; *Osyris tenuifolia* Engl.
Family: Santalaceae

Essential oil

Source: Wood
Key constituents:

Osyris tenuifolia

(*S*)-(*Z*)-Lanceol	18.0%
epi-Cyclosantalal	5.9%
2,(7Z,10Z)-Bisabolatrien-13-ol	5.6%
(–)-*epi*-α-Bisabolol	5.1%
Lanceoloxide	3.9%
β-Bisabolene	3.7%
Cyclosantalal	2.6%

(Kreipl & König 2004)

Safety summary

Hazards: None known.
Contraindications: None known.

Organ-specific effects

Adverse skin reactions: No information found.

Systemic effects

Acute toxicity: No information found.
Carcinogenic/anticarcinogenic potential: No information found.

Comments

Many of the constituents are as yet unidentified, although lanceol is the major constituent. The oil also contains various bisabolenes, bergamotenes, santalenes, tenuifolenes, cedrenes and curcumenes, each in unspecified concentrations of less than 2% (Kreipl & König 2004). East African sandalwood oils were first experimentally distilled in the 1890s (Guenther 1949–1952 vol. 5, p. 193). These, and similar species of tree, grow wild over large areas of East Africa. Oils have been produced in Kenya and Madagascar in the past, and have been used to adulterate East Indian sandalwood oil (Arctander 1960). Production was and still is centered in Tanzania, and there has recently been a revival of interest in the oil, since there is an increasing demand for all sandalwood-like materials.

Sandalwood (East Indian)

Synonyms: White sandalwood, yellow sandalwood
Botanical name: *Santalum album* L.
Family: Santalaceae

Essential oil

Source: Wood
Key constituents:

(Z)-α-Santalol	46.2–59.9%
(Z)-β-Santalol	20.5–29.0%
(Z)-Nuciferol	1.1–5.5%
epi-β-Santalol	4.1–4.3%
(Z)-α-*trans*-Bergamotol	<3.9%
α-Santalal	0.5–2.9%
β-Santalal	0.6–1.9%
(Z)-Lanceol	1.5–1.7%
(E)-β-Santalol	1.5–1.6%
β-Santalene	0.6–1.4%
Spirosantalol	<1.2%
α-Santalene	0.8–1.1%

(Lawrence 1993 p. 180–182)
Quality: East Indian sandalwood oil may be adulterated by the addition of sandalwood terpenes and fragrance chemicals (Burfield 2003). Other known adulterants include Australian sandalwood oil, East African sandalwood oil, Indian bastard sandal oil (*Erythroxylum monohynum* Roxb.), amyris oil, bleached copaiba balsam, and non-odorous materials such as polyethylene glycol, castor oil, coconut oil and DEHP.

Safety summary

Hazards: A rare but known cause of adverse skin reactions.
Contraindications: None known.
Maximum dermal use level: 2%

Our safety advice

From a total of 3,542 dermatitis patients, only 12 (0.34%) reacted to patch testing with 2% sandalwood oil. Based on this information, and because of the risk of photoallergic reactions, especially in Japanese people, we recommend a maximum use level of 2%.

Organ-specific effects

Adverse skin reactions: In a modified Draize procedure on guinea pigs, sandalwood oil was non-sensitizing when used at 5% in the challenge phase (Sharp 1978). Undiluted East Indian sandalwood oil was irritating to rabbits, was slightly irritating to mice, but produced no irritation in 18 volunteers. Tested at 10% on 25 volunteers it was not sensitizing (Opdyke 1974 p. 989–990). East Indian sandalwood oil, tested at 10% in consecutive dermatitis patients, induced allergic responses in 15 of 1,606 (0.9%) (Frosch et al 2002b), and five of 318 (1.6%) (Paulsen & Andersen 2005). Similarly tested at 2%, there were reactions in none of 387 (0%) (Rudzki et al 1976), one of 1,200 (0.08%) (Santucci et al 1987), seven of 1,606 (0.4%) (Frosch et al 2002b), and four of 318 (1.3%) (Paulsen & Andersen 2005). See Table 13.3.

In a prospective study of adverse skin reactions to cosmetic ingredients identified by patch test (1977–1980) East Indian sandalwood oil elicited contact dermatitis in two (0.4%) of

Table 13.3 Allergic reactions to East Indian sandalwood

A. Dermatitis patients

Concentration used	Percentage who reacted	Number of reactors	Reference
2%	0%	0/31	Emmons & Marks 1985
2%	0%	0/387	Rudzki et al 1976
2%	0.08%	1/1,200	Santucci et al 1987
2%	0.4%	7/1,606	Frosch et al 2002b
2%	1.3%	4/318	Paulsen & Andersen 2005
10%	0.9%	15/1,606	Frosch et al 2002b
10%	1.3%	49/3,671	Uter et al 2010
10%	1.6%	5/318	Paulsen & Andersen 2005
Various	0.4%	2/487	Eiermann et al 1982

B. Dermatitis patients suspected of cosmetic or fragrance sensitivity

Concentration used	Percentage who reacted	Number of reactors	Reference
2%	0.8%	12/1,483	Sugiura et al 2000
10%	1.8%	18/1,002	Uter et al 2010
10%	6.6%	11/167	Larsen et al 1996a
Various	0.4%	3/713	Adams & Maibach 1985

487 cosmetic-related cases (Maibach et al 1989). Of 281,100 dermatitis patients, 13,216 had contact dermatitis, and of these 713 were related to cosmetic ingredients. Of this last group, three reacted to East Indian sandalwood oil (Adams & Maibach 1985). Of 167 fragrance-sensitive dermatitis patients, 11 (6.6%) were allergic to 10% East Indian sandalwood oil on patch testing (Larsen et al 1996b). From 1990 to 1998 the average patch test positivity rate to 2% sandalwood oil in a total of 1,483 Japanese eczema patients (99% female) suspected of cosmetic sensitivity was 0.8% (Sugiura et al 2000). In a multicenter study, Germany's IVDK reported that 49 of 3,671 consecutive dermatitis patients (1.33%) and 18 of 1,002 patients suspected of fragrance allergy (1.8%) tested positive to 10% East Indian sandalwood oil (Uter et al 2010). In Japan, East Indian sandalwood oil is regarded as a high-risk skin sensitizer and potential cause of pigmented contact dermatitis (Nakayama 1998). A case of photoallergy to sandalwood oil was reported by Starke (1967) and subsequently, photoallergic reactions to 2% sandalwood oil were seen in three of 138 patients who were photopatch tested in the USA (Fotiades et al 1995). Sandalwood oil is not phototoxic (Opdyke 1974 p. 989–990).

Hepatotoxicity: Oral administration of sandalwood oil to male rats significantly reduced carbon tetrachloride-induced liver damage (Hashim et al 1992, cited in Chhabra and Rao 1993).

Systemic effects

Acute toxicity: East Indian sandalwood oil acute oral LD_{50} in rats 5.58 g/kg; acute dermal LD_{50} in rabbits >5 g/kg (Opdyke 1974 p. 989–990).

Antioxidant/pro-oxidant activity: Sandalwood oil showed moderate activity as a DPPH radical scavenger and low activity in the aldehyde/carboxylic acid assay (Wei & Shibamoto 2007a).

Carcinogenic/anticarcinogenic potential: Sandalwood oil was not genotoxic in the *B. subtilis* rec-assay, with or without S9 activation (Ishizaki et al 1985). East Indian sandalwood oil decreased DMBA-induced and TPA-promoted skin papillomas in mice, reducing papilloma incidence by 67% and multiplicity by 96%. At the same time it reduced TPA-induced ODC activity (a marker of tumor promotion) by 70% (Dwivedi & Abu-Ghazaleh 1997). These findings suggest that East Indian sandalwood oil could be an effective chemopreventive agent in skin cancer (Dwivedi & Zhang 1999). The enhancement by East Indian sandalwood oil of glutathione S-transferase activity and acid-soluble sulfydryl levels are suggestive of a chemopreventive action (Banerjee et al 1993). The oil contains no known carcinogens.

Comments

The ISO standard for East Indian sandalwood oil of >90% santalols may require re-evaluation. Specifications of >43% of (Z)-α-santalol, and >18% (Z)-β-santalol were suggested by Howes et al (2004). In 1988 an East Indian sandalwood oil produced in 1987 was compared with one produced in 1905. This comparison shows, along with other changes, increases in α- and β-santalal and α- and β-santalene, and decreases in (Z)-α-santalol (50.0% to 22.0%) and (Z)-β-santalol (20.9% to 9.8%) in the aged oil (Lawrence 1993

p. 180–182). In a report on trees, UNEP-WCMC proposed that CITES add *Santalum album* to its list of threatened plant species. Some 1,700 hectares of *Santalum album* trees are now being cultivated in Western Australia, for future production of sandalwood oil.

Sandalwood (New Caledonian)

Synonym: Pacific island sandalwood
Botanical name: *Santalum austrocaledonicum* Vieill.
Family: Santalaceae

Essential oil

Source: Wood
Key constituents:

(Z)-α-Santalol	42.3%
(Z)-β-Santalol	17.5%
(Z)-Lanceol	15.6%
(Z)-α-*trans*-Bergamotol	6.7%
(Z)-*epi*-β-Santalol	3.2%
(Z)-Nuciferol	2.4%

(Cornwell, private communication, 2004)

Safety summary

Hazards: None known.
Contraindications: None known.
Maximum dermal use level: 2%

Our safety advice

The safety profile of New Caledonian sandalwood oil is probably similar to East Indian sandalwood (see Sandalwood (East Indian) profile) as the composition of the two oils is similar.

Organ-specific effects

Adverse skin reactions: No information was found for New Caledonian sandalwood oil, or any of its constituents.

Systemic effects

Acute toxicity: No information was found for New Caledonian sandalwood oil, or any of its constituents. It is likely to be as nontoxic as East Indian sandalwood, since the chemical profile is similar.

Carcinogenic/anticarcinogenic potential: No information found. (Z)-α-santalol has anticarcinogenic effects (see Constituent profiles, Chapter 14). The oil contains no known carcinogens.

Comments

The compositional data given here are averages. This is the same species from which sandalwood Vanuatu is produced. New Caledonian sandalwood oil is the closest to East Indian sandalwood in terms of both composition and odor.

Sandalwood (Western Australian)

Botanical name: *Santalum spicatum* A. DC.
Botanical synonyms: *Santalum cygnorum* Miq; *Fusanus spicatus* R. Br.; *Eucarya spicata* Sprag. et Summ.
Family: Santalaceae

Essential oil

Source: Wood
Key constituents:

Hydrodistilled/extracted oil

(Z)-α-Santalol	13.3%
(2E,6E)-Farnesol	9.3%
(Z)-β-Curcumen-12-ol	7.2%
(Z)-β-Santalol	5.9%
(Z)-Nuciferol	5.6%
α-Bisabolol	4.9%
(Z)-α-*trans*-Bergamotol	4.7%
(Z)-γ-Curcumen-12-ol	4.4%
Bisabola-2,10-dien-6,13-diol	2.4%
Dendrolasin	2.0%
(Z)-Lanceol	2.0%
β-Bisabolol + *epi*-β-bisabolol	1.9%
(Z)-12-Hydroxy-sesquicineole	1.7%
α-Santalene	1.5%
β-Curcumene	1.4%
epi-β-Santalol	1.4%
β-Santalene	1.3%
11-*epi*-6,10-Epoxy-bisabolol-2-en-12-ol	1.0%

(Valder et al 2003)

Steam distilled oil

α-Santalol	15.3–17.0%
α-Bisabolol	12.4–15.0%
(Z)-Nuciferol	9.0–14.0%
(E,E)-Farnesol	7.9–8.4%
Dendrolasin	3.3–5.3%
(Z)-β-Santalol	4.6–4.8%
(E)-Nuciferol	2.2–4.8%
(E)-α-Bergamotol	3.8–4.6%
β-Bisabolol	2.9–4.4%
Bulnesol	1.0–3.6%
(E)-β-Santalol	2.9–3.3%
(Z)-Lanceolol	2.3–3.0%
(E)-Nerolidol	0–2.2%
Guaiol	0.4–2.0%
β-Curcumene	1.3–1.5%
epi-β-Santalol	1.0–1.4%
β-Santalene	0.5–1.0%

(Day, private communication, 2004).

Safety summary

Hazards: Drug interaction.
Cautions (oral): Drugs metabolized by CYP2D6 (Appendix B).

Organ-specific effects

Adverse skin reactions: No information found.

Systemic effects

Acute toxicity: No information found.
Carcinogenic/anticarcinogenic potential: No information found. (Z)-α-santalol displays anticarcinogenic activity (see Constituent profiles, Chapter 14). The oil contains no known carcinogens.
Drug interactions: Since α-bisabolol inhibits CYP2D6 (Table 4.11B), there is a theoretical risk of interaction between Western Australian sandalwood oil and drugs metabolized by this enzyme (Appendix B).

Comments

The commercial oil is most commonly produced by a combination of solvent extraction and steam or vacuum distillation, although extraction alone has also been used, as has steam distillation. Since hexane is the solvent of choice, traces will be present in extracted oils. As can be seen, the extracted and distilled oils are distinctly different in composition.

Sanna

Synonyms: Spiked ginger lily, kapur kachri
Botanical name: *Hedychium spicatum* Sm.
Family: Zingiberaceae

Essential oil

Source: Rhizomes
Key constituents:

1,8-Cineole	44.3%
Linalool	25.6%
T-Muurolol	4.4%
Hedycaryol	2.6%
α-Cadinol	2.3%
α-Eudesmol	2.3%
β-Eudesmol	2.2%
Ascaridole	1.9%
Eremoligenol	1.3%
β-Pinene	1.3%
Terpinen-4-ol	1.3%

(Sabulal et al 2007)

Safety summary

Hazards: May contain ascaridole. Essential oils high in 1,8-cineole can cause CNS and breathing problems in young children.

Contraindications: Do not apply to or near the face of infants or children.
Maximum adult daily oral dose: 180 mg
Maximum dermal use level: 6.3%

Our safety advice

Our oral and dermal restrictions are based on 1.9% ascaridole content with limits of 0.05 mg/kg/day and 0.12% (see Ascaridole profile, Chapter 14).

Organ-specific effects

Adverse skin reactions: No information found.

Systemic effects

Acute toxicity: No information found. Ascaridole is highly toxic. 1,8-Cineole has been reported to cause serious poisoning in young children when accidentally instilled into the nose (Melis et al 1989).
Carcinogenic/anticarcinogenic potential: No information was found for sanna oil, but it contains no known carcinogens.

Comments

Benzyl cinnamate 24.0%, benzyl acetate 16.5%, 1,8-cineole 13.0%, linalyl acetate 11.5%, and linalool 8.5% have been reported as constituents of this oil (Sinha et al 1977, cited in Burfield 2000 p264). Dutt (1940) identified ethyl *p*-methoxy cinnamate 67.8%, ethyl cinnamate 10.2% and 1,4-cineole 6.0% in sanna oil. These reports may reflect differences in varieties or chemotypes. According to Sabulal et al (2007), who analyzed *Hedychium spicatum* var. *acuminatum*, three other analyses of this same variety also identified 1,8-cineole as the major constituent (27.1–75.7%). Limited availability; the plant is reputed to be over-exploited and vulnerable in parts of India.

Saro

Synonym: Mandravasarotra
Botanical name: *Cinnamosma fragrans* Baill.
Family: Canellaceae

Essential oil

Source: Leaves
Key constituents:

1,8-Cineole	46.0–53.0%
β-Pinene	5.0–8.0%
α-Pinene	4.0–7.0%
Terpinen-4-ol	3.0–5.0%
(+)-Limonene	2.0–4.0%
α-Terpineol	1.5–4.0%
Terpinyl acetate	2.0–3.0%
Linalool	0.5–2.0%

(Behra, private communication, 2003)

Safety summary

Hazards: Essential oils high in 1,8-cineole can cause CNS and breathing problems in young children.
Contraindications: Do not apply to or near the face of infants or children.

Organ-specific effects

Adverse skin reactions: No information was found for saro oil, but judging from its composition the risk of skin reactions is likely to be low.
Reproductive toxicity: The low reproductive toxicity of camphor, 1,8-cineole, α-pinene and (+)-limonene (see Constituent profiles, Chapter 14) suggest that saro oil is not hazardous in pregnancy.

Systemic effects

Acute toxicity: No information found. 1,8-Cineole has been reported to cause serious poisoning in young children when accidentally instilled into the nose (Melis et al 1989).
Carcinogenic/anticarcinogenic potential: No information was found for saro oil, but it contains no known carcinogens. (+)-Limonene displays anticarcinogenic activity (see (+)-Limonene profile, Chapter 14).

Comments

The oil is produced in Madagascar. Limited availability.

Sassafras

Botanical names: *Sassafras albidum* (Nutt.) Nees (sassafras); *Nectandra sanguinea* Rol. Ex Rottb. (synonym: *Netandra globosa* Mez) (Brazilian sassafras); *Ocotea odorifera* (Vell.) Rohwer (synonym: *Ocotea pretiosa* (Nees) Mez) (Brazilian sassafras); *Cinnamomum porrectum* (Roxb.) Kosterm (Chinese sassafras); *Cinnamomum rigidissimum* HT Chang (Chinese sassafras)
Family: Lauraceae

Essential oil

Source: Wood and/or roots
Key constituents:

Cinnamomum porrectum (roots)
Safrole   85.5–97.0%

(Phongpaichit et al 2007)

Cinnamomum rigidissimum (wood)
Safrole	61.7%
Methyleugenol	28.6%
Elemicin	1.2%

(Zhu et al 1993)

Ocotea odorifera (wood)
Safrole	71.2–92.9%
Camphor	0.7–2.9%

| Methyleugenol | 0–2.0% |
| α-Pinene | 0.2–1.3% |

(Formacek & Kubeczka 1982; Lawrence 1989 p. 154–156)

Sassafras albidum (roots)

Safrole	82.8–88.8%
Camphor	1.2–6.8%
Methyleugenol	1.4–2.3%
1,8-Cineole	1.1%

(Zwaving & Bos 1996)
Note: Due to their compositional similarity these essential oils are treated here in one profile.

Safety summary

Hazards: Carcinogenic.
Contraindications: Should not be used, either internally or externally.

Our safety advice

Due to its high safrole content we recommend that sassafras oil is not used in therapy.

Regulatory guidelines

Sassafras oil has been prohibited in foods for many years because of its safrole content. IFRA and the EU recommend a maximum exposure level of 0.01% of safrole from the use of safrole-containing essential oils in cosmetics. IFRA recommends a maximum concentration of 0.0004% methyleugenol in leave-on products such as body lotions (IFRA 2009). The equivalent SCCNFP maximum is 0.0002% (European Commission 2002).

Organ-specific effects

Adverse skin reactions: Undiluted sassafras oil was moderately irritating to rabbits and produced mild erythema and edema in both mouse and pig skin; tested at 4% on 25 volunteers it was neither irritating nor sensitizing. It is non-phototoxic (Opdyke & Letizia 1982 p. 825–826). Undiluted Brazilian sassafras oil was moderately irritating to rabbits and was irritating to both mice and pigs; tested at 20% on 25 volunteers it was neither irritating nor sensitizing. It is non-phototoxic (Opdyke 1978 p. 831). In a study of 200 consecutive dermatitis patients, none were sensitive to 2% sassafras oil on patch testing (Rudzki et al 1976).

Systemic effects

Acute toxicity, human: A few drops of sassafras oil have been considered sufficient to kill a toddler and the US Dispensatory of 1888 records the case of a male adult who died following the ingestion of a teaspoon (∼ 5 mL) of sassafras oil; symptoms of poisoning included CNS depression (stupor, ataxia), vomiting and nausea; however the veracity of this report is in some doubt (Craig 1953). In another case, a 47-year-old ingested 5 mL and survived, suffering only vomiting and 'feeling shaky' (Grande & Dannewitz 1987). Five children all survived sassafras oil ingestion, although serious symptoms of poisoning occurred in each case. Their ages ranged from 15 months to 2½ years, and the amounts ingested from 4–60 mL (Craig 1953).

A sassafras oil overdose depresses the CNS so that respiration and blood circulation become inadequate (Craig 1953). Symptoms appear within 10–90 minutes of taking the oil and the clinical picture resembles that of eucalyptus poisoning, except that vomiting and shock are more common with sassafras, and pinpoint pupils are not seen (Grande & Dannewitz 1987).

Acute toxicity, animal: *Sassafras albidum* oil acute oral LD_{50} in rats 1.9 g/kg; acute dermal LD_{50} in rabbits >5 g/kg (Opdyke & Letizia 1982 p. 825–826). *Ocotea pretiosa* oil acute oral LD_{50} in rats 1.58 g/kg; acute dermal LD_{50} in rabbits >5 g/kg (Opdyke 1978 p. 831). The minimum lethal oral dose of safrole in the rabbit is 1.0 g/kg (Spector 1956). Safrole is highly toxic on chronic dosing; 95% lethal to rats at 10,000 ppm after 19 days' dosing (Miller 1979).

Carcinogenic/anticarcinogenic potential: Sassafras oil or safrole, given in the diet of male and female rats at 390 ppm or 1,170 ppm, produced no tumors after 22 months at either dose. At the higher level there was some evidence of kidney congestion. However, a large percentage of animals showed initial tumor development at 24 months for both safrole and sassafras oil at both doses. Significant cellular changes were observed in the kidneys, the adrenal, thyroid and pituitary glands, and in the testes or ovaries (Abbott et al 1961). Safrole and its 2′,3′-epoxy, 1′-hydroxy and 1′-sulfate metabolites can form adducts with DNA and other macromolecules in the liver (see Safrole profile, Chapter 14).

Comments

The work by Abbott et al suggests that sassafras oil is a relatively weak carcinogen requiring prolonged exposure before initiating cellular changes. It also suggests that there is little difference between the carcinogenic potential of sassafras oil and safrole. Very little oil is produced from *Sassafras albidum* in the USA. Brazilian sassafras oil is sometimes incorrectly referred to as originating from *Ocotea cymbarum* or *Ocotea pretiosa*. Chinese sassafras oil is sometimes the safrole-rich fraction of camphor oil, 'brown camphor oil', although it is also obtained from *Cinnamomum porrectum* and *Cinnamomum rigidissimum* (Zhu et al 1994). The Chinese oil has taken over from the Brazilian in the world market, because of over-logging in Brazil. Over-logging in China may now be a problem. In a report on trees it has been proposed by UNEP-WCMC that CITES add *Ocotea odifera* to its list of threatened plant species. Natural root beer, made with sassafras, used to be popular in the USA and is still made illicitly.

Satsuma

Synonym: Mikan
Botanical name: *Citrus unshiu* Marc.
Botanical synonym: *Citrus reticulata* Blanco var. *satsuma*
Family: Rutaceae

Essential oil

Source: Fruit peel, by expression

Key constituents:

(+)-Limonene	82.0–90.6%
γ-Terpinene	3.3–4.9%
Elemol	tr–2.7%
α-Farnesene	<2.5%
β-Myrcene	1.0–1.8%
Linalool	0.2–1.2%
β-Copaene	<1.2%
α-Pinene	0.5–1%

(Lawrence 1989 p. 220–222)

Safety summary

Hazards: Skin sensitization if oxidized.
Cautions: Old or oxidized oils should be avoided.

Our safety advice

Because of its (+)-limonene content we recommend that oxidation of satsuma oil is avoided by storage in a dark, airtight container in a refrigerator. The addition of an antioxidant to preparations containing it is recommended.

Regulatory guidelines

IFRA recommends that essential oils rich in limonene should only be used when the level of peroxides is kept to the lowest practical level, for instance by adding antioxidants at the time of production (IFRA 2009).

Organ-specific effects

Adverse skin reactions: No information was found for satsuma oil, but autoxidation products of (+)-limonene can cause skin sensitization (see (+)-Limonene profile, Chapter 14).
Reproductive toxicity: The low developmental toxicity of (+)-limonene in rabbits and mice (Kodama et al 1977a, 1977b) suggests that satsuma oil is not hazardous in pregnancy.

Systemic effects

Acute toxicity: No information found.
Carcinogenic/anticarcinogenic potential: Satsuma oil inhibited formation of the carcinogen NDMA in vitro by more than 70% (Sawamura 2010). (+)-Limonene displays anticarcinogenic activity (see (+)-Limonene profile, Chapter 14).

Comments

The satsuma, or mikan, is a type of mandarin, and the oil is produced in Japan. No bergapten was detected in an expressed oil from the fruit peel of *Citrus unshiu* var. *praecox*, with a detection limit of 0.1 ppm (Sawamura et al 2009). This strongly suggests that satsuma oil is not phototoxic.

Savin

Botanical name: *Juniperus sabina* L.
Family: Cupressaceae (Coniferae)

Essential oil

Source: Leaves and terminal branches
Key constituents:

(Z)-Sabinyl acetate	19.1–53.1%
Sabinene	18.3–40.8%
Elemol	tr–7.0%
β-Myrcene	3.4–3.5%
Terpinen-4-ol	1.1–3.1%
α-Pinene	1.2–2.5%
(+)-Limonene	1.4–1.6%
Terpinolene	0.6–1.5%
β-Thujone	0.2–1.5%
α-Terpineol	0.5–1.4%
γ-Terpinene	0.6–1.3%
α-Thujene	0.6–1.1%

(Lawrence 1993 p. 187)

Safety summary

Hazards: Embryo-fetotoxicity; abortifacient; hepatotoxicity.
Contraindications: Should not be used, either internally or externally.

Our safety advice

We recommend that savin oil should not be used. This is due to concerns about hepatotoxicity, and the fact that, on a risk/benefit basis, nothing much is gained by allowing use of the oil.

Regulatory guidelines

Savin oil is prohibited as a cosmetic ingredient in the EU and Canada. In the UK, *Juniperus sabina* preparations can only be sold in a pharmacy, under the supervision of a pharmacist.

Organ-specific effects

Adverse skin reactions: No information found.
Reproductive toxicity: Savin oil was given sc to pregnant mice at 15, 45 or 135 mg/kg on gestational days 6–15. All doses caused embryotoxicity, and dams on the two higher doses showed significant weight loss (Pages et al 1989b). Subcutaneously administered savin oil, containing 50% sabinyl acetate, prevented implantation in mice at 45 and 135 mg/kg, but not at 15 mg when given on gestational days 0–4. The same pattern was observed with sabinyl acetate given at 70 mg/kg. However, no antifertility effect was found when savin oil was given on gestational days 8–11, indicating that the abortifacient action of sabinyl acetate is due to inhibition of implantation (Pages et al 1996).

A fraction of Spanish sage oil containing 50% sabinyl acetate caused dose-dependent maternal toxicity and abortifacient effects in rodents, but was not fetotoxic. The abortifacient effect occurred even at very low doses (15 mg/kg) and was probably due to sabinyl acetate (Pages et al 1992). Sabinyl acetate is probably responsible for the embryotoxic and fetotoxic action of plectranthus oil (Pages et al 1988). Plectranthus oil (~60% sabinyl acetate) dramatically increased both the rate of resorption and

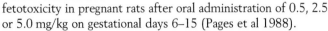

fetotoxicity in pregnant rats after oral administration of 0.5, 2.5 or 5.0 mg/kg on gestational days 6–15 (Pages et al 1988).

Hepatotoxicity: Savin oil has been reported to cause liver lesions in guinea pigs suggestive of a degenerative hepatitis (Patoir et al 1938a, 1938b). Dose-dependent hepatotoxicity (paler and smaller livers) was observed in female mice following sc savin oil administration at 15, 45 or 135 mg/kg (Pages et al 1989b).

Systemic effects

Acute toxicity: According to King's American Dispensatory (1898), 'The oil (*Oleum Sabinae*), given two or three times a day, in doses of from 10 or 15 drops on sugar, will, in most cases, cause abortion, but it is apt to violently affect the stomach and bowels at the same time, bringing life into extreme danger' (http://www.henriettesherbal.com/eclectic/kings/juniperus-sabi.html accessed August 8th 2011). A 20th century herbalist commented: 'it is a powerful emmenagogue in large doses; it is an energetic poison leading to gastroenteritis, collapse and death. It should never be used in pregnancy, as it produces abortion' (Grieve 1978). Manceau et al (1936) noted that, since the plant was so toxic, the essential oil must possess 'une valeur toxique considérable'. However, on subsequent testing in guinea pigs, this same team reported that the minimal lethal dose in the guinea pig for savin oil (presumably oral) was 3.0 g/kg. There are reports of savin oil causing convulsions, fatal poisoning, abortion, and being able to cross the placenta (Papavassiliou 1935).

Carcinogenic/anticarcinogenic potential: No information was found for savin oil, but it contains no known carcinogens. (+)-Limonene displays anticarcinogenic activity(see (+)-Limonene profile, Chapter 14).

Comments

An ether extract of *Juniperus sabina*, obtained after essential oil extraction, was responsible for a dose-dependent anti-implantation effect, showing that the essential oil is not solely responsible for the abortifacient action attributed to the plant (Chamorro et al 1990). Savin oil is sometimes confused with *Juniperus phoenicea*, or *Juniperus communis*. In the latter case this may have contributed to the belief that common juniper oil is toxic and abortifacient.

Savory

Botanical names: *Satureia hortensis* L. (summer savory); *Satureia montana* L. (winter savory)
Family: Lamiaceae (Labiatae)

Essential oil

Source: Dried aerial parts
Note: Due to their compositional similarity these two essential oils are treated here in one profile.
Key constituents:

Summer savory

Carvacrol	43.6–70.7%
γ-Terpinene	19.5–42.8%

p-Cymene	0.9–8.7%
α-Terpinene	1.8–3.5%
α-Pinene	0.7–2.7%
β-Myrcene	0.9–2.3%
α-Thujene	0–1.9%
β-Caryophyllene	0.7–1.8%
Estragole	0–0.2%

(Lawrence 1989 p. 16, 1995g p. 6)

Winter savory

Carvacrol	46.5–75.0%
γ-Terpinene	1.8–15.1%
p-Cymene	2.2–14.6%
β-Caryophyllene	0–13.6%
Thymol	1.0–8.0%
(+)-Limonene	0.2–5.7%
Bornyl acetate	0–5.1%
α-Terpineol	2.4–4.4%
Terpinen-4-ol	0–4.1%
Sabinene	0–1.9%
Citronellol	0–1.8%
α-Terpinene	0–1.5%
Linalyl acetate	0–1.4%
β-Myrcene	0–1.2%
α-Pinene	tr–1.1%
α-Copaene	0–1.1%
Methyleugenol	0–0.9%

(Lawrence 1995g p. 5, 1996f p. 55)

Safety summary

Hazards: Drug interaction; may contain methyleugenol; may inhibit blood clotting; skin irritation (low risk); mucous membrane irritation (moderate risk).
Cautions (dermal): Hypersensitive, diseased or damaged skin, children under 2 years of age.
Cautions (oral): Diabetic medication, anticoagulant medication, major surgery, peptic ulcer, hemophilia, other bleeding disorders (Box 7.1).
Maximum adult daily oral dose (winter savory): 78 mg
Maximum dermal use level (winter savory oil):

EU	0.02%
IFRA	0.04%
Tisserand & Young	1.2%

Maximum dermal use level (summer savory oil):

EU	No limit
IFRA	5.0%
Tisserand & Young	1.4%

Our safety advice

We recommend a maximum adult daily oral dose of 78 mg for winter savory oil, based on 0.9% methyleugenol and a limit of 0.01 mg/kg/day. Our dermal maximums are based on thymol and/or carvacrol content, and a dermal limit of 1% for these constituents to avoid skin irritation (see Carvacrol and Thymol profiles, Chapter 14). The EU and IFRA limits are based on estragole or methyleugenol content.

Regulatory guidelines

Has GRAS status. IFRA recommends a maximum dermal use level for estragole of 0.01% in leave-on or wash-off preparations for body and face (IFRA 2009). IFRA recommends a maximum concentration of 0.0004% methyleugenol in leave-on products such as body lotions (IFRA 2009). The equivalent SCCNFP maximum is 0.0002% (European Commission 2002).

Organ-specific effects

Adverse skin reactions: Undiluted summer savory oil was strongly irritating to both rabbits and guinea pigs; in mice it caused excoriation and 50% of the group died within 48 hours. Tested at 10% in methanol on mice, it produced edema, while 1% in methanol was non-irritating. Tested at 6% on 25 volunteers it was neither irritating nor sensitizing. It is non-phototoxic (Opdyke 1976 p. 859–860).
Cardiovascular effects: Carvacrol inhibits platelet aggregation (Enomoto et al 2001), an essential step in the blood clotting cascade. An essential oil high in carvacrol (*Satureja khuzestanica*, 93.9% carvacrol) significantly reduced plasma glucose concentrations in diabetic rats when given orally at 100 mg/kg/day for 21 days (Shahsavari et al 2009).

Systemic effects

Acute toxicity: Summer savory oil acute oral LD_{50} in rats 1.37 g/kg; acute dermal LD_{50} in rabbits 340 mg/kg (Opdyke 1976 p. 859–860).
Antioxidant/pro-oxidant activity: Both types of savory oil demonstrate potent antioxidant activity (Güllüce et al 2003; Radonic & Milos 2003).
Carcinogenic/anticarcinogenic potential: Neither summer nor winter savory oil was mutagenic in either a *Bacillus subtilis* recassay or a *Salmonella*/microsome reversion assay (Zani et al 1991). Summer savory oil protected rat lymphocytes from hydrogen peroxide-induced genotoxicity, reversing oxidative damage to the cells (Mosaffa et al 2006). The in vitro cell growth of K562 (myelogenous leukemia) cells was inhibited by both summer and winter savory oils with IC_{50} values of 85.4 and 56.15 µg/mL, respectively (Lampronti et al 2006). Estragole and methyleugenol are rodent carcinogens when exposure is sufficiently high; β-caryophyllene and (+)-limonene display antitumoral activity (see Constituent profiles, Chapter 14).
Drug interactions: Antidiabetic or anticoagulant medication, because of cardiovascular effects, above. See Table 4.10B.

Comments

Winter savory is generally grown wild, and summer savory is cultivated, but the two oils are compositionally very similar. Other chemotypes (e.g. thymol) exist, but commercially available oils are generally carvacrol-rich.

Siam wood

Synonyms: Coffin wood, peimou, pe mou, po mu
Botanical name: *Fokienia hodginsii* (Dunn) Henry et Thomas
Family: Cupressaceae

Essential oil

Source: Root bark
Composition:

(*E*)-Nerolidol	35.5%
δ-Cadinene	32.6%
Fokienol	26.4%
γ-Cadinene	15.6%
α-Muurolene	10.4%
γ-Muurolene	7.1%
β-Eudesmol	4.4%
Dauc-6(14),11-dien-5-ol	3.9%
Elemol	3.2%
γ-Eudesmol	3.0%
α-Eudesmol	2.9%
α-Cadinol	2.7%
T-Muurolol	2.3%
β-Bisabolene	1.6%
Zonarene	1.6%
Caparatriene	1.5%
α-Calacorene	1.4%
T-Cadinol	1.4%
α-Copaene	1.3%
α-Curcumene	1.1%

(Lesueur et al 2005)

Safety summary

Hazards: None known.
Contraindications: None known

Organ-specific effects

Adverse skin reactions: No information found. Nerolidol has an extremely low skin sensitization potential (see Nerolidol profile, Chapter 14).

Systemic effects

Acute toxicity: No information was found for siam wood oil, but toxicity would seem to be unlikely.
Carcinogenic/anticarcinogenic potential: No information was found for siam wood oil, but it contains no known carcinogens. Nerolidol displays anticarcinogenic activity (see Nerolidol profile, Chapter 14). α-Cadinol is active against the human colon cancer cell line HT-29 (He et al 1997a).

Comments

Limited availability. The timber was formerly used for coffins. The tree grows in China and Vietnam, and is listed as an endangered species in Vietnam by the World Conservation Monitoring Center.

Skimmia

Botanical name: *Skimmia laureola* Sieb. & Zucc. ex Walp.
Family: Rutaceae

Essential oil

Source: Leaves
Key constituents:

Linalyl acetate	55.6%
Pregeijerene	12.3%
Linalool	7.8%
Geijerene	5.0%
Geranyl acetate	2.5%
Geraniol	1.9%
α-Terpineol	1.8%
β-Phellandrene	1.6%
(*E,E*)-Farnesyl acetate	1.5%
Neryl actetate	1.1%

(Lawrence 1995g p.157)

Safety summary

Hazards: May be phototoxic.
Contraindications: None known.

Organ-specific effects

Adverse skin reactions: No information found. Bergapten has twice been reported as a component of the oil (Lawrence 1989 p. 37) but its presence in commercial oils is uncertain.

Systemic effects

Acute toxicity: No information found. Linalyl acetate acute oral LD_{50} reported as 14.5 g/kg and >10 mL/kg in rats, and 13.36 g/kg and 13.5 g/kg in mice. Acute dermal LD_{50} >5 g/kg (Letizia et al 2003b).
Carcinogenic/anticarcinogenic potential: No information was found for skimmia oil, but it contains no known carcinogens. Geraniol displays anticarcinogenic activity (see Constituent profiles, Chapter 14).

Comments

The presence of bergapten in the oil is disputed (see Ch. 5, p. 87) so there is a possible risk of phototoxicity. Produced in limited quantities in India.

Snakeroot

Synonyms: Canadian snakeroot, wild ginger
Botanical name: *Asarum canadense* L.
Family: Artistolochiaceae

Essential oil

Source: Dried roots and rhizomes

Key constituents:

Methyleugenol	36.1–44.5%
Linalyl acetate	8.0–41.4%
Geraniol	0.8–7.2%
Linalool	5.0–5.3%
Bornyl acetate	0.3–2.0%
Elemicin	<1.8%
α-Terpineol	<1.5%
α-Pinene	<1.5%
Geranyl acetate	<1.4%
Terpinen-4-ol	<1.4%
β-Pinene	<1.3%
Jujenol	<1.2%
β-Myrcene	<1.0%

(Lawrence 1989 p. 204)

Safety summary

Hazards: Potentially carcinogenic, based on methyleugenol content.
Contraindications: Should not be used, either internally or externally.

Our safety advice

Due to its high methyleugenol content, we recommend that snakeroot oil is not used in therapy.

Regulatory guidelines

IFRA recommends a maximum concentration of 0.0004% methyleugenol in leave-on products such as body lotions (IFRA 2009). The equivalent SCCNFP maximum is 0.0002% (European Commission 2002).

Organ-specific effects

Adverse skin reactions: Undiluted snakeroot oil was not irritating to rabbit, pig or mouse skin; tested at 4% on 25 volunteers it was neither irritating nor sensitizing. It is non-phototoxic (Opdyke 1978 p. 869–870).

Systemic effects

Acute toxicity: Snakeroot oil acute oral LD_{50} in rats 4.48 mL/kg; acute dermal LD_{50} in rabbits >5 g/kg (Opdyke 1978 p. 869–870).
Carcinogenic/anticarcinogenic potential: No information found. Methyleugenol is a rodent carcinogen if exposure is sufficiently high; geraniol displays anticarcinogenic activity (see Constituent profiles, Chapter 14).

Comments

Distilled from wildcrafted plants. Limited availability. Reconstituted oils have been offered.

Snowbush

Botanical name: *Eriocephalus africanus* L.
Family: Asteraceae (Compositae)

Essential oil

Source: Leaves and stem
Key constituents:

Linalyl acetate	18.0%
1,8-Cineole	4.3%
p-Cymene	3.5%
Camphene	2.8%
Linalool	2.5%
Camphor	2.4%
Sabinene	2.3%
α-Copaene	1.8%
Trideca-3,12-diene nitrile	1.5%
δ-Cadinene	1.2%
(+)-Limonene	1.1%
Terpinen-4-ol	1.0%

(Graven, private communication, 1999)

Safety summary

Hazards: None known.
Contraindications: None known.

Organ-specific effects

Adverse skin reactions: No information found.

Systemic effects

Acute toxicity: No information found.
Carcinogenic/anticarcinogenic potential: No information was found for snowbush oil, but it contains no known carcinogens.

Comments

Produced in South Africa. Limited availability.

Southernwood

Botanical name: *Artemisia abrotanum* L.
Family: Asteraceae (Compositae)

Essential oil

Source: Aerial parts
Key constituents:

1,8-Cineole	18.6%
Davanone	15.5%
Borneol	7.3%
p-Cymene	7.3%
Germacrene D	4.4%
Camphor	2.8%
(*E*)-Nerolidol	2.2%
Camphene	2.1%
α-Terpinene	1.9%
Spathulenol	1.7%
Terpinen-4-ol	1.6%
Ascaridole	0.8%

(Fakhry, private communication 2003)

Safety summary

Hazards: May contain ascaridole.
Contraindications: None known.
Maximum adult daily oral dose: 440 mg
Maximum dermal use level: 15%

Our safety advice

Our oral and dermal restrictions are based on 0.8% ascaridole content with limits of 0.05 mg/kg/day and 0.12% (see Ascaridole profile, Chapter 14).

Organ-specific effects

Adverse skin reactions: No information found.

Systemic effects

Acute toxicity: No information found. Ascaridole is very toxic (see Ascaridole profile, Chapter 14).
Carcinogenic/anticarcinogenic potential: No information found. Nerolidol and ascaridole display anticarcinogenic activity (see Constituent profiles, Chapter 14).

Comments

Thujones have been reported as major constituents of southernwood oil, but it appears that the cineole/davanone chemotype is currently the only one commercially available.

Spearmint

Botanical names: *Mentha cardiaca* G. (Scotch spearmint); *Mentha spicata* L. var. *crispa* (Bentham) Danert (native spearmint)
Botanical synonyms: *Mentha crispa* L., *Mentha viridis* L. (native spearmint)
Family: Lamiaceae (Labiatae)

Essential oil

Source: Leaves
Key constituents:

Mentha cardiaca

(−)-Carvone	60.9–71.6%
(+)-Limonene	11.4–21.2%
(Z)-Dihydrocarvone	1.0–4.9%
3-Octanol	1.3–2.6%
Menthone	0.4–1.7%
1,8-Cineole	0.8–1.5%
β-Myrcene	0.5–1.5%

(Lawrence 1995g p. 200)

Mentha spicata var. crispa

(−)-Carvone	57.2–68.4%
(+)-Limonene	9.1–13.4%
β-Myrcene	2.3–4.7%
(Z)-Dihydrocarvone	0.9–3.8%
1,8-Cineole	0.9–2.8%
3-Octanol	0.6–1.5%
Menthone	0.1–1.4%

(Lawrence 1995g p. 200)

Quality: May be adulterated with added (–)-carvone (Burfield 2003).

Safety summary

Hazards: Skin sensitization (low risk); mucous membrane irritation (low risk).
Contraindications: None known.
Maximum dermal use level: 1.7%

Our safety advice

We recommend a dermal maximum of 1.7%, based on 71.6% (−)-carvone content, and a dermal limit of 1.2%. We recommend a human daily oral maximum dose of 12.5 mg/kg for carvone isomers (see Carvone profile, Chapter 14), which is effectively not restrictive.

Regulatory guidelines

Has GRAS status. The IFRA standard for either isomer of carvone in leave-on products such as body lotions is 1.2%, for skin sensitization. The Council of Europe (1992) has set an ADI of 1 mg/kg for carvone (isomer not specified). This is equivalent to a daily dose of 90–115 mg of spearmint oil (depending on (−)-carvone content) for an adult, or approximately three drops.

Organ-specific effects

Adverse skin reactions: Undiluted spearmint oil was moderately irritating to rabbits, slightly irritating to guinea pigs and was not irritating to mice or pigs; tested at 4% on 25 volunteers it was neither irritating nor sensitizing. Spearmint oil is non-phototoxic (Opdyke 1978 p. 871–872). Spearmint oil, tested at 2% in consecutive dermatitis patients, induced allergic responses in 13 of 1,606 (0.8%) (Frosch et al 2002b), and five of 318 (1.6%) (Paulsen & Andersen 2005). Of 178 dermatitis patients who were "sensitive to fragrance", 9 (5.0%) tested positive to 5% spearmint oil (Larsen et al 2001).

Few cases of spearmint oil sensitization are recorded, suggesting that they are rare. A 64-year-old woman developed allergic lesions on one knee after applying an infusion made with fresh spearmint leaves for pain relief. She tested positive to 2% spearmint oil and 2% peppermint oil, but not to 1% menthol (Bonamonte et al 2001). There have been several cases of oral lesions linked to spearmint oil. One woman developed a sore mouth accompanied by fissuring of the lips and scaling and edema of the surrounding skin (Skrebova et al 1998). A number of similar cases were reported by both Anderson & Styles (1978) and Francalanci et al (2000). A case of allergic stomatitis to spearmint oil was reported by Clayton and Orton (2004).

Systemic effects

Acute toxicity: Spearmint oil acute oral LD_{50} in rats ~5 g/kg; acute dermal LD_{50} in rabbits >5 g/kg; acute dermal LD_{50} in guinea pigs >2 g/kg (Opdyke 1978 p. 871–872).

Carcinogenic/anticarcinogenic potential: *Mentha spicata* oil was strongly mutagenic in fruit flies (Franzios et al 1997). Spearmint oil was not mutagenic in either a CA test or an Ames test (Ishidate et al 1984). In mouse micronucleus tests, spearmint oil was not genotoxic (Hayashi et al 1988). Spearmint oil showed significant chemopreventive activity against human mouth epidermal carcinoma (KB) and mouse leukemia (P388) cell lines, with respective IC_{50} values of 65 and 61 μg/mL. The oil was more effective than three of four positive control drugs (Manosroi et al 2005). *Mentha spicata* oil was cytotoxic to human prostate cancer cells with an IC_{50} value of 0.09%, but was not cytotoxic to human lung or breast cancer cells (Zu et al 2010). Spearmint oil residues significantly induced glutathione *S*-transferase activity in mouse tissues (Lam & Zheng 1991). (+)-Limonene displays anticarcinogenic activity (see (+)-Limonene profile, Chapter 14).

Comments

(1*R*)-(+)-β-Pulegone is occasionally found in spearmint oils, at up to 1.0%, though this is not sufficient to be of concern (Farley & Howland 1980). The main producing country is the USA, and four types of oil are offered: Midwest native, Farwest native, Midwest Scotch and Farwest Scotch. Scotch spearmint was introduced to the US from Scotland, and native spearmint is believed to originate from Mitcham in England (Kubeczka 2002).

Spikenard

Synonym: Nard, Indian nard
Botanical name: *Nardostachys grandiflora* DC
Family: Valerianaceae

Essential oil

Source: Roots
Key constituents:

Nardol	10.1%
Formic acid	9.4%
α-Selinene	9.2%
Dihydro-β-ionone	7.9%
Nardol isomer*	4.8%
Selinene isomer*	3.9%
Propionic acid	3.4%
β-Caryophyllene	3.3%
Cubebol	2.9%

*Isomer not identified

α-Gurjunene	2.5%
α-Caryophyllene	2.3%
γ-Gurjunene	2.3%
Selinene isomer*	2.2%
7-Hexadecene	2.0%
(E)-Nerolidol	1.9%
Calamenene*	1.1%
Epoxy-ledene	1.0%

(Mahalwal & Ali 2002)

Safety summary

Hazards: None known.
Contraindications: None known.

Organ-specific effects

Adverse skin reactions: No information found.

Systemic effects

Acute toxicity: No information found.
Carcinogenic/anticarcinogenic potential: No information was found for spikenard oil, but it contains no known carcinogens.

Comments

Because of threatened over-exploitation, Nepal has banned the export of unprocessed *Nardostachys grandiflora*, and in recent years cultivation has been encouraged, in order to minimize the picking of wild plants. Limited availability.

Spruce (black)

Synonym: Canadian black 'pine'
Botanical name: *Picea mariana* (Mill.) Britton
Botanical synonym: *Picea nigra* Link
Family: Pinaceae

Essential oil

Source: Needles (leaves) and terminal branches
Key constituents:

Bornyl acetate	36.8%
β-Pinene	14.2%
α-Pinene	13.7%
Camphene	8.1%
(+)-Limonene	5.2%
Camphor	4.9%
δ-3-Carene	3.4%
β-Myrcene	2.8%
β-Phellandrene	2.1%
Borneol	1.4%

(Rondeau, private communication, 1999)

Safety summary

Hazards: Skin sensitization if oxidized.
Cautions: Old or oxidized oils should be avoided.

Our safety advice

Because of its combined (+)-limonene, α-pinene and δ-3-carene content we recommend that oxidation of black spruce oil is avoided by storage in a dark, airtight container in a refrigerator. The addition of an antioxidant to preparations containing it is recommended.

Regulatory guidelines

Essential oils derived from the *Pinaceae* family, including *Pinus* and *Abies* genera, should only be used when the level of peroxides is kept to the lowest practicable level, for example by the addition of antioxidants at the time of production (SCCNFP 2001a; IFRA 2009).

Organ-specific effects

Adverse skin reactions: Undiluted spruce oil was slightly to moderately irritating to rabbits, but not irritating to mice or pigs; tested at 1% on 25 volunteers it was not irritating. Spruce oil was not sensitizing when tested at 1% on two separate panels of 24 and 40 volunteers. Autoxidation products of (+)-limonene, α-pinene and δ-3-carene can cause skin sensitization (see Constituent profiles, Chapter 14). No phototoxic effects were produced in mice or swine (Ford et al 1992 p. 117S–118S).

Systemic effects

Acute toxicity: Non-toxic. For 'spruce oil' defined as deriving from several species including *Picea mariana*: acute oral LD_{50} in rats >5 g/kg; acute dermal LD_{50} in rabbits >5 g/kg (Ford et al 1992 p. 117S–118S).
Carcinogenic/anticarcinogenic potential: No information was found for black spruce oil, but it contains no known carcinogens. (+)-Limonene displays anticarcinogenic activity (see (+)-Limonene profile, Chapter 14).

Comments

A concentrated aqueous decoction of the young branches, known as essence of spruce, was used in times past in North America to make 'spruce beer', an anti-scorbutic beverage for consumption on board ships.

Spruce (hemlock)

Synonyms: Eastern hemlock, hemlock
Botanical name: *Tsuga Canadensis* (L.) Carrière
Botanical synonyms: *Pinus canadensis* L., *Picea canadensis* L.
Family: Pinaceae

*Isomer not identified

Essential oil

Source: Needles (leaves)
Key constituents:

Isobornyl acetate	34.7%
β-Pinene	20.8%
δ-3-Carene	11.5%
(+)-Limonene	9.2%
α-Pinene	8.2%
Camphene	3.8%
β-Myrcene	1.1%

(Rondeau, private communication, 1999)

Safety summary

Hazards: Skin sensitization if oxidized.
Cautions: Old or oxidized oils should be avoided.

Our safety advice

Because of its combined (+)-limonene, α-pinene and δ-3-carene content we recommend that oxidation of hemlock spruce oil is avoided by storage in a dark, airtight container in a refrigerator. The addition of an antioxidant to preparations containing it is recommended.

Regulatory guidelines

Essential oils derived from the *Pinaceae* family, including *Pinus* and *Abies* genera, should only be used when the level of peroxides is kept to the lowest practicable level, for example by the addition of antioxidants at the time of production (SCCNFP 2001a; IFRA 2009).

Organ-specific effects

Adverse skin reactions: Undiluted spruce oil was slightly to moderately irritating to rabbits, but not irritating to mice or pigs; tested at 1% on 25 volunteers it was not irritating. Spruce oil was not sensitizing when tested at 1% on two separate panels of 24 and 40 volunteers. Autoxidation products of (+)-limonene, α-pinene and δ-3-carene can cause skin sensitization (see Constituent profiles, Chapter 14). No phototoxic effects were produced in mice or swine (Ford et al 1992 p. 117S–118S).

Systemic effects

Acute toxicity: Non-toxic. For 'spruce oil' defined as deriving from several species including *Tsuga canadensis*: acute oral LD_{50} in rats >5 g/kg; acute dermal LD_{50} in rabbits >5 g/kg (Ford et al 1992 p. 117S–118S).
Subacute & subchronic toxicity: When isobornyl acetate was given to rats by gavage in doses of 15, 90 or 270 mg/kg for 13 weeks there were signs of nephrotoxicity at the two higher doses. The NOAEL was 15 mg/kg/day which is estimated to be more than 100 times greater than the maximum intake in man (Gaunt et al 1971). This NOAEL is equivalent to just over 3 g per day of hemlock spruce oil for a 70 kg adult.

Carcinogenic/anticarcinogenic potential: No information was found for hemlock spruce oil, but it contains no known carcinogens. (+)-Limonene displays anticarcinogenic activity (see (+)-Limonene profile, Chapter 14).

Comments

Should not be confused with the herb hemlock, *Conium maculatum*, which contains toxic alkaloids, and is not a source of essential oil.

Spruce (Norway)

Synonyms: Common spruce, European spruce
Botanical name: *Picea abies* L.
Botanical synonym: *Picea excelsa* Link
Family: Pinaceae

Essential oil

Source: Needles (leaves)
Key constituents:

β-Pinene	4.8–31.9%
Camphene	7.0–26.5%
α-Pinene	14.2–21.5%
(+)-Limonene	9.5–15.9%
δ-3-Carene	2.5–5.8%
β-Myrcene	3.0–5.2%
Bornyl acetate	3.0–5.1%
β-Phellandrene	1.1–5.1%
1,8-Cineole	0–4.1%
Borneol	0.4–3.0%
Tricyclene	0.7–2.7%
Camphor	0.5–2.5%
α-Terpinyl acetate	0.4–2.0%
Terpinen-4-ol	0.3–2.0%
Santene	0.5–1.2%
β-Caryophyllene	0–1.2%
α-Terpineol	0.7–1.1%

(Kubeczka & Schultze 1987)

Safety summary

Hazards: Skin sensitization if oxidized.
Cautions: Old or oxidized oils should be avoided.

Our safety advice

Because of its (+)-limonene, α-pinene and δ-3-carene content we recommend that oxidation of Norway spruce oil is avoided by storage in a dark, airtight container in a refrigerator. The addition of an antioxidant to preparations containing it is recommended.

Regulatory guidelines

Essential oils derived from the *Pinaceae* family, including *Pinus* and *Abies* genera, should only be used when the level of pcroxides is kept to the lowest practicable level, for example by the addition of antioxidants at the time of production (SCCNFP 2001a; IFRA 2009).

Organ-specific effects

Adverse skin reactions: Undiluted spruce oil was slightly to moderately irritating to rabbits, but not irritating to mice or pigs; tested at 1% on 25 volunteers it was not irritating. Spruce oil was not sensitizing when tested at 1% on two separate panels of 24 and 40 volunteers. Autoxidation products of (+)-limonene, α-pinene and δ-3-carene can cause skin sensitization (see Constituent profiles, Chapter 14). No phototoxic effects were produced in mice or swine (Ford et al 1992 p. 117S–118S).

Reproductive toxicity: The low reproductive toxicity of β-pinene, camphene, α-pinene and (+)-limonene (see Constituent profiles, Chapter 14) suggests that Norway spruce oil is not hazardous in pregnancy.

Systemic effects

Acute toxicity: Non-toxic. For 'spruce oil' defined as deriving from several species: acute oral LD_{50} in rats >5 g/kg; acute dermal LD_{50} in rabbits >5 g/kg (Ford et al 1992 p. 117S–118S).

Carcinogenic/anticarcinogenic potential: No information was found for Norway spruce oil, but it contains no known carcinogens. (+)-Limonene displays anticarcinogenic activity (see (+)-Limonene profile, Chapter 14).

Comments

One of the species most commonly used as a 'Christmas tree'.

Spruce (red)

Botanical name: *Picea rubens* Sarg.
Family: Pinaceae

Essential oil

Source: Needles (leaves)
Key constituents:

Bornyl acetate	16.4%
α-Pinene	15.4%
Camphene	12.9%
β-Pinene	11.9%
(+)-Limonene	11.5%
Camphor	6.1%
δ-3-Carene	5.4%
β-Myrcene	4.3%
β-Phellandrene	2.3%
Borneol	1.8%
1,8-Cineole	1.3%
Santene	1.3%
Terpinolene	1.1%
Tricyclene	1.1%
α-Terpineol	1.0%

(Mainguy, private communication, 2003)

Safety summary

Hazards: Skin sensitization if oxidized.
Cautions: Old or oxidized oils should be avoided.

Our safety advice

Because of its combined α-pinene, (+)-limonene and δ-3-carene content we recommend that oxidation of red spruce oil is avoided by storage in a dark, airtight container in a refrigerator. The addition of an antioxidant to preparations containing it is recommended.

Regulatory guidelines

Essential oils derived from the *Pinaceae* family, including *Pinus* and *Abies* genera, should only be used when the level of peroxides is kept to the lowest practicable level, for example by the addition of antioxidants at the time of production (SCCNFP 2001a; IFRA 2009).

Organ-specific effects

Adverse skin reactions: No information found. Autoxidation products of α-pinene, (+)-limonene and δ-3-carene can cause skin sensitization (see Constituent profiles, Chapter 14).

Systemic effects

Acute toxicity: No information found.
Carcinogenic/anticarcinogenic potential: No information was found for red spruce oil, but it contains no known carcinogens. (+)-Limonene displays anticarcinogenic activity (see (+)-Limonene profile, Chapter 14).

Comments

Limited availability.

Spruce (white)

Synonyms: Canadian spruce
Botanical name: *Picea glauca* (Moench) Voss
Botanical synonyms: *Picea alba* Link, *Picea canadensis* Mill.
Family: Pinaceae

Essential oil

Source: Needles (leaves) and terminal branches
Key constituents:

β-Pinene	23.0%
α-Pinene	16.6%
Bornyl acetate	14.1%
(+)-Limonene	13.0%
Camphene	9.9%
β-Myrcene	4.5%
δ-3-Carene	4.2%
Camphor	2.8%
Borneol	1.5%

(Rondeau, private communication, 1999)

Safety summary

Hazards: Skin sensitization if oxidized.
Cautions: Old or oxidized oils should be avoided.

Our safety advice

Because of its combined (+)-limonene, α-pinene and δ-3-carene content we recommend that oxidation of white spruce oil is avoided by storage in a dark, airtight container in a refrigerator. The addition of an antioxidant to preparations containing it is recommended.

Regulatory guidelines

Essential oils derived from the *Pinaceae* family, including *Pinus* and *Abies* genera, should only be used when the level of peroxides is kept to the lowest practicable level, for example by the addition of antioxidants at the time of production (SCCNFP 2001a; IFRA 2009).

Organ-specific effects

Adverse skin reactions: Undiluted spruce oil was slightly to moderately irritating to rabbits, but not irritating to mice or pigs; tested at 1% on 25 volunteers it was not irritating. Spruce oil was not sensitizing when tested at 1% on two separate panels of 24 and 40 volunteers. Autoxidation products of (+)-limonene, α-pinene and δ-3-carene can cause skin sensitization (see Constituent profiles, Chapter 14). No phototoxic effects were produced in mice or swine (Ford et al 1992 p. 117S–118S).

Reproductive toxicity: The low reproductive toxicity of β-pinene, α-pinene, camphene, (+)-limonene and β-myrcene (see Constituent profiles, Chapter 14) suggests that white spruce oil is not hazardous in pregnancy.

Systemic effects

Acute toxicity: For 'spruce oil' defined as deriving from several species including *Picea glauca*: acute oral LD_{50} in rats >5 g/kg; acute dermal LD_{50} in rabbits >5 g/kg (Ford et al 1992 p. 117S–118S).

Carcinogenic/anticarcinogenic potential: No information was found for white spruce oil, but it contains no known carcinogens. (+)-Limonene displays anticarcinogenic activity (see (+)-Limonene profile, Chapter 14).

Comments

Limited availability.

Styrax

Synonyms: Storax, sweetgum
Botanical names: *Liquidambar orientalis* Mill. (Asian styrax), *Liquidambar styraciflua* L. var *macrophylla* (American styrax)
Family: Hamamelidaceae

Essential oil

Source: Gum

Key constituents:

Liquidambar orientalis Mill*

Cinnamyl cinnamate	21.0%
3-Phenylpropyl cinnamate	7.5%
Cinnamic acid	4.0%
Cinnamyl alcohol	2.0%

(Hafizoglu 1982)

Liquidambar styraciflua L. var *macrophylla*

Cinnamyl cinnamate	38.0%
3-Phenylpropyl cinnamate	32.3%
Cinnamic acid	4.8%
Cinnamyl alcohol	4.1%
3-Phenylpropyl alcohol	3.1%
β-Caryophyllene	1.8%
Styrene	1.8%
Benzyl cinnamate	1.7%
δ-Cadinol	1.1%
3-Ethylphenol	1.1%

(Chalchat et al 1994a)
Quality: Some commercial styrax oils are reconstructions.

Safety summary

Hazards: Skin sensitization (moderate risk).
Cautions (dermal): Hypersensitive, diseased or damaged skin, children under 2 years of age.
Maximum dermal use level: 0.6%

Regulatory guidelines

IFRA recommends that crude gums of American and Asian styrax should not be used as fragrance ingredients. Only extracts or distillates (resinoids, absolutes and oils), prepared from exudations of *Liquidambar styraciflua* L. var. *macrophylla* or *Liquidambar orientalis* Mill., can be used and should not exceed a level of 0.6% in consumer products. This recommendation is made in order to promote good manufacturing practice for the use of styrax derivatives as fragrance ingredients. It is based on a wide variety of RIFM test data with gums, resinoids, absolutes and oils of American and Asian styrax (private communication to IFRA, IFRA 2009).

Organ-specific effects

Adverse skin reactions: There is no RIFM monograph on styrax oil, but an SCCP Opinion cites six unpublished RIFM reports on human maximation tests using four different styrax oils (two samples were tested twice) at 8%. In three of these tests there were no reactions, and the other three, which included both Asian and American styrax oils, elicited 1/25, 2/25 and 3/25 positive reactions. The collective tally was 3/154 reactions, or 1.95%. In 25 tests of crude or purified Asian or American styrax gum, the aggregate result was 62/659 reactions, or 9.4%. This suggests that styrax gum is five times more skin reactive than its essential oil. It is concluded that styrax oil has an

*Volatile fraction of the gum – the other 60% consisted of non-volatile constituents

allergenic potential, but that the quality of the data is poor. The greatest number of adverse reactions (20/25) was from a purified Asian gum (SCCP 2005d).

Systemic effects

Acute toxicity: No information found. Cinnamyl cinnamate and 3-phenylpropyl cinnamate are non-toxic (see Constituent profiles, Chapter 14).
Carcinogenic/anticarcinogenic potential: No information was found for styrax oil, but it contains no known carcinogens.

Comments

It is regrettable that RIFM have sometimes chosen not to make public the results of their tests on fragrance materials. The IFRA recommendation that the raw gum should not be used seems justified on the basis of skin sensitization risk. However, there is no obvious logic in extrapolating a maximum of 0.6% from the (still unpublished) 1970s RIFM reports, and the actual risk of adverse skin reaction from styrax oil remains unknown.

Styrene, which is named after styrax, is the precursor to polystyrene. It is widely regarded as neurotoxic. *Liquidambar orientalis* is produced in Turkey, and exists in var. *orientalis* and var. *integriloba* forms. American styrax originates from central America, mainly Guatemala and Honduras. In a report on trees it has been proposed by UNEP-WCMC that CITES add *Liquidambar styraciflua* to its list of threatened plant species.

Sugandha

Synonyms: Sugandh kokila, kokila, laurel berry
Botanical name: *Cinnamomum cecidodaphne* Meisn.
Botanical synonym: *Cinnamomum glaucescens* Nees
Family: Lauraceae

Essential oil

Source: Fruits
Key constituents:

(*E*)-Methyl cinnamate	13.7%
1,8-Cineole	13.1%
β-Caryophyllene	7.4%
α-Terpineol	6.6%
α-Copaene	4.7%
Terpinen-4-ol	4.0%
p-Cymene	3.6%
2-Undecanone	3.6%
δ-Cadinene	2.9%
Linalool	2.8%
Lauric acid	2.7%
Myristicin	2.5%
α-Santalene	2.1%
2-Nonanone	1.9%
β-Pinene	1.9%
Camphor	1.5%
α-Phellandrene	1.5%
β-Phellandrene	1.4%
α-Caryophyllene	1.3%
Decanoic acid	1.3%
α-Pinene	1.2%
β-Bisabolene	1.1%
β-Selinene	1.0%
Methyleugenol	0.6%

(Adhikary et al 1992)

Safety summary

Hazards: Potentially carcinogenic, based on methyleugenol content.
Contraindications: None known.
Maximum dermal use level:

EU	0.03%
IFRA	0.06%
Tisserand & Young	3.3%

Our safety advice

We recommend a dermal maximum of 3.3%, based on 0.6% methyleugenol content with a dermal limit of 0.02% (see Methyleugenol profile, Chapter 14).

Regulatory guidelines

IFRA recommends a maximum concentration of 0.0004% methyleugenol in leave-on products such as body lotions (IFRA 2009). The equivalent SCCNFP maximum is 0.0002% (European Commission 2002).

Organ-specific effects

Adverse skin reactions: No information found.

Systemic effects

Acute toxicity: No information found.
Carcinogenic/anticarcinogenic potential: No information found. Methyleugenol is a rodent carcinogen when exposure is sufficiently high; anticarcinogenic activity has been reported for myristicin, α-caryophyllene and β-caryophyllene (see Constituent profiles, Chapter 14).

Comments

Produced in Nepal.

Sumach (Venetian)

Synonyms: Smoke plant, smoke tree
Botanical name: *Cotinus coggyria* Scop.
Botanical synonym: *Rhus cotinus* L.
Family: Anacardiaceae

Essential oil

Source: Leaves and terminal branches

Key constituents:

α-Pinene	44.0%
(+)-Limonene	20.0%
β-Pinene	11.4%
β-Phellandrene	4.1%
Terpinolene	2.2%
δ-3-Carene	1.5%
β-Myrcene	0.1.4%
Cuminyl alcohol	1.0%

(Tsankova et al 1993)

Safety summary

Hazards: Skin sensitization if oxidized.
Cautions: Old or oxidized oils should be avoided.

Our safety advice

Because of its (+)-limonene and α-pinene content we recommend that oxidation of Venetian sumach oil is avoided by storage in a dark, airtight container in a refrigerator. The addition of an antioxidant to preparations containing it is recommended.

Regulatory guidelines

IFRA recommends that essential oils rich in limonene should only be used when the level of peroxides is kept to the lowest practical level, for instance by adding antioxidants at the time of production (IFRA 2009).

Organ-specific effects

Adverse skin reactions: No information was found for Venetian sumach oil, but autoxidation products of (+)-limonene and α-pinene can cause skin sensitization (see Constituent profiles, Chapter 14).
Reproductive toxicity: The low reproductive toxicity of α-pinene, β-pinene and (+)-limonene (see Constituent profiles, Chapter 14) and the structural similarity of monoterpenes such as β-pinene suggest that Venetian sumach oil is not hazardous in pregnancy.

Systemic effects

Acute toxicity: No information found.
Carcinogenic/anticarcinogenic potential: No information was found for Venetian sumach oil, but it contains no known carcinogens. (+)-Limonene displays anticarcinogenic activity (see (+)-Limonene profile, Chapter 14).

Comments

Produced in Bulgaria.

Sweet vernalgrass

Synonym: Flouve
Botanical name: *Anthoxanthum odoratum* L.
Family: Poaceae (Gramineae)

Essential oil

Source: Leaves
Key constituents:

Coumarin	46.8%
Methyl hexadecanoate	9.9%
Octanol	3.4%
Methyl linoleate	3.0%
p-Vinylguaiacol	1.9%
Methyl tetradecanoate	1.6%
6,10,14-Trimethyl-2-pentadecanone	1.4%
Methyl dodecanoate	1.3%
Methyl linolenate	1.2%
Methyl nonanoate	1.0%

(Tava 2001)

Absolute

Source: Leaves
Key constituents:

Coumarin	68.0%
Carvacrol	9.7%
(*E*)-β-Ionone	3.1%
2-Phenylethanol	3.1%
Ethyl methylmaleimide	3.0%
Benzyl alcohol	2.1%
Dihydroactinodiolide	2.1%
Geranyl acetone	1.3%
Neryl acetone	1.2%
Phenol	1.0%
Thymol	1.0%
Ethyl tetradecanoate	1.0%
Eugenol	1.0%
γ-Nonalactone	1.0%
Octanol	3.4%

(Lawrence 2009)

Safety summary

Hazards: Drug interaction; contains coumarin.
Cautions (oral): May interact with MAOI or SSRI antidepressants.
Maximum adult daily oral dose (sweet vernalgrass oil): 90 mg
Maximum adult daily oral dose (sweet vernalgrass absolute): 62 mg

Our safety advice

We recommend daily oral maximum doses of 90 mg for flouve oil and 62 mg for flouve absolute based on 46.8% and 68.0% coumarin, respectively, with a dose limit of 0.6 mg/kg/day (see Coumarin profile, Chapter 14).

Regulatory guidelines

Coumarin was banned by the FDA for food use in 1954.

Organ-specific effects

Adverse skin reactions: Undiluted sweet vernalgrass oil was moderately irritating to rabbits, but was not irritating to mice or pigs; tested at 4% on 25 volunteers it was neither irritating nor sensitizing. It is non-phototoxic (Opdyke 1978 p. 757).

Reproductive toxicity: Since coumarin, carvacrol and β-ionone all possess low reproductive toxicity (see Constituent profiles, Chapter 14), adverse effects from sweet vernalgrass oil or absolute are unlikely.

Hepatotoxicity: No information found. High oral doses of coumarin are hepatotoxic in animals and in a very small percentage of humans (see Coumarin profile, Chapter 14).

Systemic effects

Acute toxicity: Sweet vernalgrass oil acute oral LD_{50} in rats >4.1 g/kg; acute dermal LD_{50} in rabbits ~5 g/kg (Opdyke 1978 p. 757).

Carcinogenic/anticarcinogenic potential: No information found. Coumarin is carcinogenic in rodents, but is anticarcinogenic in humans (Felter et al 2006).

Drug interactions: Coumarin inhibits mouse brain MAO, with an IC_{50} value of 41.4 μM (6.04 mg/L) (Huong et al 2000).

Comments

Dermal application of coumarin is not hazardous (see Coumarin profile, Chapter 14). Both absolute and oil are produced in limited quantities.

Taget

Synonyms: Marigold, tagetes
Botanical names: *Tagetes minuta* L. (synonym: *Tagetes glandulifera* Schrank), *Tagetes patula* L.
Family: Asteraceae (Compositae)

Essential oil

Source: Aerial parts of flowering plant
Key constituents:

Egyptian

(Z)-β-Ocimene	31.0–43.3%
Dihydrotagetone	3.0–22.0%
(Z)-Tagetone	4.8–10.7%
(Z)-Tagetenone	4.8–10.3%
(E)-Tagetenone	4.2–7.8%
(+)-Limonene	2.9–6.8%
(E)-Tagetone	0.6–2.0%
Germacrene B	1.0–1.3%
β-Caryophyllene	0.6–1.1%

(Fakhry, private communication, 2002)

Indian

Dihydrotagetone	11.9–48.1%
(Z)-β-Ocimene	16.6–35.3%
(E)-Tagetenone + (Z)-tagetenone	8.1–32.5%

(Z)-Tagetone	18.6–27.2%
(E)-Tagetone	2.5–6.1%

(Thappa et al 1993)

South African

(Z)-β-Ocimene	40.4–69.8%
(Z)-Tagetenone	6.9–21.6%
Dihydrotagetone	5.3–17.7%
(Z)-Tagetone	1.3–12.4%
(+)-Limonene	tr–9.5%
(E)-Tagetenone	0.4–9%
(E)-Tagetone	0.4–2.4%
β-Myrcene	tr–1.4%

(Lawrence 1996e p. 64–68; Graven, private communication, 1999)

Non-volatile compounds

Psoralen	0.011%

(SCCP 2005b)

Absolute

Source: Aerial parts of flowering plant
Key constituents:

Dihydrotagetone	12.2%
(Z)-Tagetone	7.6%
(E)-Tagetenone	5.1%
(Z)-Tagetenone	4.6%
(Z)-β-Ocimene	4.2%
Linalool	3.3%
Ethyl alcohol	2.4%
(E)-Tagetone	2.3%
(+)-Limonene	1.4%

(Fakhry, private communication, 2002)

Safety summary

Hazards: Phototoxicity.
Contraindications (dermal): If applied to the skin at over maximum use level, skin must not be exposed to sunlight or sunbed rays for 12 hours.
Maximum dermal use level: 0.01% (see Regulatory Guidelines, IFRA).

Regulatory guidelines

IFRA recommends that, for application to areas of skin exposed to sunshine, taget oil or absolute is limited to a maximum 0.01% except for wash-off products (IFRA 2009). This guideline has been taken up by Health Canada. The IFRA guideline is based on unpublished research by RIFM, using both oils and absolutes from *Tagetes minuta* and *Tagetes patula*. In a June 2005 Opinion, the SCCP comment that the RIFM phototoxicity data for taget are old and largely poorly documented. The SCCP recommends that, since 'no

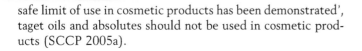
safe limit of use in cosmetic products has been demonstrated', taget oils and absolutes should not be used in cosmetic products (SCCP 2005a).

Organ-specific effects

Adverse skin reactions: Undiluted taget oil was moderately to markedly irritating to rabbits. Tested at 2% on 25 volunteers it was neither irritating nor sensitizing. In one RIFM report taget oil was non-phototoxic (Opdyke & Letizia 1982 p. 829–830). However, subsequent unpublished research by RIFM, using both oils and absolutes from *Tagetes minuta* and *Tagetes patula*, apparently did find distinct phototoxicity, and indicated similar phototoxic potential for taget oils and absolutes (IFRA 2009). A no-effect level of 0.05% for phototoxicity was determined on humans using Egyptian *T. minuta* absolute (Letizia & Api 2000). *T. patula* oil was reported to cause ACD in an aromatherapist (Bilsland & Strong 1990). However this was not an essential oil it was an acetone extract, and it was never established that the extract had even caused the reaction.

Systemic effects

Acute toxicity: Taget oil acute oral LD_{50} in rats 3.7 g/kg; acute dermal LD_{50} in rabbits >5 g/kg (Opdyke 1982 p. 829–830). Taget oil acute ip LD_{50} in rats 0.45 g/kg (Chandhoke & Ghatak 1969).

Carcinogenic/anticarcinogenic potential: No information was found for taget oil or absolute, but neither contains any known carcinogens. (+)-Limonene displays anticarcinogenic activity (see (+)-Limonene profile, Chapter 14).

Comments

There appears to be a high risk of phototoxicity, and the essential oil's content of psoralen is not sufficient to explain this. Another phototoxic compound, α-terthienyl, is found in the plant (Meynadier 1983, cited in Burfield 2004) and may be responsible for the oil's phototoxicity (Towers et al 1979). *T. patula* is also known as 'French marigold' which frequently leads to confusion with *Calendula officinalis*, the common marigold. Most commercial taget oil is *T. minuta*, but oils from *T. patula* are occasionally available.

Tana

Synonym: Issa
Botanical name: *Rhus taratana* (Baker) H. Perrier
Family: Anacardiaceae

Essential oil

Source: Leaves
Key constituents:

(+)-Limonene	25.0–30.0%
α-Pinene	16.0–23.0%
1,8-Cineole + β-phellandrene	16.0–22.0%
β-Myrcene + α-phellandrene	12.0–15.0%
β-Pinene	3.0–5.0%
Camphene	2.0–4.0%
Sabinene	1.5–3.0%
γ-Terpinene	1.5–3.0%
α-Terpinene	1.0–3.0%
p-Cymene	0.5–1.5%
Terpinolene	0.5–1.0%

(Behra, private communication, 2003)

Safety summary

Hazards: Skin sensitization if oxidized.
Cautions: Old or oxidized oils should be avoided.

Our safety advice

Because of its (+)-limonene and α-pinene content we recommend that oxidation of tana oil is avoided by storage in a dark, airtight container in a refrigerator. The addition of an antioxidant to preparations containing it is recommended.

Regulatory guidelines

IFRA recommends that essential oils rich in limonene should only be used when the level of peroxides is kept to the lowest practical level, for instance by adding antioxidants at the time of production (IFRA 2009).

Organ-specific effects

Adverse skin reactions: No information found. Autoxidation products of (+)-limonene and α-pinene can cause skin sensitization (see Constituent profiles, Chapter 14).
Reproductive toxicity: The low reproductive toxicity of α-pinene, (+)-limonene,1,8-cineole and β-myrcene (see Constituent profiles, Chapter 14) suggests that tana oil is not hazardous in pregnancy.

Systemic effects

Acute toxicity: No information found for tana oil, but none of the major constituents are toxic.
Carcinogenic/anticarcinogenic potential: No information found for tana oil, but it contains no known carcinogens. (+)-Limonene displays anticarcinogenic activity (see (+)-Limonene profile, Chapter 14).

Comments

Produced in Madagascar. Limited availability.

Tangelo

Botanical name: *Citrus reticulata* Blanco x *Citrus x paradisi* Macfady
Family: Rutaceae

Essential oil

Source: Fruit peel, by expression

Key constituents:

(+)-Limonene	73.2%
γ-Terpinene	16.8%
β-Myrcene	1.8%
α-Pinene	1.6%
β-Pinene	1.2%

(Dugo et al 1990)

Safety summary

Hazards: Skin sensitization if oxidized.
Cautions: Old or oxidized oils should be avoided.

Our safety advice

Because of its (+)-limonene content, we recommend that oxidation of tangelo oil is avoided by storage in a dark, airtight container in a refrigerator. The addition of an antioxidant to preparations containing it is recommended.

Regulatory guidelines

IFRA recommends that essential oils rich in limonene should only be used when the level of peroxides is kept to the lowest practical level, for instance by adding antioxidants at the time of production (IFRA 2009).

Organ-specific effects

Adverse skin reactions: Undiluted tangelo oil was mildly to moderately irritating to rabbits, and produced some blanching when applied to mice or pigs; tested at 8% on 25 volunteers it was neither irritating nor sensitizing. It is non-phototoxic (Opdyke & Letizia 1982 p. 831). Autoxidation products of (+)-limonene can cause skin sensitization (see (+)-Limonene profile).
Reproductive toxicity: The low developmental toxicity of (+)-limonene in rabbits and mice (Kodama et al 1977a, 1977b) suggests that tangelo oil is not hazardous in pregnancy

Systemic effects

Acute toxicity: Non-toxic. Tangelo oil acute oral LD_{50} in rats >5 g/kg; acute dermal LD_{50} in rabbits >5 g/kg (Opdyke & Letizia 1982 p. 831).
Carcinogenic/anticarcinogenic potential: No information was found for tangelo oil, but it contains no known carcinogens. (+)-Limonene displays anticarcinogenic activity (see (+)-Limonene profile, Chapter 14).

Comments

This plant is a hybrid of tangerine and grapefruit. 'Minneola' and 'Orlando' are two of the most common cultivars.

Tangerine

Botanical name: *Citrus reticulata* Blanco
Botanical synonyms: *Citrus nobilis* Andrews, *Citrus tangerine* Hort. ex Tanaka
Family: Rutaceae

Essential oil

Source: Fruit peel, by expression
Key constituents:

(+)-Limonene	87.4–91.7%
γ-Terpinene	tr–4.5%
β-Myrcene	2.2–3.2%
α-Pinene	0.8–2.0%
Sabinene	0.2–1.4%
p-Cymene	tr–1.3%
Linalool	0.3–1.2%

(Lawrence 1995g p. 41–42)
Quality: May be adulterated with synthetic dimethyl anthranilate (Singhal et al 1997).

Safety summary

Hazards: Skin sensitization if oxidized.
Cautions: Old or oxidized oils should be avoided.

Our safety advice

Because of its (+)-limonene content we recommend that oxidation of tangerine oil is avoided by storage in a dark, airtight container in a refrigerator. The addition of an antioxidant to preparations containing it is recommended.

Regulatory guidelines

Has GRAS status. In Europe, essential oils containing furanocoumarins must be used so that the total level of bergapten will not exceed: (a) 15 ppm in finished cosmetic products intended for application to skin areas likely to be exposed to sunshine, excluding rinse-off products: or (b) 1 ppm in sun protection and in bronzing products. In the presence of other phototoxic ingredients, the sum of their concentrations (expressed as % of the respective maximum levels) shall not exceed 100% (SCCNFP 2000). IFRA recommends that essential oils rich in limonene should only be used when the level of peroxides is kept to the lowest practical level, for instance by adding antioxidants at the time of production (IFRA 2009).

Organ-specific effects

Adverse skin reactions: Undiluted tangerine oil was irritating to rabbits, mice and pigs; tested at 5% on 25 volunteers it was neither irritating nor sensitizing. It is non-phototoxic (Opdyke 1978 p. 873–874). Bergapten could not be found in a sample of tangerine oil, with a detection limit of 0.00005% (Lawrence 1989 p. 43). According to IFRA, the typical bergapten content of tangerine oil is 50 ppm (0.005%). This is not sufficient to cause a phototoxic reaction, but may contribute to the total psoralen content of a mixture (IFRA 2009). Autoxidation products of (+)-limonene can cause skin sensitization (see (+)-Limonene profile).
Reproductive toxicity: The low developmental toxicity of (+)-limonene in rabbits and mice (Kodama et al 1977a, 1977b) suggests that tangerine oil is not hazardous in pregnancy.

Systemic effects

Acute toxicity: Non-toxic. Tangerine oil acute oral LD$_{50}$ in rats >5 g/kg; acute dermal LD$_{50}$ in rabbits >5 g/kg (Opdyke 1978 p. 873–874).

Carcinogenic/anticarcinogenic potential: Tangerine oil significantly induced glutathione S-transferase in mouse liver and small bowel mucosa, and inhibited B[a]P-induced neoplasia of both forestomach and lungs (Wattenberg et al 1985). The oil contains no known carcinogens. (+)-Limonene displays anticarcinogenic activity (see (+)-Limonene profile).

Comments

Assuming a bergapten content of 50 ppm, and to comply with the 15 ppm SCCNFP guideline for bergapten, tangerine oil should not be used at more than 30%. Some taxonomy sources believe that *Citrus reticulata* should now be reserved for mandarin.

Tansy

Botanical name: *Tanacetum vulgare* L.
Botanical synonyms: *Chrysanthemum tanacetum* Karsch, *Chrysanthemum vulgare* L.
Family: Asteraceae (Compositae)

Essential oil

Source: Aerial parts
Key constituents:

β-Thujone	45.2%
Artemisia ketone	10.5%
Borneol	7.8%
Bornyl acetate	7.7%
(E)-Pinocarveol	4.9%
α-Pinene	3.9%
Terpinen-4-ol	3.8%
Camphor	3.2%
p-Cymene	1.6%
γ-Terpinene	1.4%
β-Pinene	1.3%
(Z)-Chrysanthenyl acetate	1.1%
α-Thujone	1.1%

(Rondeau, private communication, 1999)

Safety summary

Hazards: Neurotoxicity.
Contraindications (all routes): Pregnancy, breastfeeding.
Maximum adult daily oral dose: 15 mg
Maximum dermal use level: 0.5%

Our safety advice

Our oral and dermal restrictions are based on 46.3% total thujone content with thujone limits of 0.1 mg/kg and 0.25% (see Thujone profile, Chapter 14).

Organ-specific effects

Adverse skin reactions: Undiluted tansy oil was slightly irritating to rabbits, but was not irritating to mice or pigs; tested at 4% on 25 volunteers it was neither irritating nor sensitizing. Tansy oil is non-phototoxic (Opdyke 1976 p. 869–871).

Neurotoxicity: There is a risk of convulsions with tansy oil (see Human toxicity, below). The thujone NOAEL for convulsions was reported to be 10 mg/kg in male rats and 5 mg/kg in females (Margaria 1963).

Systemic effects

Acute toxicity, human: Toxic signs produced by tansy oil poisoning include convulsions, irregular heartbeat, vomiting, rigid pupils, gastroenteritis, uterine bleeding, flushing, hepatitis, cramps, loss of consciousness and rapid breathing (Grieve 1978). According to King's American Dispensatory (1898), 'Oil of tansy is a poisonous agent, killing by coma and asphyxiation. The effects are different according to the amount taken. The symptoms may be chiefly gastrointestinal, or they may be spent mainly upon the nervous system. Thus vomiting and purging, with colicky pains were present in one case, the patient dying in collapse, but the mind remained clear to the last. In other cases there have been increased frequency of the pulse, pupillary dilatation, insensibility, convulsions, with frothing at the mouth, and, occasionally, death is preceded by paralysis of motion, swallowing, and respiration. Doses above 15 or 20 drops are highly dangerous' (http://www.henriettesherbal.com/eclectic/kings/tanacetum-vulg.html accessed August 8th 2011).

Acute toxicity, animal: Slightly toxic (oral), non-toxic (dermal). Tansy oil acute oral LD$_{50}$ 1.15 g/kg in rats; acute dermal LD$_{50}$ in rabbits >5 g/kg; LDLo in dogs 300 mg/kg (Opdyke 1976 p. 869–871). Both α- and β-thujone are moderately toxic, with reported oral LD$_{50}$ values ranging from 190–500 mg/kg for different species (see Thujone profile, Chapter 14).

Carcinogenic/anticarcinogenic potential: No information was found for tansy oil, but it contains no known carcinogens.

Comments

The plant has been traditionally used to stimulate menstruation and to expel worms.

Tansy (blue)

Synonyms: Moroccan Tansy, Moroccan blue chamomile
Botanical name: *Tanacetum annuum* L.
Family: Asteraceae (Compositae)

Essential oil

Source: Aerial parts of flowering plant
Key constituents:

Chamazulene	17.0–38.3%
β-Myrcene	1.1–13.8%

Camphor	3.1–12.4%
Sabinene	4.1–8.6%
β-Eudesmol	3.5–6.7%
3,6-Dihydrochamazulene	2.2–5.3%
β-Pinene	1.6–5.0%
α-Phellandrene	1.4–4.7%
Borneol	0.5–4.3%
p-Cymene	1.1–3.4%
2,5,8-Trimethylnaphthol	0.6–3.1%
Terpinen-4-ol	0.9–2.8%
7,12-Dehydro-5,6,7,8-tetrahydrochamazulene	0.7–2.7%
9-(15,16-Dihydro-15-methylenegeranyl)-p-cymene	1.2–2.6%
(+)-Limonene	0.8–2.1%
Thymol	0.8–1.8%
α-Pinene	0.7–1.8%
β-Sesquiphellandrene	0.2–1.8%
1,8-Cineole	0.4–1.7%
β-Caryophyllene	0.8–1.6%
Valencene	0.5–1.6%
Germacrene D	0.4–1.6%
α-Terpinene	0.1–1.2%
Caryophyllene oxide	0.5–1.0%
Methyl jasmonate	tr–1.0%

(Lawrence 2001a p. 48–51)

Safety summary

Hazards: Drug interaction.
Cautions (all routes): Drugs metabolized by CYP2D6 (Appendix B).
Cautions (oral): Drugs metabolized by CYP1A2 or CYP3A4 (Appendix B).

Organ-specific effects

Adverse skin reactions: No information found.

Systemic effects

Acute toxicity: No information found.
Carcinogenic/anticarcinogenic potential: No information was found for blue tansy oil, but it contains no known carcinogens.
Drug interactions: Since chamazulene inhibits CYP1A2, CYP3A4 and CYP2D6 (Table 4.11B), there is a theoretical risk of interaction between blue tansy oil and drugs metabolized by these enzymes (Appendix B).

Comments

Limited availability.

Tarragon

Synonym: Estragon
Botanical name: *Artemisia dracunculus* L.
Family: Asteraceae (Compositae)

Essential oil

Source: Aerial parts
Key constituents:

Estragole	73.3–87.3%
(Z)-β-Ocimene	tr–9.5%
(E)-β-Ocimene	tr–9.1%
(+)-Limonene	0–3.5%
α-Pinene	0.5–2.0%
Methyleugenol	0.1–1.5%

(Lawrence 1993 p. 5–6)

Safety summary

Hazards: Potentially carcinogenic, based on estragole and methyleugenol content; inhibits blood clotting.
Contraindications: Should not be taken in oral doses.
Maximum dermal use level:

EU	0.01%
IFRA	0.01%
Tisserand & Young	0.1%

Our safety advice

We recommend a dermal maximum of 0.1%, based on 87.3% estragole and 1.5% methyleugenol content with dermal limits 0.12% and 0.02%, respectively (see Constituent profiles, Chapter 14).

Regulatory guidelines

IFRA recommends a maximum dermal use level for estragole of 0.01% in leave-on or wash-off preparations for body and face (IFRA 2009). IFRA recommends a maximum concentration of 0.0004% methyleugenol in leave-on products such as body lotions (IFRA 2009). The equivalent SCCNFP maximum is 0.0002% (European Commission 2002).

Organ-specific effects

Adverse skin reactions: Undiluted tarragon oil was irritating to rabbits, mice and pigs; tested at 4% on 25 volunteers it was neither irritating nor sensitizing. It is non-phototoxic (Opdyke 1974 p. 709–710).
Cardiovascular effects: Tarragon oil inhibits platelet aggregation (Tognolini et al 2006), an essential step in the blood clotting cascade.

Systemic effects

Acute toxicity: Tarragon oil acute oral LD$_{50}$ in rats 1.9 mL/kg; acute dermal LD$_{50}$ in rabbits >5 g/kg (Opdyke 1974 p. 709–710).
Antioxidant/pro-oxidant activity: Tarragon oil generally has weak antioxidant and radical scavenging activity (Kordali et al 2005a; Lopes-Lutz et al 2008).
Carcinogenic/anticarcinogenic potential: Estragole and methyleugenol are rodent carcinogens when exposure is sufficiently high; (+)-limonene displays anticarcinogenic activity (see Constituent profiles, Chapter 14). Tarragon oil was mutagenic in the

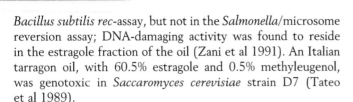

Bacillus subtilis rec-assay, but not in the *Salmonella*/microsome reversion assay; DNA-damaging activity was found to reside in the estragole fraction of the oil (Zani et al 1991). An Italian tarragon oil, with 60.5% estragole and 0.5% methyleugenol, was genotoxic in *Saccaromyces cerevisiae* strain D7 (Tateo et al 1989).

Comments

There are two forms of the tarragon plant, commonly referred to as 'Russian' and 'French'. The 'Russian' type is said to be more shrubby, and inferior in taste and odor. Only the 'French' type is used in the production of tarragon oil, which is primarily carried out in France, with some production in Hungary, Iran, New Zealand and the USA. The 'Russian' oil, is high in elemicin, sabinene and methyleugenol (Tucker & Maciarello 1987; Lawrence 1993 p. 5–6). Tarragon oil may resinify over time.

Tea leaf

Synonym: Black tea
Botanical name: *Camellia sinensis* L.
Botanical synonym: *Thea sinensis* L.
Family: Theaceae (Camelliaceae)

Absolute

Source: Leaves
Key constituents: No useful data could be found

Safety summary

Hazards: Skin sensitization (high risk).
Cautions (dermal): Hypersensitive, diseased or damaged skin, children under 2 years of age.
Maximum dermal use level: 0.2% (see Regulatory Guidelines).

Regulatory guidelines

The maximum dermal use level of 0.2% is the IFRA guideline for tea leaf absolute for category 4 (body creams, oils, lotions) (IFRA 2009).

Organ-specific effects

Adverse skin reactions: Tea leaf absolute has been found to cause sensitization in dilutions as low as 0.001% in guinea pigs; it has not been tested on humans (RIFM private communication to IFRA, 2003).

Systemic effects

Acute toxicity: No information found.
Carcinogenic/anticarcinogenic potential: No information found.

Comments

Limited availability.

Tea tree

Botanical names: *Melaleuca alternifolia* Cheel (syn. *Melaleuca linariifolia* var. *alternifolia* Maid. & Bet.)
Family: Myrtaceae

Essential oil

Source: Leaves
Key constituents:

Terpinen-4-ol	39.8%
γ-Terpinene	20.1%
α-Terpinene	9.6%
Terpinolene	3.5%
1,8-Cineole	3.1%
α-Terpineol	2.8%
p-Cymeme	2.7%
α-Pinene	2.4%
(+)-Aromadendrene	2.1%
Ledene (viridiflorene)	1.8%
δ-Cadinene	1.6%
(+)-Limonene	1.1%

(Southwell 1997)

Melaleuca *terpinen-4-ol type (ISO standard)*

Terpinen-4-ol	30.0–48.0%
γ-Terpinene	10.0–28.0%
1,8-Cineole	tr–15.0%
α-Terpinene	5.0–13.0%
α-Terpineol	1.5–8.0%
p-Cymeme	0.5–8.0%
α-Pinene	1.0–6.0%
Terpinolene	1.5–5.0%
Sabinene	tr–3.5%
(+)-Aromadendrene	tr–3.0%
δ-Cadinene	tr–3.0%
Ledene (viridiflorene)	tr–3.0%
(+)-Limonene	0.5–1.5%
Globulol	tr–1.0%
Viridiflorol	tr–1.0%

(© ISO 2004)

Quality: Tea tree oil also contains 0–0.06% methyleugenol (Southwell et al 2011). The following comments were made in an EU report (SCCP 2004a): 'The stability of tea tree oil in cosmetic formulations is questionable. A standardized method for the specification of tea tree oil is needed. Industry should develop an analytical testing method based on typical degradation products to ensure and control the stability of the material.' Since then, an RIRDC report (Southwell 2006) has addressed these issues. The findings include: that tea tree oil can remain unoxidized and undegraded for as long as 3–10 years if adequately sealed; that tea tree oil contains natural antioxidants (α-terpinene, γ-terpinene and terpinolene) that all oxidize to *p*-cymene, and that an unusually high *p*-cymene content correlates with oxidative degradation; that assessment of *p*-cymene content is simple to carry out.

Safety summary

Hazards: Skin sensitization (low risk).
Cautions (dermal): Old or oxidized oils should be avoided.
Maximum dermal use level: 15%

Our safety advice

Whether for clinical use or in personal care products, a safe and effective concentration of unoxidized tea tree oil is likely to be in the 10–20% range (Table 13.4). Therefore, we propose a 15% maximum. Oxidation of tea tree oil should be avoided by storage in a dark, airtight container in a refrigerator. The addition of an antioxidant to preparations containing it is recommended. Undiluted tea tree oil should not be used on the skin, because of the risk of sensitization.

Regulatory guidelines

Germany's Bundesinstitut für Risikobewertung (BfR), or Federal Institute for Risk Assessment, has recommended limiting the concentration of tea tree oil in cosmetic products to a maximum of 1% (Anon 2003b). COLIPA (now known as Cosmetics Europe) made a similar recommendation, and added that manufacturers should consider using antioxidants in products containing tea tree oil, and/or specific packaging to minimize exposure to light (SCCP 2004a). Tea tree oil is classed as a 'Schedule 6' poison in Australia. Substances in this category are regarded as having 'a moderate potential for causing harm, the extent of which can be reduced through the use of distinctive packaging with strong warnings and safety directions on the label.' The recommended warnings, to keep out of reach of children and to not take internally, are used by many manufacturers

Table 13.4 Adverse reactions to tea tree oil

A. Allergic reactions in dermatitis patients

Concentration	Oxidative status	Percentage who reacted	Number of ++ or +++ reactions	Country	Reference
5%	Not known	0.0%	0/160	Denmark	Veien et al 2004
5%	Unoxidized	0.14%	1/725	Italy	Lisi et al 2000
5%	Oxidized	0.3%	5/1,603[a]	N. America	Belsito et al 2006
5%	Oxidized	0.95%	10/1,058[a]	USA	Warshaw et al 2009
5%	Oxidized	1.07%	36/3,375	Germany	Pirker et al 2003
5% or 10%	Oxidized	1.38%	32/2,329	Australia	Rutherford et al 2007
10%	Not known	0.47%	1/217	Denmark	Veien et al 2004
5%, 25% or 100%	Unoxidized	0.97%	3/309[b]	Australia	Aspres & Freeman 2003
100%	Unoxidized	0.69%	5/725[a]	Italy	Lisi et al 2000
100%	Oxidized	2.4%	13/550[a]	UK	Coutts et al 2002

B. Irritation and/or sensitization reactions in clinical trials

Concentration	Condition	Number of patients	Number of reactions	Reference
5%	Acne	30	None	Enshaieh et al 2007
5%	Dandruff	63	None	Satchell et al 2002b
5%	Onychomycosis	40	None	Syed et al 1999
4% and 5%	Topical MRSA	15	None	Caelli et al 2000
5% and 10%	Topical MRSA	110	None	Dryden et al 2004
10%	Tinea pedis	37	None	Tong et al 1992
25% or 50%	Tinea pedis	158	4 (3.8%)	Satchell et al 2002a
100%	Onychomycosis	64	5 (8%)	Buck et al 1994

[a]Severity of reactions not classified
[b]Healthy individuals

on all their essential oil packaging. However, the recommended use of child-resistant closures on tea tree and other essential oils is not widely adhered to outside of Australia. Although tea tree oil is not restricted in cosmetics in the EU, it is no longer permitted as an ingredient in products making insect repellent claims (http://www.citrefine.com/eudirectives.html accessed July 31st 2011). This ruling was not made on safety grounds, but because no manufacturer registered tea tree oil as an insect repellent by the deadline set by the European Biocide Products Directive. (The European chemicals industry was successful in lobbying for registration to be onerous for natural products manufacturers.)

Organ-specific effects

Adverse skin reactions, irritation: Some irritation was noted when undiluted tea tree oil was applied to rabbits in an acute dermal LD_{50} test, and to hairless mice for phototoxicity assessment (Ford et al 1988a p. 407). When a 25% concentration of tea tree oil in liquid paraffin was applied to the shaved skin of rabbits for 30 days, there were no visible signs of irritation, but some superficial skin changes were apparent on microscopic examination (Altman 1990). The Draize irritation index for tea tree oil in rabbits was 5.0, indicating a severe irritant (Bolt 1989, cited in SCCP 2004a). When tested at 1% on 22 volunteers, tea tree oil was not irritating (Ford et al 1988a p. 407). Tested at 10% on 217 dermatitis patients, tea tree oil produced no irritant reactions (Veien et al 2004). In a study on 306 healthy human volunteers, mean Draize irritancy scores were 0.0038 for 5% tea tree in a cream base, 0.0060 for 25% tea tree in a gel base, and 0.2505 for 100% tea tree oil (Aspres & Freeman 2003). These numbers indicate a substance that can be classified as non-irritant.

It has been suggested that 1,8-cineole is primarily responsible for any irritative effects from tea tree oil, because 1,8-cineole is an irritant (Lassak & McCarthy 1983 p. 97; Williams et al 1990). However, there is no evidence to support this. Tested at concentrations ranging from 3.8% to 28.1% on 25 volunteers, 1,8-cineole was not irritating (Southwell et al 1997), nor was it irritating at 16% on 25 volunteers (Opdyke 1975 p. 105–106). When eight tea tree oils with 1,8-cineole concentrations ranging from 1.5% to 28.8% were tested for irritation at 25% on 25 panelists, there were no positive reactions (Southwell et al 1997). A gel ointment with 2% 1,8-cineole produced no histopathological signs of irritation in abdominal rat skin after 10 hours, nor was 0.05% 1,8-cineole cytotoxic to cultured human skin cells (Kitahara et al 1993).

Adverse skin reactions, sensitization: To test for sensitization, guinea pigs were given intradermal injections of tea tree oil, and challenged with a further application after two weeks. No potential for sensitization was noted (Altman 1990). Tea tree oil was not sensitizing when tested at 1% on 22 volunteers (Ford et al 1988a p. 407). In a multicenter study in Germany and Austria, 5% tea tree oil tested positive in 1.1% (36 of 3,375) dermatitis patients. Results showed great regional variations with, for example, 0% in Berlin and Vienna, 1.1% in Essen and 2.3% in Dortmund (Pirker et al 2003). In a Danish study, one of 217 consecutive dermatitis patients (0.5%) tested positive to 10% tea tree oil, and none of 160 to 5% tea tree oil (Veien et al 2004). In Italy, 725 consecutive dermatitis patients were

patch tested with 0.1%, 1% and 5% tea tree oil. Only one patient (0.15%) reacted to 1% and 5%, none reacted to 0.1% (Lisi et al 2000). In Australia, 41 of 2,320 dermatitis patients tested positive to either 5% or 10% tea tree oil (Rutherford et al 2007). In another Australian report, three of 309 volunteers (0.97%) developed allergic reactions to tea tree oil, but it was not stated which of three concentrations tested (5%, 25% and 100%) caused these reactions (Aspres & Freeman 2003). Three of 28 panelists, (11%) showed marked allergic responses to testing with a 25% concentration of tea tree oil (Southwell et al 1997).

In an onychomycosis clinical trial, 100% tea tree oil was applied twice daily to affected nails for 6 months. Adverse reactions (erythema and/or irritation) were reported in five (8%) of 64 patients (Buck et al 1994). In a clinical trial to assess the efficacy of 25% or 50% concentrations of tea tree oil in the treatment of tinea pedis, four (3.8%) of 158 patients developed moderate to severe dermatitis which rapidly improved on stopping the tea tree oil (Satchell et al 2002a). In a clinical trial for tinea pedis, there were no adverse reactions to 10% tea tree oil in a cream base in a group of 37 patients. Symptoms including inflammation, itching and burning were significantly reduced (Tong et al 1992). In a clinical trial for onychomycosis, mild inflammation was observed in four (10%) of 40 patients, after application, three times a day for 16 weeks, of a cream containing 2% butenafine and 5% tea tree oil. Each application was followed by an occlusive dressing (Syed et al 1999). A clinical trial compared 5% tea tree oil (61 patients) with 5% benzoyl peroxide (63 patients) in the treatment of acne. Side effects were reported by 79% of the benzoyl peroxide group, compared to 44% in the tea tree group. These included redness, pruritis, stinging and burning (no further details given) but the main complaint in both groups was dryness (Bassett et al 1990). In a dandruff clinical trial, a 5% tea tree oil shampoo was used daily for four weeks by 63 patients, and the same shampoo was used without tea tree oil in the placebo group of 62 patients. Mild side effects were reported by three in the treatment group, and five in the placebo group (Satchell et al 2002b).

In a clinical trial using tea tree oil for the clearance of topical MRSA colonization, 15 patients were given tea tree oil therapy, consisting of a 4% nasal ointment and a 5% tea tree oil body wash, for between three and 34 days. No adverse reactions were recorded (Caelli et al 2000). In a similar clinical trial, 110 patients had a 10% tea tree oil cream applied to their nostrils three times a day, and also to skin lesions, wounds and ulcers, and to the axillae or groin area for five days. In addition, a 5% tea tree body wash was used at least once a day on the whole body. No adverse reactions were observed. No patch testing was conducted prior to the study, but patients sensitive to tea tree oil were excluded (Dryden et al 2004). In a clinical trial for acne vulgaris, a gel with or without 5% tea tree oil was applied twice daily for 45 days, then washed off. Three of 30 patients in the treatment group, and four of 30 in the placebo group experienced mild dermal symptoms (Enshaieh et al 2007).

There are 16 reports covering a total of 31 cases of sensitization reactions to tea tree oil during the years 1991–2000 (Apted 1991; De Groot & Weyland 1992, 1993; Elliott 1993; Knight & Hausen 1994; Selvaag et al 1994, 1995; Van der Valk et al 1994; De Groot 1996; Bhushan & Beck 1997; Hackzell-Bradley et al

1997; D'Urben 1998; Rubel et al 1998; Khanna et al 2000; Varma et al 2000; Vilaplana & Romaguera 2000). In 21 cases (55%) undiluted tea tree oil was applied to the skin. One case resulted from ingestion of 'about half a teaspoonful of tea tree oil'. The 60-year-old man had a bright red rash over most of his body, and his face, hands and feet were swollen (Elliott 1993). In one case that was reported twice, analysis of the allergenic substance showed that it was not in fact tea tree oil, though this was not noted by the researchers (De Groot & Weyland 1992; Van der Valk et al 1994).

In a case of polysensitivity, an individual had marked reactions to 13 essential oils, including tea tree (Selvaag et al 1995). A man with hand eczema developed acute exudative edematous dermatitis of the face and eyelids after inhaling the hot vapors of tea tree oil several times a day for two successive days for bronchitis (De Groot 1996). A 38-year-old man experienced flushing, pruritus, throat constriction, and lightheadedness after topical application of tea tree oil. This was an immediate systemic hypersensitivity reaction, confirmed by positive wheal and flare reaction on skin testing and negative reaction to IgG and IgE assays (Mozelsio et al 2003). There is one reported case of linear immunoglobulin A (IgA) disease, which appears to have been precipitated by a contact reaction to tea tree oil. IgA disease is a rare, acquired subepidermal blistering disorder, characterized by basement membrane zone IgA deposition (Perrett et al 2003).

There is no clear consensus on the primary cause of tea tree oil allergenicity. Of seven dermatitis patients already sensitive to tea tree oil, all reacted positively to a 1% solution of the oil, six reacted to (+)-limonene, five to α-terpinene, five to (+)-aromadendrene, one to terpinen-4-ol, one to p-cymene and one to α-phellandrene, all at 1%. A few additional positive reactions were seen when the materials were tested at 5% or 10%. There were no reactions to 1,8-cineole, myrcene, α-terpineol or (+)-carvone (Knight & Hausen 1994). Of three (of 28) panelists sensitive to tea tree oil, one was sensitive to a monoterpene (α-terpinene) and all three were sensitive to sesquiterpene fractions of the oil (Southwell et al 1997). Terpinolene and α-terpinene caused moderate or strong reactions in most cases when tested on 15 dermatitis patients sensitive to tea tree oil (Harkenthal et al 2000). Some of the breakdown products of highly oxidized tea tree oil can also cause allergic reactions, including ascaridole and 1,2,4-trihydroxymenthane (Hausen et al 1999; Harkenthal et al 2000). Multidimensional gas chromatography shows these two constituents in unoxidized tea tree oil at 0.2% and 0.1%, respectively, even though neither was detectable with conventional GC (Sciarrone et al 2010).

Perhaps surprisingly, tea tree oil can reduce the edema associated with contact hypersensitivity (Brand et al 2002a, 2002b) and it significantly reduced wheal volume (but not flare area) in histamine-induced skin inflammation in volunteers (Koh et al 2002). Terpinen-4-ol, applied 10 minutes after histamine injection, inhibited the developing wheal and flare in human skin, but α-terpineol and 1,8-cineole did not (Khalil et al 2004). Undiluted tea tree oil, but not 5% tea tree oil lotion or placebo, significantly reduced the inflammatory reaction in nickel allergy. This was thought to be due to an effect on the antigen process (Pearce et al 2005). In 21 patients with ++ or +++ reactions to nickel, 20% or 50% tea tree oil reduced the severity of allergic

reaction by 40.5%, compared to clobetason butyrate (23.5%) or zinc oxide (17.4%) (Wallengren 2011). Nickel is the most common cause of skin allergy.

In a multicenter trial, a 10% tea tree oil cream was applied twice daily for four weeks to 53 dogs with chronic dermatitis. There was a good or very good response in 82% of dogs, with disappearance of major symptoms. In two cases (3.9%) there were local adverse reactions (Fitzi et al 2002). In another trial, 20 (71%) of 28 dogs were successfully treated for canine localized pruritic dermatitis with a 10% tea tree oil cream, applied twice daily for 10 days. No adverse effects related to tea tree oil were reported (Reichling et al 2004).

Adverse skin reactions, phototoxicity: Undiluted tea tree oil was not phototoxic when applied to hairless mice (Ford et al 1988a p. 407).

Mucous membrane sensitivity: In a clinical trial, there were no adverse reactions to a 2.5% tea tree oil gel applied twice daily with a toothbrush, in 16 patients with severe gingivitis (Soukoulis & Hirsch 2004). In a 4 week clinical trial for AIDS patients with oropharyngeal candidiasis, 8 of 12 who used an alcohol-based tea tree solution experienced mild to moderate oral burning, as did 2 of 13 who used an alcohol-free tea tree preparation. The burning was primarily noted in week 1, and decreased as the condition improved (Vazquez & Zawawi 2002).

Ocular toxicity: A weekly eyelid scrub with 50% tea tree oil was therapeutic in 10 of 11 patients with ocular Demodex (a parasitic mite), reducing conjunctivitis in most cases, but three patients experienced irritation (Gao et al 2007).

Auditory toxicity: In a study of ear toxicity, tea tree oil was applied to the middle ear of guinea pigs. After 30 minutes of instillation, 100% tea tree oil resulted in signs of toxicity to the cochlea (partial threshold elevation of the compound auditory nerve action potential). However, when 2% tea tree oil in saline with 0.5% surfactant (Tween-80) was instilled for the same period, there was no lasting threshold change (Zhang & Robertson 2000).

Reproductive toxicity: There is one report of a 10-year-old boy who developed gynecomastia that resolved after he had discontinued regular use of a shampoo and styling gel, both containing tea tree oil (Henley et al 2007). The products used are not named, but a subsequent website report alleges that they were manufactured by Paul Mitchell, and were analyzed by a competitor. The shampoo was said to contain 'very low concentrations' of tea tree oil, and the content in the hair gel was 'virtually undetectable' (Neustaedter 2007). Dermal absorption of fragrance from shampoo application is about 80 times less than that from body lotion (Cadby et al 2002) and tea tree oil constituents are poorly absorbed by human skin. In one study, only 3% of the essential oil volume, applied as a 20% concentration in ethanol, was absorbed in a 24 hour period (Cross & Roberts 2006).

Tea tree oil does show weak in vitro estrogenic action in MCF-7 cells (Henley et al 2007; Nielsen 2008). However, none of the tea tree oil constituents that penetrate human skin (terpinen-4-ol, α-terpineol, 1,8-cineole) are estrogenic, either singly or in combination, and α-terpineol is anti-estrogenic (Cross et al 2008; Nielsen 2008; Reichling et al 2004). Tea tree oil is not a skin penetration enhancer, and in one study reduced the quantity of other substances (benzoic acid and methiocarb) crossing the dermal barrier (Nielsen & Nielsen 2006). Whatever was responsible for this case of prepubertal gynecomastia, it was not tea tree oil.

Systemic effects

Acute toxicity, human: There are five reports of human toxicity following ingestion of tea tree oil. Three of these were children, and in four cases the doses taken were very high. A 17-month-old boy ingested less than 15 mL tea tree oil and suffered ataxia (loss of voluntary muscle coordination) and drowsiness but no mucous membrane damage and no difficulty breathing. He recovered within eight hours (Del Beccaro 1995). If the boy weighed 12 kg, this is equivalent to <0.8 mL/kg. In a comparable case, a 23-month-old boy swallowed less than 10 mL, with similar consequences and outcome; 15 g of activated charcoal was administered (Jacobs & Hornfeldt 1994). If the boy weighed 13.5 kg, this is equivalent to 1.35 mL/kg. A 4-year-old boy ingested 'a small quantity' of tea tree oil. Within 30 minutes he became ataxic, and soon progressed to unresponsiveness. After being endotracheally intubated by paramedics, his neurologic status improved gradually over 10 hours and he completely recovered (Morris et al 2003).

An adult was comatose for 12 hours and semiconscious for a further 36 hours after swallowing 'half a teacup' of tea tree oil, equivalent to approximately 0.5–1.0 mL/kg body weight. Symptoms, including diarrhea and abdominal pain, continued for a further 6 weeks (Seawright 1993). A 60-year-old man suffered a widespread rash and had an elevated white blood cell count after ingesting 'half a teaspoonful' (~2.5 mL) of tea tree oil. He had taken the same amount several times before with no ill effect, and this was probably an allergic reaction. The rash was neither itchy nor tender, but the skin over most of his body was coral pink, and there was an abnormal degree of exfoliation. Neither his spleen nor his liver were enlarged, and liver functions tests were normal; he recovered within a week (Elliott 1993). The ingested dose was much lower than in the other cases (0.04 mL/kg) and, significantly, no CNS symptoms were reported.

Acute toxicity, animal: Tea tree oil acute oral LD_{50} 1.9 g/kg in rats; acute dermal LD_{50} >5 g/kg in rabbits (Ford et al 1988a p. 407). When administered as a single oral dose to rats, tea tree oil was lethal at approximately 1.9–2.6 mL/kg; when administered dermally to rabbits at 2 g/kg, there were no apparent signs of toxicity (Altman 1990). A total of ~60 mL of undiluted tea tree oil was topically applied to three cats as a treatment for severe flea bites and to prevent further infestation. The cats had previously been shaved but there were no nicks. Later that day, one cat was hypothermic, uncoordinated and unable to stand; one was comatose with severe hypothermia and dehydration, and one was trembling and slightly ataxic. After intensive treatment two of the cats recovered and one died (Bischoff & Guale 1998).

The outcome is not surprising considering the massive amount of essential oil used, ~20 mL on each cat. Given that a typical cat weighs 3–5 kg, this is equivalent to 4.0–6.6 mL/kg. Unlike humans, cats are deficient in hepatic glucuronyl transferase, and so are not well equipped to metabolize essential oil constituents. They are therefore particularly susceptible to essential oil toxicity. The cat that died had elevated liver

enzymes, suggesting hepatotoxicity. Several cases of toxicosis are reported when tea tree oil was applied dermally to dogs and cats. In most incidents the oil was used to treat skin conditions at inappropriate, high doses. Typical signs are depression, weakness, incoordination and muscle tremors. Treatment of clinical signs and supportive care has resulted in complete recovery within 2–3 days (Villar et al 1994).

Antioxidant/pro-oxidant activity: At 0.1% in whole blood leukocytes, tea tree oil demonstrated an antioxidant, radical scavenging activity, decreasing intracellular ROS (Caldefie-Chezet et al 2004). The antioxidant activity of the oil was significant against DPPH radicals and hexanal oxidation. The relative antioxidant activity of tea tree oil constituents was α-terpinene > α-terpinolene > γ-terpinene (Kim HJ et al 2004). The same three constituents decrease in concentration when tea tree oil oxidizes.

Carcinogenic/anticarcinogenic potential: Tea tree oil was not mutagenic in the Ames test (Altman 1990). The oil had no mutagenic activity in *S. typhimurium* strains TA98 and TA100, or on *E. coli* WP2 uvrA strain, either with or without metabolic activation, but demonstrated no significant antimutagenic activity (Evandri et al 2005). None of six commercial tea tree oils were mutagenic in *S. typhimurium* TA98, TA100 or TA102, with or without metabolic activation (Fletcher et al 2005). Tea tree oil showed in vitro cytotoxic activity against five human cell lines: CTVR-1 (leukemia), Molt-4 (leukemia), K562 (myelogenous leukemia), HeLa (cervical adenocarcinoma) and Hep G2 (hepatocellular carcinoma) with IC_{50} values ranging from 0.02 to 2.7 g/L after 24 hours incubation (Hayes et al 1997). At concentrations ranging from 0.005 to 0.03%, tea tree oil inhibited the in vitro growth of human melanoma M14 WT cells and their drug-resistant counterparts M14 adriamicin-resistant cells, due to caspase-dependent apoptosis (Calcabrini et al 2004). Tea tree oil inhibited the growth of mouse cancer cell lines AE17 mesothelioma and B16 melanoma, and was significantly less toxic to normal fibroblasts (Greay et al 2010a). Applied to the skin at 10% for 10 days, tea tree oil significantly inhibited the growth of the same two aggressive, chemo-resistant cancers in mice, though only when combined with DMSO, which enhanced skin penetration of the essential oil (Greay et al 2010b).

Analysis of 128 commercial samples of tea tree oil showed methyleugenol content ranging from 0 to 0.06%. In four exhaustively distilled tea tree oils, the range of methyleugenol was 0.041–0.067% (Southwell et al 2011).

Comments

Bacterial resistance: It has been proposed that the habitual use of tea tree oil in products applied to the skin at sub-bactericidal concentrations might encourage resistant strains to develop (McMahon et al 2007, 2008). However, studies in bacteria and yeasts suggest that any resistance to tea tree oil is transient and/or negligible (Mondello et al 2006; Ferrini et al 2006). This holds true even in bacteria subcultured up to 22 times (Hammer et al 2008, 2012). In cases where they have an effect on resistance, essential oils in general tend to reduce or eliminate it, rather than increasing it. The effect of personal care products containing essential oil mixtures, with or without tea tree oil, is unknowable, since there are thousands of such products. However, the great variety of these mixtures will make it very difficult for resistance to develop.

Ingestion: There are insufficient data to establish a safe maximum oral human dose, which has led some to suggest that the oil is not safe to ingest at all. When taken orally in doses of 0.8 mL/kg or more, equivalent to over 50 mL in an adult, tea tree oil has notable CNS effects, as cited above under Acute toxicity, human. However, an oral dose of ~2.5 mL elicited no CNS toxicity in an adult male (Elliott 1993) and this is above the normal oral dose range of 0.3–1.3 mL for essential oils (Table 4.7). No neurotoxicity has been reported following the dermal application of tea tree oil in humans, even when used undiluted. Severe neurotoxic effects have occurred in cats following dermal administration, in amounts equivalent to 280–462 mL being applied to an adult human. Since a dermal dose of 2 g/kg elicited no apparent toxicity in rabbits, cats are probably more susceptible to tea tree toxicity than other species. In our opinion, the human toxicity data are more or less consistent with the rat oral LD_{50} of 1.9 g/kg, which is within the 'slightly toxic' range of 1–5 g/kg, since doses about half of this amount elicited clear signs of neurotoxicity.

Dermal application: Undiluted tea tree oil was irritating to rabbits and mice, but its irritancy to healthy human skin is negligible. In six clinical trials using tea tree oil at either 5% or 10%, there were no allergic reactions among 295 patients, 67 of them with an inflammatory skin condition (Table 13.4B). Mild reactions were not significantly greater than in placebo groups, and in some cases were less. In skin sensitization, both the concentration and the degree of oxidation need to be considered (Table 13.4A). For example, unoxidized tea tree oil at 5% produced one positive reaction in 725 dermatitis patients (Lisi et al 2000), while oxidized tea tree oil at 5% produced a seven times greater response: 36 reactions in 3,375 patients (Pirker et al 2003). Using the same patient group of 725, when 100% unoxidized tea tree oil was used, there were five reactions, an increase of five times over the 5% dilution (Lisi et al 2000). However, 100% oxidized tea tree oil produced 13/550 reactions, an increase of 3.5 times compared to the 100% unoxidized oil (Coutts et al 2002).

The oil used in the Coutts et al (2002) report was allowed to photo-oxidize in a clear glass bottle over 12 months, during which time 550 dermatitis patients were patch tested. No increase in sensitization rate was noted as the oil aged, but no assessement of peroxide value was made at any point. Of the 13 patients who reacted to 100% tea tree oil, nine were later re-tested with 5% tea tree oil. Four of these reacted, the other five did not (Clayton & Orton 2005). It is important to note that the way tea tree oil was oxidized for these tests does not reflect the quality of tea tree oil found in the marketplace, so these data do not represent real world risk. There were 614 reported adverse events from the sale of 37,135,48 products containing tea tree oil over a 10 year period in four countries, 0.0016% of products sold (Wabner et al 2006).

Unoxidized tea tree oil presents a very low risk, even in patients with compromised skin, when used at concentrations up to 10%. Undiluted tea tree oil naturally presents a greater risk than diluted oil, but there is little information on the use of concentrations between 10% and 100%. Satchell et al

(2002a) reported 3.8% of tinea pedis patients with adverse reactions to 25% or 50% tea tree oil. As an experimental treatment for contact dermatitis, 50% unoxidized tea tree oil was applied to 15 patients with nickel allergy. Since this concentration produced "some redness" in several patients, a 20% dilution was used on the remaining six patients, and there were no adverse reactions (Wallengren 2011).

According to the SCCP: "The sparse data available suggest that the use of undiluted tea tree oil as a commercial product is not safe" (SCCP 2004a). However, there is no definition of what constitutes safe or unsafe. According to Wabner et al (2006) there were 16 reported adverse events from the sale of 12,205,539 bottles of undiluted tea tree oil by an Australian company. This represents 0.00013% of bottles sold.

Misinformation: Much nonsense has been written about tea tree oil safety. About.com, for example, states that the three reported cases of breast enlargement in boys caused by tea tree oil (there was only one, with no causal link) demonstrate that the oil 'may alter hormone levels' and that therefore 'people with hormone-sensitive cancers or pregnant or nursing women should avoid tea tree oil.' The same website goes on to warn that tea tree oil 'can cause impaired immune function.' No literature is cited, but this may be in reference to research showing that the anti-inflammatory action of inhaled tea tree oil acts by inhibiting the (inflammatory) immune response in mice following induced inflammation, while having no effect on mice with no inflammation (Golab et al 2005; Golab & Skwarlo-Sonta 2007). Either that, or it is a very odd way to describe allergic reactions. To refer to either as 'impaired immune function' makes no sense.

The Consultant360 site carries a report published on July 1 2007, by Stonehouse and Studdiford, who make the claim that 'allergic contact dermatitis has been reported in about 5% of those who use tea tree oil' (http://consultant360.com/content/allergic-contact-dermatitis-tea-tree-oil, accessed August 8th 2011). However no substantive evidence is, nor could be, given to support this misleading statement.

Species: The ISO standard allows that tea tree oil may be obtained from *Melaleuca* species other than *M. alternifolia*, "provided that the oil obtained conforms to the requirements given in this International Standard". The composition of *M. dissitiflora* and *M. linariifolia* may be very similar to that of *M. alternifolia* (Cornwell et al 1999). However, the Australian Tea Tree Industry Association is not aware of any commercial oil production from these species, and there is no safety information on these oils, such as methyleugenol content. We therefore do not consider them viable sources of tea tree oil. Six chemotypes exist for *M. alternifolia*, although only the terpinen-4-ol chemotype is cultivated on a commercial scale. Of the other five, one is dominated by terpinolene, and the others are all cineole-rich, with varying concentrations of other constituents (Homer et al 2000).

Tea tree (black)

Synonyms: River tea tree oil
Botanical name: *Melaleuca bracteata* F. von Müller
Family: Myrtaceae

Essential oil

Source: Leaves
Key constituents:

Methyleugenol   97.7%
Estragole   0.3%

(Aboutabl et al 1991)

Safety summary

Hazards: Potentially carcinogenic, based on methyleugenol content.
Contraindications: Should not be used, either internally or externally.

Organ-specific effects

Adverse skin reactions: No information found.

Systemic effects

Acute toxicity: No information found.
Carcinogenic/anticarcinogenic potential: No information found. Estragole and methyleugenol are rodent carcinogens when oral exposure is sufficiently high (see Constituent profiles, Chapter 14).

Regulatory guidelines

IFRA recommends a maximum concentration of 0.0004% methyleugenol in leave-on products such as body lotions (IFRA 2009). The equivalent SCCNFP maximum is 0.0002% (European Commission 2002).

Our safety advice

Due to its high methyleugenol content, we recommend that black tea tree oil is not used in therapy.

Comments

Limited availability.

Tea tree (lemon-scented)

Synonym: Lemon tea tree
Botanical names: *Leptospermum petersonii* F. M. Bailey (syn: *Leptospermum citratum* Chall., Cheel & Penf.); *Leptospermum liversidgei* R.T. Baker & H. G. Smith
Family: Myrtaceae

Essential oil

Source: Aerial parts
Key constituents:

Leptospermum petersonii

Geranial	45.4%
Neral	31.3%
α-Pinene	12.3%
Citronellal	6.8%
Geraniol	2.7%
Isopulegol	1.3%
Linalool	1.2%
Spathulenol	1.0%

(Brophy et al 2000)

Safety summary

Hazards: Drug interaction; teratogenicity; skin sensitization.
Cautions (all routes): Drugs metabolized by CYP2B6 (Appendix B).
Cautions (oral): Diabetes medication, pregnancy.
Cautions (dermal): Hypersensitive, diseased or damaged skin, children under 2 years of age.
Maximum daily oral dose in pregnancy: 54 mg
Maximum dermal use level: 0.8%

Our safety advice

We recommend a dermal maximum of 0.8% to avoid skin sensitization, and a daily oral maximum in pregnancy of 54 mg. This is based on 77% citral content, with dermal and oral citral limits of 0.6% and 0.6 mg/kg (see Citral profile, Chapter 14).

Regulatory guidelines

IFRA recommends a dermal limit for citral of 0.6% for body oils and lotions, in order to avoid skin sensitization (IFRA 2009).

Organ-specific effects

Adverse skin reactions: No information was found for lemon-scented tea tree oil, but skin sensitization is possible due to the high citral (geranial + neral) content.
Cardiovascular effects: Gavage doses of 10, 15 or 20 mg/kg/day citral for 28 days, dose-dependently lowered plasma insulin levels and increased glucose tolerance in obese rats (Modak & Mukhopadhaya 2011).
Reproductive toxicity: Citral is dose-dependently teratogenic because it inhibits retinoic acid synthesis, and this can affect fetal development (see Citral profile, Chapter 14).

Systemic effects

Acute toxicity: No information found. Citral is slightly toxic: acute oral LD_{50} in rats 4.96 g/kg (Jenner et al 1964). Dermal LD_{50} in rabbits 2.25 g/kg (Opdyke 1979a p. 259–266).
Antioxidant/pro-oxidant activity: Leptospermum petersonii oil exhibited high radical scavenging activity in both ABTS and DPPH assays (Zhao et al 2008).
Carcinogenic/anticarcinogenic potential: No information was found for lemon-scented tea tree oil, but it contains no known carcinogens. Citral and citronellal display anticarcinogenic activity (see Constituent profiles, Chapter 14).
Drug interactions: Antidiabetic medication, because of cardiovascular effects, above. See Table 4.10B. Since citral and geraniol inhibit CYP2B6 (Table 4.11B), there is a theoretical risk of

interaction between lemon-scented tea tree oil and drugs metabolized by this enzyme (Appendix B).

Comments

The majority of growers and bulk suppliers cite *L. petersonii* as their source of lemon-scented tea tree oil. The citral CT of *L. liversidgei* has been moderately developed, and may be an occasional source of lemon-scented tea tree. It has a similar citral content to *L. petersonii*.

Tejpat

Synonym: Indian cassia
Botanical name: *Cinnamomum tamala* Buch.-Ham.
Family: Lauraceae

Essential oil

Source: Leaves
Key constituents:

Eugenol	78.0%
p-Cymene	3.2%
α-Pinene	1.5%
Eugenyl acetate	1.2%
Methyleugenol	0.5%

(Lawrence 1989 p. 75–76)

Safety summary

Hazards: Drug interaction; may contain methyleugenol; may inhibit blood clotting; skin sensitization (moderate risk); mucous membrane irritation (moderate risk).
Cautions (oral): May interact with pethidine, MAOIs or SSRIs. Anticoagulant medication, major surgery, peptic ulcer, hemophilia, other bleeding disorders (Box 7.1).
Maximum adult daily oral dose: 140 mg
Maximum dermal use level (based on methyleugenol content):

EU	0.04%
IFRA	0.08%
Tisserand & Young	4.0%

Maximum dermal use level (based on eugenol content):

EU	No legal limit
IFRA	0.6%
Tisserand & Young	0.6%

Our safety advice

We recommend a dermal maximum of 0.6%, based on 78% eugenol content and a dermal limit of 0.5% (see Eugenol profile, Chapter 14). The maximum oral dose of 140 mg/day is based on a limit of 0.01 mg/kg/day for methyleugenol (see Constituent profiles, Chapter 14).

Regulatory guidelines

IFRA recommends a dermal limit for eugenol of 0.5% for most product types, in order to avoid skin sensitization (IFRA 2009). IFRA recommends a maximum concentration of 0.0004% methyleugenol in leave-on products such as body lotions (IFRA 2009). The equivalent SCCNFP maximum is 0.0002% (European Commission 2002).

Organ-specific effects

Adverse skin reactions: No information found. Eugenol is a potential cause of skin sensitization in dermatitis patients.
Cardiovascular effects: Eugenol inhibits platelet aggregation (Janssens et al 1990), an essential step in the blood clotting cascade.

Systemic effects

Acute toxicity: The acute oral LD_{50} in mice for tejpat leaf oil was 5.36 mL/kg (Yadav et al 1999).
Carcinogenic/anticarcinogenic potential: No information found. Methyleugenol is a rodent carcinogen when oral exposure is sufficiently high; anticarcinogenic activity has been reported for eugenol (see Constituent profiles, Chapter 14).
Drug interactions: Anticoagulant medication, because of cardiovascular effects, above. Since eugenol significantly inhibits human MAO-A (Tao et al 2005), oral doses of eugenol-rich essential oils may interact with pethidine, indirect sympathomimetics, MAOIs or SSRIs (Table 4.10B).

Comments

Tejpat leaf oil is commercially available in India, and occasionally further afield.

Thorow-wax

Synonym: Shrubby hare's ear
Botanical name: *Bupleurum fruticosum* L.
Botanical synonym: *Tenoria fruticosa* Spreng.
Family: Apiaceae (Umbelliferae)

Essential oil

Source: Leaves
Key constituents:

Sabinene	39.7%
β-Phellandrene	38.7%
(+)-Limonene	5.0%
α-Pinene	2.6%
β-Myrcene	2.5%
Elemicin	2.0%
Terpinen-4-ol	1.8%
Decyl acetate	1.2%

(Manunta et al 1992)

Safety summary

Hazards: None known.
Contraindications: None known.

Organ-specific effects

Adverse skin reactions: No information found for thorow-wax oil or either of its major constituents.

Systemic effects

Acute toxicity: No information found for thorow-wax oil or either of its major constituents.
Carcinogenic/anticarcinogenic potential: No information was found for thorow-wax oil, but it contains no known carcinogens. (+)-Limonene displays anticarcinogenic activity (see (+)-Limonene profile, Chapter 14).

Comments

Limited availability.

Thuja

Synonyms: Cedar leaf, white cedar, eastern white cedar, eastern arborvitae, swamp cedar
Botanical name: *Thuja occidentalis* L.
Family: Cupressaceae

Essential oil

Source: Fresh leaves and terminal branches
Key constituents:

α-Thujone	48.7–51.5%
Fenchone	12.2–12.8%
β-Thujone	7.9–9.9%
Sabinene	1.8–4.4%
Bornyl acetate	2.3–3.2%
Camphor	2.2–2.5%
Terpinen-4-ol	1.5–2.5%
β-Myrcene	1.8–2.1%
α-Pinene	1.6–1.8%
α-Terpinyl acetate	1.0–1.8%
(+)-Limonene	1.4–1.6%
α-Fenchene	1.1–1.2%
Camphene	0–1.1%

(Yatagai et al 1985; Rondeau, private communication, 1999)

Safety summary

Hazards: Neurotoxicity.
Contraindications (all routes): Pregnancy, breastfeeding.
Contraindications: Should not be taken in oral doses.
Maximum dermal use level: 0.4%

Our safety advice

Our dermal maximum is based on 61.4% total thujone content and a dermal thujone limit of 0.25% (see Thujone profile, Chapter 14).

Organ-specific effects

Adverse skin reactions: Undiluted thuja oil was moderately irritating to rabbits, but was not irritating to mice; tested at 4% on 25 volunteers it was neither irritating nor sensitizing. It is non-phototoxic (Opdyke 1974 p. 843–844).

Systemic effects

Acute toxicity, human: A 50-year-old woman took 20 drops of thuja oil twice a day for 5 days. She was advised to take it by a 'naturologist', but did not follow instructions to dilute the oil to 1% before taking the drops. Thirty minutes after her tenth dose she suffered a tonic seizure and fell, fracturing her skull (Millet et al 1981). In Vancouver, Canada, a 2-year-old female ingested up to 15 mL of 0.1% thuja oil, and within 20 minutes had two seizures (Friesen & Phillips 2006). The type of thuja oil is not specified, nor is the preparation; there is no standard preparation consisting of 0.1% thuja oil. Thujone is mistakenly referred to as an alkaloid.

A 7-month-old child was given daily doses of a 30C homeopathic thuja preparation (made from 1% thuja oil, and then serially diluted 30 times). This would be unusual, since thuja mother tincture is normally made from the plant, not the essential oil. The child, who had a family history of seizures, had several generalized tonic-clonic convulsions over three weeks, which were attributed to the thuja preparation. The logic here is curious since, even if it was prepared initally from thuja oil, a 30C dilution would contain less than a single molecule of thujone. The child was also given a chest rub containing sage oil and camphor several times in the period prior to the seizures. Since sage oil has a high thujone content, this is a more likely cause (Stafstrom 2007).
Acute toxicity, animal: Moderately toxic (oral), slightly toxic (dermal). Thuja oil acute oral LD_{50} in rats 830 mg/kg; acute dermal LD_{50} in rabbits 4.1 g/kg (Opdyke 1974 p. 843–844). Toxic signs from thuja oil ingestion include convulsions, gastroenteritis, flatulence and hypotension. In severe cases, coma is followed by death (Leung & Foster 2003). Both α- and β-thujone are moderately toxic, with reported oral LD_{50} values ranging from 190 to 500 mg/kg for different animal species (see Thujone profile, Chapter 14).
Carcinogenic/anticarcinogenic potential: A thujone-rich fraction of *Thuja occidentalis* was cytotoxic to human melanoma (A375) cells. At 200 µg/mL it inhibited proliferation of 59% of cells and induced apoptosis, with only minimal cytotoxic effects on peripheral blood mononuclear cells (Biswas et al 2011). Thuja oil contains no known carcinogens.

Comments

Frequently sold as 'cedarleaf oil'.

Thyme (borneol CT)

Synonym: Moroccan thyme
Botanical name: *Thymus satureioides* Coss. & Bal.
Family: Lamiaceae (Labiatae)

Essential oil

Source: Aerial parts
Key constituents:

Borneol	20.0%
Carvacrol	20.0%
α-Terpineol	10.0%
Thymol	10.0%
Camphene	5.0%
Linalool	5.0%
β-Caryophyllene	4.0%
p-Cymene	4.0%
Methyl carvacrol	3.0%
Bornyl acetate	2.5%
α-Pinene	2.5%
Caryophyllene oxide	2.0%
γ-Terpinene	2.0%
(*E*)-Dihydrocarvone	1.0%

(Benjilali et al 1987)

Safety summary

Hazards: Drug interaction; may inhibit blood clotting skin irritation (low risk).
Cautions (oral): Anticoagulant medication, major surgery, peptic ulcer, hemophilia, other bleeding disorders (Box 7.1).
Maximum dermal use level: 3.3%

Our safety advice

Our dermal maximum is based on 20% carvacrol and 10% thymol content and a dermal limit of 1% for these constituents to avoid skin irritation (see Carvacrol and Thymol profiles Chapter 14).

Organ-specific effects

Adverse skin reactions: No information found. Borneol appears to be relatively non-reactive with regard to the skin (see Borneol profile, Chapter 14).
Cardiovascular effects: Thymol and carvacrol inhibit platelet aggregation (Enomoto et al 2001), an essential step in the blood clotting cascade.

Systemic effects

Acute toxicity: No information found. Borneol appears to be non-toxic (see Borneol profile, Chapter 14).
Carcinogenic/anticarcinogenic potential: No information was found for thyme oil borneol CT, but it contains no known carcinogens. Carvacrol, linalool, thymol and β-caryophyllene display antitumoral activity (see Constituent profiles, Chapter 14).
Drug interactions: Anticoagulant medication, because of cardiovascular effects, above. See Table 4.10B.

Comments

Limited availability.

Thyme (geraniol CT)

Botanical name: *Thymus vulgaris* L.
Family: Lamiaceae (Labiatae)

Essential oil

Source: Aerial parts
Key constituents:

Geranyl acetate	36.5%
Geraniol	24.9%
β-Caryophyllene	6.3%
Terpinen-4-ol	2.9%
Linalool	2.6%
Myrtenyl acetate	2.0%
Geranyl propionate	1.9%
(*Z*)-Sabinene hydrate	1.6%
γ-Terpinene	1.5%
Geranyl butyrate	1.2%

(Badoux, private communication, 2003)

Safety summary

Hazards: Drug interaction; may be choleretic.
Contraindications (oral): Cholestasis.
Cautions (oral): Drugs metabolized by CYP2B6 (Appendix B).

Regulatory guidelines

Has GRAS status.

Organ-specific effects

Adverse skin reactions: No information found. Geraniol is a low-risk skin allergen (see Geraniol profile, Chapter 14).
Gastrointestinal toxicology: Since geranyl acetate is choleretic (Trabace et al 1994), thyme oil (geraniol CT) should not be taken in oral doses by people with cholestasis (obstructed bile flow) (Fujii et al 1994).

Systemic effects

Acute toxicity: No information found. Neither geranyl acetate nor geraniol manifest any acute or subchronic toxicity (see Constituent profiles, Chapter 14).
Carcinogenic/anticarcinogenic potential: No information was found for thyme oil (geraniol CT), but it contains no known carcinogens. Geranyl acetate is not a rodent carcinogen, and geraniol displays anticarcinogenic activity (see Constituent profiles, Chapter 14).
Drug interactions: Since geraniol inhibits CYP2B6 (Table 4.11B), there is a theoretical risk of interaction between thyme oil (geraniol CT) and drugs metabolized by this enzyme (Appendix B).

Comments

Limited availability. This oil is known as thyme (geraniol CT), although logically geranyl acetate CT might make more sense.

Thyme (lemon)

Botanical name: *Thymus* × *citriodorus* (Pers.) Schreb.
Botanical synonyms: *Thymus lanuginosus* Mill. var. *citriodorum* Pers., *Thymus serpyllum* var. *citriodorus* (Hort.), *Thymus serpyllum* L. var. *vulgaris* Benth.
Family: Lamiaceae (Labiatae)

Essential oil

Source: Aerial parts
Key constituents:

Geraniol	39.2%
Carvacrol	15.4%
Geranial	9.2%
Neral	7.1%
p-Cymene	4.5%
γ-Terpinene	3.7%
1,8-Cineole	2.9%
Geranyl acetate	2.4%
Nerol	1.9%
Borneol	1.7%
(Z)-Linalool oxide	1.4%

(Horváth et al 2006)

Safety summary

Hazards: Drug interaction; teratogenicity; skin sensitization (low risk).
Cautions (oral): Drugs metabolized by CYP2B6 (Appendix B), pregnancy.
Maximum daily oral dose in pregnancy: 258 mg
Maximum dermal use level: 3.7%

Our safety advice

We recommend a dermal maximum of 3.7% to avoid skin sensitization, and a daily oral maximum in pregnancy of 258 mg. This is based on 16.3% citral content, with dermal and oral citral limits of 0.6% and 0.6 mg/kg (see Citral profile, Chapter 14).

Regulatory guidelines

IFRA recommends a maximum dermal use level for citral of 0.6% for body oils and lotions, in order to avoid skin sensitization (IFRA 2009).

Organ-specific effects

Adverse skin reactions: No information found. Citral (geranial + neral) is a potential skin sensitizer (see Citral profile, Chapter 14).
Reproductive toxicity: Citral is dose-dependently teratogenic because it inhibits retinoic acid synthesis, and this can affect fetal development (see Citral profile, Chapter 14).

Systemic effects

Acute toxicity: No information found.
Carcinogenic/anticarcinogenic potential: No information was found for lemon thyme oil, but it contains no known carcinogens. Geraniol, carvacrol and citral (geranial + neral) display anticarcinogenic activity (see Constituent profiles, Chapter 14).
Drug interactions: Since citral and geraniol inhibit CYP2B6 (Table 4.11B), there is a theoretical risk of interaction between lemon thyme oil and drugs metabolized by this enzyme (Appendix B).

Comments

This plant is a cross between *Thymus vulgaris* and *Thymus pulegioides*. Limited availability.

Thyme (limonene CT)

Botanical names: *Thymus vulgaris* L., *Thymus serpyllum* L.
Family: Lamiaceae (Labiatae)

Essential oil

Source: Aerial parts
Key constituents:

Thymus vulgaris

Thymol	27.6%
(+)-Limonene	24.2%
Carvacrol	20.5%
p-Cymene	7.0%
Linalyl propanoate	2.7%
Linalool	1.7%
Camphene	1.2%
α-Pinene	1.1%
3-Octanol	1.0%

(Juliano et al 2000)

Safety summary

Hazards: Drug interaction; may inhibit blood clotting; skin irritation (low risk); mucous membrane irritation (moderate risk).
Cautions: Old or oxidized oils should be avoided.
Cautions (oral): Anticoagulant medication, major surgery, peptic ulcer, hemophilia, other bleeding disorders (Box 7.1).
Maximum dermal use level: 2.1%

Our safety advice

Our dermal maximum is based on 48.1% total thymol and carvacrol content and a dermal limit of 1% for these constituents to avoid skin irritation (see Carvacrol and Thymol profiles, Chapter 14).

Because of its (+)-limonene content we recommend that oxidation of thyme oil (limonene CT) is avoided by storage in a dark, airtight container in a refrigerator. The addition of an antioxidant to preparations containing it is recommended. However, thymol and carvacrol are antioxidants, and may perform this role.

Regulatory guidelines

Has GRAS status. IFRA recommends that essential oils rich in limonene should only be used when the level of peroxides is kept to the lowest practical level, for instance by adding antioxidants at the time of production (IFRA 2009).

Organ-specific effects

Adverse skin reactions: No information found.
Cardiovascular effects: Thymol and carvacrol inhibit platelet aggregation (Enomoto et al 2001), an essential step in the blood clotting cascade.

Systemic effects

Acute toxicity: No information found.
Carcinogenic/anticarcinogenic potential: No information was found for thyme oil (limonene CT), but it contains no known carcinogens. Thymol, carvacrol and (+)-limonene display anticarcinogenic activity (see Constituent profiles, Chapter 14).
Drug interactions: Anticoagulant medication, because of cardiovascular effects, above. See Table 4.10B.

Comments

This oil may be confused with lemon thyme oil, as it is sometimes referred to as such. Limited availability.

Thyme (linalool CT)

Botanical names: *Thymus vulgaris* L., *Thymus zygis* L.
Family: Lamiaceae (Labiatae)

Essential oil

Source: Aerial parts
Key constituents:

Thymus zygis

Linalool	73.6–79.0%
Linalyl acetate	3.4–8.6%
α-Terpineol + borneol	1.4–4.8%
Thymol	1.0–3.8%
p-Cymene	1.5–3.3%
β-Caryophyllene	0–1.5%
Camphene	0.2–.2%
Carvacrol	1.0–1.1%
β-Myrcene	0.3–1.0%

(Lawrence 1989 p. 106; Velasco-Neguerela & Perez-Alonso 1990)

Safety summary

Hazards: None known.
Contraindications: None known.

Regulatory guidelines

Has GRAS status. According to IFRA, essential oils rich in linalool should only be used when the level of peroxides is kept to the lowest practical value. The addition of antioxidants such as

0.1% BHT or α-tocopherol at the time of production is recommended (IFRA 2009).

Organ-specific effects

Adverse skin reactions: Acute toxicity: No information found. Oxidation products of linalool may be skin sensitizing, but carvacrol and thymol possess strong antioxidant properties.
Reproductive toxicity: The virtual absence of reproductive toxicity for linalool (Politano et al 2008) suggests that thyme oil (linalool CT) is not hazardous in pregnancy.

Systemic effects

Acute toxicity: No information found. Linalool is slightly toxic (oral) and non-toxic (dermal) (see Linalool profile, Chapter 14).
Carcinogenic/anticarcinogenic potential: No information was found for thyme oil (linalool CT), but it contains no known carcinogens. Linalool, thymol, and carvacrol display anticarcinogenic activity (see Constituent profiles, Chapter 14).

Comments

Limited availability.

Thyme (spike)

Synonyms: Spiked thyme, thymbra oregano
Botanical name: *Thymbra spicata* L.
Family: Lamiaceae (Labiatae)

Essential oil

Source: Aerial parts
Key constituents:

Carvacrol	70.0%
p-Cymene	10.1%
γ-Terpinene	9.5%
β-Caryophyllene	3.7%
α-Terpinene	1.3%

(Owen, private communication, 2004)

Safety summary

Hazards: Drug interaction; may inhibit blood clotting; skin irritation (low risk); mucous membrane irritation (moderate risk).
Cautions (oral): Diabetic medication, anticoagulant medication, major surgery, peptic ulcer, hemophilia, other bleeding disorders (Box 7.1).
Maximum dermal use level: 1.4%

Our safety advice

Our dermal maximum is based on 70% carvacrol content and a dermal limit of 1% for carvacrol to avoid skin irritation (see Carvacrol profile, Chapter 14).

Organ-specific effects

Adverse skin reactions: No information found.

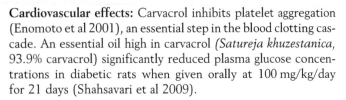

Cardiovascular effects: Carvacrol inhibits platelet aggregation (Enomoto et al 2001), an essential step in the blood clotting cascade. An essential oil high in carvacrol *(Satureja khuzestanica,* 93.9% carvacrol) significantly reduced plasma glucose concentrations in diabetic rats when given orally at 100 mg/kg/day for 21 days (Shahsavari et al 2009).

Systemic effects

Acute toxicity: No information found. Carvacrol is moderately toxic (oral), non-toxic (dermal) (see Carvacrol profile, Chapter 14).
Carcinogenic/anticarcinogenic potential: No information was found for spike thyme oil, but it contains no known carcinogens. Carvacrol displays antioxidant and anticarcinogenic activity (see Carvacrol profile, Chapter 14).
Drug interactions: Antidiabetic or anticoagulant medication, because of cardiovascular effects, above. See Table 4.10B.

Comments

The oil is produced on a small scale in Turkey.

Thyme (thujanol CT)

Botanical name: *Thymus vulgaris* L.
Family: Lamiaceae (Labiatae)

Essential oil

Source: Aerial parts
Key constituents:

(E)-4-Thujanol	39.8%
(Z)-4-Thujanol	7.5%
Myrcenol	7.4%
Linalool	6.8%
β-Myrcene	4.8%
β-Caryophyllene	4.1%
Terpinen-4-ol	4.1%
Myrtenyl acetate	4.0%
α-Terpineol	3.2%
(+)-Limonene	2.7%
γ-Terpinene	1.9%
α-Pinene	1.8%
Sabinene	1.8%
Ocimenone	1.3%
α-Terpinene	1.0%

(Badoux, private communication, 2003)

Safety summary

Hazards: None known.
Contraindications: None known.

Organ-specific effects

Adverse skin reactions: No information was found for thyme oil (thujanol CT) oil or *(E)*-4-thujanol.

Systemic effects

Acute toxicity: No information was found for thyme oil (thujanol CT) or *(E)*-4-thujanol.
Carcinogenic/anticarcinogenic potential: No information was found for thyme oil (thujanol CT), but it contains no known carcinogens. Linalool, β-caryophyllene and (+)-Limonene displays anticarcinogenic activity (see Constituent profiles, Chapter 14).

Comments

Limited availability.

Thyme (thymol CT, carvacrol CT and thymol/carvacrol CT)

Botanical names: *Thymus serpyllum* L. (wild thyme), *Thymus vulgaris* L., *Thymus zygis* L.
Family: Lamiaceae (Labiatae)

Essential oil

Source: Aerial parts
Key constituents:

Thymol CT: Thymus vulgaris

Thymol	48.3–62.5%
p-Cymene	7.2–18.9%
Carvacrol	5.5–16.3%
γ-Terpinene	5.2–6.4%
β-Caryophyllene	1.3–3.1%
Linalool	1.5–2.7%
α-Pinene	<1.0%
α-Terpinene	<1.0%

(Lawrence 1995c p. 67, 1998a p. 42–46)

Thymol CT: Thymus zygis

Thymol	30.9–74.0%
p-Cymene	10.3–37.7%
γ-Terpinene	0.9–10.1%
Linalool	0.2–9.4%
Carvacrol	tr–5.9%
(+)-Limonene	tr–3.1%
(Z)-Sabinene hydrate	0–3.1%
α-Pinene	0.3–2.5%
Terpinen-4-ol	0.1–2.3%
β-Myrcene	0.5–2.2%
α-Terpinene	0–2.2%
Camphene	tr–2.0%
Camphor	0–1.7%
α-Terpineol + borneol	0.3–1.5%
Methyl thymol	0–1.5%
Methyl carvacrol	0–1.4%
α-Terpinyl acetate	0–1.2%

(Jiménez et al 1993; Lawrence 1989 p. 106, 1993 p. 39, 111, 1995c p. 67)

Carvacrol CT: Thymus vulgaris

Carvacrol	41.8%
p-Cymene	27.4%
γ-Terpinene	10.7%
Thymol	5.0%
Carvacryl methyl ether	3.0%
Linalool	1.7%
α-Pinene	1.7%
1,8-Cineole	1.6%
β-Myrcene	1.4%
α-Terpinene	1.0%

(Lawrence 1989 p. 104-105)

Carvacrol CT: Thymus zygis

Carvacrol	43.9%
p-Cymene	20.8%
γ-Terpinene	11.9%
Linalool	4.1%
α-Terpineol + borneol	3.1%
α-Pinene	2.2%
Camphene	1.5%
β-Myrcene	1.5%
α-Terpinene	1.3%
Camphor	1.0%

(Lawrence 1989 p. 106)

Thymol/carvacrol CT: Thymus serpyllum

Carvacrol	15.6–27.8%
Thymol	16.7–25.9%
γ-Terpinene	4.4–12.3%
β-Caryophyllene	6.0–11.2%
p-Cymene	5.7–9.6%
β-Bisabolene	2.8–7.6%
Methyl thymol	7.2–7.5%
Methyl carcacrol	0.2–6.0%
Borneol	0.4–3.3%
Terpinen-4-ol	0.3–2.7%
α-Pinene	0.1–2.4%
1-Octen-3-ol	0.4–1.9%
p-Cymen-8-ol	0.6–1.8%
(*E*)-Sabinene hydrate	tr–1.6%
Germacrene D	0.4–1.5%
δ-Cadinene	0.3–1.4%
β-Myrcene	0.2–1.4%
Camphene	tr–1.4%
α-Terpinene	tr–1.4%
Linalool	0.2–1.0%

(Lawrence 1998c p. 72)

Thymol/carvacrol CT: Thymus zygis

Thymol	25.5%
Carvacrol	22.8%
p-Cymene	18.8%

γ-Terpinene	6.3%
Geranyl acetate	5.2%
Camphene	1.4%
Linalool	1.1%

(Lawrence 1998a p. 44)

Quality: Thyme oil may be adulterated with thymol, *p*-cymene, oregano oil, or other essential oils (Kubeczka 2002; Burfield 2003). There are some reconstituted thyme oils on the market, containing synthetic thymol (Milchard et al 2004). 'Red thyme oil' is often wholly synthetic (Burfield 2003).

Safety summary

Hazards: Drug interaction; may inhibit blood clotting; skin irritation (low risk); mucous membrane irritation (moderate risk).
Cautions (oral): Anticoagulant medication, major surgery, peptic ulcer, hemophilia, other bleeding disorders (Box 7.1).
Maximum dermal use level: 1.3%

Our safety advice

Our dermal maximum for these three chemotypes of thyme oil is based on 80% total thymol and carvacrol content and a dermal limit of 1% for these constituents to avoid skin irritation (see Carvacrol and Thymol profiles, Chapter 14).

Regulatory guidelines

Has GRAS status.

Organ-specific effects

Adverse skin reactions: Undiluted thyme oil was severely irritating to both mice and rabbits; tested at 8% on 25 volunteers it was neither irritating nor sensitizing. Thyme oil is non-phototoxic (Opdyke 1974 p. 1003–1004). In a study of 200 consecutive dermatitis patients, none were sensitive to 2% thyme oil on patch testing (Rudzki et al 1976). In a CAM (chorioallantoic membrane of the fertile chicken egg) assay, an established model for detecting irritants, *Origanum onites* oil with 57.4% carvacrol and 11.6% thymol was strongly irritating. This irritation was due to thymol and not to carvacrol (Demirci et al 2004). In a 48 hour occlusive patch test on 50 volunteers, the highest concentration of thymol producing no adverse reaction was 5% (Meneghini et al 1971). Two brands of thyme *absolute* produced concentration-dependent irritation at 10%, 20% and 100%, but no irritation at 2% in fragrance-sensitive volunteers (Bouhlal et al 1988b).
Cardiovascular effects: Thymol and carvacrol inhibit platelet aggregation (Enomoto et al 2001), an essential step in the blood clotting cascade.
Reproductive toxicity: When thyme oil (thymol/carvacrol CT) (0.25%, 375 mg/kg) was fed to pregnant mice for two weeks, it had no effect on embryo development (Domaracky et al 2007).
Hepatotoxicity: *Thymus zygis* oil (thymol CT) notably inhibited carbon tetrachloride-induced hepatotoxicity due to marked radical scavenging activity (Jiménez et al 1993).

Systemic effects

Acute toxicity: Slightly toxic. Thyme oil acute oral LD_{50} in rats 4.7 g/kg; acute dermal LD_{50} in rabbits >5 g/kg (Opdyke 1974 p. 1003–1004). Animal tests suggest that thyme oil is less toxic than would be expected from its content of thymol and carvacrol. This may be due to antagonism: 'Mixtures of these two phenols in levels resembling their content in the three [oregano] oils showed that the toxicity of carvacrol was reduced in the presence of thymol, thus suggesting antagonistic phenomena' (Karpouhtsis et al 1998).

Antioxidant/pro-oxidant activity: Thyme oil demonstrates significant antioxidant activity both in vitro and in vivo (Deans et al 1993; Dorman et al 1995; Recsan et al 1997). Thyme oil was given to rats in the diet at 42.5 mg/kg/day for 28 months, effectively the lifetime of a rat. Increases were seen in concentrations of the the antioxidant enzymes superoxide dismutase and glutathione peroxidase in various tissues, including the liver (Youdim & Deans 1999). A positive correlation between lifespan and and the hepatic activity of these enzymes has been reported (Barja de Quiroga et al 1992). A thyme oil with 47.9% thymol showed excellent DPPH radical scavenging activity with an IC_{50} of 0.19 µg/mL, and thyme oils displayed high antioxidant activity in various lipid systems (Bozin et al 2006; Lee and Shibamoto 2002; Sacchetti et al 2005). Carvacrol demonstrated a greater radical scavenging activity than thymol (Jiménez et al 1993).

Carcinogenic/anticarcinogenic potential: Thyme oil was not mutagenic in a chromosomal aberration test, the *Bacillus subtilis rec*-assay or the Ames test, with or without metabolic activation (Ishidate et al 1984; Zani et al 1991). It induced glutathione *S*-transferase activity to more than 2.5 times control level in mouse tissues (Lam & Zheng 1991). Thyme oil was cytotoxic to human head and neck squamous carcinoma cells, with an IC_{50} of 369 µg/mL (Sertel et al 2011a), and was cytotoxic to human prostate, lung and breast cancer cells with IC_{50} values of 0.01%, 0.01% and 0.03%, respectively (Zu et al 2010). Thymol and carvacrol display anticarcinogenic activity (see Constituent profiles, Chapter 14).

Drug interactions: Anticoagulant medication, because of cardiovascular effects, above. See Table 4.10B.

Comments

Most commercial thyme oils are thymol-rich, or thymol/carvacrol-rich. These isomeric compounds have similar safety profiles. The type of thyme oil used in the RIFM testing is identified as having thymol and carvacrol as principal constituents, and as being derived from either *T. vulgaris* or *T. zygis* (Opdyke 1974 p. 1003–1004). *T. serpyllum* (wild thyme) is included here because it is also rich in thymol and carvacrol. The source of Spanish and Turkish thyme oils of commerce is *T. zygis*. Oils from *T. vulgaris* are produced in France and other countries. Spanish *T. vulgaris* does exist; its relatively rare essential oil contains very little thymol, and is rich in (+)-limonene and 1,8-cineole. Many chemotypes have been identified for thyme including 1,8-cineole, eugenol, linalool, methyl cinnamate, α-terpineol, α-terpinyl acetate, geraniol, geranyl acetate and (*E*)-sabinene hydrate (Lawrence 1989 p. 38, p. 106; Milchard et al 2004). Most of these are not commercially

available. The so-called 'red thyme oil' is not a different species or chemotype, it is usually Spanish thymol/carvacrol CT thyme oil, containing traces of metals (principally iron from the stills used in processing the oil) which have reacted with the thymol, causing it to turn orange or red.

Tolu balsam

Synonyms: Thomas balsam, opobalsam
Botanical name: *Myroxylon balsamum* (L.) Harms var. *balsamum*
Family: Fabaceae (Leguminosae)

Resinoid

Source: Balsam resin
Key constituents:

Tolu balsam volatile compounds

Benzyl benzoate	46.6%
Benzyl alcohol	41.8%
Cinnamic acid	2.7%
Benzoic acid	2.5%
(*Z,E*)-Cinnamyl cinnamate	1.5%
Vanillin	1.4%
Ethyl cinnamate	0.8%

(Moyler 1998)

Safety summary

Hazards: Skin sensitization (low risk).
Contraindications: None known.
Maximum adult daily oral dose: 384 mg
Maximum dermal use level: 2.0%

Our safety advice

Our oral maximum is based on a limit of 5 mg/kg for 'benzoic acid equivalents', which constitute 91% of tolu balsam. Our dermal maximum is a best-practice estimate for skin safety.

Regulatory guidelines

A group ADI of 0–5 mg/kg body weight for benzoic acid, the benzoate salts (calcium, potassium and sodium), benzaldehyde, benzyl acetate, benzyl alcohol and benzyl benzoate, expressed as benzoic acid equivalents, was established by JECFA in 1996. The CIR Expert Panel considers that benzoic acid is safe to use in cosmetic formulations at concentrations up to 5% (Nair 2001a).

Organ-specific effects

Adverse skin reactions: No information was found for tolu balsam resinoid. The balsam, tested at 2.0%, was neither irritating nor sensitizing when tested on a panel of volunteers (Opdyke 1976 p. 689–690). There are occasional reports of allergy to compound tincture of benzoin, which contains tolu balsam, and reactions to tolu balsam were elicited in some of these cases (James et al 1984). Salam & Fowler (2001) report three cases of sensitivity to tolu balsam. All three patients were also sensitive to Peru balsam. Tolu balsam appears on at least one list of potential allergens (Fischer 1985). The resinoid contains several constituents for which allergic reactions have been reported. Benzyl alcohol and benzyl benzoate are low-risk allergens; benzoic and cinnamic acids may be slightly more allergenic, and benzoic acid is an irritant (see Constituent profiles, Chapter 14). According to IFRA, tolu balsam contains up to 1.7% cinnamaldehyde, also an allergen (IFRA 2009).

Reproductive toxicity: The reproductive toxicity data for benzyl benzoate, benzyl alcohol benzoic acid and cinnamic acid (Table 11.3) do not suggest any restrictions in the use of tolu balsam resinoid in pregnancy beyond those outlined above.

Systemic effects

Acute toxicity: No information was found for tolu balsam resinoid. Both the acute oral LD_{50} in rats and the acute dermal LD_{50} in rabbits of tolu balsam exceeded 5.0 g/kg (Opdyke 1976 p. 689–690).

Carcinogenic/anticarcinogenic potential: No information was found for tolu balsam resinoid, but it contains no known carcinogens. Benzyl alcohol is not a rodent carcinogen (see Benzyl alcohol profile, Chapter 14).

Comments

A resinoid (or resinoid absolute) is commonly available, generally extracted with ethanol. An essential oil, distilled from the resinoid, is occasionally produced. A commercial sample of tolu balsam contained 11.4% benzyl benzoate, 11.0% cinnamic acid, 7.8% benzoic acid and a trace of benzyl cinnamate (Harkiss & Linley 1973). From the few existing data it appears that reactions to tolu balsam are much more scarce than reactions to Peru balsam.

Tomar seed

Synonyms: Timur, wartara, winged prickly ash
Botanical name: *Zanthoxylum armatum* DC
Botanical synonym: *Zanthoxylum alatum* Steud., *Xanthoxylum alatum*
Family: Rutaceae

Essential oil

Source: Pericarp of dried fruits
Key constituents:

Linalool	72.0%
Methyl cinnamate	12.2%
(+)-Limonene	6.2%
β-Phellandrene	5.3%

(Shah 1991)

Safety summary

Hazards: None known.
Contraindications: None known.

Regulatory guidelines

According to IFRA, essential oils rich in linalool should only be used when the level of peroxides is kept to the lowest practical value. The addition of antioxidants such as 0.1% BHT or α-tocopherol at the time of production is recommended (IFRA 2009).

Organ-specific effects

Adverse skin reactions: No information found. Oxidation products of linalool may be skin sensitizing.
Reproductive toxicity: The low developmental toxicity of linalool and (+)-limonene (see Constituent profiles, Chapter 14) suggests that tomar seed oil is not hazardous in pregnancy.

Systemic effects

Acute toxicity: No information found. Linalool is non-toxic (see Linalool profile, Chapter 14).
Carcinogenic/anticarcinogenic potential: Tomar seed oil dose-dependently inhibited aflatoxin B_1-induced adducts in calf thymus DNA, in the presence of rat liver microsomes (Hashim et al 1994). Tomar seed oil significantly induced glutathione *S*-transferase in mouse liver (Banerjee et al 1994). Linalool and (+)-limonene display antitumoral activity (see Constituent profiles, Chapter 14).

Comments

Limited availability. Zanthoxylum is also spelled Xanthoxylum. The seed is ground into a powder and used as a condiment in the East.

Tonka

Botanical name: *Dipteryx odorata* (Aubl.) Willd.
Botanical synonym: *Coumarouna odorata* Aubl.
Family: Fabaceae (Leguminosae)

Absolute

Source: Dried seeds
Key constituents:

Coumarin	38.7–58.7%
Ethyl melilotate	3.9–4.3%

(Ehlers et al 1995)

Safety summary

Hazards: Contains coumarin.
Contraindications: None known.
Maximum adult daily oral dose: 71 mg

Our safety advice

Our maximum oral dose is based on 58.7% coumarin and a coumarin limit of 0.6 mg/kg/day (see Coumarin profile, Chapter 14).

455

Regulatory guidelines

Coumarin was banned by the FDA for food use in 1954.

Organ-specific effects

Adverse skin reactions: Undiluted tonka absolute was slightly irritating to the skin of both rabbits and mice; tested at 8% on 25 volunteers it was neither irritating nor sensitizing. It is non-phototoxic (Opdyke 1974 p. 1005). Unlike impure synthetic coumarin, pure, or naturally occurring coumarin is not a skin allergen (Floch et al 2002, Vocanson et al 2006).

Reproductive toxicity: Coumarin was not embryotoxic or teratogenic at 25 mg/kg in pigs (Grote et al 1977).

Hepatotoxicity: No information was found for tonka absolute. High oral doses of coumarin are hepatotoxic in animals and in a very small percentage of humans (see Coumarin profile, Chapter 14).

Systemic effects

Acute toxicity: Tonka absolute acute oral LD_{50} in rats 1.38 g/kg; acute dermal LD_{50} in rabbits 1.26 g/kg (Opdyke 1974 p. 1005).

Carcinogenic/anticarcinogenic potential: No information was found for tonka absolute. Coumarin is carcinogenic in rodents, but anticarcinogenic in humans (Felter et al 2006).

Comments

We doubt that tonka absolute is likely to be used medicinally, but the oral dose limit is given as a precaution. Dermal application of coumarin is not hazardous (see Coumarin profile, Chapter 14). The seeds are known as 'tonka beans' or 'tonquin beans'. On drying, coumarin progressively accumulates on them, appearing as a white crystalline coating.

Treemoss

Botanical name: *Pseudevernia furfuracea* (L.) Zopf.
Family: Usneaceae

Absolute

Source: Dried plant
Key constituents:

β-Sitosterol + stigmasterol	8.0%
Physodone	4.7%
Methyl β-orcinolcarboxylate	3.6%
2'-*o*-Methylphysodone	1.1%
Ethyl hematommate	1.0%
Dehydroabietic acid	0.3%
Atranol	0.3%
Chloroatranol	0.2%

(Joulain & Tabacchi 2009b)

Safety summary

Hazards: Skin sensitization (high risk).

Contraindications (dermal): Hypersensitive, diseased or damaged skin, children under 2 years of age.
Maximum dermal use level: 0.1%

Regulatory guidelines

Treemoss absolute, resinoid or concrete should not be used such that the level in finished products applied to the skin exceeds 0.1%, and the maximum concentration of combined oakmoss and treemoss extracts should not exceed 0.1% (SCCNFP 2001a; IFRA 2009). IFRA requires that treemoss extracts not contain more than 0.8% dehydroabietic acid as a marker of 2% resin acids, since oxidation products of resin acids are sensitizing.

Organ-specific effects

Adverse skin reactions: When treemoss absolute was applied to the ears of mice at concentrations ranging from 0.5% to 20% in a local lymph node assay, there were no sensitization reactions (Johnson 2004, cited in SCCP 2004b). When it was patch tested at 5% on 50 dermatitis patients who were not thought to be sensitive to fragrance there were no positive reactions. When it was tested at 5% on 20 fragrance-sensitive patients, there were six positive reactions (Larsen 1977). In two large European studies, 1% treemoss absolute produced 50/1,503 (3.3%) and 45/1,658 (2.7%) positive reactions in dermatitis patients (Heisterberg et al 2011, Schnuch et al 2007a). An RIFM monograph on treemoss *concrete* concluded that it was non-phototoxic (Opdyke 1975 p. 915–917).

Systemic effects

Acute toxicity: No information found. The acute oral LD_{50} was reported as 4.33 mL/kg for treemoss *concrete* (Opdyke 1975 p. 915–917).

Carcinogenic/anticarcinogenic potential: No information found.

Comments

The botanical source of treemoss has previously, and erroneously, been given as species of *Usnea or Parmelia*. Treemoss extracts (concretes and resinoids are also available) are produced from lichen growing predominantly on conifers in Europe, mainly *Pinus* species, and in particular *P. sylvestris*. Due to the way in which the raw material is manually collected, small quantities of pine twigs, bark and needles are also present, and these are the origin of the (allergenic) resin acid contamination (Lepoittevin & Meschkat 2000). Atranol and chloroatranol are also allergenic (see Oakmoss).

Tuberose

Botanical name: *Polianthes tuberosa* L.
Family: Agavaceae

Absolute

Source: Flowers
Key constituents:

(*E*)-Methyl isoeugenol	32.5%

Methyl salicylate	8.4%
Benzyl benzoate	8.3%
Methyl benzoate	7.8%
Hexadecanoic acid	6.6%
Oleic acid	3.6%
1,8-Cineole	3.5%
(Z)-5,11,14,17-Eicosatetraenoate methyl	3.4%
Benzyl salicylate	2.6%
(E)-Isoeugenol	2.6%
α-Terpineol	2.3%
(E,E)-Farnesol	1.7%
Methyleugenol	1.7%
(E,E)-α-Farnesene	1.6%
(Z,Z)-9,12-Octadecadienoic acid	1.1%
Benzyl cyanide	1.0%
2-Phenylethyl ester benzoic acid	1.0%

(Jones, private communication, 2002; IFRA 2009)

Safety summary

Hazards: May contain methyleugenol; skin sensitization (moderate risk).
Cautions (dermal): Hypersensitive, diseased or damaged skin, children under 2 years of age.
Maximum dermal use level:

EU	0.01%
IFRA	0.02%
Tisserand & Young	1.2%

Our safety advice

We recommend a dermal maximum of 1.2%, based on 1.7% methyleugenol content with a dermal limit of 0.02% (see Methyleugenol profile, Chapter 14).

Regulatory guidelines

IFRA recommends a maximum concentration of 0.0004% methyleugenol in leave-on products such as body lotions (IFRA 2009). The equivalent SCCNFP maximum is 0.0002% (European Commission 2002).

Organ-specific effects

Adverse skin reactions: Tested at 2%, 10% and 20% on an average of 21 volunteers with a previous history of reaction to fragrance materials, tuberose absolute produced allergic reactions in 2, 8 and 7 individuals, respectively. In this high-risk group, 0.5% was the concentration at which any observable reaction disappears (Bouhlal et al 1988b). Tuberose *concrete* dermal LD_{50} in guinea pigs reported as >5 g/kg. Skin reactions noted included severe erythema in 7 of 10 guinea pigs. No irritation occurred in 79 healthy male and female volunteers after a 1% concentration of tuberose absolute was patch tested under occlusion. The undiluted material produced one weak reaction in 25 volunteers in a patch test evaluation for skin irritation. Tested for sensitization on 25 healthy male and female volunteers at 1%, tuberose *concrete* produced one positive reaction. Tested on two further panels, each consisting of 27 volunteers, the same batch sample produced no significant irritant or allergic reactions. In a series of patch tests conducted from 1978 to 1985, tuberose produced positive reactions in 3.5% of a population with eczema or dermatitis. No details were given of concentration or type of extract, or of the vehicle used. Tuberose *concrete* was non-phototoxic in both hairless mice and human subjects. Tested at 2%, 10% and 20%, on 17, 24 and 23 individuals, respectively, it produced no photosensitization reactions in patients with a previous history of allergic reactions to Peru balsam and/or perfumes or fragrance materials (Letizia et al 2000 pS231–S233). Tuberose absolute was similarly non-phototoxic (Bouhlal et al 1988b).

Systemic effects

Acute toxicity: No information found. Acute oral LD_{50} in rats for tuberose concrete >5 g/kg (Letizia et al 2000 p. S231–S233).
Carcinogenic/anticarcinogenic potential: No information found. Methyleugenol is a rodent carcinogen if exposure is sufficiently high; anticarcinogenic activity has been reported for farnesol (see Constituent profiles, Chapter 14).

Comments

A benzyl cyanide content of 1.0%, found only in Indian tuberose absolute, would require a maximum dermal use level of 12.5%, but this is eclipsed by the need to restrict methyleugenol. Similarly, maximum dermal use levels for isoeugenol and methyl salicylate do not apply, as they are higher than that of methyleugenol. Formerly produced by the enfleurage process, tuberose absolute is now solvent extracted, usually with petroleum ether, to produce the concrete, followed by alcohol extraction to produce the absolute (Burfield 2000 p. 381).

Turmeric leaf

Botanical name: *Curcuma longa* L.
Family: Zingiberaceae

Essential oil

Source: Leaves
Key constituents:

α-Phellandrene	53.4%
Terpinolene	11.5%
1,8-Cineole	8.5%
p-Cymene	4.8%
2-Octanol	3.0%
α-Pinene	2.3%
γ-Terpinene	2.2%
(+)-Limonene	2.0%
β-Pinene	1.8%
δ-3-Carene	1.0%
Undecanol	1.0%

(Raina et al 2005)

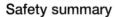

Safety summary

Hazards: None known.
Contraindications: None known.

Organ-specific effects

Adverse skin reactions: No information found. There is some suspicion that α-phellandrene might cause skin sensitization, possibly on oxidation.

Systemic effects

Acute toxicity: No information found. α-Phellandrene is non-toxic (see α-Phellandrene profile, Chapter 14).
Carcinogenic/anticarcinogenic potential: No information was found for turmeric leaf oil but it contains no known carcinogens.

Comments

Limited availability. Very similar constituents to those given above are reported by Ramachandraiah et al (1998).

Turmeric rhizome

Synonym: Curcuma, Indian saffron
Botanical name: *Curcuma longa* L.
Botanical synonym: *Curcuma domestica* Val.
Family: Zingiberaceae

Essential oil

Source: Dried, crushed rhizomes
Key constituents:

Turmerone	8.0–28.4%
ar-Turmerone	15.5–27.5%
Zingiberene	11.6–16.8%
α-Phellandrene	0.7–12.8%
β-Sesquiphellandrene	8.8–9.5%
ar-Curcumene	2.8–.3%
1,8-Cineole	0–6.9%
β-Curcumene	0–5.6%
Carlone	0–4.9%
α-Caryophyllene	0–3.9%
Terpinolene	0–3.9%
β-Bisabolene	1.8–2.2%
β-Caryophyllene	0.2–2.0%
p-Cymene	0.3–1.4%

(Toussaint 1982; Teubes, private communication, 2003)

Safety summary

Hazards: Drug interaction
Cautions (oral): Diabetes medication

Regulatory guidelines

Has GRAS status.

Organ-specific effects

Adverse skin reactions: Undiluted turmeric rhizome oil was slightly irritating to rabbits, but was not irritating to mice; tested at 4% on 25 volunteers it was neither irritating nor sensitizing. It is non-phototoxic (Opdyke & Letizia 1983 p. 839–841).
Cardiovascular effects: A turmeric oil with 45.0–58.0% *ar*-turmerone dose-dependently inhibited glucosidase enzymes more effectively than the antidiabetic drug acarbose (Lekshmi et al 2012).

Systemic effects

Acute toxicity, animal: Non-toxic. Turmeric rhizome oil acute oral LD_{50} in rats >5 g/kg; acute dermal LD_{50} in rabbits >5 g/kg (Opdyke & Letizia 1983 p. 839–841).
Subchronic toxicity, human: Turmeric rhizome oil was orally administered to eight volunteers at 0.2 mL 3 times daily for one month, followed by 1.0 mL per day in three divided doses for 2 further months. One developed a rash on the trunk on the second day; this became worse on the seventh day, and the volunteer dropped out of the study. The rash subsequently resolved. In the remaining seven volunteers, compared to baseline measurements, there were no significant changes in heart rate, blood pressure, body weight, hematological tests (hemoglobin, hematocrit, RBS, total WBC, clotting time, bleeding time, prothrombin time) liver function tests or kidney function tests. In lipid profile testing, six volunteers showed no change in fasting sugar, cholesterol, triglycerides, HDL or LDL. In one volunteer, tricglycerides and LDL were normal at 4 weeks, but elevated at 12 weeks. Levels had returned to normal one month after discontinuing the turmeric oil. There was no change in the menstrual pattern of the three female volunteers. The turmeric oil used in this study contained 59% turmerone + *ar*-turmerone, and 25% zingiberene (Joshi et al 2003).
Antioxidant/pro-oxidant activity: Turmeric rhizome oil has demonstrated significant antioxidant and DPPH radical scavenging activity (Sacchetti et al 2005; Zhao et al 2010). The essential oil counteracted oxidative stress in rats, reducing ROS in brain tissue (Rathore et al 2008).
Carcinogenic/anticarcinogenic potential: Turmeric rhizome oil was markedly antimutagenic against sodium azide in the Ames test, and showed a possibly related antioxidant activity (Jayaprakasha et al 2002). Turmeric rhizome oil was active against human mouth epidermal carcinoma (KB) cells and mouse leukemia (P388) cells, with respective IC_{50} values of 1.088 and 0.084 mg/mL (Manosroi et al 2005). Turmeric rhizome oil contains no known carcinogens. β-Sesquiphellandrene, *ar*-turmerone and α-caryophyllene display anticarcinogenic activity (see Constituent profiles, Chapter 14).
Drug interactions: Antidiabetic medication, because of cardiovascular effects, above. See Table 4.10B.

Comments

Curcumin, present in turmeric rhizomes, oleoresin and CO_2 extract, has not been reported in the essential oil. Curcumin is an orange/yellow compound possessing notable anticarcinogenic activity.

Turmeric (wild)

Botanical name: *Curcuma aromatica* Salisb.
Family: Zingiberaceae

Essential oil

Source: Rhizomes
Key constituents:

β-Curcumene	25.5–29.9%
Xanthorrhizol	16.2–25.7%
ar-Curcumene	18.6–22.1%
Germacrone	2.4–4.9%
Camphor	2.4–3.9%
Curzerenone	3.3–3.6%
Curzerene	3.2–3.3%
β-Farnesene	1.8–2.6%
ar-Turmerol	0–1.5%
α-Bergamotene	0.5–1.4%
α-Terpineol	0–1.4%
β-Elemene	1.0–1.1%
α-Zingiberene	1.0–1.1%
1,8-Cineole	0.1–1.0%

(Kojima et al 1998; Zwaving & Bos 1992)

Safety summary

Hazards: None known.
Contraindications: None known.

Organ-specific effects

Adverse skin reactions: No information was found for wild turmeric oil or its three major constituents.

Systemic effects

Acute toxicity: No information was found for wild turmeric oil or the curcumenes. Xanthorrhizol has antinephrotoxic properties (Kim et al 2005).
Carcinogenic/anticarcinogenic potential: Wild turmeric oil inhibits hepatic tumors in both rats and mice (Wu WY et al 1998b, 2000). Administered ip to rats, wild turmeric oil prevented the development of esophageal cancer through an antioxidant mechanism (Li Y et al 2009). In China, the oil has been used in the clinical treatment of liver cancers by direct infusion into the hepatic artery (Chen CY et al 2003, Cheng et al 1999, 2001). Xanthorrhizol and β-elemene display anticarcinogenic activity (see Constituent profiles, Chapter 14). Germacrone dose-dependently inhibited the growth of human breast cancer cells (MCF-7 and MDA-MB-231) in vitro (Zhong et al 2011). Curzerenone has been used as an anticancer agent in China (Hsu 1980).

Comments

Wild turmeric oil is produced in China and India.

Turpentine

Synonyms: Terebinth, yarmor
Botanical names: *Pinus ayacahuite* Ehrenb. (Mexican white pine); *Pinus caribaea* auct. (Caribbean pine); *Pinus contorta* Douglas ex Loud. var. *latifolia* Engelm. (Rocky Mountain lodgepole pine); *Pinus elliottii* Engelm. (slash pine); *Pinus halepensis* Mill. (Aleppo pine); *Pinus insularis* Endl. (syn. *Pinus kesiya* Royle ex Gordon) (Khasia pine); *Pinus latteri* Mason (Tenasserim pine); *Pinus merkusii* Jungh. & de Vriese (Merkus pine); *Pinus palustris* Mill. (longleaf pine, yellow pine); *Pinus pinaster* Aiton (maritime pine, ocean pine); *Pinus radiata* D. Don (Monterey pine); *Pinus roxburghii* Sarg. (Chir pine); *Pinus tabulaeformis* Carr. (Chinese pine, Chinese red pine); *Pinus teocote* Schiede ex Schltdl. & Cham. (twisted leaf pine); *Pinus yunnanensis* Franch. (Chinese pine, Yunnan pine)
Family: Pinaceae

Essential oil

Source: The oleoresin
Key constituents:

Pinus caribaea

α-Pinene	68.2%
β-Pinene	13.2%
β-Phellandrene	9.3%
Camphene	1.6%
β-Myrcene	1.5%

(Zhu et al 1995)

Pinus eliottii

α-Pinene	48.9%
β-Pinene	24.9%
Myrtenol	2.7%
Pinocarveol	2.6%
α Campholenal	1.3%
Umbellulone	1.3%

(Zhu et al 1995)

Pinus insularis

α-Pinene	87.8–94.3%
β-Phellandrene	1.1–4.5%
Camphene	1.0–4.5%
(+)-Limonene	0.7–2.0%
β-Pinene	0.9–1.1%

(Jantan et al 2002)

Pinus merkusii

α-Pinene	53.9–88.6%
(+)-Limonene	0.4–25.2%
β-Phellandrene	0.2–0.8%
δ-3-Carene	0.2–10.3%
α-Phellandrene	0–8.0%
β-Pinene	0.9–5.5%
Terpinolene	0.1–3.0%

β-Myrcene	0.8–2.9%

(Jantan et al 2002)

Pinus pinaster

α-Pinene	44.1–78.0%
β-Pinene	17.0–29.5%
β-Myrcene	0–4.7%
β-Caryophyllene	0.1–3.4%
δ-3-Carene	0–3.3%
(+)-Limonene	1.4–3.2%
Germacrene D	0–2.1%
α-Terpineol	0.1–1.3%
Camphene	tr-1.0%

(Kubeczka & Schultze 1987; Leseche et al 1984)

Pinus yunnanensis

α-Pinene	49.2%
β-Pinene	25.9%
β-Phellandrene	9.5%
Camphene	3.0%
δ-3-Carene	3.0%
β-Myrcene	2.9%
Terpinolene	1.4%

(Din 1983)

Safety summary

Hazards: Skin sensitization if oxidized; chronic inhalation may be asthmagenic.
Cautions: Old or oxidized oils should be avoided.
Cautions (dermal): Hypersensitive, diseased or damaged skin, children under 2 years of age.

Our safety advice

Because of its α-pinene and δ-3-carene content we recommend that oxidation of turpentine oil is avoided by storage in a dark, airtight container in a refrigerator. The addition of an antioxidant to preparations containing it is recommended.

Regulatory guidelines

The Commission E Monograph for rectified turpentine oil allows 10–50% in liquid and semisolid preparations for topical application (Blumenthal et al 1998). Essential oils derived from the *Pinaceae* family, including *Pinus* and *Abies* genera, should only be used when the level of peroxides is kept to the lowest practicable level, for example by the addition of antioxidants at the time of production (SCCNFP 2001a; IFRA 2009). The occupational exposure limit for turpentine vapors in Finland and the USA is 100 ppm, or 560 mg/m^3 (Kasanen et al 1999).

Organ-specific effects

Adverse skin reactions: Tested at 12% on 25 volunteers, turpentine oil was both non-irritant and non-sensitizing. The oil was non-phototoxic (Opdyke & Letizia 1983 p. S75). Turpentine oil is a fairly frequent cause of dermatitis, although possibly only from oxidized oils; oxidized δ-3-carene is thought to be responsible (Pirilä & Siltanen 1957, Pirilä et al 1964). Autoxidation products of α-pinene and δ-3-carene can cause skin sensitization (see Constituent profiles, Chapter 14). However, many commercial turpentine oils contain little or no δ-3-carene. Of 22 Portuguese dermatitis patients allergic to turpentine oil, 17 reacted to α-pinene, 15 to (±)-limonene (12 to both) four to δ-3-carene, three to α-terpineol and two to β-pinene (Cachao et al 1986).

Turpentine oil was a well-known contact allergen for a long time, mainly through occupational exposure (Schnuch et al 2004a). During the 1970s the incidence of turpentine oil allergy decreased considerably, following its replacement by organic solvents such as white spirit (Brun 1982, Cronin 1979). However, turpentine oil is still used in pottery, and Lear et al (1996) report 24 cases of hand dermatitis in ceramic workers, with eight sensitivities to α-pinene, four to δ-3-carene and two to turpentine peroxides. Data from Germany and Austria show a resurgence in turpentine oil allergy during a four year period, rising from 0.5% in 1992 to 3.1% in 1997 (Treudler et al 2000). Subsequent data from the same countries show an increase from 1.7% in 1996 to 4.1% 1998, then a steady drop to 1.4% in 2002. It is speculated that these trends are related to a surge in sales of essential oils and aromatherapy products, and that the turpentine oil patch test could be a surrogate marker for terpenes present in essential oils generally (Schnuch et al 2004a). Based on literature published in German, turpentine oil has been classified as category A, a significant contact allergen, by Schlede et al (2003). The topical anti-inflammatory action of turpentine oil in rats has been studied (Damas & Deflandre 1984).

Inhalation toxicity: Eight male volunteers were exposed to 450 mg/m^3 of turpentine vapors by inhalation in an exposure chamber. The subjects experienced discomfort in the throat and airways during exposure to turpentine, and airway resistance was increased after the end of exposure. Toxicokinetics and acute effects showed few, if any, interactions between α-pinene, β-pinene and δ-3-carene (Falk-Filipsson 1996). There have been two reports of occupational asthma that were reasonably attributed to chronic inhalation of turpentine vapors, although it is likely that in one case, colophony was partly responsible (Hendy et al 1985; Dudek et al 2009).

Reproductive toxicity: The low reproductive toxicity of α-pinene, β-pinene, β-myrcene, (+)-limonene and camphene (see Constituent profiles, Chapter 14) suggests that turpentine oil is not hazardous in pregnancy.

Hepatotoxicity: Inflammation and effects suggestive of hepatotoxicity were seen when turpentine, at 1:500 or 1:1,000 in olive oil, was introduced into the bile duct of rats (Martinkova et al 1990).

Systemic effects

Acute toxicity, human: A case of acute intoxication with turpentine at an estimated oral dose of more than 2 mL/kg in an 85-year-old woman was reported. On admission to hospital, she was in a coma and was not breathing. However, she made a full and rapid recovery, and suffered no apparent lung damage (Troulakis et al 1997).

Acute toxicity, animal: The acute oral LD_{50} in rats for turpentine oil was reported as 3.2 g/kg and the acute dermal LD_{50} in rabbits as 5.0 g/kg (Opdyke & Letizia 1983 p. S75).

Subchronic toxicity: When adult male rats were exposed to 300 ppm of a commercial sample of turpentine (consisting of 95% α-pinene) in the ambient air for eight weeks, α-pinene accumulated in perinephric fat and brain tissue. A number of parameters (such as brain RNA) were lower than in control brains after two weeks of exposure, but had returned to normal levels by 8 weeks. It was concluded that α-pinene accumulated in fatty tissues, even at moderate exposures to turpentine, but that no appreciable chronic effect was seen within 8 weeks (Savolainen & Pfäffli 1978).

Carcinogenic/anticarcinogenic potential: No information was found for turpentine oil, but it contains no known carcinogens. α-Pinene is antimutagenic, and is not carcinogenic in rats (see α-Pinene profile, Chapter 14).

Comments

The exudate from turpentine is a mixture of turpentine essential oil (often known simply as 'turpentine') and rosin (a solid resin), also known as colophony. Therefore the use of the word 'turpentine' in research papers is potentially ambiguous. Colophony contains resin acids, is a well-known skin allergen, and occupational exposure to colophony fumes can give rise to asthma. Turpentine is produced on a large scale, and is used as a starting material for the manufacture of many synthetic fragrance chemicals.

Good quality turpentine oils have a high α-pinene content, with a combined α- and β-pinene content of over ~70%. China is the main producer of turpentine, the principal sources being *P. yunnanensis*, *P. latteri*, *P. tabulaeformis* and *P. elliotti*. *P. pinaster* from Portugal is also a major source. *P. palustris* is the leading source of American turpentine, and *P. elliotti* is also an important source. *P. halapensis* yields Greek turpentine, *P. pinaster* French turpentine, *P. radiata* New Zealand turpentine, *P. contorta* Tasmanian turpentine, *P. roxburghii* and *P. insularisi* are sources of Indian turpentine. *P. latteri* was previously treated as synonymous with *P. merkusii*, but is now regarded as a distinct species.

Valerian (European type)

Botanical name: *Valeriana officinalis* L.
Botanical synonym: *Valeriana fauriei* Briq.
Family: Valerianaceae

Essential oil

Source: Roots
Key constituents:

Valerianol	0–33.9%
Bornyl acetate	0.9–33.5%
Valeranone	0–18.1%
Valeranal	0.5–15.9%
Camphene	0.1–14.4%
α-Kessyl acetate	0–12.6%
Elemol	0–11.7%
(+)-Limonene + β-terpinene + 1,8-cineole	0–11.1%
Myrtenyl isovalerate	0–10.5%
α-Pinene	0–10.1%
Myrtenyl acetate	tr–9.1%
β-Eudesmol	0–8.3%
Kessane	0–8.2%
Eudesma-2,6,8-triene	0–7.6%
Bicycloelemene	0–7.2%
α-Gurjunene	0–6.1%
Eugenyl hexanoate	0–4.9%
β-Pinene	tr–4.8%
Valerenic acid	0–4.7%
Drimenol	0–4.4%
δ-Elemene	0–4.4%
Myrtenol	0.1–4.0%
Cryptofauronol	0–3.9%
α-Caryophyllene	0.1–3.6%
Kessanyl acetate	0–3.5%
β-Caryophyllene	0–3.2%
Pacifigorgiol	0–3.2%
α-Guaiene	0–3.1%
Borneol	0.1–3.0%
β-Elemene	0.1–3.0%
Cryptofauronyl acetate	0–2.9%
(-)-*allo*-Aromadendrene	0.7–2.6%
β-Phellandrene	tr–2.4%
Citronellyl isovalerate	0–2.1%
Ledol	0–2.1%
epi-α-Bisabolol	0–1.9%
Palmitic acid	0–1.9%
Germacrene D	0–1.7%
(E)-Valerenyl isovalerate	0–1.7%
Nojigiku acetate	tr–1.6%
Maaliol	0–1.6%
p-Cymene	0.1–1.5%
(E)-Valerenyl acetate	0–1.5%
2,6-Dimethoxy-p-cymene	0–1.4%
β-Gurjunene	0–1.3%
Bornyl isovalerate	0–1.2%
Valerenol (Z/E)	0–1.2%
δ-Cadinene	0–1.1%
Isoeugenyl isovalerate	0–1.1%
Eugenyl isovalerate	0–1.0%
Sabinene	0–1.0%

(Lawrence 1989 p. 160–163, 1999c p. 53–56)

Safety summary

Hazards: None known.
Contraindications: None known.

Organ-specific effects

Adverse skin reactions: No information found.

Systemic effects

Acute toxicity: European valerian oil acute oral LD_{50} in rats 15,000 mg/kg; tolerated dose (highest oral dose administered daily for eight weeks to rats without noticeable injury) 2,250 mg/kg (Von Skramlik 1959). Mouse valeranone LD_{50} >3,160 mg/kg (Rücker et al 1978).

Carcinogenic/anticarcinogenic potential: No information was found for European valerian oil, but it contains no known carcinogens. (+)-Limonene and β-elemene display anticarcinogenic activity (see Constituent profiles, Chapter 14).

Comments

Valerian oils from any geographical region can be quite varied in composition, depending on factors such as cultivar, plant age and harvest time. Chinese *Valeriana officinalis* oils may be high in camphene and bornyl acetate. Because of threatened over-exploitation, Bulgaria has prohibited the collection of wild-growing *Valeriana officinalis* for commercial purposes. Plants must be cultivated for such use. Limited availability.

Valerian (Indian)

Synonym: Sugandhawal
Botanical name: *Valeriana jatamansi* Jones
Botanical synonyms: *Nardostachys jatamansi* (D. Don) DC; *Valeriana wallichii* DC, *Fedia grandiflora* Wall.; *Patrinia jatamansi* (Jones) D. Don
Family: Valerianaceae

Essential oil

Source: Roots
Key constituents:

Patchouli alcohol	40.2%
δ-Guaiene	10.7%
Seychellene	8.2%
Viridiflorol	5.2%
8-Acetoxy-patchouli alcohol	4.5%
α-Guaiene	4.3%
α-Patchoulene	4.3%
β-Pinene	2.9%
Methyl carvacrol	2.5%
Bornyl acetate	1.9%
Camphene	1.8%
α-Muurolene	1.7%
β-Caryophyllene	1.6%
α-Pinene	1.5%
Methyl thymol	1.3%
Kessane	1.2%
γ-Patchoulene	1.2%
Valencene	1.1%

(Mathela et al 2005)

Safety summary

Hazards: None known.
Contraindications: None known.

Organ-specific effects

Adverse skin reactions: No information was found for Indian valerian oil or patchouli alcohol.

Systemic effects

Acute toxicity: No information was found for Indian valerian oil or patchouli alcohol.

Carcinogenic/anticarcinogenic potential: No information was found for Indian valerian oil, but it contains no known carcinogens.

Comments

According to Mathela et al (2005) there is a second chemotype containing 64.3% maaliol, with the two chemotypes growing in separate Himalayan areas. Because of threatened over-exploitation, Nepal has banned the export of unprocessed *Valeriana jatamansi*, and cultivation has been encouraged, in order to minimize the picking of wild plants. Limited availability.

Vanilla

Botanical names: *Vanilla planifolia* Andr. (synonym: *Vanilla fragrans* Salisb.) (Bourbon vanilla); *Vanilla tahitensis* J. W. Moore (Tahitian vanilla)
Family: Orchidaceae

Absolute

Source: Seed pods (fruit)
Key constituents:

Vanilla volatile compounds

Vanillin	85.0%
4-Hydroxybenzaldehyde	8.5%
4-Hydroxybenzyl methyl ether	1.0%

(Klimes & Lamparsky 1976)

Vanilla planifolia 'extract' (presumably absolute)

Vanillin	77.2%
4-Hydroxybenzaldehyde	5.6%
Palmitic acid	4.8%
4-Hydroxy-3-methoxybenzoic acid	2.6%

(Zhu et al 1995 p. 71)

Vanilla planifolia CO_2 extract

Vanillin	12.0–95.0%
4-Hydroxybenzaldehyde	0.7–2.3%
Vanillic acid	0.3–2.2%

(Private communication from supplier)

Safety summary

Hazards: None known.
Contraindications: None known.

Regulatory guidelines

Has GRAS status.

Organ-specific effects

Adverse skin reactions: No primary irritant reactions were observed in 31 patients patch tested with vanilla (Bourbon or Tahiti) pods or extracts. Sensitivity to vanilla was found in 34 of 73 patients sensitive to Peru balsam (Opdyke & Letizia 1982 p. 849–850). Vanillin was not responsible for most cases of sensitivity to natural vanilla (Opdyke 1977a p. 633–638). One manufacturer of vanilla CO_2 extracts states that their vanilla products contain no ethyl vanillin or piperonal. However, piperonal does not appear to present a high risk of skin sensitization (see Piperonal profile, Chapter 14).

Systemic effects

Acute toxicity: For vanillin, rodent acute oral LD_{50} values range from 1.4 to 2.8 g/kg (see Vanillin profile, Chapter 14).
Carcinogenic/anticarcinogenic potential: No information was found for any type of vanilla extract. Vanillin displays anticarcinogenic activity (see Vanillin profile, Chapter 14).

Comments

There is no vanilla essential oil, but there are absolutes and CO_2 extracts made from vanilla oleoresin.

Vassoura

Synonym: Alecrim do cerrado (alecrim is 'rosemary' in Portuguese)
Botanical name: *Baccharis dracunculifolia* DC
Family: Asteraceae (Compositae)

Essential oil

Source: Leaves
Key constituents:

Nerolidol	20.0–30.0%
β-Pinene	3.8–22.0%
(+)-Limonene	4.7–18.0%
α-Pinene	1.2–16.5%
Globulol	2.5–14.5%
Spathulenol	2.6–10.0%
β-Selinene	9.9%
Bicyclogermacrene	9.6%
Farnesol	5.5%
β-Caryophyllene	5.4%
δ-Cadinene	5.1%
β-Myrcene	3.4%
(+)-Aromadendrene	1.6%

α-Terpineol	1.4%
Viridiflorol	1.3%

(Lawrence 1989 p. 123–124, 1995g p. 131; Ferracini et al 1995)

Safety summary

Hazards: None known.
Contraindications: None known.

Organ-specific effects

Adverse skin reactions: No information found.

Systemic effects

Acute toxicity: No information was found for vassoura oil, but all the major constituents are non-toxic.
Carcinogenic/anticarcinogenic potential: No information was found for vassoura oil, but it contains no known carcinogens. Anticarcinogenic activity has been reported for nerolidol, (+)-limonene farnesol and β-caryophyllene (see Constituent profiles, Chapter 14).

Comments

Limited availability.

Verbena (honey)

Synonyms: Wild verbena, greendog, zinziba
Botanical name: *Lippia javanica* Spreng.
Family: Verbenaceae

Essential oil

Source: Flowering tops
Key constituents:

Myrcenone	20.9–49.7%
(Z)-Tagetenone	24.9–39.9%
(E)-Tagetenone	11.4–20.6%
β-Myrcene	4.7–8.3%
(+)-Limonene	1.0–5.0%
(E)-Tagetone	0–4.6%
(Z)-Tagetone	1.4–2.9%
α-Pinene	0–1.5%
β-Caryophyllene	0–1.2%
Sabinene	0–1.0%

(Teubes, private communication, 2004)
Quality: The oil does not keep well, and readily resinifies.

Safety summary

Hazards: None known.
Contraindications: None known.

Organ-specific effects

Adverse skin reactions: No information was found for honey verbena oil or its three major constituents.

Systemic effects

Acute toxicity: No information was found for honey verbena oil or its three major constituents. Taget oil, which contains major constituents of similar chemical structure, is virtually non-toxic (see Taget profile, Chapter 14).

Carcinogenic/anticarcinogenic potential: No information was found for honey verbena oil, but it contains no known carcinogens. Anticarcinogenic activity has been reported for (+)-limonene (see (+)-Limonene profile, Chapter 14).

Comments

Limited availability.

Verbena (lemon)

Synonym: Verbena
Botanical name: *Aloysia triphylla* L'Hérit.
Botanical synonyms: *Aloysia citriodora* Ortega ex Pers., *Lippia citriodora* Ortega ex Pers., *Lippia triphylla* L'Hérit.
Family: Verbenaceae

Absolute

Source: Leaves
Key constituents: No useful data could be found.

Safety summary

Hazards: Skin sensitization (moderate risk).
Cautions (dermal): Hypersensitive, diseased or damaged skin, children under 2 years of age.
Maximum dermal use level: 0.2%

Regulatory guidelines

Lemon verbena absolute should be used such that the level in finished products applied to the skin does not exceed 0.2% (SCCNFP 2001a; IFRA 2009).

Organ-specific effects

Adverse skin reactions: Lemon verbena absolute is non-phototoxic. The undiluted material was slightly to moderately irritating to rabbits. Tested at 2% on 27 volunteers, and 12% on 52 volunteers it was not irritating. A mixture of 80% lemon verbena absolute and 20% (+)-limonene was not irritating when tested on 28 volunteers at 15%. Lemon verbena absolute, tested at 12% on two separate panels of volunteers, resulted in 1/26 and 2/26 sensitization reactions; when tested at 2% there were 0/27 positive reactions. A mixture of 80% lemon verbena absolute and 20% (+)-limonene at 15% produced 1/28 sensitization reactions (Ford et al 1992 p. 135S).

Systemic effects

Acute toxicity: Lemon verbena absolute acute oral LD_{50} in rats >5 g/kg; acute dermal LD_{50} in rabbits >5 g/kg (Ford et al 1992 p. 135S).

Carcinogenic/anticarcinogenic potential: No information found.

Comments

Limited availability.

Essential oil

Source: Leaves
Key constituents:

Geranial	29.5–38.3%
Neral	22.9–29.6%
(+)-Limonene	5.7–15.4%
Zingiberene	0.3–3.9%
Germacrene D	0.4–3.4%
Caryophyllene oxide	1.8–3.3%
Sabinene	0.5–2.9%
β-Caryophyllene	1.3–2.8%
(E)-β-Ocimene	1.5–2.6%
ar-Curcumene	1.1–2.2%
Spathulenol	0.1–2.2%
1,8-Cineole	0.1–1.6%
Geranyl acetate & β-bourbonene	0.8–1.3%
γ-Cadinene	0.2–1.2%
Germacrene D-4-ol	tr–1.2%
(E)-Limonene oxide	0.7–1.0%
6-Methyl-5-hepten-2-one	0.4–1.0%
(E)-Carveol	0–1.0%

(Santos-Gomes & Fernandes-Ferriera 2005)

Safety summary

Hazards: Drug interaction; teratogenicity; skin sensitization; may be mildly phototoxic.
Cautions (oral): Diabetes medication, drugs metabolized by CYP2B6 (Appendix B), pregnancy.
Cautions (dermal): Hypersensitive, diseased or damaged skin, children under 2 years of age.
Maximum daily oral dose in pregnancy: 61 mg
Maximum dermal use level: 0.9%

Our safety advice

We recommend a dermal maximum of 0.9% to avoid skin sensitization, and a daily oral maximum in pregnancy of 61 mg. This is based on 68% citral content, with dermal and oral citral limits of 0.6% and 0.6 mg/kg (see Citral profile, Chapter 14).

Regulatory guidelines

IFRA recommends that lemon verbena oil should not be used as a fragrance ingredient because of its sensitizing and phototoxic potential (IFRA 2009) and the oil is also prohibited as a fragrance ingredient in the EU (SCCNFP 2001a).

Organ-specific effects

Adverse skin reactions: Undiluted lemon verbena oil produced moderate to marked edema and erythema on rabbits, and slight to moderate edema and erythema on guinea pigs. Six different samples of lemon verbena oil, tested at 12% on a total of 159 volunteers, produced two irritation reactions. Six different samples of lemon verbena oil, tested at 12%, produced differing results in maximation tests. The six tests produced 0/30, 2/28, 4/26, 13/25, 15/25 and 18/25 sensitization reactions (Ford et al 1992 p137S–138S). Citral (geranial + neral) can induce sensitization reactions on patch testing at concentrations above 0.5% and this can allegedly be inhibited by the co-presence of (+)-limonene or α-pinene (see Constituent profiles, Chapter 14). Lemon verbena oil is moderately phototoxic. Out of six samples tested, three were phototoxic when applied undiluted; one of these was not phototoxic at 12.5%, and another was not phototoxic at 50% (Ford et al 1992 p. 137S–138S).

Cardiovascular effects: Gavage doses of 10, 15 or 20 mg/kg/day citral for 28 days, dose-dependently lowered plasma insulin levels and increased glucose tolerance in obese rats (Modak & Mukhopadhaya 2011).

Reproductive toxicity: Citral is dose-dependently teratogenic because it inhibits retinoic acid synthesis, and this can affect fetal development (see Citral profile, Chapter 14).

Systemic effects

Acute toxicity: Lemon verbena acute oral LD_{50} in rats >5 g/kg; acute dermal LD_{50} in rabbits and guinea pigs >5 g/kg. A lower dermal LD_{50} (~3.1 g/kg) has also been reported for rabbits (Ford et al 1992 p. 137S–138S).

Carcinogenic/anticarcinogenic potential: Lemon verbena oil (mistakenly referred to as from *Verbena officinalis*) and its major constituent citral, induced apoptosis in leukemic cells in blood taken from patients with chronic lymphocytic leukemia (De Martino et al 2009b). Anticarcinogenic activity has been reported for citral, (+)-limonene and β-caryophyllene (see Constituent profiles, Chapter 14).

Drug interactions: Antidiabetic medication, because of cardiovascular effects, above. See Table 4.10B. Since citral inhibits CYP2B6 (Table 4.11B), there is a theoretical risk of interaction between lemon verbena oil and drugs metabolized by this enzyme (Appendix B).

Comments

The information on skin reactions suggests either that different lemon verbena oils present radically different levels of sensitization risk, or that some of the oils tested were not genuine. Since adulteration of lemon verbena oil is common, this is plausible. The inconsistent phototoxicity results also require explanation, especially considering that lemon verbena absolute is not phototoxic. IFRA's recommendation that lemon verbena oil is not used in fragrances is presumably more due to its sensitization potential than its modest phototoxicity. However, in light of the above comments, and since only 12.0% concentrations were used in testing, the IFRA/EU guideline is unjustified. Like genuine melissa oil (previously also unjustly prohibited by IFRA)

lemon verbena oil is very costly, and may not be used by the major players in the fragrance industry that fund IFRA/RIFM.

The compositional data are for plants grown in Portugal. The total citral content varied with time of year, from 55.2% in July, to 62.5% in September.

Verbena (white)

Synonyms: Bushy lippia, white lippia, anise verbena, licorice verbena, juanilama
Botanical name: *Lippia alba* (Mill.) N.E. Brown
Botanical synonym: *Lippia geminata* Kunth.
Family: Verbenaceae

Essential oil

Source: Rhizomes
Key constituents:

(+)-Carvone	43.3–46.1%
(+)-Limonene	32.6–40.8%
Germacrene D	7.9–11.2%
β-Bourbonene	0.4–1.8%
Carvacrol	0–1.8%
Piperitenone	0–1.8%
Piperitone	0.7–1.4%

(Guilliard et al 2000; Jones, private communication, 2003)

Safety summary

Hazards: Skin sensitization if oxidized.
Cautions: Old or oxidized oils should be avoided.

Our safety advice

We agree with the IFRA guideline of 1.2% for skin sensitization, but only for (−)-carvone, and not for (+)-carvone. For toxicity, we recommend a dermal maximum of 23% for (+)-carvone, and a human daily oral maximum dose of 12.5 mg/kg for carvone isomers (see Carvone profile, Chapter 14). Therefore, white verbena oil requires no restriction in our opinion. Because of its (+)-limonene content we recommend that oxidation of white verbena oil is avoided by storage in a dark, airtight container in a refrigerator. The addition of an antioxidant to preparations containing it is recommended.

Regulatory guidelines

The IFRA standard for either isomer of carvone in leave-on products such as body lotions is 1.2%, for skin sensitization. The Council of Europe (1992) has set an ADI of 1 mg/kg for carvone (isomer not specified). This is equivalent to a daily adult dose of 150 mg of white verbena oil. IFRA recommends that essential oils rich in limonene should only be used when the level of peroxides is kept to the lowest practical level, for instance by adding antioxidants at the time of production (IFRA 2009).

Organ-specific effects

Adverse skin reactions: No information found. Autoxidation products of (+)-limonene can cause skin sensitization (see (+)-Limonene profile, Chapter 14).

Systemic effects

Acute toxicity: No information found.
Carcinogenic/anticarcinogenic potential: The carvone/limonene chemotype of white verbena oil was not genotoxic in the SOS chromotest (a modified *E. coli* PQ37 genotoxicity assay) (López et al 2011). (+)-Carvone is not a rodent carcinogen, and both carvone and (+)-limonene display anticarcinogenic activity (see Constituent profiles, Chapter 14).

Comments

Limited availability. There are a number of other chemotypes including a citral and a linalool. An absolute is occasionally produced.

Vetiver

Synonyms: Khus, khus-khus
Botanical name: *Vetiveria zizanoides* (L.) Nash
Botanical synonyms: *Andropogon muricatus* (Retz.), *Andropogon zizanoides* (L.) Urban, *Chrysopogon zizanoides* (L.) Roberty, *Phalaris zizanoides* L.
Family: Poaceae (Gramineae)

Essential oil

Source: Roots
Key constituents:

Khusimol (zizanol)	3.4–13.7%
Vetiselinenol (isonootkatol)	1.3–7.8%
Cyclocopacamphan-12-ol (epimer A)	1.0–6.7%
α-Cadinol	0–6.5%
α-Vetivone (isonootkatone)	2.5–6.4%
β-Vetivenene	0.2–5.7%
β-Eudesmol	0–5.2%
β-Vetivone	2.0–4.9%
Khusenic acid	0–4.8%
β-Vetispirene	1.5–4.5%
γ-Vetivenene	0.2–4.3%
α-Amorphene	1.5–4.1%
(*E*)-Eudesm-4(15),7-dien-12-ol	1.7–3.7%
β-Calacorene	0–3.5%
γ-Cadinene	0–3.4%
(*Z*)-Eudesm-6-en-11-ol	1.1–3.3%
γ-Amorphene	0–3.3%
Ziza-5-en-12-ol	0–3.3%
β-Selinene	0–3.1%
(*Z*)-Eudesma-6,11-diene	0–2.9%
Salvial-4(14)-en-1-one	0–2.9%
Khusinol	0–2.8%
Cyclocopacamphan-12-ol (epimer B)	1.1–2.7%
Selina-6-en-4-ol	0–2.7%
Khusian-ol	1.5–2.6%
δ-Amorphene	0–2.5%
1-*epi*-Cubenol	0–2.4%
Khusimene (ziza-6(13)-ene)	1.1–2.3%
Ziza-6(13)-en-3β-ol	0–2.3%
Ziza-6(13)-en-3-one	0–2.3%
2-*epi*-Ziza-6(13)-en-3α-ol	1.0–2.2%
12-Nor-ziza-6(13)-en-2β-ol	0–2.2%
α-Vetispirene	0–2.2%
Eremophila-1(10),7(11)-diene	0.9–2.1%
Dimethyl-6,7-bicyclo-[4.4.0]-deca-10-en-one	0–2.0%
10-*epi*-γ-Eudesmol	0–1.8%
α-Calacorene	0.4–1.7%
(*E*)-Opposita-4(15),7(11)-dien12-ol	0–1.7%
Prekhusenic acid	0–1.6%
13-Nor-eudesma-4,6-dien-11-one	0.6–1.5%
Isovalencenol	0–1.5%
Spirovetiva-1(10),7(11)-diene	0–1.5%
2-*epi*-Ziza-6(13)-en-12-al	0–1.5%
(*E*)-Isovalencenal	0.7–1.4%
Preziza-7(15)-ene	0.6–1.4%
(*Z*)-Eudesma-6,11-dien-3β-ol	0–1.4%
Intermedeol (eudesm-11-en-4-ol)	0–1.3%
Isoeugenol	0–1.3%
Isokhusenic acid	0–1.3%
Elemol	0.3–1.2%
Eremophila-1(10),6-dien-12-al	0–1.2%
Juniper camphor	0–1.2%
Khusimone	0.5–1.1%
Eremophila-1(10),4(15)-dien-2α-ol	0–1.1%
Eremophila-1(10),7(11)-dien-2β-ol	0–1.1%
(*Z*)-Isovalencenal	0–1.1%
allo-Khusiol	0–1.1%
Methyl-(*E*)-eremophila-1(10),7(11)-dien-12-ether	0–1.1%
(*E*)-2-Nor-zizaene	0–1.1%
(*Z*)-Eudesm-6-en-12-al	0–1.0%
Funebran-15-al	0–1.0%

(Champagnat et al 2006)
Quality: According to Burfield (2003) vetiver oil is not commonly adulterated, except possibly with non-odorous diluents. According to Oyen & Dung (1999 p. 168) vetiver oil may be adulterated with cheap sesquiterpenes such as caryophyllene and its derivatives, or with cyperus oil.

Safety summary

Hazards: May contain isoeugenol.
Contraindications: None known.
Maximum dermal use level (Javanese, Chinese, Brazilian and Mexican vetiver oils):

IFRA	1.5%
Tisserand & Young	15%

Our safety advice

We recommend a dermal maximum of 15%, based on 1.3% isoeugenol content with a dermal maximum of 0.2% (see Isoeugenol profile, Chapter 14).

Regulatory guidelines

Isoeugenol should not be used such that the level in finished products exceeds 0.02% (SCCNFP 2001a; IFRA 2009).

Organ-specific effects

Adverse skin reactions: In a modified Draize procedure on guinea pigs, Réunion vetiver oil was assessed as sensitizing (Sharp 1978). Undiluted vetiver oil was moderately irritating to rabbits, but was not irritating to mice; tested at 8% on 25 volunteers it was neither irritating nor sensitizing. It is non-phototoxic (Opdyke 1974 p. 1013). In a study of 200 consecutive dermatitis patients, one (0.5%) was sensitive to 2% vetiver oil on patch testing (Rudzki et al 1976). A 65-year-old aromatherapist with multiple essential oil sensitivities reacted to both 1% (weakly) and 5% vetiver oil (Selvaag et al 1995).

Systemic effects

Acute toxicity: Acute oral LD_{50} in rats >5 g/kg; acute dermal LD_{50} in rabbits >5 g/kg (Opdyke 1974 p. 1013).
Carcinogenic/anticarcinogenic potential: Vetiver oil showed significant chemopreventive activity against human mouth epidermal carcinoma (KB) cells, with an IC_{50} of 68 μg/mL, but no activity against mouse leukemia (P388) cells (Manosroi et al 2005). α-Cadinol is active against the human colon cancer cell line HT-29 (He et al 1997a). Vetiver oil contains no known carcinogens.

Comments

The composition given above is a composite of essential oils produced in nine countries. These can be divided into three subgroups, two consisting of four countries each, with Madagascar comprising a third group. Only vetiver oils from Java, China, Brazil and Mexico contain any isoeugenol. Those from Haiti, India, Reunion and El Salvador are devoid of isoeugenol, as is the oil from Madagascar. There are distinct variations in the content of khusimol, β-vetivenene and β-vetispirene between the three subgroups, but overall vetiver oils are relatively homogenous (Champagnat et al 2006). Vetiver oil is also produced in small amounts in Angola and The Seychelles. The oil is a complex mixture of over 150 sesquiterpenoid compounds, some of which have not yet been identified.

Violet leaf

Synonym: Sweet violet
Botanical name: *Viola odorata* L.
Family: Violaceae

Absolute

Source: Leaves
Key constituents:

9,12-Octadecadienoic acid	0–58.0%
2,6-Nonedienal	5.0–18.5%
Hexadecanoic acid	0–17.0%
3-pentadecenal	0–15.9%
1-Hexadecene	0.7–2.9%
1-Octadecene	0.3–10.6%
2,6,11-Trimethyldodecane	0–9.9%
Docecanol	0.4–8.6%
2,4-Dimethyldodecane	0–5.5%
2,7,11-Trimethyldodecane	0–5.5%
2,6-Nonedienol	1.7–4.8%
(3Z)-Hexen-1-ol	0–4.4%
2,5-Heptadienol	0–4.0%
7-Octen-4-ol	0–2.9%
(2E)-Hexen-1-ol	1.3–2.6%
3-Hexenyl formate	0–2.4%
Benzyl alcohol	1.0–2.1%
3,7-Dimethyloctane	0–2.0%

(Lawrence 1995g p. 134)
Quality: Violet leaf absolute may be adulterated by the addition of chrorophyll extracts, synthetic 2,6-nonedienal, and various synthetic materials not found in the absolute (Arctander 1960).

Safety summary

Hazards: None known.
Contraindications: None known.

Regulatory guidelines

Has GRAS status.

Organ-specific effects

Adverse skin reactions: In a modified Draize procedure on guinea pigs, violet leaf absolute was non-sensitizing when used at 10% in the challenge phase (Sharp 1978). Undiluted violet leaf absolute was not irritating to mice or pigs; tested at 2% on 25 volunteers it was neither irritating nor sensitizing. It is non-phototoxic (Opdyke 1976 p893). Of 167 fragrance-sensitive dermatitis patients, two (1.2%) were allergic to 2% violet leaf absolute in petrolatum, though of the 167, one (0.6%) was allergic to petrolatum (Larsen et al 1996b).

Systemic effects

Acute toxicity: No information found.
Carcinogenic/anticarcinogenic potential: No information was found for violet leaf absolute, but it contains no known carcinogens.

Comments

Violet leaf absolute is regarded as a high-risk skin sensitizer in Japan (Nakayama 1998), but we have not seen supporting evidence of this. Because of its very high cost, violet leaf absolute is particularly subject to adulteration. Violet *flower* absolute was produced on a very limited scale at one time, but has not been made for several decades.

Western red cedar

Synonyms: Pacific thuja, western arborvitae
Botanical name: *Thuja plicata* Donn ex D. Don
Family: Cupressaceae

Essential oil

Source: Needles (leaves)
Key constituents:

α-Thujone	63.5–84.0%
β-Thujone	4.9–15.2%
Sabinene	1.1–8.8%
Terpinen-4-ol	1.4–4.6%
Geranyl acetate	0.1–3.9%
β-Myrcene	0.5–3.3%
α-Pinene	0.5–2.9%
Rimuene	0.1–2.6%
γ-Terpinene	0.3–2.0%
α-Terpineol	0.3–1.8%
Beyerene	0.1–1.5%
Linalool	0.1–1.5%
(+)-Limonene	0.4–1.3%
α-Terpinene	0.1–1.2%

(Von Rudloff et al 1988)

Safety summary

Hazards: Expected to be neurotoxic, based on thujone content.
Contraindications (all routes): Pregnancy, breastfeeding.
Contraindications: Should not be taken in oral doses.
Maximum dermal use level: 0.25%

Our safety advice

Our dermal maximum is based on 99.0% total thujone content and a thujone limit of 0.25% (see Thujone profile, Chapter 14).

Organ-specific effects

Adverse skin reactions: No information found.
Neurotoxicity: No information found. There is a risk of convulsions with moderately high doses of thujone. The thujone NOAEL for convulsions was reported to be 10 mg/kg in male rats and 5 mg/kg in females (Margaria 1963).

Systemic effects

Acute toxicity: No information found. Both α- and β-thujone are moderately toxic, with reported oral LD_{50} values ranging from 190 to 500 mg/kg for different species (see Thujone profile, Chapter 14).

Carcinogenic/anticarcinogenic potential: No information was found for Western red cedar oil, but it contains no known carcinogens.

Comments

Limited availability. There is also an oil from the *wood* of *T. plicata*, though this is probably not commercially available. *T. plicata* is among the largest trees in the world, and typically reaches a height of 55–75 m (180–246 ft).

White cloud

Synonyms: White kunzea, Tasmanian spring flower, Southern spring flower, tick bush, poverty bush
Botanical name: *Kunzea ambigua* (Sm.) Druce
Family: Myrtaceae

Essential oil

Source: Leaves
Key constituents:

α-Pinene	33.2%
1,8-Cineole	14.8%
Viridiflorol	11.5%
Globulol	11.2%
Bicyclogermacrene	5.3%
α-Terpineol	4.3%
Calamenene	1.7%
Citronellol	1.6%
Spathulenol	1.6%
Ledol	1.5%
(+)-Limonene	1.2%

(Condon, private communication, 2003)

Safety summary

Hazards: Skin sensitization if oxidized.
Cautions: Old or oxidized oils should be avoided.

Our safety advice

Because of its α-pinene content we recommend that oxidation of white cloud oil is avoided by storage in a dark, airtight container in a refrigerator. The addition of an antioxidant to preparations containing it is recommended.

Organ-specific effects

Adverse skin reactions: No information was found for white cloud oil, but autoxidation products of α-pinene can cause skin sensitization (see α-Pinene profile, Chapter 14).

Systemic effects

Acute toxicity: No information found.

Carcinogenic/anticarcinogenic potential: No information was found for white cloud oil, but it contains no known carcinogens.

Comments

Limited availability.

Wintergreen

Botanical names: *Gaultheria fragrantissima* Wall.; *Gaultheria procumbens* L.
Family: Ericaceae

Essential oil

Source: Leaves
Key constituents:

Gaultheria fragrantissima (Nepalese)

Methyl salicylate   97.0–99.5%
(Vossen, private communication, 2004)

Gaultheria procumbens (Chinese)

Methyl salicylate   96.0–99.0%

(Guenther 1949–1952, vol. 4 p. 6)
Quality: Methyl salicyate may be added to, or passed off as wintergreen oil (Burfield 2003).

Safety summary

Hazards: Drug interaction; inhibits blood clotting; toxicity; high doses are teratogenic.
Contraindications (all routes): Anticoagulant medication, major surgery, hemophilia, other bleeding disorders (Box 7.1). Pregnancy, breastfeeding, children. People with salicylate sensitivity (often applies in ADD/ADHD).
Contraindications (oral): Gastroesophageal reflux disease (GERD).
Maximum adult daily oral dose: 175 mg
Maximum dermal use level: 2.4%

Our safety advice

Our oral and dermal restrictions are based on 99.5% methyl salicylate content and methyl salicylate limits of 2.5 mg/kg and 2.4% (see Methyl salicylate profile, Chapter 14). Oral use of methyl salicylate-rich essential oils should be avoided in GERD, and salicylates are contraindicated in children due to the risk of developing Reye's syndrome. Essential oils with a high methyl salicylate content should be avoided in pregnancy and lactation, and by anyone concurrently taking anticoagulant drugs. Caution is advised in those with hypersensitivity to salicylates, or dermatological conditions where the integrity of the skin is impaired.

Regulatory guidelines

An ADI for methyl salicylate was set at 0.5 mg/kg bw by the JECFA in 1967 based on a 2-year feeding study in dogs and using an uncertainty factor of 100. The same ADI, based on a two year rat study in 1963, was adopted by the Council of Europe Committee of Experts on Flavoring Substances. The Health Canada maximum for methyl salicylate is 1% in topical products (Health Canada Cosmetic Ingredient Hotlist, March 2011).

Organ-specific effects

Adverse skin reactions: No information found.
Cardiovascular effects: Methyl salicylate inhibits platelet aggregation (Tanen et al 2008), an essential step in the blood clotting cascade.
Reproductive toxicity: Large oral doses of salicylates are teratogenic in rats and monkeys, and epidemiological evidence has linked high doses of aspirin taken by pregnant women to the birth of malformed babies (Wilson 1973). It would therefore be prudent to avoid the use of any preparations containing wintergreen oil in pregnancy.

Systemic effects

Acute toxicity, human: Numerous cases of methyl salicylate poisoning have been reported, with a 50–60% mortality rate; 4–8 mL is considered a lethal dose for a child (Opdyke 1978 p. 821–825). In the years 1926, 1928 and 1939–1943, 427 deaths occurred in the US from methyl salicylate poisoning (Davison et al 1961). There may be great individual variation in the ability to handle the poison, and adults are possibly more resilient. The ingestion of 10 mL of methyl salicylate has been survived (Jacobziner & Raybin 1962b). One adult died after ingesting 15 mL; another survived ingestion of 45 mL (Stevenson 1937).

Stevenson summarizes 41 cases of wintergreen oil poisoning, between 1832 and 1935. These comprise 14 who survived and 27 who died. Of the fatalities, 17 were under three years of age. Two of the adult cases appear to have been suicides, since 200 mL and 250 mL of wintergreen oil were taken. One 2-year-old died after ingesting 4 mL, while another survived after ingesting 15 mL of the oil, but only after a severe episode involving a rapid pulse, muscle twitching, cyanosis (bluish coloration) and rapid breathing. In a fatal case, a 1-month-old girl was accidentally given 5 mL of wintergreen oil. She vomited a milky fluid 30 minutes later that smelled strongly of wintergreen and she appeared sleepy. Two hours later she vomited again, and was given peppermint water and castor oil. Her breathing was rapid and deep; her breath acidotic and she was pale but not cyanotic. She died about 24 hours after the poisoning (Stevenson 1937).

A 20-month-old child survived ingestion of ~5 ml wintergreen oil following exchange transfusion; a 3-year-old died the day after ingesting 2–3 teaspoons of wintergreen oil, and a 2-year-old died after consuming an unknown quantity of tablets containing methyl salicylate and colchicine. On admission to hospital, this last child had 72.7 mg salicylates per 100 mL of blood (Adams et al 1957). A 21-month-old infant recovered following ingestion of (presumed 4 mL) wintergreen oil. The child developed lethargy, vomiting and rapid breathing, but recovered fully and rapidly (Howrie et al 1985).

One teaspoon of wintergreen oil proved fatal to a child aged 22 months. Vomiting soon after ingestion was followed by drowsiness, labored breathing, a craving for water, and evidence in the tongue and skin of marked dehydration. Glucose and saline infusions had no effect, the child became cyanotic and hyperpyrexic, and eventually died. On autopsy, the greatest abnormalities were found in the heart muscle, the liver and the kidneys (Eimas 1938). A 3-year-old boy ingested an unknown quantity of wintergreen oil, resulting in a serum salicylate level of 118 mg/100 mL. He was treated with intermittent peritoneal dialysis and survived (Kloss & Boeckman 1967). A 44-year-old man had a seizure, and approximately 18 hours later died after being hospitalized and suffering three episodes of cardiopulmonary arrest. He had ingested about 1 oz of wintergreen oil, thinking it was castor oil (Cauthen & Hester 1989).

Common signs of methyl salicylate poisoning are: CNS excitation, rapid breathing, fever, high blood pressure, convulsions and coma. Death results from respiratory failure after a period of unconsciousness (Adams et al 1957); 0.5 mL of methyl salicylate is approximately equivalent to a dose of 21 aspirin tablets. Methyl salicylate can be absorbed transdermally in sufficient quantities to cause poisoning in humans (Heng 1987). Methyl salicylate could be 1.5–4.5 times more toxic in humans than in rodents (see Ch. 3, p. 32).

Acute toxicity, animal: No animal data was found for wintergreen oil. Reported acute oral LD_{50} values for methyl salicylate range from 887–2,800 mg/kg (see Methyl salicylate profile, Chapter 14).

Carcinogenic/anticarcinogenic potential: No information found. Methyl salicylate is not genotoxic, and does not appear to be carcinogenic (see Methyl salicylate profile, Chapter 14).

Drug interactions: Topically applied methyl salicylate can potentiate the anticoagulant effect of warfarin, causing side effects such as internal hemorrhage (Le Bourhis & Soenen 1973). It is likely that methyl salicylate administered by other routes would result in a similar potentiation. A similar interaction is possible, but by no means certain, with other anticoagulants such as aspirin and heparin.

Comments

Some commercial wintergreen oils are in fact synthetic methyl salicylate. Many liniments contain methyl salicylate or wintergreen oil. *G. fragrantissima* oil is produced in China and Nepal, and is regarded by some as a threatened species (www.vedamsbooks.com/no13185.htm, accessed August 8th 2011). *G. procumbens* oil is produced in China and North America.

Wormseed

Synonym: Chenopodium
Botanical names: *Chenopodium ambrosioides* L.; *Chenopodium ambrosioides* L. var. *anthelminticum* L (synonym: *Teloxys ambrosioides*)
Family: Chenopodiacae

Essential oil

Source: Whole plant, including fruit
Key constituents:

Spanish

Ascaridole	41.2%
(+)-Limonene	29.2%
p-Mentha-1(7),8-dien-3-ol	10.0%
(E)-Isocarveol	9.5%
(E)-Carveol	1.5%
p-Mentha-8-en-1,2-diol	1.3%
(Z)-p-Mentha-2,8-dien-1-ol	1.0%
Thymol	1.0%

(De Pascual et al 1980)

Brazilian

(Z)-Ascaridole	61.4%
(E)-Ascaridole	18.6%
Carvacrol	3.9%
p-Cymene	2.0%

(Jardim et al 2008)

Safety summary

Hazards: Toxicity; neurotoxicity.
Contraindications: Should not be used, either internally or externally.

Regulatory guidelines

IFRA recommends that wormseed oil is not used as a fragrance ingredient (IFRA 2009). Wormseed oil is prohibited as a cosmetic ingredient in the EU and Canada. In the UK, *Chenopodium ambrosioides* preparations can only be sold in a pharmacy, under the supervision of a pharmacist.

Organ-specific effects

Adverse skin reactions: Undiluted wormseed oil was slightly irritating to rabbits, and was irritating to both mice and pigs; tested at 4% on 25 volunteers it was neither irritating nor sensitizing. It is non-phototoxic (Opdyke 1976 p. 713–715).

Systemic effects

Acute toxicity, human: In the first half of the 20th century there were several reports of fatal poisoning in children due to wormseed oil being accidentally ingested or deliberately prescribed (Levy 1914; Ibrus-Määr 1932; Wolf 1935; Van Lookeren Campagne 1939; Mele 1952). Of the recorded cases of poisoning, 70% were fatal. According to King's American Dispensatory (1898), 'The essential oil, on which the vermifuge properties depend, is the best form, and is more generally employed. Its dose is from four to eight drops mixed with sugar, or in emulsion, to be given morning and evening, for four or five days successively' (http://www.henriettesherbal.com/eclectic/kings/chenopodium-ambr.html accessed August 8th 2011). If this is the kind of dosage that was being advised at that time, it is not surprising that some children died. A girl of 19 months died 24 hours after being given three one-drop doses of wormseed oil 12 hours apart (Van Lookeren Campagne 1939). A 3-year-old child was given 'several drops' of wormseed oil three times a day for 5 days, and died on the sixth day, 13 hours after admission to hospital and gastric lavage (Ibrus-Määr 1932). A 14-month-old child died following the administration of less than 5 mL of wormseed oil (Mele 1952). A 2-year-old child died after being given eight drops of wormseed oil, followed by a similar dose one week later. Autopsy showed broncho-pneumonia, liver and kidney damage, and cerebral edema (Wolf 1935).

Thirty drops of wormseed oil were fatal in a 12-year-old child, causing degeneration of the liver and kidneys, and cerebral edema; 48 drops caused the death of a 4-year-old child, with toxic signs including convulsions, bowel inflammation and generalized edema; a three-year-old child died after being given nine drops of wormseed oil, one week after having received a similar dose (Wolf 1935). It has been speculated that the damage to mucous membranes caused by the first dose allows the second dose to be more easily absorbed. There is one instance of 10–12 mL of wormseed oil having been survived in a male adult. Symptoms included slurred speech, dullness of wits, impeded motor function, and periodic lapsing into coma. A nurse was present at the time, and administered gastric lavage which undoubtedly saved his life. He did not fully recover from the episode for six months, and his mental faculties remained dulled, possibly due to permanent CNS damage (Kröber 1936).

Wormseed oil is toxic even at low doses because of its depressant action on respiration and cardiac function (Salant 1917). Toxic signs include: skin and mucous membrane irritation, headache, vertigo, tinnitus, double vision, nausea, vomiting, constipation, deafness, blindness and damage to the kidneys, liver and heart (Opdyke 1976 p. 713–715). In most cases, a major finding on autopsy has been considerable CNS damage, particularly to the brain. Wormseed oil is powerfully neurotoxic, resulting in visible edema of the brain and meninges; the oil also affects the liver and kidneys. The fatal dose is very close to the therapeutic dose, although there is a great variation in individual sensitivity (Van Lookeren Campagne 1939). Four drops of wormseed oil in a steam inhalation caused an unpleasant sensation of vertigo in the frontal part of the cranium, and caused moderate irritation of the nasal mucous membrane (author's personal experience).

Acute toxicity, animal: When 30 mg/kg/day of wormseed oil was administered ip to mice infected with *Leishmania amazonensis* for 15 days, small abcesses were found in the peritoneal cavity, and two of 12 mice died. However, oral administration of the same dose was not toxic (Monzote et al 2007). The animal data show wormseed oil to be only moderately toxic: acute oral LD_{50} 255 mg/kg in rats, 380 mg/kg in mice; acute dermal LD_{50} in rabbits 415 mg/kg (Opdyke 1976 p. 713–715); acute subcutaneous LD_{50} in mice 940 mg/kg (Essway et al 1995). Toxic signs have been reported in dogs at 280–400 mg/kg (Salant 1917).

Carcinogenic/anticarcinogenic potential: No information found. Antitumoral activity has been reported for ascaridole, carvacrol, thymol and (+)-limonene (see Constituent profiles, Chapter 14).

Comments

Our dermal maximum for ascaridole is 0.1%, so we could, on that basis, allow 0.14% of wormseed oil. However, on a risk/benefit basis, there would be no point. Wormseed is one of the most toxic essential oils. Four of the fatal cases cited above

(children aged 19 months, 2, 3 and 12 years) indicate a human fatal dose in the 10–40 mg/kg range, if average weights are ascribed to the children (Wolf 1935; Van Lookeren Campagne 1939). Therefore, wormseed oil is many times more toxic to humans than rodents, and it is in the 'very toxic' category. Toxicity is clearly due to the ascaridole content of the oil.

In the past wormseed oil was commonly employed as a remedy for intestinal parasites in children, but it is no longer used due to its toxicity. If the amount given was a mere two or three times the recommended dose of one drop per year of age, a fatal outcome was possible. In 1952 wormseed oil was described as 'one of the best-known anthelmintics, used successfully against several types of intestinal parasites in man and animals, against roundworms, tapeworms, and hookworms. However, great care must be exercised in the administration of the oil as it is very dangerous if given in excessive doses' (Mele 1952). In South America the plant is still used as an anthelmintic, and also as an emmenagogue and abortifacient (Conway & Slocumb 1979). An aqueous infusion of wormseed, containing no ascaridole, is an effective and non-toxic nematocide (MacDonald et al 2004).

A 'high-grade oil' has been described as containing a minimum of 75% ascaridole, with some oils containing up to 91% (Guenther 1949–1952, vol. 6, p161). An analysis of a commercial essential oil from Madagascar found 41.8% ascaridole, 18.1% isoascaridole, 16.2% *p*-cymene, 9.7% α-terpinene and 3.8% (+)-limonene. However, ascaridole apparently undergoes partial thermal isomerization to isoascaridole, and the actual contents were 55.3% ascaridole and 4.6% isoascaridole (Cavalli et al 2004). The essential oil of *Chenopodium ambrosioides* var. *ambrosioides* is much lower in ascaridole (0–5%) but is not commercially available. Wormseed oil can allegedly 'explode' when heated (Reynolds 1993).

Wormwood

Synonyms: Absinthe, artemisia
Botanical name: *Artemisia absinthium* L.
Family: Asteraceae (Compositae)

Essential oil

Source: Leaves and flowering tops
Key constituents:

β-*Thujone CT*

β-Thujone	33.1–59.9%
(Z)-Sabinyl acetate	18.1–32.8%
α-Thujone	2.3–3.4%
Sabinene	1.1–2.9%
(Z)-Sabinol	0.5–2.7%
Geranyl propionate	0.1–2.1%
β-Caryophyllene	1.4–1.9%
Lavandulyl acetate	0–1.8%
Linalool	1.2–1.7%
Germacrene D	0.8–1.7%
(Z)-Epoxy-ocimene	0.9–1.5%
Neryl isobutyrate	0–1.4%
β-Myrcene	1.0–1.3%

1,8-Cineole	0.6–1.0%
β-Selinene	0–1.0%

(Lawrence 1995g p. 12; Tucker et al 1993)

β-Thujone/(Z)-epoxy-ocimene CT

(Z)-Epoxy-α-ocimene	24.2–28.9%
β-Thujone	20.9–21.7%
Chrysanthendiol*	5.3–6.6%
Chrysanthenyl acetate	3.2–4.3%
Linalool	2.2–2.4%
α-Bisabolol	1.7–2.3%
Neryl acetate	0.4–2.1%
Geranyl acetate	1.4–1.6%
Sabinene	0.3–1.5%
(E)-Epoxy-α-ocimene	1.0–1.4%
Germacrene D	0.8–1.4%
Neryl butyrate	1.2–1.3%
Neryl isovalerate	1.0–1.1%

(Lawrence 1995g p. 13)

(Z)-Epoxy-ocimene CT

(Z)-Epoxy-α-ocimene	25.7–42.2%
Chrysanthenyl acetate	9.9–15.6%
Sabinyl acetate	0.3–7.4%
Neryl butyrate	1.7–3.1%
Germacrene D	2.0–2.6%
α-Bisabolol	1.5–2.5%
β-Caryophyllene	1.7–2.2%
Neryl isovalerate	1.6–2.2%
Chrysanthendiol*	1.0–1.8%
(E)-Epoxy-α-ocimene	0.8–1.6%
Linalool	0.4–.3%
Neryl isobutyrate	0.5–1.1%
Geranyl acetate	0.6–1.0%
Nerol	0.5–1.0%
β-Thujone	0.3–0.8%
α-Thujone	0–0.2%

(Lawrence 1995g p. 12)

Sabinyl acetate CT

Sabinyl acetate	31.5%
Neryl isovalerate	9.1%
Neryl butyrate	7.9%
Chrysanthenyl acetate	5.8%
Geranyl acetate	4.2%
Nerol	3.2%
Neryl isobutyrate	2.6%
Linalool	2.5%
β-Myrcene	2.1%
β-Curcumene	1.7%

Spathulenol	1.6%
β-Thujone	0.6%
α-Thujone	0.1%

(Lawrence 1995g p. 13)

Safety summary

Hazards: Neurotoxicity; embryo-fetotoxicity; abortifacient.
Contraindications (all routes): Pregnancy, breastfeeding.
Maximum use levels:

β-thujone – 0.4% (dermal maximum); no safe dose (daily adult oral maximum)

β-thujone/(Z)-epoxy-ocimene – 1.1% (dermal maximum); 32 mg (daily adult oral maximum)

(Z)-epoxy-ocimene – 25% (dermal maximum); 700 mg (daily adult oral maximum)

sabinyl acetate – 35% (dermal maximum); 1,000 mg (daily adult oral maximum)

Our safety advice

The maximum doses recommended above for the β-thujone, β-thujone/(Z)-epoxy-ocimene, (Z)-epoxy-ocimene and sabinyl acetate chemotypes of wormwood oil are based on 63.3%, 21.7%, 1.0% and 0.7% total thujone content, respectively, with dermal and oral limits of 0.25% and 0.1 mg/kg/day for thujone isomers.

Organ-specific effects

Adverse skin reactions: Undiluted wormwood oil was slightly irritating to rabbits, but was not irritating to mice; tested at 2% on 25 volunteers it was neither irritating nor sensitizing. It is non-phototoxic (Opdyke 1975 p. 721–722).

Neurotoxicity: According to King's American Dispensatory (1898), 'Physiologically both oil of wormwood and extract of absinth act upon man as nerve depressants. Less than drachm doses [1 drachm = 1/8 fluid ounce = 1.8 g] produced in rabbits and dogs tremors, spasmodic muscular action of a clonic character, intoxication, and loss of sensibility. Larger doses (from 1 to 2 drachms) produced violent epileptoid seizures, in some instances resulting fatally' (http://www.henriettesherbal.com/eclectic/kings/artemisia-absi.html accessed August 8th 2011).

In perhaps the earliest formally recorded case, a male adult ingested 'probably about half an ounce' of wormwood oil. Within minutes, he was unconscious, convulsing, foaming at the mouth with his jaw clenched. After prompt medical intervention the man survived, but he was unable to remember taking the oil (Smith 1862). In a more recent case, a 31-year-old man was hospitalized with renal failure after ingesting 10 mL of wormwood oil. He had been found by his father in an agitated, incoherent and disoriented state. Paramedics noted tonic-clonic seizures with decorticate posturing. On admission, tests revealed hypernatremia, hypokalemia and hypobicarbonatemia. On the second day he developed congestive heart failure, which was treated with diuretics, sodium restriction

*Tentative identification

and discontinuation of alkalinization. His serum creatinine peaked on the third day at 4.4 mg/dL (390 μmol/L) and then declined. He was discharged on day 8, and his serum electrolyte, creatine kinase, and creatinine concentrations were normal on day 17. He had purchased the oil through a supplier on the internet after finding a description of absinthe on an unrelated website (Weisbord et al 1997).

In 1915, the production of *absinthe* containing wormwood oil was banned in France. It was claimed that the oil acted as a narcotic in higher doses, and was habit-forming. It was, and is still, believed that the thujone in wormwood oil was largely or solely responsible for these effects. 'Absinthism', a syndrome of hallucinations, sleeplessness, tremors, convulsions and paralysis, was associated with long-term ingestion of the drink (Weisbord et al 1997). However, there is no hard evidence that absinthe is any more toxic than any other alcoholic drink nor, if it is more toxic, that this can be attributed either to wormwood or thujone. In the absinthe made 100 years ago, any toxicity could have been due to adulterants and contaminants in the beverage, which only contained <10 mg of thujone per liter of absinthe (www.feeverte.net/thujone.html accessed August 8th 2011). This concentration of thujone in an alcoholic drink is not sufficient to cause a significant psychotropic or neurotoxic effect (Dettling et al 2004).

There is a risk of convulsions with moderately high doses of thujone. The thujone NOAEL for convulsions was reported to be 10 mg/kg in male rats and 5 mg/kg in females (Margaria 1963). Sabinyl acetate is abortifacient and maternally toxicity in mice (see Constituent profiles, Chapter 14).

Systemic effects

Acute toxicity: Moderately toxic (oral), non-toxic (dermal). Wormwood oil acute oral LD_{50} in rats 960 mg/kg; acute dermal LD_{50} in rabbits >5 g/kg (Opdyke 1975 p. 721–722). Both α- and β-thujone are moderately toxic, with reported oral LD_{50} values ranging from 190–500 mg/kg for different species (see Thujone profile, Chapter 14).

Antioxidant/pro-oxidant activity: A sabinyl acetate CT of wormwood oil had only very weak DPPH radical scavenging or antioxidant activity (Lopes-Lutz 2008).

Carcinogenic/anticarcinogenic potential: No information found. None of the cited chemotypes contain any known carcinogens.

Comments

All four of the chemotypes outlined above are commercially available. There is also a chrysanthenyl acetate chemotype which may occasionally be produced. The combined risks of thujones and sabinyl acetate suggest the complete avoidance of wormwood oils in pregnancy. Wormwood oil is sometimes confused with armoise oil.

Wormwood (annual)

Synonyms: Sweet wormwood, sweet annie
Botanical name: *Artemisia annua* L.
Family: Asteraceae (Compositae)

Essential oil

Source: Flowering plant
Key constituents:

Artemisia ketone	11.9–75.9%
Artemisia alcohol	0–56.0%
Germacrene D	0–18.5%
α-Ylangene	0.16.2%
α-Pinene	0–15.7%
1,8-Cineole	0–14.7%
α-Guiaiene	0–14.7%
α-Copaene	0–12.3%
Camphor	0–11.5%
β-Caryophyllene	0–10.9%
Camphene	1.2–7.3%
Yomogi alcohol	0–6.1%
β-Pinene	0–6.0%
β-Cubebene	0–3.9%
β-Myrcene	0–3.3%
(E)-Pinovarveol	0.3–2.8%
Sabinene	0–2.8%
p-Cymene	tr–2.7%
Verbenone	0–2.6%
Pinocarvone	tr–2.2%
3-Thujen-2-ol	0–2.2%
Caryophyllene oxide	0.1–1.6%
Bicyclogermacrene	0–1.3%
γ-Cadinene	0–1.1%
(Z)-β-Farnesene	0–1.1%
(E)-β-Farnesene	0–1.0%

(Chalchat et al 1991, 1994b; Héthelyi et al 1995; Lawrence 1995b p. 52–54)

Safety summary

Hazards: None known.
Contraindications: None known.

Organ-specific effects

Adverse skin reactions: No information found.
Neurotoxicity: During LD_{50} testing (see Acute toxicity) it was noted that ip doses higher than 1,500 mg/kg caused tremors, increased motor activity and sedation in mice, while lower doses did not (Radulovic et al 2013).
Nephrotoxicity: Annual wormwood oil had no adverse effects on kidney function and produced no histopathological lesions in kidney tissue when administered ip to rats at 200 mg/kg/day for 7 days (Radulovic et al 2013).
Hepatotoxicity: Annual wormwood oil had no adverse effects on liver function and produced no histopathological lesions in liver tissue when administered ip to rats at 200 mg/kg/day for 7 days (Radulovic et al 2013).

Systemic effects

Acute toxicity: An annual wormwood oil containing 35.7% artemisia ketone, 16.5% α-pinene and 4.8% artemisia alcohol had a mouse i.p. LD_{50} of 1,832 mg/kg (Radulovic et al 2013).
Carcinogenic/anticarcinogenic potential: Annual wormwood oil induced apoptosis in cultured human hepatocarcinoma SMMC-7721 cells (Li et al 2004). The oil contains no known carcinogens.

Comments

Annual wormwood oils high in artemisia ketone appear to be virtually non-toxic. Clearly there is great variation in the composition of annual wormwood oils, but this is not likely to affect toxicity.

Wormwood (sea)

Botanical name: *Artemisia maritima* L.
Botanical synonyms: *Artemisia contra* Willd. ex Spreng., *Artemisia lercheana* Kar. & Kir., *Artemisia salina* Willd., *Seriphidium maritimum* (L.) Poljakov.
Family: Asteraceae (Compositae)

Essential oil

Source: Leaves and flowering tops
Key constituents:

α-Thujone	63.3%
Sabinene	7.8%
1,8-Cineole	6.5%
Germacrene D	2.2%
Terpinen-4-ol	1.1%
β-Caryophyllene	1.0%

(Mathela et al 1994)

Safety summary

Hazards: Expected to be neurotoxic, based on thujone content.
Contraindications: Should not be taken in oral doses.
Contraindications (all routes): Pregnancy, breastfeeding.
Maximum dermal use level: 0.4%

Our safety advice

Our dermal maximum is based on 63.3% α-thujone content and a thujone limit of 0.25% (see Thujone profile, Chapter 14).

Organ-specific effects

Adverse skin reactions: No information found.
Neurotoxicity: No information found. There is a risk of convulsions with moderately high doses of thujone. The thujone NOAEL for convulsions was reported to be 10 mg/kg in male rats and 5 mg/kg in females (Margaria 1963).

Systemic effects

Acute toxicity: No information found. Both α- and β-thujone are moderately toxic, with reported oral LD_{50} values ranging from 190–500 mg/kg for different species (see Thujone profile, Chapter 14).
Carcinogenic/anticarcinogenic potential: No information was found for sea wormwood oil but it contains no known carcinogens.

Comments

In the EU SCF report on thujone it was concluded that the available data were inadequate to establish a TDI/ADI (SCF 2003b).

Wormwood (white)

Synonyms: Armoise, desert wormwood
Botanical name: *Artemisia herba-alba* Asso
Family: Asteraceae (Compositae)

Absolute

Source: Leaves and flowering tops
Key constituents:

Thujones	<70.0%
Camphor	<7.0%
Camphene	<4.0%
(+)-Limonene	<3.0%
Linalool	<2.0%

(EFFA 2008)

Essential oil

Source: Leaves and flowering tops
Key constituents:

α-Thujone / camphor CT	
Camphor	34.0–55.0%
α-Thujone	25.7–36.8%
β-Thujone	2.0–9.0%
Camphene	0.5–9.0%
1,8-Cineole	1.5–8.0%
Pinocarvone	0.5–1.7%
Santolinyl acetate	0.4–1.4%
Artemisia alcohol	0.3–1.2%
Yomogi alcohol	0.6–1.1%
p-Cymene	0.1–1.1%
Borneol	0.5–1.0%
Bornyl acetate	0.3–1.0%

(Lawrence 1993 p. 52–54)

Safety summary

Hazards: Expected to be neurotoxic, based on camphor and thujone content.
Contraindications: Should not be taken in oral doses.
Contraindications (all routes): Pregnancy, breastfeeding.
Maximum dermal use level (oil or absolute): 0.25%

Our safety advice

Our dermal maximum is based on 95% total thujone content (see data below), and a thujone limit of 0.25% (see Thujone profile, Chapter 14).

Organ-specific effects

Adverse skin reactions: Undiluted white wormwood oil was slightly irritating to the skin of rabbits and guinea pigs, but was not irritating to mice; tested at 12% on 25 volunteers it was neither irritating nor sensitizing. It is non-phototoxic (Opdyke 1975 p. 719).
Neurotoxicity: No information found. There is a risk of convulsions with moderately high doses of thujone. The thujone NOAEL for convulsions was reported to be 10 mg/kg in male rats and 5 mg/kg in females (Margaria 1963).

Systemic effects

Acute toxicity: White wormwood acute oral LD_{50} in mice 370 mg/kg; acute dermal LD_{50} in guinea pigs >5 g/kg (Opdyke 1975 p. 719).
Carcinogenic/anticarcinogenic potential: White wormwood oil is reported to be non-genotoxic and antigenotoxic (Bakkali et al 2006). The oil contains no known carcinogens.

Comments

The low LD_{50} of white wormwood oil is likely to be a reflection of its high thujone content. The source of white wormwood oil has previously been referred to as *Artemisia vulgaris* (see common mugwort) (Arctander 1960). The correct botanical origin is *Artemisia herba-alba* (Lawrence 1989 p. 1). Seven chemotypes for *Artemisia herba-alba* have been identified:

    I: α-thujone
    II: β-thujone
    III: camphor
    IV: chrysanthenyl acetate
    V: davanone
    VI: α-thujone/camphor
    VII: α-thujone/β-thujone
(Lawrence 1993 p. 52–54)

Most commercial armoise oils contain substantial quantities of thujone and camphor, and probably derive from chemotypes I, II, III, VI or VII. Chemotypes I, II, III and VI had been previously identified (Lawrence 1989 p. 53–55). The ranges of α-thujone, β-thujone and camphor seen in commercial armoise oils have been reported as:

α-Thujone	19.5–38.6%
β-Thujone	4.3–7.5%
Camphor	36.0–40.1%

(Lawrence 1989 p. 1)

These ranges are consistent with those given for chemotypes III and VI. The ranges for these constituents in some other chemotypes are:

I α-Thujone CT

α-Thujone	36.8–82.0%
Camphor	11.0–19.0%
β-Thujone	6.0–16.2%

(Lawrence 1993 p. 52–54)

II β-Thujone CT

β-Thujone	43.4–94.0%
α-Thujone	0.5–17.0%
Camphor	2.5–15.0%

(Lawrence 1993 p. 52–54)

III Camphor CT

Camphor	40.0–70.0%
α-Thujone	2.5–25.0%
β-Thujone	0.5–7.5%

(Lawrence 1993 p. 52–54)

On this basis, we have inferred that white wormwood oil may contain up to 95% thujone. In some oils there may be a synergistic toxic effect between thujone and camphor, although this has not been demonstrated. There may be a commercially available chrysanthenyl acetate chemotype, which would be relatively non-toxic, or this essential oil may in fact be common mugwort.

Yarrow (chamazulene CT)

Synonym: Milfoil
Botanical name: *Achillea millefolium* L.
Family: Asteraceae (Compositae)

Essential oil

Source: Aerial parts of flowering plant
Key constituents:

Sabinene	26.2%
Chamazulene	19.7%
β-Myrcene	7.0%
Germacrene D	6.2%
β-Pinene	4.6%
Camphor	3.3%
Camphene	3.2%
β-Caryophyllene	2.5%
β-Phellandrene	2.0%
α-Pinene	2.0%
Borneol	1.9%
β-Thujone	1.8%
Bornyl acetate	1.7%
γ-Terpinene	1.7%
1,8-Cineole	1.5%
β-Thujone	1.1%
(+)-Limonene	1.0%

(Rondeau, private communication, 1999)

Safety summary

Hazards: Drug interaction; slight neurotoxicity.
Cautions (all routes): Drugs metabolized by CYP2D6 (Appendix B).
Cautions (oral): Drugs metabolized by CYP1A2 or CYP3A4 (Appendix B).
Maximum adult daily oral dose: 241 mg
Maximum dermal use level: 8.6%

Our safety advice

Our oral and dermal restrictions are based on 2.9% total thujone content and thujone limits of 0.1 mg/kg and 0.25% (see Thujone profile, Chapter 14).

Organ-specific effects

Adverse skin reactions: No information found.
Neurotoxicity: Since yarrow oil inhibited convulsions induced by cardazol, a GABA receptor antagonist (Kudrzycka-Bieloszabska & Glowniak 1966), the presence of thujone (a potentiator of GABA-mediated responses) in the oil may not present a risk.

Systemic effects

Acute toxicity: Yarrow oil (chamazulene CT) mouse acute LD_{50} values: 3.65 g/kg oral, 3.1 g/kg ip (Kudrzycka-Bieloszabska & Glowniak 1966).
Carcinogenic/anticarcinogenic potential: Genotoxicity in *Aspergillus nidulans* has been reported for a yarrow oil with 42.2% chamazulene, 19.7% sabinene, 5.2% terpinen-4-ol, and 4.4% β-caryophyllene (Sant'anna et al 2009).
Drug interactions: Since chamazulene inhibits CYP1A2, CYP3A4 and CYP2D6 (Table 4.11B), there is a theoretical risk of interaction between yarrow oil (chamazulene CT) oil and drugs metabolized by these enzymes (Appendix B).

Comments

Yarrow is a very polymorphic species, which may be divided into at least two subspecies, with subsp. *millefolium* being the most common (Craker & Simon 1987 p. 227).

Yarrow (green)

Synonym: Ligurian yarrow
Botanical name: *Achillea nobilis* L.
Botanical synonym: *achillea ligustica* Vis. Ex Nym.
Family: Asteraceae (Compositae)

Essential oil

Source: Aerial parts of flowering plant
Key constituents:

Camphor	13.7%
Artemisia alcohol*	9.2%
Germacrene D	8.8%
Artemisia ketone	8.7%
Viridiflorol	5.7%
Sabinyl acetate	3.7%
Borneol	3.4%
Bornyl acetate	3.4%
Terpinen-4-ol	2.9%
β-Pinene	2.7%
Camphene	2.2%
1,8-Cineole	1.9%
γ-Terpinene	1.7%
Sabinol	1.6%
α-Pinene	1.3%
Chrysanthenyl acetate	1.0%

(Badoux, private communication, 2003)

Safety summary

Hazards: May be abortifacient.
Contraindications (all routes): Pregnancy, breastfeeding.

Organ-specific effects

Adverse skin reactions: No information found.
Reproductive toxicity: No information found. Sabinyl acetate is abortifacient in rodents at 15 mg/kg, and no safe dose is known for this compound.

Systemic effects

Acute toxicity: No information found.
Antioxidant/pro-oxidant activity: Green yarrow oil demonstrates good DPPH radical scavenging activity (Tuberoso et al 2005).
Carcinogenic/anticarcinogenic potential: No information was found for green yarrow oil but it contains no known carcinogens.

Comments

Limited availability.

Ylang-ylang

Botanical name: *Cananga odorata* J. D. Hook. & T. Thompson f. *odorata*
Botanical synonym: *Cananga odorata* J. D. Hook. & T. Thompson f. *genuina*
Family: *Annonaceae*

Absolute

Source: Flowers
Key constituents:

α-Farnesene	14.9%
Linalool	13.2%
Benzyl benzoate	11.8%

*Tentative identification

δ-Cadinene	10.8%	Geranyl acetate	3.7%
β-Caryophyllene	10.0%	p-Cresyl methyl ether	3.3%
Benzyl salicylate	5.2%	(E,E)-Farnesyl acetate	2.6%
Geranyl acetate	4.0%	α-Caryophyllene	2.5%
Methyl benzoate	3.5%	(E)-Cinnamyl acetate	2.4%
α-Caryophyllene	3.3%	(E,E)-Farnesol	2.3%
p-Cresyl methyl ether	3.0%	Methyl benzoate	2.0%
Benzyl acetate	2.8%	(Z)-3-Hexen-1-yl benzoate	1.6%
γ-Cadinene	2.8%	Bicyclogermacrene	1.0%
(E,E)-Farnesol	1.8%	α-Cadinol	1.0%
Geraniol	1.7%	3-Methyl-2-buten-1-yl acetate	1.0%
Safrole	0.4%	Isoeugenol	0.2%

(Buccellato 1982)

(Jones, private communication, 2003)

Safety summary

Hazards: Skin sensitization (moderate risk).
Cautions (dermal): Hypersensitive, diseased or damaged skin, children under 2 years of age.
Maximum dermal use level: 0.8% (see Regulatory Guidelines).

Regulatory guidelines

Maximum dermal use level of 0.8% based on IFRA guidelines (IFRA 2009). IFRA recommends a maximum exposure level of 0.01% of safrole from the use of safrole-containing essential oils, but this would give a dermal maximum of 2.5%, so is redundant.

Organ-specific effects

Adverse skin reactions: No information found.

Systemic effects

Acute toxicity: No information found.
Carcinogenic/anticarcinogenic potential: No information found. Safrole is a rodent carcinogen when oral exposure is sufficiently high (see Safrole profile, Chapter 14).

Comments

The safrole content of ylang-ylang absolute oil is not sufficiently high to be of concern.

Essential oil

Source: Flowers
Key constituents:

Ylang-ylang complete

Germacrene D	28.2%
Benzyl benzoate	9.1%
(E,E)-α-Farnesene	8.6%
Benzyl acetate	7.9%
Linalool	7.4%
β-Caryophyllene	7.1%

Ylang-ylang I Madagascan

Linalool	11.7–30.0%
Benzyl benzoate	4.3–14.9%
Germacrene D	0.1–13.5%
β-Caryophyllene	1.1–11.2%
Geranyl acetate	6.2–11.0%
Methyl salicylate	1.7–10.4%
p-Cresyl methyl ether	1.1–10.4%
Benzyl acetate	3.3–8.0%
(E,E)-Farnesyl acetate	0.5–7.8%
Methyl benzoate	1.7–5.6%
γ-Cadinene + α-farnesene	0.3–4.9%
α-Caryophyllene + ε−cadinene	1.4–3.7%
Benzyl salicylate	0.3–3.4%
Geraniol	0.9–3.0%
δ-Cadinol	0.1–3.0%
δ-Cadinene	0.2–2.8%
T-Muurolol + γ-cadinol	0.1–2.4%
α-Cadinol	0.2–2.0%
(E)-Cinnamyl acetate	0.6–1.9%
γ-Muurolene	0.5–1.9%
α-Copaene	0.4–1.6%
2-Methyl-3-buten-2-ol	0.3–1.3%
α-Muurolene	0.2–1.1%

(Gaydou et al 1988)

Ylang-ylang II Madagascan

β-Caryophyllene	1.7–19.6%
Germacrene D	1.5–19.3%
γ-Cadinene + α-farnesene	1.7–12.7%
Benzyl benzoate	5.3–12.3%
Linalool	3.9–12.2%
Geranyl acetate	2.6–7.2%
(E,E)-Farnesyl acetate	0.7–6.2%
α-Caryophyllene + ε−cadinene	3.4–5.8%
p-Cresyl methyl ether	0.6–5.3%
Methyl salicylate	0.6–5.3%

δ-Cadinene	2.1–5.2%
Benzyl salicylate	1.0–3.9%
γ-Muurolene	1.5–3.8%
α-Copaene	1.9–3.6%
Benzyl acetate	0.6–3.1%
Methyl benzoate	0.6–2.3%
α-Muurolene	0.7–1.9%
α-Cadinol	0.5–1.9%
(E)-Cinnamyl acetate	0.3–1.9%
T-Muurolol + γ-cadinol	0.4–1.5%
Geraniol	0.1–1.2%
α-Pinene	0.1–1.2%
δ-Cadinol	0.2–1.0%

(Gaydou et al 1988)

Ylang-ylang III Madagascan

Germacrene D	15.1–25.1%
β-Caryophyllene	14.8–21.5%
γ-Cadinene + α-farnesene	6.5–17.4%
Benzyl benzoate	5.9–12.8%
α-Caryophyllene + ε−cadinene	3.9–5.8%
δ-Cadinene	3.1–4.8%
Linalool	1.3–4.8%
Geranyl acetate	2.0–.4%
α-Copaene	2.1–3.5%
γ-Muurolene	2.0–3.2%
(E,E)-Farnesyl acetate	1.6–3.1%
Benzyl salicylate	0.7–2.7%
p-Cresyl methyl ether	0.4–1.9%
Methyl salicylate	0.4–1.9%
Geraniol	0.1–1.7%
α-Muurolene	0.8–1.6%
α-Cadinol	0.8–1.5%
Benzyl acetate	0.4–1.2%

(Gaydou et al 1988)

Note: See Table 13.5 for composition of Comoran Ylang-ylang oils. **Quality:** Gurjun balsam oil may be used as an adulterant in ylang-ylang oil. The 'extra' quality may be adulterated with lower grades of the oil, with synthetic materials such as benzyl acetate, methyl benzoate, benzyl benzoate and p-cresyl methyl ether, and with other natural and synthetic materials (Kubeczka 2002). All ylang-ylang oils may be adulterated with cheaper ylang-ylang oils, tail fractions or reconstituted oils (Burfield 2003). The flowers of *Artabotrys uncinatus* (Lamk.) Merrill are sometimes mixed with ylang-ylang flowers as adulterants. They are fragrant and have a similar appearance (Oyen & Dung 1999 p72).

Safety summary

Hazards: Skin sensitization (moderate risk).
Cautions (dermal): Hypersensitive, diseased or damaged skin, children under 2 years of age.
Maximum dermal use level: 0.8%

Table 13.5 Ylang-ylang Comoro oil composition

Constituent	Ylang-ylang extra	Ylang-ylang I	Ylang-ylang II	Ylang-ylang III
Germacrene D	17.1%	20.1%	21.7%	21.7%
α-Farnesene	8.2%	10.7%	15.7%	23.8%
β-Caryophyllene	5.2%	8.0%	12.9%	12.4%
Benzyl acetate	12.4%	5.8%	1.7%	0.7%
Linalool	8.6%	7.3%	2.6%	0.8%
Benzyl benzoate	4.8%	5.8%	6.3%	5.4%
p-Cresyl methyl ether	8.5%	5.8%	1.2%	0.4%
Geranyl acetate	4.5%	4.3%	3.0%	1.2%
Methyl benzoate	5.0%	3.4%	–	0.2%
Cinnamyl acetate	4.0%	2.8%	1.1%	0.9%
α-Caryophyllene	1.8%	2.7%	3.4%	3.6%
Benzyl salicylate	2.4%	2.6%	3.1%	2.8%
(E,E)-Farnesyl acetate	1.7%	1.9%	2.7%	3.5%
δ-Cadinene	1.1%	1.7%	3.1%	3.7%
(Z,Z)-Farnesyl acetate	1.3%	1.6%	2.0%	1.6%
Prenyl acetate	2.3%	1.3%	–	0.02%
Isoeugenol	0.5%	0.5%	0.3%	0.4%
Estragole	0.05%	0.06%	0.05%	0.01%

Regulatory guidelines

Has GRAS status. Maximum dermal use level of 0.8% based on IFRA guidelines for category 5 (women's facial creams, hand creams) and category 4 (body creams, oils, lotions) (IFRA 2009).

Organ-specific effects

Adverse skin reactions, irritation: Undiluted ylang-ylang oil was slightly irritating to rabbits, but was not irritating to mice; tested at 10% on 25 volunteers it was not irritating (Opdyke 1974 p. 1015–1016).
Adverse skin reactions, phototoxicity: Ylang-ylang oil is non-phototoxic (Opdyke 1974 p. 1015–1016).

Adverse skin reactions, sensitization: Of four reports of maximation tests using the oil at 10%, one produced two positive reactions from 40 individuals; in the other three there were no reactions from 25, 43 and 105 volunteers (Opdyke 1974 p. 1015–1016). In an 18 month multicenter study, 18 of 1,825 dermatitis patients (1.0%) were sensitive to 20% ylang-ylang oil (De Groot et al 2000). Ylang-ylang I and ylang-ylang II, both tested at 2%, induced allergic responses in 42 (2.6%) and 41 (2.5%), respectively, of 1,606 consecutive patients (Frosch et al 2002b). The two oils, similarly tested at 10%, produced reactions in five (1.6%) and six (1.9%) of 318 patients, respectively (Paulsen & Andersen 2005). In a study of 200 consecutive patients, four (2%) were sensitive to 2% ylang-ylang oil (Rudzki et al 1976). In two multicenter studies, 1.1% of 4,893 patients, reacted to 2% ylang-ylang oil (Pratt et al 2004) and 0.7% (11/1,603) patients reacted to 2% ylang-ylang extra (Belsito et al 2006).

Of 167 fragrance-sensitive dermatitis patients, 29 (17.4%) were allergic to 10% ylang-ylang oil (Larsen et al 1996b). From 1990 to 1998 the average patch test positivity rate to 5% ylang-ylang oil in a total of 1,483 Japanese eczema patients (99% female) suspected of cosmetic sensitivity was 2.25% (Sugiura et al 2000). In a multicenter study, Germany's IVDK reported that 84 of 3,175 consecutive patients (2.65%), and 90 of 2,155 patients suspected of fragrance allergy (4.17%) tested positive to 10% ylang-ylang I or II (Uter et al 2010). Of 167 fragrance-sensitive dermatitis patients, 29 (17.4%) were allergic to 10% ylang-ylang oil (Larsen et al 1996b). The above 15 reports are summarized in Table 13.6. In a clinical trial for head lice, a preparation containing unknown concentrations of ylang-ylang oil and anise oil was applied to the heads of 70 children aged 6–14, three times over 2 weeks. No clinically detectable adverse reactions were seen (Mumcuoglu et al 2002).

A beautician with no history of atopy developed hand eczema after using a massage lotion containing ylang-ylang oil. A 2% patch test confirmed the sensitivity (Romaguera & Vilaplana 2000). A woman who filled cosmetics, some of which contained ylang-ylang oil, into containers, developed hand eczema, and tested positive to 2% ylang-ylang oil, 2% cinnamyl alcohol and 2% cinnamaldehyde (Kenerva et al 1995). A 65-year-old aromatherapist with multiple essential oil sensitivities reacted to both 1% and 5% ylang-ylang oil (Selvaag et al 1995).

Adverse skin reactions, pigmented contact dermatitis: Ylang-ylang oil is regarded as a high-risk skin sensitizer and potential cause of pigmented contact dermatitis in Japan (Nakayama 1998). In tests using guinea pigs, 20% ylang-ylang oil caused hyperpigmentation that followed contact allergy. As part of the test procedure, the animals were injected with complete adjuvant, an inflammatory substance (Imokawa & Kawai 1987).

Systemic effects

Acute toxicity: Non-toxic. Ylang-ylang oil acute oral LD_{50} in rats >5 g/kg; acute dermal LD_{50} in rabbits >5 g/kg (Opdyke 1974 p. 1015–1016).

Table 13.6 Allergic reactions to ylang-ylang oil

A. Dermatitis patients

Concentration, oil grade if stated	Percentage who reacted	Number of reactors	Reference
2% ylang-ylang extra	0.7%	11/1,603	Belsito et al 2006
2%	1.1%	54/4,893	Pratt et al 2004
2%	2%	4/200	Rudzki et al 1976
2% ylang-ylang II	2.5%	41/1,606	Frosch et al 2002b
2% ylang-ylang I	2.6%	42/1,606	Frosch et al 2002b
10%	0%	0/25	Opdyke 1974 p. 1015–1016
10%	0%	0/43	Opdyke 1974 p. 1015–1016
10%	0%	0/105	Opdyke 1974 p. 1015–1016
10% ylang-ylang I or II	2.65%	84/3,175	Uter et al 2010
10% ylang-ylang I	1.6%	5/318	Paulsen & Andersen 2005
10% ylang-ylang II	1.9%	6/318	Paulsen & Andersen 2005
10%	5%	2/40	Opdyke 1974 p. 1015–1016
20%	1%	18/1,825	De Groot et al 2000

B. Dermatitis patients with suspected cosmetic or fragrance sensitivity

Concentration, oil grade if stated	Percentage who reacted	Number of reactors	Reference
5%	2.25%	33/1,483	Sugiura et al 2000
10% ylang-ylang I or II	4.18%	90/2,155	Uter et al 2010

Antioxidant/pro-oxidant activity: In one report, ylang-ylang oil showed moderate activity as a DPPH radical scavenger (~62%) and high activity (100%) in the aldehyde/carboxylic acid assay (Wei and Shibamoto 2007a). In another report the DPPH scavenging assay for ylang-ylang oil showed identical results (Sacchetti et al 2005).

Carcinogenic/anticarcinogenic potential: No information was found for ylang-ylang oil. Estragole is a rodent carcinogen when exposure is sufficiently high. Linalool, β-caryophyllene and α-caryophyllene display anticarcinogenic acticity (see Constituent profiles, Chapter 14). α-Cadinol is active against the human colon cancer cell line HT-29 (He et al 1997a).

Comments

There are five types of ylang-ylang oil: 'extra', 'first', 'second', 'third' and 'complete'. The first four are fractional distillates which are separated in the order they are collected during distillation of the flowers. Ylang-ylang complete is a combination of all four distillates, and so is the closest to a whole essential oil. It is noteworthy from a skin safety viewpoint that isoeugenol is found in Comoran, but not Madagascan ylang-ylang. Tail fractions of ylang-ylang can contain traces of safrole. The estragole content of ylang-ylang oils is not sufficiently high to be of concern, especially considering the presence of anticarcinogenic constituents. It is interesting that methyl salicylate is found in Madagascan, and not Comoran oils, but the amounts present do not suggest a need for restriction.

There is no clear consensus on which constituent(s) of ylang-ylang oil may be responsible for skin reactions, though isoeugenol is most frequently suspected. Burfield points out that dehydrodiisoeugenol, a dimer of isoeugenol, has been identified as a potent sensitizer in ylang-ylang oil (Watanabe et al 1985, cited in: http://www.cropwatch.org/nwsletters.htm Newsletter 14 January 2009). Conversely, in a guinea pig maximation test, dehydrodiisoeugenol was less skin sensitizing than isoeugenol (Takeyoshi et al 2008).

Yuzu

Botanical name: *Citrus junos* Sieb. ex Tanaka.
Family: Rutaceae

Essential oil

Source: Fruit peel, by expression
Key constituents:

(+)-Limonene	63.1%
γ-Terpinene	12.5%
β-Phellandrene	5.4%
β-Myrcene	3.2%
Linalool	2–8%
α-Pinene	2.7%
Bicyclogermacrene	2.0%
(*E*)-β-Farnesene	1.3%
β-Pinene	1.1%

(Sawamura 2009)

Safety summary

Hazards: Skin sensitization if oxidized.
Cautions: Old or oxidized oils should be avoided.

Our safety advice

Because of its (+)-limonene content we recommend that oxidation of yuzu oil is avoided by storage in a dark, airtight container in a refrigerator. The addition of an antioxidant to preparations containing it is recommended.

Regulatory guidelines

IFRA recommends that essential oils rich in limonene should only be used when the level of peroxides is kept to the lowest practical level, for instance by adding antioxidants at the time of production (IFRA 2009).

Organ-specific effects

Adverse skin reactions: In tests of seven samples of expressed yuzu oil from Kochi Prefecture in Japan (where it is commercially produced), no bergapten was detected in four samples, and levels in the other three ranged from 0.5 to 3.8 ppm. No bergapten was found in yuzu oils produced by either steam distillation or supersonic distillation (Sawamura et al 2009). This strongly suggests that yuzu oil is not phototoxic. Autoxidation products of (+)-limonene can cause skin sensitization (see (+)-Limonene profile, Chapter 14).
Reproductive toxicity: The low developmental toxicity of (+)-limonene in rabbits and mice (Kodama et al 1977a, 1977b) suggests that yuzu oil is not hazardous in pregnancy.

Systemic effects

Acute toxicity: No information was found for yuzu oil. However, since its composition is very similar to other citrus oils it is likely to be non-toxic.
Carcinogenic/anticarcinogenic potential: Yuzu oil inhibited the formation of the carcinogen NDMA in the presence of vegetables (by 22–59%) or saliva (by 24–62%) (Sawamura et al 2005). The oil contains no known carcinogens. (+)-Limonene displays anticarcinogenic activity (see (+)-Limonene profile, Chapter 14).

Comments

Yuzu oils are produced in Japan and Korea.

Zdravetz

Synonyms: Bulgarian geranium, bigroot geranium
Botanical name: *Geranium macrorrhizum* L.
Family: Geraniaceae

Essential oil

Source: Leaves
Key constituents:

Germacrone	49.7%
Germacrene B	11.3%
γ-Curcumene	4.1%
trans-β-Elemenone	1.6%
Terpinolene	1.6%
(Z)-β-Ocimene	1.5%
γ-Terpinene	1.4%
α-Bulnesene (δ-guaiene)	1.3%
γ-Elemene	1.3%

Amorpha-4,7-dien-11-ol	1.1%
Eremophila-1(10),11-dien-9β-ol	1.1%

(Radulović et al 2010)

Safety summary

Hazards: None known.
Contraindications: None known.

Organ-specific effects

Adverse skin reactions: No information was found for zdravetz oil. In a study of 200 consecutive dermatitis patients, one (0.5%) was sensitive to 2% zdravetz *concrete* on patch testing (Rudzki et al 1976).
Hepatotoxicity: A single oral dose of 12.5, 25 or 50 mg/kg of germacrone showed dose-dependent protection against liver injury induced in mice by D-galactosamine/lipopolysaccharide or TNF-α (Morikawa et al 2002).

Systemic effects

Acute toxicity: No information was found for zdravetz oil or germacrone.
Carcinogenic/anticarcinogenic potential: No information was found for zdravetz oil, but it contains no known carcinogens. Germacrone dose-dependently inhibited the growth of human breast cancer cells (MCF-7 and MDA-MB-231) in vitro (Zhong et al 2011).

Comments

The plant has been widely used in Bulgarian folk medicine. Germacrone is reported to be odorless (Burfield 2000 p. 262).

Zedoary

Synonyms: White turmeric, hidden ginger
Botanical name: *Curcuma zedoaria* Roscoe
Family: Zingiberaceae

Essential oil

Source: Rhizomes
Key constituents:

Chinese (simultaneous steam distillation and solvent extraction)

Epicurzerenone	24.1%
Cuzerene	10.4%
Curdione	7.0%
5-Isopropylidene-3,8-dimethyl-1(5H)-azulenone	4.3%
Isocurcumenol	3.0%
Spathulenol	3.0%
Curzerenone	2.4%
1,8-Cineole	2.0%

β-Elemene	1.9%
Camphor	1.7%
Zingiberene	1.5%
Curcumol	1.4%
Eudesmol*	1.4%
α-Selinene	1.3%
β-Bisabolene	1.2%
Germacrene B	1.2%
α-Caryophyllene	1.0%
α-Curcumene	1.0%

(Mau et al 2003)

Indian (hydrodistilled)

Curzerenone	22.3%
1,8-Cineole	15.9%
Germacrone	9.0%
Camphor	7.8%
β-Pinene	5.9%
Curzerene	5.0%
α-Pinene	3.7%
Isoborneol	2.1%
Camphene	1.9%
β-Elemene	1.5%
(Z)-β-Elemenone	1.5%
Germacrene B	1.2%
(+)-Limonene	1.2%
2-Nonanol	1.0%

(Purkayastha et al 2006)

Safety summary

Hazards: May interfere with gestation.
Contraindications (all routes): Pregnancy, breastfeeding.

Regulatory guidelines

Has GRAS status.

Organ-specific effects

Adverse skin reactions: No information found.
Reproductive toxicity: Chinese zedoary oil was administered to pregnant mice on gestational days 4–6 as a 1% or 10% aqueous solution with Tween 80 as an emulsifier. Ip doses of essential oil were 156, 310 and 625 mg/kg on gestational days 2–4, and sc doses were 600 and 900 mg/kg/day on gestational days 4–6. Prevention of implantation was dose-dependently successful, ranging from 10% to 80% ip, and from 70% to 90% sc. The oil prevented 77% of pregnancies in female rats when given ip at 300 mg/kg on gestational days 7–9. It prevented 16% and 100% of pregnancies in female rabbits when administered intra-vaginally at 60 or 400 mg/kg/day on gestational days 5–9 and 2–4, respectively (An et al 1983). The oil was steam distilled, but no compositional details were given. Ethanol extracts

*Isomer not specified

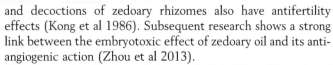

and decoctions of zedoary rhizomes also have antifertility effects (Kong et al 1986). Subsequent research shows a strong link between the embryotoxic effect of zedoary oil and its anti-angiogenic action (Zhou et al 2013).

Hepatotoxicity: Single oral doses of 12.5, 25 or 50 mg/kg of either germacrone or curcumenol showed dose-dependent protection against liver injury induced in mice by D-galactosamine / lipopolysaccharide or TNF-α (Morikawa et al 2002).

Systemic effects

Acute toxicity: No information found.

Carcinogenic/anticarcinogenic potential: A Chinese hydrodistilled zedoary oil was cytotoxic to mouse melanoma B16BL6 cells (IC$_{50}$ 41.8 µg/mL), and to human hepatoma SMMC-7721 cells (IC$_{50}$ 30.7 µg/mL). Zedoary oil also inhibited angiogenesis in mice (Chen et al 2011). The essential oil analyzed by Mau et al 2003 (see above) was cytotoxic to human leukemia HL-60 cells, with an IC$_{50}$ of 500 ppm (Lai et al 2004). α-Caryophyllene and β-elemene display anticarcinogenic activity (see Constituent profiles, Chapter 14). Germacrone dose-dependently inhibited the growth of human breast cancer cells (MCF-7 and MDA-MB-231) in vitro (Zhong et al 2011). Curzerenone has been used as an anticancer agent in China (Hsu 1980).

Comments

No NOAEL for reproductive toxicity can be extrapolated from the Chinese data cited above. We could find nothing to suggest which constituent(s) of zedoary oil might be responsible for its antifertility effect.

Constituent profiles

14

The purpose of these profiles is to provide safety information for essential oil constituents, all of which are referred to in other sections of the book, to complement the information on whole essential oils. The constituent profiles may also provide a basis for assessing the safety of an essential oil not profiled in this book. We have only included constituents for which we could find relevant data, which means that there are many compounds not profiled. These include some commonly-occurring terpenes, such as β-phellandrene, sabinene and germacrene D, and many compounds specific to only a few essential oils, such as artemisia alcohol, artemisia ketone and chrysanthenyl acetate.

Note that while some constituents present a potential risk in their isolated state, any such risk may be substantially reduced in equivalent amounts of essential oils. Examples include *p*-cresol, benzyl acetate and guaiacol. Also note that sensitization reactions can be caused, not by the principal compound being tested, but by impurities. Examples include coumarin, farnesol and nootkatone. Impurities are not necessarily sensitizing, but they are found to varying degrees in most synthesized chemicals.

We have proposed our own guidelines for some constituents that, at the time of writing, are not restricted by some regulatory agencies. In other cases we give guidelines that are less restrictive than existing ones. The reasons for this are explained in the Toxicity chapter. Table 14.1 presents a comparison of restrictions for some important toxic constituents.

In the profiles below, the percentages represent the amount of each constituent present in the corresponding aromatic material, and these cross-reference with the percentages in the essential oil profiles. In order to avoid unnecessarily long lists, some percentages are only given down to 10% or 5%, as distinct from 1% in the essential oil profiles. The materials referred to are all

essential oils, unless otherwise stated. We have not given the botanical names again, since these can be found in the essential oil profiles chapter.

The systematic names of constituents are included here together with their more common or trivial names, to clarify exactly which compounds are associated with the reported physiological actions. A systematic name is the full, unambiguous, chemical name of a compound, as opposed to the trivial name, which usually derives from the name of its source, such as 'bergamottin' (bergamot) and 'thujone' (thuja). Just as a constituent may have one or more trivial names, it may also have more than one systematic name, an example being the name recommended by the International Union of Pure and Applied Chemistry (IUPAC). Generic systematic names have been given for geometric and optical isomers which share a common connectivity between atoms. For structural isomers whose connectivity differs, one systematic name is given for each isomer. Unique Chemical Abstracts Service (CAS) registry numbers have also been included to eliminate any ambiguity relating to the identity of the compounds presented.

Although we include detailed information here about the different isomeric forms that exist for various essential oil constituents, much of the literature information presented on toxicology and pharmacology fails to mention whether specific isomers were studied. Until more precise information becomes available, these may provide an indication of the properties of the specific constituents. However, where such information is available, this is stated.

Isomers

There are many different types of isomer. In essential oils, those usually encountered are:

• *structural isomers:* isomers that have identical numbers and types of constituent atoms, but different connections between

Table 14.1 Our restrictions for toxic constituents compared to those of some regulatory agencies

Constituent	Oral maximum Tisserand & Young (mg/kg/day)	Specific gravity (g/cm^3)	Dermal maximum			
			Tisserand & Young[a]	EU	IFRA	Health Canada
Apiole (parsley)	0.4	1.2	0.76%	Not listed	Not listed	Not listed
α-Asarone	0.15	1.05	0.33%	Not listed	0.01%	Not listed
β-Asarone	0.1	1.07	0.22%	Not listed	0.01%	Not listed
Ascaridole[b]	0.05	0.99	0.12%	Not listed	Not listed	Not listed
Camphor	2.0	0.99	4.5%	Not listed	Not listed	3.0%
(+)-Carvone	12.5	0.96	23%	Not listed	1.2%[c]	Not listed
(−)-Carvone	12.5	0.96	1.2%[c]	Not listed	1.2%[c]	Not listed
Coumarin	0.6	n/a	No limit	0.001%[c,d]	1.6%[c]	Not listed
Estragole	0.05	0.97	0.12%	Not listed	0.01%	Not listed
Menthofuran	0.2	0.95	0.50%	Not listed	Not listed	Not listed
Methyleugenol	0.01	1.03	0.02%	0.0002%	0.0004%	0.0002%
Methyl salicylate	2.5	1.18	2.4%[e]	Not listed	Not listed	1.0%
Pinocamphone + isopinocamphone	0.1	0.97	0.24%	Not listed	Not listed	Not listed
β-Pulegone	0.5	0.93	1.2%	Not listed	Not listed	Not listed
Safrole	0.025	1.10	0.05%	0.01%	0.01%	—[f]
α- + β-Thujone	0.1	0.92	0.25%	Not listed	Not listed	Not listed

[a]The percentage of administered diluted oil $= (V_1) \times 100 / (V_1 + V_2)$; where V_1 = volume of essential oil and V_2 = volume of carrier oil, both in mL.

$$V_1 = \frac{\text{oral dose (mg/kg)} \times \text{weight of a human adult (kg)}}{\text{fraction of constituent(s) absorbed} \times \text{specific gravity} \times 1000}$$

These values are calculated for dermal penetration of 10%, a dilution with 30 mL of carrier oil, and a human adult weight of 70 kg.

[b]Note that wormseed oil, which contains ascaridole, is prohibited in cosmetics by IFRA, the EU, and Health Canada

[c]This limit is for skin sensitization

[d]Not a legal limit

[e]Assuming dermal penetration of 20%

[f]Safrole is prohibited by Health Canada, except 'when naturally occurring in plant extracts'

them (e.g., dill and parsley apiole). Structural isomers have different physical properties, such as boiling points

- *geometric isomers:* isomers that have identical numbers and types of constituent atoms, and the same connections between them, but different arrangements either side of a carbon–carbon double bond (e.g., nerol and geraniol, see Figure 2.3). Geometric isomers have different physical properties, such as boiling points

- *optical isomers:* pairs of molecules containing one chiral center, which have the same numbers and types of atoms and connections between them, but whose atoms are arranged differently in space. They are non-identical mirror images of one another, rather like a pair of gloves. Generally, optical isomers (also known as enantiomers) have the same chemical and physical properties, but when in solution, rotate the plane of polarized light to the same extent, but in opposite

directions. One optical isomer will rotate it clockwise (the (+)- or D-isomer), the other anti-clockwise (the (−)- or L-isomer). Despite their chemical similarities, optical isomers can have very different pharmacological and toxicological properties, as well as different tastes and odors (e.g., (+)- and (−)-carvone)

- *diastereoisomers* are similar to enantiomers, but possess more than one chiral center, and hence are usually not mirror images

Constituent profiles A–Z

Acetophenone

Synonym: Methyl phenyl ketone
Systematic name: 1-Phenylethanone

Chemical class: Benzenoid ketone
CAS number: 98-86-2

Sources >1.0%:

Cistus   0–2.2%

Note: Also found as a minor or trace component of orris, and several other essential oils.

Pharmacokinetics: The metabolism of acetophenone in animals has been extensively studied. In both rabbits and dogs it is metabolized both by reduction and oxidation (Scheline 1991 p. 114).

Adverse skin reactions: In a modified Draize procedure on guinea pigs, acetophenone was non-sensitizing when used at 20% in the challenge phase (Sharp 1978). Tested at 2% on the skin of human volunteers, acetophenone was not sensitizing (Opdyke 1978 p. 99–100).

Acute toxicity: Acute oral LD_{50} in rats 3.2 g/kg (Jenner et al 1964); acute dermal LD_{50} in guinea pigs >20 mL/kg. No rats died after exposure to an atmosphere saturated (0.45%) with acetophenone (Opdyke 1978 p. 99–100).

Subacute and subchronic toxicity: No adverse effects were observed after 1,000, 2,500 or 10,000 ppm fed to rats in the diet for 17 weeks (Hagan et al 1967).

Mutagenicity and genotoxicity: Acetophenone was not mutagenic in the Ames test (Florin et al 1980; Ishidate et al 1984).

Comments: Commercial acetophenone is extensively used as an intermediate in the fragrance, pharmaceutical and agrochemical industries. It has been used in the past as a sedative. The chemically related benzophenone is used to block UV light.

Summary: Considering its low occurrence in essential oils and lack of apparent toxicity, acetophenone is not a safety concern.

Alantolactone

Synonyms: Helenin. Elecampane camphor. Eupatal. 5,11(13)-Eudesmadien-12,8-olide
Systematic name: [3aR (3aα,5β,8aβ,9aα)]-3a,5,6,7,8,8a,9,9a-Octahydro-5,8a-dimethyl-3-methylene-naphtho[2,3-b]furan-2(3H)-one
Chemical class: Tricyclic sesquiterpenoid alkene lactone
CAS number: 546-43-0

Source:

Elecampane   52.4%

Adverse skin reactions: Sesquiterpene lactones from Compositae plants are notorious skin sensitizers (Ross et al 1993; Goulden & Wilkinson 1998). Alantolactone is a hapten that reacts with free amino acids, and with purified protein fractions taken from skin tissue (Dupuis & Brisson 1976). It elicited positive patch-test responses in sensitized guinea pigs, and four of 25 dermatitis patients were sensitized to it with a single patch test using a 1% concentration (Opdyke 1976 p. 307–308). Alantolactone was dose-dependently cytotoxic to leukocytes taken from individuals not sensitive to it (Dupuis & Brisson 1976). Based on literature published in German, alantolactone was classified as Category A, a significant contact allergen, by Schlede et al (2003).

Carcinogenic/anticarcinogenic potential: Alantolactone dose-dependently induces the detoxifying enzymes quinone reductase, glutathione reductase, glutathione S-transferase, γ-glutamylcysteine synthase and heme oxygenase (Seo et al 2008a). Alantolactone is cytotoxic in vitro against cell lines for human leukemia (IC_{50} 0.7 μM; 162 μg/L), human gastric adenocarcinoma (IC_{50} 6.9 μM; 1,600 μg/L), human uterus carcinoma (IC_{50} 6.9 μM; 1,600 μg/L), and mouse melanoma (IC_{50} 4.7 μM; 1,090 μg/L) (Lawrence et al 2001; Konishi et al 2002). Alantolactone induces apoptosis in Jurkat leukemia T cells (Dirsch et al 2001).

Comments: The propensity of alantolactone to bind with proteins is probably associated with its tendency to cause skin sensitization, to induce detoxifying enzymes, and to be toxic to cancer cells. Isoalantolacone, not profiled in this book, demonstrates similar properties.

Summary: Alantolactone is only found in one commercially available essential oil, and is partially responsible for the high risk of skin sensitization that elecampane oil presents.

Allyl isothiocyanate

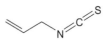

Synonyms: Allyl isosulfocyanate. 3-Isothiocyanato-1-propene
Chemical class: Aliphatic alkene thiocarbonyl compound
CAS number: 57-06-7

Sources >1.0%:

Horseradish   44.3–55.7%
Mustard   23.2–68.8%

Notes: A pale yellow, pungent, lachrymatory, irritating compound with an acrid taste. Also found in cabbage and broccoli and used in food flavorings, but in both cases at very low concentrations.

Pharmacokinetics: Allyl isothiocyanate is metabolized to mercapturic acids (Ioannou et al 1984; Mennicke et al 1983; Bollard et al 1997) and conjugated with N-acetylcysteine (Jiao et al 1994). In rats and mice ~75% was excreted in the urine, ~13–15% in the expired air and 1–5% in the feces (Ioannou et al 1984). It appears that allyl isothiocyanate can be transported around the body as inactive (−)-cysteine or glutathione conjugates and then released in the reactive form at another site, to cause damage there (Bruggeman et al 1986).

Allyl isothiocyanate stimulates liver fat production in rats (Muztar et al 1979a) and strongly depresses plasma glucose (Muztar et al 1979b). It was goitrogenic in rats at 2–4 mg po (Langer & Stolc 1965). Increases urate excretion rate (Huque & Ahmad 1975). Speeds up blood clotting in rats (Idris & Ahmad 1975).

Adverse skin reactions: A severe irritant to mucous membranes and skin (Evans & Schmidt 1980; Budavari 1989). Only two of 259 dermatitis patients (0.8%) with suspected ACD from vegetables and food had a + allergic reaction to allyl isothiocyanate, but 43 (16.6%) had a ?+reaction, which might be due to the irritancy of the compound (Lerbaek et al 2004).

Acute toxicity: Acute oral LD_{50} in rats reported as 490 mg/kg and as 340 mg/kg; mouse oral LD_{50} 310 mg/kg (Jenner et al 1964; Vernot et al 1977). Acute sc LD_{50} 80 mg/kg in mice (Klesse & Lukoschek 1955); acute dermal LD_{50} in rabbits 88 mg/kg (Vernot et al 1977). A rat oral LD_{50} value of 112 mg/kg is frequently cited on MSDS for allyl isothiocyanate, but we could find no citation for this.

Subacute and subchronic toxicity: Given to rats at 50 mg/kg in the diet for 20 days, allyl isothiocyanate caused acute to subacute stomach ulceration in all animals. At 20 mg/kg for 20 days, ulceration occurred in 50% of animals. At 50 mg/kg for 14 days, it caused thickening of the mucosal lining of the stomach in both rats and mice, and thickening of the urinary bladder wall in male mice. No gross or microscopic lesions were seen after feeding allyl isothiocyanate to rats and mice for 13 weeks at 25 mg/kg (National Toxicology Program 1982). Given to rats in the diet for 26 weeks at 1,000, 2,500 or 10,000 ppm there were no observable adverse effects (Hagan et al 1967).

Reproductive toxicity: Allyl isothiocyanate caused embryonic death and decreased fetal weight in pregnant rats when given at doses of 50 mg/kg subcutaneously on two consecutive days (Nishie & Daxenbichler 1980).

Hepatotoxicity: Orally administered allyl isothiocyanate and its glutathione and N-acetylcysteine conjugates are considerably toxic to rat liver cells. Because the glutathione conjugate is incapable of crossing cell membranes, its cytotoxicity is believed to be due to its conversion back to the parent isothiocyanate (Bruggeman et al 1986; Temmink et al 1986; Masutomi et al 2001).

Mutagenicity and genotoxicity: In the Ames test, allyl isothiocyanate has been reported as mutagenic (Eder et al 1982; Neudecker & Henschler 1985) and non-mutagenic (Eder et al 1980; Kasamaki et al 1982; Azizan & Blevins 1995; Kono et al 1995). In Neudecker & Henschler's study, modified preincubation conditions were employed which would lead to increased levels of a reactive epoxide intermediate, as well as the known mutagen, acrolein. A further report gave both positive and negative findings (Mortelmans et al 1986). Allyl isothiocyanate was weakly genotoxic in tests on Chinese hamster cells in vitro (Kasamaki et al 1982). In a bone marrow micronucleus test involving three daily ip injections, the compound was not genotoxic in mice (Shelby et al 1993).

Carcinogenic/anticarcinogenic potential: In a 2 year carcinogenesis study, food-grade allyl isothiocyanate (>93% purity) was fed at 12 or 25 mg/kg five times a week to groups of 50 rats and 50 mice of each sex. It was carcinogenic in the male rats, causing papillomas in the urinary bladder. In female rats there was equivocal evidence of subcutaneous fibrosarcomas. This effect may be attributed to chronic irritation of the bladder epithelium by high concentrations of allyl isothiocyanate and its cysteine conjugate in the bladder (Bechtel et al 1998). However, in a different assay allyl isothiocyanate was not carcinogenic in either male or female mice (National Toxicology Program 1982). Allyl isothiocyanate can cause hyperplasia and transitional cell papillomas in male rats (Dunnick et al 1982). It showed moderate chemopreventive action against nitrosamine-induced carcinogenesis in rat tissues (Chung et al 1984) and significant chemopreventive action (92.5% inhibition) against pulmonary metastasis induced by melanoma cells in mice (Manesh & Kuttan 2003).

Summary: Allyl isothiocyanate shows no clear carcinogenic action. The degree of irritancy and toxicity of the compound, and the concentrations at which it occurs in mustard and horseradish oils indicates that, with the possible exception of extremely low doses, these essential oils are not safe to use in therapy.

Regulatory guidelines: IFRA recommends that allyl isothiocyanate is not used as a fragrance ingredient (IFRA 2009). Allyl isothiocyanate is prohibited as a cosmetic ingredient in the EU and Canada (Anon 2003a; Health Canada Cosmetic Ingredient Hotlist, March 2011). In a preliminary report by an ECETOC taskforce, allyl isothiocyanate was provisionally classified as a moderate allergen (on a scale of extreme, strong, moderate and weak) likely to elicit a sensitization reaction if present at 1% or more (Kimber et al 2003).

(Z)-Ambrettolide

Synonyms: *cis*-Ambrettolide. (Z)-7-Hexadecen-16-olide. Ambrettolic acid lactone
Systematic name: (Z)-Oxacycloheptadec-8-en-2-one
Chemical class: Monocyclic sesquiterpenoid alkene lactone
CAS number: 123-69-3

Source:

Ambrette   7.6–14.7%

Adverse skin reactions: Ambrettolide was not irritating when tested full strength on rabbit skin, and was neither irritating nor sensitizing when tested at 1% on human subjects (Opdyke 1975 p. 707).
Acute toxicity: Both the acute oral LD_{50} in rats, and the acute dermal LD_{50} in rabbits exceeded 5 g/kg (Opdyke 1975 p. 707).
Summary: Limited data, but the structure of the compound does not raise any red flags.

(E)-Anethole

Synonyms: *trans*-Anethole. *p-trans*-Propenylanisole. Anise camphor
Systematic name: (E)-4-Methoxy-(1-propenyl)benzene

Chemical class: Phenylpropenoid ether
CAS number: 4180-23-8

Sources >1.0%:

Anise	75.2–96.1%
Myrtle (aniseed)	95.0%
Fennel (sweet)	58.1–92.5%
Anise (star)	71.2–91.8%
Fennel (bitter)	52.5–84.3%
Betel	0–7.8%
Damiana	1.0%

Pharmacokinetics: (E)-Anethole is distributed and metabolized in a similar way in rats, rabbits and humans (Le Bourhis 1970) with most of an orally administered dose being excreted within 48 hours in mice (Strolin-Benedetti & Le Bourhis 1972). However, it is not distributed uniformly in the body. After intravenous dosing in mice, most of the (E)-anethole accumulated in the liver, lungs and brain. In some studies it is poorly absorbed from the gastrointestinal tract, with most of an administered dose remaining in the mouse stomach (Le Bourhis 1968). In another study very good absorption after oral dosing was seen (Sangster et al 1984a). These differences may be due to the methodologies chosen. In both rats and mice given 250 mg/kg of (E)-anethole, >95% of the dose was recovered, the majority in the 0–24 hour urine, from which 18 metabolites were identified.

The metabolism and toxicity of (E)-anethole have recently been reviewed (Newberne et al 1999). (E)-Anethole undergoes biotransformation by three principle pathways: O-demethylation, N-oxidation and epoxidation. The latter, which can lead to toxic metabolites, is only a minor pathway (~3%) in humans (Sangster et al 1987; Solheim & Scheline 1973; Bounds & Caldwell 1996). In animals, (E)-anethole is metabolized differently depending on dose (Caldwell et al 1983; Sangster et al 1984b), but not in human studies (Caldwell & Sutton 1988). Rats produce metabolites from ingested (E)-anethole that other species do not (Bounds & Caldwell 1996). A study using doses of (E)-anethole close to those found in the diet revealed that the major route of excretion is via the urine; carbon dioxide is formed as a by-product and is excreted in the expired air. Nine urinary metabolites are produced, all oxidation products. Most urinary metabolites are also detected in bile, suggesting that biliary excretion is an important route for the removal of (E)-anethole (Leibman & Ortiz 1973).

Adverse skin reactions: Tested at 2% on human subjects (E)-anethole was neither irritating nor sensitizing (Opdyke 1973, p. 863–864). Of 15 dermatitis patients who tested positive to 1.0% star anise oil, five were sensitive to (E)-anethole (Rudzki & Grzywa 1976). On standing uncovered for 90 days, synthetic anethole (which generally contains 2–3% of (Z)-anethole) was found to contain (E)-anethole 90.5%, (Z)-anethole 1%, plus anisaldehyde 3.5% and anisic ketone 3.5%, which are considered products of autoxidation (Kraus & Hammerschmidt 1980). It is not known whether oxidized anethole is significantly skin sensitizing.

Acute toxicity: Acute oral LD_{50} 2.09–3.20 g/kg in rats, 1.82–5.00 g/kg in mice, 2.16 g/kg in guinea pigs (Jenner et al 1964; Newberne et al 1999). The ip and oral LD_{50} values were 650 mg/kg and 900 mg/kg, respectively, in mice, and 0.9 g/kg and 3.2 g/kg, respectively, in rats (Boissier et al 1967).

Subacute and subchronic toxicity: Given to rats in the diet at 10,000 ppm for 15 weeks (E)-anethole caused slight hydropic changes of hepatic cells in males only; at 2,500 ppm for one year there were no effects (Hagan et al 1967).

Human toxicity: In reviewing the toxicity of (E)-anethole, Newberne et al (1999) conclude that the substance poses no risk to human health when used as a food flavoring.

Cardiovascular effects: (E)-Anethole shows strong antiplatelet aggregation activity in vitro (Yoshioka & Tamada 2005).

Reproductive toxicity: (E)-Anethole has estrogen-like effects in vitro, many times weaker than endogenous estrogens (Zondek & Bergmann 1938; Albert-Puleo 1980). There is some discussion about whether this weak activity is due to (E)-anethole itself or a polymer of the compound (Albert-Puleo 1980). The anethole metabolite, 4-hydroxy-1-propenylbenzene, weakly displaced 17β-estradiol from ERα receptors with an IC_{50} value of 10^{-5} M, and promoted the proliferation of cultured human MCF-7 cells at 10^{-8}–10^{-6} M. In the latter assay, anethole had no effect up to 10^{-5} M (Nakagawa & Suzuki 2003). (E)-Anethole did bind to estrogen receptors in recombinant yeast cells, but did not have estrogenic activity in either an estrogen-responsive human cell line (below cytotoxic concentrations) or a yeast screen for androgenic and anti-androgenic compounds (Howes et al 2002). Sweet fennel tea (containing (E)-anethole) has shown in vivo estrogenic effects in humans (Türkyilmaz et al 2008).

Oral doses of 50, 70 and 80 mg/kg of (E)-anethole, given to pregnant albino Charles Foster rats on gestational days 1–10, resulted in 33.3%, 66.6% and 100% reduction in implantation, respectively. It is suggested that this may be related to a disruption of hormonal balance. Given at 80 mg/kg/day for three days, (E)-anethole caused a significant increase in uterine weight in immature female rats, suggesting an estrogenic action (Dhar 1995). These results were not supported in an earlier study, in which female Crl:CD BR rats were given (E)-anethole at 25, 175 or 350 mg/kg by gavage for 7 days prior to mating and until day four of lactation. There was no reproductive toxicity at the lower doses, while some increase in mortality, stillbirths and reduction in body weight at birth was seen in the high dose group (ARL 1992, cited in Newberne et al 1999).

In a four generation reproduction study, (E)-anethole was given at 1% in the diet to male and female rats from weaning to 3 months of age. No treatment-related adverse effects were observed in any generation (Le Bourhis 1973a, cited in Newberne et al 1999).

Hepatotoxicity: Rompelberg et al (1993) reported that 125 or 250 mg/kg/day (E)-anethole by gavage for 10 days had no effect on total CYP content of rat liver microsomes, nor on the levels of EROD and PROD. Reed & Caldwell (1992) found that 300 mg/kg/day ip of (E)-anethole for 7 days caused a 45% increase in microsomal CYP in rats, and dietary administration at 0%, 0.25%, 0.5% or 1.0% caused a dose-dependent increase which was statistically significant at the two higher doses. Considering the results of both studies, it seems that lower doses have little or no effect.

(E)-Anethole is dose-dependently cytotoxic to rat liver cells in culture, and causes glutathione depletion. Both these effects are seen at high doses, and are due to anethole 1',2'-epoxide (AE), a reactive metabolic intermediate (Marshall & Caldwell 1992, 1993). In rats, dietary (E)-anethole has no adverse effect at 0.25% in the diet, causes mild hepatic changes at 0.5%, mostly enzyme induction of no pathological consequence (Newberne et al 1989). Hepatotoxicity caused by (E)-anethole is primarily due to AE, and female Sprague Dawley rats metabolize more (E)-anethole to AE than either mice or humans. At low levels of exposure, (E)-anethole is efficiently detoxified in rodents and humans primarily by O-demethylation and omega-oxidation, respectively, while epoxidation is only a minor pathway. At high doses in rats, particularly females, a metabolic shift occurs resulting in increased epoxidation and formation of AE. Lower activity of the 'fast acting' detoxication enzyme epoxide hydrolase in females is associated with more pronounced hepatotoxicity compared to that in males (Newberne et al 1999).

Mutagenicity and genotoxicity: (E)-Anethole was mutagenic in the Ames test, but not in the *Bacillus subtilis* DNA repair assay without S9 (Sekizawa & Shibamoto 1982). It was mutagenic in a mouse lymphoma assay but not in the Ames test (Hsia et al 1979; Mortelmans et al 1986; Gorelick 1995). AE has also been reported as both mutagenic and non-mutagenic in Ames tests (Marshall & Caldwell 1993; Kim SG et al 1999). UDS assays in rat hepatocytes with (E)-anethole have been either inconclusive or negative (Müller et al 1994; Marshall & Caldwell 1996). There is, at most, a low level of genotoxic activity (Phillips et al 1984; Randerath et al 1984; Howes et al 1990) but no significant carcinogenicity (Miller et al 1983; Truhaut et al 1989). (E)-Anethole inhibited the actions of various genotoxic compounds given by gavage to mice at doses of 40–400 mg/kg, and in one case, exerted a protective effect (Abraham 2001).

Carcinogenic/anticarcinogenic potential: When (E)-anethole was fed to mice at 0.46% in the diet for 12 months, there was no increase in tumors after 18 months, unlike mice fed similar doses of safrole or estragole (Miller et al 1983). One metabolite, 3'-hydroxyanethole, is not carcinogenic (Miller et al 1983). However, AE induced hepatomas and papillomas in mice (Kim SG et al 1999). In rats, 1% dietary (E)-anethole was associated with a low level of hepatocellular neoplasms. However, the slightly increased tumor incidence was seen in only the highest dose group of female rats, not in male rats, and also not in mice. (E)-Anethole is metabolized similarly in mice and humans (Newberne et al 1989).

In a novel assay for carcinogens, groups of male rats were dosed for 2, 14 or 90 days with 0.2 or 2.0 mmol/kg/day (296 mg/kg/day) of (E)-anethole, and hepatic tissue was analyzed for precancerous changes in gene expression. The results strongly suggest that (E)-anethole is not hepatocarcinogenic in male rats (Auerbach et al 2010).

(E)-Anethole was cytotoxic to the leukemic cell lines K562 and U937, reaching 77% and 82% cell death, respectively, at 10 mM (1.48 g/L) (Duvoix et al 2004). At oral doses of 0.50 and 1.00 g/kg, (E)-anethole caused significant reductions in the size and weight of Ehrlich ascites tumors in the mouse paw (Al-Harbi et al 1995). In male and female mice given 24 ip injections of (E)-anethole in impure tricaprylin in a total dose of 2.4 or 12.0 g/kg over 24 weeks the incidence of primary lung tumors was no higher than in the control group (Stoner et al 1973). The anticarcinogenic action of (E)-anethole may be due to the promotion of detoxifying enzymes. It also targets various transcription factors that inhibit uncontrolled cell growth. For example, it inhibits TNF-induced cellular responses, such as NF-κB activation (Chainy et al 2000). The results of a gene expression study suggest potent anticarcinogenic and antimetastatic activity for (E)-anethole (Choo et al 2011).

Summary: The continuous dietary intake of high doses of (E)-anethole (i.e. cumulative exposure) induces a continuum of cytotoxicity, cell necrosis and cell proliferation in rodents. In chronic dietary studies in rats, hepatotoxicity was observed when the estimated daily hepatic production of AE exceeded 30 mg/kg body weight. In female rats, chronic hepatotoxicity and a low incidence of liver tumors were reported at a dietary intake of 550 mg (E)-anethole/kg/day. Under these conditions, daily hepatic production of AE exceeded 120 mg/kg body weight (Newberne et al 1999). (E)-Anethole inhibits platelet aggregation.

The weight of evidence supports the conclusion that (E)-anethole is not genotoxic, and that hepatocarcinogenic effects in the female rat occur via a non-genotoxic mechanism and are secondary to hepatotoxicity caused by continuous exposure to high hepatocellular concentrations of AE (Newberne et al 1999). (E)-anethole undergoes efficient metabolic detoxication in humans at low levels of exposure. There is evidence of a weak estrogenic action, but there is some doubt about what would be a safe dose in humans.

Regulatory guidelines: JECFA has set an ADI of 2 mg/kg bw for (E)-anethole (JECFA 1998). (E)-Anethole has has been given GRAS status based on its use as a flavoring agent. In reviewing the compound's GRAS status the FEMA expert panel cited, among other considerations, the (E)-anethole NOAEL of 120 mg/kg/day in the female rat reported in a 2+year study which produces a level of AE (i.e., 22 mg AE/kg body weight/day) at least 10,000 times the level (0.002 mg AE/kg body weight day) produced from the intake of (E)-anethole from use as a flavoring substance (Newberne et al 1999). However, this review does not cite the paper by Dhar (1995), in which 50 mg/kg of (E)-anethole had an anti-implantation effect in pregnant rats.

Our safety advice: We consider that there is sufficient evidence of an estrogenic action for (E)-anethole, and that administration of essential oils containing a high proportion of it should be avoided by any route in pregnancy, breastfeeding, endometriosis and estrogen-dependent cancers. Because of its antiplatelet aggregation activity, oral dosing of essential oils high in (E)-anethole is cautioned in conjunction with anticoagulant drugs, major surgery, childbirth, peptic ulcer, hemophilia or other bleeding disorders (see Box 7.1 for more detail).

(Z)-Anethole

Synonyms: *cis*-Anethole. *p-cis*-Propenylanisole
Systematic name: (Z)-4-Methoxy-(1-propenyl)benzene
Chemical class: Phenylpropenoid ether
CAS number: 25679-28-1

Sources >0.1%:

Fennel (sweet)	tr–0.7%
Anise	tr–0.5%
Anise (star)	tr–0.4%
Fennel (bitter)	tr–0.2%

Note: This isomer is significantly more toxic than the common *(E)*-isomer.

Acute toxicity: The ip LD$_{50}$ values of (Z)-anethole were 135 mg/kg in mice and 93 mg/kg in rats (Boissier et al 1967).

Carcinogenic/anticarcinogenic potential: Unlike α-asarone or β-asarone, four ip injections of 90% (Z)-anethole/10% (E)-anethole given prior to weaning did not cause hepatomas to develop in mice after 18 months (Wiseman et al 1987).

Summary: (Z)-Anethole is not regarded as a carcinogen. Its low occurrence in essential oils does not give rise to any safety concerns.

p-Anisaldehyde

Synonyms: Anisaldehyde. Anisic aldehyde
Systematic name: 4-Methoxybenzaldehyde
Chemical class: Benzenoid ether aldehyde
CAS number: 123-11-5

Sources >1.0%:

Cassie absolute	0–17.3%
Anise	0.6–2.0%
Cassia leaf	0–1.0%

Pharmacokinetics: Anisaldehyde is metabolized by glucuronide conjugation in rabbits, and is also metabolized to anisic alcohol and anisic acid in rats (Scheline 1991). Anisaldehyde prolongs the pentobarbital-induced sleeping time in rats, probably by modulating the barbiturate's metabolism by CYP (Marcus & Lichtenstein 1982).

Adverse skin reactions: Tested at 10% on human subjects, anisaldehyde was neither irritating nor sensitizing. (Opdyke 1974 p. 823–824).

Acute toxicity: Acute oral LD$_{50}$ in rats 1.51 g/kg, 1.26 in guinea pigs (Jenner et al 1964), acute dermal LD$_{50}$ in rabbits >5 g/kg (Opdyke 1974 p. 823–824).

Subacute and subchronic toxicity: Given to rats in the diet for 15 weeks, 10,000 ppm anisaldehyde produced no effects, nor did 1,000 ppm for 28 weeks (Hagan et al 1967).

Mutagenicity and genotoxicity: Anisaldehyde inhibited the mutagenic activity of compound 4-NQO in a hamster cell line at 0.2–1.0 g/L (Kim et al 2001), and was not mutagenic in the Ames test (Ishidate et al 1984; Kasamaki et al 1982; Florin et al 1980). It has been reported as non-genotoxic, weakly genotoxic and antigenotixic in tests using cultured Chinese hamster cells (Kasamaki et al 1982; Ishidate et al 1984; Imanishi et al 1990). In mouse bone marrow cells, anisaldehyde reduced CA induced by X-rays (Sasaki et al 1990).

Carcinogenic/anticarcinogenic potential: Anisaldehyde inhibited the growth of human lung, liver and stomach carcinoma cells at similar concentrations (Kim et al 2001). It also inhibited the activation of carcinogenic nitrosamines in mouse hepatic and pulmonary microsomes (Morse et al 1995).

Comments: Anisaldehyde may be an oxidation product rather than a true constituent of essential oils.

Summary: There are currently no safety concerns associated with anisaldehyde.

Anisyl alcohol

Synonyms: *p*-Anisyl alcohol. Anisalcohol. Anise alcohol. Anisic alcohol. 4-Methoxy-benzenemethanol. *p*-Methoxy benzyl alcohol
Systematic name: 4-Methoxybenzyl alcohol
Chemical class: Benzenoid ether alcohol
CAS number: 105-13-5

Sources >0.1%:

Anise	0–3.5%

Note: Can also be present in vanilla absolute.

Adverse skin reactions: In a modified Draize procedure on guinea pigs, anisyl alcohol was non-sensitizing when used at 10% in the challenge phase (Sharp 1978). There were no positive reactions when anisyl alcohol was tested at 5% on 115 dermatitis patients (Remaut 1992). In other European studies, 1/1,503, and 1/2,004 dermatitis patients (total reactions 0.06%) tested positive to 1% anisyl alcohol (Heisterberg et al 2011, Schnuch et al 2007a). Of 167 dermatitis patients suspected of fragrance sensitivity 3 (1.8%) reacted to 5% anisyl alcohol on patch testing (Larsen et al 1996b). When tested at 5% on 20 fragrance-sensitive dermatitis patients, anisyl alcohol induced 4 (20%) positive reactions (Larsen 1977).

Acute toxicity: Acute oral LD$_{50}$ values of 1.34 g/kg for rats, and 1.78 g/kg for mice have been reported (Adams et al 2005c).

Mutagenicity and genotoxicity: Anisyl alcohol was not mutagenic in *S. typhimurium* strain TA100 (Ball et al 1984).

Carcinogenic/anticarcinogenic potential: Anisyl alcohol was not carcinogenic in male mice when a total dose of 3.75 μmol (518 μg) was injected ip in increasing doses on days 1, 8, 15 and 22 prior to weaning (Miller & Miller 1983).

Comments: In a review of the data, including some not cited here, Hostýnek and Maibach (2003a) conclude that, due to various flaws in the research, there is no convincing evidence that anisyl alcohol has a significant skin sensitizing potential. Since anisyl alcohol is found in only one essential oil, at 0–3.5%, the matter is somewhat academic in our context.

Summary: Other than its controversial listing as a high-risk skin allergen, there are no safety concerns.

Regulatory guidelines: Anisyl alcohol is one of the 26 fragrance materials listed as an allergen by the EU. If present in a cosmetic product at over 100 ppm (0.01%) in a wash-off product or 10 ppm (0.001%) in a leave-on product the material must be declared on the ingredient list if sold in an EU member state. The Joint FAO/WHO Expert Committee on Food Additives commented in 2001: 'no safety concern at current levels of intake when used as a flavoring agent'. The IFRA standard for anisyl alcohol in leave-on products such as body lotions is 0.7%, for skin sensitization.

Our safety advice: We see no need for a limit on dermal exposure to anisyl alcohol for skin sensitization.

Apiole (dill)

Synonym: Dill apiol
Systematic name: 1-(2-Propenyl)-2,3-dimethoxy-4,5-methyl-enedioxybenzene
Chemical class: Bicyclic phenylpropenoid ether
CAS number: 484-31-1

Sources >0.1%:

Dill seed (Indian)	20.7–52.5%
Parsley leaf	0.2–5.2%
Piri-piri	0–1.4%

Note: Sensitive to decomposition on storage.
Mutagenicity and genotoxicity: Dill apiole has a very low level of genotoxicity (Phillips et al 1984; Randerath et al 1984).
Carcinogenic/anticarcinogenic potential: Dill apiole was not carcinogenic in male mice when a total dose of 4.75 μmol (1.05 mg) was injected ip in increasing doses on days 1, 8, 15 and 22 prior to weaning (Miller & Miller 1983).
Comments: Although there are no specific data on reproductive toxicity for dill apiole, its structural similarity to parsley apiole makes it highly suspect as being similarly hepatotoxic and hazardous in pregnancy.
Summary: There are insufficient data to draw any conclusions, but the structural similarity to parsley apiole suggests a similar toxicity.

Apiole (parsley)

Synonyms: Apiole. Parsley apiol. Parsley camphor. Apioline
Systematic name: 1-(2-Propenyl)-2,5-dimethoxy-3,4-methyl-enedioxybenzene
Chemical class: Bicyclic phenylpropenoid ether
CAS number: 523-80-8

Sources >0.1%:

Parsleyseed	11.3–67.5%

Note: Sensitive to decomposition on storage.

Pharmacokinetics: Metabolism involves extensive oxidation in both rabbits and dogs (Scheline 1991).
Acute toxicity: When 12 mice were administered a single gavage dose of 10 mL/kg parsley apiole, all died within 60 hours. There were gross and microscopic signs of liver and kidney toxicity (Amerio et al 1968).
Subacute and subchronic toxicity: The lowest total dose of parsley apiole causing death in adult humans is 4.2 g (2.1 g/day for 2 days) (D'Aprile 1928); the lowest fatal daily dose is 770 mg, which was taken for 14 days (Lowenstein & Ballew 1958); the lowest single fatal dose is 8 g (Barni & Barni 1967). At least 19 g has been survived (D'Aprile 1928). Common symptoms of parsley apiole poisoning are fever, severe abdominal pain, vaginal bleeding, vomiting and diarrhea (D'Aprile 1928; Amerio et al 1968). In the majority of cases, post-mortem examination reveals considerable damage to both liver and kidney tissue, often with gastrointestinal inflammation and sometimes damage to heart tissue (Lowenstein & Ballew 1958; Amerio et al 1968; Colalillo 1974). In one case, contamination of parsley apiole with triorthocresyl phosphate is believed to have contributed to the death of the patient (Hermann et al 1956). Such contamination was not unknown in the 1930s and 1940s, and would generally cause severe neurotoxicity (Lowenstein & Ballew 1958).
Reproductive toxicity: Parsley apiole and various preparations of parsley have been used for many years to procure illegal abortion in Italy (Barni & Barni 1967; Marozzi & Farneti 1968; Colalillo 1974). In one fatal case, a woman in her seventh month of pregnancy ingested 14 capsules of parsley apiole (300 mg of apiole per capsule) over 2 days. On the third day, she experienced violent abdominal pains with diarrhea, vomiting and vaginal bleeding. The fetus was expelled with severe menorrhagia. Her cardio-renal signs deteriorated rapidly, with signs of nephritis. The patient's cardiac function decreased, she became comatose and died (D'Aprile 1928).

Out of five cases, all of whom were between two and seven months pregnant, one aborted and later died, one did not abort but died, and three aborted and survived (D'Aprile 1928). In the case which did not abort, the fetus was dead. Post-abortive vaginal bleeding, sometimes profuse, is a feature of these cases. A cumulative effect is apparent, parsley apiole being taken daily for 3–8 days before either death or abortion ensued. One of the cases cited had traces of parsley apiole in her urine 12 days after the last ingestion. Other researchers reported similar cases of apiole intoxication, such as that of a woman who consumed 6 g of parsley apiole over 3 days, aborted, and later died, having suffered massive internal bleeding, convulsions, oliguria and pyrexia (Laederich et al 1932).

The lowest daily dose of parsley apiole that induced abortion was 900 mg taken for 8 consecutive days. The inevitable conclusion is that apiole-rich essential oils present a high risk of abortion if taken in oral doses. External use would also seem inadvisable in pregnancy. In animal studies, considerably higher doses of parsley apiole appear to be tolerated. In pregnant guinea pigs, abortion did not occur except at lethal doses, around 2 g (D'Aprile 1928). In pregnant rabbits, abortion was induced by doses of 5–14 g, with severe hemorrhage (Patoir et al 1936). In both types of animal, the dose is equivalent to ~100–200 g in a human. This is 20–40 times higher than the amount of apiole causing abortion in humans, and highlights the poor correlation between animals and humans in this area.

Carcinogenic/anticarcinogenic potential: Parsley apiole reacts only weakly with DNA and is not associated with tumor development (Phillips et al 1984). It was not carcinogenic in male mice when a total dose of 4.75 µmol (1.05 mg) was injected ip in increasing doses on days 1, 8, 15 and 22 prior to weaning (Miller et al 1983). Parsley apiole is cytotoxic to cells for myelogenous leukemia (K562, IC_{50} 24.1 µg/mL), non-small cell lung cancer (NCI-H460, IC_{50} 43.0 µg/mL) and breast cancer (MCF-7, IC_{50} 36.0 µg/mL) (Di Stefano et al 2011).

Comments: Although some apiole preparations were contaminated with triorthocresyl phosphate, a neurotoxic organophosphate, there is no evidence that this substance is abortifacient. Early preparations of apiole were not of a high or consistent purity.

Summary: In fatal or almost-fatal doses, parsley apiole is abortifacient, and toxic to the liver, kidneys, heart and digestive system. Safety thresholds have not been established.

Our safety advice: The human data suggest that apiole possesses a similar degree of oral toxicity to humans as does pulegone. The lowest single fatal dose of pennyroyal oil is one tablespoon (15 mL, corresponding to 9–12 mL of pulegone), while the lowest single fatal dose of parsley apiole is 8 g (corresponding to approximately 9 mL). Therefore, we recommend a daily oral maximum dose for parsely apiole of 0.4 mg/kg for toxicity, equivalent to 28 mg for an adult. This oral maximum is equivalent to a dermal maximum of 0.76% (Table 14.1)

Aromadendrene

Chemical class: Tricyclic sesquiterpenoid alkene
Note: Different isomers of aromadendrene exist, and the following isomer-specific information has been published.

1(10)-Aromadendrene

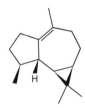

Synonyms: (+)-Ledene. Viridiflorene
Systematic name: [1aR-(1aα,7α,7aβ,7bα)]-1a,2,3,5,6,7,7a,7b-Octahydro-1,1,4,7-tetramethyl-1H-cycloprop[e]azulene
CAS number: 21747-46-6

Sources >1.0%:

Patchouli	0–3.9%
Pteronia	3.1%
Arina	3.0%
Rosalina	0.5–3.0%
Fern (sweet)	1.7%
Manuka	0.6–1.1%

(+)-Aromadendrene

Systematic name: [1aR-(1aα,4aα,7α,7aβ,7bα)]-Decahydro-1,1,7-trimethyl-4-methylene-1H-cycloprop[e]azulene
CAS number: 489-39-4

Sources >1.0%:

Rosalina	1.5–4.0%
Tea tree	tr.–3.0%
Rose (Japanese)	2.5%
Manuka	1.6–2.2%
Eucalyptus globulus	0.1–2.2%
Rambiazana	2.0%
Eucalyptus maidenii	1.7%
Vassoura	1.6%
Eucalyptus camaldulensis	0.6–1.4%
Cangerana	1.1%

(−)-allo-Aromadendrene

Systematic name: [1aR-(1aα,4aβ,7α,7aβ,7bα)]-Decahydro-1,1,7-trimethyl-4-methylene-1H-cycloprop[e]azulene
CAS number: 25246-27-9

Sources >1.0%:

Gurjun	4.0–6.0%
Patchouli	0–5.0%
Cubeb	1.7–4.2%
Cardamon (black)	3.2%
Phoebe	2.4–2.6%
Valerian (European)	0.7–2.6%
Chaste tree seed	0–2.1%
Eucalyptus polybractea (cryptone CT)	2.0%
Chaste tree leaf	0–2.0%
Copaiba	0–1.8%
Cistus	0–1.2%
Katrafay	0.2–1.0%

Adverse skin reactions: Of seven dermatitis patients already sensitive to tea tree oil, five were sensitive to (+)-aromadendrene tested at 1% (Knight & Hausen 1994). Tested at 5%, (+)-aromadendrene was not sensitizing to 11 dermatitis patients sensitive to tea tree oil (Hausen et al 1999).

Mutagenicity and genotoxicity: (+)-Aromadendrene was not mutagenic in *S. typhimurium* strains TA98 and TA100 with or without S9 (Gonçalves et al 2011).

Summary: Sparse data, but there are no structural red flags.

α-Asarone

Synonyms: (E)-Asarone. *trans*-Asarone
Systematic name: (E)-2,4,5-Trimethoxy-1-(1-propenyl)benzene
Chemical class: Phenylpropenoid ether
CAS number: 2883-98-9

Sources >0.1%:

Calamus (tetraploid form)	1.3–6.8%
Cubeb	0.9–3.7%

Pharmacokinetics: The major metabolite of α-asarone in rabbits is 2,4,5-trimethoxycinnamic acid, which is non-toxic (Antunez-Solis et al 2009). This compound, in addition to unchanged α-asarone (at 11–1,150 µg/L in five of seven individuals) and a hydroxylated metabolite were detected in human urine after ingestion of varying amounts of calamus oil (Björnstad et al 2009). It has been suggested that α-asarone 1,2-oxide may be a metabolite (Kim SG et al 1999). In rats given ip injections of α-asarone, small amounts of three ninhydrin-positive substances were detected in the urine (Oswald et al 1969). This is a test for amines, and SCF (2002a) suggests that these could possibly be phenylisopropylamines or amphetamines.

Acute toxicity: Mouse acute oral LD$_{50}$ 418 mg/kg, acute ip LD$_{50}$ 310 mg/kg (Belova et al 1985), rat ip LD$_{50}$ 300 mg/kg (Sharma & Dandiya 1962).

Subacute and subchronic toxicity: Oral administration of α-asarone to rats for 28 days at 10 or 50 mg/kg produced no apparent toxicity (Chamorro et al 1993).

Cardiovascular effects: An iv dose of 10 mg/kg α-asarone caused a prompt fall in blood pressure of 50 mmHg in anesthetized dogs, with a return to normal after 45 minutes; 3 mg/kg had no significant effect (Sharma & Dandiya 1962).

Neurotoxicity: A single ip dose of 25 mg/kg α-asarone reduced the average duration of electroshock seizures from 5.6 seconds to 3.5 seconds in rats (Dandiya & Menon 1963).

At 50 mg/kg ip, α-asarone was not convulsant in rats; it protected animals against metrazol-induced seizures, and only slightly exacerbated picritoxin-induced seizures (Dandiya & Sharma 1962). However 50% of rats given single ip doses of 300 mg/kg experienced mild to moderate clonic convulsions in the hind limbs, 30 minutes after injection. Most animals showed ataxia and loss of righting reflex at 100–300 mg/kg doses (Sharma & Dandiya 1962). Mice given a single ip dose of α-asarone exhibited signs of CNS depression at 100 mg/kg, but doses of 60 or 22 mg/kg were non-toxic. These lower doses inhibited magnesium-deficiency audiogenic seizures in mice, and delayed the onset of seizures induced by picritoxin, pentylenetetrazole or pilocarpine. It is suggested that the protective effect of α-asarone may be due to antioxidant/neuroprotective mechanisms. The induction of antioxidant enzymes in the brain was reported (Pages et al 2010).

Reproductive toxicity: Male mice were given 0, 10 or 30 mg/kg α-asarone by gavage for 5 consecutive days, and sperm motility, concentration and shape were assessed for eight weeks. Shape was not affected, concentration was reduced only in the 30 mg/kg group, and motility was reduced at both doses. However, the effects on motility were not dose-dependent. In the high dose group, the relative weights of testis and epididymis were not affected, but seminal vesicle weight was reduced. When separate groups of male mice given 0, 10 or 30 mg/kg of α-asarone mated with females, there was a dose-dependent increase in post-implantation loss on gestational days 13–15, even though there was no apparent effect on pregnancy incidence. The authors suggested that genotoxicity of α-asarone might have caused non-viable eggs (Chamorro et al 1998).

In a subsequent study using the same species of mouse, daily oral doses of 0, 10 and 20 mg/kg of α-asarone 5 days per week for 8 weeks were given to males, which mated with untreated females, and to females, which mated with untreated males. There was no decrease in fertility, no germinal mutations in male or female mice, and in male mice there were no adverse effects on sperm count or shape. DNA repair processes were considered responsible for the lack of adverse effects at these doses (Chamorro et al 1999). When administered by gavage to pregnant mice at 60 mg/kg/day on gestation days 6–15, α-asarone induced fetal malformations and significantly reduced maternal weight gain (Salazar et al 1992).

Hepatotoxicity: Exposure of adult rat hepatocytes to micromolar concentrations of α-asarone (10–50 µg/mL) in vitro for one or two weeks, causes morphological and ultrastructural changes, fat accumulation and inhibition of protein synthesis which would be associated with gross pathology if seen in vivo (López et al 1993).

Antioxidant/pro-oxidant activity: α-Asarone, given orally at 10 mg/kg/day, protected rat temporal cortex and hippocampus tissue from neuronal damage induced by amyloid-β through an antioxidant mechanism (Limón et al 2009). Given ip at 3, 6 or 9 mg/kg/day, α-asarone similarly protected rat cerebral cortex from oxidative stress induced by noise (Manikandan & Devi 2005).

Mutagenicity and genotoxicity: α-Asarone was not mutagenic in the Ames test with S9 (Hsia et al 1979), but a putative metabolite, α-asarone 1,2-oxide, was dose-dependently mutagenic in the three *S. typhimurium* strains tested: TA1535, TA100 and TA98 (Kim SG et al 1999). α-Asarone induced a slight but consistent increase in SCE in mouse bone marrow in vivo, and human lymphocytes in vitro, in the absence of metabolic activation (Morales-Ramírez et al 1992). α-Asarone was genotoxic in rat hepatocytes, possibly due to a novel, but CYP-dependent activation mechanism (Hasheminejad & Caldwell 1994). A previous study had also found that α-asarone induced UDS in rat hepatocytes, and that it elicited strand breaks (Ramos-Ocampo 1988).

Carcinogenic/anticarcinogenic potential: α-Asarone increased hepatoma incidence in male mice (no females were tested) given four ip injections over four days prior to weaning totaling 4.8 µmol/g (998 µg/g) bw; tumors were found on autopsy at 13 months (Wiseman et al 1987). Single ip injections of 0.25 or 0.5 µmol/g (52 or 104 µg/g) bw α-asarone given to 12 day-old mice dose-dependently increased hepatoma incidence at 10–11 months. Injections of 0.125, 0.25 or 0.5 µmol/g (26, 52 or 104 µg/g) bw α-asarone 1,2-oxide (a putative metabolite) increased hepatoma incidence, but only at the highest dose. Asarone was five times more toxic than its oxide. Topical application of 5 µmol (1.03 mg) α-asarone or α-asarone 1,2-oxide once weekly for 3 weeks had no effect on skin papilloma incidence in female mice (Kim SG et al 1999).

Comments: In reproductive toxicity testing, there was one report of adverse effects on sperm motility, but since this effect was not dose-dependent it may be unreliable, and a subsequent study by the same group found no adverse effects.

The discrepancy between the Ames test result and the genotoxicity testing is probably because the S9 used does not fully replicate metabolism. This is supported by the positive result in an Ames test for α-asarone 1,2-oxide. However, there is no definitive evidence that the oxide is a metabolite of α-asarone, and even if it is, such oxides are generally detoxified so rapidly in humans that they cause no harm. It is notable that α-asarone has only shown carcinogenic action when administered by ip injection to infant mice, and it has been suggested that hepatoma formation in this scenario could arise from local liver damage (SCF 2002a). There are no studies of oral dosing, and short-term topical application seems to be non-toxic. There is no evidence that either α-asarone, or an essential oil containing it, has ever caused tumor formation in humans by any route.

Summary: There are indications of neurotoxicity, reproductive toxicity, hepatotoxicity, genotoxicity and carcinogenicity for α-asarone. In mice, 60 mg/kg is fetotoxic, 30 mg/kg marginally reduces male fertility, and 10 mg/kg can be taken as the oral NOAEL for reproductive toxicity.

Regulatory guidelines: α-Asarone is permitted in the US as a pharmaceutical ingredient. IFRA recommends that α-asarone should not be used as a fragrance ingredient, and that the level of asarone in consumer products containing calamus oil should not exceed 0.01% (IFRA 2009).

Our safety advice: No NOAEL for carcinogenicity can be derived from the data. However, the NOAEL for oral β-asarone in rats is 20 mg/kg, and β-asarone is 1.5–1.6 times more potent a carcinogen than α-asarone in mice (Wiseman et al 1987). Therefore, the NOAEL for α-asarone carcinogenicity could be 30 mg/kg. There are insufficient data to compare the human metabolism of α-asarone with either rat or mouse. If we adopt the standard uncertainty factor of 10 for interspecies differences, this reduces the NOAEL dose from 30 to 3 mg/kg. We can compare the carcinogenicity of α-asarone with that of estragole. The average number of hepatomas per mouse per μmol test substance per g bw was 8.8 for estragole and 2.7 for α-asarone (Wiseman et al 1987). This suggests that α-asarone is 3.3 times less potent a carcinogen than estragole. The estimated human NOAEL for estragole is 1.2 mg/kg, and so we might estimate the human NOAEL for α-asarone to be 4 mg/kg. This is close to our earlier estimate of 3 mg/kg. If we then apply the same uncertainty factor used for estragole of 20 to allow for interindividual differences and drug interactions, we arrive at a safe dose of 0.15 mg/kg/day. This is equivalent to a dermal maximum of 0.33% (Table 14.1).

β-Asarone

Synonyms: (Z)-Asarone. *cis*-Asarone
Systematic name: (Z)-2,4,5-Trimethoxy-1-(1-propenyl)benzene
Chemical class: Phenylpropenoid ether
CAS number: 5273-86-9

Sources >0.1%:

Calamus (tetraploid form)	42.5–78.4%
Calamus (triploid form)	8.0–19.0%

Pharmacokinetics: The major metabolite of β-asarone in rat hepatocytes is 2,4,5-trimethoxycinnamic acid (Hasheminjad & Caldwell 1994). Formation of the epoxide has also been proposed (Unger & Melzig 2012). The serum half-life of orally administered β-asarone in rats was 54 minutes, with a peak serum concentration of 3.2 mg/L after 12 minutes (Wu & Fang 2004).

Acute toxicity: Rat oral LD_{50} 1,010 mg/kg, mouse ip LD_{50} 184 mg/kg (JECFA 1981), rat ip LD_{50} 122 mg/kg (Sharma & Dandiya 1962).

Subacute and subchronic toxicity: In rats given 100 mg/kg/day β-asarone ip for 5 days, there was weight loss and decreased food consumption. Heart and thymus weights were reduced, and adrenal weights increased. There were no effects on hematology, and liver function tests were normal (Ramos-Ocampo & Hsia 1987). In a study looking for potential therapeutic effects in Alzheimer's disease, oral administration of β-asarone to rats for 28 days at 12.5, 25 or 50 mg/kg/day produced no apparent toxicity (Geng et al 2010; Liu et al 2010).

Cardiovascular effects: An iv dose of 3 mg/kg β-asarone caused a prompt fall in blood pressure of 50 mmHg in anesthetized dogs, with a return to normal after 45 minutes (Sharma & Dandiya 1962).

Neurotoxicity: An ip dose of 25 mg/kg β-asarone increased the average duration of electroshock seizures from 5.6 seconds to 11 seconds in rats (Dandiya & Menon 1963). At 50 mg/kg ip, β-asarone caused generalized seizures of moderate severity, and did not protect rats from metrazole-induced seizures (Dandiya & Sharma 1962). Rats given single doses of 100–200 mg/kg ip β-asarone experienced generalized seizures, and doses over 170 mg/kg induced severe clonic seizures. There was no ataxia or loss of righting reflex at any dose (Sharma & Dandiya 1962).

Reproductive toxicity: When chicken eggs were injected with 0.04 mg β-asarone, 43% survived, while none survived after a 4 mg dose (JECFA 1981).

Mutagenicity and genotoxicity: β-Asarone was not mutagenic to any *Salmonella* strain in the Ames test with S9 (Hsia et al 1979). In another Ames test it was mutagenic to TA100, though only with S9, and there was no mutagenicity in TA1535, TA1537, TA1538 or TA98, with or without S9 (Göggelmann & Schimmer 1983). β-Asarone tested positive in the SOS chromotest (a modified *E. coli* PQ37 genotoxicity assay) with S9 activation (Kevekordes et al 1999). It was also genotoxic both in human lymphocytes with metabolic activation, and in the human hepatoma cell line HepG2 (Kevekordes et al 2001). The genotoxicity of β-asarone may be due to a novel, but CYP-dependent activation mechanism (Abel 1987a; Hasheminjad & Caldwell 1994). When tested in rat hepatocytes, β-asarone was not genotoxic, and in fact significantly reduced UDS, possibly due to cytotoxicity (Ramos-Ocampo & Hsia 1987).

Chronic toxicity and carcinogenic/anticarcinogenic potential: β-Asarone produced malignant liver tumors in mice given four ip injections totaling 4.8 μmol/g bw (984 μg/g bw) prior to weaning; tumors were found on autopsy at 13 months (Wiseman et al 1987). When male and female rats (five animals per group) were given dietary β-asarone at 400, 800 or

2,000 ppm (equivalent to 20, 40 and 100 mg/kg bw) for 2 years, none of the high-dose rats survived beyond 84 weeks, and mortality was also increased in the 800 ppm group. Dose-dependent malignant tumors occurred in the small intestine of male rats only, and in the low-dose group incidence was no greater than the control group. These were leiomyosarcomas, an unusual type of cancer, and they were also found in two female control rats in unspecified organs, but not small intestine. Other pathological signs included fluid in the pleural and abdominal cavities, atrophy and fatty degeneration of cardiac muscle, hepatic necrosis and depressed body weight (Taylor 1981, private report cited in JECFA 1981). By contrast, β-asarone suppressed the growth of human LoVo colon cancer cells and induced apoptosis in vitro and in vivo in a dose- and time-dependent manner at doses ranging from 0.05–0.8 mM (Zou et al 2012). It also inhibited colon cancer formation in an in vivo mouse model, and in vitro in human colorectal HT29 and SW480 cells at doses of 10–100 nM for 24–72 hours (Liu et al 2013).

Comments: The absence of liver tumors on oral dosing of β-asarone suggests the possibility that those caused in infant mice from ip dosing were due to local liver damage (SCF 2002a). It is notable that, in three studies involving oral administration of the tetraploid form of calamus oil (42.5–78.4% β-asarone) for 2 years, the only tumors seen were leiomyosarcomas in the small intestine and the only report of hepatocellular carcinomas was from the triploid form of calamus oil (8.0–19.0% β-asarone). Estragole, methyleugenol and safrole all target the liver on oral dosing, and they are all alkenybenzenes that are bioactivated via 1′-hydroxylation, whereas β-asarone is a propenylbenzene, and little is known about its metabolism.

Summary: There are indications of neurotoxicity, genotoxicity, carcinogenicity and anticarcinogenicity for β-asarone. On oral dosing, β-asarone was carcinogenic to rats in doses of 40 mg/kg/day or higher, and the NOAEL was 20 mg/kg.

Regulatory guidelines: β-Asarone is not permitted in the US as a pharmaceutical ingredient. The Council of Europe lists it under 'substances which are suspected to be genotoxic carcinogens and therefore no MDI can be set' (Council of Europe 2003). Both the UK and EU 'standard permitted proportion' of β-asarone in food flavorings is 0.1 mg/kg (European Community Council 1988, Anon 1992b). IFRA recommends that β-asarone should not be used as a fragrance ingredient, and that the level of asarone in consumer products containing calamus oil should not exceed 0.01% (IFRA 2009).

Our safety advice: The rat NOAEL for β-asarone-induced cancer is 20 mg/kg. There are insufficient data to compare the human metabolism of β-asarone with either rat or mouse, but if we adopt the standard uncertainty factor of 10 for interspecies differences, this reduces the NOAEL dose from 20 to 2 mg/kg. There is one study that directly compares the toxicity of β-asarone with that of another carcinogenic essential oil constituent: estragole. The average number of hepatomas per mouse per μmol test substance per g bw was 8.8 for estragole and 4.2 for β-asarone (Wiseman et al 1987). This suggests that β-asarone could be 2.1 times less potent a carcinogen than estragole. The estimated human NOAEL for estragole is 1.2 mg/kg, and so we might estimate the human NOAEL for β-asarone to be about 2.5 mg/kg. This is close to our earlier estimate of 2 mg/kg. If we then apply the same uncertainty

factor used for estragole of 20, to allow for inter-individual differences and drug interactions, we arrive at a safe dose of 0.1 mg/kg/day. This is equivalent to a dermal maximum of 0.22% (Table 14.1).

Ascaridole

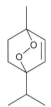

Synonym: Ascarisin
Systematic name: 1-Methyl-4-(1-methylethyl)-2,3-dioxabicyclo[2.2.2]oct-5-ene
Chemical class: Tricyclic monoterpenoid alkene peroxide
CAS number: 512-85-6

Sources >0.1%:

Wormseed	41.2–80.0%
Boldo	21.25%
Sanna	1.9%
Southernwood	0.8%

Notes: Different isomers of ascaridole exist. Ascaridole is prone to explode when heated or mixed with organic acids (Reynolds 1993).

Pharmacokinetics: Ascaridole caused an 83-fold increase in the permeation of 5-fluorouracil across human skin, suggesting its importance as a skin permeation enhancer (Williams and Barry 1991). This may also point to the efficient skin permeation of ascaridole itself, which could indicate a high potential for dermal toxicity.

Adverse skin reactions: Ascaridole was patch tested on two groups of consecutive patients suspected of cosmetic or fragrance allergy. When tested at 1% on 602 patients, it produced one irritant response and nine allergic reactions. When tested at 5% on 144 patients, there were five irritant and 21 allergic reactions. None of the reactions were +++ in severity (Bakker et al 2011).

Tested at 5%, ascaridole was sensitizing to 9 of 11 dermatitis patients sensitive to tea tree oil (Hausen et al 1999).

Acute toxicity: Rat oral LD_{50} 200 mg/kg, mouse oral LD_{50} 400 mg/kg, dog LDlo 250 mg/kg (References cited in http://www.lookchem.com/Ascaridole, accessed February 24th 2011). A dose of 100 mg/kg of ascaridole produced hypothermia and reduced locomotor activity in mice, and at 300 mg/kg it was fatal (Okuyama et al 1993). Wormseed oil, which primarily consists of ascaridole, is very toxic to humans, with an oral fatal dose in the 10–40 mg/kg range (see Wormseed oil profile, Chapter 13). Ascaridole is more toxic than wormseed oil (Salant & Nelson 1915; Livingston 1922).

Carcinogenic/anticarcinogenic potential: Ascaridole was cited as having carcinogenic activity by Van Duuren (1965). However, ascaridole, extracted from wormseed oil, exhibited cytotoxic activity towards two human leukemia cell lines (HL60 and CCRF-CEM), one human breast cancer cell line (MDA-MB-231) and their multidrug-resistant counterparts MDR1, MRP1 and BCRP (Efferth et al 2002b). Ascaridole was cytotoxic to human cell lines for colon cancer and leukemia, and inhibited connective tissue cancer in mice at 10 or 20 mg/kg, with little damage to normal tissue (Bezerra et al 2009).

Comments: Ascaridole may be formed in highly oxidized tea tree oil (Hausen et al 1999), and it has been detected at 0.2% in unoxidized tea tree oil (Sciarrone et al 2010).

Summary: There are few hard data on this compound, though it is generally regarded as highly toxic, and is more toxic to humans than rodents. It may be anticarcinogenic.

Our safety advice: We recommend a daily maximum adult dose of 0.05 mg/kg ascaridole, equivalent to a dermal concentration of 0.12% (Table 14.1). This is based on an estimated rodent NOAEL of 1–10 mg/kg, with human toxicity being 10–20 times greater than rodent.

Benzaldehyde

Synonyms: Benzoic aldehyde. Benzenecarbaldehyde. Formyl benzene

Chemical class: Benzenoid aldehyde

CAS number: 100-52-7

Sources >1.0%:

Almond (bitter, FFPA)	98%
Almond (bitter, unrectified)	95.0%
Cassia leaf	1.1–6.3%
Cistus	0–2.8%
Cassia bark	0.4–2.3%
Cinnamon bark	tr–2.2%

Notes: Also a minor component of several other oils. A yellowish liquid with an almond smell and burning aromatic taste. Fairly water-soluble. Benzaldehyde slowly oxidizes to benzoic acid in the presence of oxygen.

Pharmacokinetics: The major metabolic pathway (~90%) involves oxidation to benzoic acid which is excreted as free benzoic acid and as hippuric acid following conjugation with glycine; the relative quantities vary with species. Rabbits were also found to excrete ~10% of the dose as benzoyl glucuronide and <0.01% as benzylmercapturic acid. Inhaled benzaldehyde appears to be entirely excreted in the urine by rats, <90% as hippuric acid (Scheline 1991). Inhaled benzaldehyde is rapidly absorbed in rats, with only 0.8% of the administered dose in the lungs after 1.5 minutes. Subsequent clearance from the tissues was rapid and paralleled the removal from the blood (Kutzman et al 1980). Benzaldehyde is metabolized to benzoic acid in the skin (Andersen 2006a).

Adverse skin reactions: Tested at 4% on two separate panels of volunteers benzaldehyde was neither irritating nor sensitizing (Opdyke 1976 p. 693–698). Three of 747 dermatitis patients

suspected of fragrance allergy (0.4%) reacted to 5% benzaldehyde (Wöhrl et al 2001). Based on literature published in German, benzaldehyde was classified as category C, not significantly allergenic, by Schlede et al (2003). In a CIR report on benzaldehyde, it was considered not to be a contact sensitizer (Andersen 2006a). In an in vitro assay, benzaldehyde was non-phototoxic (Placzek et al 2007).

Acute toxicity: Acute oral LD_{50} in rats 1.3 g/kg, 1.0 g/kg in guinea pigs (Jenner et al 1964). Another report gives acute rat oral LD_{50} as 2.85 g/kg; acute dermal LD_{50} <1.25 g/kg in rabbits. The oral fatal dose in humans has been estimated as 50–60 mL (Opdyke 1976 p. 693–698).

In a short-term clinical study, there was no evident toxicity from oral doses of 200–400 mg (Kleeberg 1959).

Subacute and subchronic toxicity: Fed to rats for 14 days at 10,000 ppm benzaldehyde decreased both body and liver weight gains. Rats given 10 mg benzaldehyde orally every second day for 12 weeks had normal nitrogen and lipid levels, normal liver enzyme activity and normal ascorbic acid content in the adrenal glands (Opdyke 1976 p693–698). In a 16 day gavage study, male and female rats and mice received 0, 200, 400, 800 or 1,600 mg/kg benzaldehyde. No gross treatment-related lesions were seen, and there were no effects on body weight at doses of 400 mg/kg or less in any rodents (National Toxicology Program 1990b).

Benzaldehyde had no adverse effect on rats when given in the diet at at 10,000 ppm for 16 weeks, or 1,000 ppm for 27–28 weeks (Hagan et al 1967). In a 90 day gavage study, male and female rats were dosed with 0, 50, 100, 200, 400 or 800 mg/kg, and male and female mice were dosed with 0, 75, 150, 300, 600 or 1,200 mg/kg benzaldehyde. In rats, the highest dose caused some deaths, and gross signs of toxicity in the brain, liver, kidneys and forestomach. There was no detectable toxicity at <400 mg/kg. In mice, there were some male fatalities at 1,200 mg/kg, and some mean body weight reduction and kidney toxicity at >600 mg/kg. The NOAELs from these studies were 400 mg/kg in male and female rats, 300 mg/kg in male mice, and 600 mg/kg in female mice (Kluwe et al 1983; National Toxicology Program 1990b).

Inhalation toxicity: The RD_{50} value for benzaldehyde is 363 ppm (Steinhagen & Barrow 1984). Repeated inhalation of benzaldehyde vapor produced eye and nose irritation at 500 ppm, and death at 750 ppm in rabbits (Andersen 2006a).

Neurotoxicity: In a 90 day gavage study, necrotic and degenerative lesions were found in the cerebellar and hippocampal regions of rats dosed with benzaldehyde at 800 mg/kg; inactivity, tremors or hyperexcitability were observed in rats at this dose. However, neither the clinical signs nor the neuronal lesions were seen in mice at doses up to 1,200 mg/kg, nor in rats at <400 mg/kg (Kluwe et al 1983).

Hepatotoxicity: Intraperitoneal injection of 500 mg/kg benzaldehyde in rats caused a significant increase in the rate of ROS formation in hepatic mitochondrial fractions (Mattia et al 1993). Benzaldehyde was subsequently found to weakly inactivate the antioxidant enzyme glutathione peroxidase with a K_i value of 15 mM (1.59 g/L) (Tabatabaie & Floyd 1996). When benzaldehyde was administered orally to rats at 435 mg/kg/day for 4 days, livers appeared normal with no macroscopic lesions (Taylor et al 1964).

Mutagenicity and genotoxicity: Benzaldehyde was non-mutagenic in the Ames test, both with and without metabolic activation (Sasaki & Endo 1978; Florin et al 1980; Kasamaki et al 1982; Haworth et al 1983; Nohmi et al 1985; Heck et al 1989). It was non-mutagenic in fruit flies (Woodruff et al 1985), was not mutagenic in a rec-assay (Oda et al 1978) and was not genotoxic in primary rat hepatocytes (Heck et al 1989). In one study, it did not cause SCE in Chinese hamster ovary cells (Sasaki et al 1989), but in another it did (Galloway et al 1987), and in a third it induced SCE in human lymphocytes (Jansson et al 1988). Chromosomal aberrations in Chinese hamster ovary cells were induced in one report (Sofuni et al 1985), were only weakly induced in another (Kasamaki et al 1982) and were not induced in third (Galloway et al 1987). Benzaldehyde was positive in two mouse lymphoma assays (Heck et al 1989; McGregor et al 1991). It was genotoxic in the wing somatic mutation and recombination test (SMART) of fruit flies (Demir et al 2008), but did not cause sex-linked recessive lethal mutations in male fruit flies (Woodruff et al 1985). In a comet assay, benzaldehyde was genotoxic at 10 and 25 mM (1.06 and 2.65 g/L), but not at 1, 5 or 50 mM (106, 530 or 5,300 mg/L), and the effect was therefore not dose-dependent (Demir et al 2010).

Carcinogenic/anticarcinogenic potential: In 2 year oral dosing studies, benzaldehyde was non-toxic to rats (at 200–400 mg/kg/day) and very weakly carcinogenic to mice, with increased incidences of squamous cell papillomas and forestomach hyperplasia (National Toxicology Program 1990b). Benzaldehyde caused slight hyperkeratosis of the forestomach in rats fed large amounts in the diet (Feron et al 1991). Benzaldehyde is a mouse-specific carcinogen (Battershill & Fielder 1998).

Benzaldehyde demonstrates anticarcinogenic activity, even in mice. Pulmonary metastasis was significantly reduced in mice treated with benzaldehyde, due to an augmentation of natural killer cell activity (Ochiai et al 1986; Masuyama et al 1987, 1988). It inhibited the activation of carcinogenic nitrosamines in mouse hepatic and pulmonary microsomes and the growth of human cervical cancer cells in vitro (Petterson et al 1983; Morse et al 1995). In dogs, even at the very low dose of 10 mg/kg/day, some response was seen in cases of oral cancers, and one dog's oral melanoma stabilized for 8 weeks (MacEwen 1986). In preclinical evaluations, benzaldehyde showed mixed results. It failed to inhibit the growth of various cancer cell lines in vitro, or the in vivo growth of two human xenografted cancers. However, when tested against human colony-forming cells from 30 patients with solid tumors, significant inhibition of colony growth (>70%) was seen in six patients (Taetle & Howell 1983).

Ninety patients with inoperable carcinoma in the terminal stages and 12 patients in serious condition with other tumor types were given benzaldehyde in the form of β-cyclodextrin benzaldehyde inclusion compound (CDBA) orally or rectally at a daily dose of 10 mg/kg divided into four doses. Toxic effects, including hematologic or biochemical disturbances, were not seen during long-term successive administration of CDBA. Fifty-seven of the patients treated were evaluable; 19 patients responded completely and 10 responded partially (greater than 50% regression). Longer response durations were associated with longer CDBA treatment periods (Kochi et al 1980).

Summary: Benzaldehyde is not a dermal irritant or allergen, but the vapor can cause respiratory irritation. Benzaldehyde is considered a mouse-specific, non-genotoxic carcinogen. This may explain the conflicting mutagenicity data. The compound is neurotoxic and hepatotoxic in elevated doses. Rat NOAEL values are 400 mg/kg/day over 90 days, and 200 mg/kg/day over 2 years. Since oral benzaldehyde was not toxic in humans when taken long-term at 10 mg/kg, this is therefore a safe dose.

Regulatory guidelines: A group ADI of 0–5 mg/kg body weight for benzoic acid, the benzoate salts (calcium, potassium and sodium), benzaldehyde, benzyl acetate, benzyl alcohol and benzyl benzoate, expressed as benzoic acid equivalents, was established by JECFA in 1996 and confirmed in 2001 (JECFA 2001a). The IFRA standard for benzaldehyde in leave-on products such as body lotions is 0.27%, for skin sensitization. The CIR recommended maximum for benzaldehyde in cosmetics is 0.5%. Benzaldehyde is listed under the FDA Controlled Substances Act as a 'List 1 chemical', one that can be used in the manufacture of illegal drugs (http://www.fda.gov/regulatoryinformation/legislation/ucm148726.htm#cntlsba accessed August 5th 2012).

Our safety advice: We support the JECFA <5 mg/kg as a daily oral dose maximum for benzaldehyde. We see no need for a limit on dermal exposure to benzaldehyde for skin sensitization.

Benzoic acid

Synonym: Benzenecarboxylic acid
Chemical class: Benzenoid carboxylic acid
CAS number: 65-85-0

Sources >1.0%:

Benzoin	0.1–18.4%
Peru balsam	1.4–6.3%
Tolu balsam	2.5%

Notes: Odorless crystalline solid, used for the topical treatment of ringworm and as a preservative in foodstuffs and soft drinks. Excreted by most vertebrates except fowl. Being a weak acid, benzoic acid may be corrosive to tissues.

Pharmacokinetics: Benzoic acid is rapidly absorbed in many species. Two days after applying [^{14}C]benzoic acid to human abdominal skin in vitro, a median of 44.9% of the dose was absorbed (Franz 1975). In pregnant rats, [^{3}H]benzoic acid penetrated the placental and fetal blood–brain barriers (Maickel & Snodgrass 1973). Benzoic acid is primarily metabolized by conjugation with glycine (in the kidney in most species) to form hippuric acid (40–100% in man) (Select Committee on GRAS Substances 1973). It is also conjugated with glucuronic acid in some species, especially at higher doses (Wan & Riegelman 1972).

Adverse skin reactions: Tested at 2% on 25 volunteers, benzoic acid was not irritating (Opdyke 1979a p. 715–722). In a retrospective multicenter study in Finland, there were 21 irritant (5.0%) reactions in 417 dermatitis patients (Kanerva et al 2001a). There were 43 (39%) irritation reactions to 5% benzoic acid in 110 dermatitis patients (Lahti 1980). Of 80 women, none with known perfume allergy, 76 (95%) had erythematous reactions of varying severity to 2% benzoic acid, with 17 (21%) showing symptoms of itching, stinging, burning or irritation (Safford et al 1990).

Non-immune immediate contact reactions (NIICR) to urticants (also known as contact urticaria, or hives) are concentration dependent, and in this respect benzoic acid is similar to cinnamaldehyde (Kligman 1990). At a sufficiently high concentration these agents produce a reaction in a majority of people without any previous sensitization. Benzoic acid induced NIICR in the majority of 200 volunteers (Basketter and Wilhelm 1996). Lahti (1980) reported that the lowest concentration of benzoic acid needed to elicit a wheal and flare reaction was 0.05% in water or 0.1% in petrolatum. However, the following year Lahti & Hannuksela (1981) reported that benzoic acid and a placebo (lactose) produced an equally high incidence of urticarial reactions in dermatology patients, assessed both objectively and subjectively.

Benzoic acid was not sensitizing when tested at 2% on 25 volunteers (Opdyke 1979a p. 715–722). Applied to the skin of 10 benzoyl peroxide-sensitive subjects at 5%, there were no allergic reactions to benzoic acid (Leyden & Kligman 1977). Of 627 dermatitis patients, eight (1.3%) tested positive to 5% benzoic acid (De Groot et al 1986). In a retrospective multicenter study in Finland, there were 18 allergic (4.3%) reactions to benzoic acid in 417 dermatitis patients (Kanerva et al 2001a). Of 5,202 patients with possible atopic dermatitis, 34 (0.66%) tested positive to benzoic acid. An allergic reaction was noted in one of 155 patients (0.7%) with cosmetic allergy (Broeckx et al 1987). Of 102 dermatitis patients sensitive to Peru balsam, 20 tested positive to 5% benzoic acid (Hausen 2001).

Acute toxicity: Acute oral LD_{50} reported as 1.7, 2.0–2.5 and 2.53 g/kg in rats (Fassett 1963; FASEB 1973; NIOSH 1977), 2.0 g/kg in dogs and cats (NIOSH 1977), and 1.25, 2.0 and 2.37 g/kg in mice (NIOSH 1977; Adams et al 2005b). Given ip to mice, the LD_{50} was 1.46 g/kg (NIOSH 1977), and transdermally in rabbits was 5 g/kg (Opdyke 1979a p. 715–722). In humans, the low toxic dose to skin was 6 mg/kg, and the low lethal oral dose was estimated to be 500 mg/kg (NIOSH 1977). The corresponding low lethal dose in rabbits was 2,000 mg/kg po and sc, 1,400 mg/kg ip in guinea pigs and 100 mg/kg sc in frogs (NIOSH 1977).

Subacute and subchronic toxicity: In cats, daily oral doses of 130–300 mg/kg benzoic acid given for 3–30 days had no effect at lower doses, but caused mild CNS disturbance with recovery at the higher doses. Doses of 300–900 mg/kg given for 1–3 days led to CNS disturbance and death (Bedford & Clarke 1972). In the longer term, benzoic acid could be fed at up to 200 mg/kg, with damage to liver and possibly kidney cells only at higher doses. Hyperesthesia, depression, apprehension and sometimes death were noted (Bedford & Clarke 1972). Benzoic acid has since been discontinued as a preservative in cat food.

When 100 mice (50 of each sex) were fed 80 mg/kg/day benzoic acid by oral intubation for 3 months there was a significant reduction in weight gain compared to controls, although feed intake was similar (Shtenberg & Ignatev 1970). In rats, no changes to liver microsomal protein or CYP levels, N-demethylation of aminopyrine or aniline p-hydroxylation were detected when 362 ppm benzoic acid was given in the diet (Corthay

et al 1977). The rat dietary NOAEL was estimated to be 10,000 ppm (1%), equivalent to 500 mg/kg bw (JECFA 1974).
Chronic toxicity: Forty rats (20 of each sex) received dietary 0.5% or 2% benzoic acid for one year. A slight reduction of growth rate was noted at 2%, but no effects were observed at 0.5% (Ohno et al 1978). When four generations of rats were dosed with 0.5% or 1% benzoic acid in feed for 1 year (~250 or ~500 mg/kg/day) there were no adverse effects at any dose, but a significant increase in lifespan was noted in the 0.5% group (Kieckebusch & Lang 1960). When 20 female and 30 male rats were dosed with 1.5% benzoic acid for 18 months decreased feed intake and reduced growth occurred (Marquardt 1960).
Human toxicity: No adverse effects were detected following ingestion of 100 mg/day (82 doses in 86 days) 500 or 1,000 mg/day (for 44 days) or 1,000 mg/day (88 doses in 92 days) in an unknown number of volunteers (FASEB 1973). Benzoic acid was ingested by 12 volunteers for 20 days at 1,000, 1,500, 2,000 and 2,500 mg/day, taking each dose for five days. Three of the participants took the entire dose of 35 g, and experienced nausea, indigestion, headache, weakness and esophageal burning (Wiley & Bigelow 1908). Orally administered benzoic acid provoked weak hypersensitivity in < 5% asthmatics (Rosenhall and Zetterström 1974, 1975). Hereditary hepatic porphyria was exacerbated in a patient by oral ingestion of a mouthwash containing benzoic acid (Bickers et al 1975).
Reproductive toxicity: Benzoic acid was not estrogenic, either in a yeast human estrogen receptor assay, or a uterotrophic assay (test for increase in uterine weight) in female rats and mice (Ashby et al 1997). When pregnant rats were given a single gavage dose of 510 mg/kg benzoic acid on gestation day nine, there was no increase in resorption rates or malformations (Kimmel et al 1971). Benzoic acid depleted pregnant rats of glycine at high doses and thus increased their sensitivity to teratogenicity from salicylic acid and aspirin (Davis 1970; Kimmel et al 1971). In a four-generation reproductive toxicity study, benzoic acid dosing at 375 or 750 mg/kg/day resulted in no adverse effects in rats (Cosmetic Ingredient Review Expert Panel 2011).
Mutagenicity and genotoxicity: Benzoic acid was non-mutagenic in SCE assays (Jansson et al 1988; Oikawa et al 1980) and the Ames test (Litton Bionetics Inc 1975; McCann et al 1975; Cotruvo et al 1977; Anderson & Styles 1978; Ishidate et al 1984; Fujita & Sasaki 1986; Zeiger et al 1988), but produced marginal CA in Chinese hamster fibroblasts (Ishidate et al 1984). Benzoic acid was slightly genotoxic in the wing somatic mutation and recombination test (SMART) of *Drosophila melanogaster* (Demir et al 2008) and was not mutagenic in *S. cereveisiae* (Cotruvo et al 1977). It was not genotoxic in the *S. typhimurium* TA135/pSK1002 umu test (Nakamura et al 1987). In a comet assay, benzoic acid was genotoxic at 5 mM (610 mg/L), but not at 0.05, 0.1, 0.5 or 1.0 mM (6.1, 12.2, 61 or 122 mg/L) (Demir et al 2010). Benzoic acid was not genotoxic in a micronucleus test in mouse lymphoma cells with or without metabolic activation (Nesslany & Marzin 1999).
Summary: Benzoic acid has been much studied as it is used as a preservative in foods. It is a dose-dependant skin irritant, but is not a significant contact allergen. In animal studies, toxic effects were seen at dietary doses of >1% benzoic acid. Multigenerational feeding studies in rats indicate a NOAEL of 500 mg/kg/day. A 92 day study in humans concluded that daily

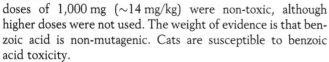

doses of 1,000 mg (~14 mg/kg) were non-toxic, although higher doses were not used. The weight of evidence is that benzoic acid is non-mutagenic. Cats are susceptible to benzoic acid toxicity.

Regulatory guidelines: A group ADI of 0–5 mg/kg body weight for benzoic acid, the benzoate salts (calcium, potassium and sodium), benzaldehyde, benzyl acetate, benzyl alcohol and benzyl benzoate, expressed as benzoic acid equivalents, was established by JECFA in 1996 and confirmed in 2001 (JECFA 2001a). The same ADI was proposed by the SCCNFP, who considered that a NOAEL of 500 mg/kg could be taken from the long-term and multigenerational studies, and a 100-fold uncertainty factor was then applied. The CIR Expert Panel has determined that benzoic acid is safe to use in cosmetic formulations at concentrations up to 5% (Nair 2001a).

Our safety advice: We support the JECFA <5 mg/kg as a daily oral dose maximum, and we support the CIR limit of 5% in cosmetics for benzoic acid.

Benzo[a]pyrene

Synonyms: 3,4-Benzpyrene. B[a]P
Chemical class: Fused pentacyclic benzenoid hydrocarbon
CAS number: 50-32-8

Sources:

Cade (unrectified)	~8 ppm
Cade (rectified)	<20 ppb

Pharmacokinetics: Many polynuclear hydrocarbons, including B[a]P, are readily bioactivated by the liver's CYP enzyme system to highly reactive and genotoxic compounds, often epoxides, which are potent initiators and promoters of cancer. The instillation of B[a]P into the nasal cavities of rats resulted in the transport of B[a]P and/or B[a]P metabolites along the olfactory neurons to the olfactory bulb (Persson et al 2002).

Mutagenicity and genotoxicity: B[a]P was mutagenic in the Ames test (Haworth et al 1983) and in the *S. typhimurium* TA135/pSK1002 umu test (Nakamura et al 1987). Benzo[a]pyrene-7,8-dihydrodiol-9,10-epoxide (BPDE) is the major mutagenic and carcinogenic metabolite (Huberman et al 1976; Meehan & Bond 1984).

Carcinogenic/anticarcinogenic potential: B[a]p induced tumors in the mammary glands, forestomach, lungs, skin, trachea, bronchi, liver, abdomen and uterus of several species, according to the route of administration (National Toxicology Program 2005).

Comments: Benzo[a]pyrene is probably the best-known example of the carcinogenic polynuclear hydrocarbons typically found in cigarette smoke and tar. It is used in animal testing to induce cancers, in order to evaluate the antitumoral potency of other substances.

Summary: B[a]P is a carcinogen. Exposure to it in essential oils must be greatly limited.

Regulatory guidelines: B[a]p is listed under 'Substances known to be human carcinogens' by the NTP (National Toxicology Program 2005). Rectified cade oil, in which most of the polynuclear hydrocarbons are removed by fractional distillation, is regarded by IFRA as safe for use in fragrances (IFRA 2009).

Benzyl acetate

Synonyms: Acetic acid benzyl ester. Acetic acid phenylmethyl ester
Systematic name: Phenylmethyl ethanoate
Chemical class: Benzenoid ester
CAS number: 140-11-4

Sources >1.0%:

Jasmine absolute	15.0–24.5%
Ylang-ylang	0.4–12.4%
Narcissus absolute	9.5–9.6%
Hyacinth absolute	8.1%
Jasmine sambac absolute	4.3%
Champaca absolute (orange)	0.1–4.0%
Ylang-ylang absolute	2.8%
Jonquil absolute	1.0%

Pharmacokinetics: Benzyl acetate is rapidly and almost completely metabolized via benzyl alcohol to benzoic acid in man, and excreted as hippuric acid (Scheline 1991). After dermal application of benzyl acetate in rats, virtually all the absorbed dose is excreted within 24 hours, with the water-soluble metabolites (glucuronide conjugate, benzoic acid and hippuric acid) detectable in the urine (Chidgey et al 1987).

In a study comparing similar doses administered by gavage or in feed, considerable toxicokinetic differences were seen in rats and mice. Gavage administration at 500 mg/kg/day in F344/N rats, or 1,000 mg/kg/day in mice, resulted in high benzoic acid plasma concentrations. These were much lower from feed administration at 615 mg/kg/day for rats and 850 mg/kg/day for mice. Bolus gavage administration was found to saturate the benzoic acid elimination pathway, while feed administration did not (Yuan et al 1995). Blood levels of benzoic acid in a gavage study were up to 300 times higher than those in a feed study (National Toxicology Program 1986, 1993b).

Adverse skin reactions: Tested at 8% on 25 volunteers, benzyl acetate was not sensitizing (Opdyke 1973 p. 875–876). There were no irritant or allergic reactions in 100 consecutive dermatitis patients tested with 5% benzyl acetate (Frosch et al 1995a). None of 70 patients with contact dermatitis reacted to 1% benzyl acetate (Nethercott et al 1989). In Japan, three of 155 cosmetic-sensitive patients (1.9%) had positive allergic reactions to benzyl acetate (Itoh 1982). In an in vitro assay, benzyl acetate was non-phototoxic (Placzek et al 2007).

Mucous membrane irritation: Benzyl acetate vapors can be irritating to the mucous membranes, eyes and respiratory passages (Opdyke 1973 p. 875–876).

Acute toxicity: The acute oral LD_{50} has been reported as 2.49 and 3.69 g/kg in rats, and as 2.64 in rabbits (Jenner et al 1964; Adams 2005b). Acute dermal LD_{50} in rabbits >5 g/kg (Opdyke 1973 p. 875–876). Can cause vomiting and diarrhea if ingested (Budavari 1989).

Subacute and subchronic toxicity: In a 28 day study, benzyl acetate was fed to male F344/N rats at 2%, 3.5% or 5% in the diet. There was no evidence of toxicity in the 2% group. Toxic signs in the higher dose groups included increased body weight loss, increased mortality, and neuronal necrosis in the cerebellum, hippocampus and pyriform cortex. Outward signs of neurotoxicity included ataxia and convulsions. Benzyl acetate toxicity was attenuated by concurrent glycine administration, suggesting that neurodegeneration is mediated by glycine depletion (Abdo et al 1998). The doses used are equivalent to approximately 860, 1,500 and 2,150 mg/kg/day.

In a 90 day study in F344/N rats, 10 of each sex of animal received 0, 62.5, 125, 250, 500 or 1,000 mg/kg benzyl acetate by corn oil gavage. The only clinical signs attributed to benzyl acetate dosing were in male and female rats on 1,000 mg/kg, and in females on 500 mg/kg. These included trembling, sluggishness and ataxia. Thickened stomach walls were seen in 2/9 males and 4/10 females on 1,000 mg/kg. No histopathological effects were observed (National Toxicology Program 1986).

In a 90 day mouse study, 10 of each sex of animal received 0, 125, 250, 500, 1,000 or 2,000 mk/kg bw benzyl acetate by corn oil gavage. Eight of the ten female mice receiving 2,000 mg/kg died. There were several deaths in other groups, attributed to 'gavage error'. Clinical signs seen in high-dose mice included trembling, inactivity, labored breathing and depressed body temperature. No treatment-related gross or microscopic effects were observed (National Toxicology Program 1986).

Reproductive toxicity: In a developmental toxicity study based on OECD guidelines, benzyl acetate was orally administered to pregnant rats at 0, 10, 100, 500 or 1,000 mg/kg/day on gestational days 6–15. Based on increases in the number of fetuses with skeletal and other malformations, and reductions in body weight gain at 1,000 mg/kg/day, the fetal NOAEL was determined to be 500 mg/kg/day. Even the high dose was not maternally toxic (Ishiguro et al 1993).

Mutagenicity and genotoxicity: Benzyl acetate was not mutagenic in the Ames test, with or without S9 (Florin et al 1980; Mortelmans et al 1986; Tennant et al 1987). Benzyl acetate was mutagenic in a mouse lymphoma assay (MLA) without S9 (McGregor et al 1988). In another MLA, it was mutagenic with S9, but not without S9 (Caspary et al 1988). The MLA has been criticized for having a very high incidence of false positive results (Caldwell 1993). In a subsequent study, nine chemicals that were positive in the MLA were re-evaluated in an in vitro CA assay using Chinese hamster lung cells. Three of the nine, including benzyl acetate, proved negative in this assay (Matsuoka et al 1996). Benzyl acetate was positive in one rec assay and negative in another (Oda et al 1978; Yoo 1986).

Benzyl acetate was not genotoxic in Chinese hamster ovary cells, with or without metabolic activation (Galloway et al 1987). In a mouse bone marrow micronucleus test, the compound showed no genotoxic effect (Shelby et al 1993). Benzyl acetate was not genotoxic either in human lymphocytes or in the human hepatoma cell line HepG2 (Kevekordes et al 2001). In the SOS chromotest (a modified E. coli PQ37 genotoxicity assay) benzyl acetate was not genotoxic, with or without S9 activation (Kevekordes et al 1999). Benzyl acetate was not genotoxic in Saccharomyces cerevisiae except at cytotoxic concentrations, and even then only a weak effect was seen (Zimmermann et al 1989). In a comet assay, benzyl acetate was very weakly genotoxic at 50 mM (7.5 g/L), but not at 1, 5, 10 or 25 mM (150, 750, 1,500 or 3,750 mg/L) (Demir et al 2010).

Benzyl acetate did not induce UDS in rat hepatocytes (Mirsalis et al 1983), and when rats were injected ip with 150, 500 or 1,500 mg/kg benzyl acetate, no DNA damage was evident in pancreatic cells after one hour (Longnecker et al 1990). However, in a comet assay, benzyl acetate was genotoxic in 4 of 8 mouse tissues, and 6 of 8 rat tissues (Sekihashi et al 2002). The compound was moderately genotoxic in the wing somatic mutation and recombination test (SMART) of fruit flies (Demir et al 2008) but did not cause sex-linked recessive lethal mutations in male fruit flies (Woodruff et al 1985).

Carcinogenic/anticarcinogenic potential: In a 2 year NTP study, benzyl acetate was given by corn oil gavage to F344/N rats at 0, 250 or 500 mg/kg/day, and to mice at 0, 500 or 1,000 mg/kg/day. There were no adverse effects on mean body weights. There was increased incidence of acinar cell adenoma of the exocrine pancreas in male rats, but not female rats or mice of either sex. Even in the control group of male rats, 22/50 had pancreatic tumors. In the low dose group, 27/50 had tumors, and in the high dose group, 37/49. In mice of both sexes (but not rats) there were statistically significant increases in liver and forestomach tumors. These were more numerous in males than in females (Abdo et al 1985; National Toxicology Program 1986).

In a subsequent NTP study, benzyl acetate was given in feed to groups of F344/N rats and B6C3F$_1$ mice for 2 years with no resulting carcinogenicity. Doses were 3,000, 6,000, or 12,000 ppm in rats, equivalent to 130, 260, 510 mg/kg/day for males and 145, 280, 575 mg/kg/day for females. In mice, doses were 330, 1,000, or 3,000 ppm, equivalent to 35, 110, 345 mg/kg/day for males, and 40, 130, 375 mg/kg/day for females (National Toxicology Program 1993b).

In a further 2-year study, benzyl acetate was given at 0.8% (8,000 ppm) in the diet to male F344/N rats. There were no adverse effects on growth or survival, but 3/38 rats developed pancreatic carcinomas, which was considered marginally significant. Benzyl acetate weakly promoted exocrine pancreatic acinar tumors in rats, when the animals had been previously exposed to the carcinogen azaserine (Longnecker et al 1990). When male Lewis or F344/N rats were given benzyl acetate either by gavage (500 mg/kg/day, 5 days per week) or at 0.9% in the diet, both until weaning, there was no evidence of pancreatic tumors, nor was there any significant tumor increase in rats given azaserine (Longnecker et al 1986).

A retrospective analysis of NTP data found that there was an increased incidence of pancreatic acinar cell adenoma in male rats receiving corn oil by gavage, compared to untreated controls (Haseman et al 1985). Similarly, azaserine-initiated male Lewis rats had an increased incidence of pancreatic tumors after four months on a 20% fat diet high in essential fatty acids (Roebuck et al 1985).

Summary: In 90 day studies, dietary doses of 500 mg/kg/day were neurotoxic in female rats, but no toxicity was apparent at 250 mg/kg/day. In cancer studies, questions have been raised about increased toxicity from corn oil gavage administration, principally in regard to forestomach tumors, since benzyl acetate is a gastric irritant, especially to mice (Ashby 1994). The consensus of opinion is that tumors found in benzyl acetate gavage studies are largely gavage-related. The general lack of genotoxicity, except in a minority of assays, suggests that benzyl

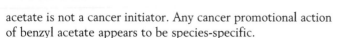

acetate is not a cancer initiator. Any cancer promotional action of benzyl acetate appears to be species-specific.

Regulatory guidelines: A group ADI of 0–5 mg/kg body weight for benzoic acid, the benzoate salts (calcium, potassium and sodium), benzaldehyde, benzyl acetate, benzyl alcohol and benzyl benzoate, expressed as benzoic acid equivalents, was established by JECFA in 1996 and confirmed in 2001 (JECFA 2001a). In 1999 the IARC concluded that there was '*limited evidence*' in experimental animals for the carcinogenicity of benzyl acetate' (Anon 1999).

Our safety advice: We support the JECFA <5 mg/kg as a daily oral dose maximum for benzyl acetate.

Benzyl alcohol

Synonyms: Benzenemethanol. Phenylcarbinol. α-Hydroxytoluene
Systematic name: Phenylmethanol
Chemical class: Benzenoid alcohol
CAS number: 100-51-6

Sources >1.0%:

Tolu balsam	41.8%
Benzoin	38.8–43.4%
Hyacinth absolute	40.0%
Narcissus absolute	1.7–4.8%
Violet leaf absolute	1.0–2.1%
Champaca absolute (orange)	0.3–2.0%
Bakul absolute	1.6%
Jasmine sambac absolute	1.3%

Note: Used as an excipient in numerous topical formulations. Benzyl alcohol is slowly oxidized to benzoic acid on exposure to air.

Pharmacokinetics: The human organism readily oxidizes benzyl alcohol to benzoic acid which, after conjugation with glycine, is rapidly eliminated as hippuric acid (Scheline 1991). Hippuric acid formation is deficient in preterm neonates, confirming that the benzyl alcohol/benzoic acid detoxification process is poorly developed in premature newborns (LeBel et al 1988).

Adverse skin reactions: In a modified Draize procedure on guinea pigs, benzyl alcohol was non-sensitizing when used at 10% in the challenge phase (Sharp 1978). Undiluted benzyl alcohol was moderately irritating to guinea pig skin; tested at 10% on 25 volunteers it caused no allergic reactions (Opdyke 1973 p. 1011–1013).

When tested at 5%, one of 4,195 (0.025%) eczema patients reacted to benzyl alcohol (Mitchell et al 1982). In 20 eczema patients and in 34 patients suspected of suffering from cosmetic dermatitis (54 individuals) there were no reactions to 10% benzyl alcohol on patch testing (Malten et al 1984). When benzyl alcohol was patch tested at 5% on 50 dermatitis patients who were not thought to be sensitive to fragrances there were no positive reactions (Larsen 1977). Of 241 dermatitis patients tested with 5% benzyl alcohol, there were no positive reactions (Ferguson & Sharma 1984). None of 70 patients with contact dermatitis reacted to 5% benzyl alcohol (Nethercott et al 1989). In two HRIPT studies, there were two sensitization

reactions in 101 subjects tested with 5% benzyl alcohol, and no sensitization reactions in 107 subjects tested with 3% benzyl alcohol (RIFM 2005a, RIFM 2004c, cited in Scognamiglio et al 2012). The results of two European studies are reported in Table 5.10.

There were four positive reactions among 242 patients (1.7%) with atopic dermatitis of varying origins (Van Joost et al 1985). In 5,202 patients with possible atopic dermatitis 48 (0.9%) tested positive to benzyl alcohol (Broeckx et al 1987). Of 182 dermatitis patients suspected of contact allergy to cosmetics, three (1.6%) tested positive to 10% benzyl alcohol (Malten et al 1984). Of 167 dermatitis patients suspected of fragrance sensitivity two (1.2%) were allergic to 1% benzyl alcohol (Larsen et al 1996b). In 578 dermatitis patients known to be sensitized to cosmetics, three (0.5%) tested positive to benzyl alcohol (Adams & Maibach 1985). Benzyl alcohol was responsible for two cases (0.4%) of contact dermatitis of 487 cosmetic-related cases (Eiermann et al 1982). Of 713 cosmetic dermatitis patients, three reacted to benzyl alcohol (Adams & Maibach 1985). When patch tested at 5% on 20 dermatitis patients who were sensitive to fragrant substances, benzyl alcohol induced three (15%) positive reactions (Larsen 1977). Of 102 dermatitis patients sensitive to Peru balsam, eight tested positive to 5% benzyl alcohol (Hausen 2001).

Tested at 5%, benzyl alcohol was the causative agent in a 46-year-old man who developed acute eczema of the penis and in a 63 year-old woman with a three year history of vulval dermatitis (Li & Gow 1995; Corazza et al 1996).

Based on literature published in German, benzyl alcohol was classified as Category C, not significantly allergenic, by Schlede et al (2003).

Acute toxicity: The acute oral LD50 in rats has been reported as 1.23, 1.57, 2.08, 3.0 and 3.1 g/kg in rats, 1.58 g/kg in mice, and 1.94 g/kg in rabbits (Adams et al 2005b). Acute dermal LD_{50} in guinea pigs <5 mL/kg (Opdyke 1973 p. 1011–1013). When doses of undiluted benzyl alcohol ranging from 0.025–0.4 mL/kg were administered iv to mice, convulsions, dyspnea and reduced mobility were observed at all doses except for the lowest (Montaguti et al 1994). Fatal doses of 0.055 mL/kg in dogs produced respiratory and cardiac arrest, but no convulsions were seen (Kimura et al 1971). A lack of effect on blood pressure following iv administration of 1 mL/kg of a 0.9% solution of benzyl alcohol to dogs was noted by Kimura et al (1971).

In early 20th century reports, benzyl alcohol apparently caused respiratory failure, hypotension and convulsions in experimental animals (MMWR 1982). Respiratory difficulties from high doses are noted in later research, but not hypotension, and there is no consensus on convulsions.

Subacute and subchronic toxicity: In 16 day studies, all five male and five female rats and mice dosed with 2,000 mg/kg benzyl alcohol died. Two of five male and 3/5 female rats and 1/5 male and 2/5 female mice dosed with 1,000 mg/kg died. In the two highest dose groups rats and mice of each sex were lethargic after dosing, and there was subcutaneous, urinary and gastrointestinal hemorrhaging. Animals administered lower doses of benzyl alcohol (125, 250, or 500 mg/kg) had no compound-related histologic lesions (National Toxicology Program 1989a). On reviewing this report the EPA determined that the NOAEL was ≦250 mg/kg for male mice and ≦500 mg/kg for female mice (Environmental Protection Agency 1989).

In 13 week corn oil gavage studies, rats and mice were dosed with 0, 50, 100, 200, 400, and 800 mg/kg of benzyl alcohol. Eight of 10 male rats at 800 mg/kg died during weeks 7 and 8; four of these deaths were considered gavage related. Rats dosed with 800 mg/kg exhibited clinical signs indicative of neurotoxicity including staggering, respiratory difficulty, and lethargy, but no convulsions. Hemorrhages occurred around the mouth and nose, and there were histologic lesions in the brain, thymus, skeletal muscle, and kidney. In mice, deaths were scattered among all doses, but none occurred in vehicle controls; all deaths but one were considered gavage related. Staggering after dosing also occurred during the first two weeks of the studies in mice dosed with 800 mg/kg. There were reductions in relative weight gain in 800 mg/kg male rats, in female rats dosed with 200 mg/kg or more, in 400 or 800 mg/kg male mice, and in female mice dosed with 200 mg/kg or more. No notable changes in body weight gain or compound-related histopathologic lesions were observed in rats or mice from the lower dose groups (National Toxicology Program 1989a). On reviewing these data the EPA determined that the 90 day NOAEL for female rats was 143 mg/kg. Using this level, and applying an uncertainty factor of 100 (10 for interspecies difference and 10 to protect unusually sensitive individuals) gave a rounded down human reference dose of 1 mg/kg/day (Environmental Protection Agency 1989).

Inhalation toxicity: When 18 rats were exposed to 2,000 ppm of benzyl alcohol vapor, nine died within 14 days (Carpenter et al 1949). Inhalation of 1,000 ppm of benzyl alcohol vapor for 8 hours resulted in the death of three of six rats within 14 days (Smyth et al 1951). It was concluded that rats could inhale air saturated with benzyl alcohol for a maximum of two hours, and that the vapor was a moderate hazard. Inhalation of benzyl alcohol vapor by mice decreases their motility (Buchbauer et al 1991). Benzyl alcohol vapors can penetrate intact skin (Jones, 1967, cited in Opdyke 1973 p. 1011–1013). Benzyl alcohol is a highly volatile compound, but its volatility is notably reduced as a constituent of absolutes and resinoids. Inhalation toxicity, therefore, cannot be extrapolated from the pure substance to these materials.

Human toxicity: Because of its antibacterial action and good safety record, 0.9% benzyl alcohol has been used as a preservative in injected drugs for decades (Novak et al 1972). Sixteen cases of pre-term neonatal death were thought to be caused by benzyl alcohol used as a bacteriostatic agent (9 mg/mL) in isotonic saline used to flush intravascular catheters. No deaths have occurred since the two institutions concerned changed to flush solutions without benzyl alcohol. Review of the medical records of affected infants resulted in estimates of daily intake of benzyl alcohol ranging from 99–405 mg/kg (Gershanik et al 1981; Brown et al 1982). Retrospective reviews of patient records in two neonatal intensive care units showed significant improvement in the survival rate of infants weighing less than 1 kg following the discontinuation of benzyl alcohol solutions (Menon et al 1984; Hiller et al 1986). Benzyl alcohol has also been associated with delay of mental development, and other neurological deficits in low birth weight infants (Benda et al 1986; Sreenan et al 2001).

Toxic symptoms displayed by the infants included metabolic acidosis, hypotension and respiratory distress progressing to gasping respirations. Many infants also had central neural depression, seizures or intracranial hemorrhage. Although many of these clinical features commonly occur in neonates seriously ill from other causes, the evidence for benzyl alcohol toxicity was considered convincing (Anon 1982). Toxic effects of benzyl alcohol previously observed include convulsions and respiratory failure. In a comparison of 9 pre-term and 14 term infants receiving phenobarbital containing benzyl alcohol, there was greater accumulation of benzoic acid in the serum of preterm compared to the term neonates. In addition, larger concentrations of benzyl alcohol were found in urine as benzoic acid in preterm babies, while less hippuric acid appeared in their urine than term newborns. Hippuric acid formation is therefore deficient in preterm neonates, confirming the suspected immaturity of the benzoic acid detoxification process in premature newborns (LeBel et al 1988).

Reproductive toxicity: When 50 pregnant mice were dosed with 750 mg/kg/day benzyl alcohol by gavage on gestational days 7–14, there were 19 deaths attributable to benzyl alcohol. A significant day 18 mean body weight decrease was noted, as was a decrease in mean litter pup weight, but there was no reduction in litter viability or in reproductive or gestational indices (Inveresk Research International Ltd. 1983). In a similar study, 50 pregnant mice were dosed with 750 mg/kg/day benzyl alcohol by gavage on gestational days 6–13. Nineteen of the dosed mice died before delivery compared to none of the controls. Viability in the benzyl alcohol group was 21 of 22 litters (compared to 29/29 in the control group). There was no significant change in maternal weight, but birth weight and 3 day weight gain were significantly less in the benzyl alcohol group (Hardin et al 1987).

When 50 pregnant mice were dosed with 550 mg/kg/day benzyl alcohol by gavage on gestational days 6–15 no differences between the dosed group and control group were noted with respect to maternal status, length of gestation, reproductive index, postnatal survival, litter weight or pup weight (Environmental Health Research and Testing Inc 1986). In an ex vivo assay, benzyl alcohol did not bind to estrogen receptors in female rat uterus tissue (Blair et al 2000). Also see Human toxicity, above.

Hepatotoxicity: Intraperitoneal injection of 500 mg/kg benzyl alcohol in rats caused a significant increase in the rate of ROS formation in hepatic mitochondrial fractions (Mattia et al 1993).

Antioxidant/pro-oxidant activity: Benzyl alcohol exhibited a strong antioxidant activity, inhibiting monaldehyde formation by 32% at 400 µg/mL (Lee & Shibamoto 2001). Benzyl alcohol is oxidized to benzoic acid on exposure to air.

Mutagenicity and genotoxicity: Benzyl alcohol was not mutagenic in the Ames test, with or without metabolic activation (Florin et al 1980; Ball et al 1984; Ishidate et al 1984; Mortelmans et al 1986; Rogan et al 1986; Heck et al 1989; National Toxicology Program 1989a; Zeiger et al 1990). In two reports, benzyl alcohol was both non-mutagenic and antimutagenic in *E. coli* WP2*uvr*A (Kuroda et al 1984a; Yoo 1986). Benzyl alcohol was mutagenic in two *B. subtilis* rec assays, and not in a third (Oda et al 1978; Kuroda et al 1984b;

Yoo 1986). Benzyl alcohol was genotoxic in the wing somatic mutation and recombination test (SMART) of *Drosophila melanogaster* (Demir et al 2008). It was not genotoxic in Chinese hamster fibroblasts (Ishidate et al 1984) but showed some genotoxicity in Chinese hamster ovary cells (Anderson et al 1990). In a mouse micronucleus test, benzyl alcohol was not genotoxic (Hayashi et al 1988). In a comet assay, it was very weakly genotoxic at 25 and 50 mM (2.7 and 5.4 g/L), but not at 1, 5 or 10 mM (108, 540 or 1,080 mg/L), and the effect was not dose-dependent (Demir et al 2010).

In cytogenetic assays with Chinese hamster ovary cells, treatment with benzyl alcohol produced an increase in SCE which was considered equivocal both with and without S9; an increase in CA was seen after exposure to benzyl alcohol in the presence, but not the absence, of S9. In a mouse lymphoma assay, benzyl alcohol induced an increase in trifluorothymidine-resistant cells in the absence, but not in the presence, of S9; the effect was associated with toxicity (National Toxicology Program 1989a). Similarly equivocal or weakly positive SCE induction and aberrations were obtained by Anderson et al (1990).

Carcinogenic/anticarcinogenic potential: Benzyl alcohol was not carcinogenic in male mice when a total dose of 3.75 μmol (405 μg) was injected ip in increasing doses on days 1, 8, 15 and 22 prior to weaning (Miller et al 1983). There was no evidence of carcinogenic activity in male or female rats dosed with 200 or 400 mg/kg benzyl alcohol for 2 years, nor in male or female mice dosed with 100 or 200 mg/kg benzyl alcohol for two years (National Toxicology Program 1989a).

Comments: Considering the overall low level of skin reactions to benzyl alcohol, it cannot be regarded as an important sensitizer in an aromatherapy context. It is difficult to understand why benzyl alcohol has been classed as a high-risk allergen by the EU. The neurotoxic action of benzyl alcohol in premature neonates highlights the risks of intensive application of essential oils to this high-risk group, in which detoxification mechanisms are poorly developed.

Summary: Out of 6,776 patch tests on dermatitis patients not known to be cosmetic- or fragrance-sensitive, there were a total of 7 or 8 reactions to benzyl alcohol (0.1%). Little can be extrapolated from the high-concentration inhalation toxicity tests in rodents, except that there may be a risk to humans at some level. Benzyl alcohol is not safe to use on premature or low birth weight neonates. Benzyl alcohol is not carcinogenic, and there are some false-positive results for genotoxicity (Kirkland et al 2005).

Regulatory guidelines: Based on the current intake of benzyl alcohol as a flavoring agent, JECFA stated in 2001 that there was 'no safety concern' (SCF 2002b). A group ADI of 0–5 mg/kg body weight for benzyl alcohol, benzoic acid, benzoate salts (calcium, potassium and sodium), benzaldehyde, benzyl acetate and benzyl benzoate, expressed as benzoic acid equivalents, was established by JECFA in 1996 and confirmed in 2001 (JECFA 2001a). The FDA has recommended that benzyl alcohol should not be used in intravascular flush solutions or other medications for neonates.

Benzyl alcohol is one of 26 fragrance materials listed as an allergen by the EU. If present in a cosmetic product at over 100 ppm (0.01%) in a wash-off product or 10 ppm (0.001%) in a leave-on product the material must be declared on the ingredient list if sold in an EU member state. The CIR Expert Panel

has determined that benzyl alcohol is safe to use in cosmetic formulations at concentrations up to 5% (Nair 2001a). The IFRA standard for benzyl alcohol in leave-on products such as body lotions is 2.7%, for skin sensitization. In Europe, benzyl alcohol is permitted at up to 1% as a preservative.

Our safety advice: We support the JECFA <5 mg/kg as a daily oral dose maximum for benzyl alcohol. We see no need for a limit on dermal exposure to benzyl alcohol for skin sensitization.

Benzyl benzoate

Synonyms: Benzyl benzenecarboxylate. Benzoic acid. Benzyl ester. Benzoic acid phenylmethyl ester
Systematic name: Phenylmethyl benzenecarboxylate
Chemical class: Benzenoid ester
CAS number: 120-51-4

Sources >1.0%:

Peru balsam	59.0–86.2%
Tolu balsam	46.6%
Benzoin	39.3–50.7%
Jasmine absolute	8.0–20.0%
Ylang-ylang	4.3–14.9%
Carnation absolute	5.0–14.6%
Massoia	8.1–13.4%
Ylang-ylang absolute	11.8%
Narcissus absolute	0.7–8.9%
Tuberose absolute	8.3%
Hyacinth absolute	6.0%
Jonquil absolute	4.4%
Cinnamon leaf	tr–4.1%
Ginger lily absolute	2.9%
Cassia leaf	tr–2.9%
Cananga	2.0%
Bakul absolute	1.1%
Cassia bark	tr–1.0%
Cinnamon bark	tr–1.0%

Note: Widely used for the topical treatment of scabies.
Adverse skin reactions: When tested at 30% on 25 volunteers benzyl benzoate elicited no sensitization reactions. Cross-sensitization reactions have been reported in subjects sensitized to Peru balsam, and four cases of dermatitis have been attributed to benzyl benzoate (Opdyke 1973 p. 1015–1016). Used on 980 patients in the treatment of scabies, benzyl benzoate produced no incidents of dermatitis. A 20% emulsion of benzyl benzoate was applied to each patient, from neck to soles of feet, by an attendant using a 2.5 inch paintbrush (Graham 1943).

Tested at at 5%, there was one allergic reaction to benzyl benzoate from 658 people (0.15%) with hand eczema (Heydorn et al 2003b). Of 241 dermatitis patients tested with 2% benzyl benzoate, one (0.4%) had a positive reaction (Ferguson & Sharma 1984). When tested at 2%, three of 284 (1%) and none of 335 dermatitis patients reacted to benzyl benzoate (Mitchell et al 1982). The results of two European studies are reported in Table 5.10.

Tested at 5%, benzyl benzoate produced no allergic reactions in 45 cosmetic dermatitis patients (Itoh 1982). Of 487 cosmetic-related cases, benzyl benzoate was responsible for one (0.2%) of contact dermatitis (Eiermann et al 1982). One of 713 cosmetic dermatitis patients (0.14%) reacted to benzyl benzoate (Adams & Maibach 1985). Of 102 dermatitis patients sensitive to Peru balsam, four tested positive to 5% benzyl benzoate (Hausen 2001). One of 20 fragrance-sensitive patients (5%) reacted to 5% benzyl benzoate (Larsen 1977).

Benzyl benzoate was not phototoxic when tested on guinea-pigs at 10%, 30% or 50% (Cosmetic Ingredient Review Expert Panel 2011).

Acute toxicity: Acute oral LD_{50} reported as 1.9 and 2.8 g/kg in rats, 1.68 and 2.0 g/kg in rabbits, 1.57 g/kg in mice, 1.1 g/kg in guinea pigs and 2.24 g/kg in cats (Adams et al 2005b). Acute dermal LD_{50} in rabbits 4 mL/kg (Opdyke 1973 p. 1015–1016).

Reproductive toxicity: Charles and Darbre (2009) reported that benzyl benzoate produced estrogenic responses and increased the proliferation of MCF-7 cells at 10^{-4} M (21.2 mg/L). However, Hashimoto et al (2003) reported no estrogenic activity in MCF-7 cells at concentrations ranging from 10^{-9}–10^{-4} M. Benzyl benzoate had no estrogenic activity in a *Xenopus* hepatocyte assay, suggesting that any in vitro estrogenic activity does not take place in vivo, perhaps due to metabolic inactivation (Nomura et al 2006). In a retrospective study, the safety of a 25% benzyl benzoate lotion (applied 1–3 times as a treatment for scabies) was assessed in 444 pregnant women and 1,776 matched controls. There were no significant differences in any of the assessed outcomes: proportion of abortions, congenital abnormalities, neonatal deaths, stillbirths and premature births (Mytton et al 2007).

Dietary benzyl benzoate produced no fetotoxic effects when given to female rats at 0.04% or 1.0% (~24 or 595 mg/kg/day) from day 0 to to day 21 post-parturition. However in a similar study there was an increase in skeletal anomalies in pups born to animals in the high dose group (Cosmetic Ingredient Review Expert Panel 2011). The high dose is equivalent to a 70 kg human ingesting 41.7 g per day for 3 weeks.

Mutagenicity and genotoxicity: Benzyl benzoate was not mutagenic in the Ames test (Florin et al 1980).

Carcinogenic/anticarcinogenic potential: Benzyl benzoate completely inhibited the growth of ascites sarcoma BP8 cells (a rat cell line) at a concentration of 1.0 mM (212 mg/L) (Pilotti et al 1975).

Comments: Considering the overall low level of adverse skin reactions to benzyl benzoate, it cannot be regarded as an important sensitizer and it is difficult to understand why it has been classed as a high-risk allergen by the EU.

Summary: In dermatitis patients not known to be fragrance-sensitive, skin reactions ranged from 0% to 1.0% of those tested, which indicates that considerably less than 1% of the general population is likely to react to benzyl benzoate. Massive doses given to rats caused borderline fetotoxicity, but a dose equivalent to 1.7 g in an adult human was not fetotoxic.

Regulatory guidelines: A group ADI of 0–5 mg/kg body weight for benzoic acid, benzoate salts (calcium, potassium and sodium), benzaldehyde, benzyl acetate, benzyl alcohol and benzyl benzoate, expressed as benzoic acid equivalents, was established by JECFA in 1996 and confirmed in 2001 (JECFA 2001a). Benzyl benzoate is one of the 26 fragrance materials listed as an allergen by the EU. If present in a cosmetic product at over 100 ppm (0.01%) in a wash-off product or 10 ppm (0.001%) in a leave-on product the material must be declared on the ingredient list if sold in an EU member state. The IFRA standard for benzyl benzoate in leave-on products such as body lotions is 26.7%, for skin sensitization.

Our safety advice: We support the JECFA <5 mg/kg as a daily oral dose maximum for benzyl benzoate. We see no need for a limit on dermal exposure to benzyl benzoate for skin sensitization.

Benzyl cinnamate

Synonyms: Benzyl-β-phenylacrylate. Cinnamic acid benzyl ester
Systematic name: Phenylmethyl 3-phenylprop-2-enoate
Chemical class: Phenylpropenoid benzenoid ester
Note: Different isomers of benzyl cinnamate exist, and the following isomer-specific information has been published.

(2Z)-Benzyl cinnamate

Synonym: *cis*-Benzyl cinnamate
CAS number: Not found

(2E)-Benzyl cinnamate

Synonyms: *trans*-Benzyl cinnamate. Cinnamein
CAS number: 103-41-3

Sources >1.0%:

Peru balsam	0.4–30.1%
Styrax (American)*	1.7%

Adverse skin reactions: Tested at 8% on 25 volunteers, benzyl cinnamate was neither irritant nor sensitizing. The undiluted compound produced mild irritant effects in rabbits patch-tested for 24 hours under occlusion (Opdyke 1973 p. 1017–1018). In a human repeat insult patch test, 4% benzyl cinnamate produced no reactions in 25 male and 76 female volunteers. UV spectral data suggest that benzyl cinnamate has no potential for phototoxicity or photoallergy (Belsito et al 2007). In 20 dermatitis patients suspected of suffering from contact sensitivity to cosmetics, there were no reactions to 8% benzyl cinnamate. Of 182 dermatitis patients suspected of contact allergy to cosmetics, six (3.3%) tested positive to 8% benzyl

*Isomer not specified

503

cinnamate (Malten et al 1984). Three of 747 dermatitis patients suspected of fragrance allergy (0.4%) reacted to 5% benzyl cinnamate (Wöhrl et al 2001). Of 102 dermatitis patients sensitive to Peru balsam, three tested positive to 2% benzyl cinnamate (Hausen 2001). The results of two further European studies are reported in Table 5.10.

Acute toxicity: Acute oral LD_{50} reported as 3.76 g/kg in guinea pigs and 3.28 g/kg in rats. Acute dermal LD_{50} in rabbits >3 g/kg (Opdyke 1973 p. 1017–1018).

Subacute and subchronic toxicity: When 10,000 ppm of benzyl cinnamate was fed to rats in the diet for 19 weeks there were no macroscopic effects, and the NOAEL was 500 mg/kg/day (Hagan et al 1967).

Mutagenicity and genotoxicity: Benzyl cinnamate was not mutagenic in a *Bacillus subtilis* rec assay (Yoo 1986).

Comments: Considering that there is only one peer-reviewed report of benzyl cinnamate eliciting any skin reactions it is difficult to understand why it has been classed as a high-risk fragrance allergen by the EU. The question of whether or not to impose a limit in relation to essential oils is somewhat redundant, since both Peru balsam oil and styrax oil are already subject to dermal limits.

Summary: Low toxicity, irritancy and allergenicity.

Regulatory guidelines: Benzyl cinnamate is one of the 26 fragrance materials listed as an allergen by the EU. If present in a cosmetic product at over 100 ppm (0.01%) in a wash-off product or 10 ppm (0.001%) in a leave-on product the material must be declared on the ingredient list if sold in an EU member state. Based on literature published in German, benzyl cinnamate was classified as Category B, moderately allergenic, by Schlede et al (2003). The IFRA standard for benzyl cinnamate in leave-on products such as body lotions is 2.1%, for skin sensitization.

Our safety advice: We see no need for a limit on dermal exposure to benzyl cinnamate for skin sensitization.

Benzyl cyanide

Synonyms: Benzeneacetonitrile. Phenylacetonitrile. α-Tolunitrile. ω-Cyanotoluene

Chemical class: Benzenoid nitrile

CAS number: 140-29-4

Sources >0.1%:

Karo karoundé absolute	4.8%
Nasturtium absolute	2.0%
Ginger lily absolute	1.3%
Orange flower absolute	1.0%

Pharmacokinetics: In rats given benzyl cyanide either orally or ip, cyanide ions were slowly liberated from the dosed nitrile and excreted as cyanide and thiocyanate, the proportion of the former increasing with increasing ip dose and with the highest oral dose (Guest et al 1982). Administered orally to rats at 150 mg/kg, benzyl cyanide led to markedly increased urinary thiocyanate levels, which equated to 61% of the dose for males and 89% for females (Potter et al 2001a). When benzyl cyanide was applied dermally to rats at 150 mg/kg and maintained under occlusion for 24 hours, there was a marked increase in urinary thiocyanate levels, attributable to the release of cyanide in vivo. The amount of thiocyanate recovered was equivalent to 37% of the dose for males and 32% for females (Potter et al 2001b). Rat liver, but not the nose, contains at least two CYP isozymes involved in the metabolism of benzyl cyanide to cyanide ions. Inhaled benzyl cyanide is substantially detoxified in the nasal cavity (Dahl & Waruszewski 1989).

Adverse skin reactions: According to Lewis (1992), benzyl cyanide is an irritant. However, we could find no concrete information to support this view.

Acute toxicity: Lethal doses of benzyl cyanide in rats were 0.64 mmol/kg (75 mg/kg) (ip), 1.8 and 2.6 mmol/kg (211 and 304 mg/kg) (oral) for females and males, respectively. Sublethal oral doses were nephrotoxic, causing increased excretion of protein, amino acids and glucose (Guest et al 1982). Lewis (1992) gives the rat oral LD_{50} for benzyl cyanide as 270 mg/kg and states that it is a poison by ingestion, inhalation, skin contact, subcutaneously or intraperitoneally.

Comments: Unlike inorganic cyanides such as hydrocyanic acid, organic cyanides like benzyl cyanide do not ionize in solution to release highly toxic cyanide ions. Although some of the toxicity of benzyl cyanide is attributable to cyanide ions formed during metabolism, its presence in certain absolutes at less than 5% is not of great concern. The rat acute oral LD_{50} of karo karoundé absolute, for instance, is 1.4 g/kg (Ford et al 1988a p. 61S).

Summary: Although benzyl cyanide is nephrotoxic, its use is, if anything, over-restricted.

Regulatory guidelines: IFRA recommends that benzyl cyanide is not used as a fragrance ingredient; exposure from oils and extracts is not significant and their use is authorized so long as the level of benzyl cyanide in the finished product does not exceed 100 ppm (0.01%) (IFRA 2009). Benzyl cyanide is prohibited as a fragrance ingredient in the EU and Canada (Anon 2003a; Health Canada Cosmetic Ingredient Hotlist, March 2011). Benzyl cyanide is listed under the FDA Controlled Substances Act as a 'List 1 chemical', one that can be used in the manufacture of illegal drugs (http://www.fda.gov/regulatoryinformation/legislation/ucm148726.htm#cntlsba accessed August 5th 2012).

Benzyl isothiocyanate

Synonyms: Isothiocyanatomethylbenzene. Isothiocyanic acid benzyl ester. Benzyl mustard oil

Chemical class: Benzenoid thiocarbonyl compound

CAS number: 622-78-6

Source:

Nasturtium absolute	72.3%

Pharmacokinetics: Benzyl isothiocyanate reacts rapidly with glutathione to form the conjugate, which is degraded to the cysteine conjugate and then acetylated to give the corresponding mercapturic acid N-acetyl-S-(N-benzylthiocarbamoyl)-(−)-cysteine. This compound is the major urinary metabolite in both rat (40% of an oral dose) and man (~54% of an oral dose) (Scheline 1991).

Adverse skin reactions: Intensely irritating (Lewis 2000).

Acute toxicity: Poison by ip and sc routes. LDLo 100 mg/kg ip rat; LDLo 100 mg/kg ip mouse; LD$_{50}$ 150 mg/kg sc mouse (Lewis 2000).

Reproductive toxicity: Benzyl isothiocyanate was administered orally to female rats both pre- and post-implantation at 12.5, 25 or 50 mg/kg. A dose-dependant increase in early fetal resorptions was seen in rats treated prior to implantation, but this was not statistically significant. There was no significant fetal loss at any dose, but both fetal and placental weights in the 25 and 50 mg/kg groups were significantly lower than in controls. In addition, there were three maternal deaths in the high dose group, with signs of toxicity including hypo-activity, peri-nasal staining and weight loss (Adebiyi et al 2004).

Hepatotoxicity: Benzyl isothiocyanate was considerably more toxic to rat RL-4 hepatocytes than its glutathione and N-acetylcysteine conjugates. The glutathione conjugate, unlike the N-acetylcysteine conjugate, cannot cross cell membranes, and its toxicity is believed to be due to conversion back to the parent isothiocyanate (Bruggeman et al 1986, Masutomi et al 2001).

Mutagenicity and genotoxicity: Using human hepatoma G2 cell gel electrophoresis, there was no evidence for a protective effect of benzyl isothiocyanate against DNA damage caused by B[a]P or (±)-anti-benzo[a]pyrene-7,8-dihydrodiol-9,10-epoxide, its ultimate genotoxic metabolite. On the contrary, at up to 1.25 μM (186 μg/L), benzyl isothiocyanate potentiated B[a]P-induced DNA damage, and at 5 μM (745 μg/L) and above, it alone caused DNA damage (Kassie et al 2003).

Carcinogenic/anticarcinogenic potential: There was an increased incidence of bladder hyperplasia and cancer in male rats fed 0.1% benzyl isothiocyanate for 32 weeks, especially in animals previously dosed with cancer promoting substances (Hirose et al 1998). Epithelial cell inflammation, due to cytotoxicity and irritation, leads to continuous cell proliferation, and this seems to play an important role in the early stages of carcinogenesis (Akagi et al 2003).

Benzyl isothiocyanate was cytotoxic to four human ovarian carcinoma cell lines and one human lung carcinoma cell line in the range 0.86–9.4 μM (128–1,400 μg/L) (Pintao et al 1995). It was cytotoxic to human leukemia HL60 cells with an IC$_{50}$ of 4.62 μg/mL (Nibret & Wink 2010). In rat liver RL34 cells, benzyl isothiocyanate induced apoptosis at 20 μmol (2.98 mg), and modified mitochondrial respiration and the release of cytochrome c (Nakamura et al 2002). Benzyl isothiocyanate also stimulates apoptosis in human colon adenocarcinoma LS-174 and Caco-2 cell lines, and is thus thought to afford protection against DNA damage when present in the diet (Bonnesen et al 2001). Benzyl isothiocyanate in the diet may inhibit the development of preneoplastic lesions while having little effect on normal cells (Musk et al 1995).

Benzyl isothiocyanate was moderately chemopreventive against nitrosamine-induced carcinogenesis in rat tissues (Chung et al 1984). Other workers have found evidence of a significant chemopreventive action. Rat bladder cell dysplasia, papilloma and carcinoma induced by N-butyl-N-(4-hydroxybutyl)nitrosamine were dramatically reduced by simultaneous treatment with benzyl isothiocyanate (at 10, 100 and 1,000 ppm in the diet). This finding contrasts with the weak carcinogenic activity observed for the isothiocyanate alone (Okazaki et al 2002).

Benzyl isothiocyanate inhibited lung tumorigenesis in A/J mice when induced by the polycyclic aromatic hydrocarbons benzo[a]pyrene, 5-methylchrysene or dibenzo[a,h]anthracene, or the nitrosamine NNK. Induction of apoptosis and activation of mitogen-activated protein kinase, AP-1 transcription factors and p53 phosphorylation were proposed as possible mechanisms (Hecht 1995; Hecht et al 2002; Yang et al 2002). Fifteen minutes after administering benzyl isothiocyanate (6.7 μmol [1.00 mg] or 13.4 μmol [2.00 mg]) by gavage, mice received the carcinogens by gavage once weekly for 8 weeks. Nineteen weeks after the last dose, lung tumor multiplicity had significantly reduced in all groups by 63.5–90.6% (Hecht et al 2002). Under these conditions, benzyl isothiocyanate was more potent than the known chemopreventive compounds butylated hydroxyanisole and sulforaphane.

Similar results were found when benzyl isothiocyanate (9 μmol [1.34 mg] or 12 μmol [1.79 mg]), phenylethyl isothiocyanate 12 μmol (1.96 mg), or a combination of the two were given by gavage 2 hours before each of 8 weekly gavage treatments of a mixture of benzo[a]pyrene and NNK (3 μmol each [756 μg and 621 μg, respectively]). Daily dosing benzyl isothiocyanate in the diet was more effective than weekly dosing by gavage (Hecht et al 2000). In the mouse forestomach, benzyl isothiocyanate-induced increases in glutathione S-transferase activity were accompanied by a reduced incidence of benzo[a]pyrene-induced tumor formation. Benzyl isothiocyanate also inhibited DMBA-induced mammary neoplasia when administered subsequently (Wattenberg 1983).

Summary: Benzyl isothiocyanate demonstrates some hepatotoxicity and reproductive toxicity. The reproductive toxicity NOAEL in rats is 12.5 mg/kg. There is one report of mutagenicity, and it is carcinogenic in male rat bladder, in part due to irritation. However, it is cytotoxic to human cancer cell lines, and there are seven reports of chemopreventive activity. Benzyl isothiocyanate is regarded as a promising therapeutic agent for lung cancer (Akagi et al 2003).

Benzyl salicylate

Synonyms: Salicylic acid benzyl ester. o-Hydroxybenzoic acid benzyl ester
Systematic name: Phenylmethyl 2-hydroxybenzoate
Chemical class: Phenolic ester
CAS number: 118-58-1

Sources >1.0%:

Ylang-ylang absolute	5.2%
Carnation absolute	3.9%
Ylang-ylang	0.3–3.9%
Tuberose absolute	2.6%

Note: Being a substituted phenol, benzyl salicylate is a weak acid which may be corrosive to tissues.

Adverse skin reactions: In a modified Draize procedure on guinea pigs, benzyl salicylate was non-sensitizing when used at 2% in the challenge phase (Sharp 1978). Tested at 30% on the skin of 25 volunteers, benzyl salicylate was not sensitizing (Opdyke 1973 p. 1029–1030). The potential of benzyl salicylate to induce hypersensitivity or to elicit reactions to pre-existing hypersensitivity in the general population was evaluated by analysing patch-test data. No induced or elicited responses directly attributable to benzyl salicylate were observed in 35 patch tests of 10% benzyl salicylate in ethanol, or in 10,503 patch tests of consumer products containing <2% benzyl salicylate. From this study it was concluded that benzyl salicylate has a very low potential to induce hypersensitivity ('induced' reactions) or to elicit reactions attributable to pre-existing sensitization ('elicited' reactions). People with any active skin disease were excluded from this survey (Kohrman et al 1983).

There were two allergic reactions to benzyl salicylate (0.3%) when it was tested at 5% in 658 people with hand eczema (Heydorn et al 2003b). When benzyl salicylate was patch tested at 2% on 50 dermatitis patients who were not thought to be sensitive to fragrance materials there were no positive reactions (Larsen 1977). In 100 consecutive dermatitis patients there were no irritant or allergic reactions to 1% benzyl salicylate, and there was one irritant reaction and no allergic reactions to 5% (Frosch et al 1995a). None of 70 patients with contact dermatitis reacted to 2% benzyl salicylate (Nethercott et al 1989). In a multicenter study, 10 of 1,825 dermatitis patients (0.5%) were sensitive to 2% benzyl salicylate (De Groot et al 2000). The results of two further European studies are reported in Table 5.10.

Of 713 cosmetic dermatitis patients, one (0.14%) reacted to benzyl salicylate (concentration not reported) (Adams & Maibach 1985). In 578 cases of eczema patients known to be sensitized to cosmetics, one (0.17%) tested positive to benzyl salicylate (concentration not reported) (Adams & Maibach 1985). Of 167 dermatitis patients suspected of fragrance sensitivity five (3%) were allergic to 2% benzyl salicylate on patch testing (Larsen et al 1996b). Three of 747 dermatitis patients suspected of fragrance allergy (0.4%) reacted to 1% benzyl salicylate (Wöhrl et al 2001). When benzyl salicylate was tested at 2% on 20 fragrance-sensitive dermatitis patients, there were two positive reactions (Larsen 1977). Of 102 dermatitis patients sensitive to Peru balsam, three tested positive to 2% benzyl salicylate (Hausen 2001).

Based on literature published in German, benzyl salicylate was classified as category C, not significantly allergenic, by Schlede et al (2003). Benzyl salicylate is thought to be a more common cause of skin sensitization in Japan than in the USA or Europe (Larsen et al 1996b), and the patch testing data support this view. In 11 Japanese reports, 2% benzyl salicylate produced allergic reactions in a total of 173 of 5,087 dermatitis patients, or 3.4%. In seven European and North American studies, including some of fragrance-sensitive individuals, the corresponding incidence was 20 of 2,640 dermatitis patients, or 0.76% (Lapczynski et al 2007a). In a Korean study, benzyl salicylate produced no sensitization reactions in 422 patients with suspected contact allergy (An et al 2005).

Acute toxicity: Acute oral LD_{50} in rats 2.23 g/kg; acute dermal LD_{50} in rabbits 14.15 g/kg (Opdyke 1973 p. 1029–1030).

Reproductive toxicity: Salicylates in general are known to dose-dependently inhibit growth and cause congenital abnormalities in experimental animals (Wilson 1973; Karabulut et al 2000), though benzyl salicylate is not normally included in the salicylates tested. However, it probably does not occur in any essential oil or absolute in quantities sufficient to be teratogenic. Benzyl salicylate increased proliferation of MCF-7 breast cancer cells at 10^{-5} M (2.28 mg/L), suggesting estrogenic activity, but at 10^{-4} M (22.8 mg/L) it had the opposite effect (Hashimoto et al 2003). Curiously, Charles & Darbre (2009) reported that benzyl salicylate produced estrogenic responses and increased the proliferation of MCF-7 cells at 10^{-4} M.

Mutagenicity and genotoxicity: Benzyl salicylate was not mutagenic in the Ames test (Zeiger et al 1987).

Comments: Excluding cosmetic- and frangrance-sensitive patients, a total of 14/4,744 dermatitis patients (0.30%) reacted to 1%, 2% or 5% benzyl salicylate. One of the most telling recent reports is that only two of 2,041 European dermatitis patients (0.1%) tested positive to 1% benzyl salicylate (Schnuch et al 2007a), since this indicates that 1% represents a negligible risk. It therefore makes no sense to restrict naturally occurring benzyl salicylate to concentrations 1,000 times less than this in Europe.

Summary: Benzyl salicylate is a probable moderate-risk skin allergen in people of Japanese origin. Minimal equivalent risk in people of other ethnicities.

Regulatory guidelines: Benzyl salicylate is one of the 26 fragrance materials listed as an allergen by the EU. If present in a cosmetic product at over 100 ppm (0.01%) in a wash-off product or 10 ppm (0.001%) in a leave-on product the material must be declared on the ingredient list if sold in an EU member state. The IFRA standard for benzyl salicylate in leave-on products such as body lotions is 8.0%, for skin sensitization.

Our safety advice: We see no need for a limit on dermal exposure to benzyl salicylate for skin sensitization.

Bergamottin

Synonyms: 5-Geranoxypsoralen. 5-GOP. 5-Geranoxy-6,7-furanocoumarin

Systematic name: 5-((E)-3,7-Dimethyl-2,6-octadien-1-yloxy)-furano[3,2-g]benzopyran-7-one

Chemical class: Furanocoumarin alkene ether

CAS number: 7380-40-7

Sources:

Lime expressed	1.7–3.0%
Bergamot (expressed)	0.68–2.75%
Bergamot (FCF)	0–1.625%
Lemon (expressed)	0.16–0.54%
Grapefruit	< 0.11%

Pharmacokinetics: Bergamottin inhibits CYP3A, with an IC_{50} value of 22 µM (7.44 mg/L) (Guo et al 2000) and inhibits CYP3A4 with an IC_{50} value of 13.63 µM (4.61 mg/L) (Modarai et al 2011). It is also a potent inhibitor of CYP1A1 and CYP1A2 (Wen et al 2002; Baumgart et al 2005). Bergamottin metabolism may be different in rats and humans (Le Goff-Klein et al 2004).

Adverse skin reactions: Bergamottin photosensitizes mamallian cells in tissue culture, and irradiation with black light or fluorescent ceiling lights produced at least four photobiologically active degradation products (Ashwood-Smith et al 1992). However, in vivo studies, in which bergamottin was applied to the skin, showed no phototoxicity (Naganuma et al 1985, Zaynoun et al 1977b). Bergamottin is only marginally phototoxic, which shows up in in vitro testing using V79 cells (Lohr et al 2010; Messer et al 2012), but the effect is not strong enough to produce a positive result in vivo (Bode et al 2005).

Mutagenicity and genotoxicity: Bergamottin was not mutagenic in five strains of *S. typhimurium* without S9 mix either in presence or absence of UVA (Ballantyne 2002). However, the SCCNFP expressed reservations about the integrity of this report (SCCNFP 2003a). Bergamottin was not mutagenic in an HPRT assay and was not photomutagenic. Similarly, it was neither genotoxic nor photogenotoxic in a micronucleus assay (Lohr et al 2010). Bergamottin does not interact with DNA after UV irradiation (it is not photomutagenic) and its action may involve ROS (Aubin et al 1994, Bode et al 2005, Morlière et al 1991). Bergamottin reduced the formation of B[*a*]P metabolites (including phenols, diols and tetraols) in cultured mouse keratinocytes, and inhibited the formation of adducts induced by B[*a*]P or DMBA (Cai et al 1997a). Given topically five minutes prior to an initiating dose of B[*a*]P, bergamottin dose-dependantly decreased covalent binding of B[*a*]P to DNA 24 hours after treatment, a 400 nmol (135 µg) dose causing a 72% reduction (Cai et al 1997b).

Carcinogenic/anticarcinogenic potential: Bergamottin was a potent inhibitor of tumor initiation by B[*a*]P (Cai et al 1997b). It prevented B[*a*]P- and DMBA-induced adduct formation in the human breast MCF-7 adenocarcinoma cell line via inhibition of multiple human CYPs (Kleiner et al 2002). Bergamottin suppressed tumor promotion in mammalian cells through inhibition of superoxide and nitric oxide generation (Miyake et al 1999).

Comments: Bergamottin is one of many psoralens found in citrus fruit oils. The existing data indicate that it is neither phototoxic nor photomutagenic, but the SCCNFP has reservations about its safety in this respect. The matter is of some consequence, since bergamottin is present in substantial concentrations in several citrus fruit oils; a restriction on total psoralens has different repercussions to a restriction on only those proven to be photomutagenic. A recent report confirms that bergamottin is not photomutagenic (Lohr et al 2010). The ability of bergamottin to inhibit DNA adducts, and to inhibit the metabolic activation of B[*a*]P, may be due to the inhibition of CYP enzymes.

Summary: Bergamottin is phototoxic but is not photomutagenic. It demonstrates some in vitro and in vivo antitumoral activity.

Regulatory guidelines: In its report on bergamottin the SCCNFP concluded that there are insufficient data for evaluation of its safety in relation to photomutagenicity and photocarcinogenicity (SCCNFP 2003a). For tanning products, the SCCNFP set a maximum of 1 ppm for 'furocoumarin-like substances' in 1995, later reviewed and confirmed (SCCNFP 2003b). This has now been extended to apply to all cosmetic products, and bergamottin is specifically included (SCCP 2005b).

Bergapten

Synonyms: 5-Methoxypsoralen. 5-MOP. Psoraderm. Heraclin
Systematic name: 5-Methoxyfurano[3,2-*g*]benzopyran-7-one
Chemical class: Furanocoumarin ether
CAS number: 484-20-8

Sources >0.0001%:

Lime expressed	0.17–0.33%
Bergamot (expressed)	0.11–0.33%
Orange (bitter)	0.035–0.073%
Lemon (expressed)	0.0001–0.035%
Grapefruit	0.012–0.019%
Rue	0.018%
Bergamot (FCF)	0–0.0091%
Angelica root	0.0078%
Mandarin leaf	0.005%
Tangerine	0–0.005%
Parsley leaf	0.002%
Mandarin	0–0.0003%
Skimmia	Uncertain

Pharmacokinetics: Bergapten is an inducer of CYP1A1 (Diawara et al 1999). It strongly inhibited CYP3A4, with IC_{50} values of 19 µM (4.1 mg/L) and 36 µM (7.8 mg/L) in two different human livers (Ho et al 2001).

Adverse skin reactions: Bergapten is phototoxic (Zaynoun et al 1977a, 1977b). It may increase the DNA-damaging effects of ultraviolet light, although it can also protect against them (see Carcinogenic potential, below).

Cardiovascular effects: Bergapten shows strong antiplatelet aggregation activity in vitro (Chen IS et al 1996).

Reproductive toxicity: Bergapten was given in the diet to pregnant female rats for 39–49 days (until the day before expected parturition) at 0, 1,250 or 2,500 ppm, corresponding to 0, ~100 mg/kg and ~200 mg/kg, respectively. Numbers of implantation sites and of pups per female were lower in the dosed groups, and uterine weight was reduced in the high-dose group. Circulating 17β-estradiol levels were dose-dependently reduced, and liver mRNAs for CYP1A1 and UGT1A6 were significantly induced. Enhanced metabolism of estrogens may explain the reproductive toxicity of bergapten in female rats (Diawara et al 1999; Diawara & Kulkosky 2003).

When male rats were given dietary bergapten at 0, 1,250 or 2,500 ppm (corresponding to 0, ~75 or ~150 mg/kg, respectively) for 8 weeks, treated males had smaller pituitary and prostate glands. Sperm counts were reduced in the high-dose group and more breeding attempts were required to impregnate females. Dosing significantly elevated testosterone, and relative liver weight; body weight gain was reduced in the high-dose group (Diawara et al 2001).

Hepatotoxicity: Dietary administration of 1,000 ppm (~100 mg/kg) of bergapten for four weeks reduced total CYP levels in female mice, but not in males. In both sexes there was hypertrophy of the centrilobular hepatocytes (Diawara et al 2000).

Mutagenicity and genotoxicity: There are many reports showing bergapten to be photogenotoxic (Abel 1987b; Averbeck et al 1990; Schimmer & Kühne 1990). These are summarized in SCCNFP (2003b). The lowest dose inducing a genotoxic response was ~1 ppm or lower. The treatment of human blood cultures with bergapten, followed by UVA exposure, resulted in chromosome damage; even a concentration as low as 0.001 µg/mL was clastogenic, while 0.0001 µg/mL was not (Youssefi et al 1994). The formation of photoadducts in cellular DNA is similar exposure to UVA after bergapten or methoxsalen treatment. The primary photoproducts are 4,5-monoadducts, which crosslink on subsequent radiation (Amici & Gasparro 1995). A recent report found bergapten to be 'strongly' photomutagenic in an HPRT assay (Lohr et al 2010).

Carcinogenic/anticarcinogenic potential: In studies using hairless albino mice, with 0, 5, 15 or 50 ppm bergapten applied 5 days a week for 65 or 75 weeks, bergapten was phototumorigenic even at 5 ppm. The addition of sunscreens afforded total protection at 5 and 15 ppm (Young et al 1990). Using bergapten in a sunscreen at 15, 30 or 45 ppm dose-dependently induced melanogenesis by 2.5–5.0-fold, and increased stratum corneum thickness by 10–40% compared to sunscreen without bergapten. This protects against subsequent UV-induced DNA damage, especially in individuals who tan poorly (Young et al 1988). The protection begins after three to five daily exposures, reaches a peak at eight days and some protection remains for up to 14 weeks after ceasing application (Chadwick et al 1994). DNA damage in similar tests was measured directly using a monoclonal antibody to thymine dimers (a major category of DNA lesion induced by UV radiation) (Potten et al 1993). In similar human tests of skin types I–V (there are six skin types, lightest to darkest) skin biopsies showed that UDS was significantly reduced in skin types I and II when bergapten was used (Young et al 1991).

Topical application of a bergapten-containing sunscreen five days a week for 20 weeks, each application followed by UV radiation, resulted in the eventual development of squamous cell carcinomas in hairless mice (Cartwright & Walter 1983). These findings are at odds with the human studies cited above, which may be due to differences in duration of study. In the human trials bergapten and UV radiation was applied for a maximum of two weeks, compared to 20 weeks or, in the case of Young et al (1990), 65 or 75 weeks in the rodent studies. In addition, mice are much less capable than humans of repairing DNA damage from UV radiation (Hosomi & Kuroki 1985; Cleaver & Crowley 2002; Yarosh et al 2002).

Bergapten is cytotoxic to the human hepatocellular carcinoma cell line; it kills cells directly, induces apoptosis, and inhibits proliferation (Lee et al 2003).

Comments: There are IFRA guidelines addressing phototoxicity for all the above listed essential oils except for *Skimmia laureola*. No regulatory agency has addressed bergapten's reproductive toxicity, probably because it is not likely to

cause such toxicity at the very low levels required to avoid phototoxicity.

Summary: Bergapten is phototoxic. When combined with UV radiation, bergapten may be carcinogenic in humans when used at more than extremely low doses/concentrations. This applies to both oral and dermal routes of administration. However, there is no evidence that bergapten is otherwise carcinogenic. Bergapten is reproductively toxic to both male and female mice, and inhibits platelet agegration in vitro.

Regulatory guidelines: IFRA recommends that the total bergapten content in leave-on products should not exceed 0.0015% (15 ppm) (IFRA 2009). For sun protection and bronzing products, the SCCNFP set a maximum of 1 ppm for 'furocoumarin-like substances' in 1995, and this was later reviewed and confirmed (SCCNFP 2003b). An IARC report concluded, as of 1998, that there was sufficient evidence for the carcinogenicity of bergapten to experimental animals when combined with UV radiation, but there was inadequate evidence for carcinogenicity either to experimental animals in the absence of UVA radiation, or to humans. However, bergapten plus UV was thought to be 'probably carcinogenic to humans' (IARC 1986a).

α-Bisabolol

Synonym: 2,10-Bisaboladien-7-ol
Systematic names: (R*,R*)-α,4-Dimethyl-α-(4-methyl-3-pentenyl)-3-cyclohexene-1-methanol, 6-Methyl-2-(4-methyl-3-cyclohexen-1-yl)-5-hepten-2-ol
Chemical class: Monocyclic sesquiterpenoid alkene alcohol
Note: Different isomers of α-bisabolol exist, and the following isomer-specific information has been published.

(+)-α-Bisabolol

Synonyms: (6R,7R)-Bisabolol. Bisabolol. Camilol
CAS number: 23178-88-3

(−)-α-Bisabolol

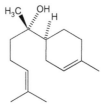

Synonyms: (6S,7S)-Bisabolol. Levomenol
CAS number: 23089-26-1

Sources >1.0%:

Chamomile (blue)	1.6–60.1%
Balsam poplar	27.4%
Sandalwood (W. Australian)	4.9–15.0%
Phoebe	3.3–3.6%
Chaste tree leaf	0–2.7%

Wormwood ((Z)-epoxy ocimene CT) 1.5–2.5%
Wormwood (β-thujone /
(Z)-epoxy ocimene CT)   1.7–2.3%
Chaste tree seed   0–1.8%
Myrtle (bog)   1.0%

(+)-epi-α-Bisabolol

CAS number: 76738-75-5

(−)-epi-α-Bisabolol

Synonym: Anymol
CAS number: 78148-59-1

Sources >1.0%:

Sage (blue mountain)   27.1%
Sandalwood (E. African)   5.1%
Valerian (European)   0–1.9%

Pharmacokinetics: In the presence of α-bisabolol, 5-fluorouracil was 17 times better absorbed transdermally in human skin, and triamcinolone acetonide was 73 times more permeable (Kadir & Barry 1991).

Adverse skin reactions: α-Bisabolol was not phototoxic when tested on guinea pigs at 3% and 15% (CIR 1999).

Acute toxicity: α-Bisabolol acute oral LD_{50} 15.25 mL/kg in rats and 15.1 mL/kg in mice (Habersang et al 1979). Acute rat oral LD_{50} also reported as >5 g/kg. Mouse acute ip LD_{50} 633 mg/kg, with gross signs of hepatic toxicity (CIR 1999).

Subacute and subchronic toxicity: In 28 day gavage studies, α-bisabolol was administered to groups of rats and dogs at 2 mL/kg and 3 mL/kg. In rats there was dose-dependent motor agitation and urinary ketone body reaction; rats on the higher dose had decreased body weight gain and a 20% mortality rate, and some abnormal liver function tests in females. The dogs on 3 mL/kg had their dose increased to 4 mL/kg for the second 2 weeks. In two of six dogs on the lower dose, reduced appetite and vomiting were seen. In the higher dose dogs, body weight gain was reduced, some liver function parameters were abnormal, and liver weight relative to body weight was significantly increased. In a 6 week study, 1 mL/kg of α-bisabolol was administered by gavage to male and female rats, and no adverse signs or symptoms were observed (Habersang et al 1979).

Pure α-bisabolol (87.5%) was applied daily for 28 days to the clipped skin of male and female rats at 1%, 4% or 20% in olive oil, with a semiocclusive dressing, resulting in doses of 50, 200 or 1,000 mg/kg bw. No treatment-related adverse effects were seen in the low and mid-dose groups. In the high-dose groups, a significant decrease in mean absolute liver weight was noted in females, and an increase in mean relative testes weight in males (CIR 1999).

Reproductive toxicity: No teratogenic effect was observed at doses up to 1 mL/kg when α-bisabolol was administered by gavage to pregnant rats and rabbits on gestational days 6–15. At 3 mL/kg, there was a reduction in fetal numbers in both species (Habersang et al 1979).

Mutagenicity and genotoxicity: α-Bisabolol was not mutagenic in Ames tests, with or without S9 (CIR 1999, Gomes-Carneiro

et al 2005b, Gonçalves et al 2011). It did not induce CA in Chinese hamster V79 cells, with or without S9 (CIR 1999). In fruit flies, α-bisabolol was not genotoxic, and protected against genotoxicity induced by hydrogen peroxide (Anter et al 2011).

Carcinogenic/anticarcinogenic potential: α-Bisabolol had a strong time- and dose-dependent cytotoxic effect on human and rat glioma (brain cancer) cells, while normal rat glial cells were not affected. Cytotoxicity was due to the induction of apoptosis and mitochondrial damage (Cavalieri et al 2004, Darra et al 2007). α-Bisabolol was highly toxic in vitro to human pancreatic cancer cells (Darra et al 2008) and moderately cytotoxic to human leukemia (HL-60) cells (Anter et al 2011). The increased toxicity of α-bisabolol to malignant cells is due to greater cellular uptake than in normal cells (Cavalieri et al 2009).

Summary: We could find no relevant dermal data. α-Bisabolol is not mutagenic and shows antitumoral activity. In both acute and subacute toxicity studies there are signs of hepatotoxicity with elevated doses, and high doses are also fetotoxic. The lowest NOAEL is 200 mg/kg.

Borneol

Synonyms: Bornyl alcohol. 2-Bornanol. Camphol. Borneo camphor. Malayan camphor. Sumatra camphor
Systematic name: 1,7,7-Trimethylbicyclo[2.2.1]heptan-2-ol
Chemical class: Bicyclic monoterpenoid alcohol
Note: Different isomers of borneol exist, and the following isomer-specific information has been published.

(+)-Borneol

Synonyms: (1R,2S)-Borneol. (1R)-endo-Borneol
CAS number: 464-43-7
Note: (+)-Borneol, which predominates in nature, occurs in the oil from Dryobalanops aromatica Gaertn. and in many other plants (Budavari 1989).

(−)-Borneol

Synonyms: (1S,2R)-Borneol. (1S)-endo-Borneol. Linderol. Ngai camphor
CAS number: 464-45-9
Note: (−)-Borneol is found in the oil from Blumea balsamifera (L.) DC (Budavari 1989).

(−)-Isoborneol

Synonyms: (1R,2R)-Borneol. (1R)-exo-Borneol
CAS number: 10334-13-1

(+)-Isoborneol

Synonyms: (1S,2S)-Borneol. (1S)-exo-Borneol
CAS number: 16725-71-6
Sources >5.0%:

Sage (Dalmatian)   1.5–23.9%
Thyme (borneol CT)   20.0%
Rosemary (borneol CT)   15.6%

Inula	15.3%
African bluegrass	6.4–9.5%
Rosemary (camphor CT)	2.0–9.0%
Rosemary (bornyl acetate CT)	5.0–8.4%
Camphor (Borneo)	8.3%
Tansy	7.8%
Southernwood	7.3%
Citronella (Sri Lankan)	0–6.6%
Sage (Spanish)	1.5–6.4%
Marjoram (Spanish)	3.8–5.9%
Chamomile (Roman)	0–5.0%

Pharmacokinetics: Both (+)-borneol and (−)-borneol are largely excreted as bornyl glucuronides in rabbits (~22%), dogs (50–75%) and man (~80%) after oral ingestion (Scheline 1991).

Adverse skin reactions: Tested at 20% (−)-borneol was not irritating in 23 male volunteers. (−)-Borneol was non-sensitizing in 25 volunteers at 8% and in 23 volunteers at 20%. In a third panel, there were two mild sensitization reactions in 25 volunteers (various RIFM reports, cited in Bhatia et al 2008f).

Acute toxicity: (−)-Borneol acute oral LD_{50} in rats 6.5 g/kg, acute dermal LD_{50} in rabbits >2 g/kg (Opdyke, 1978 p. 655–656). Acute mouse oral LD_{50} for borneol (isomer not specified) reported as 1.06 g/kg (Horikawa & Okada 1975).

Neurotoxicity: According to Budavari (1989) borneol 'may cause nausea, confusion, dizziness and convulsions' but no reference or further information is given. A convulsant effect is highly unlikely, since both (+)-borneol and (−)-borneol have a significant GABAergic action (Granger et al 2005).

Mutagenicity and genotoxicity: Borneol was not mutagenic in the Ames test, both with and without S9 activation (Simmon et al 1977; Azizan & Blevins 1995). It was also not mutagenic in *E. coli* (Yoo 1986), nor was any genotoxicity (DNA strand breaks) detected in human VH10 fibroblasts (Slamenová et al 2009). At the relatively high doses of 0.5–2.0 mM (77–308 mg/L), borneol protected rat hepatocytes against DNA damage (strand breaks) induced by hydrogen peroxide, but at 2.5 or 3.0 mM (385 or 462 mg/L) borneol increased hydrogen peroxide genotoxicity. The latter concentrations were also cytotoxic, which is often taken as an indication that the substance is not truly genotoxic. In rats given 1 or 2 mM (154 or 308 mg/L) of borneol in drinking water for 7 days, hydrogen peroxide genotoxicity was reduced in hepatic and testicular cells (Horváthová et al 2009).

Summary: The limited data on borneol suggest that it presents very little risk of toxicity.

Bornyl acetate

Synonyms: *endo*-Borneol acetate. *endo*-Bornyl ethanoate. Acetic acid bornyl ester
Systematic name: *endo*-1,7,7-Trimethylbicyclo[2.2.1]hept-2-yl ethanoate
Chemical class: Bicyclic monoterpenoid ester
Notes: Isomeric with isobornyl acetate. Different isomers of bornyl acetate exist, and the following isomer-specific information has been published:

(+)-Bornyl acetate

Synonyms: (1R,2S)-Bornyl acetate. (1R)-*endo*-Bornyl acetate
CAS number: 20347-65-3

(−)-Bornyl acetate

Synonyms: (1S,2R)-Bornyl acetate. (1S)-*endo*-Bornyl acetate
CAS number: 5655-61-8

Sources >5.0%:

Inula	46.1%
Spruce (black)	36.8%
Valerian (European)	0.9–33.5%
Fir needle (Siberian)	31.0%
Fir needle (Japanese)	27.9%
Goldenrod	19.5%
Spruce (red)	16.4%
Fir needle (Canadian)	4.9–16.2%
Coleus	15.0%
Rosemary (bornyl acetate CT)	11.5–14.3%
Spruce (white)	14.1%
Pine (grey)	12.5–12.6%
Silver fir (cones)	1.3–12.5%
Fir (Douglas)	10.0%
Larch needle	7.9%
Pine (dwarf)	1.0–7.9%
Tansy	7.7%
Rosemary (verbenone CT)	2.0–7.6%
Hinoki leaf	7.2%
Bee balm	1.5–5.7%
Sage (Dalmatian)	0.3–5.7%
Boswellia frereana	0–5.6%
Spruce (Norwegian)	3.0–5.1%
Savory (winter)	0–5.1%

Adverse skin reactions: Tested at 2% on human subjects (−)-bornyl acetate was neither irritating nor sensitizing (Opdyke 1973 p. 1041–1042).

Acute toxicity: (−)-Bornyl acetate acute oral LD_{50} in rats >5 g/kg, acute dermal LD_{50} in rabbits >10 mL/kg (Opdyke 1973 p. 1041–1042).

Summary: The limited data on bornyl acetate suggests that it presents little risk of toxicity.

3-Butyl phthalide

Synonyms: 3-*n*-Butyl phthalide. 3-*n*-Butylphthalic acid lactone. 1,3-Dihydro-3-butylisobenzofuran-1-one
Systematic name: 1,3-Dihydro-3-butylbenzo[c]furan-1-one
Chemical class: Bicyclic benzenoid furanoid lactone
CAS number: 6066-49-5

Sources >1.0%:

Celery leaf	6.2%
Celery seed	2.1–3.0%

Adverse skin reactions: When applied undiluted to rabbit skin for 24 hours under occlusion, 3-butyl phthalide was moderately irritating. Tested at 2% on 30 volunteers it was neither irritating nor sensitizing (Opdyke 1979a p. 251).

Acute toxicity: Acute oral LD_{50} in rats 2.45 g/kg; acute dermal LD_{50} in rabbits >5 g/kg (Opdyke 1979a p. 251).

Carcinogenic/anticarcinogenic potential: 3-Butyl phthalide induced glutathione *S*-transferase in mouse liver and small intestine, and reduced the incidence of forestomach cancer (Zheng et al 1993b).

Summary: Limited data suggests that 3-butyl phthalide presents minimal risk in terms of adverse skin reactions, toxicity or carcinogenicity.

3-Butylidene phthalide

Systematic name: 1,3-Dihydro-3-butylidenebenzo[*c*]furan-1-one
Chemical class: Bicyclic benzenoid furanoid lactone
CAS number: 551-08-6
Note: Different isomers of 3-butylidene phthalide exist, and the following isomer-specific information has been published:

(*E*)-3-Butylidene phthalide

Synonym: *trans*-3-Butylidene phthalide

Sources >1.0%:

Angelica root (Himalayan)	0.4–2.3%

(*Z*)-3-Butylidene phthalide

Synonym: *cis*-3-Butylidene phthalide

Sources >1.0%:

Angelica root (Himalayan)	11.3–20.5%
Lovage root	1.5%

3-Butylidene phthalide (isomer not specified)

Sources >1.0%:

Celery seed	2.3–8.0%

Adverse skin reactions: Tested at 2% on the skin of 25 volunteers, 3-butylidene phthalide was neither irritating nor sensitizing. The undiluted material produced slight irritant effects in rabbits patch-tested for 24 hours under occlusion (Opdyke & Letizia 1983 p. 659–660).

Acute toxicity: Acute oral LD_{50} in rats reported as 1.85 g/kg and 2.42 g/kg; acute dermal LD_{50} in rabbits >5 g/kg. (Opdyke & Letizia 1983 p. 659–660).

Carcinogenic/anticarcinogenic potential: 3-Butylidene phthalide was dose-dependently cytotoxic to human colorectal cancer HT-29 cells (Kan et al 2008).

Summary: Limited data suggests that 3-butylidene phthalide presents minimal risk in terms of adverse skin reactions or toxicity.

Cadinene

Chemical class: Bicyclic sesquiterpenoid alkene
Note: Different isomers of cadinene exist, and the following isomer-specific information has been published:

γ-Cadinene

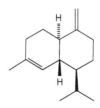

Synonym: Cadina 4,10(15)-diene
Systematic name: [1*R*-(1*a*,4aβ,8a*a*)]-1,2,3,4,4a,5,6,8a-Octahydro-7-methyl-4-methylene-(1-methylethyl)-naphthalene
CAS number: 1460-97-5

Sources >5.0%:

Siam wood	15.6%
Hinoki wood	12.5%
Hop	5.5%
Copaiba	0–5.5%
Pine (Scots)	tr–5.4%
Katrafay	1.0–5.0%

δ-Cadinene

Synonym: Cadina 1(10),4-diene
Systematic name: (1*S*-*cis*)-1,2,3,5,6,8a-Hexahydro-4,7-dimethyl-1-(1-methylethyl)-naphthalene
CAS number: 483-76-1

Sources >5.0%:

Siam wood	32.6%
Cade (rectified)	24.2%
Cedrela	11.7%
Hinoki wood	10.8%
Ylang-ylang absolute	10.8%
Cubeb	tr–9.5%
Pine (Scots)	tr–9.5%
Pepper (pink)	4.7–9.1%
Rhododendron	9.1%
Cedarwood (Port Orford)	8.2%
Copaiba	1.7–7.7%
Cangerana	7.4%
Peta	7.4%
Manuka	4.8–7.2%
Balsam poplar	6.9%
Muhuhu	6.5%

Cananga	6.0%
Ylang-ylang	0.2–5.2%
Chamomile (blue)	0–5.2%
Vassoura	5.1%

Notes: Other isomers have also been reported, namely γ_1-, γ_2-, ε-, σ-, τ- and ω-cadinene. ω-Cadinene was originally named δ-cadinene, which may cause some confusion. The δ- and γ- forms of cadinene together occur in over 150 essential oils. σ-Cadinene occurs in evodia and conifer wood oils; and τ-cadinene in ylang ylang.

Pharmacokinetics: Cadinene was found to induce CYP2B1 and CYP3A2 (Hiroi et al 1995).

Adverse skin reactions: Tested at 10% on 25 volunteers, cadinene was neither irritating nor sensitizing (Opdyke 1973 p. 1045).

Acute toxicity: Acute oral LD_{50} in rats >5 g/kg, acute dermal LD_{50} in rabbits > 5 g/kg (Opdyke 1973 p. 1045).

Carcinogenic/anticarcinogenic potential: δ-Cadinene exhibited moderate in vitro cytotoxicity against two human carcinoma cell lines (Kubo & Morimitsu 1995).

Summary: Limited data suggests that cadinene isomers present minimal risk in terms of adverse skin reactions or toxicity.

Camphene

Synonyms: 3,3-Dimethyl-2-methylenenorcamphane. 3,3-Dimethyl-2-methylenenorbornane
Systematic name: 2,2-Dimethyl-3-methylenebicyclo[2.2.1]heptane
Chemical class: Bicyclic monoterpenoid alkene
Note: Different isomers of camphene exist, and the following isomer-specific information has been published:

(+)-Camphene

Synonym: (1R)-Camphene
CAS number: 5794-03-6

(−)-Camphene

Synonym: (1S)-Camphene
CAS number: 5794-04-7

Sources >5.0%:

Spruce (Norwegian)	7.0–26.5%
Fir needle (Siberian)	24.2%
Fir needle (Japanese)	18.5%
Fir (Douglas)	16.7%
Silver fir (needles)	14.8%
Valerian (European)	0.1–14.4%
Spruce (red)	12.9%
Pine (grey)	2.8–12.1%
Sage (Spanish)	4.6–10.6%
Cistus	1.1–10.3%
Rosemary (α-pinene CT)	7.0–10.0%
Rosemary (camphor CT)	2.8–10.0%
Spruce (white)	9.9%

Fir needle (Canadian)	3.5–9.7%
Pine (Scots)	1.6–9.4%
Sage (Dalmatian)	0–8.6%
Spruce (black)	8.1%
Silver fir (cones)	5.8–8.0%
Citronella (Sri Lankan)	0.1–8.0%
Feverfew	5.4–7.7%
Wormwood (annual)	1.2–7.3%
Rosemary (bornyl acetate CT)	5.9–7.0%
Labdanum	1.4–7.0%
Pine (dwarf)	1.3–6.7%
Sage (African wild)	6.5%
Marjoram (Spanish)	4.3–6.0%
Chamomile (Roman)	0–6.0%
Lavender (Spanish)	2.8–5.5%
African bluegrass	3.6–5.4%
Pine (white)	5.2%
Thyme (borneol CT)	5.0%

Pharmacokinetics: The main metabolic pathway is that of epoxidation and hydration. In rabbits the glucuronide conjugate of a hydroxy derivative (camphenol) and the monoglucuronide of camphene glycol are excreted (Scheline 1991). When 0.6 µg camphene/kg body weight was injected iv into a human subject, 3.6% was eliminated unchanged in the expired air within three hours, the majority within five minutes (Römmelt et al 1974).

Adverse skin reactions: Tested at 4% on 25 volunteers camphene produced no sensitization reactions (Opdyke 1975 p. 735–738).

Acute toxicity: Acute oral LD_{50} in rats >5 g/kg; acute dermal LD_{50} in rabbits >2.5 g/kg (Opdyke 1975 p. 735–738).

Reproductive toxicity: In a developmental toxicity study, pregnant rats were given oral doses of 250 or 1,000 mg/kg camphene on gestational days 6–15. No teratogenic effects were reported in offspring and the developmental NOAEL was therefore 1,000 mg/kg/day. At the high dose, dams experienced temporary reduced motor activity, and therefore the maternal NOAEL was 250 mg/kg/day (Hoechst AG 1992, cited in Environmental Protection Agency 2006).

Mutagenicity and genotoxicity: Camphene was not mutagenic in the Ames test (Connor et al 1985), nor was (±)-camphene genotoxic in Chinese hamster ovary cells (Sasaki et al 1989).

Carcinogenic/anticarcinogenic potential: The proliferation of mouse B16 melanoma cells was very weakly inhibited by camphene with an IC_{50} value of 178 mM (24.2 g/L) (Tatman & Huanbiao 2002).

Summary: Limited data suggest that camphene isomers present minimal risk in terms of adverse skin reactions, toxicity or carcinogenicity.

Camphor

Synonyms: 2-Bornanone. 2-Camphanone
Systematic name: 1,7,7-Trimethylbicyclo[2.2.1]heptan-2-one
Chemical class: Bicyclic monoterpenoid ketone
Note: Different isomers of camphor exist, and the following isomer-specific information has been published:

(+)-Camphor

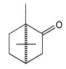

Synonyms: (1*R*,4*R*)-(+)-Camphor. Japan camphor
CAS number: 464-49-3

(−)-Camphor

Synonym: (1*S*,4*S*)-(−)-Camphor
CAS number: 464-48-2

Sources >1.0%:

Ho leaf (camphor CT)	42.0–84.1%
Lavender (Spanish)	16.4–56.2%
Wormwood (white)	34.0–55.0%
Sage (Dalmatian)	7.3–50.2%
Feverfew	28.0–44.2%
Sage (Spanish)	12.9–36.1%
Basil (Madagascan)	24.0–30.0%
Rosemary (camphor CT)	17.0–27.3%
Lavender (spike)	10.8–23.2%
Mugwort (common, camphor/thujone CT)	20.8%
Rosemary (α-pinene CT)	6.6–20.7%
Finger root	16.9%
Fenugreek	16.3%
Rosemary (borneol CT)	15.3%
Rosemary (verbenone CT)	11.3–14.9%
Rosemary (cineole CT)	7.4–14.9%
Galangal (greater)	5.0–14.0%
Yarrow (green)	13.7%
Tansy (blue)	3.1–12.4%
Lavandin Grosso	6.6–12.2%
Mugwort (great)	11.8%
Wormwood (annual)	0–11.5%
Mango ginger	11.2%
Lanyana	11.0%
Lavandin Abrialis	7.0–11.0%
Rosemary (bornyl acetate CT)	9.9–10.4%
Marjoram (Spanish)	5.5–8.9%
Zedoary	1.7–7.8%
Coriander seed	1.6–7.7%
Sassafras albidum	1.2–6.8%
Spruce (red)	6.1%
Cedarwood (Port Orford)	5.9%
Lavandin Super	4.5–5.3%
Spruce (black)	4.9%
Rosemary (β-myrcene CT)	2.1–4.4%
Turmeric (wild)	2.4–3.9%

Yarrow (chamazulene CT)	3.3%
Tansy	3.2%
Camphor (brown)	<3.0%
Ocotea odorifera	0.7–2.9%
Sage (Greek)	2.8%
Southernwood	2.8%
Spruce (white)	2.8%
Sage (blue mountain)	2.7%
Lavender cotton	1.5–2.6%
Thuja	2.2–2.5%
Spruce (Norwegian)	0.5–2.5%
Camphor (white)	2.4%
Snowbush	2.4%
Thymus zygis (thymol CT)	0–1.7%
Sugandha	1.5%
Cinnamon bark	tr–1.4%
Sage (white)	1.3%
Lavender absolute	1.2%
Peta	1.2%
Artemisia vestita	1.1%
Galangal (lesser)	1.0%
Thymus zygis (carvacrol CT)	1.0%
Basil (estragole CT)	tr–1.0%

Pharmacokinetics: In rabbits, camphor is metabolized by hydroxylation (Robertson & Hussein 1969; Leibman & Ortiz 1973). It can be both oxidized and reduced (to borneol) in liver preparations from the dog and rabbit (Horning et al 1974). There are distinct inter-species differences. Urine analysis of two men following ingestion of 6–10 g camphor revealed six metabolites. The main metabolic pathways were hydroxylation in the 3-, 5-, 8-, and 9- positions, with subsequent oxidation to a corresponding ketone and carbonic acid (Köppel et al 1982). Camphor is porphyrigenic and so is especially hazardous to those with defects in hepatic heme synthesis (Bonkovsky et al 1992).

Significant increases were seen in the activities of hepatic CYP, glutathione *S*-transferase, b₅, and aryl hydrocarbon hydroxylase in female mice given camphor at 300 mg/kg/day for 20 days, but not at 50 or 150 mg/kg/day (Banerjee et al 1995). Camphor is readily absorbed through mucous membranes, and crosses the placenta freely (Opdyke 1978 p. 665–671). Camphor is primarily metabolized by oxidation to 5-*exo*-hydroxycamphor by human liver microsomal CYP enzymes, primarily CYP2A6. There are species-related differences in the metabolism of camphor in rats, rabbits and humans (Gyoubu & Miyazawa 2007).

The human systemic exposure to camphor from application in commercial skin patches was relatively low (Martin et al 2004).

Adverse skin reactions: Camphor was patch tested at 10% in two patients who had developed acute eczema following topical application of a camphor-containing spray; neither reacted (Aguirre et al 1994). Camphor may be a skin irritant when applied in excessive amounts or too vigorously (http://www.inchem.org/documents/pims/pharm/camphor.htm, accessed August 8th 2011).

Mucous membrane irritation: Camphor may have contributed to the intense pain when preparations for topical use containing it were instilled into the eyes (Blanchard 1989). Camphor is an eye irritant, may irritate mucous membranes and cause a burning pain in the mouth or throat (http://www.inchem.org/documents/pims/pharm/camphor.htm, accessed August 8th 2011).

Acute toxicity: Acute oral LD_{50} reported as 1.31 g/kg in mice, >5 g/kg in rats; acute ip lethal dose 400 mg/kg in cats; acute dermal LD_{50} in rabbits >5 g/kg (Opdyke 1978 p. 665–671).

Inhalation toxicity: According to Reynolds (1993) camphorated oils or ointments should not be placed into or close to the nostrils of infants, since this can lead to respiratory collapse. We could not substantiate this. Camphor can cause convulsions, congestion, damage to the kidneys and brain, and changes in the GI tract in animals exposed for prolonged periods to a level of 6 mg/m^3 (Flury & Zernicke 1931). Inhalatory LD_{50} in mice is 450 mg/m^3 (72 ppm), and in rats 500 mg/m^3 (80 ppm) (www.epa.gov/opprd001/inerts/camphor.pdf accessed August 9th 2011). In a camphor packaging plant, workers exposed to 30–40 mg/m^3 of camphor experienced slight, transient eye irritation and transient olfactory fatigue. No adverse symptoms occurred with a concentration of 2 ppm (Gronka et al 1969). All the inhalation data are for (±)-camphor.

Human toxicity: Camphor is classified as very toxic and the probable human lethal dose has been estimated at be 5–20 g (Spector 1956) and 50–550 mg/kg (Opdyke 1978 p. 665–671). Although as much as 42 g has been ingested by adults who have recovered, the ingestion of 2 g generally produces toxic effects, and 4 g can be fatal. In children, ingestions of 700–1,000 mg of camphor have proven fatal, and 70 mg/kg can be fatal in infants. If a product containing 5% camphor is ingested, 20 mL, or 4 teaspoons, is a potentially lethal dose (Committee on Drugs 1994). The only retrospective review covered 182 cases of camphor exposure over a three year period from two poison centers. Of 81 cases of camphor ingestion of 2 mg/kg or more, 73 (90%) remained asymptomatic, three (4%) developed minor symptoms and five (6%), all ingesting over 59 mg/kg, developed major symptoms. There were no fatalities. In six fatal cases the mean lethal dose was 199 mg/kg (range 64–570 mg). All patients ingesting less than 2 mg/kg remained asymptomatic (Geller et al 1984).

Toxic effects may follow a pattern of CNS stimulation (delirium, seizures) followed by depression (lack of coordination, respiratory depression, coma (Budavari 1989). Neurologic symptoms can include anxiety, depression, confusion, headache, dizziness and hallucinations (Siegel & Wason 1986; Committee on Drugs 1994). Initial symptoms of camphor toxicity have occurred in 5–15 minutes of ingestion. With mild poisoning, GI tract effects such as burning of the mouth, nausea, vomiting, and diarrhea are more frequently reported than neurologic effects. Seizures may be associated with apnea and asystole (Committee on Drugs 1994). In fatal cases, death results from respiratory depression (apnea) or complications of status epilepticus (Committee on Drugs 1994). Autopsy results indicate that camphor can damage the liver, kidneys and the brain (Smith & Margolis 1954; Siegel & Wason 1986).

There are many cases where camphorated oil ingestion (20% pure camphor in cottonseed oil) has caused serious poisoning, usually in young children. Cottonseed oil is non-toxic (Anon 2001a). In 1973, 500 cases of camphor intoxication were reported to the medical authorities in the USA (Aronow 1976). From 1985 to 1989, 32,362 human exposures to camphor were reported to the American Association of Poison Control Centers. There were no childhood fatalities, but life-threatening toxicity was reported in 33 children following ingestion. In 18 of these cases the products consumed contained between 6% and 11% of camphor, and major toxic events occurred in seven cases where products containing less than 5% of camphor were ingested (Committee on Drugs 1994).

An earlier analysis reveals that 45% of cases of symptomatic camphor poisoning in children under five suffered convulsions (Verhulst et al 1961). There have been reports of instant collapse in infants following the local application of camphor to their nostrils (Reynolds 1993). There is one report of hepatotoxity in a child of two months following dermal application of a camphor-containing cold remedy (Uc et al 2000). Manoguerra et al (2006) reviewed camphor poisoning and its management.

Cardiovascular effects: Camphor can cause a transient fall, followed by a rise in blood pressure when given to cats; it increased heart rate in the isolated rabbit heart, via a direct effect on heart muscle (Christensen & Lynch 1937). In humans, the predominant effect on the heart appears to be depressant. However, at least one report suggests that camphor can sensitize the heart to adrenaline (Saratikov et al 1957).

Neurotoxicity: The potential for camphor to produce convulsions is well known (Merkulova 1957). Subcutaneously injected camphor induced seizures in mice at 600 mg/kg (Wenzel & Ross 1957). However, humans are more susceptible to camphor intoxication than rodents.

In 1924 a fatal case was reported in which one teaspoon of camphorated oil had been consumed by a 16-month-old boy. Signs of intoxication included frequent fits, constriction of the pupils, rapid pulse and an extremely high respiratory rate. Gross damage to the CNS was noted on autopsy (Smith & Margolis 1954). Ingestion of 70 mL of a camphor, menthol and eucalyptus-containing ointment by a 15-month-old child resulted in seizures, foaming at the mouth, delirium and dyspnea (Gouin & Patel 1996). A 3-year-old girl suffered a generalized convulsion two hours after ingesting 700 mg of camphor (Phelan 1976). A 2-year-old suffered tonic-clonic seizures after swallowing 9.5 mL camphorated oil containing perhaps 1 mL camphor and was successfully managed on oral phenobarbital (Gibson et al 1989).

Two cases of intoxication by a 19-year-old and a 72-year-old with 1 oz of camphorated oil (~6 g camphor) were survived with no serious consequences following generalized seizures (Reid 1979). A 22-year-old female experienced two violent epileptiform convulsions following the ingestion of 12 g of camphor (Klingensmith 1934). A man attempted suicide by ingesting 150 mL of camphorated oil (~30 g camphor). He had peripheral circulatory shock and severe dehydration because of vomiting. Severe and prolonged grand-mal seizures occurred, but he survived after intensive treatment. This is one of the largest camphor overdoses to be survived (Vasey & Karayannoppoulos 1972).

Camphor does not have to be ingested to initiate seizures. A 15-month-old child suffered ataxia and seizures after crawling through camphorated oil spilled by a sibling. He recovered fully, but one year later had another seizure immediately after inhaling a preparation containing 4.8% camphor. This case shows an unusual sensitivity to camphor (Skoglund et al 1977). A child with a heavy cold was soaked in camphorated oil by the parents for 80 hours before a doctor was called. The child was hyperpyrexic, had a rash all over and was delirious and hallucinating. Removal of all traces of camphor from the house prompted a full recovery (Summers 1947). A 9-month-old child fitted three times, the first 24 hours after a dressing containing ~15 g of camphor was administered to thoracic burns. The level of camphor in the blood was 2.6 mg/L at the time of the seizures. It is assumed that most of the camphor was absorbed percutaneously (Joly et al 1980).

Reproductive toxicity: Camphor was fed daily at 0, 100, 400 or 800 mg/kg to pregnant rats during gestational days 6–15. There was a dose-related increase in liver weight, but this did not exceed 10% of control values. Food consumption was temporarily suppressed at the two higher doses, and maternal weight gain was reduced in all treatment groups, notably at the highest dose. No adverse effects were observed on any index of fetal growth, viability or morphological development, even at 800 mg/kg/day, and there was no maternal mortality. At 1.25 g/kg/day camphor caused 90% maternal mortality (National Toxicology Program 1992a).

When 0, 100, 400 or 800 mg/kg/day (+)-camphor was administered orally to pregnant rats on gestational days 6–15, maternal toxicity was observed in the mid and high dose groups, but not in the low dose group. No effect on fetal growth, viability or morphological development was seen in any of the treatment groups. Similarly, when (+)-camphor was administered po at 0, 216, 464 or 1,000 mg/kg/day to pregnant rats on gestational days 6–17, or to groups of pregnant rabbits at 0, 50, 100 or 400 mg/kg/day on gestational days 6–19, or at 0, 147, 316 or 681 mg/kg/day on gestational days 6–18, there was some dose-dependent maternal toxicity but no embryotoxicity or teratogenicity (Leuschner 1997).

Pregnant rabbits were fed 0, 50, 200 or 400 mg/kg of camphor during gestational days 6–19. A slight, dose-related suppression of weight gain was seen in the treatment groups, but food consumption was not altered. No adverse effects were observed on fetal growth, viability or morphological development, even at 400 mg/kg/day, and there was no maternal mortality. At 500 mg/kg/day camphor caused 60% maternal mortality (National Toxicology Program 1992b).

In a study group of 50,282 mother–child pairs, 168 women said they had used camphor during months 1–4 of pregnancy. Of these, 10 had given birth to infants with malformations, which was less than expected. There were 13 malformed children out of 763 women who had used camphor at some time during pregnancy, while 13.65 were expected (Heinonen et al 1977).

There have been four reported cases of (usually accidental) substantial camphorated oil ingestion by pregnant women. In one case, a 32-year-old woman was hospitalized during the third month of gestation with a threatened abortion, manifested by uterine cramps and bleeding. Two days later she was accidentally given 45 mL of camphorated oil by a nurse. The woman vomited several times almost immediately, then had a convulsion and became unconscious. Further convulsions followed, as did therapy, including gastric lavage, and she recovered consciousness one hour later. A normal infant was born six months later (Blackmon & Curry 1957). This case strongly suggests that camphor is not abortifacient.

In a second case, a woman who was 40 weeks pregnant ingested 2 oz (about 57 mL) of camphorated oil (containing about 10 g camphor), also while in hospital. Gastric lavage was initiated 20 minutes later, and although the woman was severely intoxicated by the camphor, she recovered fully. Her baby was stillborn 36 hours later. To quote from the report: 'Several factors may have contributed to the death of this infant...Whether or not the camphor precipitated these difficulties is problematical'. It seems likely that the camphor at least contributed to the infant's death; camphor was detected in its liver, brain and kidneys (Riggs et al 1965).

In a third case, the baby was also a full-term infant. The mother ingested 2 oz (about 57 mL) of camphorated oil, and had the first of three seizures 20 minutes later. She was admitted to hospital, and gastric lavage was performed. Spontaneous labour commenced the following morning, and her baby, smelling distinctly of camphor, was born without complication. The baby was closely monitored for three days, and camphor was just detectable in its blood. The mother's blood, collected 24 hours after ingestion, contained large amounts of camphor (Weiss & Catalano 1973).

The baby in the third case was some 1.5 kg heavier than the second case infant, and there were no complications. Otherwise the two cases are remarkably similar, except that one infant died and the other survived. In a fourth case a 16-year-old girl ingested 30 g of camphor dissolved in 250 mL wine in order to induce abortion. She started vomiting 45 minutes after ingestion, which may have saved her life. She did not abort. It is suggested that camphor ingestion may lead to abortion because camphor crosses the placenta, and fetuses lack the enzymes to hydroxylate and conjugate with glucuronic acid (Rabl et al 1997).

After crossing the placenta, camphor evidently passes into fetal lung, liver, brain and kidney tissue. It also destroys the placenta, causing hemorrhage (Phelan 1976). A non-pregnant woman survived the combined ingestion of 7.5 mL Vicks Va-Tro-Nol drops, containing camphor and aspirin, but suffered delirium, amnesia and convulsions (Seife & Leon 1954).

Mutagenicity and genotoxicity: (±)-Camphor was non-mutagenic in the Ames test, both with and without metabolic activation (Anderson & Styles 1978; Gomes-Carneiro et al 1998). (±)-Camphor was antimutagenic through competitive inhibition of PROD, with an IC_{50} of 7.89 μM (1.20 mg/L) (De Oliveira et al 1997). Camphor inhibited UV-induced mutations in both E. coli and S. cerevisiae (Vuković-Gačić et al 2006). A single ip injection of 76 mg/kg camphor was given to four mice, resulting in a significant increase in the frequency of SCE in bone marrow (Goel et al 1989). Camphor was also genotoxic in the wing somatic mutation and recombination test (SMART) of Drosophila melanogaster (Pavlidou et al 2004).

Carcinogenic/anticarcinogenic potential: In male and female mice given 24 ip injections of (+)-camphor in tricaprylin in a total dose of 3.6 or 18.0 g/kg over 24 weeks the incidence of primary lung tumors was no higher than in the control group (Stoner et al 1973).

Comments: Camphor is found in many essential oils. It is also present at concentrations of 3.0–11.0% in many over-the-counter preparations, which may present a risk to health, especially in children (Love et al 2004). Considering its neurotoxicity and lethality, camphor is surprisingly non-teratogenic.

Summary: There is little published information on skin and mucous membrane irritation, or on skin sensitization. Some irritancy is suspected. Camphor is neurotoxic, and is also toxic to the liver and kidneys in ways that have not been studied. It is not reproductively toxic or abortifacient except in almost fatal doses. Camphor has been reported as mutagenic, non-mutagenic and anti-mutagenic; it is not regarded as a carcinogen. Camphor is a CNS stimulant and its toxic effects range from mild excitation to grand-mal convulsions. It is not clear whether camphor toxicity is due to the parent compound, a metabolite, or both (Kresel 1982). The lowest lethal dose of camphor in humans, including infants, is reported as 50 mg/kg, and the mean human lethal dose as 200 mg/kg. Compared to mice (LD_{50} =1.31 g/kg), this suggests that camphor is approximately 6.5 times more toxic in humans.

Regulatory guidelines: In 1982 the FDA ruled that camphorated oil could no longer be sold in the US, and that the concentration of camphor in products should not exceeed 11% (Food and Drug Administration 1983). The Health Canada maximum for camphor is 3% in topical products (Health Canada Cosmetic Ingredient Hotlist, March 2011). In the USA the OSHA permissible exposure limit (PEL) by inhalation is 2 mg/m³ (0.3 ppm) averaged over an eight-hour work shift (known as a time-weighted average, or TWA) (http://www.cdc.gov/niosh/pel88/76-22.html accessed August 9th 2011). In most of Europe the eight-hour TWA is 2 ppm (12 mg/m³). The Commission E Monograph for camphor gives an average daily oral dose of 30–300 mg, and a topical concentration of 10–20% in semisolid preparations (Blumenthal et al 1998).

Our safety advice: Even at relatively high doses, there is little evidence in animal studies of teratogenicity or developmental toxicity. No adverse fetal effects were seen from feeding pregnant rats at 1,000 mg/kg/day, or pregnant rabbits at 681 mg/kg/day. Maternal toxicity was seen in rats at 400 mg/kg/day, but not at 100 mg/kg/day. In a 70 kg adult human, the rat NOAEL of 100 mg/kg/day would extrapolate to 7 g/day. However, observations on symptom-free human exposure (Geller et al 1984), imply that this would overestimate the safe dose by a factor of some 50-fold. This suggests a human daily oral maximum dose of 2 mg/kg/day, or 140 mg per 70 kg adult, equivalent to a dermal exposure of 4.6% (Table 14.1).

δ-3-Carene

Synonyms: 3-Carene. δ³-Carene. Isodiprene
Systematic name: 3,7,7-Trimethylbicyclo[4.1.0]hept-3-ene
Chemical class: Bicyclic monoterpenoid alkene
Note: Different isomers of δ-3-carene exist, and the following isomer-specific information has been published:

(1S)-*cis*-3-Carene

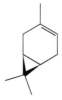

Synonym: $(+)$-δ^3-Carene
CAS number: 498-15-7

(1R)-*trans*-3-Carene

Synonym: $(-)$-δ^3-Carene
CAS number: 20296-50-8

Sources >5.0%:

Sage (blue mountain)	38.1%
Blackcurrant bud	15.0–35.0%
Pine (Scots)	0.4–31.8%
Pine (dwarf)	0.5–30.1%
Fir needle (Canadian)	0–27.3%
Pepper (white)	25.2%
Cypress	15.2–21.5%
Blackcurrant bud absolute	12.6–19.0%
Pine (ponderosa)	17.2%
Boswellia rivae	15.7%
Pepper (black)	tr–15.5%
Larch needle	14.0%
Angelica root	4.5–13.0%
Pine (grey)	7.3–12.7%
Fir needle (Siberian)	12.2%
Galbanum	2.0–12.1%
Spruce (hemlock)	11.5%
Basil (pungent)	0–10.9%
Turpentine	0–10.3%
Boswellia serrata	3.6–9.6%
Narcissus absolute	6.6–8.4%
Pine (red)	4.2–7.3%
Spruce (Norwegian)	2.5–5.8%
Spruce (red)	5.4%
Ravensara leaf	4.9–5.0%

Pharmacokinetics: δ-3-Carene is primarily metabolized by hydroxylation in rabbits (Scheline 1991). In rabbits, δ-3-carene was metabolized to $(-)$-*m*-mentha-4,6-dien-8-ol, 3-caren-9-ol, $(-)$-3-carene-9-carboxylic acid and 3-carene-9,10-dicarboxylic acid (Ishida et al 1981). δ-3-Carene-10-ol and δ-3-carene epoxide were identified as metabolites in an in vitro assay using human liver and lung microsomes (Duisken et al 2005). Human volunteers inhaled 10, 225 and 450 mg/m³ of δ-3-carene, and a pulmonary uptake of ~70% was observed for the higher exposure levels. Total uptake increased linearly with increasing exposure. About 3% of the total uptake was eliminated unchanged through the lungs while less than 0.001% was eliminated in the urine.

A long half-life in blood was observed in the terminal phase, suggesting a high affinity for adipose tissue (Falk et al 1991a).

Adverse skin reactions: Tested at 10% on 25 volunteers δ-3-carene was neither irritating nor sensitizing (Opdyke 1973 p. 1053–1054). However, its autoxidation products can be sensitizing. Patch tests were performed on 28 dermatitis patients who were not sensitive to turpentine oil with various concentrations of freshly distilled, unoxidized δ-3-carene. Concentrations of 70–80% were irritating in most patients, at 50% weak reactions were obtained 'in some cases' while no reactions were observed at 25–30% (Pirilä et al 1964).

Terpenes including δ-3-carene, fractionated from turpentine oil, were allergenic only after autoxidation in light and air. The presence of antioxidants inhibited the formation of sensitizing agents. Tests with δ-3-carene showed stronger allergenic effect relative to its peroxide content than did α-pinene (Pirilä & Siltanen 1955). Peroxides of δ-3-carene are believed to be primarily responsible for the allergenic effect of turpentine oil (Pirilä & Siltanen 1955, 1956, 1957, 1958; Pirilä & Pirilä 1964). In 106 patients sensitized to turpentine oil the allergenic effect paralleled the concentration of δ-3-carene or δ-2-carene present (Pirilä et al 1969).

Based on literature published by Schlede et al (2003), δ-3-carene and its oxidation products have been classified as category A, significant contact allergens.

Acute toxicity: Acute oral LD_{50} in rats 4.8 g/kg, acute dermal LD_{50} in rabbits > 5 g/kg (Opdyke 1973 p. 1053–1054).

Inhalation toxicity: When inhaled, δ-3-carene caused dose-dependent decreases in mouse respiratory frequency due to sensory irritation; no histopathological changes in lung tissue were found (Kasanen et al 1999). δ-3-Carene caused bronchoconstriction in guinea pig lungs at 1,900 mg/m^3 (Låstbom et al 2003). In humans there was statistically significant divergence between ratings of irritation between 225 ppm and 450 ppm of δ-3-carene in inhaled air (Falk et al 1991a).

Reproductive toxicity: (+)-δ-3-Carene dose-dependently antagonized oxytocin-induced contractions in rat uterus, with an IC_{50} of 0.8 μM (108 μg/L) (Ocete et al 1989).

Summary: δ-3-Carene is non-toxic, but may cause irritation when inhaled. Due to the formation of sensitizing peroxides on autoxidation, there is a risk of dermal sensitization from old or poorly stored batches of essential oils rich in δ-3-carene.

Regulatory guidelines: The Swedish occupational exposure limit to inhaled terpenes such as δ-3-carene is 150 mg/m^3 (Eriksson et al 1997).

Our safety advice: In order to prevent oxidation the use of antioxidants in combination with δ-3-carene-rich essential oils is recommended. Such oils should be stored in a refrigerator in a sealed container. Commercial products containing δ-3-carene will keep longer in light-tight packaging.

Carvacrol

Synonyms: Antioxine. *p*-Cymen-2-ol. 2-Hydroxy-*p*-cymene. Isothymol

Systematic name: 2-Methyl-5-(1-methylethyl)phenol

Chemical class: Monoterpenoid phenol

CAS number: 499-75-2

Sources >1.0%:

Oregano	61.6–83.4%
Marjoram wild (carvacrol CT)	76.4–81.0%
Savory (winter)	46.5–75.0%
Savory (summer)	43.6–70.7%
Thyme (spike)	70.0%
Thymus zygis (carvacrol CT)	43.9%
Thymus vulgaris (carvacrol CT)	41.8%
Thymus serpyllum	15.6–27.8%
Oregano (Mexican)	0.5–24.8%
Marjoram wild (linalool CT)	23.3%
Thymus zygis (thymol/carvacrol CT)	22.8%
Thyme (limonene CT)	20.5%
Thyme (borneol CT)	20.0%
Ajowan	1.0–16.4%
Thymus vulgaris (thymol CT)	5.5–16.3%
Thyme (lemon)	15.4%
Thymus zygis (thymol CT)	tr–5.9%
Black seed	0.5–4.2%
Verbena (white)	0–1.8%
Eucalyptus polybractea (cryptone CT)	1.1%
Thyme (linalool CT)	1.0–1.1%

Notes: Isomeric with thymol. Being a substituted phenol, carvacrol is a weak acid which may be corrosive to tissues.

Pharmacokinetics: Carvacrol is rapidly excreted in the urine primarily as a tertiary alcohol derivative formed on oxidation of the isopropyl group (Scheline 1991).

Adverse skin reactions: Undiluted carvacrol was severely irritating to rabbit skin. Tested at 4% on human volunteers, carvacrol was neither irritating nor sensitizing. Tested at 0.1% and 1% it was irritating to a patient with dermatitis; patients allergic to thyme oil also reacted to carvacrol (Opdyke 1979a p. 743–745). There were two reactions (1.1%) to 5% carvacrol in 179 dermatitis patients suspected of allergy to cosmetics (De Groot et al 1985).

Acute toxicity: Rat acute oral LD_{50} 810 mg/kg (Jenner et al 1964), rabbit oral lethal dose 100 mg/kg, acute dermal LD_{50} in rabbits >5 g/kg (Opdyke 1979a p. 743–745). Dog iv lethal dose 310 mg/kg (Caujolle & Franck 1944a).

Cardiovascular effects: Carvacrol shows strong antiplatelet aggregation activity in vitro (Enomoto et al 2001). *Satureja khuzestanica* oil (93.9% carvacrol) significantly reduced plasma glucose concentrations in diabetic rats when given orally at 100 mg/kg/day for 21 days (Shahsavari et al 2009).

Reproductive toxicity: During gestational days 0–15, pregnant rats received drinking water containing 100, 500 or 1,000 ppm of *Satureja khuzestanica*, an essential oil consisting of 93.9% carvacrol. There were no signs of maternal toxicity or teratogenicity at any dose, and in the two higher dose groups there was a significant increase in the number of implantations and live fetuses (Abdollahi et al 2003; Abdollahi, private communication, 2004).

Hepatotoxicity: At 73 mg/kg ip, carvacrol was not hepatotoxic in rats, and protected against hepatotoxicity induced by ischemia-reperfusion (Canbek et al 2008). At 125 mg/kg ip, carvacrol protected rats from CCl_4-induced hepatotoxicity, and demonstrated marked radical scavenging activity (Jiménez et al 1993).

Antioxidant/pro-oxidant activity: Significant antioxidant activity for carvacrol has been observed by Vardar-Unlu et al (2003) and by Aeschbach et al (1994), who reported that it decreased peroxidation of phospholipid liposomes in the presence of iron (III) and ascorbate. Carvacrol dose-dependently inhibited LDL oxidation in human aortic endothelial cells at 1.25–10 μM (188–1,500 μg/L) (Pearson et al 1997).

Mutagenicity and genotoxicity: Carvacrol was non-mutagenic in the Ames test, with and without metabolic activation (Kono et al 1995). Carvacrol was not mutagenic, and was in fact antimutagenic, in *S. typhimurium* strains TA98 and T100, with and without S9 (Ipek et al 2005). When given to *Drosophila* larvae in food at 0.005%, 0.1% or 0.2%, carvacrol was strongly antimutagenic in the presence of urethane, an indirect-acting mutagen (Mezzoug et al 2007). In human peripheral blood lymphocytes, carvacrol did not induce SCE, and inhibited SCE induction by mitomycin C (Ipek et al 2003). Carvacrol protected K562 leukemic cells from DNA damage induced by hydrogen peroxide, with an IC$_{50}$ of 175 μM (26.3 mg/L) (Horváthová et al 2007). At lower concentrations (0.0005–0.05 mM; 0.075–7.5 mg/L) carvacrol was not genotoxic in human lymphocytes, and over the range 0.00005–0.5 mM (0.0075–75 mg/L) it protected them from DNA damage. However, at higher concentrations (0.1–2 mM; 15–300 mg/L) carvacrol was genotoxic, causing significant increases in DNA damage (Aydin et al 2005). In a comet assay, carvacrol was not genotoxic at any of the three concentrations used: 1, 5 or 25 μM (150, 750 or 3,750 μg/L) (Ündeger et al 2009). The genotoxic potential of carvacrol is considered to be very weak, although the possibility of action at the DNA level could not be excluded (Stammati et al 1999; Nafisi et al 2004). When rats were injected ip with 10, 30, 50 or 70 mg/kg bw of carvacrol, it was dose-dependently genotoxic to their bone marrow cells (Azirak & Rencuzugullari 2008). However, carvacrol reduced hydrogen peroxide-induced DNA damage to rat hepatocytes and testicular cells when given in drinking water at 30 or 60 mg/kg/day for seven days, or at 15 or 30 mg/kg/day for 14 days (Slamenová et al 2008).

Carcinogenic/anticarcinogenic potential: Carvacrol inhibited the proliferation of human metastatic breast cancer cells, with an IC$_{50}$ of 100 μM (15 mg/L), and induced apoptosis (Arunasree 2010). A population of mouse B16(F10) melanoma cells were inhibited by carvacrol with an IC$_{50}$ value of 120 M (18 mg/L) (He et al 1997b). Carvcrol inhibited the in vitro cell growth of human myelogenous leukemia (K562) cells, with an IC$_{50}$ of 112.5 μM (16.9 mg/L) (Lampronti et al 2006). Rat leiomyosarcoma (smooth muscle cancer) growth was dose-dependently inhibited in vitro by carvacrol. In vivo, it reduced tumor incidence from 100% to 70% (Karkabounas et al 2006). Carvacrol inhibited the growth of mouse myoblast cells, and prevented DNA synthesis, even after the activation of mutated N-ras oncogene (Zeytinoglu et al 2003). Carvacrol was a potent inhibitor of growth in a human non-small cell lung carcinoma (A549) cell line (Koparal & Zeytinoglu 2003). Carvacrol (99.3% purity, extracted from *Origanum onites*) administered ip over eight days, inhibited DMBA-induced lung cancer in rats (Zeytinoglu et al 1998). Essential oil of *Thymus broussonetti*, consisting of 83.2% carvacrol, was cytotoxic in vitro to tumor cells resistant to chemotherapy, and had a significant antitumor effect in mice (Ait M'barek et al 2007b).

Comments: Phenols in general tend to be strong antibacterial agents and also tend to be corrosive to tissues. These features may be related to their high chemical reactivity. In justifying the CIR maximum of 0.5% for carvacrol, Andersen (2006b) explains: 'It may be that…thymol…and carvacrol do not cause chemical leukoderma at concentrations higher than 0.5%, but data are not available to support that possibility.' However, the only reference given to suggest that carvacrol might cause skin depigmentation is Mathias et al (1988), and this report does not mention thymol or carvacrol. It states that common causes of toxic vitiligo (chemical leukoderma) 'include *para*-substituted phenols and catechols'. Carvacrol is neither of these. Our 1% maximum for carvacrol is based on substantial clinical evidence that thymol is non-irritant at 1% (see Thymol profile) and evidence that carvacrol is likely to be less irritant than thymol (Demirci et al 2004; Fachini-Queiroz et al 2012).

Summary: There is little information on adverse skin reactions, but carvacrol does not appear to present a high risk. There are no concerns in regard to reproductive toxicity or hepatotoxicity. Carvacrol has been reported to be genotoxic, very weakly genotoxic, non-genotoxic and antigenotoxic. This may be dose-related, with only high concentrations presenting a risk. Some in vitro anticarcinogenic activity is evident. Carvacrol inhibits platelet aggregation.

Regulatory guidelines: The CIR recommended maximum for carvacrol in cosmetics is 0.5%.

Our safety advice: In order to avoid skin irritation, we recommend a maximum dermal use level of 1% for carvacrol. Essential oils high in carvacrol should be used with caution in oral doses by diabetics taking drugs to control blood glucose. Because of its antiplatelet aggregation activity, oral dosing of essential oils high in carvacrol is cautioned in conjunction with anticoagulant drugs, major surgery, childbirth, peptic ulcer, hemophilia or other bleeding disorders (see Box 7.1 for more detail).

Carvone

Synonym: *p*-Mentha-6,8-dien-2-one
Systematic name: 2-Methyl-5-(1-methylethenyl)-2-cyclohexene-1-one
Chemical class: Monocyclic monoterpenoid alkene ketone
Note: Different isomers of carvone exist, and the following isomer-specific information has been published:

(S)-(+)-Carvone

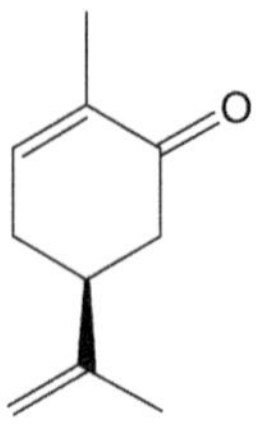

CAS number: 2244-16-8

Sources >5.0%:

Caraway	47.3–59.5%
Dill seed (European)	27.3–53.3%
Verbena (white)	43.3–46.1%
Dill weed	31.6–42.4%
Dill seed (Indian)	17.4–23.1%

(R)-(−)-Carvone

CAS number: 6485-40-1

Sources >5.0%:

Spearmint	57.2–71.6%
Balsamite	51.5%

Note: (+)-Carvone has the odor of caraway; (−)-carvone has the odor of spearmint.

Pharmacokinetics: Carvone is metabolized by oxidation and glucuronide conjugation in rabbits (Scheline 1991). (+)-Carvone is metabolized to (+)-carveol by different CYP enzymes in rats and humans, and rat metabolism is approximately five times more active than human metabolism (Shimada et al 2002). When incubated with rat or human liver microsomes (R)-(−)-carvone was converted to (4R,6S)- (−)-carveol, while (S)-(+)-carvone was converted to (4S,6S)-(+)-carveol (Jäger et al 2000). Only the former metabolite underwent glucuronidation in each preparation. V_{max} values were higher in rat than human microsomes. After being given separately to human subjects at doses of 300 mg topically, rapid uptake was followed by stereoselective metabolism of the (R)-(−)-isomer, while no metabolism of the (S)-(+)-isomer could be detected (Jäger et al 2001).

When (−)-carvone was given orally to rats at 600 mg/kg/day for 3 days, no effects were observed on the levels of either CYP or cytochrome b_5 (Moorthy et al 1989a). Both (+)- and (−)-carvone prolong the pentobarbital-induced sleeping time in rats, probably by modulating the barbiturate's metabolism by CYP (Marcus & Lichtenstein 1982).

Adverse skin reactions: (−)-Carvone is skin sensitizing to guinea-pigs (Karlberg et al 2001; Nilsson et al 2004). When applied undiluted to rabbit skin, (+)-carvone produced erythema lasting 24 hours. Tested at 2% on 25 healthy human volunteers, it was neither irritating nor sensitizing (Opdyke 1978 p. 673–674). Tested at 1% on 25 volunteers (−)-carvone was similarly neither irritating nor sensitizing (Opdyke 1973 p. 1057–1058). When (−)-carvone was tested at 5% on 541 dermatitis patients, there were allergic reactions in 15 (2.8%) (Paulsen et al 1993a). Tested at 5%, neither (−)-carvone nor (+)-carvone was sensitizing to 11 dermatitis patients sensitive to tea tree oil (Hausen et al 1999). (−)-Carvone has been identified as one of the skin-sensitizing oxidation products of limonene (Karlberg et al 1992). In a 58-year-old woman suffering from chronic erosive cheilitis, a correlation was established with (−)-carvone in toothpaste. After changing to a product containing no (−)-carvone, her condition resolved (Worm et al 1998). An intolerance to carvone was indicated by patch testing in a patient with oro-facial granulomatosis, a condition characterized by swelling of the lips and lower face (Patton et al

1985). Carvone was the probable cause of a woman's allergic reaction to a hair conditioner with a 'mint' scent. Patch testing for carvone was positive (Quertermous & Fowler 2010). Only (−)-carvone smells minty.

Acute toxicity: For carvone the acute oral LD_{50} was 1,640 mg/kg in rats and 766 mg/kg in guinea pigs (Jenner et al 1964); the acute subcutaneous LD_{50} was 2,675 mg/kg in mice (Wenzel & Ross 1957). For (+)-carvone, the acute oral LD_{50} was 3,710 mg/kg in rats, and the rabbit dermal LD_{50} was 3,860 mg/kg (Opdyke 1978 p. 673–674). In mice, the acute ip LD_{50} values were 484 mg/kg for (+)-carvone, and 426 mg/kg for (−)-carvone (De Sousa et al 2007).

Subacute, subchronic and chronic toxicity: Carvone was administered to rats for 14 days at 1% in the diet, corresponding to ~500 mg/kg/day. Increased serum cholesterol and triacylglycerol levels were observed in the dosed rats, as were body weight gain and decreased food consumption. Groups of only three or four rats were used in this study (Imaizumi et al 1985). Given to rats in the diet at 10,000 ppm (~500 mg/kg/day) for 16 weeks, carvone caused growth retardation and testicular atrophy, while no effect was seen at 1,000 ppm (~50 mg/kg/day) over 27–28 weeks, nor at 2,500 ppm (~125 mg/kg/day) for one year (Hagan et al 1967). In groups of male and female rats fed 93, 187, 375, 750 or 1,500 mg/kg (+)-carvone for 13 weeks, 59 of the 60 rats on 750 or 1,500 mg/kg died before the end of the study period. In the 750 mg/kg males, there was testicular degeneration and a reduction in sperm. Atrophy of the thymic cortex was seen in 750 mg/kg rats of both sexes. In the 187 and 375 mg/kg groups, the relative weights of various organs, and the relative body weights, were significantly different to controls. The NOAEL in this study was 93 mg/kg (National Toxicology Program 1990c).

Mutagenicity and genotoxicity: Carvone was not mutagenic in the Ames test (Florin et al 1980) but was genotoxic in fruit flies (Franzios et al 1997). (+)-Carvone was not mutagenic in the Ames test (Haworth et al 1983; Mortelmans et al 1986; National Toxicology Program 1990c; Stammati et al 1999) but was genotoxic in Chinese hamster ovary cells (Gallaway 1985; National Toxicology Program 1990c). (+)-Carvone also gave a positive response in the E. coli DNA repair test, indicating a direct reaction with DNA (Stammati et al 1999). Both (+)- and (−)-carvone were very weakly genotoxic in Saccharomyces cerevisiae (Zimmermann et al 1989).

Carcinogenic/anticarcinogenic potential: There was no evidence of carcinogenic activity in 50 male and 50 female mice fed 375 or 750 mg/kg of (+)-carvone, 5 days per week for 2 years (National Toxicology Program 1990c). Carvone significantly inhibited the growth of cultured mouse sarcoma BP8 cells. At a concentration of 0.1 μM (15 μg/L) the growth inhibition was 13%, and at 1.0 μM (150 μg/L) it was 100% (Pilotti et al 1975). In male and female mice given 24 ip injections of either (+)-carvone or (−)-carvone in impure tricaprylin in a total dose of 1.2 or 6.0 g/kg over 24 weeks the incidence of primary lung tumors for both compounds was no higher than in controls (Stoner et al 1973). Carvone had no effect on tumor growth in lung metastasis induced by melanoma cells in mice (Raphael & Kuttan 2003a). (+)-Carvone induced glutathione S-transferase in several mouse target tissues

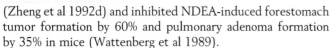

(Zheng et al 1992d) and inhibited NDEA-induced forestomach tumor formation by 60% and pulmonary adenoma formation by 35% in mice (Wattenberg et al 1989).

Comments: The carvone isomers smell quite different, they are metabolized differently after application to the skin, (+)-carvone is anticonvulsant while (−)-carvone is not (De Sousa et al 2007), and only (−)-carvone is associated with skin sensitization. Reports of allergic reactions to spearmint oil are consistent with its content of (−)-carvone, but there are no reports of allergenicity for essential oils high in (+)-carvone.

Summary: (−)-Carvone may be moderately allergenic, but there is no information on the allergenicity of (+)-carvone. In doses of 500 mg/kg (+)-carvone is reproductively toxic in male rats, but not at 375 mg/kg. In spite of several reports of genotoxicity for (+)-carvone, it is not carcinogenic. Rat NOAEL values of 93 mg/kg for (+)-carvone (given over 13 weeks) and 125 mg/kg for 'carvone' (given over 12 months) have been reported.

Regulatory guidelines: An ADI of 1 mg/kg for carvone has been set by the Council of Europe (1992). This is based on the rat 13 week NOAEL of 93 mg/kg, with an uncertainty factor of 100. The IFRA standard for either isomer of carvone in leave-on products such as body lotions is 1.2%, for skin sensitization.

Our safety advice: We agree with the IFRA guideline of 1.2% for skin sensitization, but only for (−)-carvone, and not for (+)-carvone. We recommend a human daily oral maximum dose of 12.5 mg/kg for carvone isomers, based on the one year rat NOAEL of 125 mg/kg, with an uncertainty factor of ten (five for interspecies, five for interindividual differences). This is equivalent to a dermal limit of 23% (Table 14.1).

α-Caryophyllene

Synonym: α-Humulene
Systematic name: (1E,4E,8E)-2,6,6,9-Tetramethyl-1,4,8-cycloundecatriene
Chemical class: Monocyclic sesquiterpenoid alkene
CAS number: 6753-98-6
Note: α-Caryophyllene exists as more than one isomer.

Sources >5.0%:

Hop	36.7%
Cananga	9.2%
Hemp	4.5–7.4%
Lantana	6.2%
Copaiba	2.7–6.1%
Geranium	0–6.0%
Pilocarpus microphyllus	1.7–5.4%
Rosemary (cineole CT)	0.1–5.4%

Antioxidant/pro-oxidant activity: α-Caryophyllene protected astrocytes from hydrogen peroxide-induced cell death in vitro (Elmann et al 2009).

Carcinogenic/anticarcinogenic potential: α-Caryophyllene significantly induced glutathione S-transferase in mouse liver and small intestine (Zheng et al 1992c). The compound was very weakly active against against the human solid tumor cell lines MCF-7, PC-3, A-549, DLD-1, M4BEU and CT-26, with GI$_{50}$ values of 55–73 mM (11.2–14.9 g/L). α-Caryophyllene

induced dose- and time-dependent glutathione depletion and an increase of ROS in the tumor cells (Legault et al 2003). In other research, it was not active against MCF-7 (human breast cancer) cells, but was highly active against human hormone-dependent prostate cancer (LNCaP) cells in vitro, with an IC$_{50}$ value of 11.24 μg/mL (Loizzo et al 2007).

Summary: α-Caryophyllene protects glial cells from oxidative stress from ROS, yet it is capable of increasing ROS damage in tumor cells.

β-Caryophyllene

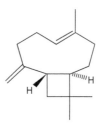

Synonyms: *trans*-Caryophyllene. (E)-(1R,9S)-(−)-Caryophyllene. Caryophyllene
Systematic name: [1R-(1R*,4E,9S*)]-4,11,11-Trimethyl-8-methylenebicyclo[7.2.0]undec-4-ene
Chemical class: Bicyclic sesquiterpenoid alkene
CAS Number: 87-44-5
Note: 4,11,11-Trimethyl-8-methylenebicyclo[7.2.0]undec-4-ene also exists as other isomers.

Sources >5.0%:

Copaiba	24.7–53.3%
Pilocarpus microphyllus	23.9–40.6%
Cananga	38.2%
Pepper (black)	9.4–30.9%
Cangerana	28.6%
Catnip	6.2–24.6%
Fern (sweet)	24.5%
Pepper (white)	23.4%
Ylang-ylang	1.1–21.5%
Hemp	13.7–19.4%
Melissa	0.3–19.1%
Camphor (Borneo)	18.1%
Fenugreek	14.6%
Blackcurrant bud absolute	9.0–14.0%
Savory (winter)	0–13.6%
Clove stem	3.5–12.4%
Clove bud	0.6–12.4%
Lantana	12.0%
Pine (black)	5.3–11.8%
Thymus serpyllum	6.0–11.2%
Myrtle (bog)	11.0%
Wormwood (annual)	0–10.9%
Mugwort (common, camphor/thujone CT)	10.6%
Ylang-ylang absolute	10.0%

Basil (hairy)	4.3–10.0%
Hop	9.8%
Sage (Dalmatian)	0.2–9.7%
Chaste tree seed	0.8–9.3%
Chaste tree leaf	2.3–8.9%
Niaouli (nerolidol CT)	0.5–8.7%
Ravensara leaf	1.5–8.4%
Longoza	0.8–8.0%
Betel	0–7.8%
Boswellia sacra (α-pinene CT)	1.9–7.5%
Sugandha	7.4%
Curry leaf	7.3%
Pimento berry	4.0–6.6%
Clove leaf	3.5–6.4%
Thyme (geraniol CT)	6.3%
Rosemary (cineole CT)	0.5–6.3%
Cade (rectified)	6.1%
Katrafay	3.0–6.0%
Lavender	1.8–5.9%
Cinnamon bark	1.3–5.8%
Carrot seed	0.7–5.6%
Sage (Greek)	5.5%
Vassoura	5.4%
Fir needle (Himalayan)	5.3%
Helichrysum italicum	5.0%
Pimento leaf	4.1–5.0%

Pharmacokinetics: In rabbits the major metabolite (80%) was 14-hydroxycaryophyllene-5,6-oxide, and a second metabolic pathway involved epoxidation (Asakawa et al 1986).

Adverse skin reactions: Undiluted β-caryophyllene was irritating to rabbit skin; tested at 4% on 25 volunteers, it was neither irritating nor sensitizing (Opdyke 1973 p. 1059–1060). Tested at 5%, β-caryophyllene induced allergic responses in 10 (0.6%) of 1,606 consecutive dermatitis patients (Frosch et al 2002b). In a multicenter study involving 1,511 consecutive dermatitis patients, 8 (0.5%) tested positive to 3% oxidized β-caryophyllene, containing 25% β-caryophyllene and 75% caryophyllene oxide. There was one positive reaction to 3% oxidized β-caryophyllene in 21 dermatitis patients hypersensitive to fragrance materials, and there were none in 66 hand eczema patients (Matura et al 2005). Sköld et al (2005) found that β-caryophyllene oxidized readily when air exposed, although no hydroperoxides were produced. After 6 weeks, only 50% of the original compound remained, with caryophyllene oxide as the major oxidation product. When air exposed for 10 weeks, β-caryophyllene showed only a weak sensitizing capacity in a local lymph node assay.

Acute toxicity: Acute oral LD_{50} in rats >5 g/kg, acute dermal LD_{50} in rabbits >5 g/kg (Opdyke 1973 p. 1059–1060).

Mutagenicity and genotoxicity: β-Caryophyllene was not mutagenic in *S. typhimurium* strains TA98 and TA100, and was antimutagenic in several assays (Di Sotto et al 2008, Gonçalves et al 2011). β-Caryophyllene was not genotoxic in the mouse bone marrow micronucleus test, nor was it cytotoxic to bone marrow erythrocytes (Molina-Jasso et al 2009). It was also not genotoxic in Chinese hamster ovary cells (Sasaki et al 1989).

Carcinogenic/anticarcinogenic potential: β-Caryophyllene significantly induced glutathione S-transferase in mouse liver and small intestine (Zheng et al 1992c) and was moderately cytotoxic to cell lines for human breast and cervical cancer, and to human and mouse melanoma cells (Kubo et al 1996). Kubo & Morimitsu (1995) reported similar results for two human carcinoma cell lines. Proliferation of mouse B16 melanoma cells was very weakly inhibited by β-caryophyllene with an IC_{50} value of 190 mM (38.8 mg/mL) (Tatman & Huanbiao 2002). β-Caryophyllene inhibited the growth of myelogenous leukemia cells (IC_{50} 98.0 μM; 20.4 μg/mL), human leukemia HL60 cells (IC_{50} 19.31 μg/mL), human melanoma cells (IC_{50} 20.10 μg/mL) and renal cell adenocarcinoma cells (IC_{50} 21.81 μg/mL) (Lampronti et al 2006; Loizzo et al 2007, 2008; Nibret & Wink 2010). In mice with ascites tumors, survival was significantly increased after four daily ip doses of 20 mg/kg β-caryophyllene. This was associated both with a direct action on the tumor cells, and a restoration of natural killer cell activity to normal levels (Da Silva et al 2007).

Summary: β-Caryophyllene is a weak skin allergen, and oxidation does not increase its allergenicity. It is non-toxic, non-mutagenic and antitumoral.

β-Caryophyllene oxide

Synonyms: 6,7-Epoxy-3(15)-caryophyllene. Epoxycaryophyllene. *trans*-Caryophyllene oxide

Systematic name: $1R$-($1\alpha,4\beta,6\alpha,10\beta$)]-4,12,12-Trimethyl-9-methylene-5-oxatricyclo[8.2.0.0^{4,6}]dodecane

Chemical class: Bicyclic sesquiterpenoid alkene epoxide

CAS number: 1139-30-6

Note: β-Caryophyllene oxide exists as more than one isomer.

Sources >1.0%:

Catnip	14.3–19.4%
Pilocarpus microphyllus	2.7–15.4%
Piri-piri	4.6–13.7%
Melissa	0.8–10.0%
Hemp	2.0–5.8%
Pine (Scots)	0–4.9%
Labdanum	0–4.4%
Angelica root (Himalayan)	2.0–4.0%
Verbena (lemon)	1.8–3.3%
Hyssop (linalool CT)	1.7–3.2%
Echinacea	3.0%
Carrot seed	0.3–2.8%
Helichrysum italicum	2.6%
Damiana	2.5%
Chaste tree seed	0–2.5%
Inula	2.2%
Feverfew	1.0–2.1%
Thyme (borneol CT)	2.0%
Palmarosa	0.1–1.8%
Wormwood (annual)	0.1–1.6%
Betel	0–1.6%

Lemongrass (East Indian)	0–1.6%	Cade (rectified)	<15.0%
Fern (sweet)	1.5%	Cade (unrectified)	<15.0%
Mugwort (common)	1.2–1.5%	Cedarwood (Chinese)	2.1%
Boswellia sacra (α-pinene CT)	0–1.4%		
Rosemary (verbenone CT)	0.3–1.3%		
Phoebe	1.0–1.1%		
Mastic	tr–1.1%		
Tansy (blue)	0.5–1.0%		
Pimento leaf	0.2–1.0%		

Pharmacokinetics: In rabbits the major metabolite of β-caryophyllene oxide (60%) was 14-hydroxycaryophyllene-5,6-oxide (Asakawa et al 1986).

Acute toxicity: Acute oral LD_{50} in rats >5 g/kg, acute dermal LD_{50} in rabbits reported as >2.0 kg/kg and >5 g/kg (Opdyke & Letizia 1983 p. 661–662).

Adverse skin reactions: Patch tested for 48 hours at 4% on volunteers, β-caryophyllene oxide was not irritating. When applied full strength to rabbit skin for 24 hours under occlusion it was moderately irritating. Neither a maximation test with 4% β-caryophyllene oxide on 28 volunteers nor a repeated insult patch test on 50 healthy subjects with 20% β-caryophyllene oxide produced any sensitization reactions. No photoirritant or photoallergic reactions were produced by 20% β-caryophyllene oxide tested on 20 human volunteers (Opdyke & Letizia 1983 p. 661–662). In a multicenter study involving 1,511 consecutive dermatitis patients, only two (0.14%) tested positive to 3.9% β-caryophyllene oxide. β-Caryophyllene oxide is an allergen of only moderate strength (Sköld et al 2005). There were no positive reactions to 3.9% β-caryophyllene oxide in 21 dermatitis patients hypersensitive to fragrance materials or in 66 hand eczema patients (Matura et al 2005).

Mutagenicity and genotoxicity: There was no evidence of mutagenic potential in the Ames test with metabolic activation (Opdyke & Letizia 1983 p. 661–662).

Carcinogenic/anticarcinogenic potential: β-Caryophyllene oxide strongly induced glutathione *S*-transferase in mouse liver and small intestine (Zheng et al 1992c). When tested in vitro against six cancer cell lines, it showed significant activity in all six (Sibanda et al 2004).

Summary: The dermal allergenic potency of β-caryophyllene oxide is negligible. It is non-toxic, non-mutagenic and anticarcinogenic.

α-Cedrene

Synonyms: 8-Cedrene. Cedr-8-ene
Systematic name: [3*R*-(3α,3aβ,7β,8aα)]-2,3,4,7,8,8a-Hexahydro-3,6,8,8-tetramethyl-1*H*-3a,7-methanoazulene
Chemical class: Tricyclic sesquiterpenoid alkene
CAS number: 469-61-4
Note: α-Cedrene exists as more than one isomer.

Sources >1.0%:

Cedarwood (Virginian)	21.1–38.0%
Cedarwood (Texan)	22.6–30.7%
Cedarwood (Himalayan)	15.8%

Adverse skin reactions: Tested at 5% on 25 volunteers α-cedrene was neither irritant nor sensitizing (Opdyke 1978 p. 679–680).

Acute toxicity: Both the acute oral LD_{50} in rats and the acute dermal LD_{50} in rabbits exceeded 5 g/kg for α-cedrene (Opdyke 1978 p. 679–680).

Subacute and subchronic toxicity: Cedrene (isomer not specified) whether administered ip, orally or inhalationally, significantly induced both CYP and ethylmorphine *N*-demethylase (EMND). Oral administration of 200 mg/kg once daily for 3 days produced a 160% increase in ethylmorphine metabolism, and a 40% increase in CYP content. Inhalational administration, in a dose of 60 mg/kg/day to rats for either 2 or 6 days, resulted in a 180% increase in ethylmorphine *N*-demethylase activity and a 30% increase in CYP content (Hashimoto et al 1972).

Reproductive toxicity: Gavage doses of acetyl cedrene, a similar compound, were given to pregnant rats at 25, 50 or 100 mg/kg/day on gestational days 7–17. Maternal and developmental NOAEL values were 50 and 100 mg/kg/day, respectively (Lapczynski et al 2006).

Mutagenicity and genotoxicity: α-Cedrene was not mutagenic in *S. typhimurium* strains TA98 and TA100 with or without S9 (Gonçalves et al 2011).

Carcinogenic/anticarcinogenic potential: α-Cedrene was cytotoxic to human leukemia HL60 cells with an IC_{50} of 22.20 μg/mL (Nibret & Wink 2010).

Comments: The increase in EMND activity may interfere with the action of opioid analgesics.

Summary: Limited data suggests that α-cedrene presents minimal risks in terms of irritancy, allergenicity and toxicity. There is a theoretical possibility of drug interaction with opioid analgesics from exposure to essential oils high in α-cedrene.

β-Cedrene

Synonyms: 8(15)-Cedrene. Cedr-8(15)-ene
Systematic name: [3*R*-(3α,3aβ,7β,8aα)]-Octahydro-3,8,8-trimethyl-6-methylene-1*H*-3a,7-methanoazulene
Chemical class: Tricyclic sesquiterpenoid alkene
CAS number: 546-28-1
Note: β-Cedrene exists as more than one isomer.

Sources >1.0%:

Juniperus virginiana	8.2–9.2%
Juniperus ashei	5.5%
Hinoki leaf	4.7%
Cedarwood (Himalayan)	1.4%

Subacute and subchronic toxicity: Cedrene (isomer not specified) whether administered ip, orally or inhalationally, significantly induced both CYP and ethylmorphine *N*-demethylase (EMND). Oral administration of 200 mg/kg once daily for 3 days produced a 160% increase in ethylmorphine metabolism, and a 40% increase in CYP content. Inhalational administration, in a dose of 60 mg/kg/day to rats for either 2 or 6 days, resulted in a 180% increase in ethylmorphine N-demethylase activity and a 30% increase in CYP content (Hashimoto et al 1972).

Comments: The increase in EMND activity may interfere with the action of opioid analgesics.

Summary: Limited data suggests that α-cedrene presents minimal risks in terms of irritancy, allergenicity and toxicity. There is a theoretical possibility of drug interaction with opioid analgesics from exposure to essential oils high in β-cedrene.

α-Cedrol

Synonyms: 3-Cedranol. (+)-Cedrol. 8βH-Cedran-8-ol. Cedar camphor. Cypress camphor

Systematic name: [3R-(3α,3aβ,6α,7β,8aα)]-Octahydro-3,6,8,8-tetramethyl-1H-3a,7-methanoazulen-6-ol

Chemical class: Tricyclic sesquiterpenoid alcohol

CAS number: 77-53-2

Sources >1.0%:

Cedarwood (Virginian)	12.3–22.2%
Cedarwood (Texan)	12.2–19.1%
Cypress	2.0–7.0%
Copaiba	0–4.8%
Cedarwood (Himalayan)	1.3%

Adverse skin reactions: Tested at 8% on 25 volunteers α-cedrol was neither irritating nor sensitizing (Opdyke 1975 p. 745–746).

Acute toxicity: Acute dermal LD_{50} in rabbits >5 g/kg (Opdyke 1975 p. 745–746).

Subacute and subchronic toxicity: In a 28 day oral toxicity study, male and female rats were dosed with 8.4 mg/kg/day α-cedrol by gavage. In female rats, there were decreases in absolute brain weight and in brain-to-body and ovary-to-body weight, but there were no associated clinical changes (Bhatia et al 2008c). In this study, the only dose given was considered as the male and female rat NOAEL for α-cedrol, though this conclusion seems premature.

Carcinogenic/anticarcinogenic potential: α-Cedrol inhibited the in vitro growth of human melanoma C32 cells and renal cell adenocarcinoma ACHN cells with IC_{50} values of 44.36 and 41.06 μg/mL, respectively (Loizzo et al 2008).

Summary: Limited data suggests that α-cedrol presents minimal risks in terms of irritancy, allergenicity and toxicity.

Chamazulene

Synonyms: Dimethulene. 1,4-Dimethyl-7-ethylazulene

Systematic name: 1,4-Dimethyl-7-ethylbicyclo[0.3.5]deca-1,3,5,7,9-pentaene

Chemical class: Bicyclic sesquiterpenoid polyalkene

CAS number: 529-05-5

Sources >1.0%:

Tansy (blue)	17.0–38.3%
Chamomile (blue)	3.4–23.4%
Mugwort (great)	22.4%
Yarrow (chamazulene CT)	19.7%
Cypress (blue)	5.6%
Chamomile (Roman)	0–4.4%
Pine (Scots)	0–1.7%

Antioxidant/pro-oxidant activity: Chamazulene is a powerful antioxidant. It inhibited lipid peroxidation in a concentration and time dependent manner, presenting an IC_{50} of 18 μM (3.31 μg/mL) after 45 minutes incubation. It also weakly inhibited the autoxidation of DMSO (33 mM; 6.07 mg/mL) by 76% at 25 mM (4.60 mg/mL) (Rekka et al 1996). In two antioxidant assays, deoxyribose degradation and non-enzymatic lipid peroxidation, chamazulene had IC50 values of 0.042 μL/mL and 0.0021 μL/mL, respectively (Burits et al 2001).

Summary: We could find no toxicity data for chamazulene.

1,4-Cineole

Synonyms: Isocineole. 1,4-Epoxy-p-menthane

Systematic name: 1-Methyl-4-(1-methylethyl)-7-oxabicyclo [2.2.1]heptane

Chemical class: Bicyclic monoterpenoid ether

CAS number: 470-67-7

Sources >1.0%:

Lime (distilled, Mexican)	2.0–3.0%
Lime (distilled, Persian)	1.8%
Cedarwood (Port Orford)	1.3%

Pharmacokinetics: 1,4-Cineole was given orally to rabbits at 2 g per animal. Four neutral metabolites and one acidic metabolite were isolated from the urine. These were 9-hydroxy-1,4-cineole (the most abundant metabolite) and its oxidized derivative 1,4-cineole-9-carboxylic acid, the allylic alcohol derivative 1,4-cineole-8-en-9-ol, and the two diols 3,8-dihydroxy-1,4-cineole, 8,9-dihydroxy-1,4-cineole (Asakawa et al 1988). CYP3A4 enzymes in rat and human liver microsomes also give rise to 2-exo-hydroxy-1,4-cineole as a major metabolite (Miyazawa et al 2001a).

Adverse skin reactions: Tested at 16% on 25 volunteers 1,4-cineole was neither irritiating nor sensitizing (Ford et al 1988a p. 291).

Acute toxicity: Acute oral LD_{50} in rats 3.1 g/kg; acute dermal LD_{50} in rabbits <5 g/kg (Ford et al 1988a p. 291).

Summary: Limited data suggests that 1,4-cineole presents minimal risk in terms of adverse skin reactions or toxicity.

1,8-Cineole

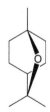

Synonyms: Cineole. Eucalyptol. Cajeputol. 1,8-Epoxy-p-menthane

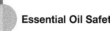

Systematic name: 1,3,3-Trimethyl-2-oxabicyclo[2.2.2]octane
Chemical class: Bicyclic monoterpenoid ether
CAS number: 470-82-6

Sources >10.0%:

Eucalyptus plenissima	85.0–95.0%
Eucalyptus polybractea	88.7–91.9%
Eucalyptus globulus	65.4–83.9%
Eucalyptus camaldulensis	46.9–83.7%
Eucalyptus smithii	77.5%
Eucalyptus maidenii	76.8%
Cajuput	41.1–70.8%
Sage (white)	68.4%
Niaouli (cineole CT)	55.0–65.0%
Eucalyptus radiata	60.4–64.5%
Ho leaf (cineole CT, Madagascan)	56.7–63.7%
Cardamon (black)	61.3%
Sage (Greek)	59.0%
Marjoram (Spanish)	45.1–58.6%
Rosemary (cineole CT)	39.0–57.7%
Saro	46.0–53.0%
Ho leaf (cineole CT, Chinese)	50.0%
Galangal (lesser)	49.6%
Rambiazana	47.4%
Cardamon	26.5–44.6%
Sanna	44.3%
Laurel leaf	38.1–43.5%
Sage (Spanish)	12.0–40.3%
Myrtle	18.9–37.5%
Chaste tree leaf	15.6–35.2%
Niaouli (viridiflorol CT)	30.0–35.0%
Lavender (spike)	28.0–34.9%
Galangal (greater)	30.2–33.6%
Fragonia	31.0–33.0%
Eucalyptus macarthurii	28.9–29.0%
Rosalina	18.0–26.0%
Rosemary (α-pinene CT)	15.0–25.1%
Chaste tree seed	8.4–23.3%
Rosemary (camphor CT)	17.0–22.5%
Tana (+β-phellandrene)	16.0–22.0%
Sage (Dalmatian)	1.8–21.7%
Boldo	21.1%
Rosemary (borneol CT)	20.0%
Lanyana	19.1%
Southernwood	18.6%
Basil (holy)	12.6–16.5%
Eucalyptus polybractea (cryptone CT)	16.1%
Zedoary	2.0–15.9%
Sage (African wild)	15.5%
Tea tree	tr.–15.0%
Hyssop (linalool CT)	12.3–14.9%
White cloud	14.8%
Wormwood (annual)	0–14.7%
Lavender (Spanish)	3.6–14.5%
Oregano (Mexican)	1.8–14.0%
Rosemary (bornyl acetate CT)	6.8–13.6%
Ho leaf (linalool CT)	0.2–13.3%
Sugandha	13.1%
Damiana	11.4%
Lavandin abrialis	6.0–11.0%
Lavandin grosso	5.2–10.2%

Note: 1,8-Cineole is also found in over 200 essential oils, generally in concentrations less than 10%.

Pharmacokinetics: 1,8-Cineole reached the arterial circulation in mice after the inhalation of rosemary oil vapor and produced increased physical activity whether given to the animals orally or by inhalation (Kovar et al 1987). Prolonged inhalation in humans results in a peak plasma concentration after approximately 18 minutes. Elimination from the blood is biphasic, with a mean distribution half-life of 6.7 minutes and an elimination half-life of 104.6 minutes (Jäger et al 1996). Animal studies have shown that numerous metabolites are formed from 1,8-cineole following hydroxylation and glucuronide conjugation (Scheline 1991).

When a human volunteer ingested 19 μg/kg bw of 1,8-cineole, the urinary metabolites detected over 10 hours were 20.9% 2-hydroxy-1,8-cineole, 17.2% 9-hydroxy-1,8-cineole, 10.6% 3-hydroxy-1,8-cineole and 3.8% 7-hydroxy-1,8-cineole. The 2-hydroxy isomer was the predominant plasma metabolite at 86 nmol/L, followed by the 9-hydroxy isomer at 33 nmol/L (Horst & Rychlik 2010). 1,8-Cineole is primarily metabolized to 2-hydroxy-1,8-cineole by CYP3A4 in both rats and humans, with human metabolism being 2.7 times greater than rat (Miyazawa et al 2001b).

1,8-Cineole caused a 95-fold increase in the permeation of 5-fluorouracil across human skin, suggesting its importance as a skin permeation enhancer (Williams & Barry 1991). When a subcutaneous dose of 500 mg/kg was administered to pregnant rats, 1,8-cineole penetrated placental tissue and reached a concentration in fetal blood sufficient to stimulate hepatic enzyme activity. However, similar studies showed that 1,8-cineole would not cross the blood–milk barrier in sufficient concentration to affect hepatic enzymes in the offspring (Jori & Briatico 1973).

Drug interactions: Single subcutaneous doses of 250 or 500 mg/kg 1,8-cineole increased the activity of drug-metabolizing enzymes in rats, but 125 mg/kg had no effect (Jori et al 1969, 1972). When administered to rats as a continuous aerosol for 3, 6 or 9 days (22 of each 24 hour period), 1,8-cineole significantly induced CYP in liver microsomes, but not in the lungs (Madyastha & Chadha 1986). This finding explains the compound's ability to reduce plasma and/or brain levels of several drugs in vivo in rats (Jori et al 1970). In a later study, 1,8-cineole was found to induce CYP2B1 and CYP3A2 (Hiroi et al 1995). Overall, these very high exposures (and the lack of effect of 125 mg/kg sc) do not suggest a need for caution at therapeutic doses of essential oils high in 1,8-cineole.

Adverse skin reactions: 1,8-Cineole has been used in counter-irritant ointments (Reynolds 1993) and it has been claimed that it is a skin irritant (Lassak & McCarthy 1983 p. 97; Williams et al 1990). However, patch testing reveals no evidence of this. Tested at 16% on 25 volunteers 1,8-cineole was not irritating (Opdyke 1975 p. 105–106). When tested at concentrations ranging from 3.8% to 28.1% in petrolatum on 25 volunteers, 99.5% pure 1,8-cineole was not irritating. When eight tea tree oils with 1.5% to 28.8% 1,8-cineole were tested for irritation at 25% on 25 panelists, there were no positive reactions (Southwell et al 1997). A gel ointment with 2% 1,8-cineole produced no histopathological signs of irritation in abdominal rat skin after 10 hours, nor was 0.05% 1,8-cineole cytotoxic to cultured human skin cells (Kitahara et al 1993).

In a modified Draize procedure on guinea pigs, 1,8-cineole was non-sensitizing when used at 50% in the challenge phase (Sharp 1978). In a similar test, 1,8-cineole was non-sensitizing when used at concentrations ranging from 3.125% to 25.0% in the challenge phase (Ohsumi et al 1996). 1,8-Cineole was not allergenic in 11 tea tree oil sensitive patients, when tested at 5% (Hausen et al 1999). Of seven dermatitis patients already sensitive to tea tree oil, none was sensitive to 1,8-cineole tested at 5% (Knight & Hausen 1994). Tested at 16% on 25 volunteers 1,8-cineole was not sensitizing (Opdyke 1975 p. 105–106).

There are five recorded cases of 1,8-cineole allergy. One dermatitis patient sensitive to tea tree oil was also sensitive to 1,8-cineole, and not to six other constituents of the oil. This case has been reported twice (De Groot & Weyland 1992; Van Der Valk 1994). In another case, an athlete developed eczema on his toes after two years of using a topical cream. He tested positive to 1% 1,8-cineole, and to no other ingredient of the cream (Vilaplana and Romaguera 2000). Tested at concentrations ranging from 3.8% to 28.1% on 28 volunteers, 1,8-cineole was sensitizing to three panelists also allergic to tea tree oil (Southwell et al 1997).

1,8-Cineole increased the skin permeability of haloperidol, but not chlorpromazine (Almirall et al 1996). In an uptake study of human skin, 26.2% of the 1,8-cineole applied was found in the stratum corneum (Cornwell et al 1996). 1,8-Cineole changes the dynamics of the stratum corneum, but does not denature stratum corneum proteins, a finding that is consistent with a non-irritant (Anjos et al 2007).

1,8-Cineole produced an edema response when injected into rat paw, and when tested in vitro it caused degranulation of rat peritoneal mast cells at a concentration of 0.3 µL/mL (Santos & Rao 1997). Subcutaneous injection of 1,8-cineole in mice produced mast cell-mediated scratching behavior (Santos & Rao 2002). However, (cineole-rich) *Eucalyptus globulus* oil was anti-inflammatory, inhibiting induced rat paw edema when subsequently injected (Silva et al 2003).

Mucous membrane irritation: Pre-treatment with 1,8-cineole by rectal instillation at 200 or 400 mg/kg significantly attenuated chemically induced colonic damage in rats, and caused repletion of glutathione (Santos et al 2004). In rats, 1,8-cineole protected against ethanol-induced mucosal stomach damage when dosed at 50–200 mg/kg; the action was thought to be related to an antioxidant effect (Santos & Rao 2001). Similarly, cardamon oil (26.5–44.6% 1,8-cineole) significantly inhibited gastric irritation and ulcerative lesions induced by ethanol and aspirin in rats (Jamal et al 2006). These data indicate a distinct lack of mucous membrane irritancy on the part of 1,8-cineole.

Acute toxicity: 1,8-Cineole acute oral LD_{50} in rats 2.48 g/kg (Jenner et al 1964) acute dermal LD_{50} in rabbits >5 g/kg. Low oral toxicity according to some sources (Baker 1960) but 1 mL has caused transient coma. Recovery has occurred after ingestion of 30 mL. Poisoning produces severe gastrointestinal and CNS effects.

Subacute and subchronic toxicity: Groups of ten male Wistar rats were given 0, 500, or 1000 mg/kg bw/day by gavage for 28 days. Significant decreases in body weight, and increases in relative liver and kidney weights were found in both dose groups. No macroscopical changes were seen. There were no significant histopathological changes in the brain or the liver. In the kidneys, a dose-related accumulation of eosinophilic protein droplets containing α2u-globulin was induced (Kristiansen & Madsen 1995).

Groups of six male and six female rats received 1,8-cineole at for 28 days either by stomach tube on 5 days a week at doses of 150, 300, 600 and 1,200 mg/kg bw or in encapsulated form with the diet at concentrations of 3,750, 7,500, 15,000 and 30,000 mg/kg, equivalent to 381–3,342 mg/kg bw/day for the male rats and to 353–3,516 mg/kg/day for the female rats. At doses of 600 mg/kg and higher, there was a decrease in body weight gain and absence of a normal degree of hepatic centrilobular cytoplasmic vacuolization was observed in male rats. In addition, other dose-related lesions in the liver, kidneys and parotid salivary glands were found at all doses in male rats fed encapsulated 1,8-cineole (Wolff et al 1987a).

Groups of six male and six female mice were fed 1,8-cineole for 28 days either by stomach tube on 5 days a week at doses of 150, 300, 600 and 1200 mg/kg bw or in encapsulated form at concentrations of 3,750, 7,500, 15,000 and 30,000 mg/kg, equivalent to 600–5607 mg/kg bw/day for male and 705–6777 mg/kg/day for female mice. The liver weight/body weight ratio in males was increased at all but the lowest dose given in encapsulated form as was the brain weight/body weight ratio in females at the highest dose. Microscopic examination revealed a minimal hypertrophy of centrilobular hepatocytes in animals of both sexes fed the encapsulated compound, especially at the two highest doses (Wolff et al 1987b).

Human toxicity: Instillation of 1,8-cineole into the nose, or introducing by drops, results in a combination of oral ingestion and inhalation. There are reports from Belgium, France and the UK of non-fatal, but serious toxicity in children who have had solutions containing either menthol (four cases), niaouli (one case), Olbas Oil (one case) or 1,8-cineole (nine cases) instilled into their noses (Melis et al 1989; Wyllie et al 1994; Decocq et al 1996). The ages ranged from 1 month to 3 years and 9 months. The effects of poisoning included irritated mucous membranes, tachycardia, dyspnea, nausea, vomiting, vertigo, muscular weakness, drowsiness and coma (Melis et al 1989; Reynolds 1993). 1,8-Cineole may have contributed to the intense pain when preparations for topical use containing it have been instilled into the eyes (Blanchard 1989).

However, 1,8-Cineole can be of benefit in respiratory disorders. In a double-blind, placebo-controlled trial, 200 mg/day of 1,8-cineole taken orally by asthma patients showed an anti-inflammatory effect on the airways, allowing a reduction in oral steroid dosage (Juergens et al 2003). This effect is thought to be related to the inhibition by 1,8-cineole of cytokines and arachidonic acid pathways (Juergens et al 1998a, 1998b).

Neurotoxicity: In in vitro tests on rat brain slices, 1,8-cineole altered brain sodium and potassium concentrations in a similar way to camphor, and in a way consistent with increased susceptibility to convulsions (Steinmetz et al 1987). However, Zibrowski et al (1998) observed that bursts of fast wave activity (~20 Hz) in the brains of rats inhaling 1,8-cineole were not kindling-induced, seizure-like reactions. While CNS depression and coma are notable in LD$_{50}$ tests in rats given 1,8-cineole, convulsions are not (Jenner et al 1964). CNS depression, rather than stimulation, is supported by evidence that in rats, iv 1,8-cineole was dose-dependently hypotensive at 0.3–10 mg/kg and decreased heart rate at the highest dose (Lahlou et al 2002a).

Seizures were not reported in any of the subchronic toxicity studies cited above, and have only been reported in very few cases of human poisoning with 1,8-cineole-rich eucalyptus oil (see Eucalyptus profile, Chapter 13). However, the CNS depression (extreme drowsiness) seen in animal toxicity tests sometimes does manifest in children exposed to moderate amounts of eucalyptus oil (Darben et al 1998; Waldman 2011).

Reproductive toxicity: 1,8-Cineole crosses the placenta in sufficient quantity to affect the activity of fetal liver enzymes when given by sc injection to pregnant rats at a dose of 500 mg/kg for four days (Jori & Briatico 1973). Eucalyptus oil (~75% 1,8-cineole) showed no embryotoxicity or fetotoxicity when tested on mice (injected sc at 135 mg/kg on gestational days 6–15) and had no effect on birth weight or placental size (Pages et al 1990). Niaouli oil (50.6% 1,8-cineole) was maternally toxic and fetotoxic when injected ip to pregnant rats for 18 days at 1,350 mg/kg (Laleye et al 2004). Extrapolating from the above information, in pregnant rodents, 1,8-cineole at 101 mg/kg sc for 10 days had no adverse effect, at 500 mg/kg sc for four days it affected fetal liver enzymes (i.e. it was fetotoxic), and at 682 mg/kg ip for 18 days it was maternally toxic and fetotoxic. This suggests an oral NOAEL for reproductive toxicity greater than 100 mg/kg/day.

1,8-Cineole was not estrogenic in an in vitro assay using MCF-7 cells (Nielsen 2008). In an ex vivo assay, 1,8-cineole did not bind to estrogen receptors in female rat uterus tissue (Blair et al 2000).

Hepatotoxicity: A single dose of 400 mg/kg 1,8-cineole protected mice against chemically induced hepatotoxicity (Santos et al 2001). 1,8-Cineole was not hepatotoxic when given orally to male rats at 200, 400 or 800 mg/kg/day for 3 days. These doses induced CYP2B1, CYP2B2, CYP3A1 and CYP3A2, and the metabolic activation of 1,8-cineole potentiated the hepatotoxicity of thiocetamide (Kim NH et al 2004). However, the lowest dose is 25 times greater than the oral dose equivalent of 600 mg for eucalyptus oil. At 100 mg/kg/day for 60 days, gavage doses of 1,8-cineole protected rat liver from chemically induced oxidative stress (Ciftçi et al 2011).

Antioxidant/pro-oxidant activity: Antioxidant acivity has been reported for 1,8-cineole (Perry et al 2001; Saito et al 2004). DPPH radical scavenging activity was observed by Mimica-Dukic et al (2003) but not by Kordali et al (2005b).

Mutagenicity and genotoxicity: 1,8-Cineole was not mutagenic in the Ames test (Haworth et al 1983; Gomes-Carneiro et al 1998; Vuković-Gačić et al 2006), and suppressed UV-induced mutations (Vuković-Gačić et al 2006). At nanomolar concentrations, 1,8-cineole suppressed t-butyl hydroperoxide induced genotoxicity, both in bacteria and cultured human cells. This was predominantly mediated by radical scavenging activity (Mitić-Culafić et al 2009). 1,8-Cineole was not genotoxic, either in Chinese hamster ovary cells (Sasaki et al 1989) or in the wing somatic mutation and recombination test (SMART) of Drosophila melanogaster (Pavlidou et al 2004).

Carcinogenic/anticarcinogenic potential: 1,8-Cineole showed moderate in vitro cytotoxic activity against five human cell lines: CTVR-1 (leukemia), Molt-4 (leukemia), K562 (myelogenous leukemia), HeLa (cervical adenocarcinoma) and HepG2 (hepatocellular carcinoma) with IC$_{50}$ values ranging from 0.1–6.7 g/L after 24 hours incubation (Hayes et al 1997). Specific induction of apoptosis by 1,8-cineole was observed in human leukemia Molt 4B and HL-60 cells, but not in human stomach cancer KATO III cells. The fragmentations of DNA by 1,8-cineole were concentration- and time-dependent in Molt 4B and HL-60 cells, but not in KATO III cells (Moteki et al 2002).

In male and female mice given 24 ip injections of cineole in tricaprylin in a total dose of 2.4 or 12.0 g/kg over 24 weeks the incidence of primary lung tumors was no higher than in the control group (Stoner et al 1973). 1,8-Cineole did not significantly reduce the average number of tumors per rat or the median tumor latency period in a DMBA-induced rat mammary carcinogenesis model (Russin et al 1989). Topically applied essential oil of Salvia libanotica, which contains 47.4–57.7% 1,8-cineole, strongly inhibited tumor promotion in mouse skin, with a 50% concentration reducing tumor weight by 75% (Gali-Muhtasib & Affara 2000; Farhat et al 2001).

Comments: 1,8-Cineole does not appear to be as toxic as is often believed, although elevated oral doses certainly are toxic, and children are susceptible to cineole toxicity. The long-held belief that it is a skin irritant may be based on animal data from injected 1,8-cineole which is neither relevant to dermal application, nor is it borne out by studies in humans. The instillation of 1,8-cineole into the noses of young children is clearly not a sensible procedure, but this should not be taken to mean that any preparation containing 1,8-cineole is highly dangerous to children per se. Safe doses for 1,8-cineole-containing products intended for both children and adults need to be established. The protein droplet nephropathy reported in rats can be a precursor to renal carcinoma but, as with (+)-limonene, this effect is specific to male rats, and similar nephropathy is very unlikely to occur in humans (Hard et al 1993).

Summary: 1,8-Cineole presents a low risk of both skin irritation and sensitization. It is non-mutagenic and shows no evidence of carcinogenesis or teratogenesis in rodents. It is non-fetotoxic in normal doses. Rodent data demonstrates that only negligible toxicity results from subchronic dosing at under 500 mg/kg bw. Although a few cases of seizure have been reported from eucalyptus oil, 1,8-cineole does not appear to be a convulsant. 1,8-Cineole neurotoxicity manifests primarily as depression and coma. Instillation of 1,8-cineole into the nose of children up to four years of age results in non-fatal but serious toxicity, and may interfere with respiration.

Regulatory guidelines: The Council of Europe lists 1,8-cineole under 'substances which are suspected to be potent toxicants and for which, due to insufficient existing toxicological data, it was not possible to set an MDI' (Council of Europe 2003). The CEFS of the Council of Europe has allocated a provisional TDI of 0.2 mg/kg bw for 1,8-cineole. This was derived from assuming a minimum lethal dose of 60 mg/kg for children, and applying a safety factor of 300 (Council of Europe 2000). In contrast, the joint FAO/WHO committee expressed 'no safety concern' about 1,8-cineole as a food additive in 2003 (http://www.inchem.org/documents/jecfa/jecmono/v52je16.htm accessed November 24th 2012).

Cinnamaldehyde

Synonyms: Cinnamal. Cinnamic aldehyde. β-Phenylacrolein
Systematic name: 3-Phenyl-2-propenal
Chemical class: Phenylpropenoid aldehyde
Note: Different isomers of cinnamaldehyde exist, and the following isomer-specific information has been published:

(2*E*)-Cinnamaldehyde

Synonym: *trans*-Cinnamic aldehyde
CAS number: 14371-10-9

Sources >0.1%:

Cassia leaf	54.6–90.1%
Cassia bark	73.2–89.4%
Cinnamon bark	63.1–75.7%
Bakul absolute	1.3%
Cinnamon leaf	0.6–1.1%

(2*Z*)-Cinnamaldehyde

Synonym: *cis*-Cinnamic aldehyde
CAS number: 57194-69-1

Sources >0.1%:

Cassia bark	0.8–12.3%
Cassia leaf	0.4–10.5%

Pharmacokinetics: Cinnamaldehyde distributes primarily to the GI tract (75–85%) after oral administration to rats, with small amounts being distributed to blood (~2%), muscle (~2%), liver (~1%), kidneys (~0.3%) fat (~0.2%) and other tissues after 30–60 minutes. The major metabolic pathway for single and multiple doses of 5 or 50 mg/kg was degradation to benzoic acid through beta-oxidation and excretion in the urine mainly as hippuric acid (81.6–84.8%), with much smaller amounts of benzoic acid (3.4–5.1%) and cinnamic acid (1.0–1.6%). Multiple oral doses of 500 mg/kg cinnamaldehyde in rats are metabolized by a very different route compared to single doses of 500 mg/kg, or lower multiple doses. This results in 7.6% urinary hippuric acid, along with 2.1% cinnamic acid and 73.3% benzoic acid (Sapienza et al 1993). Urinary excretion of

hippuric acid follows conjugation with glucuronic acid or glycine (Scheline 1991 p. 95).

Cinnamaldehyde is metabolized to cinnamic alcohol and cinnamic acid in human skin (Weibel & Hansen 1989b). When 10 μL of cinnamaldehyde was applied to excised female human skin from the breast or abdomen which was then occluded, 9.4% was absorbed over 24 hours. This was detected as 2.6% cinnamaldehyde, 2.4% cinnamyl alcohol and 4.4% cinnamic acid (Smith et al 2000).

Adverse skin reactions: In a modified Draize procedure on guinea pigs, cinnamaldehyde was sensitizing when used at 20% in the challenge phase (Sharp 1978). A modified mouse local lymph node assay supports the classification of cinnamaldehyde as a moderately potent sensitizer (Karrow et al 2001). After a 48 hour closed-patch test on volunteers 3% cinnamaldehyde produced no irritation, but when similarly tested at 8% it proved to be severely irritating (Opdyke 1976 p. 253–258). Of 1,200 dermatitis patients patch tested, there were no irritant reactions to 2% cinnamaldehyde. In a second group of 1,500 dermatitis patients there were no irritant reactions to 1% cinnamaldehyde (Santucci et al 1987).

Tested at 2%, cinnamaldehyde produced positive sensitization reactions in one of 34 males (2.9%) and 5 of 55 females (9.1%) (Schorr 1975). Tested at 0.1, 0.3, 1, 3, and 10% on eight volunteers, cinnamaldehyde was not sensitizing at the two lowest concentrations, produced one positive reaction at 1% (12.5%) and five at 3% and 10% (62.5%) (Nater et al 1977). Tested on 25 volunteers, the compound produced two reactions (8%) at 0.5% and 11/25 (44%) reactions at 2% (Opdyke 1976 p. 253–258). The results of testing on dermatitis patients at 1%, 2% or 5% are shown in Table 14.2A.

In a prospective study of adverse skin reactions to cosmetic ingredients identified by patch test (1977–1980) cinnamaldehyde was responsible for five cases (1%) of contact dermatitis of 487 cosmetic-related cases (Eiermann et al 1982). Of 713 cosmetic dermatitis patients, six reacted to cinnamaldehyde (Adams & Maibach 1985).

In a European multicenter study, 10 of 78 (12.8%) dermatitis patients known to be sensitive to fragrance materials tested positive to 1% cinnamaldehyde (Wilkinson et al 1989). Of 167 dermatitis patients suspected of fragrance sensitivity 24 (14.4%) were allergic to 1% cinnamaldehyde on patch testing (Larsen et al 1996b). When patch tested at 1% on 20 dermatitis patients who were sensitive to fragrance materials, cinnamaldehyde induced six (30%) positive reactions (Larsen 1977). Of 182 dermatitis patients suspected of contact allergy to cosmetics 3.7% (presumably either six or seven) tested positive to 8% cinnamaldehyde (Malten et al 1984). Of 180 dermatitis patients suspected of contact allergy to cosmetics, four (2.2%) tested positive to 0.5% cinnamaldehyde (Malten et al 1984). In 18 eczema patients known to be sensitive to 2% cinnamaldehyde, 13 (72%) reacted to 0.8%, three (17%) reacted to 0.1%, one (6%) reacted to 0.02%, and none reacted to 0.01% (Johansen et al 1996a).

The prevalence of allergy to cinnamaldehyde in patients suspected of having contact dermatitis, reported by the North American Contact Dermatitis Group, steadily reduced over a 13 year period: 5.9% (1984–1985), 3.1% (1985–1989), 2.7% (1992–1994) and 2.4% (1994–1996) (Storrs et al 1989; Nethercott et al 1991; Marks et al 1995, 1998). A 1% concentration was used in each study except for Storrs et al (1989), in

Table 14.2 Allergic reactions to cinnamaldehyde in different groups

A. Dermatitis patients

Concentration used	Percentage who reacted	No. of reactors	Reference
1%	0.0%	0/50	Larsen 1977
1%	0.14%	1/702	Frosch et al 1995b
1%	0.2%	3/1,500	Santucci et al 1987
1%	0.95%	10/1,072	Frosch et al 1995a
1%	1.0%	21/2,063	Schnuch et al 2007a
1%	1.3%	20/1,503	Heisterberg et al 2011
1%	1.7%	27/1,603	Belsito et al 2006
1%	2.4%	75/3,112	Marks et al 1998
1%	2.7%	95/3,528	Marks et al 1995
1%	3.1%	123/3,964	Nethercott et al 1991
1%	3.3%	8/241[a]	Ferguson & Sharma 1984
2%	0.75%	9/1,200	Santucci et al 1987
2%	5.4%	24/441	Mitchell et al 1982
2%	5.9%	62/1,048	Storrs et al 1989
2%	18.7%	45/241[a]	Ferguson & Sharma 1984
5%	29.2%	24/82	Opdyke 1979a p. 253–258

B. Fragrance-sensitive dermatitis patients

Concentration used	Percentage who reacted	No. of reactors	Reference
0.5%	2.2%	4/180	Malten et al 1984
1%	12.8%	10/78	Wilkinson et al 1989
1%	14.4%	24/167	Larsen et al 1996b
1%	30%	6/20	Larsen 1977

[a]Same group of patients

which 2% was used. A similar pattern is seen in the UK. From a total of 25,545 dermatitis patients patch tested from January 1980 to December 1996, there was a reduction of 18% per year in the frequency of sensitivity to cinnamaldehyde. The authors surmise that this is probably due to a reduction in the concentrations of cinnamaldehyde used in personal care products (Buckley et al 2000).

The majority of workers in a Danish company exposed to high concentrations during the manufacture of cinnamon spice substitutes developed cinnamaldehyde sensitivity (Collins & Mitchell

1975). A preparation containing cinnamaldehyde produced bullous lesions in a man using it which completely regressed on stopping (Manzur et al 1995). An 82-year-old female developed cheilitis from using cinnamaldehyde-containing lipstick and toothpaste, and tested positive to 1% cinnamaldehyde. When she stopped using both products her cheilitis cleared in three weeks (Maibach 1986). Other single cases of cinnamaldehyde allergy have been reported (Drake & Maibach 1976; Decapite & Anderson 2004; Hoskyn & Guin 2005).

The only recorded instance of anaphylaxis to an essential oil constituent was to cinnamaldehyde. A 42-year-old woman was being tested with the fragrance mix constituents which were applied for 20 minutes. A strong urticarial reaction was seen to cinnamaldehyde, and 40 minutes after the test the patient developed widespread pruritis and erythema. Five minutes later she started to feel faint, and her blood pressure was unrecordably low. She was treated with 10 mg chlorphenamine maleate and 1 mg intramuscular epinephrine (adrenaline), and made a good recovery (Diba & Statham 2003).

Results of studies involving a total of 4,117 patch tests indicated that cinnamaldehyde contained in consumer products and fragrance blends at concentrations up to 0.6%, and patch-tested at concentrations up to 0.008%, had no detectable potential to induce hypersensitivity. When tested alone, cinnamaldehyde induced a dose-related hypersensitivity response. When tested alone or as part of a mixture in subjects in the general population, no pre-existing hypersensitivity reactions to the fragrance material were observed in any of the 4,117 patch tests that constituted the survey. It was concluded that cinnamaldehyde, at the concentrations contained in consumer products and fragrances, has a very low potential to induce hypersensitivity ('induced' reactions) or to elicit sensitization reactions ('elicited' reactions) in the general population (Danneman et al 1983).

The mechanism of cinnamaldehyde sensitization (interaction with proteins in the skin) has been investigated (Majeti & Suskind 1977; Weibel & Hansen 1989a). Cinnamaldehyde may be markedly less allergenic in aged preparations, where it has oxidized to cinnamic acid, and in mixtures in which it can react with alcohols and/or amines to form non-allergenic compounds (Fisher & Dooms-Goosens 1976). A North American study revealed a decline in incidence of reactions to cinnamaldehyde over the period 1970–2002 (Nguyen et al 2008).

Cinnamaldehyde has produced phototoxic effects in some in vitro assays, and not in others. Of 76 patients with photodermatoses, four exhibited photo-patch reactions to cinnamaldehyde (Plazcek et al 2007).

Acute toxicity: Acute oral LD$_{50}$ reported as 2.22, 3.4 and 3.35 g/kg in rats, and 1.16 g/kg in guinea pigs (Jenner et al 1964; Sporn et al 1965; Adams et al 2004). LD$_{100}$ 940 mg/kg/day in rats, 2,620 mg/kg/day in mice (Hébert et al 1994). Acute ip LD$_{50}$ in mice reported as 200 mg/kg by Opdyke (1979 p. 253–258) and as 2,320 mg/kg by Sporn et al (1965). Acute dermal LD$_{50}$ in rabbits 590 mg/kg (Opdyke 1979a p. 253–258).

Subacute and subchronic toxicity: Forestomach hyperplasia was seen at dietary doses of 1.25% or over in 2- or 3-week toxicity studies in rats; doses of 0.625% or less were not toxic (Hébert et al 1994). Groups of ten male and ten female rats were maintained for 16 weeks on diets containing 0.1%, 0.25% or 1.0% cinnamaldehyde (approximately 50, 125 and 500 mg/kg/day). No effects were seen at 0.1% or 0.25%; at 1.0% slight hepatic cell swelling was observed, and slight hyperkeratosis of the squamous portion of the stomach (Hagan et al 1967). Cinnamaldehyde caused forestomach hyperkeratosis in rats fed 1% in diet for 16 weeks (Feron et al 1991). The MTD for five mice receiving six ip injections over 14 days was 250 mg/kg cinnamaldehyde (Stoner et al 1973). Given in doses of 10 or 50 mg ip on alternate days to rats on normal or low-protein diets, cinnamaldehyde did not affect growth, liver weight and ascorbic acid content, or the activity of aspartic-glutamic transaminase, but liver aldolase activity increased dose-dependently (Sporn et al 1965).

Male and female rats were given 0, 1.25%, 2.5%, 5.0% or 10.0% microencapsulated cinnamaldehyde in the diet for 13 weeks, corresponding to daily intakes of 0, 625, 1,250, 2,500 or 5,000 mg/kg. There were no clinical or hematological signs of cinnamaldehyde-related toxicity, and there were no morphological alterations to the liver. However, mean body weight values decreased in animals on the three higher doses (NTP 1995, unpublished report, cited in Adams et al 2004). Groups of rats and mice were dosed with microencapsulated (E)-cinnamaldehyde for 15 weeks at daily doses up to 4,000 mg/kg (rats) and 5,475 mg/kg (mice). There was considerable weight loss and reduction in feed consumption in higher dose groups, and significant incidence of forestomach lesions, including squamous epithelial hyperplasia. This toxicity may be partly due to saturation of the primary metabolic pathway for cinnamaldehyde at these very high doses (Hooth et al 2004, National Toxicology Program 2004).

Cytotoxicity: Cinnamaldehyde was not cytotoxic to mouse (RAW 264.7) macrophages, at concentrations up to 200 μM (26.4 mg/L) (Tung et al 2008). It was not cytotoxic to mouse (J774A.1) macrophages at 24 μM or 80 μM (3.17 or 10.6 mg/L), but it slightly reduced cell proliferation at concentrations above 40 μM (5.3 mg/L) (Chao et al 2008).

Cardiovascular effects: Cinnamaldehyde shows strong antiplatelet aggregation activity in vitro and in vivo (Huang J et al 2007a). At oral doses of 5, 10 or 20 mg/kg/day for 45 days, cinnamaldehyde dose-dependently decreased plasma glucose concentrations in streptozotocin-diabetic male rats, and 20 mg/kg markedly increased plasma insulin levels (Babu et al 2007).

Nephrotoxicity: Rats were dosed by gavage with 2.14, 6.96, 22.62 or 73.5 mg/kg of cinnamaldehyde for 10, 30 or 90 days. There were histological changes in the kidneys of rats dosed at 73.5 mg/kg for 90 days, proteinuria and creatinuria, and increased activities of renal, serum and urinary enzymes. Other groups of animals were not affected (Gowder & Devaraj 2008). An increased toxicity of gavage dosing in rats with cinnamaldehyde observed by Hébert et al (1994) is not acknowledged or discussed. The increased enzyme activity is consistent with a dose that saturates detoxification mechanisms, which is more likely to occur with gavage dosing. When rats were given microencapsulated cinnamaldehyde in the diet for three months at doses equivalent to 275, 625, 1,300 or 4,000 mg/kg, urinary creatinine and total protein levels were altered only at 1,300 mg/kg or higher (National Toxicology Program 2004).

Reproductive toxicity: Using chick embryos at 72 hours of incubation, Forschmidt (1979) determined that cinnamaldehyde had a teratogenic value of 43.05% relative to a control value of 7.9%. The implications of this for humans is unknown. Cinnamaldehyde was administered by gavage at 1,200 mg/kg/day to 49 pregnant mice on gestational days 6–13. None of the dosed mice died before delivery, and viability in the cinnamaldehyde group was 34 of 34 litters, compared to 39/46 in the control group. There were no significant effects on maternal weight gain or in birth weight compared to controls (Hardin et al 1987). When pregnant rats were given gavage doses of 5, 25 or 250 mg/kg cinnamaldehyde there was a reduction of maternal weight gain in the two higher dose groups. There was no reduction in fertility or live births; in fact cinnamaldehyde dosing significantly increased fertility. Some fetal abnormalities were seen, but these were not dose-dependent, and their significance is difficult to assess from this study (Mantovani et al 1989). Administered to pregnant rats, sc injections of to 50, 75 or 100 mg/kg of cinnamaldehyde in DMSO inhibited fetal malformations induced by 5-azacytidine. Cinnamaldehyde alone, even at 100 mg/kg, did not increase fetal mortality (Kurishita & Ihara 1990).

Every second day 2 mg of cinnamaldehyde po was administered to two generations of rats for 223 days and 210 days, respectively. There were no changes in body weight of adults or offspring, number of pregnant females, development and viability of young, liver protein content or activity of hepatic aldolase. However, hepatic lipid content increased by 20% in the first generation and 22% in the second (Sporn et al 1965).

When female rats and mice were injected with an unspecified dose of cinnamaldehyde, no estrogenic action was observed (Zondek & Bergmann 1938).

Hepatotoxicity: Following ip administration to rats of 0.5 mL/kg cinnamaldehyde, hepatic glutathione was lowered to 53% of control values after 30 minutes and to 35% after two hours (Boyland & Chasseaud 1970). When cinnamaldehyde was administered ip to rats daily for seven days at 25 or 50 mg/kg, glutathione S-transferase activity reduced to ~57% of control values, but glutathione levels were not reduced (Choi et al 2001). In rat hepatocytes, dose-dependent glutathione depletion by cinnamaldehyde occurred to a minimum of 20% of control values, mostly within one hour (Swales & Caldwell 1992). Similar results were observed in Chinese hamster lung fibroblast V79 cells by Glaab et al (2001). However, about fivefold higher concentrations were required to induce similar glutathione depletion in primary human colon cells or in CaCo-2 (human colon tumor) cells. Following rapid hepatocyte glutathione depletion by cinnamaldehyde, ROS were formed and lipid peroxidation was induced, although non-cytotoxic concentrations decreased ROS formation (Niknahad et al 2003).

Antioxidant/pro-oxidant activity: When mouse or human macrophages were incubated with 24 or 80 μM (3.17 or 10.6 mg/L) cinnamaldehyde it was not cytotoxic, but inhibited LPS-induced hydrogen peroxide release and production of the pro-inflammatory cytokines IL-6 and IL-2. Cinnamaldehyde does not scavenge hydrogen peroxide, but rather prevents its generation (Chao et al 2008). This demonstrates both antioxidant and related anti-inflammatory effects that might not be expected from a potential skin sensitizer.

Mutagenicity and genotoxicity: DEREK, a structure-activity model, predicts with 'moderate' confidence that cinnamaldehyde will be mutagenic, as a result of the α,β-unsaturated aldehyde functionality, which may lead to electrophilic and hence DNA reactivity (Marchant 1996). However, the toxicity to bacteria associated with lipophilic compounds of this type may impede adequate mutagenicity testing in *Salmonella* (Eder et al 1992). Ishidate (1984) reported cinnamaldehyde to be mutagenic in the Ames test, but seven similar studies found no mutagenicity (Sasaki & Endo 1978; Kasamaki et al 1982; Lutz et al 1982; Prival et al 1982; Marnett et al 1985; Mortelmans et al 1986; Azizan & Blevins 1995). An NTP report found that cinnamaldehyde was not mutagenic in the Ames test, with and without S9, in strains TA98, TA102, TA104, TA1535 and TA1537, but tested positive in TA100 with mouse S9 (National Toxicology Program 2000). Dillon et al (1998) had previously reported weak mutagenicity in the TA100 strain, but several other workers found no evidence of mutagenicity using this strain (Lijinsky & Andrews 1980; Lutz et al 1982; Sekizawa & Shibamoto 1982; Neudecker et al 1983; Eder et al 1991).

Cinnamaldehyde was mutagenic in a *Bacillus subtilis* DNA repair test assay (Sekizawa & Shibamoto 1982). It was negative in a bacterial reversion test with TA100 and TA98, but gave a positive response in a *E. coli* DNA repair test, indicating a direct reaction with DNA (Stammati et al 1999).

Cinnamaldehyde showed significant antimutagenic activity against some mutagens, but not others. The promotion of a DNA repair system by cinnamaldehyde is suspected, possibly by interfering with an inducible error-prone DNA repair pathway (Ohta et al 1983a, 1983b). Cinnamaldehyde was significantly antimutagenic in *S. typhimurium* strains TA104, but not in TA98 or TA100. This effect was observed at GC sites, but not AT sites. Cinnamaldehyde was thought to reduce mutation through enhancing recombinational repair, and not via an antioxidant action (Shaughnessy et al 2001). Cinnamaldehyde was antimutagenic in gamma-induced mutagenesis *S. typhimurium* strain TA2638 and in UV-induced mutagenesis in *E. coli* WP2s. The action against gamma-induced mutagenesis could be due to radical scavenging (Motohashi et al 2001). Cinnamaldehyde may cause a type of mutagenicity that elicits recombinational repair, which fixes not only the damage caused by cinnamaldehyde, but also other DNA damage. Antimutagenic effects have been seen in both *E. coli* and human colon cancer cells (Shaughnessy et al 2006; King et al 2007).

There are also mixed results in genotoxicity tests. Hayashi et al (1988) reported cinnamaldehyde as non-genotoxic in micronucleus tests in mice, while Mereto et al (1994) observed marginal increases in micronucleated hepatocytes in rats and mice, but a lack of genotoxicity in other assays. In assays using Chinese hamster cells, cinnamaldehyde was negative in two studies, weakly positive in one study, and positive in two studies (Kasamaki et al 1982; Imanishi et al 1990; Fiorio & Bronzetti 1994; Glaab et al 2001; National Toxicology Program 2004). Cinnamaldehyde can cause lethal mutations at high doses in fruit flies (Woodruff et al 1985). In mouse bone marrow cells, cinamaldehyde reduced CA induced by X-rays (Sasaki et al 1990).

Carcinogenic/anticarcinogenic potential: In a two year toxicology and carcinogenesis study, groups of 50 male and 50 female rats were given diets containing 0, 1,000, 2,100 or 4,100 ppm microencapsulated (*E*)-cinnamaldehyde, delivering average daily doses of 0, 50, 100 or 200 mg/kg. Survival of the high dose males was greater than that of controls, and mean body weights and feed consumption in the high dose groups were less than controls. Groups of male and female mice were given the same dietary concentrations, delivering average daily doses of 125, 270 or 550 mg/kg. Feed consumption was similar to that of controls, but mean body weights in the two higher dose groups were generally less than controls. Survival of males in the 2,100 ppm group was lower than controls. There was no evidence of cinnamaldehyde-related carcinogenesis in any of the groups of rodents, nor was there any increase in the incidence of non-neoplastic lesions. In fact, there was a statistically significant *decrease* in the incidence of hepatocellar adenomas and carcinomas in some of the treated mouse groups compared to controls. The primary metabolic pathway was not saturated during the 24 months of exposure (Hooth et al 2004; National Toxicology Program 2004).

Concentrations of 5.0%, 1.0% and 0.1% cinnamaldehyde, painted on 50-day-old mice for three consecutive days, did not suppress non-specific esterase activity in the sebaceous glands of the skin (Barry et al 1972). Suppression of esterase activity has been correlated with carcinogenesis. In male and female mice given 16 ip injections of cinnamaldehyde in impure tricaprylin in a total dose of 0.8 or 4.0 g/kg over 24 weeks the incidence of primary lung tumors was no higher than in the control group (Stoner et al 1973). Dietary cinnamaldehyde at 0.5% for 28 weeks significantly reduced the incidence of lung tumors previously induced with ip injections of NNK in two strains of mouse (Imai et al 2002). Unlike α-asarone or β-asarone, four ip injections of cinnamaldehyde given prior to weaning did not cause hepatomas to develop in mice after 18 months (Wiseman 1987).

Cinnamaldehyde inhibited human melanoma cell proliferation in vitro, and inhibited the proliferation and invasiveness of human melanoma xenografts in mice (Cabello et al 2009). At the high dose of 200 μM (26.4 mg) cinnamaldehyde inhibited the proliferation of DLD-1 human colon cancer cells (Duessel et al 2008). Cinnamaldehyde completely inhibited the growth of ascites sarcoma BP8 cells (a rat cell line), but at the high concentrations of 1.0 and 0.1 mM (132 and 13.2 mg/L) (Pilotti et al 1975). Cinnamaldehyde had a powerful antiproliferative effect on human PLC/PRF/5 hepatoma cells, inducing apoptosis (Wu SJ et al 2004d).

Cinnamaldehyde was cytotoxic to L1210 mouse leukemia cells, inhibiting their growth by 50%. The terminal aldehyde group of the molecule was responsible, and it is thought to operate by blocking protein synthesis in the cell (Moon & Pack 1983). Cinnamaldehyde induced apoptosis in human promyelocytic leukemia cells. The apoptotic signal was transduced via ROS generation, thereby inducing mitochondrial permeability transition and resultant cytochrome c release (Ka et al 2003). Cinnamaldehyde was cytotoxic to K562 human leukemia cells through very similar mechanisms that included intracellular glutathione depletion (Huang T-C et al 2007b). Cinnamaldehyde was cytotoxic to human leukemia HL60 cells with an IC_{50} of 32.62 μg/mL (Nibret & Wink 2010).

Comments: Cinnamaldehyde inhibits ROS generation in macrophages, yet promotes it in leukemia cells and colon cancer cells, demonstrating selective toxicity. The glutathione-depleting action of cinnamaldehyde is not a problem in normal doses of cinnamaldehyde-rich essential oils. Cinnamaldehyde does not quite produce the steady, linear increase in skin reactions correspondent with an increase in concentration, and a small increase can cause a surge in reactions. However, safe levels for dermal application can be extrapolated from the data.

Summary: Cinnamaldehyde is a concentration-dependent skin irritant and sensitizer. In overdose it depletes hepatic glutathione, and subchronic and reproductive toxicity studies describe changes in the liver and kidneys on chronic dosing. The observation that multiple doses of >500 mg/kg are metabolized differently to lower or single doses may partly explain the toxicity seen on chronic dosing. Three investigations have failed to reveal any carcinogenesis, and in several studies the compound showed in vitro cytotoxicity towards cancer cells. Setting aside toxicity related to gavage dosing, the lowest rodent NOAEL was 100 mg/kg in rats, in a two-year study. There are signs of possible reproductive toxicity, but the data are inconclusive. Cinnamaldehyde inhibits platelet aggregation.

Regulatory guidelines: An ADI of 1.25 mg/kg for cinnamaldehyde has been set by the Council of Europe (1992). Cinnamaldehyde is one of the 26 fragrance materials listed as an allergen by the EU. If present in a cosmetic product at over 100 ppm (0.01%) in a wash-off product or 10 ppm (0.001%) in a leave-on product the material must be declared on the ingredient list if sold in an EU member state. The concentration of cinnamaldehyde in the finished cosmetic product should not exceed 0.1% (SCCNFP 2001a). IFRA recommends a maximum dermal use level for cinnamaldehyde of 0.05% for most product types (IFRA 2009). Based on literature published in German, cinnamaldehyde was classified as Category A, a significant contact allergen, by Schlede et al (2003). In a preliminary report by an ECETOC taskforce, cinnamaldehyde was provisionally classified as a moderate allergen (on a scale of extreme, strong, moderate and weak) likely to elicit a sensitization reaction if present at 1% or more (Kimber et al 2003).

Our safety advice: We agree with the IFRA guideline of 0.05% for dermal use of cinnamaldehyde. Essential oils high in cinnamaldehyde should be used with caution in oral doses by diabetics taking drugs to control blood glucose. Because of its antiplatelet aggregation activity, oral dosing of essential oils high in cinnamaldehyde is also cautioned in conjunction with anticoagulant drugs, major surgery, childbirth, peptic ulcer, hemophilia or other bleeding disorders (see Box 7.1 for more detail).

Cinnamic acid

Synonym: β-Phenylacrylic acid
Systematic name: 3-Phenyl-2-propenoic acid
Chemical class: Phenylpropenoid carboxylic acid
Note: Different isomers of cinnamic acid exist, and the following isomer-specific information has been published:

(2E)-Cinnamic acid

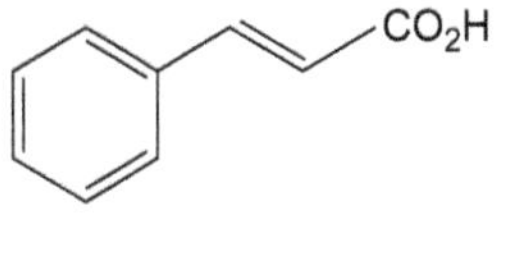

Synonym: *trans*-Cinnamic acid
CAS number: 140-10-3

Sources >1.0%:

Peru balsam	0–5.8%
Styrax (American)	4.8%
Boronia absolute	4.3%
Styrax (Asian)	4.0%
Tolu balsam	2.7%
Benzoin	tr–1.4%
Labdanum	0–1.4%

(2Z)-Cinnamic acid

Synonym: *cis*-Cinnamic acid
CAS number: 102-94-3

Sources >1.0%:

Boronia absolute	1.9%

Pharmacokinetics: Cinnamic acid is produced in vivo by oxidation of cinnamaldehyde (Spector 1956). The majority is excreted in the urine as hippuric acid; dogs, cats, rats and rabbits excrete 39–74%. In man 50–87% is excreted as hippuric acid, and 1–6% as cinnamoyl glucuronide (Scheline 1991). In mice, depending on administered ip dose, 44.2–69.9% was excreted as hippuric acid (increasing with dose size) and 2.4–28.6% as cinnamoylglycine (decreasing with dose size) (Nutley et al 1994).

Drug interactions: Cinnamic acid is a very weak inhibitor of mouse brain monoamine oxidase, with an IC_{50} of 252. µM (37.4 mg/L) (Huong et al 2000).

Adverse skin reactions: Tested at 4% on 25 volunteers cinnamic acid was neither irritating nor sensitizing; positive reactions to 5% cinnamic acid were reported in 32 of 128 patients (25%) previously sensitized to Peru balsam (Opdyke 1978 p. 687–690). Of 102 dermatitis patients sensitive to Peru balsam, 33 tested positive to 5% cinnamic acid (Hausen 2001). Of 184 Japanese dermatitis patients, none was sensitive to 2% cinnamic acid, but one was sensitive to 5% (Ishihara 1978).

Acute toxicity: Acute oral LD_{50} reported as 2.5 g/kg, 3.4 g/kg and 4.45 g/kg in rats, and >5.0 g/kg in rat, mouse and guinea pig; acute dermal LD_{50} in rabbits >5 g/kg (Zaitsev & Rakhmanina 1974; Opdyke 1978 p. 687–690; Adams et al 2004).

Reproductive toxicity: Cinnamic acid was administered to pregnant rats in oral doses of 5 or 50 mg/kg throughout the course of pregnancy. No embryotoxic effects were observed, and offspring were normal with regard to body weight, size, survival, and general development (Zaitsev & Maganova 1975). In an ex vivo assay, cinnamic acid did not bind to estrogen receptors in female rat uterus tissue (Blair et al 2000).

Hepatotoxicity: Cinnamic acid does not deplete hepatic glutathione (Swales & Caldwell 1992).

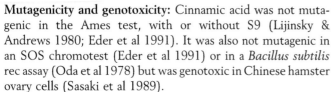

Mutagenicity and genotoxicity: Cinnamic acid was not mutagenic in the Ames test, with or without S9 (Lijinsky & Andrews 1980; Eder et al 1991). It was also not mutagenic in an SOS chromotest (Eder et al 1991) or in a *Bacillus subtilis* rec assay (Oda et al 1978) but was genotoxic in Chinese hamster ovary cells (Sasaki et al 1989).

Summary: Cinnamic acid may be allergenic to fragrance-sensitive individuals. It possesses 'slight' acute toxicity, is not reproductively toxic, and there is one report of mutagenicity.

Cinnamyl acetate

Systematic name: 3-Phenyl-2-propenyl ethanoate
Chemical class: Phenylpropenoid ester
Note: Different isomers of cinnamyl acetate exist, and the following isomer-specific information has been published:

(2*E*)-Cinnamyl acetate

Synonym: *trans*-Cinnamyl acetate
CAS number: 21040-45-9

(2*Z*)-Cinnamyl acetate

Synonym: *cis*-Cinnamyl acetate
CAS number: 77134-01-1

Sources >1.0%:

Cassia leaf	1.4–12.5%
Cinnamon bark	0.3–10.6%
Cassia bark	0.1–5.4%
Cinnamon leaf	0.8–4.6%
Ylang-ylang	0.3–4.0%
Bakul absolute	1.2%
Boswellia sacra (α-pinene CT)	0–1.0%

Adverse skin reactions: Undiluted cinnamyl acetate was non-irritant when tested on pigs, was mildly irritant to guinea pigs, and moderately irritant to rabbits. A semi-occluded patch test with 32% cinnamyl acetate on 50 male volunteers was assessed as mildly irritating. There were no irritant or allergic reactions when it was tested at 5% on 25 human volunteers (Bhatia et al 2007a).

Acute toxicity: Rat acute oral LD_{50} 3.3 g/kg, rabbit acute dermal LD_{50} >5 g/kg (Opdyke 1973 p. 1063). Mouse ip LD_{50} 1.2 g/kg (Powers et al 1961).

Mutagenicity and genotoxicity: Cinnamyl acetate was not mutagenic in an Ames test (RIFM 2003, cited in Bhatia et al 2007b), and was not genotoxic in Chinese hamster ovary cells (Sasaki et al 1989).

Summary: Cinnamyl acetate is virtually non-irritating to the skin, is non-mutagenic, and there are no acute toxicity concerns.

Cinnamyl alcohol

Synonym: Cinnamic alcohol
Systematic name: 3-Phenyl-2-propen-1-ol
Chemical class: Phenylpropenoid alcohol

Note: Different isomers of cinnamyl alcohol exist, and the following isomer-specific information has been published:

(2*E*)-Cinnamyl alcohol

Synonym: *trans*-Cinnamyl alcohol
CAS number: 4407-36-7

Sources >0.1%:

Bakul absolute	13.7%
Hyacinth absolute	11.0%
Styrax (American)	4.1%
Narcissus absolute	0.8–2.9%
Styrax (Asian)	2.0%
Cinnamon leaf	0–0.6%
Cassia leaf	0–0.2%

(2*Z*)-Cinnamyl alcohol

Synonym: *cis*-Cinnamyl alcohol
CAS number: 4510-34-3

Pharmacokinetics: The most significant urinary metabolites after ip dosing in rats are hippuric acid (the glycine conjugate of benzoic acid), 3-hydroxy-3-phenylpropanoic acid and a glutathione conjugate. Some unchanged cinnamyl alcohol was also found. In rabbits, cinnamic acid and benzoic acid were the chief urinary metabolites following oral administration, as well as some 3-phenylpropanol and unchanged cinnamyl alcohol (Scheline 1991 p. 42). Topically applied cinnamyl alcohol is converted by enzymes in the skin to cinnamic acid and cinnamaldehyde. The conversion to the latter compound is thought to be primarily responsible for any skin sensitizing action of cinnamyl alcohol (Smith et al 2000; Cheung et al 2003).

Adverse skin reactions: A patch test using undiluted cinnamyl alcohol for 24 hours produced no irritation reactions in 20 human subjects (Katz 1946). In tests using various excipients, 10% cinnamyl alcohol produced no irritation reactions in a total of 476 male and female volunteers (Letizia et al 2005). In a 48 hour occlusive patch test on 50 volunteers, the highest concentration of cinnamyl alcohol producing no adverse reaction was 10%. Similarly tested at 0.5%, it produced one reaction in 414 eczema patients (Meneghini et al 1971). In a similar test, cinnamyl alcohol produced reactions in 21 of 577 Japanese patients with dermatoses (3.6%) when tested at 0.2% (Fujii et al 1972). Cinnamyl alcohol produced one irritation reaction in 24 Japanese Americans at when tested at 4% (RIFM 1979b, cited in Letizia et al 2005).

Tested at 4% on 25 volunteers cinnamyl alcohol was not sensitizing (Opdyke 1974 p. 855–856). Tested at 10% in 21 panels of volunteers, cinnamyl alcohol produced 71 sensitization reactions in a total of 527 maximation tests (13.47%). In human repeat insult patch tests, cinnamyl alcohol was sensitizing in 7 of 259 volunteers (2.7%) (Letizia et al 2005). In a modified Draize procedure on guinea pigs, cinnamyl alcohol was non-sensitizing when used at 10% in the challenge phase (Sharp 1978).

When cinnamyl alcohol was patch tested at 5% on 50 dermatitis patients who were not thought to be sensitive to fragrance there were no positive reactions (Larsen 1977). When tested at 5%, 34 of 441 (7.7%) eczema patients reacted to cinnamyl alcohol (Mitchell et al 1982). Of 241 patients tested with 2% cinnamyl alcohol, nine (3.7%) had a positive reaction (Ferguson & Sharma 1984). Of 1,200 dermatitis patients patch tested, there were no irritant reactions and nine allergic reactions (0.75%) to 3% cinnamyl alcohol. In a second group of 1,500 dermatitis patients there were no irritant reactions and five allergic reactions (0.33%) to 1% cinnamyl alcohol (Santucci et al 1987). In a European multicenter study six of 1,072 dermatitis patients (0.56%) reacted to 1% cinnamyl alcohol (Frosch et al 1995a). Four of 702 dermatitis patients (0.57%) tested positive to 1% cinnamyl alcohol (Frosch et al 1995b). The results of two further European studies are reported in Table 5.10.

In a prospective study of adverse skin reactions to cosmetic ingredients identified by patch test (1977–1980) cinnamyl alcohol was responsible for 14 cases (2.9%) of contact dermatitis of 487 cosmetic-related cases (Eiermann et al 1982). Of 713 cosmetic dermatitis patients, 17 reacted to cinnamyl alcohol (Adams & Maibach 1985). Of 18,747 dermatitis patients, 1,781 had contact dermatitis and one (0.005% of dermatitis patients and 0.06% of contact dermatitis patients) was allergic to cinnamyl alcohol. Of the 1,781 patients 75 were allergic to cosmetic products, so the one reaction constituted 1.4% of this group (De Groot 1987).

In 20 eczema patients suspected of suffering from contact sensitization to cosmetics, there were no reactions to 5% cinnamyl alcohol on patch testing. Of 182 dermatitis patients suspected of contact allergy to cosmetics, 19 (10.5%) tested positive to 5% cinnamyl alcohol (Malten et al 1984). Of 167 dermatitis patients suspected of fragrance sensitivity 11 (6.6%) were allergic to 5% cinnamyl alcohol on patch testing (Larsen et al 1996b).

Cinnamyl alcohol tested positive in 6 of 156 (3.8%) eczema patients with contact allergy to cosmetics (Broneck et al 1987). Of 119 eczema patients with contact allergy to cosmetics 2 (1.7%) were allergic to 5% cinnamyl alcohol (De Groot et al 1988). In 578 cases of eczema patients known to be sensitized to cosmetics, 17 (3%) tested positive to cinnamyl alcohol (Adams & Maibach 1985). There were positive reactions to cinnamyl alcohol in 26 of 144 patients (18%) already sensitized to Peru balsam (Opdyke 1974 p. 855–856). Of 102 dermatitis patients sensitive to Peru balsam, 38 tested positive to 5% cinnamyl alcohol (Hausen 2001). When patch tested at 5% on 20 dermatitis patients who were sensitive to fragrance, cinnamyl alcohol induced 15 (75%) positive reactions (Larsen 1977).

Although cinnamyl alcohol itself can induce concentration-dependent hypersensitivity, data from a total of 16,530 patch tests indicates that, as present in consumer products and fragrance blends, cinnamyl alcohol has no detectable potential to induce hypersensitivity (Steltenkamp 1980b). From a total of 25,545 dermatitis patients patch tested from January1980 to December 1996 in the UK, a significant and steady reduction (9% per year) could be deduced in the frequency of sensitivity to cinnamyl alcohol (Buckley et al 2000).

Acute toxicity: Rat acute oral LD$_{50}$ reported as 2.68 g/kg and 2.0 g/kg, rabbit acute dermal LD$_{50}$ >5 g/kg (Opdyke 1974 p. 855–856; Zaitsev & Rakhmanina 1974).

Reproductive toxicity: Using chick embryos at 72 hours of incubation, Forschmidt (1979) determined that cinnamyl alcohol had a teratogenic value of 29.6% relative to a control value of 7.9%. The implications of this for humans are unknown. Cinnamyl alcohol was orally administered to female rats at 0 or 535 mg/kg either on day 4 or days 10–12 of pregnancy, and fetuses were examined on day 20. There were no differences between test and control animals in respect to survival, body weight and hepatic nucleic acids, nor in respect to malformations of the eyes, brain, or internal organs. However there was a slight reduction in skeletal ossification of the extremities. In a second study, cinnamyl alcohol was administered orally to female rats at 0 or 53.5 mg/kg on gestational days 1–20 (i.e., throughout pregnancy). Some fetuses were examined on day 20, and there were no treatment-related effects on survival, body weight, bone development, structural abnormalities or hepatic nucleic acids. The remaining fetuses were delivered normally, and were observed at birth and at one month. Using the same parameters no adverse effects were seen at either time point, and general development was considered to be normal (Zaitsev & Maganova 1975).

Mutagenicity and genotoxicity: Cinnamyl alcohol was not mutagenic in the Ames test, but was positive in the *Bacillus subtilis* DNA repair test (Sekizawa & Shibamoto 1982). Eder et al (1980) found cinnamyl alcohol negative in five strains of *S. typhimurium*. Cinnamyl alcohol did not induce SCE in cultured Chinese hamster ovary cells (Sasaki et al 1989). Cinnamyl alcohol was not mutagenic in one *Bacillus subtilis* rec assay (Oda et al 1978), but was mutagenic in another (Yoo 1986).

Carcinogenic/anticarcinogenic potential: In male and female mice given 14 ip injections of cinnamyl alcohol in impure tricaprylin in a total dose of 1.4 or 7.0 g/kg over 24 weeks the incidence of primary lung tumors was no higher than in the control group (Stoner et al 1973).

Comments: With only 0.33–0.56% of dermatitis patients reacting to a 1% concentration, and considering the low levels of cinnamyl alcohol in essential oils and absolutes (it is not likely to be present at more than 0.25%) it carries a low risk of skin sensitization in an aromatherapy context. The rat reproductive toxicity findings suggest a NOAEL somewhere between 53.5 and 535 mg/kg/day.

Summary: Synthetic cinnamyl alcohol is a moderate risk allergen, possesses moderate acute toxicity, and is not teratogenic or mutagenic.

Regulatory guidelines: Cinnamyl alcohol is one of the 26 fragrance materials listed as an allergen by the EU. If present in a cosmetic product at over 100 ppm (0.01%) in a wash-off product or 10 ppm (0.001%) in a leave-on product the material must be declared on the ingredient list if sold in an EU member state. Cinnamyl alcohol should not be used at more than 0.8% in cosmetic products in the EU (SCCNFP 2001a), and it should not be used such that the level in consumer products exceeds 0.4% in most product types (IFRA 2009). This recommendation is based on test results showing a weak sensitizing potential for the individual ingredient (private communication to IFRA) and the absence of sensitizing reactions in tests of a considerable number of formulations containing cinnamic alcohol (Steltenkamp et al 1980b).

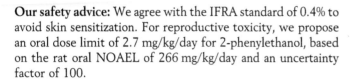

Our safety advice: We agree with the IFRA standard of 0.4% to avoid skin sensitization. For reproductive toxicity, we propose an oral dose limit of 2.7 mg/kg/day for 2-phenylethanol, based on the rat oral NOAEL of 266 mg/kg/day and an uncertainty factor of 100.

Cinnamyl cinnamate

Synonym: 3-Phenylallyl cinnamate
Systematic name: 3-Phenyl-2-propen-1-yl 3-phenyl-2-propenoate
Chemical class: Phenylpropenoid ester
Note: Different isomers of cinnamyl cinnamate exist, and the following isomer-specific information has been published:

(*E,E*)-Cinnamyl cinnamate

Synonym: *trans, trans*-Cinnamyl cinnamate
CAS number: 40918-97-6

(*Z,E*)-Cinnamyl cinnamate

Synonym: *cis, trans*-Cinnamyl cinnamate
CAS number: 61019-10-1

(*E,Z*)-Cinnamyl cinnamate

Synonym: *trans, cis*-Cinnamyl cinnamate
CAS number: Not found

(*Z,Z*)-Cinnamyl cinnamate

Synonym: *cis, cis*-Cinnamyl cinnamate
CAS number: Not found

Sources >1.0%:

Styrax (American)	38.0%
Styrax (Asian)	21.0%

Adverse skin reactions: Undiluted cinnamyl cinnamate was non-irritant to rabbits, and was neither irritant nor sensitizing when tested at 4% on human volunteers (Opdyke 1975 p. 753–754). Of 102 dermatitis patients sensitive to Peru balsam, 20 tested positive to 5% cinnamyl cinnamate (Hausen 2001). UV spectral data suggest that cinnamyl cinnamate has no potential for phototoxicity or photoallergy (Belsito et al 2007).
Acute toxicity: Rat acute oral LD$_{50}$ 4.2 g/kg, rabbit acute dermal LD$_{50}$ >5 g/kg (Opdyke 1975 p. 753–754).
Summary: Cinnamyl cinnamate is non-irritant, and is only allergenic in some fragrance-sensitive individuals. It is only minimally toxic.

Citral

Systematic name: 3,7-Dimethyl-2,6-octadienal
Chemical class: Aliphatic monoterpenoid alkene aldehyde

Notes: Citral occurs naturally as a mixture of the two geometric isomers, geranial (citral a, (*E*)- or α-citral) and neral (citral b, (*Z*)- or β-citral). Commercial citral typically contains 60–65% geranial and 35–40% neral. Although citral is not a single compound, it is included here because it has been the subject of very much more research than either of its isomers. Since citral is a mixture of two isomers, both of which are subject to variation, we cannot accurately state precise ranges in essential oils.
CAS number: 5392-40-5

Sources >1.0%:

Myrtle (lemon)	<90.0%
Lemongrass (East Indian)	~83.0% (<90%)*
Lemongrass (West Indian)	~77.0% (<90%)*
Tea tree (lemon-scented)	~77%
May chang	<74.0% (<78%)*
Verbena (lemon)	<68.0%
Myrtle (honey)	~66.5%
Melissa	<64.4%
Lemon leaf	<50.0% (<26%)*
Basil (lemon)	<42.2 %
Lemon balm (Australian)	~17.6%
Thyme (lemon)	~16.3%
Lime (expressed)	~4.0% (<6.5%)*
Bergamot (wild)	~3.0%
Lemon (distilled)	~2.5% (<3%)*
Lemon (expressed)	~2.5% (<3%)*
Orange (sweet)	<1.5%
Palmarosa	~1.2%

Pharmacokinetics: In rats, citral is rapidly and completely absorbed from the GI tract and then redistributed equally to all the tissues. Within 24 hours 61% is excreted in the urine, 17% in the feces and 20% in the expired air. Rats and mice can eliminate all of a single oral dose of citral (up to 1 g/kg) within 72 hours and 120 hours, respectively (Phillips et al 1976). Citral is significantly (27%) eliminated in the bile by rats, although most of its metabolites are lost in the urine (Diliberto et al 1988a, 1988b). In rabbits, citral is regioselectively oxidized and a (*E*)-methyl group was carboxylated (Ishida et at 1989). In rabbits, geranic acid and 8-carboxygeranic (Hildebrandt) acid are excreted in the urine (Scheline 1991).

Citral potently inhibited the high affinity form of rat mitochondrial aldehyde dehydrogenase in vitro, an enzyme formerly suggested to be involved in its oxidation. This finding may have important consequences for the oxidation of endogenous aldehydes (Boyer & Petersen 1991). Citral induced rat microsomal CYP4A1 (Roffey et al 1990).
Adverse skin reactions: In a cumulative irritation study, with patches being replaced every day for 21 days, citral was tested on eight volunteers in concentrations of 1, 4 and 8%. The 8% concentration was marginally irritant. There were no irritation reactions in twelve different panels of volunteers when numerous samples of citral were closed-patch tested for 48 hours at concentrations ranging from 1% to 8% (Opdyke 1979a p. 259–266). In 100

*IFRA values

consecutive dermatitis patients tested with 1% citral there were two irritant reactions and no allergic reactions (Frosch et al 1995a). Some irritancy is only evident at raised temperatures: citral causes contact dermatitis when the skin is exposed to hot cleaning solutions containing it (Rothenborg et al 1977).

In panels averaging 25 volunteers, maximation tests were conducted using samples of different types of citral (e.g., from lemongrass oil, synthetic, 'refined', 'pure') at various concentrations. One sample tested at 8% resulted in eight (32%) positive reactions. Five samples tested at 5% produced 8, 10, 12, 14 and 16 positive rections (32%, 40%, 48%, 56%, 64%, respectively). Six samples tested at 4% resulted in 3, 3, 4, 5, 5 and 9 positive reactions (12%, 16%, 20%, 36%, respectively). Maximation tests were also conducted in panels with citral at 2%, 0.5% and 0.1%, which resulted in 2/24, 2/25 and 1/25 reactions, respectively (8.3%, 8% and 4%) (Opdyke 1979a p. 259–266).

Of 115 dermatitis patients suspected of contact allergy to cosmetics 12 (10.5%) tested positive to 8% citral. Five of 182 dermatitis patients suspected of cosmetic sensitivity (2.6%) tested positive to 2% citral (Malten et al 1984). In a multicenter study conducted from September 1988 to April 1989, 19 of 1,825 dermatitis patients (1.0%) were sensitive to 2% citral (De Groot et al 2000). There were six positive reactions to 1.0% (0.36%) and 12 to 2.0% citral (0.7%) in 1,701 dermatitis patients (Frosch et al 2005a). Tested at 1% on 228 dermatitis patients, citral produced four (1.7%) positive results (Mitchell et al 1982). Tested on 658 people with hand eczema at three concentrations, citral produced 28 reactions (4.25%) at 2%, three reactions (0.46%) at 1%, and one reaction (0.15%) at 0.5% (Heydorn et al 2003b). The results of two further European studies are reported in Table 5.10.

A total of 22 induced sensitizations occurred in 174 tests conducted with 1% to 5% citral in ethanol, while no inductions occurred at the 0.5% level in 82 test subjects. No subject demonstrated pre-existing sensitization to any of the personal care products containing citral in 10,660 patch tests, and none of these products induced hypersensitivity that could be attributed to citral. In tests where citral was applied alone in solvent at concentrations of 1% or greater hypersensitivity was observed. Induction of sensitization to citral appears to be dose related, since there were no confirmed reactions to citral in 2,098 patch tests with fragrance blends containing it at concentrations below 0.5%. There were seven cases of sensitization but the causative agent was not identified (Steltenkamp et al 1980a). A bartender with hand dermatitis was allergic to lemon peel, and patch testing resulted in a positive reaction to citral (Cardullo et al 1989).

Sensitization to citral can be reduced by the co-presence of (+)-limonene or α-pinene (Opdyke 1976 p. 197–198; Hanau et al 1983). Lemon leaf oil (~41.0% citral) was not sensitizing to a panel of 25 volunteers when tested at 10% (Opdyke 1978 p. 807) nor was may chang oil (~68.0% citral) when tested similarly at 8% (Opdyke 1982). This is equivalent to citral not causing sensitization at concentrations of 4.1% and 5.4%, possibly due to the presence of 19.4% and 15.5% of limonene, respectively, in those two essential oils. Very small amounts of α-pinene are also present.

A receptor-mediated mechanism may be responsible for citral's reported ability to cause sebaceous gland proliferation when applied for 90 days to the backs of male rats (Sandbank et al 1988). Essential oils high in citral have been known to turn the skin a yellow color if applied in concentrated amounts.

Acute toxicity: Acute oral LD$_{50}$ in rats 4.96 g/kg (Jenner et al 1964). The maximum non-lethal dose in mice was reported as 900 mg/kg orally and 250 mg/kg ip (Le Bourhis & Soenen 1973). Dermal LD$_{50}$ in rabbits 2.25 g/kg (Opdyke 1979a p. 259–266).

Subacute and subchronic toxicity: Given to Wistar rats either orally or ip for three days, citral increased by 25% the activity of CYP, glucuronyl transferase, 4-nitrobenzoate reductase and biphenyl 4-hydroxylase (Parke & Rahman 1969; Roffey et al 1990). Given to Osborne-Mendel rats for 13 weeks, there was no observable adverse effect from citral at doses of 1,000, 2,500 or 10,000 ppm in the diet (Hagan et al 1967). In a 14 week study, groups of 20 F344/N rats and 10 B6C3F1 mice of each sex were fed microencapsulated citral at 3,900, 7,800, 15,600 or 31,300 ppm. Microencapsulation was used to minimize evaporation of citral. At the highest dose, all the rats and four of the ten male mice died and in rats only, forestomach and kidney lesions were seen. At the highest two doses, lesions occurred in bone marrow, thymus and testes in rats, and ovaries in female mice (Ress et al 2003). NOAEL values of 10,000 ppm (500 mg/kg) for rats, and 7,800 ppm (905 mg/kg) for mice can be extrapolated from the above findings.

There is conflicting evidence concerning citral and ocular tension. In one study, a very low daily oral dose (2–5 µg) produced an increase in intra-ocular pressure within two weeks in monkeys, and 5 µg/kg was said to produce a long-standing elevation of intra-ocular pressure in rabbits after one or two days (Leach & Lloyd 1956a). However a later study failed to find any such effect after giving rabbits doses of 10 µg/kg for 5 days, then either 25, 50, 250 or 500 µg/kg for 12 days, followed by 1,000 µg/kg for a further six days (Berggren 1957). In a clinical study of citral as a treatment for bladder cancer, 44 patients took 4 mL citral daily for varying periods of time. Three of these were randomly selected, and underwent opthalmological examinations pre- and post-treatment. There were no signs that citral dosing had any adverse effect on their eyes (Morrow 1960).

Cardiovascular toxicity: Gavage doses of 10, 15 or 20 mg/kg/day citral for 28 days, dose-dependently lowered plasma insulin levels and increased glucose tolerance in obese rats (Modak & Mukhopadhaya 2011).

Reproductive toxicity: Using chick embryos at 72 hours of incubation, Forschmidt (1979) determined that citral had a teratogenic value of 60.1% relative to a control value of 7.9%. Citral has produced malformations in chick embryos when injected into fertilized hen's eggs (Aydelotte 1963; Abramovici 1972). It often induces abnormal eye development (Abramovici et al 1978). Citral impaired reproductive performance in female Wistar rats by reducing the number of normal ovarian follicles. This was apparent after a series of six monthly ip injections at 300 mg/kg, or after topical administration for 60 or 100 days at 460 mg/kg/day. There was no apparent endocrine effect, since neither the estrus cycle nor the histology of the uterus were affected (Toaff et al 1979).

Meiosis and early fetal development are stimulated by endogenous retinoic acid, and citral is an inhibitor of the enzyme ALDH1A1 that catalyzes the synthesis of retinoic acid from retinaldehyde. Using cultured human fetal ovary tissues, a dose of 55 µM citral partially prevented the initiation of meiosis (Le Bouffant et al 2010). When treated sub-blastodermally with high doses of citral (100–200 mM), chick embryos developed caudal neural tube defects in 51.4% of recovered embryos. This was prevented by co-administering retinoic acid. However, there was no increase in mortality (Griffith & Zile 2000). When *Xenopus* embryos were treated with 60 mM citral at various stages of development, a range of effects were seen, from a dose-dependent reduction in embryo length to embryo death. However, citral reversed the teratogenic effects caused by high levels of retinoic acid when administered at the late blastula/early gastrula stage (Schuh et al 1993).

Tooth development was totally blocked in 7/10 CD-1 Swiss mouse embryonic mandible explants when exposed to 1.75 µM citral for 24 hours. The remaining explants developed only to the bud stage after two weeks in culture. Retinoic acid administration restored odontogenesis to varying degrees (Kronmiller et al 1995). In the developing ICR mouse cranial base, a dose of 1 mg/mL citral (6.6 mM) caused a reduction in the thickness of the hypertrophic zone and retarded inhibition of size-enlargement of the hypertrophic chondrocytes. It also increased programmed cell death of chondrocytes within the spheno-occipital synchondrosis region (Kwon et al 2011). Intra-abdominal injections of citral into pregnant BALB/c mice at below 1 µL/g (~6 µmol/g) had no effect on embryos, whilst doses higher than 6 µL/g (~35 µmol/g) (maximum not stated) resulted in transient retardation of normal fetal cranial bone formation and tooth development. However, no noticeable effects were apparent by adulthood. The authors concluded that citral is safe for the public at these doses (Koussoulakou et al 2011).

Studies in pregnant Sprague–Dawley rats suggest that citral is non-fetotoxic by inhalation. Animals were exposed to 10, 34 or 68 ppm citral for six hours per day on gestational days 6–15, and there were no adverse effects on the number of corporea lutea, implantations, reporptions, fetal viability, litter size or sex ratio, and no visceral or skeletal malformations were seen (Gaworski et al 1992). However, oral dosing seems to be more toxic. Citral was given by corn oil gavage to pregnant Wistar rats on gestational days 6–15 at 60, 125, 250 500 or 1,000 mg/kg. Decreases in weight gain indicated some maternal toxicity over the dose range tested and a slight but statistically significant increase in resorptions per implantation occurred with 60 and 125 mg/kg. Doses higher than 125 mg/kg reduced dose-dependently the ratio of pregnancy per mated female, and signs of slight teratogenicity were found in doses higher than 60 mg/kg (Nogueira et al 1995). Since adverse effects at 60 mg/kg were not significant, the rat NOAEL for citral embryofeto-toxicity is 60 mg/kg.

In male Wistar rats, dermal administration of 185 mg/kg/day of citral for three months produced benign prostatic hyperplasia (Abramovici et al 1985) which may be testosterone-dependent (Servadio et al 1986). Later studies suggested that citral could act synergistically with testosterone (Engelstein et al 1996). Other work suggests that the effect occurs via competition with estrogen receptors and that citral has an estrogenic effect in causing vaginal hyperplasia in rats (Geldof et al 1992). Female animals were given 27 mg of citral vaginally for four days, 62 mg was applied to the backs of male rats three times a week for one

or two weeks. Further work demonstrated that the Wistar and Sprague–Dawley strains were susceptible to developing BPH, but that the F344 and Acl/Ztm rat strains remained resistant to treatment with citral (Scolnik et al 1994a). Citral-induced BPH may therefore be mediated via a non-specific inflammatory reaction, and not an endocrine one (Scolnik et al 1994b).

Citral displaced [^{3}H]17β-estradiol from isolated human ERα and ERβ receptors at concentrations 4–5 orders of magnitude higher than estradiol. However, citral lacked estrogenic or anti-estrogenic activity in either an estrogen-responsive human cell line (below cytotoxic concentrations) or a yeast screen for androgenic and anti-androgenic compounds. In yeast cell-expressed human estrogen receptors, citral showed very weak agonist activity (Howes et al 2002).

Mutagenicity and genotoxicity: Citral was not mutagenic the Ames test, with or without S9 (Lutz et al 1982; Ishidate et al 1984; Zeiger et al 1987; Gomes-Carneiro et al 1998; National Toxicology Program 2003). Citral was antimutagenic through concentration-dependent, competitive inhibition of PROD, with an IC$_{50}$ of 1.19 µM (181 µg/L) (De-Oliveira et al 1997). Ishidate et al (1984) reported that citral was not genotoxic in Chinese hamster cells. In the same test, the National Toxicology Program (2003) reported no CA, but did observe SCE. In a mouse micronucleus test, citral was not genotoxic (National Toxicology Program 2003). In another mouse micronucleus test, citral inhibited the clastogenic activity of nickel chloride, and scavenged superoxide radicals with an IC$_{50}$ of 19 µg/mL (Rabbani et al 2006).

Chronic toxicity and carcinogenic/anticarcinogenic potential: Citral dose- and time-dependently induces glutathione S-transferase, and neral is primarily responsible for this activity (Nakamura et al 2003). Citral inhibits the oxidation of retinol to retinoic acid in mouse epidermis, and thereby interferes with tissue morphogenesis and tumor production (Connor 1991; Tanaka et al 1996). There is one report of citral causing hemolysis in vitro via a free radical mechanism (Tamir et al 1984) and another that it can quicken the neoplastic response of hamster trachea in vitro to benzo[a]pyrene (Crocker & Sanders 1970).

Thomas & Pasternak (1969) found that citral (21 µM; 3.19 mg/L) inhibited the growth of P815Y mast-cell tumors by 50% and Zolotovich et al (1967, 1969) reported the aldehyde's marked cytotoxic effect on HeLa cells. The proliferation of mouse B16 melanoma cells was very weakly inhibited by citral with an IC$_{50}$ of 30 mM (4.56 g/L) (Tatman & Huanbiao 2002). Citral induced apoptosis in human leukemia (HL-60) cells (Hata et al 2003). It also induced apoptosis in two mouse and two human leukemia cell lines, with no toxicity to normal spleen cells. Apoptosis was associated DNA fragmentation and caspase-3 induction, and was dependent on the α,β-unsaturated group in the molecule (Dudai et al 2005).

Citral produced an (unquantified) retardation of tumor growth in mice given 10 mg per day (Boyland & Mawson 1938). It significantly inhibited the growth of spontaneous carcinomas and, to a lesser extent, of grafted sarcomas when fed to mice at 25 mg per day (Boyland 1940). Treatment of tumor-bearing rats and mice with citral produced cytotoxic changes in the nuclear membrane, chromatin and nucleolus of Yoshida ascites sarcoma and Ehrlich ascites hepatoma cells (Osato et al 1961). Citral (5% emulsion given im) and citronellal (given orally) together were used to treat 121 cases of advanced carcinoma. Of these six (5%) were said to be cured, having been followed up for 10–15 years (Osato 1965).

In a clinical study of citral as a treatment for bladder cancer, 44 patients with progressive, uncontrolled disease, took 4 mL citral daily; 18 of them for less than 4 months, and 26 for more than 4 months. Six of the 26 experienced significant tumor regression over time. Liver function test results were not affected by citral dosing, and there was no evidence of bone marrow depression. Mild skin rashes developed in four patients on the face and/or limbs, and were considered to be due to citral. They first appeared 2–5 months after the commencement of therapy, and disappeared when citral dosing was reduced or discontinued (Morrow 1960).

In 2-year feed studies, citral was not carcinogenic to male or female F344/N rats exposed to 1,000, 2,000, or 4,000 ppm (equivalent to approximately 50, 100 and 210 mg/kg/day). It was also not carcinogenic to male B6C3F1 mice ingesting 500, 1,000, or 2,000 ppm citral (equivalent to approximately 60, 120 and 260 mg/kg/day). There was equivocal evidence of carcinogenic activity in female mice based on increased incidences of malignant lymphoma. However, incidences were within the NTP historical control range, and could not be definitively linked to citral dosing. There were no other clinical findings in either rats or mice that suggested adverse effects at any dose (National Toxicology Program 2003; Ress et al 2003).
Comments: We do not support the IFRA QRA approach for citral. A critique of QRA can be found on Ch. 5, p. 94. However, we agree with 0.6% as a guideline dermal maximum for citral. The work by Leach & Lloyd (1956b) on ocular tension and cardiovascular damage should be regarded with circumspection. The weight of evidence strongly suggests that citral is not estrogenic in humans.
Summary: Citral has a clear potential to elicit skin sensitization, although there is debate about whether some of the reactions to citral may have been due to irritation (Heydorn et al 2003a). Citral is not sensitizing at concentrations of 0.5% or less, and higher concentrations may not be sensitizing in the co-presence of quenching agents. Therefore, for general use, a maximum dermal use level of 0.6% citral seems reasonable, in the absence of specific data for an essential oil. According to some sources, limonene can reduce the severity of sensitization elicited by citral, although the validity of this phenomenon has been questioned. Citral may be a female mouse-specific carcinogen. It has been reported to be non-mutagenic, antimutagenic, genotoxic, non-genotoxic and antigenotoxic. NOAEL values of 500 mg/kg for rats and 950 mg/kg for mice suggest that no dose limitation is required for citral (except in pregnancy). Citral is slightly teratogenic on oral dosing, due to inhibition of retinoic acid synthesis, but inhalation appears to be non-teratogenic. High doses of citral cause BPH in some rat strains, and not others. It is likely that citral has no estrogenic action.
Regulatory guidelines: JECFA has set a group ADI of 0 to 0.5 mg/kg bw (expressed as citral) for citral, citronellol, geranyl acetate, linalool and linalyl acetate (JECFA 1999a). Citral is one of the 26 fragrance materials listed as an allergen by the EU. If present in a cosmetic product at over 100 ppm (0.01%) in a wash-off product or 10 ppm (0.001%) in a leave-on product the material must be declared on the ingredient list if sold in

an EU member state. In a preliminary report by an ECETOC taskforce, citral was provisionally classified as a weak allergen (on a scale of extreme, strong, moderate and weak) only likely to elicit a sensitization reaction if present at 3% or more (Kimber et al 2003). The IFRA standard for citral in leave-on products such as body lotions is 0.6%, for skin sensitization.
Our safety advice: For reproductive toxicity, we propose an oral dose limit of 0.6 mg/kg/day, based on the female rat NOAEL of 60 mg/kg/day, and an uncertainty factor of 100. We agree with the IFRA standard of 0.6% for skin sensitization, and this is more than enough to guard against reproductive toxicity from external use. Essential oils high in citral should be used with caution in oral doses by diabetics taking drugs to control blood glucose.

β-Citronellal

Synonyms: Citronellal. 2,3-Dihydrocitral
Systematic name: 3,7-Dimethyl-6-octenal
Chemical class: Aliphatic monoterpenoid alkene aldehyde
Note: Different isomers of β-citronellal exist, and the following isomer-specific information has been published:

(3R)-(+)-β-Citronellal

CAS number: 2385-77-5

(3S)-(−)-β-Citronellal

CAS number: 5949-05-3

Sources >1.0%:

Lemon-scented gum	66.9–86.2%
Combava leaf	58.9–81.5%
Citronella (Sri Lankan)	5.2–46.8%
Citronella (Javanese)	34.8–42.8%
Combava fruit	0.4–16.8%
Melissa	4.5–13.3%
Tea tree (lemon-scented)	6.8%
Lemon leaf	1.5–2.9%

Pharmacokinetics: In rabbits citronellal is largely conjugated with glucuronic acid (~25%) and a proportion is excreted as a dicarboxylic acid (Scheline 1991 p. 87).
Adverse skin reactions: Tested at 4% on 25 volunteers citronellal was neither irritating nor sensitizing. However, it is also reportedly a mild irritant, it can cause occasional sensitization, and is believed to be the cause of eczematous irritation from citronella oil (Opdyke 1975 p. 755–756). None of 70 patients with contact dermatitis reacted to 1% citronellal (Nethercott et al 1989). There have been several reports of contact dermatitis from citronella oil; in two instances patch testing showed that citronellal was responsible (Keil 1947; Davies et al 1978). In an in vitro assay, citronellal was non-phototoxic (Placzek et al 2007).
Acute toxicity: Acute oral LD_{50} in rats >5 g/kg, acute dermal LD_{50} in rabbits 2.5 g/kg (Opdyke 1975 p. 755–756).
Reproductive toxicity: Citronellal produced malformations in chick embryos when injected into fertilized hen's eggs (Aydelotte 1963; Abramovici 1972). Using chick embryos at 72 hours of incubation, Forschmidt (1979) determined that

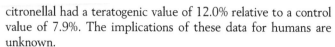

citronellal had a teratogenic value of 12.0% relative to a control value of 7.9%. The implications of these data for humans are unknown.

Mutagenicity and genotoxicity: No mutagenic activity was found for citronellal in the Ames test (Kasamaki et al 1982; Gomes-Carneiro et al 1998). It shows antimutagenic activity through concentration-dependent, competitive inhibition of PROD, with an IC_{50} of 1.56 μM (240 μg/L) (De-Oliveira et al 1997a). In one report, citronellal was weakly genotoxic in Chinese hamster cells (Kasamaki et al 1982); in another it was not (Sasaki et al 1989).

Carcinogenic/anticarcinogenic potential: Citral (5% emulsion given by intramuscular injection) and citronellal (given orally) together were used to treat 121 human cases of advanced carcinoma. Of these six (5%) were said to be cured, having been followed up for 10–15 years (Osato 1965).

Comments: Considering that aldehydes have a tendency to be skin reactive, citronellal has not been very comprehensively tested in this area.

Summary: Citronellal has been classified as both a weak and a moderate skin allergen. It presents minimal acute toxicity. There is one report of weak genotoxicity, which is not unusual in aldehydes.

Regulatory guidelines: Based on literature published in German, citronellal was classified as category B, moderately allergenic, by Schlede et al (2003). In a preliminary report by an ECETOC taskforce, citronellal was provisionally classified as a weak allergen (on a scale of extreme, strong, moderate and weak) only likely to elicit a sensitization reaction if present at 3% or more (Kimber et al 2003). In a 2003 report, JECFA stated that the committee had "no safety concern" about citronellal, based on current intake as a food flavoring (http://www.inchem.org/documents/jecfa/jecmono/v52je27.htm accessed August 8th 2011).

Citronellic acid

Synonym: Rhodinolic acid
Systematic name: 3,7-Dimethyl-6-octenoic acid
Chemical class: Aliphatic monoterpenoid alkene carboxylic acid
Note: Different isomers of citronellic acid exist, and the following isomer-specific information has been published:

(3*R*)-(+)-Citronellic acid

CAS number: 18951-85-4

(3*S*)-(−)-Citronellic acid

CAS number: 2111-53-7

Sources >1.0%:

Cypress (emerald)	24.3%
Chaste tree leaf	0–6.6%
Cypress (jade)	1.6%

Adverse skin reactions: Undiluted citronellic acid was moderately irritating to rabbit skin. Tested at 2% on 25 volunteers,

it was neither irritating nor sensitizing (Opdyke 1982 p. 653–654).

Acute toxicity: Acute oral LD_{50} in rats 2.61 g/kg; acute dermal LD_{50} in rabbits 450 mg/kg (Opdyke 1982 p. 653–654).

Summary: Limited data suggest that citronellic acid is 'slightly' toxic, and presents a minimal risk of skin reactivity.

β-Citronellol

Synonyms: Citronellol. Cephrol. 2,3-Dihydrogeraniol
Systematic name: 3,7-Dimethyl-6-octen-1-ol
Chemical class: Aliphatic monoterpenoid alkene alcohol
Note: Different isomers of β-citronellol exist, and the following isomer-specific information has been published:

(3*R*)-(+)-β-Citronellol

CAS number: 1117-61-9

(3*S*)-(−)-β-Citronellol

CAS number: 7540-51-4

Sources >1.0%:

Rose (Japanese)	44.5%
Rose (Damask)	16.0–43.5%
Citronella (Sri Lankan)	3.0–21.8%
Rose absolute (Provencale)	8.8–12.0%
Citronella (Javanese)	9.7–11.5%
Lemon-scented gum	0–5.4%

β-Citronellol (isomer not specified)

Sources >1.0%:

Geranium	18.6–47.7%
Grindelia	1.0–5.0%
Angelica root (Himalayan)	1.5–3.0%
Combava fruit	2.9%
Cedarwood (Port Orford)	2.3%
Fir (Douglas)	2.1%
Savory (winter)	0–1.8%
White cloud	1.6%

Pharmacokinetics: Citronellol is largely metabolized by oxidation (Scheline 1991).

Adverse skin reactions: Undiluted (±)-citronellol was not irritating, either when tested on 20 volunteers for five days, or on 30 volunteers for 4 hours and assessed for up to 3 days (Katz 1946; Basketter et al 2004). In a 48 hour closed-patch test, 20% (±)-citronellol produced no irritation reactions in 35 volunteers (Fujii et al 1972). When tested at 25% in 3:1 DEP/ethanol, (±)-citronellol was not irritating in one group of 22 volunteers, but produced 6 reactions in 12 volunteers when tested at 25% in 1:3 DEP/ethanol (RIFM 2002, cited in Lapczynski et al 2008b). Tested at 6% on 25 volunteers (±)-citronellol was not sensitizing (Opdyke 1975 p. 757–758). Out of a further 101 volunteers

Table 14.3 Citronellol reactions in dermatitis patients

Concentration used	Percentage who reacted	No. of reactors	Reference
0.5%	0.12%	2/1,701[a]	Frosch et al 2005a
1%	0.07%	1/3,506	Heisterberg et al 2011
1%	0.24%	4/1,701[a]	Frosch et al 2005a
1%	0.4%	7/1,855	Frosch et al 2002a
1%	0.5%	10/2,003	Schnuch et al 2007a
1%	1.0%	1/100	Frosch et al 1995a
5%	0.0%	0/100	Frosch et al 1995a
5%	0.0%	0/50	Larsen 1977
5%	0.0%	0/45	Itoh 1982
5%	0.0%	0/291	Lapczynski et al 2008b
5%	0.0%	0/194	Ishihara et al 1979
5%	0.0%	0/315	Heydorn et al 2002
5%	0.3%	2/658	Heydorn et al 2003b
Unstated	0.005%	1/18,747	De Groot 1987

[a]Same group of patients

($\pm$)-citronellol caused no sensitization reactions when tested at 25% (RIFM 2005a, cited in Belsito et al 2008).

There were two sensitization reactions to 0.5% (0.12%) and four to 1.0% ($\pm$)-citronellol (0.24%) in 1,701 dermatitis patients (Frosch et al 2005a). In two groups of 100 consecutive dermatitis patients there was one irritant and one allergic reaction to 1% ($\pm$)-citronellol, and two irritant and no allergic reactions to 5% ($\perp$)-citronellol (Frosch et al 1995a). When citronellol was patch tested at 5% on 50 dermatitis patients who were not thought to be sensitive to fragrance there were no positive reactions (Larsen 1977). There were no sensitization reactions in 45 Japanese dermatitis patients to 5% (+)-citronellol (Itoh 1982) nor to 5% (−)-citronellol in a total of 291 Japanese dermatology patients (Lapczynski et al 2008b). ($\pm$)-Citronellol at 5% similarly elicited no reactions in 194 Japanese dermatology patients and 21 control subjects (Ishihara et al 1979).

Of 18,747 dermatitis patients, 1,781 had contact dermatitis and one (0.005% of dermatitis patients and 0.06% of contact dermatitis patients) was allergic to citronellol. Of the 1,781 patients 75 were allergic to cosmetic products, so the one reaction constituted 1.4% of this group (De Groot 1987). In a multicenter study in Europe, seven of 1,855 consecutive dermatitis patients (0.4%) tested positive to 1% ($\pm$)-citronellol (Frosch et al 2002a). In two groups of hand eczema patients, 0/315 and 2/658 tested positive to 5% ($\pm$)-citronellol (Heydorn et al 2002, 2003b). The results of the previous 10 reports, and of two further European studies, are listed in Table 14.3. These represent dermatitis patients not noted as fragrance-sensitive.

Two of 119 dermatitis patients (1.7%) sensitive to cosmetics were allergic to 2% ($\pm$)-citronellol (De Groot et al 1988). When patch tested at 5% on 20 dermatitis patients who were sensitive to fragrance, citronellol induced seven (35%) positive reactions (Larsen 1977). In two separate worldwide multicenter studies of dermatitis patients with proven sensitization to fragrance materials, 10 of 178 (5.6%) tested positive to 5% (−)-citronellol and 19 of 218 (8.7%) tested positive to 5% ($\pm$)-citronellol (Larsen et al 2001, 2002). A patch test using 1% citronellol gave a moderate positive reaction in two of three people sensitive to citronella oil (Keil 1947).

In an in vitro assay, citronellol was non-phototoxic (Placzek et al 2007).

Acute toxicity: Acute oral LD_{50} in rats 3.45 g/kg, acute dermal LD_{50} in rabbits 2.65 g/kg (Opdyke 1975 p. 757–758).

Inhalation toxicity: When mice were exposed for one minute to ($\pm$)-citronellol vapors, the dose causing a 25% reduction in respiratory rate (i.e. irritation) was 990 µg/L (Lapczynski et al 2008b).

Mutagenicity and genotoxicity: Citronellol was non-mutagenic in the Ames test, with and without metabolic activation (Rockwell & Raw 1979; Kono et al 1995). ($\pm$)-Citronellol was negative in a *Bacillus subtilis* rec-assay (Oda et al 1978).

Carcinogenic/anticarcinogenic potential: Marginal antitumor activity has been reported for citronellol (Fang et al 1989, Wattenberg 1991). In a 'COMPACT' evaluation, citronellol was evaluated as unlikely to be carcinogenic (Lewis et al 1994).

Comments: Synthetic citronellol is a clear risk to people who are sensitive to fragrance materials. In contrast, the level of risk to dermatitis patients in general is remarkably low. Between 1977 and 1995, there were two allergic reactions out of 19,136 dermatitis patients tested, not including those hypersensitive to cosmetics or fragrance. Looking at the data from 2000 onwards, only 0.34% (23/6,823) tested positive to 1%, or 5% citronellol. Since this is only slightly more than the 0.3% that react to petrolatum, citronellol cannot be regarded as a high-risk allergen. In skin irritation tests, citronellol was not irritating in 107 volunteers when tested at 20%, 25% or 100%, but produced six reactions in one group of 12 volunteers, which seems highly inconsistent.

Summary: Citronellol may be a skin irritant, and is a low-risk allergen. It is 'slightly' toxic, and is unlikely to be a carcinogen.

Regulatory guidelines: JECFA has set a group ADI of 0 to 0.5 mg/kg bw for citral, citronellol, geranyl acetate, linalool and linalyl acetate (JECFA 1999a). Citronellol is one of the 26 fragrance materials listed as an allergen by the EU. If present in a cosmetic product at over 100 ppm (0.01%) in a wash-off product or 10 ppm (0.001%) in a leave-on product the material must be declared on the ingredient list if sold in an EU member state. Based on literature published in German, citronellol was classified as category B, moderately allergenic, by Schlede et al (2003). The IFRA standard for citronellol in leave-on products such as body lotions is 13.3%, for skin sensitization.

Our safety advice: We see no need for a limit on dermal exposure to citronellol for skin sensitization.

β-Citronellyl acetate

Synonyms: Citronellol acetate. Acetic acid citronellyl ester
Systematic name: 3,7-Dimethyl-6-octen-1-yl ethanoate
Chemical class: Aliphatic monoterpenoid alkene ester

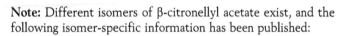

Note: Different isomers of β-citronellyl acetate exist, and the following isomer-specific information has been published:

(3*R*)-(+)-β-Citronellyl acetate

CAS number: 20425-54-1

(3*S*)-(−)-β-Citronellyl acetate

CAS number: 67601-05-2

Sources >1.0%:

Lemon-scented gum	tr–9.7%
Chaste tree leaf	0.3–7.8%
Citronella (Sri Lankan)	0.9–7.3%
Chaste tree seed	0.2–6.0%
Combava leaf	0.9–5.1%
Angelica root (Himalayan)	2.2–3.4%
Rose (Damask)	0.2–2.8%
Citronella (Javanese)	1.0–2.0%
Combava fruit	0.5–1.5%

Adverse skin reactions: Acute dermal LD_{50} in rabbits, >2 g/kg. Applied undiluted to rabbit skin for 24 hours under occlusion citronellyl acetate was irritating. Tested at 4% on 25 volunteers it was mildly irritating and was not sensitizing (Opdyke 1973 p. 1069).

Acute toxicity: Rat acute oral LD_{50} 6.8 g/kg (Opdyke 1973 p. 1069).

Carcinogenic/anticarcinogenic potential: In a two year carcinogenesis study, food-grade geranyl acetate (71% geranyl acetate, 29% citronellyl acetate) was fed to 50 male and 50 female rats at 0, 1,000 or 2,000 mg/kg, and to 50 male and 50 female mice at 0, 500 or 1,000 mg/kg five times a week. It was not considered to be carcinogenic to rats or mice of either sex. A marginal (but not significant) increase was observed in squamous cell papillomas of the skin, and tubular cell adenomas of the kidney in the male rats at the higher doses (National Toxicology Program 1987). 'Marginal antitumor activity' has been reported for citronellyl acetate (Fang et al 1989).

Summary: β-Citronellyl acetate is slightly irritating to the skin, is non-toxic and non-carcinogenic.

β-Citronellyl formate

Synonyms: Citronellol formate. Formic acid citronellyl ester
Systematic name: 3,7-Dimethyl-6-octen-1-yl methanoate
Chemical class: Aliphatic monoterpenoid alkene ester
Note: Different isomers of β-citronellyl acetate exist, and the following isomer-specific information has been published:

(3*R*)-(+)-β-Citronellyl formate

CAS number: 93919-91-6

(3*S*)-(−)-β-Citronellyl formate

CAS number: 93919-93-8

Sources >1.0%:

Geranium	4.8–12.4%

Adverse skin reactions: Acute dermal LD_{50} in rabbits, >2 g/kg. Applied undiluted to rabbit skin for 24 hours under occlusion citronellyl formate was irritating. Tested at 4% on 25 volunteers the material was mildly irritating and was not sensitizing (Opdyke 1973 p. 1073).

Acute toxicity: Rat acute oral LD_{50} 8.4 g/kg (Opdyke 1973 p. 1073).

Carcinogenic/anticarcinogenic potential: 'Marginal antitumor activity' has been reported for citronellyl formate (Fang et al 1989).

Summary: β-Citronellyl formate is slightly irritating to the skin and is non-toxic. Being an ester, this compound is unlikely to be carcinogenic.

β-Citronellyl propionate

Synonyms: Citronellol propanoate. Propionic acid citronellyl ester
Systematic name: 3,7-Dimethyl-6-octen-1-yl propanoate
Chemical class: Aliphatic monoterpenoid alkene ester
Note: Different isomers of β-citronellyl propionate exist, and the following isomer-specific information has been published:

(3*R*)-(+)-β-Citronellyl propionate

CAS number: 94086-40-5

(3*S*)-(−)-β-Citronellyl propionate

CAS number: 89460-13-9

Sources >1.0%:

Geranium	0–2.5%
Khella	1.2%

Adverse skin reactions: Acute dermal LD_{50} in rabbits >5 g/kg. The undiluted material was not irritating to rabbits patch-tested for 24 hours under occlusion. Tested at 4% on the skin of 25 volunteers, citronellyl propionate was neither irritating nor sensitizing (Opdyke 1975 p. 759).

Acute toxicity: Acute oral LD_{50} in rats >5 g/kg (Opdyke 1975 p. 759).

Summary: β-Citronellyl propionate is non-irritant and non-toxic. Being an ester, this compound is unlikely to be carcinogenic.

Citropten

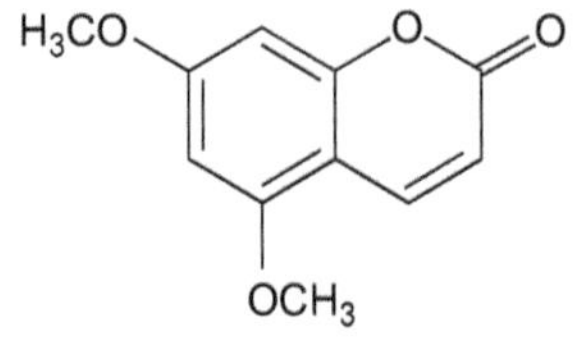

H₃CO / O / O / OCH₃

Synonyms: 5,7-Dimethoxycoumarin. Limettin
Systematic name: 5,7-Dimethoxy-2*H*-1-benzopyran-2-one
Chemical class: Coumarin ether
CAS number: 487-06-9

Sources >0.0001%:

Lime (expressed)	0.4–2.2%
Bergamot (expressed)	0.01–0.35%
Lemon (expressed)	0.05–0.17%
Bergamot (FCF)	0–0.0052%

Adverse skin reactions: Citropten is both phototoxic and photomutagenic (Ashwood-Smith et al 1983).
Carcinogenic/anticarcinogenic potential: Dietary citropten inhibited rat mammary carcinogenesis, but had no effect on forestomach carcinogenesis in female mice (Wattenberg et al 1979).
Mutagenicity and genotoxicity: Citropten forms single-strand photoadducts with DNA, but does not form cross-links (Ou et al 1978).
Comments: Citropten has not been tested for photocarcinogenicity.
Summary: Citropten is phototoxic and photomutagenic.

Coniferyl benzoate

Synonym: [(Z)-3-(4-Hydroxy-3-methoxyphenyl)allyl] benzoate
Systematic name: Benzoic acid (Z)-3-(4-hydroxy-3-methoxyphenyl)-2-propen-1-yl ester
Chemical class: Phenolic phenylpropenoid ester
CAS number: Not found.

Sources:

Benzoin resinoid	Traces?
Peru balsam	Traces?

Note: Being a substituted phenol, coniferyl benzoate is a weak acid which may be corrosive to tissues. It is a major constituent of raw Peru balsam and gum benzoin.
Adverse skin reactions: In tests on guinea pigs, a number of compounds were rated as strong, moderate or weak sensitizers. Coniferyl benzoate was a moderate sensitizer (Hausen et al 1992). Of 102 dermatitis patients sensitive to Peru balsam, 29 tested positive to 1% coniferyl benzoate (Hausen 2001). It has been suggested that coniferyl alcohol esters are the most important allergens in Peru balsam, since 70 of 82 Peru balsam-sensitive patients (85.4%) reacted to coniferyl benzoate (Hjorth 1961).
Summary: Coniferyl benzoate is a moderate skin allergen.

Costunolide

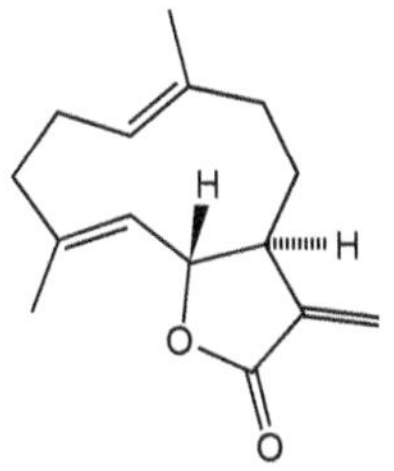

Synonyms: Costus lactone. 1(10), 4, 11(13)-Germacratrien-12,6-olide
Systematic name: [3aS-(3aR*,6E,10E,11aS*)]-3a,4,5,8,9,11a-Hexahydro-6,10-dimethyl-3-methylene-cyclodeca[b]furan-2(3H)-one

Chemical class: Bicyclic sesquiterpenoid polyalkene lactone
CAS number: 553-21-9

Source:

Costus	11.0%

Adverse skin reactions: Costunolide is considered a sensitizer (Benezra & Epstein 1986), and sesquiterpene lactones from Compositae plants are notorious skin sensitizers (Ross et al 1993; Goulden & Wilkinson 1998). An individual known to be allergic to oakmoss had a +++ reaction to 0.1% costunolide in acetone (Benezra et al 1978).
Cardiovascular effects: Costunolide reduced VEGF-induced neovascularization in vivo in mice at 100 mg/kg/day ip, and inhibited umbilical vein endothelial cell proliferation in vitro with an IC50 value of 3.4 mM (Jeong et al 2002).
Carcinogenic/anticarcinogenic potential: Costunolide was dose- and time-dependently cytotoxic to human cell lines for breast cancer (MCF-7 and MDA-MB-231) (Bocca et al 2004, Choi et al 2005b), in addition to liver (HepG2), ovary (OVCAR-3) and cervical (HeLa) cancer (Sun et al 2003). It was also toxic to human leukemia cell lines HL-60 and U937 (Choi et al 2002; Hibasami et al 2003), and to RAW 264.7, a mouse leukemia cell line (Kang et al 2004). Costunolide has demonstrated chemopreventive activity in rat colon carcinogenesis induced by azoxymethane (Mori et al 1994; Kawamori et al 1995) and in DMBA-induced hamster cheek pouch carcinogenesis (Ohnishi et al 1997).
Comments: Based on literature published in German, costunolide was classified as category A, a significant contact allergen, by Schlede et al (2003).
Summary: Costunolide is a skin allergen. We could find no acute toxicity data. Costunolide has demonstrated anticarcinogenic activity. Its antiangiogenic activity suggests caution in pregnancy.

Coumarin

Synonyms: 1,2-Benzopyrone. Tonka bean camphor
Systematic name: 2H-1-Benzopyran-2-one
Chemical class: Benzenoid lactone
CAS number: 91-64-5

Sources >1.0%:

Sweet vernalgrass absolute	68.0%
Tonka absolute	38.7–58.7%
Sweet vernalgrass	46.8%
Deertongue absolute	< 25.0%
Hay absolute	< 8.0%
Lavender absolute	4.3%
Lavandin absolute	3.0%
Cassia leaf	0.03–2.5%
Cassia bark	tr–1.9%
Narcissus absolute	0–1.2%

Pharmacokinetics: Coumarin is rapidly and extensively absorbed from the skin of both humans and rats, and is readily distributed and excreted. Peak plasma concentrations were achieved at, or before, one hour after application of 0.2 mg/cm^2

541

to the skin, and mean plasma half-lives were 1.7 hours and five hours, respectively (Ford et al 2001).

Coumarin is largely subject to first-pass metabolism by the liver after oral administration and is excreted mainly as the glucuronide. Some biotransformation may also occur in the gut (Ritschel et al 1977, 1979). Metabolites of coumarin, especially o-hydroxyphenylacetic acid and o-hydroxyphenyl lactic acid were found to inhibit glucose 6-phosphatase in the liver. This may be an important factor in liver toxicity (Feuer et al 1966). After oral administration, the main excretion products in man are 7-hydroxycoumarin as its glucuronide and sulfate conjugates (Ford et al 2001). There are significant qualitative and quantitative interspecies differences in the way coumarin is metabolized (Booth et al 1959; Shilling et al 1969; Gangolli et al 1974; Cohen 1979; Born et al 2000a; Ford et al 2001). For example, the percentage of orally administered coumarin excreted in the urine as 7-hydroxycoumarin was 1% in guinea pigs, 3% in dogs, 19% in cats, 60% in baboons (Gangolli et al 1974), and 79% in humans (Shilling 1969). In rodents, coumarin 3,4-oxide formation predominates, leading to several potentially toxic metabolites (Lake 1999).

However, some individuals metabolize coumarin to 3-hydroxycoumarin, due to a single amino acid substitution in their CYP2A6 (Hadidi et al 1997). After testing 103 individuals one was identified who was 7-hydroxylation deficient (Hadidi et al 1998). In another report, there was no correlation between individuals with elevated liver enzymes (after 90 mg coumarin in 231 German patients) and those with variant CYP2A6*2 or CYP2A6*3 (Burian et al 2003). Further study seems to confirm that genetic polymorphism of CYP2A6*9 results in a decrease of coumarin 7-hydroxylase metabolism (Kiyotani et al 2003).

Ring fission appears to be more important in man than in rats (Piller 1977), and formation of hepatotoxic coumarin 3,4-oxide in man is considerably less important than in the rat and mouse (Born et al 2000a). The situation is, however, complicated by dose-dependency in the mode of excretion.

Drug interactions: Coumarin inhibits mouse brain monoamine oxidase, with an IC_{50} of 41.4 µM (6.04 mg/L) (Huong et al 2000). This suggests the probability of oral doses of coumarin-rich essential oils interacting with MAOI or SSRI drugs.

Adverse skin reactions: Tested at 8% on 25 volunteers coumarin was not sensitizing (Opdyke 1974 p. 385–388). When it was patch tested at 5% on 50 dermatitis patients thought not to be sensitive to fragrance there were no positive reactions (Larsen 1977). There were no irritant or allergic reactions in 100 consecutive dermatitis patients tested with 5% coumarin (Frosch et al 1995a). Of 14,000 consecutive dermatitis patients tested with 5% (the majority) or 8% coumarin 58 (0.4%) were positive (Kunkeler et al 1998).

In a prospective study of adverse skin reactions to cosmetic ingredients identified by patch test (1977–1980), coumarin elicited contact dermatitis in four (0.8%) of 487 cosmetic-related cases (Eiermann et al 1982). In a multicenter study, 13 of 1,825 dermatitis patients (0.7%) were sensitive to 5% coumarin on patch testing (De Groot et al 2000). Of 713 cosmetic dermatitis patients, four reacted to coumarin (Adams & Maibach 1985). There were no positive reactions to 5% coumarin in 1,701 dermatitis patients (Frosch et al 2005a). In 658 people with hand eczema, three (0.46%) reacted to 5% coumarin (Heydorn et al 2003b). The results of two further European studies are reported in Table 5.10.

Of 182 dermatitis patients suspected of contact allergy to cosmetics, 12 (6.7%) tested positive to 8% coumarin (Malten et al 1984). Of 167 dermatitis patients suspected of fragrance sensitivity two (1.2%) were allergic to 5% coumarin on patch testing (Larsen et al 1996b). Of 241 dermatitis patients tested with 5% coumarin, two (0.8%) had a positive reaction (Ferguson & Sharma 1984). Of 119 eczema patients with contact allergy to cosmetics one (0.8%) was allergic to 5% coumarin (De Groot et al 1988). In 20 eczema patients suspected of cosmetic dermatitis, there were no reactions to 1% coumarin (Malten et al 1984). When tested at 5% on 20 dermatitis patients who were sensitive to fragrance, coumarin induced two (10%) positive reactions (Larsen 1977).

Floch et al (2002) maintain that most of the data on coumarin skin allergy are unreliable since they do not indicate a clear purity of the material used: 'This is an important point as indicated in Hausen (1989), because some derivatives in the coumarin family could have weak-to-moderate sensitizing properties. . .further to purity, one can raise questions on concentration and irritation (homogeneity and stability of suspension in petrolatum), and cases of cross-reaction to allergens for which coumarin may only be a detector reagent.' The authors further claim that the statistics in these papers are not significant. They then go on to detail their own research, in which none of 100 dermatitis patients reacted to 1% and 10% of a stable, homogeneous suspension of coumarin in petrolatum. Similarly, Vocanson et al (2006) found only 1 of 512 dermatitis patients allergic to to 2% or 10% of a stable, homogeneous suspension of pure coumarin, and showed that coumarin allergy is due to impurities, not coumarin itself.

Acute toxicity: Coumarin oral LD_{50} has been reported as 196 mg/kg in mice, 202 mg/kg in guinea pigs and 293 mg/kg and 680 mg/kg in rats (Jenner et al 1964; Opdyke 1974 p. 385–388). Coumarin was hepatotoxic to rats after single ip or oral doses of 125–500 mg/kg, producing necrosis of centrilobular cells, the severity of which is dose-related. Toxic metabolites produced by CYP-mediated oxidation seem to be responsible (Lake 1984).

Subacute and subchronic toxicity: Oral administration (90 days) of coumarin produced severe liver damage at a level of 2,500 ppm in the diet of rats and 100 mg/kg per day for dogs (Hazleton et al 1956). In rats fed 10,000 ppm coumarin for 4 weeks marked growth retardation, testicular atrophy and mild to moderate liver damage were seen (Hagan et al 1967).

Cardiovascular toxicity: Although coumarin derivatives are used as anticoagulant drugs (e.g., warfarin, dicoumarin), coumarin itself is not anticoagulant (Feuer 1974).

Reproductive toxicity: Pregnant mice were fed 0.05%, 0.1% or 0.25% coumarin in the diet on gestational days 6–17. No abnormalities were found in the offspring, but the 0.25% dose led to increased ossification, and increased mortality up to three weeks of life was seen at all levels (Roll & Bär 1967). In a study on 17 pregnant miniature pigs, 25 mg/kg/day coumarin, and 150 mg/kg/day troxerutin (a mixture of flavanoids), were administered orally on gestational days 6–30. Pathological histological, and morphological examinations of uteri and fetuses revealed no indications of embryotoxic or teratogenic effects (Grote et al 1977).

Hepatotoxicity: Changes in the activity of rat hepatocyte enzymes have been reported following subcutaneous coumarin administration (Feuer et al 1965). In the 1970s, however, the relevance of animal data to humans was being questioned. One study, giving coumarin to baboons at 50 ppm and 100 ppm (3 weeks at each dose) did find histological damage in the liver (Gangolli et al 1974). In another, coumarin was administered to baboons for between 16 and 24 months at 2.5, 7.5, 22.5 or 67.5 mg/kg/day. At the highest dose only, an increase in liver weight was noted, and ultrastructural examination revealed dilatation of the endoplasmic reticulum (Evans et al 1979). Because of major interspecies differences in the bioavailability, metabolism and excretion of coumarin, the relevance of animal toxicity to man was in doubt (Fentem & Fry 1993).

This last report indicates a NOAEL of 22.5 mg/kg/day, equivalent to ~1.6 g/day for a 70 kg human. This dose is over 30 times higher than the 50 mg/day received by many of the cancer patients for two years. In clinical trials using coumarin as an anticancer agent only 0.37% of patients developed (reversible) abnormal liver function. The majority of 2,173 patients were given 100 mg/day of coumarin for one month, followed by 50 mg/day for two years. (The other patients took between 25 mg/day and 2,000 mg/day.) Of the total, eight patients developed elevated liver enzyme levels, which returned to normal on stopping the coumarin (Cox et al 1989). On this evidence, coumarin cannot be regarded as hepatotoxic in humans (Egan et al 1990). However, inter-individual variation in levels of coumarin 7-hydroxylase, the enzyme responsible for coumarin metabolism, is a complicating factor in assessing risk (Yamano et al 1990; Rautio et al 1992; Pelkonen et al 1993; Van Iersel et al 1994; Hadidi et al 1997).

Mutagenicity and genotoxicity: In Ames tests, Haworth et al (1983) reported that coumarin was mutagenic, Florin et al (1980) that it was not, and Edenharder & Tang (1997) that it was antimutagenic. In the SOS chromotest (a modified *E. coli* PQ37 genotoxicity assay) coumarin was not genotoxic, with or without S9 activation (Kevekordes et al 1999). Coumarin did not induce UDS in rat hepatocytes after oral doses of up to the minimum tolerated dose of 320 mg/kg (Edwards et al 2000). When tested in an in vivo mouse micronucleus assay, no evidence could be found for genotoxicity of coumarin at single oral doses of up to 200 mg/kg (Api 2001b). Coumarin also had no effect in human liver slices, suggesting that it is not genotoxic in this organ (Beamand et al 1998). On the contrary, it protected against aflatoxin B_1-induced genomutation in the presence of chick embryo liver S9, although marked interspecies differences were found (Goeger et al 1998). When human liver S9 was used, coumarin exhibited co-mutagenicity with aflatoxin B_1 (Goeger et al 1999). Coumarin was antigenotoxic in human hepatoma (HepG2) cells and Chinese hamster V79 cells (Imanishi et al 1990; Sanyal et al 1997). However, Kevekordes et al (2001) reported coumarin to be genotoxic in HepG2 cells.

Chronic toxicity and carcinogenic/anticarcinogenic potential: In rats fed 1,000, 2,500 or 5,000 ppm in the diet for two years, no effect was seen at 1,000 ppm, but at the higher doses there was growth retardation and hepatotoxicity. In dogs fed 25 mg/kg for 133–330 days, 50 mg/kg for 35–277 days, or 100 mg/kg for 9–16 days, there was jaundice, liver damage, emaciation and pathological changes in the gall bladder, spleen and bone marrow. At 10 mg/kg for 297–350 days there was no observable adverse effect. Bile duct carcinomas were found in rats fed

coumarin at 5,000 ppm for 18 months (Bär & Griepentrog 1967). Coumarin was fed for up to two years to male and female rats at 0, 25, 50 or 100 mg/kg, and to male and female mice at 0, 50, 100 or 200 mg/kg. There was an increase in renal adenomas in male rats, with only a marginal increase in female rats. There was evidence of alveolar/bronchiolar adenomas in male mice and there was clear carcinogenic activity in lung and liver tissue of female mice (National Toxicology Program 1993a). In short-term studies, dietary coumarin inhibited carcinogenesis in both rats (mammary) and mice (forestomach) (Wattenberg et al 1979).

Coumarin is used in the treatment of lymphedema, has been tried as a treatment for various cancers, and is reported to be an immunostimulant (Reynolds 1993). In a meta-analysis of clinical trials for the treatment of lymphedema with high-dose oral coumarin, it was concluded that side effects are minor, most being gastrointestinal, and largely prevented by the use of enteric-coated tablets or delayed release capsules (Casley-Smith 1999).
Comments: Coumarin is one of the most controversial aromatic compounds. This is perhaps not surprising since it is so clearly carcinogenic in rodents, and yet it is not carcinogenic in humans. Coumarin also suffers from being incorrectly associated with the effects of similar compounds, 'coumarin derivatives', including warfarin and dicoumarin (anticoagulant in humans), herniaren (allergic and photoallergic in humans) and bergapten (photosensitizing and phototoxic in humans) (Clark 1995). (Coumarin derivatives, not coumarin, are used as rat poisons.) However, coumarin itself is not anticoagulant, nor does it manifest any of these side effects.

Coumarin allergy is due to impurities in the compound used for testing, and poor testing procedures (Floch et al 2002; Vocanson et al 2006). The classification of naturally-occurring coumarin as an allergen by the EU is therefore fallacious and unsound. Felter et al (2006) have suggested a reference dose (acceptable daily exposure level for a lifetime) of 0.64 mg/kg/day, based on 16 mg/kg/day NOAEL in female rats, with a total uncertainty factor of 25. They describe this as a conservative value, protective for all health endpoints, including cancer and non-cancer.
Summary: Coumarin is metabolized primarily to (carcinogenic) 3-hydroxycoumarin in rodents, and primarily to (non-carcinogenic) 7-hydroxycoumarin in man, but in some individuals, elevated liver enzymes and hepatotoxicity are evident on oral dosing. This phenomenon may be related to the 0.37% of individuals who reacted badly to coumarin therapy (Cox et al 1989). It remains to be resolved what percentage of the general population may be at risk from oral coumarin. It has been suggested that, since it is so effective, coumarin could be reinstated as an accepted treatment for lymphedema by excluding those with non-functional CYP2A6 (Farinola & Piller 2005).

In reviewing the available data for coumarin in humans, it has been concluded that a normal daily intake in food and/or cosmetic products of 0.06 mg/kg/day does not represent a risk to health (Lake 1999; Born et al 2000a). Toxicity, which has been observed in rats and mice has been rationalized in terms of a predominant metabolic pathway involving 3,4-epoxidation and the formation of toxic metabolites including *o*-hydroxyphenylacetaldehyde and *o*-hydroxyphenylacetic acid (Lake 1999; Born et al 2000b). In humans this pathway is less important than 7-hydroxylation, which leads to detoxification.

A more recent review of coumarin safety observed that 'coumarin is not DNA-reactive and…the induction of tumors at high doses in rodents is attributed to cytotoxicity and regenerative hyperplasia.' Rats are said to be particularly susceptible to liver effects from coumarin, and mice to lung effects. Coumarin is, it is concluded, safe as used in the human diet, and as a perfume in personal care products, no adverse liver effects having been reported in humans following coumarin exposure via dietary sources or dermal application (Felter et al 2006). Similarly, Casley-Smith (1999) points out that only high-dose oral coumarin may cause idiosyncratic hepatitis (3 per 1,000) and that topical coumarin does not.

Coumarin is found in a small number of absolutes, and even fewer essential oils. While there is a small risk of hepatotoxicity from high oral doses, and of possible drug interactions, humans are not at risk from externally applied coumarin, and no toxic effects have been reported for any coumarin-containing essential oil or absolute. Even therapeutic doses of externally-applied coumarin (in 12 clinical trials for lymphedema) do not disturb hepatic enzymes, and the transdermal route seems to avoid all adverse reactions (Casley-Smith 1999, Felter et al 2006).

Regulatory guidelines: Coumarin is one of the 26 fragrance materials listed as an allergen by the EU. If present in a cosmetic product at over 100 ppm (0.01%) in a wash-off product or 10 ppm (0.001%) in a leave-on product the material must be declared on the ingredient list if sold in an EU member state. The IFRA standard for coumarin in leave-on products such as body lotions is 1.6%, for skin sensitization. Based on the animal data known at the time, the FDA prohibited the use of coumarin in food in 1954, and similar prohibitions currently exist in Japan and India. In many countries the use of coumarin in food is restricted to a concentration limit. Both the UK and EC 'standard permitted proportion' of coumarin in food flavorings is 2 mg/kg (European Community Council 1988; Anon 1992b).

Our safety advice: Because of its MAO inhibiting action, essential oils high in coumarin should be used with caution in oral doses by anyone taking MAOIs, SSRIs, pethidine, and indirect sympathomimetics (see Table 4.10 for more detail). We recommend a daily oral maximum of 0.6 mg/kg/day for coumarin, rounded down from the 0.64 mg/kg/day reference dose proposed by Felter et al (2006). We see no need for a coumarin dermal limit, either for toxicity or skin sensitization.

Cresol

Synonyms: Hydroxytoluene. Methylphenol
Chemical class: Phenol
Note: Different isomers of cresol exist, and the following isomer-specific information has been published:

o-Cresol

Synonyms: 2-Cresol. 2-Methyl phenol. 2-Hydroxytoluene. *o*-Hydroxytoluene. *o*-Methylphenol. *o*-Toluol. *o*-Tolyl alcohol
Systematic name: 1-Hydroxy-2-methylbenzene
CAS number: 95-48-7

m-Cresol

Synonyms: 3-Cresol. 3-Methyl phenol. 3-Hydroxytoluene. *m*-Hydroxytoluene. *m*-Methylphenol. *m*-Toluol. *m*-Tolyl alcohol
Systematic name: 1-Hydroxy-3-methylbenzene
CAS number: 108-39-4

p-Cresol

Synonyms: 4-Cresol. 4-Methyl phenol. 4-Hydroxytoluene. *p*-Hydroxytoluene. *p*-Methylphenol. *p*-Toluol. *p*-Tolyl alcohol
Systematic name: 1-Hydroxy-4-methylbenzene
CAS number: 106-44-5

Sources:

Birch tar	Major constituent (isomer not specified)
Cade (unrectified)	< 2.5% (mixed cresols)

Notes: Being substituted phenols, cresol isomers are weak acids which may be corrosive to tissues. Minor amounts may be present in ylang-ylang oils. It is not known which cresol isomer is present in birch tar oil and the isomers can be difficult to distinguish from each other.

Adverse skin reactions: Undiluted *p*-cresol was irritating to rabbit skin; tested at 4% it was neither irritating nor sensitizing in human subjects (Opdyke 1974 p. 389–390). It is a severe skin and eye irritant (National Toxicology Program 2000).

Acute toxicity: The rat oral LD_{50} values for cresol isomers are *o*-cresol 121 mg/kg, *m*-cresol 242 mg/kg and *p*-cresol 207 mg/kg. The rabbit dermal LD_{50} values are 890 mg/kg (*o*-cresol), 2,830 mg/kg (*m*-cresol) and 300 mg/kg (*p*-cresol). *p*-Cresol oral LD_{50} 344 mg/kg in mice; dermal LD_{50} 750 mg/kg in rats; subcutaneous LD_{50} 150 mg/kg in mice, 200 mg/kg in guinea pigs. Exposure can cause irritation to the eyes, nose and throat, severe eye damage, vomiting, sleeplessness and damage to the lungs, liver, kidneys, blood, nervous system and respiratory system. It can cause corrosion of all tissues (Vernot et al 1977; National Toxicology Program 2001).

Subacute and subchronic toxicity: Rats and mice of both sexes were given *p*-cresol at concentrations ranging from 300 to 30,000 ppm in the diet for 28 days. All rats survived but some mice given 10,000 or 30,000 ppm died before the end of the study. Feed consumption was depressed during the first study week in all high-dose groups and weight gains were generally less than controls in groups given 10,000 or 30,000 ppm. Increased relative liver weights and kidney weights were noted in both rats and mice given as little as 3,000 ppm. However, there were no consistent microscopic changes associated with these weight changes. Bone marrow hypoplasia and uterus, ovary and occasional mammary gland atrophy were seen primarily at the highest dietary concentration. Atrophy and regenerative changes in the nasal epithelia and forestomach, presumably a direct result of the irritant effects of the chemical or its vapors, were noted (National Toxicology Program 1991).

Human toxicity: Cresols may cause gastrointestinal corrosive injury, central nervous system and cardiovascular disturbances, and renal and hepatic injury following intoxication. A 44-year-old male was found unconscious after ingesting 300 mL of 50% cresol-soap solution in a suicide attempt. He had dermal burns, esophageal and gastric erosion, pneumonia, mixed metabolic acidosis and respiratory alkalosis, renal and liver function impairment, leukocytosis and dark urine. Acute renal failure and hemolysis developed, but he recovered after hemodialysis and intensive supportive care. Urine levels of o-cresol, m-cresol, p-cresol and phenol were respectively 125, 2059, 2083 and 68 mg/g creatinine at 7 hours post-ingestion. Although the amount of cresol the man claimed to have ingested (150 g) far exceeded the reported lethal dose of 30–60 g, and although multiple complications developed, he recovered (Wu ML et al 1998a).

In an earlier case, a 46-year-old male ingested approximately 100 mL of 50% cresol-soap solution and survived, probably only because of medical intervention. The total serum concentration of cresol was 117 µg/g (Yashiki et al 1990). In a fatal case, a 65-year-old male drank at least 240 mL of 50% cresol-soap solution, and died within 15 minutes. Free m-cresol and p-cresol levels of 957.3 and 458.8 µg/mL, respectively, were detected in the heart blood, and 250 mL of fluid smelling of cresol were found in his stomach. A lethal dose of 50% cresol-soap solution is considered to be 60–120 mL, with fatal blood levels being 71–190 µg/mL of total cresols (Monma-Ohtaki et al 2002).

Reproductive toxicity: In a yeast screen for estrogenic activity, o-cresol was considered inactive, while p-cresol was considered active (Nishihara et al 2000).

Hepatotoxicity: p-Cresol is hepatotoxic to rat liver in vitro, with an LC_{50} value of 1.32 mM (142 mg/L). It rapidly depletes rat hepatic intracellular glutathione, and is more potently hepatotoxic than the o- and m- isomers (Thompson et al 1994, 1996).

Nephrotoxicity: p-Cresol is a well-known uremic toxin (De Smet et al 2003).

Mutagenicity and genotoxicity: p-Cresol was not mutagenic in the Ames test, with or without metabolic activation (Florin et al 1980, Haworth et al 1983, National Toxicology Program 2008b). p-Cresol was not mutagenic in E. coli strain WP2, with or without metabolic activation. A 60/40 mix of m-/p-cresol was not genotoxic to mouse peripheral blood leukocytes (micronucleus test) after 13 weeks of exposure in the diet (National Toxicology Program 2008b). The quinone methide derivative of p-cresol is a reactive intermediate leading to the formation of DNA adducts in HL-60 cells treated with p-cresol. The levels of DNA adducts formed were dependent on concentrations of p-cresol and treatment time (Gaikwad & Bodell 2003).

Carcinogenic/anticarcinogenic potential: The proliferation of mouse B16 melanoma cells was weakly inhibited by 'cresol' with an IC_{50} value of 200 mM (21.6 g/L) (Tatman & Huanbiao 2002). In a 2-year carcinogenesis study using mixed cresols (60% m-cresol, 40% p-cresol), male rats were fed 1,500, 5,000 or 15,000 ppm, equivalent to average daily doses of 70, 230 or 720 mg/kg bw, and female mice were fed 1,000, 3,000 or 10,000 ppm, equivalent to daily doses of 100, 300 or 1,040 mg/kg bw. There were no adverse effects on survival in any group compared to controls. In the male rats, there was a marginal increase in renal tubule adenoma incidence, only in the high dose group (3 of 50 rats); this was not statistically significant. There were non-malignant lesions in the kidneys, liver and nose. In the female mice there was an increase in squamous cell papilloma of the forestomach in the high dose group (10 of 50 mice), and there were non-malignant lesions in the thyroid, liver, nose and lungs (National Toxicology Program 2008b).

Comments: The non-malignant respiratory and nasal lesions mentioned above were dose-dependent, and are thought to be due to chronic irritation caused by inhalation of the cresols while feeding. The renal lesions in male rats, both malignant and non-malignant, were not statistically significant, except for hyperplasia of the renal pelvis epithelium at the high dose. It is notable that renal failure occurs in cases of human overdose. Cresols are significantly more irritant than other phenols found in essential oils such as eugenol, thymol and carvacrol. The slight tendency to cause malignant tumors in rodents may be more a reflection of the irritancy of high doses in those species than a true carcinogenic action. Although the quinone methide derivative of p-cresol leads to the formation of DNA adducts, its formation in vivo is likely to be negligible. A comparison of animal and human lethality suggests that cresols are less orally toxic to humans than rodents.

Cresols are used in disinfectants, wood preservatives and other consumer products. Low levels of cresols naturally occur in smoked fish, cow's milk, cheese, whiskey, fried bacon and other foods. p-Cresol is formed in the human gut from tyrosine metabolism (Sanders et al 2009).

Summary: Cresols (especially p-cresol) are highly corrosive and toxic compounds. Chronic inhalation of large amounts may cause adverse effects in the respiratory system, and chronic oral ingestion or overdose is likely to be hepatotoxic and/or nephrotoxic. Currently, there is insufficient information to establish a safe dose threshold. Fortunately, cresols only occur very rarely in essential oils.

Regulatory guidelines: The CIR recommended maximum for o-cresol and m-cresol in cosmetics is 0.5%. Mixed cresols are prohibited as a cosmetic ingredient in Canada, because they "pose a risk to consumers" (Health Canada Cosmetic Ingredient Hotlist, March 2011).

p-Cresyl methyl ether

Synonyms: 4-Methoxytoluene. 4-Methylanisole
Systematic name: 1-Methyl-4-methoxybenzene
Chemical class: Benzenoid ether
CAS number: 104-93-8

Sources >1.0%:

Ylang-ylang	0.4–10.4%
Ylang-ylang absolute	3.0%
Cananga	2.6%

Adverse skin reactions: Tested at 2% on 25 volunteers, p-cresyl methyl ether was neither irritating nor sensitizing (Opdyke 1974 p. 393).

Acute toxicity: Acute dermal LD_{50} in rabbits, >5 g/kg ; acute oral LD_{50} in rats reported as 1.92 g/kg (Opdyke 1974 p. 393) and 207 mg/kg (Sweet 1987, cited in Thompson 1994).

Summary: p-Cresyl methyl ether appears to be non-irritant and non-sensitizing, but it does possess moderate toxicity.

Cuminaldehyde

Synonyms: Cuminal. Cuminic aldehyde
Systematic name: 4-(1-Methylethyl)benzaldehyde

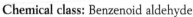

Chemical class: Benzenoid aldehyde
CAS number: 122-03-2

Sources >1.0%:

Cumin	19.8–40.0%
Eucalyptus polybractea (cryptone CT)	3.3%
Labrador tea	1.6%

Pharmacokinetics: Oral cuminaldehyde is oxidized in rabbits to hydroxyl and carboxyl derivatives of *p*-isopropylbenzoic acid (cumic acid). Some reduction to *p*-cumyl alcohol also occurs (Scheline 1991 p. 90).
Adverse skin reactions: Tested at 4% on 25 volunteers cuminaldehyde was neither irritating nor sensitizing. Applied full strength, it was not irritating to mouse skin, but was irritating to rabbit skin (Opdyke 1974 p. 395–396). There were three reactions to 15% cuminaldehyde (1.7%) in 179 dermatitis patients suspected of allergy to cosmetics (De Groot et al 1985).
Acute toxicity: Acute oral LD_{50} in rats 1.39 g/kg (Jenner et al 1964); acute dermal LD_{50} in rabbits 2.8 g/kg (Opdyke 1974 p. 395–396).
Mutagenicity and genotoxicity: Cuminaldehyde was not mutagenic in *S. typhimurium* strains T98 and T100 (Rockwell & Raw 1979) and was not genotoxic in Chinese hamster ovary cells (Sasaki et al 1989).
Carcinogenic/anticarcinogenic potential: Cuminaldehyde reduced the incidence of spontaneous carcinomas in mice by 45% when given at 5 mg per day (Boyland 1940).
Summary: Cuminaldehyde may be slightly irritating or allergenic to the skin; it is only slightly toxic. It possesses some non-mutagenic and anticarcinogenic activity.

Cuminyl alcohol

Synonyms: Cuminic alcohol. *p*-Isopropylbenzyl alcohol
Systematic name: 4-(1-Methylethyl)benzyl alcohol
Chemical class: Benzenoid alcohol
CAS number: 536-60-7

Sources >0.1%:

Cumin	0.2–2.2%
Venetian sumach	1.0%

Adverse skin reactions: Cuminyl alcohol was moderately irritating to rabbit skin when applied undiluted for 24 hours under occlusion. Tested at 4% on 24 volunteers the material was neither irritating nor sensitizing (Opdyke 1974 p. 871).
Acute toxicity: Acute oral LD_{50} in rats 1.02 g/kg; acute dermal LD_{50} in rabbits 2.5 g/kg (Opdyke 1974 p. 871).
Summary: Cuminyl alcohol appears to be non-irritant and non-allergenic to the skin; it is only slightly toxic.

p-Cymene

Synonyms: 4-Isopropyl toluene. Dolcymene
Systematic name: 1-Methyl-4-(1-methylethyl)benzene
Chemical class: Benzenoid monoterpenoid hydrocarbon
CAS number: 99-87-6
Note: *p*-Cymene also exists as other isomers.

Sources >5.0%:

Black seed	14.7–38.0%
Thymus zygis (thymol CT)	18.9–37.7%
Oregano (Mexican)	7.7–28.0%
Thymus vulgaris (carvacrol CT)	27.4%
Camphor (white)	24.2%
Ajowan	20.8–24.0%
Thymus zygis (carvacrol CT)	20.8%
Thymus vulgaris (thymol CT)	7.2–18.9%
Thymus zygis (thymol/carvacrol CT)	18.8%
Eucalyptus polybractea (cryptone CT)	18.3%
Cascarilla (Bahamian)	10.0–18.0%
Cumin	5.9–17.5%
Blackcurrant bud absolute	1.9–15.4%
Savory (winter)	2.2–14.6%
Boswellia frereana	0.7–11.7%
Pepper (pink)	2.9–11.5%
Pteronia	11.3%
Bee balm	2.1–11.0%
Oregano	3.0–10.9%
Lime expressed (Persian)	0.4–10.4%
Thyme (spike)	10.1%
Angelica root	3.5–9.8%
Thymus serpyllum	5.7–9.6%
Boswellia neglecta	9.5%
Savory (summer)	0.9–8.7%
Boldo	8.6%
Narcissus absolute	1.3–8.5%
Coriander seed	0–8.4%
Tea tree	0.5–8.0%
Elemi	1.4–7.7%
Fir cone (silver)	0.1–7.5%
Boswellia sacra (α-pinene CT)	0–7.5%
Southernwood	7.3%
Boswellia rivae	7.1%
Thyme (limonene CT)	7.0%
Pine (dwarf)	0.4–6.9%
Cajuput	0.7–6.8%
Labdanum	2.1–6.3%
Rosemary (verbenone CT)	1.8–6.3%
Eucalyptus dives	6.1%
Marjoram wild (carvacrol CT)	5.2–6.0%
Rosemary (β-myrcene CT)	2.4–6.0%
Marjoram (sweet)	2.2–5.3%

Pharmacokinetics: There are significant interspecies differences in the metabolism of *p*-cymene, and a total of 23 metabolites have been identified, though not all in any one species. The major metabolite in rats is cumic acid, and in guinea pigs it is cuminuric acid. *p*-Cymen-8-ol and *p*-cymen-9-ol are important minor metabolites in both species (Walde et al 1983). In rabbits, *p*-cymene was metabolized to myrcene-3(10)-glycol, uroterpenol and *p*-cymene-9-carboxylic acid (Ishida et al 1981). Several further rabbit metabolites have been identified (Matsumoto et al 1992).

Adverse skin reactions: Tested at 4% on 25 volunteers, *p*-cymene was neither irritating nor sensitizing, but it has been reported as a primary irritant, and was moderately irritating when applied undiluted to rabbit skin (Opdyke 1974 p. 401–402). Of seven dermatitis patients already sensitive to tea tree oil one was sensitive to 1% *p*-cymene (Knight & Hausen 1994). Tested at 5%, *p*-cymene caused no reactions in 11 dermatitis patients sensitive to tea tree oil (Hausen et al 1999).

Acute toxicity: *p*-Cymene acute oral LD_{50} in rats 4.75 g/kg (Jenner et al 1964). Acute dermal LD_{50} in rabbits >5 g/kg (Opdyke 1974 p. 401–402).

Comments: As well as being a normal essential oil constituent, *p*-cymene is often found as a degradation product.

Summary: *p*-Cymene may be slightly irritant or allergenic; it appears to be non-toxic.

Decanoic acid

Synonyms: Capric acid. Decylic acid
Chemical class: Aliphatic carboxylic acid
CAS number: 334-48-5

Sources >1.0%:

Blue chamomile (α-bisabolol oxide A / (*E*)-β-farnesene CT)	1.3%
Sugandha	1.3%

Adverse skin reactions: Decanoic acid was moderately-to-severely irritating to rabbit skin when applied undiluted for 24 hours under occlusion. Tested at 1% on 28 volunteers the material was neither irritating nor sensitizing (Opdyke 1979a p. 735–741).

Acute toxicity: Acute oral LD_{50} in rats 3.73 g/kg; acute dermal LD_{50} in rabbits >5 g/kg (Opdyke 1979a p. 735–741).

Carcinogenic/anticarcinogenic potential: Decanoic acid had no antitumoral effect on Ehrlich ascites carcinoma in mice (Nishikawa et al 1976). However, it demonstrated tumor-inhibiting activity when mixed with tumor cells of 6C3HED, Ehrlich and TA_3 strains before injection into mice (Tolnai & Morgan 1962).

Summary: Decanoic acid appears to be non-irritant and non-allergenic to the skin; it is only slightly toxic, and may possess antitumoral activity.

2-Decenal

Synonym: Decenaldehyde
Systematic name: 2-Decen-1-al
Chemical class: Aliphatic alkene aldehyde
CAS number: 3913-71-1

Source:

Coriander leaf	26.8–46.5%

Adverse skin reactions: 2-Decenal was severely irritating to rabbits when applied undiluted for 24 hours under occlusion.

Tested at 4% on 25 volunteers it was neither irritating nor sensitizing (Opdyke 1979a p. 761).

Acute toxicity: Acute oral LD_{50} in rats ~5 g/kg; acute dermal LD_{50} in rabbits 3.4 g/kg (Opdyke 1979a p. 761).

Summary: 2-Decenal may cause skin irritation if used in high concentrations. It presents minimal risk of toxicity.

Decyl acetate

Synonyms: *n*-Decyl acetate. Acetic acid decyl ester
Systematic name: Decyl ethanoate
Chemical class: Aliphatic ester
CAS number: 112-17-4

Sources >1.0%:

Ambrette	0–5.6%
Thorow-wax	1.2%

Adverse skin reactions: Decyl acetate was slightly irritating to rabbit skin when applied undiluted for 24 hours under occlusion. Tested at 8% on 25 volunteers it was neither irritating nor sensitizing (Opdyke 1975 p. 689–690).

Acute toxicity: Acute oral LD_{50} in rats >5 g/kg; acute dermal LD_{50} in rabbits >5 g/kg (Opdyke 1975 p. 689–690).

Summary: Decyl acetate appears to be non-irritant, non-allergenic and non toxic. As an ester, it is very unlikely to be a carcinogen.

Dehydrocostuslactone

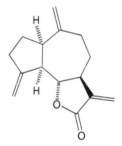

Synonym: 4(15),10(14),11(13)-Guaiatrien-12,6-olide
Systematic name: [3a*S*-(3aα,6aα,9aα,9bβ)]-Decahydro-3,6,9-tris(methylene)-azuleno[4,5-*b*]furan-2(3*H*)-one
Chemical class: Sesquiterpenoid lactone
CAS number: 477-43-0

Source:

Costus	6.0%

Adverse skin reactions: A dermal sensitizer (Benezra & Epstein 1986). Four of ten patients reacted positively to 0.033% dehydrocostuslactone (Paulsen et al 1998). Sesquiterpene lactones from Compositae plants are notorious skin sensitizers (Ross et al 1993; Goulden & Wilkinson 1998). Patch testing in 250 selected gardeners showed Compositae allergy in 25 (17 females and 8 males). Of these, 24 were possibly occupationally sensitized (Paulsen et al 1998).

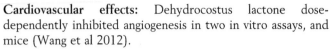

Cardiovascular effects: Dehydrocostus lactone dose-dependently inhibited angiogenesis in two in vitro assays, and mice (Wang et al 2012).

Carcinogenic/anticarcinogenic potential: Dehydrocostus lactone was dose- and time-dependently cytotoxic against selected human cancer cell lines (Sun et al 2003).

Summary: The limited data points to dehydrocostuslactone being a possibly potent skin allergen. Its antiangiogenic actions suggests caution in pregnancy.

Diallyl disulfide

Synonyms: Allyl disulfide. Garlicin. 4,5-Dithia-1,7-octadiene
Systematic name: Di-(2-propenyl) disulfide
Chemical class: Aliphatic alkene disulfide
CAS number: 2179-57-9

Sources:

Garlic	25.2–46.8%
Mustard	0–4.1%

Pharmacokinetics: After ip injection of [^{35}S]-diallyl disulfide in mice, more than 80% of the radioactivity was found in the liver cytosol fraction after two hours, along with about 8% of unchanged compound (Scheline 1991 p. 480). Diallyl disulfide is mainly converted to allyl mercaptan and allyl methyl sulfide in primary rat hepatocytes (Sheen et al 1999b). It is also reduced to diallyl sulfide in the isolated perfused rat liver (Egen-Schwind et al 1992).

Adverse skin reactions: Undiluted diallyl disulfide was irritating to rabbit skin. Tested at 1% on 31 volunteers it was not sensitizing, and produced one irritant reaction (Ford et al 1988a p. 297–298). Diallyl disulfide produced 18 positive reactions in 23 garlic-sensitive individuals (78%) when tested at 5%, but none when tested at 0.5% (Papageorgiou et al 1983). It has been known to induce photoallergic contact dermatitis (Scheman & Gupta 2001; Alvarez et al 2003) and systemic contact dermatitis (Pereira et al 2002).

Acute toxicity: Acute mouse oral LD$_{50}$ 145 mg/kg (male) and 130 mg/kg (female) (Nutrition International 1990). Acute rat oral LD$_{50}$ 260 mg/kg, acute rabbit dermal LD$_{50}$ in 3.6 g/kg (Ford et al 1988a p. 297–298).

Cardiovascular effects: Diallyl disulfide shows strong antiplatelet aggregation activity in vitro (Chan et al 2002).

Hepatotoxicity: Diallyl disulfide was cytotoxic to isolated rat hepatocyte membranes at 2 mM (292 mg/L) (Sheen et al 1999a). Doses of 80 mg/kg of the compound given orally to rats 3 times per week for 6 weeks caused significant increases in glutathione reductase and glutathione S-transferase activity, but decreased glutathione peroxidase activity (Wu et al 2001). At concentrations of 0.5 and 1.0 mM (73 and 146 mg/L), diallyl disulfide protected isolated rat hepatocytes against aflatoxin B$_1$-induced DNA damage, and this has been rationalized by increases in glutathione S-transferase and glutathione peroxidase activities (Sheen et al 2001). Diallyl disulfide, administered orally to rats at 100 µmol/kg (14.6 mg/kg) for 14 consecutive days, significantly reduced the hepatic injury caused by carbon tetrachloride in rats (Fukao et al 2004).

Mutagenicity and genotoxicity: Diallyl disulfide strongly induced CA and SCE in Chinese hamster ovary cells. The addition of S9 reduced the induction of SCEs, but enhanced CA generation (Musk et al 1997). In a comet assay, diallyl disulfide did not increase the number of strand breaks in HepG2 cells at 5–100 µM. In the same concentration range, diallyl disulfide protected HepG2 cells from DNA damage induced by aflatoxin B1, hydrogen peroxide and benzo[a]pyrene (Belloir et al 2006). Diallyl disulfide was antimutagenic against three mutagens in vivo in rats, which was closely associated with the induction of phase II enzymes (Guyonnet et al 2001). It also protected against aflatoxin B$_1$ genotoxicity in rat liver (Guyonnet et al 2002).

Carcinogenic/anticarcinogenic potential: Diallyl disulfide significantly increased the glutathione content of red blood cells and the activity of glutathione S-transferase in rats when given orally at 80 mg/kg (Wu et al 2001). However, it dose-dependently reduced intracellular glutathione in canine mammary tumor cells, while inhibiting their growth (Sundaram & Milner 1993). Diallyl disulfide potently induces the detoxifying enzymes quinone reductase, glutathione peroxidase and glutathione S-transferase (Munday & Munday 2001; Fukao et al 2004). Diallyl disulfide had a promotion-inhibiting action in rats (Guyonnet et al 2004). Human colorectal HCT-116 cells exposed to 4.6 and 23 µM (0.67 and 3.36 mg/L) diallyl dispulphide showed a 1.9 and 2.9-fold increase in apoptosis, respectively, which appeared to be p53-dependant (Bottone et al 2002). It significantly inhibited the proliferation of human hepatoma cell line HepG2, human leukemia CCRF-CEM cell lines (including multidrug-resistant strains), and has been chemopreventive in cancers of the breast, colon, lung and skin (Knowles & Milner 1998; Nakagawa et al 2001; Efferth et al 2002a; Kwon et al 2002). Diallyl disulfide reduced NDEA-induced forestomach tumor formation by 90%, and pulmonary adenoma formation by 30% in mice (Wattenberg et al 1989).

Summary: Diallyl disulfide is moderately toxic in rodent oral studies, and this may be linked to hepatotoxicity. However, there is also evidence of a hepatoprotective action. There may be a risk of skin irritation or sensitization, but probably not at 0.5% or less. Diallyl disulfide inhibits platelet aggregation.

Diallyl sulfide

Synonyms: Allyl sulfide. Thioallyl ether. 3,3'-Thiobis-1-propene
Systematic name: Di-(2-propenyl) sulfide
Chemical class: Aliphatic alkene sulfide
CAS number: 592-88-1

Sources:

Mustard	0–5.5%
Garlic	1.1–2.4%

Pharmacokinetics: Diallyl sulfide is mainly converted to allyl methyl sulfide in primary rat hepatocytes (Sheen et al 1999b).

Adverse skin reactions: Tested at 0.5% on 22 volunteers, diallyl sulfide was neither irritating nor sensitizing. The undiluted compound was extremely irritating to rabbit skin. Tested at 0.5% on human subjects, and at 5% on 23 garlic-sensitive patients, diallyl sulfide produced no sensitization reactions (Ford et al 1988a p. 299–300).

Acute toxicity: Acute oral LD_{50} in 2.03 g/kg in male mice, and 1.81 g/kg in female mice (Nutrition International 1990). Acute oral LD_{50} in rats 2.98 g/kg, acute dermal LD_{50} in rabbits >5 g/kg (Musk et al 1997).

Cardiovascular effects: Diallyl sulfide shows strong antiplatelet aggregation activity in vitro (Chan et al 2002).

Hepatotoxicity: Diallyl sulfide offers some protection against paracetamol-induced hepatotoxicity, probably by inhibiting the transformation of paracetamol to more toxic metabolites (Hu et al 1996). At concentrations of 0.5 and 2.0 mM (57 and 228 mg/L), diallyl sulfide protected isolated rat hepatocytes against aflatoxin B_1-induced DNA damage, and this has been rationalized by increases in glutathione S-transferase and glutathione peroxidase activities (Sheen et al 2001). Diallyl sulfide is much less cytotoxic to rat hepatocyte membranes than diallyl disulfide (Sheen et al 1999a).

Mutagenicity and genotoxicity: Diallyl sulfide weakly induces CA and SCE in Chinese hamster ovary cells (Musk et al 1997). However, it is weakly antimutagenic against two mutagens in vivo in rats (Guyonnet et al 2001), protects against aflatoxin B(1) genotoxicity in rat liver (Guyonnet et al 2002) and is a weak inducer of the detoxifying enzymes quinone reductase and glutathione S-transferase (GST) (Munday & Munday 2001). The compound slightly but significantly increased CYP2E1 activity (Fukao et al 2004) and at 200 mg/kg it significantly increased PROD activity (Wu et al 2002). In a comet assay, diallyl sulfide did not increase the number of strand breaks in HepG2 cells at 5–100 μM. In the same concentration range, diallyl sulfide protected HepG2 cells from DNA damage induced by aflatoxin B1, hydrogen peroxide or benzo[a]pyrene (Belloir et al 2006).

Carcinogenic/anticarcinogenic potential: An oral dose of 200 mg/kg of diallyl sulfide had a significant chemopreventive effect in female mice given 20 mg/kg ip 1,2-dimethylhydrazine (Nutrition International 1990). Diallyl sulfide inhibited benzo[a]pyrene-induced neoplasia of the forestomach and lung in female mice when given prior to the carcinogen challenge (Sparnins et al 1988). Diallyl sulfide reduced incidence of NNK-induced lung tumors in mice from 100% to 37.9%, and reduced the number of tumors per mouse from 7.2 to 0.6 (Hong et al 1992). A significant protection from skin carcinogenesis in mice occurred when diallyl sulfide was applied topically either one hour before or one hour after the administration of either DMBA or B[a]P (Singh & Shukla 1998).

Diallyl sulfide can act as a tumor promoter in rat liver, but has no co-promoting effect (Guyonnet et al 2004). It totally inhibited NMBA-induced esophageal papillomas and squamous cell carcinomas in rats, and substantially reduced hepatic microsomal metabolism of the carcinogen (Wargovich et al 1988). It also inhibited 2-amino-3-methylimidazo[4,5-f] quinoline-induced hepatocarcinogenesis, and DMBA-induced mammary cancer in rats (Ip et al 1992; Tsuda et al 1994). In rats, diallyl sulfide increased the expression of GST 12-fold, and reversed the GST-depleting effect of the mammary carcinogen diethylstilbestrol (Green et al 2007a). Diallyl sulfide induces the expression of nucleotide excision repair enzymes in female rats exposed to diethylstilbestrol, enhancing the ability of breast tissue to repair DNA damage (Green et al 2007b).

Summary: There are no reports of skin reactions in humans, and diallyl sulfide is less likely than diallyl disulfide to cause skin reactions. Diallyl sulfide is also less acutely toxic in rodent studies, and there is no evidence of hepatotoxicity. Diallyl sulfide has significant chemopreventive activity. Diallyl sulfide inhibits platelet aggregation.

Diallyl trisulfide

Synonyms: Allitridin. 4,5,6-Trithia-1,8-nonadiene
Systematic name: Di-(2-propenyl) trisulfide
Chemical class: Aliphatic alkene trisulfide
CAS number: 2050-87-5

Sources:

Garlic	18.0–48.8%
Mustard	0–9.7%

Pharmacokinetics: Diallyl trisulfide, administered orally to rats at 10 μmol/kg (1.78 mg/kg) for 14 consecutive days, significantly increased the activities of quinone reductase, glutathione peroxidase and glutathione S-transferase (Fukao et al 2004). Munday & Munday (2001) similarly found that diallyl trisulfide increased the activities of quinone reductase and glutathione S-transferase in a variety of rat tissues. Given orally to rats at 70 mg/kg three times a week for 6 weeks, diallyl trisulfide lowered N-nitrosodimethylamine demethylase activity, and did not affect the activity of ethoxyresorufin O-deethylase or erythromycin demethylase. However, glutathione S-transferase activity was significantly increased (Wu CC et al 2002).

Cardiovascular effects: Diallyl trisulfide shows strong antiplatelet aggregation activity in vitro (Chan et al 2002).

Hepatotoxicity: Cultured primary rat hepatocytes were treated with 0, 0.025, 0.05 or 0.25 mM (0, 4.45, 8.90 or 44.5 mg/L) diallyl trisulfide for 0, 4, 8 or 24 hours. At 0.025 or 0.05 mM, diallyl trisulfide enhanced antioxidation and detoxification capabilities by increasing the intracellular glutathione level and the activity of glutathione peroxidase, glutathione reductase, or glutathione S-transferase. However, 0.05 and 0.25 mM diallyl trisulfide might adversely affect the viability of hepatocytes since these concentrations increased LDH leakage (Wu CC et al 2004a). Diallyl trisulfide, administered orally to rats at 10 μmol/kg/day (1.78 mg/kg/day) for 14 consecutive days, significantly reduced the hepatic injury caused by carbon tetrachloride in rats (Fukao et al 2004). Similarly, 30 mg/kg/day diallyl trisulfide attenuated oxidative stress-mediated liver injury in mice, reversing ALT and AST leakage, and inhibiting both lipid peroxidation and the depletion of glutathione and other antioxidant enzymes (Zeng et al 2008).

Carcinogenic/anticarcinogenic potential: Diallyl trisulfide is significantly cytotoxic to cell lines for human cancers of the bladder, bone, breast, lungs and stomach, in each case with strong evidence of apoptosis (Li & Lu 2002; Malki et al 2009; Wang et al 2010; Xiao et al 2009, Zhang et al 2009). The mechanisms of diallyl trisulfide cytotoxicity in relation to brain, liver and prostate cancers has been reviewed by Powolny & Singh (2008). Diallyl trisulfide inhibited benzo[a]pyrene-induced neoplasia of the forestomach in female mice when given

96 hours prior to the carcinogen challenge (Sparnins et al 1988). Antitumoral effects have also been seen in mouse studies involving cancers of the liver and prostate, using xenografted human cancer cells (Xiao et al 2006, Zhang et al 2007). The lack of weight loss in either case suggests minimal collateral toxicity.

Summary: Diallyl trisulfide is a potent inducer of antioxidant enzyme systems. This partly explains its antitumoral action, and is largely responsible for its hepatoprotective effect. Diallyl trisulfide inhibits platelet aggregation.

Dimethyl anthranilate

Synonym: Methyl *N*-methylanthranilate
Systematic name: Methyl 2-methylaminobenzoate
Chemical class: Benzenoid amine ester
CAS number: 85-91-6

Source:

Mandarin leaf	43.2–51.9%

Adverse skin reactions: Undiluted dimethyl anthranilate was not irritating to rabbit skin; tested at 10% on human subjects, it was neither irritating nor sensitizing (Opdyke 1975 p. 791). Dimethyl anthranilate was phototoxic in eight of ten human volunteers at 5.0%, with a NOAEL of 0.5%; at 5.0% it was not photoallergenic (Opdyke 1979a p. 273).

Acute toxicity: Acute oral LD_{50} in rats reported as 3.7 mL/kg, and between 2.25 and 3.38 g/kg; acute dermal LD_{50} in rabbits >5 g/kg (Opdyke 1975 p. 791).

Subacute and subchronic toxicity: In a study in rats over 90 days, the NOAEL for dimethyl anthranilate was between 300 and 1200 ppm. A further study in rats over 12 weeks suggested a NOAEL of 20.3 mg/kg (Opdyke 1975 p. 791).

Summary: Dimethyl anthranilate does not appear to be irritant or allergenic, but it is phototoxic at concentrations over 0.5%. The 12 week rat NOAEL was 20.3 mg/kg.

Regulatory guidelines: For applications on areas of skin exposed to sunshine, excluding bath preparations, soaps and other products which are washed off the skin, dimethyl anthranilate should not be used such that the level in the consumer product exceeds 0.1% (SCCNFP 2001; IFRA 2009). The level comprises the fragrance ingredient added as such, as well as contributions from mandarin leaf oil. This recommendation is based on the phototoxic potential of dimethyl anthranilate referred to above. In addition this compound did not cause photoallergy at 0.5% in human subjects (private communication from RIFM).

Dimethyl disulfide

Synonyms: Methyl disulfide. 2,3-Dithiabutane
Chemical class: Aliphatic disulfide
CAS number: 624-92-0

Source:

Garlic	0.4–1.2%

Inhalation toxicity: Exposing two male and two female rats to 250 ppm dimethyl disulfide for 6 hours per day for 13 days resulted in lethargy, respiratory difficulty, low weight gain, and congested organs. After 20 days of 6 hour exposures at 100 ppm there were no toxic signs or organ abnormalities in two male and two female rats (Gage 1970). In a 90 day study, male and female rats were exposed to dimethyl disulfide vapors at 0, 5, 25 or 125 ppm for 6 hours/day. The NOAEL for male rats was 5 ppm, and for female rats the NOAEL was 25 ppm (Kim HY et al 2006).

Summary: The inhalational NOAEL for dimethyl disulfide was 5 ppm.

1-Dodecanal

Synonyms: *n*-Dodecanal. *n*-Dodecyl aldehyde. Lauraldehyde. Lauryl aldehyde. Laurenobiolide
Systematic name: 1-Oxo-dodecane
Chemical class: Aliphatic aldehyde
CAS number: 112-54-9

Sources >0.1%:

Kesom	44.1%
Betel	0–7.1%
Coriander leaf	1.0–1.7%
Cistus	0–1.1%

Adverse skin reactions: Tested at 5% on 25 volunteers 1-dodecanal was not sensitizing (Opdyke 1973 p. 483).

Acute toxicity: Acute oral LD_{50} in rats 23.1 g/kg; acute dermal LD_{50} in rabbits >2 g/kg (Opdyke 1973 p. 483).

Summary: Limited data suggest that 1-dodecanal is not allergenic, and it is non-toxic.

2-Dodecenal

Synonym: β-Octyl acrolein
Systematic name: 1-Oxo-dodec-2-ene
Chemical class: Aliphatic alkene aldehyde
CAS number: 4826-62-4

Source:

Coriander leaf	2.7–10.3%

Adverse skin reactions: Applied full strength to rabbit skin for 24 hours under occlusion 2-dodecenal was severely irritating. Tested at 1% on 25 volunteers it was neither irritating nor sensitizing (Opdyke & Letizia 1983 p. 849).

Acute toxicity: Acute oral LD_{50} in rats >5 g/kg; acute dermal LD_{50} in rabbits <5 g/kg (Opdyke & Letizia 1983 p. 849).

Inhalation toxicity: Dodecanal vapors may cause eye irritation (Cometto-Muñiz et al 2007).

Summary: Limited data suggest that 2-dodecenal may be irritant in high concentrations, is not allergenic, and is non-toxic.

Dodecyl acetate

Synonyms: *n*-Dodecyl acetate. Lauryl acetate. Acetic acid dodecyl ester

Systematic name: *n*-Dodecyl ethanoate
Chemical class: Aliphatic ester
CAS number: 112-66-3

Sources >1.0%:

Ambrette	0.2–4.0%
Boronia absolute	3.8%

Adverse skin reactions: Dodecyl acetate was slightly irritating to rabbit skin when applied undiluted for 24 hours under occlusion. Tested at 20% on 25 volunteers the material was neither irritating nor sensitizing (Opdyke 1976 p. 667–668).
Acute toxicity: Acute oral LD_{50} in rats >5 g/kg; acute dermal LD_{50} in rabbits >5 g/kg (Opdyke 1976 p. 667–668).
Subacute and subchronic toxicity: Following DMBA initiation, repeated application of high doses of undiluted dodecyl acetate promoted skin tumors in three of 15 mice; no tumors developed in 15 mice similarly treated with a 33% solution in acetone, or in mice not initiated with DMBA (Sicé et al 1957).
Summary: Limited data suggest that dodecyl acetate is neither irritant not allergenic, and it is non-toxic.

β-Elemene

Synonyms: Elemene. 1,3,11-Elematriene
Systematic name: 1-Ethenyl-1-methyl-2,4-bis-(1-methylethenyl)-cyclohexane
Chemical class: Monocyclic sesquiterpenoid polyalkene
CAS number: 11029-06-4
Note: Different isomers of β-elemene exist, and the following isomer-specific information has been published:

(−)-β-Elemene

Synonyms: [1S-(1α,2β,4β)]-Elemene. (1S,2R,4R)-Elemene
CAS number: 515-13-9

Sources >1.0%:

Atractylis	18.0%
Myrrh	8.7%
Katrafay	3.0–6.0%
Copaiba	0–4.4%
Citronella (Javanese)	1.9–3.2%
Valerian (European)	0.1–3.0%
Mango ginger	2.8%
Betel	0–2.6%
Magnolia leaf	2.4%
Magnolia flower	2.3%
Arina	2.1%
Cascarilla (Bahamian)	1.6–2.0%
Zedoary	1.5–1.9%
Manuka	0.6–1.6%
Basil (linalool CT)	0.9–1.5%
Pilocarpus jaborandi	0–1.5%
Cangerana	1.3%
Boswellia frereana	0–1.3%

Patchouli (Chinese)	0–1.3%
Elecampane	1.2%
Cubeb	1.0–1.2%
Catnip	0–1.2%
Turmeric (wild)	1.0–1.1%
Ravensara leaf	tr–1.1%
Ginger	<1.2%
Cascarilla (El Salvadorian)	1.0%
Cedarwood (Port Orford)	1.0%
Finger root	1.0%
Juniperberry	0–1.0%

Pharmacokinetics: In rats, β-elemene was absorbed and eliminated rapidly and distributed widely in the body after ip or iv administration. Protein binding was high. Only small amounts of unchanged β-elemene were found in the urine, feces and bile (Wang & Su 2000). Also in rats, one biliary metabolite was identified: 1-methyl-1-ethenyl-2,4-diisopropenyl aldehydohexamethylene (Li et al 2000).
Cardiovascular effects: β-Elemene inhibited the expression of VEGF in B16F10 melanoma cells at 20 and 50 mg/kg/day sc for 21 days in mice, and inhibited VEGF-induced sprouting of rat aortic ring vessels in chick embryo chorioallantoic membranes at 20 and 50 μM in vitro (Chen et al 2011). β-Elemene attenuated angiogenesis in gastric cancer stem-like cells at 50 and 100 mg/kg ip (Yan et al 2013).
Carcinogenic/anticarcinogenic potential: β-Elemene is dose-dependently cytotoxic to human K562 leukemia cells, this effect being due to apoptosis (Zheng et al 1997; Yuan et al 1999; Zou et al 2001). The IC_{50} values of elemene for promyelocytic leukemia HL-60 cells and erythroleukemia K562 cells were 27.5 μg/mL and 81 μg/mL, respectively, while the IC_{50} for peripheral blood leukocytes was 254.3 μg/mL (Yang et al 1996).

β-Elemene selectively targeted human non-small-cell lung cancer cells, triggering apoptosis (Wang et al 2005). Similarly, the growth of human ovarian cancer cells was inhibited by β-elemene, while normal ovary cells were only marginally affected. This effect was also seen in cells resistant to the anticancer drug cisplatin, and the mechanism by which β-elemene overcame this resistance was outlined (Li et al 2005). β-Elemene inhibited the growth of human laryngeal cancer cells in vitro, inducing apoptosis, and laryngeal tumors transplanted to mice were inhibited in vivo (Tao et al 2006). Treatment with β-elemene inhibited the growth of cells for cancers of the brain, breast, cervix, lung, colon and prostate, with IC_{50} values ranging from 47 to 95 μg/mL (Li et al 2010).

In a clinical trial, β-elemene was effective in the management of malignant pleural and peritoneal effusions. There was no bone marrow, liver, cardiac or renal toxicity, while major adverse effects were fever, local pain and gastrointestinal disturbance (Wang et al 1996). In a second trial of 40 brain cancer cases, β-elemene therapy reduced mean tumor size by 61%, and there were four cases of complete recovery. The response to β-elemene was better than in the control group of 29 patients, who received conventional chemotherapy (Tan et al 2000). In China, β-elemene is used for the treatment of various cancers, including lung, brain, liver and esophagus. In 1993 it was designated as a Chinese national Class II new drug, and in 1994 its anticancer effect was officially recognised by the Chinese health authority. **Summary:** We could find no toxicity or dermal data for β-elemene. It has demonstrated in vitro, in vivo and clinical antitumoral effects. The antiangionenic action suggests caution in pregnancy.

Elemicin

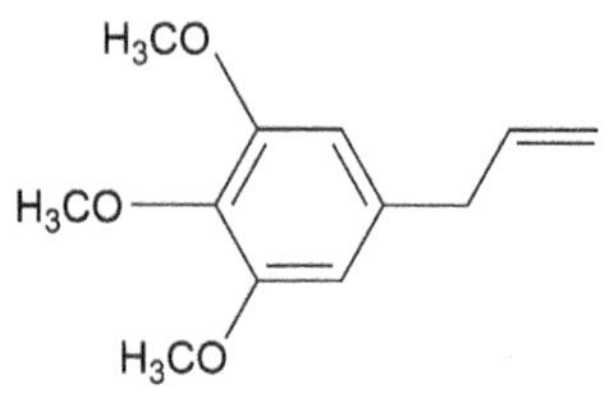

Synonym: 3,4,5-Trimethoxy-1-allylbenzene
Systematic name: 3,4,5-Trimethoxy-1-(2-propenyl)benzene
Chemical class: Phenylpropenoid ether
CAS number: 487-11-6

Sources >1.0%:

Elemi	1.8–10.6%
Parsleyseed	0–8.8%
Nutmeg (E. Indian)	0.1–4.6%
Mace (Indian)	3.1%
African bluegrass	1.8–2.7%
Thorow-wax	2.0%
Mace (East Indian)	0.2–2.0%
Snakeroot	< 1.8%
Nutmeg (W. Indian)	1.2–1.4%
Cinnamomum rigidissimum	1.2%

Pharmacokinetics: Elemicin undergoes two main biotransformations in rats: oxidation to 3-(3,4,5-trimethoxyphenyl)-propionic acid and 3-(3,4,5-trimethoxyphenyl)-propane-1,2-diol. Small amounts of the epoxide of the 3-O-demethylated derivative of elemicin were also found (Solheim & Scheline 1980). O-demethyl elemicin and O-demethyl dihydroxy elemicin were present in human urine after nutmeg ingestion (Beyer et al 2006). 1'-Hydroxyelemicin has not been detected as a metabolite.

Neurotoxicity: Elemicin may be partially responsible for nutmeg's hallucinogenic properties. A myriticin- and elemicin-rich fraction of nutmeg oil has been reported to be reproduce many of the psychotropic characteristics of ground nutmeg (Truitt 1967). A metabolic pathway has been proposed which could convert myristicin and elemicin to TMA (3,4, 5-trimethoxyamphetamine) (Weil 1965, 1966) or MMDA (3-methoxy-4,5-methylenedioxyamphetamine) (Weil 1965), both known hallucinogens. Further work has confirmed that myristicin and elemicin are potentially convertible to chemicals similar to hallucinogens (Kalbhen 1971). However, myristicin and elemicin *per se* are insufficiently potent to explain the psychotropic effects of nutmeg (Truitt 1967).

Mutagenicity and genotoxicity: Elemicin was antimutagenic in the *S. typhimurium* TA135/pSK1002 umu test, due to inhibition of the metabolic activity of S9 (Miyazawa and Kohno 2005). Two studies reported a low to moderate level of genotoxicity for elemicin (Phillips et al 1984; Randerath et al 1984) while in a third it was considered significantly genotoxic (Hasheminejad & Caldwell 1994).

Carcinogenic/anticarcinogenic potential: Neither elemicin nor 1'-hydroxyelemicin was carcinogenic in male mice when a total dose of 4.75 µmol (1.0 mg and 1.1 mg, respectively) was injected ip in increasing doses on days 1, 8, 15 and 22 prior to weaning (Miller et al 1983). However, in a similar study using a total dose of 9.5 µmol (2.13 mg) 1'-hydroxyelemicin, the average number of hepatomas per male mouse was 0.8, compared to 0.1 in the control group. Similarly, a single ip injection of 0.1 or 0.25 µmol/g of 1'-hydroxyelemicin at 12 days of age resulted in 0.3 and 0.4 (respectively) hepatomas per male mouse, compared to 0.2 in the control group. Tumors were assessed at 13 months (Wiseman et al 1987). Antiproliferative activity has been reported for elemicin against various isolated tumor cells, with ED_{50} values of 4.5 µg/mL (MK-1) 2.0 µg/mL (HeLa) and 2.6 µg/mL (B16F10) (Ikeda et al 1998).

Comments: The data suggest a weak carcinogenic potential in male $B6C3F_1$ mice for 1'-hydroxyelemicin. In the only test using elemicin, it was not carcinogenic. There are no chronic dosing studies for elemicin, nor are there studies using rats or female mice, which would be required to properly assess carcinogenicity. A number of essential oil constituents show selective hepatocarcinogenicity in male mice, and these effects are usually marginal or not dose-dependent.

Summary: Currently there are insufficient data to regard elemicin as either neurotoxic or carcinogenic.

Regulatory guidelines: The Council of Europe lists elemicin under 'substances which are suspected to be genotoxic carcinogens and therefore no MDI can be set' (Council of Europe 2003).

Estragole

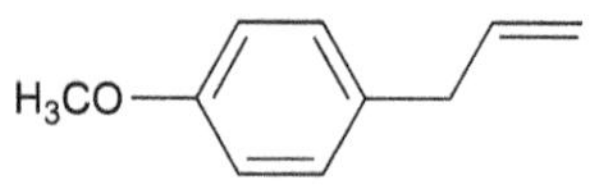

Synonyms: O-Methyl chavicol. 4-Allyl anisole. 4-Methoxyallylbenzene
Systematic name: 4-Methoxy-1-(2-propenyl)benzene
Chemical class: Phenylpropenoid ether
CAS number: 140-67-0

Sources >0.1%:

Ravensara bark	90.0–95.0%
Tarragon	73.3–87.3%
Basil (estragole CT)	73.4–87.4%
Marigold (Mexican)	84.7%
Chervil	49.9–81.3%

Basil (Madagascan)	45.0–50.0%
Pine (ponderosa)	22.0%
Basil (holy)	9.7–12.9%
Ravensara leaf	2.4–11.9%
Anise (star)	0.3–6.6%
Fennel (bitter)	2.8–6.5%
Fennel (sweet)	1.1–4.8%
Betel	0–4.8%
Myrtle (aniseed)	4.4%
Anise	0.3–4.0%
Basil (linalool CT)	0.2–2.0%
Myrtle	0–1.4%
Basil absolute (linalool CT)	1.0%
Basil (methyl cinnamate CT)	tr–0.8%
Damiana (+ myrtenol)	0.4%
Basil (hairy)	0.3–0.4%
Boswellia serrata	0–0.4 %
Tea tree (black)	0.3%
Basil (pungent)	0.2%
Savory (summer)	0–0.2%
Bay (West Indian)	tr–0.1%

Pharmacokinetics: After oral administration to rats, estragole is extensively O-demethylated to the phenol derivative, chavicol, most of which is excreted as such (Solheim & Scheline 1973). Other routes involve oxidation of the allylic side chain (by CYP) to give the potentially genotoxic metabolites, 1′-hydroxyestragole and estragole 2′,3′-oxide. 1′-Hydroxyestragole is further converted to its genotoxic sulfate conjugate in rats, 1′-sulfooxyestragole. Estragole 2′,3′-oxide and related epoxides may form briefly and have the potential to form DNA adducts, but the epoxides are rapidly deactivated by efficient detoxification reactions in rats (Delaforge et al 1980, Luo & Guenthner 1995, 1996). Moreover, the 2′,3′-oxide is hydrolyzed much more rapidly in human liver than in rat liver, thus allowing for a wide margin of safety in humans (Guenthner & Luo 2001). The estragole → 1′-hydroxyestragole → 1′sulfooxyestragole pathway remains a potential route to DNA adducts and carcinogenesis (Rietjens et al 2005a).

At lower doses, estragole is detoxified much more efficiently by enzyme systems than at higher doses. The amount of 1′-hydroxyestragole formed from estragole increased from 0.9% to 8.0% in rats, and from 1.3% to 9.5% in mice as the dosage given was increased from 0.05 mg/kg to 1,000 mg/kg (Zangouras et al 1981). In a later study, at the same two doses, the percentage of 1′-hydroxyestragole formed rose from 1.3% to 13.7% in rats, and from 1.3% to 9.4% in mice (Anthony et al 1987). In in vitro preparations of various rat tissues, O-demethylation of estragole to (non-carcinogenic) 4-allylphenol is the major metabolic route at low doses, and occurs mainly in the lungs and kidneys. Saturation of this metabolic pathway occurs at higher doses, leading to the formation of 1′-hydroxyestragole, primarily in the liver (Punt et al 2008).

In vitro tests suggest that CYP1A2, 2A6, 2C19, 2D6 and 2E1 can all metabolize estragole to 1′-hydroxyestragole in human liver; at physiologically relevant concentrations of estragole, CYP1A2 and 2A6 are the most important of these enzymes (Jeurissen et al 2007). In a comparison of species differences, sulfonation

of estragole to 1′-sulfooxyestragole, was about 30 times more efficient in rat liver than either male mouse liver or mixed sex human liver, suggesting that data from male mice may provide a reasonable estimate of the cancer risk in humans (Punt et al 2007). The formation of 1′-hydroxyestragole glucuronide is a major pathway of estragole metabolism, and accounts for as much as 24% and 33% of the estragole urinary metabolites in rats and mice, respectively. In human liver cells about 12.5% of estragole was converted to 1′-hydroxyestragole in 24 hours (Nath et al 2001, unpublished data). In humans, the amount of 1′-hydroxyestragole found in excreted urine has been reported as 0.3% and 0.4% of ingested estragole (Sangster et al 1987; Zeller et al 2009).

Research using human liver microsomes taken from 27 individuals, suggests three ways in which there could be a greater risk of estragole toxicity in some individuals than in others, due to differences in metabolism. These center on three uridine diphosphate glucuronosyltransferase (UGT) isoforms that are proposed to catalyze the glucuronidation (and hence, detoxification) of 1′-hydroxyestragole - UGT2B7, UGT1A9 and UGT2B15. Firstly, certain drugs are metabolized by UGT2B7 (for example, ibuprofen) and some are metabolized by UGT1A9. Hence, people taking these drugs chronically may be more at risk from estragole toxicity because of competition. Secondly, constituents of certain foods compete for these enzymes. For example, fatty acids are metabolized by UGT2B7, and flavonoids are metabolized by UGT1A9. Therefore, differences in diet may lead to different capacities for detoxification of 1′-hydroxyestragole. Thirdly, two isoforms of the enzyme UGT2B7 have been found, designated H and Y, and these may be expressed to different extents in humans according to genetic and environmental factors. In the liver tissue from the 27 individuals tested, there was a tenfold variation in 1′-hydroxyestragole glucuronidation (Iyer et al 2003).

Estragole prolongs the pentobarbital-induced sleeping time in rats, probably by modulating the barbiturate's metabolism by CYP (Marcus & Lichtenstein 1982).

Adverse skin reactions: Tested at 3% on 25 volunteers estragole was neither irritating nor sensitizing. Estragole was moderately irritating when applied undiluted to rabbit skin (Opdyke 1976 p. 603).

Acute toxicity: Acute oral LD$_{50}$ in mice 1.25 g/kg, in rats 1.82 g/kg (Opdyke 1976 p. 603). Estragole induced CNS depression when given to experimental animals in very high doses (Shipochliev 1968).

Subacute and subchronic toxicity: Estragole of 99% purity was given to groups of ten male and female rats and mice at doses of 37.5, 75, 150, 300 or 600 mg/kg/day 5 days per week for 90 days by corn oil gavage. The NOAEL for male mice was 37.5 mg/kg/day, but no NOAEL could be established for female mice or for rats of either sex. Most signs of toxicity were seen in the liver and bile duct, but some toxic effects were also seen in the glandular stomach, kidneys and nose of rats, the pituitary gland and testes of male rats, and the nose of both sexes of mice, and the stomach of females. At 600 mg/kg, all female mice died during week 1, and one male mouse died during week 9. In all animals on 300 or 600 mg/kg/day, mean body weights were reduced, and liver weights increased (National Toxicology Program 2008a).

Cardiovascular effects: Estragole shows strong antiplatelet aggregation activity in vitro and is reported to be as effective as aspirin (Yoshioka & Tamada 2005).

Reproductive toxicity: In the above mentioned study, all males in the 300 mg/kg and 600 mg/kg groups had marked bilateral degeneration of the germinal epithelium in the testes, and bilateral hypospermia in the epididymides. Testicular weights were reduced in these groups. Such adverse effects are suggestive of male reproductive toxicity at high doses.

Hepatotoxicity: Slight, microscopic liver lesions in rats were seen after oral administration of estragole at 605 mg/kg/day for four days (Taylor et al 1964). A single ip injection of 300 mg/kg estragole in mice is hepatotoxic to adult females, but not to adult males or to suckling offspring of either sex. Administration of estradiol benzoate decreases the resistance of castrated males to estragole toxicity (Vasil'ev et al 2005). When estragole was given to groups of ten male and female rats and mice at doses of 37.5, 75, 150, 300 or 600 mg/kg/day 5 days per week for 90 days by corn oil gavage, there were occurrences of bile duct and oval cell hyperplasia at the lowest dose in rats, oval cell hyperplasia in female mice at 75 mg/kg and male mice at 300 mg/kg, and some liver function tests were abnormal at 75 mg/kg or higher in rats. Bile duct hyperplasia and liver function were not tested in mice (National Toxicology Program 2008a).

Antioxidant/pro-oxidant activity: Estragole demonstrated no capacity for scavenging DPPH radicals (Tominaga et al 2005).

Mutagenicity and genotoxicity: Conflicting mutagenicity results have been obtained for estragole. It was not mutagenic in one *Bacillus subtilis* DNA repair test (Sekizawa & Shibamoto 1982), yet was dose-dependently mutagenic in another (Zani et al 1991). Estragole has been reported as non-mutagenic in the Ames test (Sekizawa & Shibamoto 1982; Zeiger et al 1987). However, positive results were reported for estragole in strain TA135, with the addition of a sulfation cofactor (To et al 1982), and to strain TA100, in the presence of liver extract S13 (Swanson et al 1979). It is believed that activation of estragole requires several metabolic steps, and that S9 might be an incomplete activation system.

Estragole demonstrates clear genotoxicity in rat hepatocytes (Phillips et al 1984; Randerath et al 1984; Howes et al 1990; Müller et al 1994,), but it was not genotoxic in V79 cells, with or without metabolic activation (Müller et al 1994). This again can be explained because estragole adduct formation requires 1'hydroxylation, followed by sulfation, and DNA adducts are found in V79 cells in the presence of a human sulfotransferase (Wakazono et al 1998). Estragole formed DNA adducts in human hepatoma cells (Zhou et al 2007). Estragole-DNA adducts were found in the livers of adult and newborn mice given ip injections of estragole, and they persisted longer in the neonates. This is probably related to the greater sensitivity of newborn mice to tumor induction by estragole (Phillips et al 1984). In mouse liver, estragole-DNA adducts decreased by 85% over three days after a single dose, and then reduced much more gradually (Phillips et al 1981b).

A physiologically based biodynamic (PBBD) model for rats using in vitro data predicts a linear increase in adduct formation in reponse to dose, both above and below carcinogenic amounts. It predicts the formation of 2 and 12.8 estragole-DNA adducts per 100 million nucleotides from dosing of, respectively, 0.01 and 0.07 mg/kg estragole (Paini et al 2010). This is 10 to 100 times less than the background level of DNA damage that is considered of no consequence (Williams 2008).

Carcinogenic/anticarcinogenic potential: Hepatocellular carcinomas developed by about 12 months of age when single or multiple intraperitoneal injections of estragole were administered to male or female mice prior to weaning (Miller et al 1983; Wiseman et al 1987). Similar tumors were found when estragole was administered subcutaneously to preweanling male mice on days 1, 8, 15 and 22, the doses totaling either 650 or 770 μg (Drinkwater et al 1976). A newborn mouse weighs about 1 g, and at weaning (3 weeks) a mouse weighs about 10 g. A total dose of 700 μg is equivalent to 140 mg/kg for a mouse weighing 5 g.

Hepatocellular carcinomas developed when estragole was consumed by female mice in the diet at 0.23% or 0.46% for 12 months (Miller et al 1983). When estragole was given to groups of ten male and female rats and mice at doses of 37.5, 75, 150, 300 or 600 mg/kg/day 5 days per week for 90 days by corn oil gavage, two male rats on 600 mg/kg/day developed bile duct cancer in the liver, and a third developed hepatocellular carcinoma. All males had fibrosis of the bile ducts, which is considered a pre-cancerous state (National Toxicology Program 2008a).

The carcinogenicity of estragole is primarily due to metabolism to 1'-hydroxyestragole and its sulfate ester (Swanson et al 1981). 1'-Hydroxyestragole is a more potent carcinogen than estragole when administered sc or ip to preweanling male mice (Drinkwater et al 1976, Miller & Miller 1983). The same metabolic process is believed to occur in humans (Sangster et al 1987).

Estragole carcinogenicity has been reviewed (De Vincenzi 2000b, McDonald 1999, Smith et al 2002). A RIFM evaluation of the toxicological and exposure data for methyleugenol and estragole concludes: 'The currently available metabolic, biochemical and toxicological data found for methyleugenol in laboratory species provide clear evidence of non-linearity in the dose–response relationships for methyleugenol and estragole with respect to metabolic activation and mechanisms associated with the carcinogenic effects. Consideration of this data indicates, that in all probability, a No-Observed-Effect-Level (NOEL) for methyleugenol in the rat exists in the dose-range of 1–10 mg/kg body weight/day...In the case of estragole there is metabolic evidence that the NOEL is likely to be significantly higher, perhaps in the region of 10–100 mg/kg...'.The panel concluded that, based on the available data, 'neither methyleugenol nor estragole is likely to present a human cancer risk at current levels of exposure resulting from their addition to fragranced products (added as such or from essential oils)' (RIFM 2001).

In a novel assay for carcinogens, groups of male rats were dosed for 2, 14 or 90 days with 0.2 or 2.0 mmol/kg/day (30 or 296 mg/kg/day) of estragole, and then hepatic tissue was analyzed for precancerous changes in gene expression. The results strongly suggest a dose- and duration-dependent hepatocarcinogenic action for estragole, although a safe dose cannot be extrapolated from the data (Auerbach et al 2010). Similarly, 15 μM (2.22 mg/L) estragole was a threshold for hepatotoxicity in isolated primary rat hepatocytes, with higher concentrations being cytotoxic and lower ones not (Paini et al 2010).

Comments: The weight of evidence suggests that low exposure to estragole entails negligible risk to humans. In addition, it should not be assumed essential oils containing estragole will present a level of risk proportionate to their estragole content. Holy basil oil, which contains ~11% estragole, has demonstrated anticarcinogenic effects against stomach cancer in mice, and against cell lines for human mouth cancer and mouse leukemia (Aruna & Sivaramakrishnan 1996; Manosroi et al 2005). Kaledin et al (2009) present the hypothesis that only female mice are susceptible to estragole-induced cancers. However, Wiseman et al (1987) reported that in two strains of mice, males were much more susceptible to 1'-hydroxyestragole carcinogenicity than were females. Kaledin et al also assert that estragole is not carcinogenic in rats, but there is no meaningful evidence to support this assertion.

Summary: Estragole is hepatocarcinogenic in male and female mice and in male rats through bioactivation to 1'-hydroxyestragole and its sulfate ester. 1'-Sulfooxyestragole readily binds to DNA and is primarily responsible for the hepatocarcinogenicity of estragole in mice. Gene expression data suggest that estragole is also hepatocarcinogenic in male rats, depending on dose and duration. Estragole is metabolized to 1'-hydroxyestragole glucuronide more efficiently in rat liver than human liver, but metabolism in mouse and human liver is similar. This pathway is still a major human route of detoxification, and therefore it is probably carcinogenic in humans if exposure is sufficiently high. At low doses, estragole is essentially non-toxic, as it mainly undergoes O-demethylation, but at higher doses 1'-hydroxylation is a major pathway. Because of genetic and environmental factors, some individuals may be at greater risk than others. Females may be more susceptible to hepatotoxicity, and therefore subsequent carcinogenicity, than males. Estragole inhibits platelet aggregation, and shows signs of reproductive toxicity in male rats.

Regulatory guidelines: The expert panel of FEMA determined that exposure to estragole from the consumption of food and spices does not pose a significant cancer risk (Smith at al 2002). However, the EU Scientific Committee on Food's report on estragole (SCF 2001b) concluded that, since estragole is genotoxic and carcinogenic, 'reductions in exposure and restrictions in use levels are indicated.' It has been suggested that a limit of 0.05 mg/kg should be applied to the use of estragole in food (De Vincenzi et al 2000b).

In 1999, estragole was added to the list of carcinogenic chemicals known to the State of California (McDonald 1999). The Council of Europe lists estragole under 'substances which are suspected to be genotoxic carcinogens and therefore no MDI can be set' (Council of Europe 2003). However, the CEFS of the Council of Europe recommended an exposure limit of 0.05 mg/kg, until full carcinogenicity studies in rats and mice of both sexes had been conducted (CEFS 2000). The current IFRA guideline for estragole is 0.01% in leave-on or rinse-off consumer products.

Our safety advice: Taking the PBBD model for rats, doses of 0.1 and 0.7 mg/kg were predicted to be non-genotoxic. Taking the median of 0.4 mg/kg, the rat NOAEL could be estimated at ten times less, 0.04 mg/kg. Since estragole toxification is some 30 times more efficient in rats than humans (Punt et al 2007), the human NOAEL can be estimated at 1.2 mg/kg (0.04 × 30). Factoring in an uncertainty factor of 10 for inter-individual differences (Iyer et al 2003) and a further factor of 2 to allow for drug interactions gives an approximate safe dose of 0.05 mg/kg/day. This is equivalent to a dermal maximum of 0.12% (Table 14.1). Because of its antiplatelet aggregation activity, oral dosing of essential oils high in estragole is cautioned in conjunction with anticoagulant drugs, major surgery, childbirth, peptic ulcer, hemophilia or other bleeding disorders (see Box 7.1 for more detail).

Ethyl acetate

Synonyms: Acetoxyethane. Acetic acid ethyl ester. Acetic ether
Systematic name: Ethyl ethanoate
Chemical class: Aliphatic ester
CAS number: 141-78-6

Source:

| Mustard | 3.8% |

Pharmacokinetics: Ethyl acetate is hydrolyzed to ethanol, which is then partly excreted unchanged in the expired air and urine. The rest is metabolized (Opdyke 1974 p. 711–712).
Adverse skin reactions: Tested at 10% on the skin of human subjects, ethyl acetate was neither irritant nor sensitizing (Opdyke 1974 p. 711–712).
Acute toxicity: Acute oral LD_{50} in rats 5.6 g/kg; acute inhalational LC_{50} in rats 1,600 ppm after 8 hours (Opdyke 1974 p. 711–712).
Neurotoxicity: Male and female rats were exposed to inhalation of 350, 750 or 1,500 ppm of ethyl acetate for 13 weeks, 6 hours per day, 5 days per week. Some signs of neurotoxicity were evident in the two higher dose groups, but these were reversible on cessation of the exposure, and caused no neuro-physiological damage. A neurotoxic LOEL of 1,500 ppm was based on transient reduction of motor activity in females (Christoph et al 2003).
Mutagenicity and genotoxicity: In micronucleus tests in mice, ethyl acetate showed no genotoxicity (Hayashi et al 1988).
Summary: Ethyl acetate appears to be non-irritant and non-allergenic, and has minimal oral toxicity. The US inhalational threshold limit is 400 ppm.
Regulatory guidelines: In 1973 an inhalational threshold limit value for ethyl acetate was set at 400 ppm by the US Governmental Industrial Hygienists. Above this level it can produce nose and throat irritation and has a mild narcotic action (Opdyke 1974 p. 711–712).

(E)-Ethyl cinnamate

Synonyms: *trans*-Ethyl cinnamate. Ethyl cinnamate. *trans*-Cinnamic acid ethyl ester. Ethyl β-phenylacrylate
Systematic name: (E)-Ethyl 3-phenylpropenoate
Chemical class: Phenylpropenoid ester
CAS number: 103-36-6

Sources >1.0%:

Maraba	13.2–16.5%
Narcissus absolute	0.5–5.6%
Bakul absolute	1.9%
Benzoin	0.8–1.0%
Tolu balsam	0.8%

Adverse skin reactions: Non-irritant when tested full strength on rabbit skin, neither irritant nor sensitizing when tested at 4% on human subjects (Opdyke 1974 p. 721–722). In patch tests using undiluted ethyl cinnamate there was one positive reaction of 22 individuals (Katz 1946). UV spectra data suggest that ethyl cinnamate has no potential for phototoxicity or photoallergy (Belsito et al 2007).

Acute toxicity: Rat acute oral LD_{50} reported as 4.0 g/kg and 7.8 g/kg, rabbit acute dermal LD_{50} >5 g/kg (Opdyke 1974 p. 721–722, Zaitsev & Rakhmanina 1974).

Reproductive toxicity: In an ex vivo assay, ethyl cinnamate did not bind to estrogen receptors in female rat uterus tissue (Blair et al 2000).

Mutagenicity and genotoxicity: Ethyl cinnamate was not mutagenic in the Ames test but produced marginal CA in Chinese hamster fibroblasts (Ishidate et al 1984) and was genotoxic in Chinese hamster ovary cells (Sasaki et al 1989). It was not mutagenic in a *Bacillus subtilis* rec assay (Oda et al 1978).

Summary: Ethyl cinnamate appears to be non-irritant, non-allergenic, non-toxic and non-estrogen modulating. There is some evidence of mutagenicity.

β-Eudesmol

Synonyms: (+)-β-Eudesmol. β-Selinenol. Eudesm-4(14)-en-11-ol
Systematic name: [2R-(2α,4aα,8aβ)]-Decahydro-8-methylene-α,α,4a-trimethyl-2-naphthylmethanol
Chemical class: Bicyclic sesquiterpenoid alkene alcohol
CAS number: 473-15-4
Note: β-Eudesmol exists as more than one isomer.

Sources >1.0%:

Atractylis	26.0%
Araucaria	25.9%
Cypress (blue)	14.4%
Phoebe	6.8–8.4%
Valerian (European)	0–8.3%
Amyris	3.2–7.9%
Tansy (blue)	3.5–6.7%
Hinoki leaf	6.5%
Eucalyptus smithii	6.3%
Cypress (emerald)	5.7%
Vetiver	0–5.2%
Siam wood	4.4%
Cascarilla (Bahamian)	<3.0%
Arina	2.2%
Sanna	2.2%
Galangal (greater)	0.4–1.1%
Artemisia vestita	1.0%

Acute toxicity: β-Eudesmol acute oral LD_{50} in mice >2 g/kg (Chiou et al 1997).

Cardiovascular effects: β-Eudesmol displays considerable in vitro antiplatelet activity (Wang et al 2000). β-Eudesmol inhibited angiogenesis in granuloma tissue in mice at 0.90 mol/kg (202 g/kg) ip (Tsuneki et al 2005).

Hepatotoxicity: Significant anti-hepatotoxic effects were exhibited by β-eudesmol against carbon tetrachloride-induced cytotoxicity in rat hepatocytes (Kiso et al 1983).

Carcinogenic/anticarcinogenic potential: β-Eudesmol inhibited the in vitro growth of human liver cancer cells, and doses of 2.5–5.0 mg/kg suppressed hepatoma and sarcoma growth in mice (Ma et al 2008). Both in vitro and in vivo antiangiogenic activity has been observed for β-eudesmol, its action being due at least in part to blocking of the ERK signaling pathway (Tsuneki et al 2005).

Summary: We could find no dermal data for β-eudesmol. It has minimal acute toxicity, inhibits platelet aggregation in vitro, and has demonstrated antiangiogenic and antitumoral effects.

Our safety advice: Because of its antiplatelet aggregation activity, oral dosing of essential oils high in β-eudesmol is cautioned in conjunction with anticoagulant drugs, major surgery, childbirth, peptic ulcer, hemophilia or other bleeding disorders (see Box 7.1 for more detail). The antiangiogenic action of β-eudesmol suggests caution in pregnancy.

γ-Eudesmol

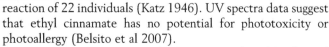

Synonyms: 4-Eudesmen-11-ol. 4-Selinen-11-ol. Uncineol
Systematic name: (2R)-(Z)-1,2,3,4,4a,5,6,7-Octahydro-α,α,4a,8-tetramethyl-2-naphthalenemethanol
Chemical class: Bicyclic sesquiterpenoid alkene alcohol
CAS number: 1209-71-8

Sources >1.0%:

Araucaria	19.0%
Coleus	12.5%
Cypress (blue)	9.1%
Hinoki leaf	8.3%
Amyris	6.6–8.0%
Siam wood	3.0%
Cypress (emerald)	2.4%

Carcinogenic/anticarcinogenic potential: γ-Eudesmol displayed moderate activity against the human hepatoma cell line G2, with an IC_{50} of 1.5 µg/mL, and potent activity against Hep 2,2,15 (HepG2 cell line transfected with hepatitis B virus) with an IC_{50} of 0.01 µg/mL (Hsieh et al 2001).

Summary: We could find no toxicity or dermal data for γ-eudesmol. It has demonstrated in vitro antitumoral effects.

Eugenol

H_3CO
HO

Synonyms: 2-Methoxy-4-allylphenol. 4-Allylguaiacol. Eugenic acid

Systematic name: 2-Methoxy-4-(2-propenyl)phenol
Chemical class: Phenylpropenoid phenolic ether
CAS number: 97-53-0

Sources >1.0%:

Clove bud	73.5–96.9%
Clove leaf	77.0–88.0%
Cinnamon leaf	68.6–87.0%
Clove stem	76.4–84.8%
Pimento leaf	66.0–84.0%
Pimento berry	67.0–80.0%
Tejpat	78.0%
Basil (pungent)	62.9%
Bay (West Indian)	44.4–56.2%
Basil (holy)	31.9–50.4%
Basil absolute (linalool CT)	33.7%
Betel	20.5–33.2%
Basil (linalool CT)	9.4–15.2%
Cinnamon bark	2.0–13.3%
Carnation absolute	1.7–3.6%
Laurel leaf	1.2–3.0%
Jasmine absolute	1.1–3.0%
Rose absolute (Provencale)	0.7–2.8%
Citronella (Javanese)	1.1–2.5%
Cistus	0–2.3%
Ginger lily absolute	1.4%
Rose (Damask)	tr–1.3%
Basil (estragole CT)	tr–1.2%
Rose (Japanese)	1.0%
Pine (huon)	0.5–1.0%

Note: being a substituted phenol, eugenol is a weak acid which may be corrosive to tissues.

Pharmacokinetics: In experimental animals, eugenol is redistributed rapidly to the blood and kidneys following oral administration. Over 70% of an oral dose of eugenol was excreted in the urine of rabbits (Schröder & Vollmer 1932). In man eugenol was rapidly absorbed and metabolized. Following an oral dose (150 mg), 95% was excreted in the urine, with ~55% as glucuronide and sulfate conjugates. Only 0.1% of unchanged eugenol was detected in man (Fischer et al 1990). Glucuronidation of eugenol has been seen with UDP-glucuronosyltransferase 2B17 (Turgeon et al 2003). Eugenol dose-dependently increased the levels of hepatic UDP-glucuronyltransferase when given in the diet at 1%, 3% or 5% for 23 days (Yokota et al 1988).

Work with rat hepatocytes in culture demonstrated that eugenol is metabolized to toxic compounds including eugenol 2′,3′-oxide and 1′-hydroxyeugenol in an analogous manner to acetaminophen (paracetamol) in acetaminophen poisoning (Scheline 1991). However, although the 2′,3′-oxide is very reactive and therefore potentially genotoxic, its rate of metabolism is much greater than its rate of formation in rat liver. Moreover, the epoxide is hydrolysed much more rapidly in human liver than in rat liver, thus allowing for a wide margin of safety in humans (Guenthner & Luo 2001). The epoxidation and 1′-hydroxylation of eugenol are significantly less important than

for safrole and estragole (Swanson et al 1981; Zangouras et al 1981; Sutton et al 1985; Anthony et al 1987; Burkey et al 2000).

Drug interactions: Eugenol dose-dependently inhibited human MAO-A with a K_i value of 26 µM, and inhibited human MAO-B to a much lesser extent (Tao et al 2005). This suggests the probability of oral doses of eugenol-rich essential oils interacting with MAOI or SSRI drugs.

Adverse skin reactions: A patch test with undiluted eugenol for 24 hours produced no irritation in 20 volunteers (Katz 1946). Tested at 8% in petrolatum, eugenol produced one mild irritation in a 48 hour closed-patch test in 25 volunteers (Opdyke 1975 p. 545–547). Tested at 8.0% in petrolatum on 25 volunteers, eugenol produced no sensitization reactions (Greif 1967). When 5% eugenol was tested in 100 volunteers there were no reactions (De Groot et al 1993). From a total of 11,632 patch tests with consumer products containing eugenol or clove leaf oil, one instance of induced hypersensitivity at 0.05%, and one instance of pre-existing sensitization at 0.09% were noted. It was concluded that eugenol alone, or as part of clove leaf oil, has a very low potential either to elicit pre-existing sensitization or to induce hypersensitivity (Rothenstein et al 1983). This is in spite of the widespread use of eugenol, which has been detected in 57% of deodorants and 27% of household products (Rastogi et al 1998, 2001).

In a retrospective multicenter study in Finland, there were 15 irritant reactions (0.6%) and 10 allergic reactions (0.4%) to eugenol in 2,527 dermatitis patients (Kanerva et al 2001a).

Of 1,200 dermatitis patients tested, there were no irritant reactions and eight allergic reactions (0.67%) to 3% eugenol. In a second group of 1,500 dermatitis patients there were no irritant reactions and nine allergic reactions (0.6%) to 1% eugenol (Santucci et al 1987). These, and other reports of reactions in dermatitis patients, are listed in Table 14.4B.

Of 713 cosmetic dermatitis patients, four reacted to eugenol (Adams & Maibach 1985). In a prospective study of adverse skin reactions to cosmetic ingredients identified by patch test (1977–1980) eugenol elicited contact dermatitis in four (0.8%) of 487 cosmetic-related cases (Eiermann et al 1982). Of 182 dermatitis patients suspected of contact allergy to cosmetics, 20 (11.1%) tested positive to 8% eugenol, as did three of 66 (4.6%) similar patients (Malten et al 1984). Of 167 dermatitis patients suspected of fragrance sensitivity 13 (7.8%) were allergic to 5% eugenol on patch testing (Larsen et al 1996b). Of 119 dermatitis patients with contact allergy to cosmetics four (3.4%) were allergic to 5% eugenol (De Groot et al 1988). When patch tested at 2% on 20 dermatitis patients who were sensitive to fragrance, eugenol induced four (20%) positive reactions (Larsen 1977). Of 102 dermatitis patients sensitive to Peru balsam, 19 tested positive to 2% eugenol (Hausen 2001).

There was no significant change in the frequency of allergic reactions to eugenol from a total of 25,545 dermatitis patients patch tested from January 1980 to December 1996 in the UK (Buckley et al 2000).

On the basis of the guinea pig maximation test, eugenol was classified as a mild skin sensitizer. This conclusion was supported by local lymph node assay data (Takeyoshi et al 2004). In a predictive endpoints assay for contact sensitizers,

Table 14.4 Allergic reactions to eugenol in different groups

A. Individuals with healthy skin

Concentration used	Percentage who reacted	Number of reactors	Reference
5%	0.0%	0/100	De Groot et al 1993
8%	0.0%	0/25	Greif 1967
Various	0.02%	2/11,632	Rothenstein et al 1983

B. Dermatitis patients

Concentration used	Percentage who reacted	Number of reactors	Reference
1%	0.0%	0/107[a]	Frosch et al 1995a
1%	0.27%	4/1,502	Heisterberg et al 2011
1%	0.4%	8/2,065	Schnuch et al 2007a
1%	0.6%	9/1,500	Santucci et al 1987
1%	0.7%	5/702	Frosch et al 1995b
1%	1.2%	13/1,072	Frosch et al 1995a
2%	0.0%	0/50	Larsen 1977
2%	2.0%	5/241	Ferguson & Sharma 1984
3%	0.67%	8/1,200	Santucci et al 1987
4%	1.38%	14/1,016	Storrs et al 1989
5%	1.9%	2/107[a]	Frosch et al 1995a
5%	2.0%	13/658	Heydorn et al 2003b
Unstated	0.4%	10/2,527	Kanerva et al 2001a

C. Dermatitis patients suspected of cosmetic or fragrance sensitivity

Concentration used	Percentage who reacted	Number of reactors	Reference
5%	3.4%	4/119	De Groot et al 1988
5%	7.8%	13/167	Larsen et al 1996b
8%	11.1%	20/182	Malten et al 1984
8%	4.6%	3/66	Malten et al 1984
Various	0.8%	4/487	Eiermann et al 1982
Various	0.56%	4/713	Adams & Maibach 1985

D. Fragrance-sensitive dermatitis patients

Concentration used	Percentage who reacted	Number of reactors	Reference
2%	19.4%	19/102	Hausen 2001
2%	20.0%	4/20	Larsen 1977

[a]Same group of patients

eugenol was classed as a moderate contact sensitizer (Ashikaga et al 2002).

Paradoxically, sensitization to cinnamaldehyde can be reduced by the co-presence eugenol. In ten people who developed urticaria after cinnamaldehyde had been applied to the skin, six had a greatly diminished reaction when it was applied combined with eugenol (Allenby et al 1984). This may be due to competition at receptor sites, or to an anti-inflammatory action of eugenol where there is sensitization to cinnamaldehyde and not to eugenol. Eugenol, administered intraperitoneally, totally prevented anaphylaxis in rats by inhibiting mast cell release of histamine and TNF-α (Kim et al 1997).

Mucous membrane irritation: Applied undiluted for five minutes to the tongues of dogs, eugenol caused erythema and occasionally ulcers (Lilly et al 1972). The application of undiluted eugenol to rat labial mucosa, observed for up to 6 hours, caused swelling, cell necrosis and vesicle formation (Kozam & Mantell 1978). The authors commented that eugenol progressively destroys the cells of the mucosal epithelium, and causes an acute inflammatory response. Even when eugenol was left for 1 minute only, and then removed as far as possible, a severe reaction occurred. When eugenol was applied to the mucous membranes of mice it caused severe hyperkeratosis, parakeratosis, cellular edema and patchy chronic inflammation (Fujisawa et al 2001). It should be emphasized that the undiluted compound was used in these studies.

The stomachs of rats and guinea pigs, given 150 mg eugenol per animal, showed histological damage, consisting of desquamation of the epithelium and punctate hemorrhages in the pyloric and glandular regions (Hartiala et al 1966). However, given orally pre-treatment at 10–100 mg/kg, eugenol reduced the number of ulcers and the gravity of lesions induced by either ethanol or platelet activating factor (Capasso et al 2000). Similarly, doses of 5–50 μg/kg eugenol reduced tongue edema in mice (Dip et al 2004). It appears that lower concentrations of eugenol have the opposite effect to higher ones on mucous membranes. This idea is given support by Markowitz et al (1992) who reported that low concentrations of eugenol exerted anti-inflammatory and local anesthetic effects on dental pulp, but high concentrations were cytotoxic, and could cause extensive tissue damage.

Cytotoxicity: Clove oil was cytotoxic to human fibroblasts at concentrations as low as 0.03%, with up to 73% of this effect attributable to eugenol (Prashar et al 2006). At a concentration higher than 3 mM (492 mg/L), eugenol was cytotoxic to oral mucosal fibroblasts, and decreased cellular ATP. Cell death was associated with intracellular depletion of glutathione. Eugenol also inhibited lipid peroxidation. No DNA strand break activity for eugenol was found at concentrations between 0.5 and 3 mM (82 and 492 mg/L). At a concentration less than 1 mM (164 mg/L), eugenol might protect cells from the genetic attack of ROS via inhibition of xanthine oxidase activity and lipid peroxidation (Jeng et al 1994a).

Acute toxicity: Eugenol acute oral LD_{50} 2.13 g/kg in guinea pigs, 2.68 g/kg in rats and 3.0 g/kg in mice (Jenner et al 1964). Maximal dose not causing death or any other toxic signs in male Swiss mice was 750 μg/kg po, 50 μg/kg ip, and 25 μg/kg iv (Dip et al 2004). Intravenous infusion of 4 μL and 8 μL of undiluted eugenol in rats causes hemorrhagic pulmonary edema, which may be partly mediated by a pro-oxidant action (Wright et al 1995).

Inhalation toxicity: Groups of rats inhaled submicron aerosols of eugenol at 0.77, 1.37 or 2.58 mg/L for four hours, followed by a 14 day observation period. The estimated maximum total dose was 240 mg/kg, and the mean aerosol particle size was 0.8 μm in diameter. During exposure, there were dose-dependent signs of increased salivation and restlessness (indicative of irritation) and abnormal breathing patterns. There were marked reductions in food and water intake and there was weight loss compared to control animals. There were no deaths, and no eugenol-related pulmonary abnormalities. All rats had recovered fully, and were normal in all respects by the end of day one of the observation period (Clark 1988).

Subacute and subchronic toxicity: Administration of eugenol at 1,000 ppm or 10,000 ppm in the diet of rats for 19 weeks had no observable adverse effect. Dietary administration of 1.4 g/kg, increased gradually to 4.0 g/kg over 34 days, caused 8/20 deaths within the time period. Moderate damage was observed in the forestomach, slight enlargement of liver and adrenals was noted, as was a small degree of osteoporosis (Hagan et al 1965). When eugenol was fed in the diet for 13 weeks to rats at doses ranging from 800 to 12,500 ppm, and to mice at doses ranging from 400–6,000 ppm, no animals died, and no dose-related histopathological effects were seen (National Toxicology Program 1983).

Cardiovascular effects: Eugenol demonstrates a dose-dependent anti-platelet activity ex vivo at 10 mg/mL and 100 mg/mL of rabbit blood (Rasheed et al 1984; Janssens et al 1990). Eugenol inhibits cardiovascular calcium channels, which suggests that it may be hypotensive and may reduce heart rate (Teuscher et al 1989). Eugenol decreased the expression of VEGF and VEGF1 in induced tumors in rats at 100 mg/kg po (Manikandan et al 2010).

Neurotoxicity: Eugenol protected neuronal cells from neurotoxicity induced by NMDA, xanthine, or oxygen-glucose deprivation (Wie et al 1997).

Reproductive toxicity: Administration of 0.2–0.5 mg/kg/day eugenol by intramuscular injection in sodium hydroxide solution to male rats for ten days caused degeneration of the seminal vesicle secretory cells (Vanithakumari et al 1998). The muscle used is not stated. The results of an in vitro test, the embryonic stem cell test (EST), suggest that eugenol has a potential for embryotoxicity (Chen et al 2010). However, oral administration of 100 mg/kg eugenol to pregnant mice on gestational days 0–18 (the full gestational period) caused no increase in resorption, and no detectable fetal defects. In a parallel study, the same eugenol dosing protocol significantly reduced the teratogenic effects of a single gavage dose of retinoic acid on the tenth day of gestation (Amini et al 2003). The EST does not appear to be predictive in this instance. Isoeugenol (an isomer of eugenol) was not developmentally toxic at 500 mg/kg/day in rats (George et al 2001). In an ex vivo assay, eugenol did not bind to estrogen receptors in female rat uterus tissue (Blair et al 2000).

Hepatotoxicity: Deteriorating liver function was a feature in a case of near fatal poisoning after ingestion of 5–10 mL of clove oil by a 2-year-old boy (Hartnoll et al 1993). Similarly, a 15-month-old boy developed acute liver failure after ingesting 10–20 mL of clove oil (Janes et al 2005). It has been proposed that the toxic effects of eugenol are mediated by a reactive quinine methide oxidation product that can bond covalently with protein or glutathione residues, and that the latter leads to depletion of cytoprotective thiols including glutathione. Pretreatment with N-acetylcysteine prevents glutathione loss and hence cell death (Thompson et al 1990, 1991, 1998). Eugenol hepatotoxicicty is only evident in high doses.

At 600 mg/kg, orally dosed eugenol caused hepatic damage in mice whose livers had been experimentally depleted of glutathione (Mizutani et al 1991). Slight liver toxicity was seen in rats with normal livers given four daily oral doses of ∼900 mg/kg eugenol, but none occurred in rats fed eugenol at 1.0% in the diet for four months (Taylor et al 1964). Oral administration of 1,000 mg/kg to rats did not deplete the hepatoprotective enzymes glutathione peroxidase, glutathione reductase, superoxide dismutase and catalase, and the activity of glutathione S-transferase increased significantly after 15 and 90 days of treatment (Vidhya & Devaraj 1999). Similarly, eugenol induced hepatic glutathione S-transferase when given to rats in the diet at 1%, 3% or 5% for 90 days, though feeding and body weight were adversely affected in rats at the 5% level (Yokota et al 1988).

A daily oral dose of 100 mg/kg eugenol for 10 days protected rats from the lipid peroxidation and hepatic toxicity of a subsequent high dose of iron (Reddy & Lokesh 1996). At 10.7 mg/kg ip for 14 days, eugenol inhibited carbon tetrachloride-induced hepatotoxicity in rats by acting as an in vivo antioxidant, and inhibiting the decrease of protective enzymes such as glutathione S-transferase (Kumaravelu et al 1995). In carbon tetrachloride-induced hepatotoxicity in rats, eugenol was most effective when given concurrently or soon after CCl_4 administration (Nagababu & Lakshmaiah 1994; Nagababu et al 1995).

Antioxidant/pro-oxidant activity: Eugenol is a potent antioxidant and radical scavenger (Tsujimoto et al 1993; Lee et al 2000; Teissedre & Waterhouse 2000; Lee & Shibamoto 2001; Fujisawa et al 2002; Kelm et al 2002; Park et al 2003; Chericoni et al 2005; Tominaga et al 2005). Administered to rats at 10.7 mg/kg ip, eugenol protected against the loss of functional integrity and membrane lipid alterations induced by oxidative stress, and it protected red blood cells from hemolysis by binding to the cell membranes (Kumaravelu et al 1996). At the high concentration of 100 mM (16.4 g/L), eugenol protected thymocytes from oxidative damage and apoptosis caused by gamma-ray irradiation. This was thought to be primarily due to antioxidant-mediated protection of the cell membranes (Pandey and Mishra 2004). Eugenol inhibits lipid peroxidation at concentrations below 1 mM (164 mg/L), while being cytotoxic to oral mucosal fibroblasts above 3 mM (492 mg/L), causing depletion of cellular glutathione (Jeng et al 1994a).

Mutagenicity and genotoxicity: Eugenol was mutagenic in the *Bacillus subtilis* DNA repair test assay without S9 (Sekizawa & Shibamoto 1982) and in the mouse micronucleus test (Woolverton et al 1986; Ellahueñe et al 1994). It was not mutagenic in any Ames test (Dorange et al 1977; Green & Savage 1978; Swanson et al 1979; Florin et al 1980; Eder et al 1982; Pool & Lin 1982; Haworth et al 1983; Ishidate et al 1984; Azizan & Blevins 1995; Kono et al 1995). Eugenol significantly inhibited tobacco-induced mutagenesis, and DMBA-induced mutagenesis, both evaluated using the Ames test (Amonkar et al 1986, Sukumaran & Kuttan 1994). It was similarly antimutagenic against four of five further mutagens, two of these with metabolic activation, in the *S. typhimurium* TA135/pSK1002 umu test, and was antimutagenic against *tert*-butyl hydroperoxide-induced mutagenesis in *E. coli* (Ramos et al 2003). According to To et al (1982) metabolites of eugenol are only weakly mutagenic.

Eugenol caused strong genotoxic effects in human VH10 fibroblasts and moderate effects in Caco-2 cells, but had no effect in HepG2 cells. These differences have been explained by the presence or absence of suitable enzymes for detoxifying eugenol-induced radicals (Slamenová et al 2009). Eugenol was genotoxic in Chinese hamster fibroblasts both in the presence and absence of rat liver S9, and also in Syrian hamster embryo cells (Ishidate et al 1984; Hikiba et al 2005; Maralhas et al 2006). It was also genotoxic in *Saccharomyces cerevisiae* (Schiestl et al 1989). Eugenol was not genotoxic in the DNA alkaline elution technique, the granuloma pouch essay or the bone marrow micronucleus test in rats (Maura et al 1989; Shelby et al 1993). It was not genotoxic in Chinese hamster ovary cells (Sasaki et al 1989). Eugenol showed no genotoxicity in one mouse micronucleus test, and some antigenotoxic activity in another (Hayashi et al 1988, Rompelberg et al 1995). No antimutagenic or antigenotoxic action could be demonstrated in vivo in mice (Rompelberg et al 1996b). In rats, assessment of four endpoints failed to find any evidence of genotoxicity in vivo (Allavena et al 1992).

Eugenol has consistently failed to bind to mouse liver DNA, unlike safrole, estragole and methyleugenol (Randerath et al 1984; Phillips et al 1984; Phillips 1990), and is not genotoxic in rat hepatocytes (Howes et al 1990). Eugenol was cytotoxic, but not genotoxic to human dental pulp fibroblasts, nor was it genotoxic in lymphocytes taken from human blood (Jansson et al 1988; Chang et al 2000). Eugenol inhibited the actions of various known genotoxic compounds in vivo in mice at gavage doses of 40–400 mg/kg (Abraham 2001). Eugenol may decrease the mutagenicity of some carcinogens such as benzo[*a*]pyrene (B[*a*]P) by decreasing their conversion to reactive epoxides (Yokota et al 1986). In humans, however, no significant antigenotoxic effects were found after ingestion of 150 mg eugenol per day for seven days (Rompelberg et al 1996c).

Carcinogenic/anticarcinogenic potential: In a 2-year study, female rats were fed dietary eugenol at 6,000 or 12,500 ppm, and male and female mice were fed 3,000 or 6,000 ppm. No tumors were detected in any female rodents, but there was an increased incidence of liver tumors, both benign and malignant. Interestingly, this was only seen in the *low* dose group (National Toxicology Program 1983). When eugenol was fed to mice at 0.5% in the diet for 12 months, there was no increase in liver tumors after 18 months, unlike mice fed similar doses of safrole or estragole (Miller et al 1983). Maintained on a diet containing 0.8% eugenol for 12 months, rats pretreated with the potent carcinogens 1,2-dimethylhydrazine and 1-methyl-1-nitrosourea showed enhanced development of hyperplasia and papillomas in the forestomach (Imaida et al 1990). In a novel assay for carcinogens, groups of male rats were dosed for 2, 14 or 90 days with 0.2 or 2.0 mmol/kg/day (33 or 328 mg/kg/day) of eugenol, and then hepatic tissue was analyzed for precancerous changes in gene expression. The results strongly suggest that eugenol is not hepatocarcinogenic in male rats (Auerbach et al 2010).

Eugenol inhibited the degranulation of rat liver microsomes by the chemical carcinogen diethyl nitrosamine through an unknown mechanism (Selvi & Niranjali 1998). The proliferation of mouse B16 melanoma cells was very weakly inhibited by eugenol with an IC_{50} value of 163 mM (26.7 g/L) (Tatman & Huanbiao 2002). Eugenol inhibited proliferation of human melanoma cells in vitro (Ghosh et al 2005). At 0.38 mM (62.3 mg/L), eugenol was cytotoxic to human myeloid leukemia (HL-60) cells, inducing apoptosis (Okada et al 2005). Eugenol extracted from clove bud oil induced apoptosis in HL-60 cells (with an IC_{50} of 23.7 μM; 3.89 mg/L) via ROS generation, depleting intracellular glutathione and reducing mitochondrial membrane potential (Yoo et al 2005). Eugenol was similarly toxic to human HepG2 hepatoma cells with a midpoint cytotoxicity concentration of 0.26 mM (42.6 mg/L). Depletion of intracellular glutathione was noted (Babich et al 1993). Eugenol showed significant activity as an inducer of glutathione *S*-transferase in mouse liver and small intestine (Zheng et al 1992c). Moderate in vitro activity was shown by eugenol in an androgen-independent, highly metastatic human prostate cancer cell line (Ghosh et al 2009).

At an oral dose of 15.2 µM (2.49 mg/L), eugenol inhibited B[*a*]P-induced forestomach tumors in mice by 55% (Bhide et al 1991a). Eugenol partially inhibited B[*a*]P carcinogenicity in mouse skin when applied concurrently (Van Duuren & Goldschmidt 1976). Prior application of eugenol reduced the number of DMBA-induced papillomas in mice by 84%, and there was a considerable decrease in the number of animals bearing tumors and their onset. Radical scavenging activity was thought to be responsible for this chemopreventive action (Sukumaran et al 1994). Eugenol very effectively inhibited DMBA-induced squamous cell skin cancer in mice when given orally at 1.25 mg/kg twice a week for 14 weeks after DBMA application (Pal et al 2010). Using the same dose regimen but administered ip, eugenol showed a dramatic anticarcinogenic action against malignant melanoma in female mice, inducing apoptosis, decreasing tumor size, completely preventing metastasis, and resulting in no deaths, compared to 50% of deaths in the control group. Eugenol significantly inhibited DMBA-induced skin cancers in mice pre-treated with 30 µL, due to antioxidant and pro-apoptotic activities (Kaur et al 2010). Eugenol inhibited nitrosamine-induced gastric cancer in rats through down-regulation of NF-κB (Manikandan et al 2011).

Comments: The occurrence of liver tumors only in male mice, and the lack of a dose-related action, is a pattern also seen in isoeugenol. Considering the otherwise anticarcinogenic action of eugenol this can be considered a sex-specific and species-specific effect. The lack of dose-dependency has yet to be explained. The adverse effect reported on male rat seminal vesicles may not translate to a very toxic action by non-intramuscular routes. On oral dosing, the similar compound isoeugenol was not reproductively toxic to male rats at 230 mg/kg/day (NTP Report RACB97004, July 10 2002).

Summary: Eugenol is a mild dermal irritant. There is a concentration-dependent risk of skin sensitization in dermatitis patients but, when applied to intact skin, the risk appears to be negligible. Eugenol, patch tested at various concentrations, caused reactions in a total of 59 of 9,356 dermatitis patients (0.63%). Oral eugenol can cause hepatotoxicity at 900 mg/kg, may possibly be hepatotoxic at 600 mg/kg, but is hepatoprotective at 100 mg/kg. At 3% (120–240 mg/kg) eugenol had a positive effect on hepatic glutathione enzyme levels. The dose-dependent nature of eugenol is particularly striking. Low concentrations are hepatoprotective, antioxidant and anti-inflammatory, while in high concentrations eugenol acts as a pro-oxidant, and is capable of hepatotoxicity, cytotoxicity and tissue damage. There is strong evidence of antiplatelet activity at moderate doses, and there is weak evidence of a depressant effect on the heart. In spite of some evidence of mutagenicity, eugenol is not a rodent carcinogen (except possibly in male mice), and there is evidence of antimutagenic, antiangiogenic and anticarcinogenic activity.

Regulatory guidelines: JECFA has set an ADI of 2.5 mg/kg bw for eugenol (JECFA 1982). Eugenol is one of the 26 fragrance materials listed as an allergen by the EU. If present in a cosmetic product at over 100 ppm (0.01%) in a wash-off product or 10 ppm (0.001%) in a leave-on product the material must be declared on the ingredient list if sold in an EU member state. In a preliminary report by an ECETOC taskforce, eugenol was provisionally classified as a weak allergen (on a scale of extreme, strong, moderate and weak) only likely to elicit a sensitization reaction if present at 3% or more (Kimber et al 2003). The IFRA standard for eugenol in leave-on products such as body lotions is 0.5%, for skin sensitization.

Our safety advice: For general use, a maximum dermal use level of 0.5% seems reasonable, in the absence of specific data for an essential oil. Because of its MAO inhibiting action, essential oils high in eugenol should be used with caution in oral doses by anyone taking MAOIs, SSRIs, pethidine, and indirect sympathomimetics (see Table 4.10 for more detail). Because of its antiplatelet aggregation activity, oral dosing of essential oils high in eugenol is cautioned in conjunction with anticoagulant drugs, major surgery, childbirth, peptic ulcer, hemophilia or other bleeding disorders (see Box 7.1 for more detail).

Eugenyl acetate

Synonyms: Eugenol acetate. Acetyleugenol. 4-Allyl-2-methoxyphenyl acetate
Systematic name: 2-Methoxy-4-(2-propenyl)phenyl ethanoate
Chemical class: Phenylpropenoid ether ester
CAS number: 93-28-7

Sources >1.0%:

Clove bud	0.5–10.7%
Cinnamon leaf	1.0–8.1%
Clove stem	0.4–8.0%
Tejpat leaf	1.2%
Clove leaf	tr–1.2%

Adverse skin reactions: Undiluted eugenyl acetate was moderately irritating to rabbit skin; tested at 20% on 25 volunteers it was neither irritating nor sensitizing (Opdyke 1974 p. 877–878).
Acute toxicity: Acute oral LD_{50} in rats 1.67 g/kg (Jenner et al 1964).
Subacute and subchronic toxicity: Neither 1,000, 2,500 nor 10,000 ppm fed to rats in the diet for 19 weeks produced any observable effect (Hagan et al 1967).
Summary: Eugenyl acetate appears to be non-irritant and non-allergenic, and possesses minimal acute and subchronic toxicity.

Farnesol

Systematic name: 3,7,11-Trimethyl-2,6,10-dodecatrien-1-ol
Chemical class: Aliphatic sesquiterpenoid polyalkene alcohol

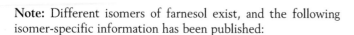

Note: Different isomers of farnesol exist, and the following isomer-specific information has been published:

(2E,6E)-Farnesol

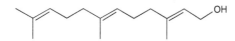

Synonym: *trans, trans*-Farnesol
CAS number: 106-28-5

Sources >1.0%:

Ambrette	3.4–39.0%
Sandalwood (W. Australian)	7.9–9.3%
Neroli	0–3.2%
Ylang-ylang absolute	1.8%
Tuberose absolute	1.7%
Rose (Damask)	0–1.5%
Rose absolute (Provencale)	0.5–1.3%

(2E,6Z)-Farnesol

Synonym: *trans, cis*-Farnesol
CAS number: 3879-60-5

Sources >1.0%:

Palmarosa	0.5–6.1%
Neroli	0–1.6%

(2Z,6E)-Farnesol

Synonym: *cis, trans*-Farnesol
CAS number: 3790-71-4

Sources >1.0%:

Ambrette	0.3–3.3%

(2Z,6Z)-Farnesol

Synonym: *cis, cis*-Farnesol
CAS number: 16106-95-9

Sources >1.0%:

Palmarosa	0.1–1.0%

Farnesol (isomer not specified)

Sources >1.0%:

Orange flower absolute	tr–7.7%
Vassoura	5.5%
Rose (Japanese)	3.8%
Galangal (greater)	0–3.1%
Cabreuva	2.5%

Note: The (2E,6E)- isomer occurs exclusively in many essential oils, but is found with (2E,6Z)-farnesol in orange leaf and some other oils (Budavari 1989).

Pharmacokinetics: When rats ingested a mixture of farnesol isomers with 39% (2E,6E)-farnesol, 24% (2E,6Z)-farnesol, 25% (2Z,6E)-farnesol and 11% (2Z,6Z)-farnesol, 80% of the farnesol recovered in plasma was (2E,6E)-farnesol. Oral administration of farnesol isomers to rats for 28 days the activities of the following hepatic enzymes were significantly increased: CYP1A, CYP2A1-3, CYP2B1/2, CYP2C11/12, CYP2E1, CYP3A1/2, CYP4A1-3, glutathione reductase, NADPH/quinone oxidoreductase and UGT. The activity of glutathione *S*-transferase was increased in the kidney (Horn et al 2005).

Adverse skin reactions: There were no irritation reactions in a total of 226 individuals patch tested with 10% or 12% farnesol for 48 hours (Belsito et al 2008). During the induction phase of human repeated insult patch tests, 5% farnesol was applied to three groups of 101, 103 and 108 volunteers for 24 hour periods, 3 days per week for 3 weeks. There were no irritation reactions. Following the challenge phase, there were also no sensitization reactions in any of the three groups. In maximation tests, 5% of healthy individuals (16/322) had allergic reactions to 10% or 12% farnesol. Undiluted farnesol caused reactions in 11/75 individuals (14.7%) (Belsito et al 2008). In both human and animal studies, 10% farnesol was neither phototoxic nor photoallergic (Lapczynski et al 2008d).

In a multicenter European study, 10 of 1,855 consecutive dermatology patients (0.54%) reacted to 5% farnesol (Frosch et al 2004). During a 6 month period in 2003, 2,021 consecutive dermatology patients (1,243 females and 778 males) were tested with 5% farnesol. Of these 22 (1.1%) had a positive reaction (Schnuch et al 2004b). There were four positive reactions to 2.5% (0.2%) and five to 5% farnesol (0.4%) in 1,701 dermatitis patients (Frosch et al 2005a). The results of two further European studies are reported in Table 5.10.

In 20 dermatitis patients suspected of suffering from contact sensitization to cosmetics, there were no reactions to 4% farnesol on patch testing. Of 182 dermatitis patients suspected of contact allergy to cosmetics, 2 (1.1%) tested positive to 4% farnesol (Malten et al 1984). Of 102 dermatitis patients sensitive to Peru balsam, four tested positive to 5% farnesol (Hausen 2001). Among 230 Danish patients sensitive to Peru balsam, one (0.4%) tested positive to farnesol (Hjorth 1961).

In Japan, 5 (1.1%) of 466 dermatitis patients tested positive to farnesol at either 5% or 10%, and 1 (0.2%) of the same group reacted to the compound at 2% (Sugai 1994). From 1990 to 1998 the average patch test positivity rate to 5% farnesol in a total of 1,483 Japanese eczema patients (99% female) suspected of cosmetic sensitivity was 0.95% (Sugiura et al 2000). Seven of 573 (1.2%) cosmetic dermatitis or eczema patients tested positive to 20% farnesol over a 2.5 year period (Hirose et al 1987).

Theoretically, and experimentally in guinea pigs, farnesol is regarded as a weak sensitizer, and farnesol allergy is not likely to be common (Hemmer et al 2000). Farnesol is sometimes used as a bacteriostat, as well as a fragrance material in deodorants, and positive skin reactions have been reported in young women using deodorant products. In one case a 30-year-old female presented with an itchy erythema in both axillae, and she tested positive to 5% farnesol (Goossens & Merckx 1997). In a second case of long-standing axillary dermatitis a 23-year-old female tested positive to 5% farnesol (Hemmer et al 2000).

Acute toxicity: Farnesol acute oral LD_{50} in rats >5 g/kg; acute oral LD_{50} in mice 8.76 g/kg acute dermal LD_{50} in rabbits >5 g/kg; acute ip LD_{50} in mice 327 mg/kg (Lapczynski et al 2008d).

Subacute and subchronic toxicity: A mixture of all four farnesol isomers (see Pharmacokinetics above) was administered orally to male and female rats for 28 days at 500 or 1,000 mg/kg/day, followed by a recovery period of 28 days. No clinical evidence of toxicity was observed. There were dose-related increases in kidney and liver weights, which were considered to be due to the induction of drug metabolizing enzymes (Horn et al 2005).

Mutagenicity and genotoxicity: Farnesol was not mutagenic in Ames tests, with or without S9 (Rupa et al 2003; RIFM 1989, cited in Lapczynski et al 2008d; Gonçalves et al 2011). Farnesol was not mutagenic in the *Salmonella/E. coli* assay, and was not genotoxic in Chinese hamster ovary cells or in the mouse micronucleus assay (Doppalapudi et al 2007). Oral farnesol suppressed cadmium-induced renal genotoxicity and oxidative stress in mice, restoring antioxidant status (Jahangir et al 2005). Similarly, oral farnesol inhibited benzo[a]pyrene-induced genotoxicity in mice, and restored depleted levels of antioxidant enzymes (Jahangir & Sultana 2008).

Carcinogenic/anticarcinogenic potential: A population of mouse B16(F10) melanoma cells were significantly inhibited by farnesol with an IC_{50} value of 50 μM (11.1 mg/L) (He et al 1997b). Farnesol completely inhibited the growth of ascites sarcoma BP8 cells (a rat cell line) at a concentration of 1.0 mM (222 mg/L) (Pilotti et al 1975). Farnesol reduced both pre-cancerous cell proliferation and DNA damage during the initial phases of liver carcinogenesis in rats (Ong et al 2006). Farnesol induced apoptosis in human pancreatic tumor BxPC3 cells, and decreased incidence of pancreatic carcinoma in hamsters (Burke et al 2002). At 30 mM (6.66 g/L), farnesol preferentially inhibited proliferation and induced apoptosis of tumor cells taken from patients with acute myeloid leukemia, but was not toxic to normal white blood cells (Rioja et al 2000). At 30, 50 or 60 mM (6.66, 11.1 or 13.3 g/L), farnesol inhibited the proliferation of human oral squamous cell carcinoma cells in vitro by up to 56.25%, and induced apoptosis (Scheper et al 2008).

Comments: The composition of farnesol isomers used in patch testing is not specified, but mixed isomer farnesols of 90%, 95% and 96% purity are commercially available. We would surmise that the patch test data in dermatitis patients suggest a maximum use level in the region of 3–5%, however the relevance of these data to the risk of using essential oils containing farnesol is unclear. A review by Gilpin & Maibach (2010) concludes that predictive human testing of farnesol indicates a low potential for skin sensitization, and that the human patch test data is not definitive 'in pointing to a causative relationship between farnesol and contact dermatitis.'

Summary: The real-world risk of an adverse skin reaction from farnesol in an essential oil is low. Farnesol has low oral toxicity, is not mutagenic, and demonstrates in vitro and in vivo anticarcinogenic activity. It may induce drug metabolizing enzymes, and

substantial oral doses may therefore interact with certain medications.

Regulatory guidelines: Farnesol is one of the 26 fragrance materials listed as an allergen by the EU. If present in a cosmetic product at over 100 ppm (0.01%) in a wash-off product or 10 ppm (0.001%) in a leave-on product the compound must be declared on the ingredient list if sold in an EU member state. The IFRA standard for farnesol in leave-on products such as body lotions is 1.2%, for skin sensitization. IFRA recommends that farnesol should only be used as a fragrance ingredient if it contains a minimum of 96% of farnesol isomers as determined by GLC. This is based on the results of tests conducted by RIFM on the sensitizing potential of farnesol samples containing variable amounts of impurities (IFRA 2009).

Our safety advice: There are insufficient clinical data to set a limit for dermal exposure to farnesol.

Farnesyl acetate

Synonym: Acetic acid farnesyl ester
Systematic name: 3,7,11-Trimethyl-2,6,10-dodecatrien-1-yl ethanoate
Chemical class: Aliphatic sesquiterpenoid polyalkene ester
Note: Different isomers of farnesyl acetate exist, and the following isomer-specific information has been published:

(2E,6E)-Farnesyl acetate

Synonym: *trans, trans*-Farnesyl acetate
CAS number: 4128-17-0

Sources >1.0%:

Ambrette	30.0–65.3%
Ylang-ylang	0.5–7.8%
Skimmia	1.5%

(2E,6Z)-Farnesyl acetate

Synonym: *trans, cis*-Farnesyl acetate
CAS number: 24163-98-2

(2Z,6E)-Farnesyl acetate

Synonym: *cis, trans*-Farnesyl acetate
CAS number: 40266-29-3

Sources >1.0%:

Ambrette	2.6–5.8%

(2Z,6Z)-Farnesyl acetate

Synonym: *cis, cis*-Farnesyl acetate
CAS number: 24163-97-1

Sources >1.0%:

Ylang-ylang	0–2.0%

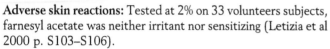

Adverse skin reactions: Tested at 2% on 33 volunteers subjects, farnesyl acetate was neither irritant nor sensitizing (Letizia et al 2000 p. S103–S106).

Acute toxicity: Acute oral LD_{50} in both rats and mice >5 g/kg; acute dermal LD_{50} >5 g/kg in both rabbits and guinea pigs (Letizia et al 2000 p. S103–S106).

Summary: Farnesyl acetate appears to be non-irritant and non-allergenic, and possesses minimal acute toxicity.

Fenchone

Synonyms: 1,3,3-Trimethyl-2-norbornanone. 1,3,3-Trimethyl-2-norcamphanone

Systematic name: 1,3,3-Trimethylbicyclo[2.2.1]heptan-2-one

Chemical class: Bicyclic monoterpenoid ketone

Note: Different isomers of fenchone exist, and the following isomer-specific information has been published:

(1*R*,4*S*)-(−)-Fenchone

CAS number: 7787-20-4

(1*R*,4*S*)-(+)-Fenchone

CAS number: 4695-62-9

Sources >1.0%

Lavender (Spanish)	14.9–49.1%
Fennel (bitter)	4.0–24.0%
Thuja	12.2–12.8%
Fennel (sweet)	0.2–8.0%
Cedarwood (Port Orford)	4.7%
Labdanum	1.4–2.3%
Pine (Scots)	0–2.1%
Sage (African wild)	1.4%
Cistus	0–1.1%

Note: (−)-Fenchone is found in thuja oil, (+)-fenchone in Spanish lavender and bitter and sweet fennel oils.

Pharmacokinetics: In both dogs and rabbits (+)-fenchone is metabolized by hydroxylation. 4-Hydroxyfenchone and 5-hydroxyfenchone have been found in dog urine, while 8-hydrohyfenchone, 9-hydrohyfenchone and 10-hydrohyfenchone appeared in rabbit urine (Scheline 1991).

Adverse skin reactions: Tested at 4% on human subjects fenchone was neither irritating nor sensitizing (Opdyke 1976 p. 769–771).

Acute toxicity: Acute oral LD_{50} in rats 6.16 g/kg (Jenner et al 1964); acute dermal LD_{50} in rabbits >5 g/kg (Opdyke 1976 p. 769–771).

Neurotoxicity: Subcutaneously injected fenchone produced clonic convulsions in mice at 1,133 mg/kg, but not at 500 mg/kg (Wenzel & Ross 1957). Orally administered to dogs for 16 days, (+)-fenchone was convulsant and lethal at 1,400 mg/kg/day, produced transient tremors at 750 mg/kg/day, and had no apparent effects at 210–420 mg/kg/day (Rimini 1901).

Mutagenicity and genotoxicity: Fenchone was not mutagenic in *S. typhimurium* strains TA97, TA98, TA100 or TA1535, with or without S9. In a rat bone marrow micronucleus test fenchone was not genotoxic, though at the highest dose (2,500 mg/kg ip for 3 days) the results were considered equivocal (National Toxicology Program 2011).

Comments: The very high dose used by Wenzel & Ross (1957) is not representative of therapeutic doses of fenchone-rich oils. Since a dose of 500 mg/kg did not cause seizures, fenchone does not appear to possess significant convulsant properties. Fenchone has only been convulsant in mice, and only at a very high dose. There are no recorded cases of seizures in humans from fenchone-rich essential oils. The French legislation is not based on any toxicological data, and is a legislative response to what was perceived in 1915 as absinthe toxicity.

Summary: Fenchone appears to be non-irritant, non-allergenic, and non-toxic. There is no evidence that it can cause seizures in therapeutic doses.

Regulatory guidelines: In France, fenchone is limited, in absinthe or similar alcoholic beverages, to 5 mg/L (Lachenmeier et al 2008). This is a November 1988 update of legislation first passed in March 1915.

(*E*)-Geranial

Synonyms: (*E*)-Citral. *trans*-Citral. α-Citral. Citral a

Systematic name: (2*E*)-3,7-Dimethyl-2,6-octadienal

Chemical class: Aliphatic monoterpenoid alkene aldehyde

CAS number: 141-27-5

Note: Geranial is an isomer of neral, and a component of citral

Sources >1.0%:

Myrtle (lemon)	46.1–60.7%
Lemongrass (West Indian)	36.7–55.9%
Lemongrass (East Indian)	45.1–54.5%
Tea tree (lemon-scented)	45.4%
May chang	37.9–40.6%
Lemon leaf	10.9–39.0%
Verbena (lemon)	29.5–38.3%
Melissa	12.5–38.3%
Myrtle (honey)	37.5%
Basil (lemon)	23.3–25.1%
Lemon balm (Australian)	9.9%
Thyme (lemon)	9.2%
Fenugreek	4.8%
Lemon (expressed)	0.5–4.3%
Lime (expressed, Persian)	2.2–3.9%
Lime (expressed, Mexican)	2.4%
Lemon (distilled)	0.7–2.2%
Palmarosa	0.5–1.9%
Orange (sweet)	<1.8%
Bergamot (wild)	1.2–1.6%
Finger root	1.5%

Note: We could find no safety data for geranial, but see citral, of which geranial is a naturally-occurring constituent.

(E)-Geraniol

Synonyms: (E)-Geraniol. *trans*-Geraniol. Geranyl alcohol. Lemonol
Systematic name: (2E)-3,7-Dimethyl-2,6-octadien-1-ol
Chemical class: Aliphatic monoterpenoid alkene alcohol
CAS number: 106-24-1
Note: Geraniol is an isomer of linalool and nerol

Sources >1.0%:

Bergamot (wild)	86.8–93.2%
Jamrosa	54.0–85.0%
Palmarosa	74.5–81.0%
Thyme (lemon)	39.2%
Geranium	7.3–30.3%
Citronella (Sri Lankan)	16.8–29.1%
Rose (Damask)	2.1–25.7%
Citronella (Javanese)	22.1–25.4%
Thyme (geraniol CT)	24.9%
Finger root	20.8%
Lemon leaf	0.5–15.0%
Rose (Japanese)	12.8%
Orange flower & leaf water absolute	10.0%
Melissa	1.0–8.1%
Snakeroot	0.8–7.2%
Osmanthus absolute	1.2–7.1%
Lemongrass (West Indian)	0–6.7%
Rose absolute (Provencale)	4.9–6.4%
Coriander seed	0.3–5.3%
Davana	5.0%
Basil (lemon)	4.3–4.7%
Lemongrass (East Indian)	0.2–3.8%
Lemon balm (Australian)	3.7%
Neroli	0.8–3.6%
Myrtle (honey)	3.4%
Eucalyptus macarthurii	1.9–3.3%
African bluegrass	1.7–3.2%
Orange leaf (Paraguayan)	2.1–3.0%
Ylang-ylang	0–3.0%
Eucalyptus radiata	0.2–2.8%
Tea tree (lemon-scented)	2.7%
Betel	0–2.5%
Boswellia serrata	0–2.4%
Orange leaf (bigarade)	1.4–2.3%
Carrot seed	0–2.2%
Skimmia	1.9%
Ylang-ylang absolute	1.7%
Cistus	0–1.7%
May chang	0.5–1.6%
Cananga	1.5%
Hop	1.5%
Orange flower absolute	<1.5%
Ghandi root	1.4%
Clary sage	<1.2%
Cardamon	0.3–1.1%
Galangal (greater)	0.3–1.1%
Linaloe wood	1.0%

Pharmacokinetics: In rabbits, geraniol is extensively metabolized to a dicarboxylic acid derivative (Scheline 1991). Geraniol is metabolized to 8-carboxygeranic acid by the liver, and excreted as such in the urine (Asano & Yamakasa 1950). A significant increase in the concentration of CYP in rat liver was observed after three days dosing with geraniol (Chadha & Madyastha 1984).

Adverse skin reactions: Geraniol caused no adverse reactions when photopatch tested at 5% on 111 patients, or at 1% on 41 patients suspected clinical photosensitivity (Nagareda et al 1992). In a modified Draize procedure on guinea pigs, geraniol was non-sensitizing when used at 10% in the challenge phase (Sharp 1978). In modified Draize tests, 10% geraniol caused two allergic reactions in a total of 177 volunteers. Patch tested at 6%, geraniol produced one allergic reaction in a total of 75 volunteers (Belsito et al 2008). There were no positive reactions to 5% geraniol tested on 100 volunteers (De Groot et al 1993). There were no reactions to 5% geraniol in a total of 237 volunteers patch tested in Japan (Itoh et al 1986, 1988). Tested at concentrations ranging from 2% to 12.5%, HRIPT testing with geraniol resulted in three questionable reactions in a total of 412 volunteers (Belsito et al 2008).

Geraniol produced six allergic reactions in 658 people (0.9%) with hand eczema (Heydorn et al 2003b). Of 1,200 dermatitis patients tested, there were no irritant reactions and four allergic reactions (0.34%) to 3% geraniol. In a second group of 1,500 dermatitis patients there were no irritant reactions and four allergic reactions (0.27%) to 1% geraniol (Santucci et al 1987). There were no irritant or allergic reactions in a group of 100 consecutive dermatitis patients tested with 1% geraniol. In Japan, 5% geraniol elicited reactions in a total of 0.48% (10/2,069) of patients (Itoh et al 1986, 1988; Nagareda et al 1992; Nishimura et al 1984). These, and other reports of reactions in dermatitis patients, are listed in Table 14.5A.

In a prospective study of adverse skin reactions to cosmetic ingredients identified by patch test (1977–1980) geraniol elicited contact dermatitis in five (1%) of 487 cosmetic-related cases (Eiermann et al 1982). Of 713 cosmetic dermatitis patients, eight (1.1%) reacted to geraniol (Adams & Maibach 1985). Of 18,747 dermatology patients, 1,781 had contact dermatitis and one (0.005% of dermatitis patients and 0.06% of contact dermatitis patients) was allergic to geraniol. Of the 1,781 patients 75 were allergic to cosmetic products, so the one reaction constituted 1.4% of this group (De Groot 1987).

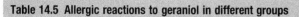

Table 14.5 Allergic reactions to geraniol in different groups

A. Dermatitis patients

Concentration used	Percentage who reacted	Number of reactors	Reference
0.1%	0.0%	0/106	Frosch et al 1995a
1%	0.0%	0/100	Frosch et al 1995a
1%	0.0%	0/1,502	Heisterberg et al 2011
1%	0.27%	4/1,500	Santucci et al 1987
1%	0.4%	8/2,063	Schnuch et al 2007a
1%	0.43%	3/702	Frosch et al 1995b
1%	0.75%	8/1,072	Frosch et al 1995a
2%	0.13%	3/2,227	Hagvall et al 2012
2%	0.28%	7/2,461	Calnan et al 1980
3%	0.34%	4/1,200	Santucci et al 1987
5%	0.0%	0/50	Larsen 1977
5%	0.4%	3/756	Itoh et al 1988
5%	0.44%	3/680	Itoh et al 1986
5%	0.57%	3/522	Nishimura et al 1984
5%	0.9%	1/111	Nagareda et al 1992
5%	0.9%	6/658	Heydorn et al 2003b
Unstated	0.06%	1/1,781	De Groot 1987
Unstated	0.21%	11/5,202	Broeckx et al 1987
Unstated	0.3%	59/19,546	Angelini et al 1997

B. Dermatitis patients suspected of cosmetic or fragrance sensitivity

Concentration used	Percentage who reacted	Number of reactors	Reference
1%	0.0%	0/20	Malten et al 1984
1%	1.6%	3/182	Malten et al 1984
5%	0.34%	5/1,483	Sugiura et al 2000
5%	0.6%	1/155	Itoh 1982
5%	1.7%	2/119	De Groot et al 1988
5%	3.0%	5/167	Larsen et al 1996b
10%	6.1%	11/179	De Groot et al 1985
Unstated	1.3%	1/75	De Groot 1987

C. Cosmetic-sensitive or fragrance-sensitive dermatitis patients

Concentration used	Percentage who reacted	Number of reactors	Reference
1%	5.1%	4/78	Wilkinson et al 1989
1%	7.17%	67/934	Buckley et al 2000
5%	30%	6/20	Larsen 1977
10%	13.3%	2/15	Opdyke 1974 p. 881–882
Unstated	1.0%	5/487	Eiermann et al 1982
Unstated	1.1%	8/713	Adams & Maibach 1985

From 1990 to 1998 the average patch test positivity rate to 5% geraniol in a total of 1,483 Japanese eczema patients (99% female) suspected of cosmetic sensitivity was 0.34% (Sugiura et al 2000). Similarly, only one of 155 suspected cosmetic cases was allergic to geraniol (Itoh 1982).

There were 11 reactions to 10% geraniol (6.1%) in 179 dermatitis patients suspected of allergy to cosmetics (De Groot et al 1985). Of 167 dermatitis patients suspected of fragrance sensitivity 5 (3%) were allergic to 5% geraniol on patch testing (Larsen et al 1996b). Of 119 eczema patients with contact allergy to cosmetics two (1.7%) were allergic to 5% geraniol (De Groot et al 1988). In 20 eczema patients suspected of suffering from contact sensitization to cosmetics, there were no reactions to 1% geraniol on patch testing. Of 182 dermatitis patients suspected of contact allergy to cosmetics, three (1.6%) tested positive to 1% geraniol (Malten et al 1984).

At 10%, geraniol tested positive in two of 15 individuals (13.3%) sensitive to Peru balsam (Opdyke 1974 p. 881–882). When patch tested at 5% on 20 dermatitis patients who were sensitive to fragrance materials, geraniol induced six (30%) positive reactions (Larsen 1977). Of two cases of contact dermatitis in which geraniol was patch tested at 1%, one was negative and the other was mildly positive (Keil 1947); a third case, tested at 2%, produced a moderate positive response (Guerra et al 1987). A bartender with dermatitis of the hand had allergic contact sensitivity to lemon peel, and patch testing resulted in a positive reaction to geraniol (Cardullo 1989).

There was no significant change in the frequency of allergic reactions to geraniol in a total of 25,545 dermatitis patients patch tested from January 1980 to December 1996 in the UK (Buckley et al 2000). In a subsequent seven year multicenter study (1996–2002) only 5.9% of fragrance-mix positive individuals also reacted to geraniol (Schnuch et al 2004a). This is in spite of the widespread use of geraniol in deodorants (76% of 73 deodorants analysed) and household products (41% of 59 analysed) (Rastogi et al 1998, 2001).

Acute toxicity: Acute oral LD_{50} in rats reported as 3.6 g/kg (Jenner et al 1964) and 4.8 g/kg (Opdyke 1974 p. 881–882).

Subacute and subchronic toxicity: There were no observable adverse effects from feeding geraniol to rats at 1,000 ppm for 28 weeks or at 10,000 ppm for 16 weeks (Hagan et al 1967).

Reproductive toxicity: Geraniol produced malformations in chick embryos when injected into fertilized hen's eggs (Aydelotte 1963; Abramovici 1972). Using chick embryos at 72 hours of incubation, Forschmidt (1979) determined that geraniol had a teratogenic value of 11.3% relative to a control value of 7.9%. The implications of these data for humans are unknown. Since geraniol is an isomer of linalool, their degree of reproductive toxicity may be similar. When gavage doses of linalool were given to pregnant rats at 250, 500 or 1,000 mg/kg/day, on gestational days 7–17, no fetal toxicity or teratogenicity was seen at any dose. Since there was some maternal increase in relative body weight and feed consumption in the high dose group, the NOAEL for maternal toxicity was 500 mg/kg/day (Politano et al 2008).

Antioxidant/pro-oxidant activity: Geraniol has marked DPPH scavenging activity (Choi et al 2000).

Mutagenicity and genotoxicity: Geraniol was not mutagenic in the Ames test with and without S9 (Florin et al 1980; Eder et al 1982; Ishidate et al 1984; Rupa et al 2003) but was marginally genotoxic in Chinese hamster fibroblasts (Ishidate et al 1984). It was not mutagenic in the *Salmonella/E. coli* assay, and was not genotoxic in the mouse micronucleus assay; the results in Chinese hamster ovary cells were inconclusive (Doppalapudi et al 2007). In another report, geraniol was not genotoxic in Chinese hamster ovary cells (Sasaki et al 1989).

Carcinogenic/anticarcinogenic potential: Geraniol concentration-dependently slowed the growth of mouse P388 leukemia cells and B16 melanoma cells. Mice given 0.1% dietary geraniol for 14 days prior to and following P388 cell transfer survived significantly longer than controls (Shoff et al 1991). Geraniol inhibited the proliferation of mouse B16(F10) melanoma cells with an IC_{50} value of 150 µM (23.1 mg/L); HMG-CoA reductase activity was suppressed at the same time (He et al 1997b). Geraniol significantly suppressed the growth of hepatomas and melanomas transplanted to rats and mice, respectively (Yu et al 1995a). In rats, it reduced both DNA damage and pre-cancerous cell proliferation, increasing apoptosis, during the initial phases of induced liver carcinogenesis. Animals were given 250 mg/kg/day of geraniol by gavage for eight weeks (Ong et al 2006). Geraniol also inhibited the promotional stage of liver cancer in rats given the same dose for five weeks (Cardozo et al 2011).

At the high dose of 400 mM (61.6 g/L), geraniol caused a 70% inhibition of cell growth in human colon cancer (Caco-2) cells, and a concomitant inhibition of DNA synthesis. It increased the survival time of mice grafted with the human colorectal tumor cells TC118, and induced apoptosis in human pancreatic tumor BxPC3 cells (Burke et al 2002; Carnesecchi et al 2004). The proliferation of MCF-7 human breast cancer cells was suppressed by geraniol in vitro (Duncan et al 2004). Geraniol had a significant chemopreventive action on DMBA-induced mammary carcinogenesis in rats and induced glutathione S-transferase in mouse tissues (Zheng et al 1993a). Geraniol activated the intracellular catabolism of polyamines (which are enhanced in cancer growth) through a 50% decrease in ornithine decarboxylase activity (Carnesecchi et al 2001).

Comments: In studies collectively totaling 11,875 dermatitis patients, only 50 (0.42%) reacted to geraniol tested at 1–5% (Table 14.5A). In this context it is difficult to understand why it has been flagged as a high-risk skin allergen by the EU. There has been a call from dermatologists to treat geraniol less restrictively (Schnuch et al 2004a).

Summary: Geraniol is a very weak skin sensitizer, and possesses minimal acute and subchronic toxicity. Reports on mutagenicity are either negative or inconclusive. Geraniol has demonstrated in vitro and in vivo antitumoral effects.

Regulatory guidelines: Geraniol is one of the 26 fragrance materials listed as an allergen by the EU. If present in a cosmetic product at over 100 ppm (0.01%) in a wash-off product or 10 ppm (0.001%) in a leave-on product the compound must be declared on the ingredient list if sold in an EU member state. Based on literature published in German, geraniol was classified as category B, moderately allergenic, by Schlede et al (2003). The IFRA standard for geraniol in leave-on products such as body lotions is 5.3%, for skin sensitization.

Our safety advice: We agree with the IFRA standard of 5.3% for geraniol.

(E)-Geranyl acetate

Synonyms: *trans*-Geranyl acetate. Acetic acid *trans*-geranyl ester
Systematic name: (2E)-3,7-Dimethyl-2,6-octadien-1-yl ethanoate
Chemical class: Aliphatic monoterpenoid alkene ester
CAS number: 105-87-3

Sources >1.0%:

Thyme (geraniol CT)	36.5%
Jamrosa	18.0–25.0%
Eucalyptus macarthurii	18.8–21.8%
Ylang-ylang	1.2–11.0%
Palmarosa	0.5–10.7%
Thymus zygis (thymol/carvacrol CT)	5.2%
Citronella (Javanese)	2.9–5.1%
Rose (Damask)	0–4.7%
Orange leaf (Paraguayan)	2.9–4.5%
Geranium	0–4.4%
Wormwood (sabinyl acetate CT)	4.2%
Neroli	0.7–4.1%
Lemon balm (Australian)	4.0%
Ylang-ylang absolute	4.0%
Lemongrass (East Indian)	0.1–4.0%
Lemon leaf	tr–4.0%
Western red cedar	0.1–3.9%
Carrot seed	0–3.7%
Linaloe wood	3.5%
Orange leaf (bigarade)	1.9–3.4%
Citronella (Sri Lankan)	2.1–3.4%
Melissa	0.7–3.3%
Coriander seed	0–3.1%
Myrtle	1.4–2.9%
Lavender absolute	2.7%
Skimmia	2.5%
Thyme (lemon)	2.4%
Lemongrass (West Indian)	0.4–1.9%
Orange flower & leaf water absolute	1.8%
Mint (bergamot)	0.7–1.8%
Orange leaf absolute	1.6%
Wormwood (β-thujone/(Z)-epoxy-ocimene CT)	1.4–1.6%
Cananga	1.5%
Snakeroot	<1.4%
Clary sage	<1.2%
Lavandin Grosso	0–1.2%
Pine (ponderosa)	1.1%
Combava fruit	1.0%
Myrtle (honey)	1.0%
Wormwood ((Z)-epoxy-ocimene CT)	0.6–1.0%

Adverse skin reactions: Tested at 4%, geranyl acetate was not sensitizing in 25 volunteers (Opdyke 1974 p. 885–886). Two cases of contact dermatitis in which geranyl acetate was patch tested at 1% both produced a mild positive response (Keil 1947).

Acute toxicity: Acute oral LD_{50} in rats 6.33 g/kg (Jenner et al 1964).
Subacute and subchronic toxicity: No adverse effects were seen from feeding geranyl acetate to rats at 1,000, 2,500 and 10,000 ppm for 17 weeks (Hagan et al 1967).
Mutagenicity and genotoxicity: Geranyl acetate was not mutagenic in the Ames test (Mortelmans et al 1986). It was mutagenic in mouse lymphoma cells with S9, but was not in human lymphoblast cells, with or without S9 (Caspary et al 1988). Geranyl acetate was not genotoxic in Chinese hamster ovary cells, with or without metabolic activation (Galloway et al 1987). In a mouse micronucleus test, geranyl acetate showed no genotoxic effect (Shelby et al 1993).
Carcinogenic/anticarcinogenic potential: In a two year carcinogenesis study, food-grade geranyl acetate (71% geranyl acetate, 29% citronellyl acetate) was fed to 50 male and 50 female rats at 0, 1,000 or 2,000 mg/kg, and to 50 male and 50 female mice at 0, 500 or 1,000 mg/kg 5 times a week. It was not considered to be carcinogenic to rats or mice of either sex. A marginal but not significant increase was observed in squamous cell papillomas of the skin, and tubular cell adenomas of the kidney in the male rats at the higher doses (National Toxicology Program 1987). The proliferation of mouse B16 melanoma cells was very weakly inhibited by geranyl acetate with an IC_{50} value of 185 mM (36.3 g/L) (Tatman & Huanbiao 2002).
Summary: Geranyl acetate is a very weak skin sensitizer. It is neither toxic nor carcinogenic.
Regulatory guidelines: JECFA has set a group ADI of 0 to 0.5 mg/kg bw for citral, citronellol, geranyl acetate, linalool and linalyl acetate (JECFA 1999a).

(E)-Geranyl acetone

Synonyms: *trans*-Geranylacetone. α,β-Dihydropseudoionone
Systematic name: (5E)-6,10-Dimethyl-5,9-undecadien-2-one
Chemical class: Aliphatic monoterpenoid alkene ketone
CAS number: 3796-70-1

Sources >1.0%:

Cascarilla (Bahamian)	<2.2%

Adverse skin reactions: Geranyl acetone was moderately irritating to rabbit skin when applied undiluted for 24 hours under occlusion. Tested at 10% on 22 volunteers the material was neither irritating nor sensitizing (Opdyke 1979a p. 787).
Acute toxicity: Acute oral LD_{50} in rats >5 g/kg; acute dermal LD_{50} in rabbits >5 g/kg (Opdyke 1979a p. 787).
Carcinogenic/anticarcinogenic potential: The proliferation of mouse B16 melanoma cells was very weakly inhibited by geranyl acetone with an IC_{50} value of 171 mM (33.2 g/L) (Tatman & Huanbiao 2002).
Summary: Geranyl acetone appears to be non-irritant, non-allergenic, and non-toxic.

(E)-Geranyl formate

Synonyms: *trans*-Geranyl formate. Formic acid *trans*-geranyl ester

Systematic name: (2E)-3,7-Dimethyl-2,6-octadien-1-yl methanoate
Chemical class: Aliphatic monoterpenoid alkene ester
CAS number: 105-86-2

Sources >1.0%:

Geranium	1.6–7.6%
Citronella (Sri Lankan)	0–4.2%

Adverse skin reactions: In a modified Draize procedure on guinea pigs, geranyl formate was non-sensitizing when used at 20% in the challenge phase (Sharp 1978). Tested at 2% on 25 volunteers geranyl formate produced a mild irritation but was not sensitizing; applied full strength to rabbit skin for 24 hours under occlusion it was not irritating (Opdyke 1974 p. 893).
Acute toxicity: The acute oral LD_{50} in rats exceeded 6 g/kg, and the acute dermal LD_{50} in rabbits exceeded 5 g/kg (Opdyke 1974 p. 893).
Summary: Geranyl formate appears to be slightly irritant, non-allergenic, and non-toxic.

Geranyl linalool

Synonym: 1,6,10,14-Phytatetraen-3-ol
Systematic name: 3,7,11,15-Tetramethyl-1,6,10,14-hexadeca-tetraen-3-ol
Chemical class: Aliphatic diterpenoid polyalkene alcohol
Note: Different isomers of geranyl linalool exist, and the following isomer-specific information has been published:

(R,E,E)-Geranyl linalool

Synonym: (E,E)-Geranyl linalool
CAS number: 1113-21-9

Sources >1.0%:

Jasmine sambac absolute	0–8.0%
Jasmine absolute	2.5–5.0%
Khella	4.1%

Adverse skin reactions: Tested at 1% on 29 volunteers, geranyl linalool was neither irritating nor sensitizing. The undiluted material was irritating to rabbit skin when applied for 24 hours under occlusion (Bhatia et al 2008f).
Acute toxicity: Rat acute oral LD_{50} >5 g/kg; mouse acute oral LD_{50} 14.6 g/kg; mouse acute ip LD_{50} >2.0 g/kg; rabbit acute dermal LD_{50} >5 g/kg (Bhatia et al 2008f).
Inhalation toxicity: None of 12 rats died after being exposed to an atmosphere saturated with geranyl linalool for up to 7 hours (Bhatia et al 2008f).
Summary: Geranyl linalool appears to be non-allergenic and non-toxic.

(E)-Geranyl propionate

Synonyms: *trans*-Geranyl *n*-propanoate. Propionic acid *trans*-geranyl ester
Systematic name: (2E)-3,7-Dimethyl-2,6-octadien-1-yl propanoate

Chemical class: Aliphatic monoterpenoid alkene ester
CAS number: 105-90-8

Sources >1.0%:

Wormwood (β-thujone CT)	0.1–2.1%
Thyme (geraniol CT)	1.9%
Geranium	0.1–1.7%

Adverse skin reactions: Tested at 4% on volunteers geranyl propionate was neither irritating nor sensitizing. Applied undiluted to rabbit skin for 24 hours under occlusion it was not irritating (Opdyke 1974 p. 897).
Acute toxicity: Acute oral LD_{50} in rats >5 g/kg. The acute dermal LD_{50} in rabbits exceeded 5 g/kg (Opdyke 1974 p. 897).
Summary: Geranyl propionate appears to be non-irritant, non-allergenic, and non-toxic.

(E)-Geranyl tiglate

Synonyms: *trans*-Geranyl tiglate. Tiglic acid *trans*-geranyl ester
Systematic name: (2E)-3,7-Dimethyl-2,6-octadien-1-yl (2E)-2-methyl-butenoate
Chemical class: Aliphatic monoterpenoid polyalkene ester
CAS number: 7785-33-3

Sources >1.0%:

Geranium	0.2–3.0%

Adverse skin reactions: Tested at 6% on 25 volunteers, geranyl tiglate was neither irritating nor sensitizing (Opdyke 1974 p. 899).
Acute toxicity: Acute oral LD_{50} in rats >5 g/kg; acute dermal LD_{50} in rabbits >5 g/kg (Opdyke 1974 p. 899).
Summary: Geranyl tiglate appears to be non-irritant, non-allergenic, and non-toxic.

Guaiacol

Synonyms: O-Methyl catechol. 2-Methoxyphenol. Anastil
Systematic name: 1-Hydroxy-2-methoxybenzene
Chemical class: Phenolic ether
CAS number: 90-05-1

Sources >1.0%:

Birch tar	Major constituent
Cade (unrectified)	<1.5%
Eucalyptus macarthurii	0.8–1.0%

Note: Being a substituted phenol, guaiacol is a weak acid which may be corrosive to tissues.
Pharmacokinetics: In rabbits, guaiacol is largely excreted in the urine as the sulfate and glucuronide conjugates, while some unchanged compound is excreted via the lungs. In rats, O-demethylation also occurs, leading to catechol conjugates (Scheline 1991 p. 56).
Adverse skin reactions: Undiluted guaiacol was moderately-to-severely irritating to rabbit skin; tested at 2% on 25 volunteers it was neither irritating nor sensitizing (Opdyke 1982 p. 697–701).

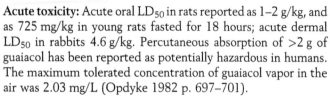

Acute toxicity: Acute oral LD$_{50}$ in rats reported as 1–2 g/kg, and as 725 mg/kg in young rats fasted for 18 hours; acute dermal LD$_{50}$ in rabbits 4.6 g/kg. Percutaneous absorption of >2 g of guaiacol has been reported as potentially hazardous in humans. The maximum tolerated concentration of guaiacol vapor in the air was 2.03 mg/L (Opdyke 1982 p. 697–701).

Human toxicity: The lowest dose causing death in humans is 50 mg/kg (3.5 g in a 70 kg adult); guaiacol ingestion in humans has been associated with irritation, burning pain with vomiting, cardiovascular collapse and possibly bloody diarrhea. The ingestion of 5 mL of guaiacol caused the death of a 9-year-old girl (Opdyke 1982 p. 697–701).

Antioxidant/pro-oxidant activity: In common with most penolic compounds, guaiacol is a scavenger of superoxide radicals (Tsujimoto et al 1993).

Mutagenicity and genotoxicity: Guaiacol was not mutagenic in the Ames test, with or without metabolic activation (Ferretti et al 1977; Pool & Lin 1982), but was genotoxic in several assays. It has induced SCE (Jansson et al 1988; Miyachi & Tsutsui 2005), morphological transformation (Yamaguchi & Tsitsui 2003) and CA (Hikiba et al 2005). It has also induced UDS, though only with metabolic activation (Hamaguchi & Tsitsui 2000). Guaiacol was cytotoxic, but not genotoxic to human dental pulp fibroblasts (Chang et al 2000).

Carcinogenic/anticarcinogenic potential: Wood creosote is a mixture of phenolic compounds, principally guaiacol, creosol, o-cresol, and 4-ethylguaiacol, and is derived from beech, not coal tar. In a 96–103 week gavage study in rats, it was dosed at 20, 50, or 200 mg/kg. There were signs of toxicity at the high dose, and several rats died (possibly due to the chosen method of dosing) but wood creosote was not carcinogenic (Kuge et al 2001). Guaiacol reduced the weight of sarcoma 180 tumors in mice (Murakami and Yamafuji 1969, cited in Opdyke 1982 p. 697–701).

Comments: It is probable that guaiacol is more toxic in humans than other species.

Summary: Guaiacol is probably irritating to human skin at some level. It is significantly toxic in humans. It is mutagenic, but appears to be non-carcinogenic.

Regulatory guidelines: Wood creosote, which includes guaiacol, is prohibited as a cosmetic ingredient in Canada (Health Canada Cosmetic Ingredient Hotlist, March 2011). Guaiacol is neither prohibited nor restricted as such.

Guaiazulene

Synonyms: 7-Isopropyl-1,4-dimethylazulene. 1,4-Dimethyl-7-(1-methylethyl)azulene. Eucazulen
Systematic name: 1,4-Dimethyl-7-(1-methylethyl)-bicyclo[5.3.0]deca-1,3,5,7,9-pentaene
Chemical class: Bicyclic sesquiterpenoid polyalkene
CAS number: 489-84-9

Sources >1.0%:

Boldo	8.8%
Cypress (blue)	6.2%

Pharmacokinetics: Guaiazulene inhibits the activity of several CYP isoforms in rats, and has a protective effect in paracetamol toxicity (Kourounakis et al 1997a, 1997b).

Mucous membrane irritation: Five patients suffering from inflamed lips after using the same toothpaste were weakly sensitive to guaiazulene on patch testing (Angelini & Vena 1984).

Antioxidant/pro-oxidant activity: Guaiazulene inhibits lipid peroxidation in rat liver, and effectively scavenges hydroxyl radicals and DPPH (Kourounakis et al 1997b).

Mutagenicity and genotoxicity: Guaiazulene was not mutagenic in *S. typhimurium* strains TA98 and TA100 with or without S9 (Gonçalves et al 2011).

Summary: We could find no dermal or toxicity data for guaiazulene. There is one report of weak oral sensitization. It appears to have an antioxidant and hepatoprotective action.

3-Hexenol

Synonym: 3-Hexen-1-ol
Chemical class: Aliphatic alkene alcohol
Note: Different isomers of 3-hexanol exist, and the following isomer-specific information has been published:

(3E)-Hexen-1-ol

Synonym: *trans*-3-Hexenol
CAS number: 928-97-2

(3Z)-Hexen-1-ol

Synonyms: Leaf alcohol. *cis*-3-Hexenol
CAS number: 928-96-1

Sources >1.0%:

Cistus	0–6.8%
Violet leaf absolute	0–4.4%
Mustard	3.3%

Adverse skin reactions: Acute dermal LD$_{50}$ in rabbits >5 g/kg. Applied full strength to rabbit skin for 24 hours under occlusion (3Z)-hexen-1-ol was not irritating. Tested at 4% on 25 volunteers it was neither irritating nor sensitizing (Opdyke 1974 p. 909–910).

Acute toxicity: (3Z)-Hexen-1-ol acute oral LD$_{50}$ in rats 4.7 g/kg (Opdyke 1974 p. 909–910).

Subacute and subchronic toxicity: In a 90 day study, rats were given dietary (3Z)-hexen-1-ol at 310, 1,250 and 5,000 ppm. No effects were seen at the lower two levels, but at 5,000 ppm the relative kidney weight was increased in male rats, and the urine collected was more concentrated (Opdyke 1974 p. 909–910).

Summary: (3Z)-Hexen-1-ol appears to be non-irritant, non-allergenic, and non-toxic.

3-Hexenyl benzoate

Synonym: Benzoic acid 3-hexenyl ester
Systematic name: 3-Hexen-1-yl benzoate
Chemical class: Benzenoid ester
Note: Different isomers of 3-hexenyl benzoate exist, and the following isomer-specific information has been published:

(3*E*)-Hexen-1-yl benzoate

Synonym: *trans*-3-Henexyl benzoate
CAS number: 75019-52-2

(3*Z*)-Hexen-1-yl benzoate

Synonym: *cis*-3-Henexyl benzoate
CAS number: 25152-85-6

Source >1.0%:

Jasmine sambac absolute	2.3%

Adverse skin reactions: (3*Z*)-Hexen-1-yl benzoate was moderately irritating to rabbit skin when applied undiluted for 24 hours under occlusion. Tested at 10% on 32 volunteers the compound was neither irritating nor sensitizing (Opdyke 1978 p. 773).
Acute toxicity: (3*Z*)-Hexen-1-yl benzoate acute oral LD_{50} in rats >5 g/kg; acute dermal LD_{50} in rabbits >5 g/kg (Opdyke 1978 p. 773).
Summary: (3*Z*)-Hexen-1-yl benzoate appears to be non-irritant, non-allergenic, and non-toxic.

3-Hexenyl formate

Synonyms: 3-Hexenyl methanoate. Formic acid 3-hexenyl ester
Systematic name: 3-Hexen-1-yl methanoate
Chemical class: Aliphatic alkene ester
Note: Different isomers of 3-hexenyl formate exist, and the following isomer-specific information has been published:

(3*E*)-Hexen-1-yl formate

Synonym: *trans*-3-Henexyl formate
CAS number: 56922-80-6

(3*Z*)-Hexen-1-yl formate

Synonym: *cis*-3-Henexyl formate
CAS number: 33467-73-1

Sources >1.0%:

Violet leaf absolute	0–2.4%

Adverse skin reactions: 3-Hexenyl formate was moderately irritating to rabbit skin when applied undiluted for 24 hours under occlusion. Tested at 10% on 25 volunteers the compound was neither irritating nor sensitizing (Opdyke 1979a p. 797).
Acute toxicity: Acute oral LD_{50} in rats >5 g/kg; acute dermal LD_{50} in rabbits >5 g/kg (Opdyke 1979a p. 797).
Summary: 3-Hexenyl formate appears to be non-irritant, non-allergenic, and non-toxic.

Hexyl butyrate

Synonym: Butyric acid hexyl ester
Systematic name: Hexyl butanoate
Chemical class: Alpihatic ester
CAS number: 2639-63-6

Sources >1.0%:

Chamomile (Roman)	0–3.9%

Adverse skin reactions: Hexyl butyrate was slightly irritating to rabbit skin when applied undiluted for 24 hours under occlusion. Tested at 12% on 30 volunteers the compound was neither irritating nor sensitizing (Opdyke 1979a p. 815).
Acute toxicity: Acute oral LD_{50} in rats >5 g/kg; acute dermal LD_{50} in rabbits >5 g/kg (Opdyke 1979a p. 815).
Summary: Hexyl butyrate appears to be non-irritant, non-allergenic, and non-toxic.

Hydrocyanic acid

Synonyms: Hydrogen cyanide. Prussic acid
Chemical class: Inorganic acid
CAS number: 74-90-8

Source:

Almond (bitter, unrectified)	2.0–4.0%

Notes: A gas at room temperature. Released from amygdalin during distillation of bitter almond oil and present in the unrectified oil. Very weak acid with characteristic almond odor (which cannot therefore be used to detect contaminated samples of bitter almond oil). Removed during the production of bitter almond oil FFPA (free from prussic acid).
Acute toxicity: The acute dermal LD_{50} of hydrocyanic acid in rabbits was 0.26 mmol/kg (7.0 mg/kg) for intact skin and 0.087 mmol/kg (2.3 mg/kg) for abraded skin. High cyanide concentrations were measured in whole blood, serum, heart, liver, kidney, spleen, lung, brain and spinal cord (Ballantyne 1994). The acute sc LD_{50} in mice was 8.4 mg/kg (Yamamoto 1995).
Human toxicity: Poisoning may occur from inhalation, ingestion or dermal absorption. Poisoning produces rapid and labored breathing (causing increased intake), paralysis, unconsciousness, convulsions and death. The fatal dose for man is considered to be about 50 mg (Reynolds 1993). This would equate to a human lethal dose of ~0.8 mg/kg. Exposure to 150 ppm for 30 to 60 minutes may endanger life, and death may result from a few minutes exposure to 300 ppm (Budavari 1989). A dose of 250–325 mg of sodium or potassium cyanide (equivalent to 100–180 mg of hydrocyanic acid) is considered lethal in humans (Timbrell 2000).
Summary: Hydrocyanic acid is extremely toxic by any route of exposure, and has caused many human fatalities. Exposure to it is tightly controlled.
Regulatory guidelines: Hydrocyanic acid is prohibited as a cosmetic ingredient in the EU and Canada. Both the UK and EC 'standard permitted proportion' of hydrocyanic acid in food flavorings is 1 mg/kg food, or 1 ppm (European Community Council 1988, Anon 1992b). In Great Britain, the maximum inhalation exposure limit of hydrocyanic acid is 10 mg/m^3 short term and 5 mg/m^3 long term (Reynolds 1993).

Indole

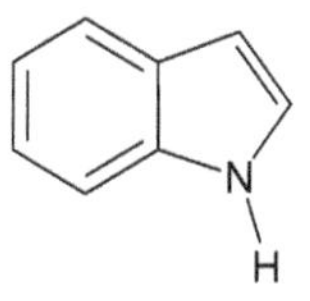

Synonyms: 1*H*-Indole. 2,3-Benzopyrrole
Systematic name: Benzo[*b*]pyrrole
Chemical class: Bicyclic nitrogen heterocycle
CAS number: 120-72-9

Sources >1.0%:

Jasmine sambac absolute	14.1%
Champaca absolute (orange)	2.9–12.0%
Ginger lily absolute	7.0%
Jasmine absolute	0.7–3.5%
Honeysuckle absolute	3.3%
Jonquil absolute	1.7%
Narcissus absolute	0–1.5%
Orange flower absolute	0.1–1.0%

Pharmacokinetics: In rats indole is metabolized by hydroxylation, and is excreted partly as the glucuronide, but mainly as the sulfate conjugate. After oral dosing in rats, ~80% is excreted in the urine, ~10% in the feces and ~2% in the expired air. The major urinary metabolite (50% of the dose) was indoxyl sulfate (Scheline 1991).
Adverse skin reactions: Tested at 1% on 25 volunteers indole was not sensitizing; it was reported as not irritating to rabbit skin (Opdyke 1974 p. 925–926).
Acute toxicity: Acute oral LD_{50} in rats 1 mL/kg; single skin-penetration LD_{50} in rabbits 0.79 mL/kg (Opdyke 1974 p. 925–926).
Carcinogenic/anticarcinogenic potential: Indole was not mutagenic in the Ames test (Florin et al 1980).
Summary: Limited data suggests that indole is non-irritant and non-allergenic. It possesses 'moderate' acute toxicity, and appears to be non-mutagenic.

α-Ionone

Synonyms: Parmone. 4,7-Megastigmadien-9-one
Systematic name: (3*E*)-4-(2,6,6-Trimethyl-2-cyclohexen-1-yl)-3-buten-2-one
Chemical class: Monocyclic monoterpenoid alkene ketone
Notes: 'Ionone' is sometimes used to describe a mixture consisting mainly of α-ionone and β-ionone. Different isomers of α-ionone exist, and the following isomer-specific information has been published:

(*R,E*)-α-Ionone

CAS number: 24190-29-2

Sources >1.0%:

Osmanthus absolute	tr–2.3%
Champaca absolute (orange)	0.1–1.6%

Pharmacokinetics: Metabolism involves oxidation, reduction and glucuronide conjugation (Ide & Toki 1970). α-Ionone induced CYP1A and CYP2B (Jeong HG et al 2002).
Adverse skin reactions: In a modified Draize procedure on guinea pigs, α-ionone was non-sensitizing when used at 30% in the challenge phase (Sharp 1978). Tested on 25 volunteers,

undiluted ionone (a mixture of α and β isomers) was not irritating, and an 8% concentration was not sensitizing (Opdyke 1975 p. 549–550). When a 48 hour closed patch test was conducted on 50 male volunteers using α-ionone at 32% in acetone, moderate irritation was seen (Motoyoshi et al 1979). When tested at 1% there were no irritant or allergic reactions to α-ionone in 100 consecutive dermatitis patients; when similarly tested at 5% there was one questionable irritant reaction but no allergic reactions (Frosch et al 1995a).
Acute toxicity: α-Ionone acute oral LD_{50} in mice reported as 6.6 g/kg and 7.0 g/kg (RIFM 1967, 1980, cited in Lalko et al 2007a). Acute oral LD_{50} in rats 4.59 g/kg for 'ionone standard' (60% α-ionone, 40% β-ionone) (Jenner et al 1964); subcutaneous mouse LD_{50} 2.6 g/kg for 'ionone' (Wenzel & Ross 1957).
Subacute and subchronic toxicity: In a 90 day study, dietary α-ionone was fed to male and female rats at 10 or 100 mg/kg/day. Renal function and hematological studies were carried out throughout the study, and a number of abnormalities were seen in the high dose group. Some changes also took place in the low dose group, but these were presumably not considered significant, as 10 mg/kg was established as the NOAEL in this study (RIFM 1983, cited in Lalko et al 2007a).

In a 17 week feeding study 1,000, 2,500 and 10,000 ppm of 'ionone standard' produced dose-dependent microscopic liver changes in rats (Hagan et al 1967). In a 12 week feeding study in rats, the NOAEL was 10.6 mg/kg for α-ionone (Bär & Griepentrog 1967). When α-ionone was consumed by male rats at 11.8 mg/kg/day, and by female rats at 11.1 mg/kg/day in the diet for 90 days, no significant adverse effects were observed on growth, food consumption, hematology, blood chemistry, liver weight, kidney weight, or the microscopic or gross appearance of major organs (Oser et al 1965).
Mutagenicity and genotoxicity: α-Ionone was non-mutagenic in the Ames test, but was weakly genotoxic in tests on Chinese hamster cells (Kasamaki et al 1982). It was not genotoxic in a mouse micronucleus test (RIFM 2006, cited in Lalko et al 2007a).
Carcinogenic/anticarcinogenic potential: The proliferation of mouse B16 melanoma cells was very weakly inhibited by α-ionone with an IC_{50} value of 190 mM (36.5 g/L) (Tatman & Huanbiao 2002).
Summary: α-Ionone appears to be non-sensitizing and virtually non-irritating. Acute toxicity is not a concern, and the 90 day NOAEL was 10 mg/kg.

β-Ionone

Synonyms: Boronione. 5,7-Megastigmadien-9-one
Systematic name: (3*E*)-4-(2,6,6-Trimethyl-1-cyclohexen-1-yl)-3-buten-2-one
Chemical class: Monocyclic monoterpenoid alkene ketone
CAS number: 79-77-6

Note: 'Ionone' is sometimes used to describe a mixture consisting mainly of α-ionone and β-ionone.

Sources >1.0%:

Osmanthus absolute	7.6–33.8%
Boronia absolute	14.9%
Champaca absolute (orange)	0.2–3.4%

Pharmacokinetics: β-Ionone metabolism involves oxidation, reduction and glucuronide conjugation (Ide & Toki 1970; Scheline 1991). β-Ionone is a relatively potent inhibitor of rat liver microsomal pentoxy resorufin O-depentilase in vitro, suggesting that it might alter the biotransformation of drugs and toxic substances (De-Oliveira et al 1999). Treatment of rats with β-ionone resulted in an increase in activity of CYP of 50–75% (Parke & Rahman 1969). Jeong et al (2002) reported that β-ionone induced CYP1A and CYP2B.

Adverse skin reactions: Tested on 25 volunteers, undiluted ionone (a mixture of α and β isomers) was not irritating, and an 8% concentration was not sensitizing (Opdyke 1975 p. 549–550). When tested at 1% there were no irritant or allergic reactions to β-ionone in 100 consecutive dermatitis patients; when similarly tested at 5% there were two questionable irritant reactions and no allergic reactions (Frosch et al 1995a).

Acute toxicity: β-Ionone acute oral LD_{50} in mice reported as 2.0 g/kg (gavage dosing) and 5.33 g/kg (oral dosing) (RIFM 1967, 1980, cited in Lalko et al 2007b). Acute oral LD_{50} in rats 4.59 g/kg for 'ionone standard' (60% α-ionone, 40% β-ionone) (Jenner et al 1964); subcutaneous mouse LD_{50} 2.6 g/kg (Wenzel & Ross 1957).

Subacute and subchronic toxicity: In a 90 day study, dietary β-ionone was fed to male and female rats at 10 or 100 mg/kg/day. Renal function and hematological studies were carried out throughout the study, and a number of abnormalities were seen in the high dose group. Some changes also took place in the low dose group, but these were presumably not considered significant, as 10 mg/kg was established as the NOAEL (RIFM 1983, cited in Lalko et al 2007b).

In a 17 week feeding study 1,000, 2,500 and 10,000 ppm of 'ionone standard' produced dose-dependent microscopic liver changes in rats (Hagan et al 1967). In a 12 week feeding study in rats, the NOAEL was 11.4 mg/kg for β-ionone (Bär & Griepentrog 1967). When β-ionone was consumed by male rats at 11.6 mg/kg/day, and by female rats at 13.1 mg/kg/day in the diet for 90 days, no significant adverse effects were observed on growth, food consumption, hematology, blood chemistry, liver weight, kidney weight, or the microscopic or gross appearance of major organs (Oser et al 1965).

Reproductive toxicity: At 1,000 mg/kg, oral β-ionone caused a high proportion of resorptions in rats. However, given 45 minutes previously, at 250, 500 or 750 mg/kg it attenuated cyclophosphamide-induced embryolethality and teratogenicity (Gomes-Carneiro et al 2003). A single gavage dose of 48, 240 or 480 mg/kg β-ionone was administered on day eight of gestation to pregnant hamsters. Examinations took place on day 14. There were no clinical signs of toxicity, including maternal weight gain, incidence of abnormal litters, or mean litter fetal body weight (Willhite 1986).

Mutagenicity and genotoxicity: β-Ionone was not mutagenic in the Ames test (Florin et al 1980; Mortelmans et al 1986;

Gomes-Carneiro et al 2006). The compound inhibited the mutagenicity of cyclophosphamide and aflatoxin B1, possibly via inhibition of CYP2B1 (Gomes-Carneiro et al 2006).

Carcinogenic/anticarcinogenic potential: The proliferation of mouse B16(F10) melanoma cells was inhibited by β-ionone with an IC_{50} value of 140 µM (26.9 mg/L) (He et al 1997b). β-Ionone completely inhibited the growth of ascites sarcoma BP8 cells (a rat cell line) at a concentration of 1.0 mM (192 mg/L) (Pilotti et al 1975). β-Ionone exhibited moderate in vitro cytotoxicity against two human carcinoma cell lines (Kubo & Morimitsu 1995) and had a significant chemopreventive action on DMBA-induced mammary carcinogenesis in rats (Yu et al 1995b). The proliferation of MCF-7 human breast cancer cells was dose-dependently suppressed by β-ionone in vitro, with 80% cell growth inhibition at 500 µM (96.0 mg/L) (Duncan et al 2004).

Summary: β-Ionone appears to be non-sensitizing and virtually non-irritating. Acute toxicity is not a concern, and the 90 day NOAEL was 10 mg/kg. Single oral doses of 750 mg/kg in rats, and 480 mg/kg in hamsters were not reproductively toxic. β-Ionone appears to be non-mutagenic and anticarcinogenic.

α-Irone

Systematic name: 4-(2,5,6,6-Tetramethyl-2-cyclohexen-1-yl)-3-buten-2-one
Chemical class: Monocyclic monoterpenoid alkene ketone
Note: Different isomers of α-irone exist, and the following isomer-specific information has been published:

(−)-(E)-α-Irone

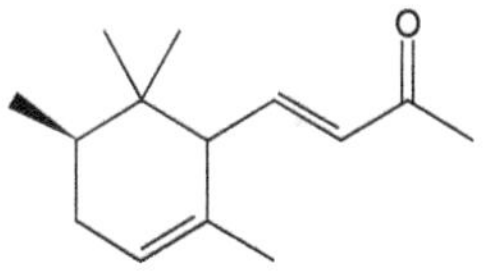

Synonyms: (−)-trans-α-Irone. (1R,5R)-α-Irone
CAS number: 35124-14-2

(+)-(E)-α-Irone

Synonyms: (+)-trans-α-Irone. (1S,5S)-α-Irone
CAS number: Not found

(−)-(Z)-α-Irone

Synonyms: (−)-cis-α-Irone. (1R,5S)-α-Irone
CAS number: Not found

(+)-(Z)-α-Irone

Synonyms: (+)-cis-α-Irone. (1S,5R)-α-Irone
CAS number: Not found

(E)-α-Irone

Iris pallida absolute	4.7–5.0%
Iris pallida	3.7–4.8%
Iris germanica absolute	1.7–3.9%
Iris germanica	0.5–2.7%

(Z)-α-Irone

Iris germanica	57.6–66.2%
Iris germanica absolute	58.4–62.7%
Iris pallida	26.0–40.6%
Iris pallida absolute	34.9–39.8%

Adverse skin reactions: Tested at 10% on 25 volunteers α-irone was neither irritating nor sensitizing (Opdyke 1975 p. 551). Also at 10%, α-irone induced allergic responses in 5 (0.3%) of 1,606 consecutive dermatitis patients (Frosch et al 2002b).

Acute toxicity: Acute oral LD_{50} in rats >5 g/kg; acute oral LD_{50} in mice 7.4 g/kg; acute dermal LD_{50} in rabbits >5 g/kg (Lalko et al 2007a)

Subacute and subchronic toxicity: Male and female mice received six ip injections of α-irone over 14 days, and were observed for a further 4–6 weeks. A maximum tolerated dose was determined at 400 mg/kg (Stoner et al 1973). When α-irone was consumed by male rats at 5.2 mg/kg/day, and by female rats at 5.9 mg/kg/day in the diet for 90 days, no significant adverse effects were observed on growth, food consumption, hematology, blood chemistry, liver weight, kidney weight, or the microscopic or gross appearance of major organs (Oser et al 1965).

Carcinogenic/anticarcinogenic potential: In male and female mice given 24 ip injections of α-irone in impure tricaprylin in a total dose of 1.95 or 9.6 g/kg over 24 weeks the incidence of primary lung tumors was no higher than in the control group (Stoner et al 1973).

Summary: α-Irone appears to be non-irritant, non-allergenic, and of minimal acute toxicity. The rat 90 day NOAEL was 5.2 mg/kg/day or greater.

Isoamyl isovalerate

Synonyms: Isopentyl isovalerate. Isovaleric acid isoamyl ester
Systematic name: 1-Ethylpropyl 3-methylbutanoate
Chemical class: Aliphatic ester
CAS number: 659-70-1

Sources >0.1%:

Khella	3.1%

Adverse skin reactions: Isoamyl isovalerate was moderately irritating to rabbit skin when applied undiluted for 24 hours under occlusion. Tested at 2% on 30 volunteers, it was neither irritating nor sensitizing (Opdyke 1978 p. 789).

Acute toxicity: Acute oral LD_{50} in rats >5 g/kg; acute dermal LD_{50} in rabbits >5 g/kg (Opdyke 1978 p773).

Mutagenicity and genotoxicity: Isoamyl isovalerate oil did not produce CA in Chinese hamster lung cells (Ishidate et al 1988).

Summary: Limited data suggest that isoamyl isovalerate is non-irritant, non-allergenic, non-toxic, and non-mutagenic.

Isobornyl acetate

Synonyms: exo-Bornanyl acetate. exo-2-Camphanyl acetate. Acetic acid isobornyl ester
Systematic name: exo-1,7,7-Trimethylbicyclo[2.2.1]heptan-2-yl ethanoate

Chemical class: Bicyclic monoterpenoid ester
Notes: Isomeric with bornyl acetate. Different isomers of bornyl acetate exist, and the following isomer-specific information has been published:

(−)-Isobornyl acetate

Synonyms: (1R,2R)-Bornyl acetate. (1R)-exo-Bornyl acetate
CAS number: 125-12-2

(+)-Isobornyl acetate

Synonyms: (1S,2S)-Bornyl acetate. (1S)-exo-Bornyl acetate
CAS number: Not found

Sources >1.0%:

Spruce (hemlock)	34.7%

Adverse skin reactions: Undiluted isobornyl acetate was mildly irritating to rabbit skin. Tested at 10% on 25 volunteers it was not sensitizing (Opdyke 1975 p. 552). Tested at 5% isobornyl acetate produced no irritant or allergic reactions in a group of 100 consecutive dermatitis patients (Frosch et al 1995a).

Acute toxicity: Acute oral LD_{50} in rats >10 g/kg; acute dermal LD_{50} in rabbits >20 g/kg (Opdyke 1975 p. 552).

Subacute and subchronic toxicity: When isobornyl acetate was given to rats by gavage in doses of 15, 90 or 270 mg/kg for 90 days there were signs of nephrotoxicity at the two higher doses. The NOAEL was 15 mg/kg/day (Gaunt et al 1971).

Summary: Isobornyl acetate is non-irritant and non-allergenic. It possesses minimal acute toxicity, and the rat 90 day NOAEL was 15 mg/kg/day.

Isobutyl butyrate

Synonyms: Isobutyl butanoate. Butyric acid isobutyl ester
Systematic name: 2-Methylpropyl butanoate
Chemical class: Aliphatic ester
CAS number: 539-90-2

Source:

Chamomile (Roman)	0–20.5%

Adverse skin reactions: Tested at 12% on 25 volunteers isobutyl butyrate was neither irritating nor sensitizing (Opdyke 1979a p. 833).

Acute toxicity: Both the acute oral LD_{50} in rats and the acute dermal LD_{50} in rabbits exceeded 5 g/kg (Opdyke 1979a p. 833).

Summary: Minimal data suggest that isobutyl butyrate is non-irritant, non-allergenic and non-toxic.

Isoeugenol

Synonyms: 2-Methoxy-4-(2-methylvinyl)phenol. 4-Propenyl-guaiacol
Systematic name: 2-Methoxy-4-(1-propenyl)phenol
Chemical class: Phenylpropenoid phenolic ether
Note: Different isomers of isoeugenol exist, and the following isomer-specific information has been published:

(1*E*)-Isoeugenol

Synonym: *trans*-Isoeugenol
CAS number: 5932-68-3

(1*Z*)-Isoeugenol

Synonym: *cis*-Isoeugenol
CAS number: 5912-86-7

Sources >0.1%:

Calamus (tetraploid form)	2.3–25.0%
Ginger lily absolute	18.4%
Betel	0–10.6%
Tuberose absolute	2.6%
Basil (pungent)	2.4%
Vetiver	0–1.3%
Karo karoundé absolute	0.5%
Ylang-ylang	0–0.5%
Clove stem	0.1–0.4%
Clove bud	0.1–0.2%
Mace	0–0.1%

Notes: Isomeric with eugenol. Being a substituted phenol, isoeugenol is a weak acid which may be corrosive to tissues.

Pharmacokinetics: Administered orally to rats, more than 85% of isoeugenol was excreted in the urine, primarily as sulfate or glucuronide metabolites, by 72 hours. Approximately 10% was recovered in the feces, and less than 0.1% was recovered as CO_2 or expired organics. At 72 hours less than 0.25% of the dose remained in the tissues (Badger et al 2002).

Adverse skin reactions: The irritation potential of isoeugenol was determined to be moderate, after 48 hour patch testing with 32% isoeugenol in acetone, on 50 male adult volunteers with no known allergies (Motoyoshi et al 1979). In a closed-patch test at 5%, primary irritation (erythema) was produced in three out of 35 volunteers (9%); isoeugenol was non-sensitizing when tested on 25 volunteers at 8% (Opdyke 1975 p. 815–817). Further research by RIFM showed isoeugenol to be sensitizing at 8% and 10% (IFRA 2009). There were no positive reactions to 5% isoeugenol tested on 100 volunteers (De Groot et al 1993) or to 0.2% isoeugenol tested on 20 volunteers (Johansen et al 1996b).

Of 1,200 dermatitis patients patch tested, there were no irritant reactions and 14 allergic reactions (0.42%) to 5% isoeugenol. In a second group of 1,500 dermatitis patients there were no irritant reactions and 12 allergic reactions (0.8%) to 1% isoeugenol (Santucci et al 1987). When isoeugenol was tested at 2% on 50 dermatitis patients who were not thought to be sensitive to fragrance materials there were no positive reactions (Larsen 1977). Of 241 dermatitis patients tested with 2% isoeugenol, 13 (5.4%) had a positive reaction (Ferguson & Sharma 1984). Seventeen of 702 dermatitis patients (2.4%) tested positive to 1% isoeugenol (Frosch et al 1995b). In a European multicenter study 20 of 1,072 dermatitis patients (1.86%) reacted to 1% isoeugenol (Frosch et al 1995a). Similarly, 1.8% (40 of 2,261) dermatitis patients reacted to 1% isoeugenol in a European multicenter study nine years later (Tanaka et al

2004). In other European studies, 14/1,502 and 26/2,063 dermatitis patients tested positive to 1% cinnamaldehyde (Schnuch et al 2007a; Heisterberg et al 2011).

In a prospective study of adverse skin reactions to cosmetic ingredients identified by patch test (1977–1980) isoeugenol elicited contact dermatitis in 10 (2%) of 487 cosmetic-related cases (Eiermann et al 1982). Of 713 cosmetic dermatitis patients, 10 reacted to isoeugenol (Adams & Maibach 1985).

There were 36 reactions (20.1%) to 8% isoeugenol in 179 dermatitis patients suspected of allergy to cosmetics (De Groot et al 1985). Of 167 dermatitis patients suspected of fragrance sensitivity 23 (13.8%) were allergic to 4% isoeugenol on patch testing (Larsen et al 1996b). Of 119 eczema patients with contact allergy to cosmetics two (1.7%) were allergic to 3% isoeugenol (De Groot et al 1988). Of 102 dermatitis patients sensitive to Peru balsam, 28 tested positive to 2% isoeugenol (Hausen 2001). In a European multicenter study, 16 eczema patients (20.5%) of 78 known to be allergic to fragrance materials reacted to 2% isoeugenol (Wilkinson et al 1989). When patch tested at 2% on 20 dermatitis patients who were sensitive to fragrance materials, isoeugenol induced 5 (25%) positive reactions (Larsen 1977). A group of 19 eczema patients known to be allergic to fragrance materials were tested with eight serial dilutions of isoeugenol, from 0.8% to 0.01%. Of the 19, 4 (21%) still reacted positively at the 0.01% concentration. As the concentration of isoeugenol was reduced, so did the percentage of patients who reacted (Johansen et al 1996b).

Results from a total of 6,512 patch tests (involving approximately 5,850 dermatitic and non-dermatitic subjects) demonstrated that hypersensitivity induced by isoeugenol was concentration dependent. All but two of the reactions occurring in this survey were at exposure concentrations greater than or equal to 0.8% isoeugenol, and no induced reactions occurred in the 1,004 patch tests reported at isoeugenol concentrations between 0.03 and 0.5%. From this report it was concluded that isoeugenol has a very low potential for either eliciting pre-existing sensitization reactions ('elicited' reactions) or inducing hypersensitivity ('induced' reactions) in subjects exposed to consumer products containing this ingredient (Thompson et al 1983). Calamus oil (tetraploid form), which contains 2.3–25% isoeugenol, elicited no skin reactions in 200 dermatitis patients when tested at 2% (Rudzki et al 1976). This is equivalent to 0.05–0.5% isoeugenol.

A moderate increase in the frequency of allergic reactions to isoeugenol was observed in 25,545 dermatitis patients patch tested from January 1980 to December 1996 in the UK (Buckley et al 2000).

Acute toxicity: Acute oral LD_{50} 1.56 g/kg in rats, 1.41 in guinea pigs (Jenner et al 1964).

Subacute and subchronic toxicity: There was no observable effect in rats given 10,000 ppm in the diet for 16 weeks (Hagan et al 1967). In a 14 week gavage study, groups of male and female rats and mice were dosed with isoeugenol at 37.5, 75, 150, 300 or 600 mg/kg/day five days per week. The NOAEL for all endpoints in all animals was 75 mg/kg, with one exception. In male mice, there was a dose-dependent increase in relative liver weight in all dosed groups. A similar increase was apparent in female mice at 600 mg/kg, and in female rats at

300 and 600 mg/kg, but male rats were not affected in this way (National Toxicology Program 2010a).

Cardiovascular effects: Isoeugenol shows in vitro antiplatelet aggregation activity (Janssens et al 1990).

Nephrotoxicity: Isoeugenol, a potent free radical scavenger, was active against cisplatin-induced cytotoxicity in vero cells as well as in rat renal cortical slices, although it was not able to arrest the reduction of the glutathione content induced by cisplatin in either the vero cells or the renal cortical slice model. Treatment with 10 mg/kg ip of isoeugenol one hour before 3 mg/kg ip cisplatin resulted in partial but significant protection against cisplatin-induced reduction of body weight, and elevation of blood urea, nitrogen and serum creatinine in rats, the protection being 34%, 46%, and 62%, respectively (Rao M et al 1999b).

Reproductive toxicity: Pregnant rats were given 250, 500 or 1,000 mg/kg/day isoeugenol by gavage on gestational days 6–19. Prenatal viability was not affected, but at the highest dose a reduction in fetal body weight gain was noted, as was a skeletal variation. The NOAEL for developmental toxicity was therefore 500 mg/kg/day. Maternal toxicity was noted at all three doses, so a NOAEL was not established (George et al 2001). When isoeugenol was administered by gavage to male and female rats at 0, 70, 230 or 700 mg/kg/day for two generations some non-reproductive toxicity was seen at all doses (hyperkeratosis and hyperplasia in the non-glandular stomach and decreased body weight) and mild reproductive toxicity (decreased number of male pups) was seen at the highest dose (NTP Report RACB97004, July 10 2002). The non-reproductive toxic effects were likely due to gavage dosing. In an ex vivo assay, mixed isomer isoeugenol did not bind to estrogen receptors in female rat uterus tissue (Blair et al 2000).

Antioxidant/pro-oxidant activity: Isoeugenol demonstrates potent antioxidant and radical scavenging activity (Rauscher et al 2001, Tominaga et al 2005).

Mutagenicity and genotoxicity: Isoeugenol was not mutagenic in *Saccharomyces cerevisiae* (Nestmann & Lee 1983) nor in the Ames test, with or without S9 (Hsia et al 1979; Florin et al 1980; Sekizawa & Shibamoto 1982; Mortelmans et al 1986; National Toxicology Program 2010a). Isoeugenol was mutagenic in the *Bacillus subtilis* DNA repair test (Sekizawa & Shibamoto 1982) and was genotoxic in human lymphocytes (Jansson et al 1988). After three months of gavage dosing, isoeugenol was not genotoxic in male mice, and was very slightly genotoxic in female mice (National Toxicology Program 2010a). It was not genotoxic in Chinese hamster ovary cells (Sasaki et al 1989; National Toxicology Program 2010a). Unlike safrole, isoeugenol was not genotoxic in a 'SMART' fruit fly test (Munerato et al 2005). And, unlike methyleugenol and safrole, isoeugenol did not induce UDS in rats or mice. It has been suggested that the compound is extensively detoxified by glucuronidation and sulfation at the free hydroxyl group (Burkey et al 2000).

Carcinogenic/anticarcinogenic potential: In a novel assay for carcinogens, groups of male rats were dosed for 2, 14 or 90 days with 0.2 or 2.0 mmol/kg/day (33 or 328 mg/kg/day) of isoeugenol, and then hepatic tissue was analyzed for precancerous changes in gene expression. The results strongly suggest that isoeugenol is not hepatocarcinogenic in male rats (Auerbach et al 2010). In a 2-year gavage study, groups of male and female rats and mice were dosed with isoeugenol at 75, 150 or 300 mg/kg/day 5 days per week. In the high-dose male rat group (48 animals), one had a benign thymus tumor and another had a malignant thymus tumor. None were seen in any other group of rats or mice. No malignancies were seen in any other tissues of rats or female mice. However in male mice, hepatocellular carcinomas occurred in 18, 19 and 18 of 50 animals in the three dosed groups, compared to 8/50 controls. Although not dose-dependent, this strongly suggests carcinogenicity for isoeugenol in male mice, and there was a similar pattern of increased incidence of benign hepatic tumors (National Toxicology Program 2010a).

Comments: The gene expression study by Auerbach et al (2010) correctly predicted a lack of hepatocarcinogenicity for isoeugenol in male rats. In the National Toxicology Program (2010a) study, the increase in relative liver weight noted in the 14 week study for male mice correlates with the increased incidence of liver tumors seen in male mice in the 2-year study. This suggests that the tumors were directly related to chronic hepatotoxicity. Why this should only occur in male mice and not in female mice or in rats, and whether it indicates a material risk for humans, are questions to be addressed. However, the increase in liver weight, combined with a lack of definitive genotoxicity and sex or species differences, is a pattern typical in chemicals that are mildly or moderately carcinogenic in some rodents but not humans. The increased liver weight is a function of a higher metabolic rate (Monro 1992, 1993). The absence of a dose-dependent action adds to the weakness of the case for isoeugenol being carcinogenic. Isoeugenol is one of the most allergenic fragrance materials, and restrictions for dermal application seem justified, although this will have only a minimal impact on the use of essential oils in aromatherapy.

Summary: As with all fragrance materials, skin reactions to isoeugenol vary with the concentration of the material and the status of dermal health of the individuals being patch tested. Reactions in volunteers to 5% isoeugenol varied from 0% to 9%, and in dermatitis patients reactions to 1% isoeugenol varied from 0.8% to 1.8%. Among fragrance-sensitive patients, a significant number reacted to 0.01% isoeugenol. The 90 day rodent LOAEL is 75 mg/kg. Isoeugenol is hepatocarcinogenic in male mice. Isoeugenol inhibits platelet aggregation.

Regulatory guidelines: Isoeugenol is one of the 26 fragrance materials listed as an allergen by the EU. If present in a cosmetic product at over 100 ppm (0.01%) in a wash-off product or 10 ppm (0.001%) in a leave-on product the compound must be declared on the ingredient list if sold in an EU member state (SCCNFP 2001a). The current IFRA guideline requires that isoeugenol is not used in most product types at more than 0.02% (IFRA 2009). This recommendation is based on test results showing sensitization reaction at 8% and no sensitization when tested as such at 0.5%; other data on mixtures indicate a NOAEL in the region of 0.2% (private communication to IFRA, IFRA 2004). For non skin-contact products, a maximum use level of 0.2% is recommended by IFRA. In a preliminary report by an ECETOC taskforce, isoeugenol was provisionally classified as a moderate allergen (on a scale of extreme, strong, moderate and weak) only likely to elicit a sensitization reaction if present at 1% or more (Kimber et al 2003).

Our safety advice: We recommend a maximum dermal use level of 0.2% for isoeugenol in essential oils, for skin sensitization.

Isomenthone

Synonyms: 2-Isopropyl-5-methylcyclohexanone. *p*-Menthan-3-one
Systematic name: 2-(1-Methylethyl)-5-methylcyclohexanone
Chemical class: Monocyclic monoterpenoid ketone
Note: Different isomers of isomenthone exist, and the following isomer-specific information has been published:

(−)-Isomenthone

Synonyms: (2*S*)-*cis*-2-Isomenthone. (2*S*,5*S*)-2-Isomenthone
CAS number: 18309-28-9

(+)-Isomenthone

Synonyms: (2*R*)-*trans*-2-Isomenthone. (2*R*,5*S*)-2-Isomenthone
CAS number: 1196-31-2

Sources >1.0%:

Pennyroyal (N. American)	0.8–31.0%
Buchu (diosphenol CT)	4.6–29.1%
Buchu (pulegone CT)	3.6–27.6%
Cornmint	6.8–12.1%
Pennyroyal (Turkish)	11.1%
Geranium	3.4–9.8%
Peppermint	2.0–8.7%
Pennyroyal (European)	0.8–8.6%
Calamint (lesser)	0–2.8%
Cistus	0–2.3%

Notes: Isomeric with menthone. The (rare) isomenthone CT of *Agathosma betulina* leaf oil contains 39–49% of isomenthone.
Pharmacokinetics: (+)-Isomenthol was the major, and possibly the only urinary metabolite of isomenthone detected in rabbit urine (Scheline 1991).
Adverse skin reactions: Tested at 8% on 25 volunteers isomenthone was neither irritating nor sensitizing (Opdyke 1976 p. 315).
Acute toxicity: Acute dermal LD$_{50}$ in rats >5 g/kg (Opdyke 1976 p. 315).
Antioxidant/pro-oxidant activity: Isomenthone demonstrated significant radical scavenging activity against DPPH and OH radicals (Mimica-Dukic et al 2003).
Summary: Minimal data suggest that isomenthone is non-irritant, non-allergenic and non-toxic.

Isopimpinellin

Synonyms: 5,8-Dimethoxypsoralen. 5,8-Dimethoxy-6,7-furanocoumarin
Systematic name: 5,8-Dimethoxyfurano[3,2-*g*]benzopyran-7-one
Chemical class: Furanocoumarin ether
CAS number: 482-27-9

Sources:

Lime (expressed)	0.1–1.3%
Rue	0.02%
Lemon (expressed)	0–0.011%

Pharmacokinetics: Isopimpinellin is a potent inhibitor of CYP1A1 (Baumgart et al 2005).
Adverse skin reactions: Isopimpinellin, confirmed to contain as impurities only trace quantities at most of psoralen, bergapten and methoxsalen, is not phototoxic when tested in a chick skin bioassay system. These findings are at variance with earlier studies showing isopimpinellin to be phototoxic in chick skin and support the conclusion that isopimpinellin is photobiologically inactive. The reports of isopimpinellin photoactivity are most likely attributable to contamination by small amounts of highly active psoralens such as bergapten or methoxsalen (Ivie & Beier 1996). Hudson et al (1987) found that isopimpinellin was not phototoxic in viruses or cells, and Lohr et al (2010) also found a total lack of phototoxicity, in V79 cells.
Mutagenicity and genotoxicity: Isopimpinellin appears to have negligible photomutagenic activity (Schimmer & Kühne 1990). Isopimpinellin was not mutagenic in an HPRT assay, and was not photomutagenic. Similarly, it was neither genotoxic nor photogenotoxic in a micronucleus assay (Lohr et al 2010).
Carcinogenic/anticarcinogenic potential: Isopimpinellin reduced overall binding of DMBA to epidermal DNA by 52% when applied topically at a dose of 400 nmol (98 µg). It also inhibited benzo[a]pyrene (B[a]P)-DNA adduct formation at a similar dose, but to a lesser extent (Cai et al 1997a). When given orally (70 mg/kg per os, 4 successive daily doses) isopimpinellin significantly blocked EROD and PROD activities in the epidermis at 1 and 24 hours after oral dosing, and significantly inhibited PROD activities in lung and forestomach at 1 hour after the final dose (Kleiner et al 2001). Orally administered isopimpinellin at 70 mg/kg inhibited B[a]P-DNA adduct formation in mouse skin by 37%, and in a second, dose–response study, 35, 70 and 150 mg/kg blocked DMBA-DNA adduct formation by 23, 56 and 69%, respectively. At the same three doses, isopimpinellin reduced the mean number of papillomas per mouse by 49, 73 and 78%, respectively (Kleiner et al 2002). Isopimpinellin prevents B[*a*]P- and DMBA-induced adduct formation in the human breast MCF-7 adenocarcinoma cell line via inhibition of multiple human CYPs (Kleiner et al 2003).
Comments: Since isopimpinellin is known to be neither phototoxic nor photomutagenic, the SCCP guideline should be revised.
Summary: Isopimpinellin is neither phototoxic nor photomutagenic. It has demonstrated significant in vitro and in vivo anti-tumoral activity.
Regulatory guidelines: For tanning products, the SCCNFP set a maximum of 1 ppm for 'furocoumarin-like substances' in 1995, later reviewed and confirmed (SCCNFP 2003b). This has now been extended to apply to all cosmetic products, and specifically includes isopimpinellin (SCCP 2005b).

Isopinocamphone

Synonym: 3-Pinanone
Systematic name: 2,6,6-Trimethylbicyclo[3.1.1]heptan-3-one
Chemical class: Bicyclic monoterpenoid ketone

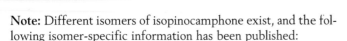

Note: Different isomers of isopinocamphone exist, and the following isomer-specific information has been published:

(−)-Isopinocamphone

Synonyms: (1S,2S,5R)-3-Pinanone. (Z)-Pinocamphone. *cis*-Pinocamphone.
CAS number: 14575-93-0

(+)-Isopinocamphone

Synonym: (1R,2R,5S)-3-Pinanone
CAS number: 473-62-1
Note: Isomeric with pinocamphone.

Sources >1.0%:

Hyssop (pinocamphone CT)	30.9–39.2%
Rosemary (verbenone CT)	1.2–2.9%
Cistus	0–2.5%
Hyssop (linalool CT)	1.0–1.5%

Pharmacokinetics: Isopinocamphone is metabolized in vitro and in vivo primarily by CYP enzymes to hydroxylated derivatives. This has been proposed as a probable detoxification pathway (Höld et al 2002).
Acute toxicity: Acute ip LD_{50} in mice 175 mg/kg (Höld et al 2002).
Neurotoxicity: Isopinocamphone is partly responsible for the neurotoxicity of hyssop oil (Millet et al 1980). In ip LD_{50} testing, mice exhibited neurological signs 1–2 minutes after injection of isopinocamphone, and these progressed to generalized, unremitting convulsions, followed by either death or recovery. Isopinocamphone acts as a GABA-gated chloride channel blocker, and its convulsant activity can be reversed by administration of diazepam (Höld et al 2002). The lowest known convulsant dose of pinocamphone isomers in humans was ~210 mg (10 drops of hyssop oil containing ~70% pinocamphone and isopinocamphone); this is equivalent to 3 mg/kg (Millet 1981).
Comments: The structurally similar cyclic monoterpenoid ketone, thujone, shares many of the properties of isopinocamphone. Both are convulsant, both noncompetitively inhibit $GABA_A$ receptor-mediated responses, and both are metabolized by CYP enzymes to less toxic hydroxyl derivatives (Höld et al 2002). They also seem to have similar toxicities in humans, the lowest known convulsant dose of pinocamphone isomers being 3 mg/kg (Millet 1981), and the equivalent dose for thujone isomers being 2.2–2.9 mg/kg (Burkhard et al 1999).
Summary: Isopinocamphone is neurotoxic, high doses causing convulsions in mice, rats and humans. The ip LD_{50} data in mice suggest that isopinocamphone is 1.4 times more toxic than pinocamphone (175 mg/kg and >250 mg/kg. respectively).
Regulatory guidelines: In France, pinocamphone is limited, in absinthe or similar alcoholic beverages, to 20 mg/L (Lachenmeier et al 2008). Isopinocamphone is not specified, but the intent seems to be to limit both isomers of pinocamphone.
Our Safety Advice: Due to the similarities noted in Comments above, we have applied the same limits to isopinocamphone as we have for thujone, i.e. a daily maximum oral dose of 0.1 mg/kg/day, which is equivalent to 7 mg per adult, and a dermal exposure of 0.24% (Table 14.1).

Isopulegol

Synonym: *p*-Menth-8-en-3-ol
Systematic name: 2-Isopropenyl-5-methylcyclohexanol
Chemical class: Monocyclic monoterpenoid alkene alcohol
CAS number: 7786-67-6
Note: Different isomers of isopulegol exist.

Sources >1.0%:

Combava leaf	0.3–4.9%
Lemon-scented gum	0–4.0%
Citronella (Sri Lankan)	0.5–2.1%
Juniper (Phoenician)	tr–1.6%
Cedarwood (Port Orford)	1.4%
Cornmint	0.9–1.4%
Tea tree (lemon-scented)	1.3%
Jamrosa	1.0%

Adverse skin reactions: Undiluted isopulegol was severely irritating to rabbits, while at 50% it was not irritating to guinea pigs. Tested at 8%, it was not irritating to 10 human volunteers, nor was it sensitizing to 25. In a 48 hour closed-patch test, neither 10% nor 20% isopulegol produced any irritant reactions in 15 male and 15 female volunteers. Dilutions of isopulegol up to 50% were not phototoxic in guinea pigs (RIFM 1999, cited in Bhatia et al 2008e).
Acute toxicity: Isopulegol acute oral LD_{50} in rats 1.03 g/kg, with noted ataxia and CNS depression, and slight pulmonary hyperemia. Acute dermal LD_{50} in rabbits ~3 mL/kg (RIFM 1971, cited in Bhatia et al 2008e).
Mutagenicity and genotoxicity: Isopulegol was not mutagenic in *S. typhimurium* strains TA98, TA100, TA1525 and TA1537, with or without S9. It was also not mutagenic in *E. coli* WP2*uvr*A (RIFM 1999, cited in Bhatia et al 2008e). 'Pulegonol' (assumed to denote isopulegol) was not genotoxic in Chinese hamster ovary cells (Sasaki et al 1989).
Summary: Isopulegol appears to be non-irritant and non-allergenic in humans, and it is not mutagenic. It possesses 'slight' acute toxicity, which will not present any problems considering the low concentrations of isopulegol found in essential oils.

Isosafrole

Systematic name: 1-Propenyl-3,4-methylenedioxybenzene
Chemical class: Phenylpropenoid ether
Note: Isomeric with safrole. Different isomers of cresol exist, and the following isomer-specific information has been published:

(*E*)-Isosafrole

Synonym: *trans*-Isosafrole
CAS number: 4043-71-4

(Z)-Isosafrole

Synonym: *cis*-Isosafrole
CAS number: 17627-76-8

Source: Sometimes found in trace amounts in ylang-ylang oil.

Pharmacokinetics: Isosafrole induced the formation of a novel form of CYP in rats (Dickins et al 1978). In rats, isosafrole is mainly (~79%) O-demethylenated to the catechol derivative, some of which is further converted to O-methylated and side-chain-reduced products. Only relatively little of the methylenedioxy group survives, to give the 1′,2′-diol (ca. 2%) and 3′-alcohol (Scheline 1991 p. 73). Isosafrole is a potent inducer of cytochromes P450 and P448 (Ioannides et al 1985).
Acute toxicity: Acute oral LD_{50} 1.34 g/kg in rats, 2.47 g/kg in mice (Jenner et al 1964).
Mutagenicity and genotoxicity: Isosafrole is not mutagenic in the Ames test (Eder et al 1980, 1982). It has been reported both as weakly genotoxic and non-genotoxic (Randerath et al 1984; Howes et al 1990).
Carcinogenic/anticarcinogenic potential: Fed to rats at 5,000 ppm for two years and 10,000 ppm for 11 weeks, isosafrole caused growth retardation, enlargement of the liver, and slight microscopic liver damage at both doses. At the lower dose, 5/50 rats had primary hepatic tumors (two had adenomas, three had carcinomas) and there was an increased incidence of chronic nephritis and of interstitial cell tumors in the testes; slight hyperplasia of the thyroid was observed. At the higher dose, none of the rats survived beyond 11 weeks (Hagan et al 1967). In a novel assay for carcinogens, groups of male rats were dosed for 2, 14 or 90 days with 0.2 or 2.0 mmol/kg/day (32 or 324 mg/kg/day) of isosafrole, and then hepatic tissue was analyzed for precancerous changes in gene expression. The results suggest that isosafrole is weakly hepatocarcinogenic in male rats (Auerbach et al 2010).
Summary: The report on isosafrole of the EU Scientific Committee on Food concludes: '*Isosafrole is a weak rodent hepatocarcinogen; the carcinogenicity is probably mediated by a non-genotoxic mechanism. Isosafrole metabolites may give rise to only very low binding to liver DNA in mice. It cannot be excluded that high exposure to isosafrole may give rise to isomerization of 3′-hydroxy- isosafrole to 1′-hydroxysafrole, the proximate carcinogen metabolite of safrole. However, generally the exposure to isosafrole is estimated to be very low. A clear NOEL could not be demonstrated for hepatic effects in the long-term studies. Therefore, the Committee could not establish a TDI. The Committee notes that isosafrole occurs together with safrole, but at much lower concentrations. Any measure to restrict exposure to safrole in food would also cover isosafrole'* (SCF 2003a).
Regulatory guidelines: IFRA makes no recommendation on isosafrole itself, but recommends that the total concentration of safrole, isosafrole and dihydrosafrole should not exceed 0.01% (IFRA 2009). Both the UK and EC 'standard permitted proportion' of isosafrole in food flavorings is 0.001 g/kg (European Community Council 1988; Anon 1992b). See safrole. Isosafrole is listed under the FDA Controlled Substances Act as a 'List 1 chemical', one that can be used in the manufacture of illegal drugs

(http://www.fda.gov/regulatoryinformation/legislation/ucm148726.htm#cntlsba accessed August 5th 2012).

(Z)-Jasmone

Synonym: *cis*-Jasmone
Systematic name: (Z)-3-Methyl-2-(2-pentenyl)-2-cyclopenten-1-one
Chemical class: Monocyclic monoterpenoid alkene ketone
CAS number: 488-10-8

Sources >1.0%:

Jasmine absolute	1.5–3.3%
Ginger lily absolute	1.2%

Adverse skin reactions: Undiluted (Z)-jasmone was moderately-to-severely irritating to rabbit skin; tested at 8% on 25 volunteers, it was neither irritating nor sensitizing (Opdyke 1979a p. 845).
Acute toxicity: Acute oral LD_{50} in rats ~5 g/kg, acute dermal LD_{50} in rabbits >5 g/kg (Opdyke 1979a p. 845).
Mutagenicity and genotoxicity: (Z)-jasmone was genotoxic in Chinese hamster ovary cells (Sasaki et al 1989).
Carcinogenic/anticarcinogenic potential: (Z)-Jasmone dose-dependently inhibited the proliferation of two human lung cancer cell lines in vitro, and apoptosis was observed (Yeruva et al 2006). It also inhibited the proliferation of human prostate PC-3 (but not HTB-81) cancer cells in vitro (Samaila et al 2004). Jasmonates such as (Z)-jasmone act directly and selectively on mitochondria derived from cancer cells, by-passing premitochondrial apoptotic blocks (Rotem et al 2005).
Summary: There is no evidence of skin reactivity in humans, and (Z)-jasmone is non-toxic. The only mutagenicity test was positive, but the anticancer data suggest that (Z)-jasmone is not carcinogenic.

Lavandulyl acetate

Synonyms: Lavandulyl ethanoate. Acetic acid lavandulyl ester
Systematic name: 5-Methyl-2-(1-methylethenyl)-4-hexen-1-yl ethanoate
Chemical class: Aliphatic monoterpenoid alkene ester
Note: Different isomers of lavandulyl acetate exist, and the following isomer-specific information has been published:

(+)-Lavandulyl acetate

Synonym: (S)-Lavandulyl ethanoate
CAS number: 144831-70-9

(−)-Lavandulyl acetate

Synonym: (R)-Lavandulyl ethanoate

CAS number: 20777-39-3

Sources >1.0%:

Lavender	1.0–5.0%
Lavandin Grosso	2.3–2.4%
Lavandin Abrialis	1.0–2.0%
Wormwood (β-thujone CT)	0–1.8%
Lavandin super	1.5–1.7%

Adverse skin reactions: Tested at 10% on 25 volunteers, lavandulyl acetate was neither irritating nor sensitizing (Opdyke 1978 p. 805).
Acute toxicity: Acute oral LD_{50} in rats >5 g/kg; acute dermal LD_{50} in rats >5 g/kg (Opdyke 1978 p. 805).
Summary: Lavandulyl acetate is non-toxic, and the limited dermal data suggest that it is not skin reactive.

(+)-Limonene

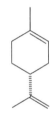

Synonyms: *d*-Limonene. (*R*)-(+)-Limonene. *p*-Mentha-1,8-diene. 1,8-*p*-Menthadiene. Cinene
Systematic name: (*R*)-(+)-1-Methyl-4-(1-methylethenyl)cyclohexene
Chemical class: Monocyclic monoterpenoid alkene
CAS number: 5989-27-5

Sources >10.0%:

Orange (sweet)	83.9–95.9%
Grapefruit	84.8–95.4%
Clementine	94.8–95.0%
Orange (bitter)	89.7–94.7%
Tangerine	87.4–91.7%
Satsuma	82.0–90.6%
Lemon (expressed)	56.6–76.0%
Celery seed	68.0–75.0%
Mandarin	65.3–74.2%
Tangelo	73.2%
Lemon (distilled)	64.0–70.5%
Dill seed (European)	35.9–68.4%
Pilocarpus jaborandi	0–67.0%
Elemi	26.9–65.0%
Palo santo	58.6–63.3%
Yuzu	63.1%
Lime expressed (Persian)	51.5–59.6%
Fleabane	56.4%

Lime distilled (Persian) (+ 1,8-cineole)	55.6%
Fir needle (silver)	54.7%
Bergamot (expressed)	27.4–52.0%
Lime distilled (Mexican) (+ 1,8-cineole)	40.4–49.4%
Caraway	36.9–48.8%
Lime expressed (Mexican)	48.2%
Bergamot (FCF)	28.0–45.0%
Dill seed (Indian)	5.9–45.0%
Pepper (Sichuan)	44.4%
Camphor (white)	44.2%
Verbena (white)	32.6–40.8%
Angelica seed	2.3–38.7%
Pine (dwarf)	6.1–37.1%
Fir cone (silver)	28.5–34.1%
Lemon leaf	8.1–30.7%
Lemon balm (Australian) (+β-phellandrene)	30.5%
Gingergrass	30.1%
Tana	25.0–30.0%
Fir needle (Himalayan)	29.6%
Wormseed	29.2%
Buchu (diosphenol CT)	11.6–28.2%
Boswellia rivae	28.0%
Turpentine	0–25.2%
Dill weed	22.5–24.9%
Pepper (black)	16.4–24.4%
Thyme (limonene CT)	24.2%
Pepper (white)	22.6%
May chang	8.4–22.6%
Ravensara leaf	13.9–22.5%
Boswellia sacra (α-pinene CT)	6.0–21.9%
Spearmint	9.1–21.2%
Fennel (sweet)	0.2–21.0%
Sumach (Venetian)	20.0%
Vassoura	4.7–18.0%
Neroli	6.0–17.9%
Goldenrod	17.8%
Buchu (pulegone CT)	2.1–17.2%
Boswellia frereana	0–17.0%
Eucalyptus macarthurii	9.8–16.2%
Spruce (Norwegian)	9.5–15.9%
Fir needle (Canadian)	1.8–15.6%
Verbena (lemon)	5.7–15.4%
Combava fruit	5.3–13.8%
Angelica root	6.0–13.2%
Ahibero	0.5–13.2%
Rhododendron	13.3%
Spruce (white)	13.0%
Myrtle	5.1–12.7%
Niaouli (cineole CT)	6.0–12.0%
Mandarin leaf	7.2–11.7%
Spruce (red)	11.5%

Citronella (Sri Lankan)	2.6–11.3%
Eucalyptus camaldulensis	0–11.2%
Pine (grey)	7.1–10.9%
Juniperberry	0–10.9%
Helichrysum italicum subsp. *microphyllum*	10.7%
Rosemary (β-myrcene CT)	2.4–10.6%
Blackcurrant bud	0.8–10.0%

Notes: (−)-Limonene and ψ-limonene (*psi*-limonene) are also found as very minor constituents of some essential oils. There is a separate profile on (−)-limonene below.

Pharmacokinetics: When (+)-limonene was given to rabbits by oral administration, 72% of it was excreted in the urine within 72 hours, with 7% appearing in the feces, via biliary excretion and non-absorption from the gastrointestinal tract. No unchanged (+)-limonene was found in the urine. The substance was completely metabolized to oxidation products and water-soluble conjugates (Kodama et al 1974). Similar products are seen if (+)-limonene is given orally to rats (Regan & Bjeldanes 1976). There are differences between rats and humans in the way that (+)-limonene is oxidized by CYP2B enzymes (Miyazawa et al 2001a). (+)-Limonene was converted to carveol, perillyl alcohol and carvone by dogs, rabbits and guinea pigs. However, in mice, rats, monkeys and humans, carveol and perillyl alcohol were produced, but no carvone (Shimada et al 2002).

(+)-Limonene undergoes rapid distribution and extensive metabolism in humans (Falk-Filipsson et al 1993). In human liver microsomes the principal metabolites were (+)-(*E*)-carveol and (+)-perillyl alcohol (Miyazawa et al 2001a). The (+)-(*E*)-carveol is further transformed to (+)-carvone (Shimada et al 2002). In a phase I clinical trial and pharmacokinetic study, the predominating circulating metabolites of (+)-limonene were, in descending order of predominance: perillic acid, dihydroperillic acid, limonene-1,2-diol, uroterpenol and an isomer of perillic acid (Vigushin et al 1998). A similar study established that the perillyl alcohol is biotransformed to perillic acid and dihydroperillic acid (Ripple et al 2000). The main human urinary metabolites are (+)-limonene 8,9-diol, perillic acid and their derivatives (Concise International Chemical Assessment Document No 5, 1998). Other urinary metabolites of limonene in humans include numerous hydroxylated monoterpenes, such as carveol (*p*-mentha-1,8-diene-6-ol) and uroterpenol (*p*-menth-1-ene-8,9-diol) (Crowell et al 1992).

In animal studies (+)-limonene increased the transdermal penetration of indomethacin (Okabe et al 1989) and haloperidol, but not chlorpromazine (Almirall et al 1996). In an uptake study of human skin, 8.9% of the (+)-limonene applied was found in the stratum corneum (Cornwell et al 1996).

(+)-Limonene induces CYP enzymes (Parke & Rahman 1969) and reduces the activity of HMGCoA reductase in birds (Qureshi et al 1988). Single oral doses of 200–1,200 mg/kg/day (+)-limonene in rats did not affect hepatic enzymes, but at 400 mg/kg/day for 30 days, there were increases in total CYP enzymes (31%), cytochrome *b*5 (30%), aminopyrine demethylase (26%) and aniline hydroxylase (22%) (Ariyoshi et al 1975).

Adverse skin reactions: Tested at 20% on 20 dermatitis patients, 98% pure (+)-limonene was not irritating (Christensson et al 2009). Undiluted (+)-limonene was moderately irritating to rabbit skin; tested at 8% on 25 healthy human volunteers, it produced no sensitization reactions (Opdyke 1975 p. 825–826). Patch tests were performed on 28 dermatitis patients who were not sensitive to turpentine oil with various concentrations of freshly distilled, unoxidized (+)-limonene. Concentrations of 70–80% were irritating in most patients, at 50% weak reactions were obtained 'in some cases' while no reactions were observed at 25–30% (Pirilä et al 1964).

In a group of 100 consecutive dermatitis patients tested with 1% (+)-limonene there was one irritant reaction and no allergic reactions (Frosch et al 1995a). Of 1,200 dermatitis patients patch tested, there were no irritant reactions and three (0.25%) allergic reactions to 2% (+)-limonene (Santucci et al 1987). Tested at 3%, (+)-limonene induced allergic responses in nine (0.56%) of 1,606 consecutive dermatitis patients (Frosch et al 2002b). The results of two further European studies are reported in Table 5.10.

There were two reactions to 10% (+)-limonene (1.1%) in 179 dermatitis patients suspected of allergy to cosmetics (De Groot et al 1985). Of seven dermatitis patients already sensitive to tea tree oil, six reacted positively to [oxidized?] (+)-limonene at 1% (Knight & Hausen 1994). Tested at 5%, (+)-limonene was slightly sensitizing to 1 of 11 dermatitis patients sensitive to tea tree oil (Hausen et al 1999). Dermal exposure to (+)-limonene in one subject caused burning, itching, aching and a longstanding purpuric rash (Falk et al 1991b). ACD has been reported in workers picking plants containing (+)-limonene, and who reacted to (+)-limonene on patch testing (Guarneri et al 2008; Wei et al 2006).

In a modified Draize procedure on guinea pigs, (+)-limonene ex citrus oil was non-sensitizing when used at 20% in the challenge phase (Sharp 1978). Other studies in guinea pigs suggest that oxidation products in older samples of (+)-limonene are the primary cause of sensitization rather than (+)-limonene itself. (+)-Limonene of high purity elicited no significant allergic reactions in guinea pigs, while (+)-limonene exposed to the air for two months was sensitizing (Karlberg et al 1991). No significant response was obtained to unoxidized (+)-limonene even if the animals were sensitized to oxidized (+)-limonene (Karlberg et al 1992).

Of the five oxidation products that were identified, (−)-carvone, and a mixture of (*Z*)- and (*E*)- isomers of (+)-limonene 1,2-oxide were potent sensitizers, while (*Z*)- and (*E*)-carveol were not (Karlberg et al 1992). Two further oxidation products, the (*Z*)- and (*E*)- isomers of limonene-2-hydroperoxide, were also potent contact allergens in guinea pigs (Karlberg et al 1994a). However, antioxidants such as ascorbic acid and α-tocopherol can reduce the sensitizing effect of limonene-2-hydroperoxide (Gafvert et al 2002). A total of 22 oxidation products of (+)-limonene were identified by Nilsson et al (1996). In descending order of concentration, the four most prolific compounds after three months of oxidation were (−)-carvone, limonene 1,2-oxide, (*E*)-carveol and *p*-menth-8-ene-1,2-diol.

Two of 88 dermatitis patients (2.3%) tested positive to 2% oxidized (+)-limonene (Chang et al 1997). Of 2,273 consecutive patients patch tested at four dermatology clinics in Europe, 63 (2.8%) reacted positively to 3% oxidized (+)-limonene (Matura et al 2002). A 42-year-old male mechanic with chronic hand eczema tested positive to 1% and 2% oxidized (+)-limonene. His hand eczema resolved in discontinuing his (+)-limonene-based hand cleanser (Chang et al 1997).

Two batches of oxidized (+)-limonene were tested, both at 3%, on groups of consecutive dermatitis patients in both Stockholm and Leuven. The first batch was oxidized for 10 weeks, and the second for 20 weeks. The (+)-limonene was 96% pure, and was stored in open flasks at room temperature (about 20 °C) and stirred for one hour four times each day. In Stockholm, there was an increase from the first batch of (+)-limonene (1.9% of patients reacting) to the second batch (2.6%). However, in Leuven there was a decrease from the 10 week oil (1.6%) to the 20 week oil (0.9%). Since there were 150–400 patients in each group, this suggests a lack of correlation between the degree of oxidation of (+)-limonene and the incidence of skin sensitization (Karlberg & Dooms-Goossens 1997). Oxidized (+)-limonene produced five allergic reactions in 658 people (0.76%) with hand eczema when tested at 3% (Heydorn et al 2003b).

Cold (4–6 °C) and dark storage of (+)-limonene in closed vessels prevents any significant autoxidation for 12 months. The addition of BHT (butylated hydroxytoluene, an antioxidant) to (+)-limonene prevents significant autoxidation for periods which depend on the purity of the materials and the ambient temperature, but in two of the tests it prevented significant oxidation in air-exposed (+)-limonene for 34 and 43 weeks. In these tests, the (+)-limonene was oxidized as described in the previous paragraph. There was no direct correlation between the amount of BHT used and the time before the onset of oxidation could be detected, and after the BHT was consumed oxidation proceeded at about the same rate as for (+)-limonene without BHT (in the tests using BHT, once oxidation commenced, the (+)-limonene content was reduced from 95–99% to ~20% in less than 20 weeks). The concentration of sensitizing oxidation products reached a peak after 10–20 weeks of air oxidation, and then declined due to polymerization of the oxidation products. After 48 weeks the identified oxidation products constituted 14% of the material (Karlberg et al 1994b).

In in vitro testing, unoxidized (+)-limonene significantly inhibited mast cell activation and degranulation in the skin, showing an anti-allergic action (Cariddi et al 2011).

Acute toxicity: (+)-Limonene acute oral LD_{50} in rats >5 g/kg; acute dermal LD_{50} in rabbits >5 g/kg (Opdyke 1975 p. 825–826). Acute oral LD_{50} in male mice was 6.3 mL/kg and in female mice was 8.1 mL/kg (Tsuji et al 1974). A single dose of limonene at at 100 mg/kg was non-toxic in seven healthy humans (Crowell et al 1994a). There is no indication that (+)-limonene is toxic to humans or indeed most experimental animals (Regan & Bjeldanes 1976; Webb et al 1990).

Subacute and subchronic toxicity: Groups of male and female rats were administered 0, 277, 554, 1,385 or 2,770 mg/kg/day (+)-limonene orally for 30 days. A general decrease in food intake and a dose-related decrease in body weight were seen in males, but there was little or no effect on absolute or relative organ weights. No significant changes were seen in urinalysis, haematology or biochemical values. The following tissues were examined histopathologically: adrenals, duodenum, heart,

kidneys, liver, lungs, lymph nodes, pancreas, pituitary, spleen, stomach, testes/ovaries, thymus and thyroids. No significant changes were noted except that granular casts were seen in the kidneys of most male rats (Tsuji et al 1975a). When (+)-limonene was administered by corn oil gavage to male rats for 90 days at 0, 2, 5, 10, 30 and 75 mg/kg/day, there were no changes in body weight, food consumption or absolute liver or kidney weights at any dose (Webb et al 1989). Relative kidney and liver weights significantly increased at the 75 mg/kg dose only, and (+)-limonene nephrotoxicity is well known in male rats (see Nephrotoxicity below). Because of this, and the method of dosing, the relevance to humans of male rat toxicity at this dose is uncertain.

Inhalation toxicity: When volunteers inhaled 10, 225 or 450 mg^3 (+)-limonene for two hours, the high dose was associated with a 2% decrease in lung vital capacity compared to the low dose. This was statistically but not clinically significant (Falk-Filipsson et al 1993). The reported sensory irritation threshold for inhaled limonene in humans is above 80 ppm, while the NOAEL was estimated to be 100 ppm in mice (Larsen et al 2000). (+)-Limonene can react with ozone to form significant concentrations of submicron particles in indoor air (Wainman et al 2000). A reaction mixture of (+)-limonene and ozone was strongly irritating to mouse airways (Clausen et al 2001). Since ozone is produced for example by photocopiers, this may have relevance for indoor air quality. However, inhaled (+)-limonene significantly prevented bronchial obstruction in rats constantly exposed to 125 ppm of (+)-limonene for seven days (Keinan et al 2005).

The effect of limonene 1,2-epoxide on human lung cells was studied, and it was determined that this is not the active compound in limonene toxicity. At cell culture conditions most similar to the in vivo situation, oxygen did not increase the toxicity of limonene beyond an additive effect. The mechanism of action of limonene on biological systems and particularly in combination with oxidative compounds remains to be elucidated. Experimental evidence suggests that detoxification of limonene in human lung cells occurs primarily by mechanisms not involving the glutathione system (Rolseth et al 2002).

Nephrotoxicity: (+)-Limonene may be nephrotoxic to male Wistar rats but only at excessive oral doses (~1 g/kg) (Dietrich & Swenberg 1991; Kristiansen & Madsen 1995). In adult male rats, (+)-limonene caused renal accumulation of a soluble protein, α_{2u}-globulin with associated microscopic abnormalities and chronic nephrosis (Kanerva et al 1987; Kanerva & Alden 1987; Lehman-McKeeman et al 1989; Saito et al 1991). This nephrotic effect is specific to male rats, and so conspicuously absent in studies on humans and other mammals, evidence that no related caution is required in using (+)-limonene-rich essential oils (Webb et al 1990; Hard & Whysner 1994). According to Webb et al (1989) the major metabolite associated with α_{2u}-globulin is (+)-limonene-1,2-oxide. Male rats have high levels of α_{2u}-globulin in their kidneys, and metabolize (+)-limonene to (E)-carveol and perillyl alcohol in greater amounts than female rats (Miyazawa et al 2001b).

Reproductive toxicity: The developmental toxicity of (+)-limonene has been investigated in rabbits, mice and rats. In the rabbit study, 10–18 pregnant rabbits were administered

0, 250, 500, or 1,000 mg/kg/day (+)-limonene by gavage on gestation days 6–18. In the two higher dose groups there was maternal toxicity (reductions in food consumption and body weight, deaths at highest dose) but developmental toxicity was not seen at any dose (Kodama et al 1977b).

In the mouse study, 15 pregnant animals per group were administered 0, 591, or 2,363 mg/kg/day (+)-limonene by gavage on gestation days 7–12. Maternal toxicity (reduction in body weight) and developmental toxicity (increase in the number of fetuses with skeletal anomalies and delayed ossification) were seen in the 2,363 mg/kg/day group. No maternal or fetal effects occurred at 591 mg/kg/day (Kodama et al 1977a).

In the rat study, pregnant animals were given 2,869 mg/kg/day on gestation days 9–15. There was maternal toxicity (decreased body weight, fatalities) and fetal growth retardation (delayed ossification, decreased total body and organs weights) but no teratogenic effects were seen (Tsuji et al 1975b).

When frog embryos were exposed to (+)-limonene in concentrations ranging from 0.00114 ppm to 114 ppm, there was no effect on survival. Teratogenicity was seen only at the lowest dose, suggesting that (+)-limonene is not a teratogen (Holck et al 1991). When (+)-limonene was co-administered with B[a]P to pregnant mice, it inhibited the formation of B[a]P-DNA adducts in the liver and lungs of the fetuses (Chae et al 1997). This suggests that (+)-limonene crosses the placenta, and that it may have beneficial effects on fetal health, for example in smokers.

Mutagenicity and genotoxicity: (+)-Limonene inhibited gap-junctional intercellular communication in keratinocytes, which suggests a mutagenic action (Jansen & Jongen 1996). However, it was not mutagenic or genotoxic in 12 other reports. (+)-Limonene was not mutagenic in the Ames test (Florin et al 1980; Haworth et al 1983; Connor et al 1985). (+)-Limonene can be oxidized to various epoxides by the liver, but these are not mutagenic (Watabe et al 1980, 1981; Von der Hude et al 1990). (+)-Limonene was not mutagenic either in a mouse lymphoma assay, or in the mouse spot test (Fahrig 1982; Myhr et al 1990). (+)-Limonene demonstrated strong antimutagenic activity through concentration-dependent, competitive inhibition of PROD, with an IC_{50} of 0.19 µM (25.8 µg/L) (De-Oliveira et al 1997a). It significantly inhibited the mutagenic activity of compound 4-NQO in a hamster cell line at 0.2–1.0 g/L (Kim et al 2001). In a comet assay, (+)-limonene was not genotoxic in any of the eight tissues studied in both rats and mice; brain, bone marrow, bladder, colon, kidney, lung, liver and stomach (Sekihashi et al 2002). (+)-Limonene was not genotoxic in Syrian hamster embryo cells (Pienta 1980; Oshiro et al 1998) or in Chinese hamster ovary cells (Sasaki et al 1989; Anderson et al 1990).

Carcinogenic/anticarcinogenic potential: (+)-Limonene renal carcinogenicity has been seen only in one strain of male rat. In this case oral (+)-limonene was carcinogenic to male F344/N rats in two year chronic oral dosing studies (National Toxicology Program 1990a). In a similar study, male rat renal pre-carcinogenic changes were detectable as early as 28 days into the protocol (Elcombe et al 2002). (+)-Limonene was not mutagenic in male big blue rat kidney and liver tissue, indicating a non-genotoxic mechanism to this toxicity (Turner et al

2001). (+)-Limonene was non-toxic even at high oral doses in other rat studies (Ariyoshi et al 1975).

In early tests using various undiluted citrus oils on mouse skin, orange, lime, lemon and grapefruit oils all produced tumors at the site of application (Roe 1959; Roe & Peirce 1960; Peirce 1961; Roe & Field 1965). These tumors only appeared in mice primed with a cancer initiator, and the essential oils did not give rise to tumors on their own. Some of the tumors were malignant, some were benign. One paper concluded that 'Anatomical differences and considerations of dosage render it unlikely that the citrus oils are a serious tumor-promoting hazard for man' (Field & Roe 1965).

(+)-Limonene was suspected of causing these tumors. Orange oil was found to weakly promote both benign and malignant tumors when applied dermally, but (+)-limonene only promoted benign ones. It was therefore concluded that the promoting substance was not in fact (+)-limonene, and was either a minor constituent terpene or a contaminant. Neither orange oil nor (+)-limonene had promotional activity when given in the diet (Elegbede et al 1986a). Earlier research strongly suggested that the problem was caused by oxidation products of (+)-limonene (Homburger & Boger 1968).

More recent and extensive research has demonstrated that (+)-limonene itself prevents malignant tumors in rodents primed with cancer initiators. (+)-Limonene is chemopreventive in rat mammary cancer (Elegbede et al 1984, 1986b; Elson et al 1988; Maltzman et al 1989; Russin et al 1989; Haag et al 1992), in rat stomach cancer (Uedo et al 1999), in pancreatic cancer in hamsters (Nakaizumi et al 1997), in mouse lung metastasis induced by melanoma cells, in human gastric cancer implanted in mice (Lu XG et al 2004a), and in human lung, liver (Hep 3B) and stomach carcinoma cells (Kim et al 2001). Other workers have observed similar anticarcinogenic effects (Homburger et al 1971; Wattenberg et al 1989; Wattenberg 1990; Wattenberg & Coccia 1991). The human consumption of citrus peel, a major dietary source of (+)-limonene, has been correlated with a significant reduction in occurrence of squamous cell carcinoma of the skin (Hakim et al 2000).

The early tests, it is assumed, must have all used oxidized citrus oils or oxidized (+)-limonene. In male and female mice given 24 ip injections of (+)-limonene in tricaprylin in a total dose of 4.8 or 24.0 g/kg over 24 weeks the incidence of primary lung tumors was no higher than in the control group (Stoner et al 1973). (+)-Limonene induced glutathione S-transferase in several mouse target tissues (Zheng et al 1992d, 1993b). It maintained hepatic glutathione S-transferase at 92% of control values in mice given high doses of acetaminophen (paracetamol) (Reicks & Crankshaw 1993). (+)-Limonene also induced CYP and epoxide hydratase activity in rats, and reduced DMBA-DNA adducts in rat liver, lung, kidney and spleen by 50% (Maltzman et al 1991).

(+)-Limonene inhibits the activation of the tobacco-specific carcinogen NNK in mouse pulmonary and hepatic microsomes (Morse & Toburen 1996). Lung metastasis induced by melanoma cells in mice was reduced by 65% following ip administration of (+)-limonene (Raphael & Kuttan 2003a). (+)-Limonene is cytotoxic to human (BGC-823) gastric cancer cells, and induces apoptosis (Lu et al 2003). Bicas et al (2011) reported cytotoxic activity against cells for K562 (myeloid leukemia), MCF-7 (breast cancer), NCI-ADR/RES (multidrug resistant breast adenocarcinoma), PC-3 (prostate cancer) and NCI-H460 (non-small cells lung cancer). (+)-Limonene inhibits hepatocarcinogenesis in rats, probably by inhibiting cell proliferation and enhancing apoptosis (Kaji et al 2001). (+)-Limonene had an EC_{50} of 35 μg/mL on lymphoma cells, and an EC_{50} of 72 μg/mL on normal mouse lymphocytes (Manuele et al 2008). Metabolites of (+)-limonene that have demonstrated chemopreventive or chemotherapeutic activity include carveol and uroterpenol (Crowell et al 1992), limonene 1,2-oxide (Morse & Toburen 1996), perillic acid (Bardon et al 2002; Raphael & Kuttan 2003a) and perillyl alcohol.

Comments: There appear to be no data on how long (+)-limonene will remain unoxidized if an antioxidant is added and the product is not exposed to the air. We know that significant air-oxidation of (+)-limonene will be apparent within 10–20 weeks, and that once oxidation begins it progresses rapidly. We also know that BHT-preserved, air-exposed (+)-limonene will show significant oxidation within 34–43 weeks in comparative tests, which would seem to indicate a factor of 3 or 4. Since cold and dark storage of (+)-limonene effectively prevented oxidation for 12 months, the addition of an antioxidant might feasibly extend this time period to three or four years. However this is speculative, especially in regard to (+)-limonene-rich essential oils, which will contain other pro-oxidant or antioxidant constituents.

Summary: (+)-Limonene is not acutely toxic, nephrotoxic or carcinogenic, but it is possible that oxidized (+)-limonene may carry some toxicity. The 90 day rat NOAEL was 30 mg/kg/day. Reproductive toxicity NOAELs were 591 mg/kg/day in mice and 250 mg/kg/day in rabbits. Unoxidized limonene, tested at 2% or 3%, was allergenic in 17/8,997 (0.2%) of dermatitis patients; oxidized limonene, tested at 2% or 3%, was allergenic in 101/5,116 (2.0%) of dermatitis patients. While these data cannot be directly compared, they suggest that the oxidation of (+)-limonene could increase its allergenicity tenfold. A reaction mixture of (+)-limonene and ozone may be inhalationally irritating, but (+)-limonene may also protect against respiratory irritation.

Regulatory guidelines: (+)-Limonene is one of the 26 fragrance materials listed as an allergen by the EU. If present in a cosmetic product at over 100 ppm (0.01%) in a wash-off product or 10 ppm (0.001%) in a leave-on product the compound must be declared on the ingredient list if sold in an EU member state. Limonene, and natural products containing substantial amounts of it, should only be used when the level of peroxides is kept to the lowest practical level, for instance by adding antioxidants at the time of production. Such products should have a peroxide value of less than 20 mmol peroxide per liter, determined according to the FMA method (SCCNFP 2001, IFRA 2009). Based on literature published in German, (+)-limonene was classified as Category B, moderately allergenic, by Schlede et al (2003).

Our safety advice: In order to prevent oxidation the use of antioxidants in combination with limonene-rich essential oils is recommended. Such oils should be stored in a refrigerator in a closed container. Commercial products containing limonene will keep longer in light-proof packaging.

(−)-Limonene

Synonyms: (S)-(−)-Limonene. p-Mentha-1,8-diene. 1,8-p-Menthadiene
Systematic name: (S)-(−)-1-Methyl-4-(1-methylethenyl)cyclohexene
Chemical class: Monocyclic monoterpenoid alkene
CAS number: 5989-54-8

Sources: A minor component of a few pine, mint and other oils.
Pharmacokinetics: Differences have been found between rats and humans in the way that (−)-limonene is oxidized by CYP2B enzymes (Miyazawa et al 2001a).
Adverse skin reactions: Tested at 4% on 25 volunteers (−)-limonene was neither irritating nor sensitizing (Opdyke 1978 p. 809). Of 1,200 dermatitis patients patch tested, there were no irritant or allergic reactions to 2% (−)-limonene (Santucci et al 1987). Oxidized (−)-limonene produced six allergic reactions in 658 people (0.9%) with hand eczema (Heydorn et al 2003b).
Acute toxicity: Acute oral LD_{50} in rats >5 g/kg; acute dermal LD_{50} in rabbits >5 g/kg (Opdyke 1978 p. 809).
Nephrotoxicity: (−)-Limonene caused protein droplet nephropathy in male rats when given by gavage at 800 or 1,600 mg/kg/day for 28 days (Kristiansen & Madsen 1995). This may be a precursor to renal carcinoma. However, male rats have high levels of α2u-globulin in their kidneys, and metabolize (−)-limonene to (E)-carveol and perillyl alcohol in greater amounts than female rats (Miyazawa et al 2001b). Differences have been found between rats and humans in the way that (−)-limonene is oxidized by CYP2B enzymes (Miyazawa et al 2001a). As with (+)-limonene, the nephrotoxicity of (−)-limonene is specific to male rats.
Summary: Pure (−)-limonene is not skin reactive, but oxidized (−)-limonene can be. (−)-Limonene is not acutely toxic. It is nephrotoxic, but only to certain species of male rat.
Regulatory guidelines: (−)-Limonene, and natural products containing substantial amounts of it, should only be used when the level of peroxides is kept to the lowest practical level, for instance by adding antioxidants at the time of production. Such products should have a peroxide value of less than 20 mmol peroxide per liter, determined according to the FMA method (SCCNFP 2001, IFRA 2009).

Linalool

Synonym: Linalol
Systematic name: 3,7-Dimethyl-1,6-octadien-3-ol
Chemical class: Aliphatic monoterpenoid alkene alcohol
Note: Different isomers of linalool exist, and the following isomer-specific information has been published:

(S)-(+)-Linalool

Synonym: Coriandrol
CAS number: 126-90-9

(R)-(−)-Linalool

Synonym: Licareol
CAS number: 126-91-0

Sources >10.0%:

Ho wood	95%
Ho leaf (linalool CT)	66.7–90.6%
Rosewood	82.3–90.3%
Coriander seed	59.0–87.5%
Thyme (linalool CT)	73.6–79.0%
Magnolia leaf	78.9%
Champaca absolute (white)	76.3%
Honeysuckle absolute	75.0%
Bee balm	64.5–74.2%
Tomar seed	72.0%
Magnolia flower	69.9%
Marjoram wild (linalool CT)	67.7%
Ghandi root	62.1%
Basil (linalool CT)	53.7–58.3%
Mint (bergamot)	24.9–55.2%
Rosalina	35.0–55.0%
Neroli	31.4–54.3%
Hyssop (linalool CT)	48.0–51.7%
Orange flower & leaf water absolute	51.6%
Basil (hairy)	31.7–50.1%
Lavender	25.0–45.0%
Lavender (spike)	27.2–43.1%
Orange leaf absolute	42.5%
Lavandin Abrialis	30.0–38.0%
Basil absolute (linalool CT)	34.4%
Lavandin Super	29.4–32.7%
Orange flower absolute	30.0–32.0%
Linaloe wood	30.0%
Ylang-ylang	0.8–30.0%
Ginger lily absolute	29.3%
Khella	28.8%
Lavender absolute	28.0%
Lavandin Grosso	22.5–28.0%
Basil (methyl cinnamate CT)	17.3–27.3%
Sanna	25.6%
Orange leaf (Paraguayan)	20.8–25.2%
Lavandin absolute	25.0%
Orange leaf (bigarade)	12.3–24.2%
Niaouli (linalool CT)	23.9%
Bergamot (expressed)	1.7–20.6%
Bergamot (FCF)	4.0–20.0%
Clary sage	9.0–19.3%
Jonquil absolute	17.8%
Coriander leaf	4.3–17.5%
Helichrysum italicum subsp. *Microphyllum*	17.3%
Sage (wild mountain)	15.0%
Ho leaf (camphor CT)	0.5–15.0%
Jasmine sambac absolute	13.9%
Geranium	0.5–13.8%
Ylang-ylang absolute	13.2%
Fragonia	11.7–12.4%
Narcissus absolute	0.6–11.7%
Sage (Spanish)	0.2–11.2%

Notes: Isomeric with geraniol and nerol. Linalool is found in some 200 essential oils.

Pharmacokinetics: Following an intragastric dose of 500 mg/kg of linalool in rats, 96% was excreted within 72 hours following rapid absorption from the stomach. Of the dose, 58% was excreted in the urine, 23% in the expired air (principally as CO_2) and 15% in the feces (much of this following excretion into the bile). Of the remaining linalool, 0.5% was found in the liver, 0.6% in the gut, 0.8% in the skin and 1.2% in the skeletal muscle (Parke et al 1974b). Linalool is oxidized by CYP before being conjugated to a glucuronide (Powers & Beasley 1985). After one hour of inhaling 5 mg/L linalool, serum levels in mice were 7–9 ng/mL (Jirovetz et al 1991).

Linalool increases the activity of rat liver enzymes (Roffey et al 1990). It induces liver CYP activity by ~50% after oral administration of 600 mg/kg/day for 3 days, but the activity decreased to control values after 6 days (Chadha & Madyastha 1984). Linalool increases the activity of cytochrome b5 (Parke et al 1974a), which is part of the enzyme chain by which cells respire, but only at 500 mg/kg/day for 30 days. It can induce β-oxidation in the liver, which is a part of the process by which fat molecules are metabolized (Roffey et al 1990). Linalool did not induce p-nitroanisole O-demethylase or aniline hydroxyalse in rat liver (Letizia et al 2003a).

Adverse skin reactions: Tested at 20% on two separate panels of 25 healthy human volunteers linalool was not irritating (Fujii et al 1972; Opdyke 1975 p. 827–832). Tested at 40% on 20 dermatitis patients, 97% pure linalool was not irritating (Christensson et al 2009). Linalool was not irritating when tested at 0.4% on the forearms of 84 male and female dermatitis patients (Fujii et al 1972). Linalool has been reported as having mildly irritant effects on the skin, producing an eczematous reaction in some people (Powers & Beasley 1985). During the induction phase of human repeated insult patch tests, 12.7% linalool was applied to 119 volunteers for 24 hour periods, 3 days per week for 3 weeks. There were no irritation reactions. Following the challenge phase, there were also no sensitization reactions (Lapczynski et al 2008g). Tested at 8% and 20% on two separate panels of volunteers, linalool was not sensitizing (Opdyke 1975 p. 827–832). There were no positive reactions to 97% pure linalool tested at 20%, or to oxidized linalool tested at 1%, either in 21 dermatitis patients hypersensitive to fragrance, or in 66 hand eczema patients (Matura et al 2005). In a modified Draize procedure on guinea pigs, linalool was not sensitizing when used at 10% in the challenge phase (Sharp 1978).

In a local lymph node assay, pure linalool showed no sensitizing potential (Sköld et al 2004). A commercial grade of linalool (97% pure) was a weak sensitizer, and the following compounds were present: dihydrolinalool (1.92%), linalool oxide (0.66%), 3-hexenyl butyrate (0.18%), epoxylinalool (0.14%) and 3,7-dimethyl-1,7-octadiene-3,6-diol. Neither linalool nor dihydrolinalool are protein-reactive compounds, and the sensitization potency of repurified linalool was considerably reduced (Basketter et al 2002b). After being oxidized for a period of 10 weeks linalool, now only 80% pure, formed oxidation products, including linalool hydroperoxide (7-hydroperoxy-3,7-dimethylocta-1,5-diene-3-ol) and was sensitizing (Sköld et al 2002). Hydroperoxides, formed on oxidation, were the strongest allergens of the oxidation products tested by Sköld et al (2004). Epoxylinalool is not a significant skin sensitizer (Bezard et al 1997). In a multicenter study involving 1,511 consecutive dermatitis patients, 20 (1.3%) tested positive to 2% oxidized linalool (containing 30% linalool and 16% linalool hydroperoxide), and 16 (1.9%) tested positive to 0.5% linalool hydroperoxides. It is notable that the majority of these reactions were + and the rest were ++; no +++ reactions were seen (Matura et al 2005). Linalool has antioxidant properties (Celik & Ozkaya 2002).

Of 1,200 dermatitis patients patch tested, there were no irritant reactions and no allergic reactions to 5% linalool (Santucci et al 1987). There was one irritant but no allergic reactions in a group of 100 consecutive dermatitis patients (36 males and 64 females) tested with 5% linalool (Frosch et al 1995a). These, and other results from testing on dermatitis patients, are shown in Table 14.6A.

Of 18,747 dermatitis patients, 1,781 had contact dermatitis and one (0.005% of dermatitis patients and 0.06% of contact dermatitis patients) was allergic to linalool. Of the 1,781 patients 75 (4%) were allergic to cosmetic products, so the one reaction constituted 1.4% of this group (De Groot 1987). In a worldwide multicenter study, of 218 dermatitis patients with proven sensitization to fragrance materials, none was sensitive to 5% linalool (Larsen et al 2002). There were no reactions to 30% linalool in 179 dermatitis patients suspected of allergy to cosmetics (De Groot et al 1985). Of 119 patients with contact allergy to cosmetics products 1 (0.9%) reacted to 10% linalool (De Groot et al 1988). Patch testing with 5% linalool elicited no reactions in 99 patients with non-cosmetic dermatitis, nor in 60 patients with cosmetic dermatitis (Itoh et al 1986, 1988).

A 52-year-old man with a rash in the beard area was allergic to his after-shave and to two of its ingredients, hydroxycitronellal and linalool. The problem resolved after discontinuing the after-shave and use of topical steroids (De Groot & Liem 1983). A 53-year-old patient with relapsing eczema who frequently used essential oils in his home tested positive to 2% linalool. Sensitization was thought to be due to previous exposure to lavender, jasmine and rosewood (Schaller & Korting 1995). In six cases of dermatitis none of the individuals was sensitive to linalool on patch testing (Letizia et al 2003a).

Linalool does not absorb UV light in the range of 290–400 nm and therefore would not have the potential to elicit photoirritation or photoallergy (Bickers et al 2003b).

Acute toxicity: The acute oral LD_{50} has been reported as 2.79 g/kg in rats (Jenner et al 1964) and 2.2, 3.5 and 3.92 g/kg in mice (Letizia et al 2003a). Acute dermal LD_{50} in rabbits 5.61 g/kg (Opdyke 1975 p. 827–832). Acute ip LD_{50} reported as 307 and 687 mg/kg in rats, and 200, 340 and 495 mg/kg in mice. An MTD of 125 mg/kg has also been reported (Letizia et al 2003a). Acute toxicity from high doses presents as ataxia and narcosis (Powers & Beasley 1985).

Subacute and subchronic toxicity: Linalool was administered once daily for 13 weeks to the shaved backs of male and female rats in doses of 0.25, 1.0 or 4.0 g/kg. There were no changes at the lowest dose, except for transient erythema and depressed

activity. At 1.0 g/kg it produced decreased weight gain, decreased activity and erythema. At the high dose, decreased body weight and increased liver weight was observed, and nine females and two males died from a total of 120 animals (Letizia et al 2003a).

Reproductive toxicity: Linalool was administered by gavage to pregnant rats at 250, 500 or 1,000 mg/kg/day, on gestational days 7–17. No fetal toxicity or teratogenicity was seen at any dose. Since there was some maternal increase in relative body weight and feed consumption in the high dose group, the NOAEL for maternal toxicity was 500 mg/kg/day (Politano et al 2008).

Table 14.6 Allergic reactions to linalool in different groups

A. Dermatitis patients

Concentration used	Percentage who reacted	No. of reactors	Reference
5%	0.0%	0/99	Itoh et al 1986
5%	0.0%	0/100	Frosch et al 1995a
5%	0.0%	0/1,200	Santucci et al 1987
10%	0.0%	0/70	Nethercott et al 1989
10%	0.07%	1/1,397	Heisterberg et al 2011
10%	0.5%	4/792	Fregert & Hjorth 1969
10%	0.2%	5/2,401	Schnuch et al 2007a
20%	0.17%	3/1,825	De Groot et al 2000
Various	0.005%	1/18,747	De Groot 1987

B. Dermatitis patients suspected of cosmetic or fragrance sensitivity

Concentration used	Percentage who reacted	No. of reactors	Reference
5%	0.0%	0/60	Itoh et al 1988
10%	0.9%	1/119	De Groot et al 1988
30%	0.0%	0/179	De Groot et al 1985

C. Fragrance-sensitive dermatitis patients

Concentration used	Percentage who reacted	No. of reactors	Reference
5%	0.0%	0/218	Larsen et al 2002

Mutagenicity and genotoxicity: Linalool was not mutagenic in Ames tests with and without S9 (Rockwell & Raw 1979; Eder et al 1980, 1982; Ishidate et al 1984; Heck et al 1989; Di Sotto et al 2008), nor was it mutagenic in CA tests (Ishidate et al 1984; Letizia et al 2003a), or in a mouse micronucleus assay (Letizia et al 2003a). Rat urinary metabolites of linalool were also non-mutagenic (Rockwell & Raw 1979). Linalool was mutagenic in one *Bacillus subtilis* rec assay (Yoo 1986), produced questionable results in a second (Kuroda et al 1984b) and was not mutagenic in a third (Oda et al 1978). Several studies have failed to detect any antimutagenic effect for linalool (Ohta et al 1986; Yoo 1986; Ohta 1995; Di Sotto et al 2008), but a strong antimutagenic action was reported by Berić et al (2007), who noted that this was linked to antioxidant activity.

Linalool was not genotoxic in a mouse bone marrow micronucleus test (RIFM 2001b, cited in Belsito et al 2008). Linalool did not induce SCE in cultured Chinese hamster ovary cells (Sasaki et al 1989) nor did it induce UDS in primary rat hepatocytes (Heck et al 1989; RIFM 1986c, cited in Belsito et al 2008). At nanomolar concentrations, linalool suppressed t-butyl hydroperoxide induced genotoxicity, both in bacteria and cultured human cells. This was predominantly mediated by radical scavenging activity (Mitić-Culafić et al 2009).

Carcinogenic/anticarcinogenic potential: A single application of DMBA in 0.2 mL acetone was made to the clipped skin of albino mice. After three weeks 20% linalool in acetone was dermally applied once a week for 33 weeks, and this elicited a weak tumor-promoting reponse compared to controls (Roe & Field 1965). In contrast to this finding, mice treated topically with 10% linalool in acetone from three days before to three days after DMBA treatment had an average number of 10.4 papillomas per mouse compared to an average of 15 for the acetone control (Gould et al 1987).

In male and female mice given 24 ip injections of linalool in tricaprylin in a total dose of 0.6 or 3.0 g/kg over 24 weeks the incidence of primary lung tumors was no higher than in the control group (Stoner et al 1973). An ip injection of 0.6 g/kg or 3 g/kg linalool 3 times a week for 8 weeks produced no increase in primary lung tumor induction in mice (Powers & Beasley 1985). ($\pm$)-Linalool did not significantly reduce the average number of tumors per rat or the median tumor latency period in a DMBA-induced rat mammary carcinogenesis model (Russin et al 1989). Linalool was active against human amelanotic melanoma and renal cell adenocarcinoma cell lines, with IC_{50} values of 23.16 and 23.77 µg/mL, respectively (Loizzo et al 2007). Linalool was active against all of nine carcinoma cell lines tested, with the most potent activity against cancers of the cervix (HeLa, IC_{50} 0.37 µg/mL), stomach (AGS, IC_{50} 14.1 µg/mL), skin (BCC-1/KMC, IC_{50} 14.9 µg/mL) lung (H520, IC_{50} 21.5 µg/mL) and bone (U$_2$OS, IC_{50} 21.7 µg/mL). The other cancers were mouth, kidney, lung (H661), and bladder (Cherng et al 2007).

In HepG2 cells, reductions of 50% and 100% in viability were obtained with 0.4 µM (61.6 µg/L) and 2.0 µM (308 µg/L), respectively, of linalool, with intracellular increases in ROS generation (Usta et al 2009). Linalool showed significant activity against histiocytic lymphoma U937 cells and Burkitt lymphoma P3HR1 cells (human cell lines) with IC_{50} values of 3.51 and 4.21 µg/mL, respectively. It was also active against human leukemia K562 cells (Chiang et al 2003). Linalool preferentially inhibited growth and induced apoptosis in six types of human leukemia cells, but spared normal hematopoietic cells. It was less active against six further types of leukemia cell (Gu et al 2010).

Comments: Linalool seems incapable of eliciting any allergic reactions in healthy individuals, and even when tested at 20% in dermatitis patients elicited reactions in either 0% or 0.17% of those tested. The reports from Basketter et al (2002b) and Sköld et al (2002) indicate that only oxidized linalool was skin sensitizing. Although it can be oxidized, and oxidized linalool can be sensitizing, we do not know how readily linalool oxidizes in essential oil mixtures, fragrances or personal care products, especially those containing antioxidants. The oxidation data has been used by the SCCNFP to justify its opinion that linalool should be listed as an allergen (SCCNFP 2003d). However, as the SCCNFP also states: 'antioxidants can in most cases minimize the oxidation'. This should be efficacious in minimizing reactions to linalool, since even the oxidized material elicited a majority of mild reactions, and not a single severe reaction.

In a comprehensive review of ACD to linalool, Hostýnek & Maibach (2008) conclude that linalool is only a weak sensitizer, and that 'It is most probable that autoxidation of linalool is well controlled during the normal lifetimes and under forseeable usage conditions of cosmetics and household products…Regardless of the possibility that autoxidation may enhance the allergenic potential of this substance, it is not yet documented as a major fragrance allergen.'

Taking into account all the clinical data cited above for skin reactions, a total of nine dermatitis patients out of 23,430 (0.04%) were allergic to linalool when tested at concentrations ranging from 5% to 30%. However, linalool is rarely, if ever, used in such high concentrations in commercial preparations, and is estimated to occur at a maximum of 4.3% (Bickers et al 2003b). The risk to the general population is therefore negligible.

Linalool is one of the most common fragrance materials to be found in nature, and occurs in over 200 commercial essential oils, in at least 40 instances at concentrations of 10% or more. It is also widely used as a single compound in fragrances. One survey found it in 61% (36 of 59) of household products (Rastogi et al 2001). If allergy was a concern with linalool there would surely be a great many recorded cases, but in fact there are very few. In a preliminary report by an ECETOC taskforce, linalool was provisionally classified as a weak allergen (on a scale of extreme, strong, moderate and weak) only likely to elicit a sensitization reaction if present at 3% or more (Kimber et al 2003). While this is consistent with the clinical data, it does not correlate well with the EU guideline of 0.01% in wash-off products and 0.001% in leave-on products. Such a low maximum is not supported by any scientific data.

Summary: Linalool is not acutely toxic in rodents, and shows negligible toxicity at 250 g/kg subchronically. Linalool is not carcinogenic, and demonstrates broad spectrum anticancer activity in cell lines. It possesses enzyme inducing and sedative properties. Linalool presents an extremely low risk of skin sensitization.

Regulatory guidelines: JECFA has set a group ADI of 0 to 0.5 mg/kg bw for citral, citronellol, geranyl acetate, linalool and linalyl acetate (JECFA 1999a). Linalool is one of the 26 fragrance materials listed as an allergen by the EU. If present in a cosmetic product at over 100 ppm (0.01%) in a wash-off product or 10 ppm (0.001%) in a leave-on product the compound must be declared on the ingredient list if sold in an EU member state. The 38th Amendment to the IFRA Standard states that 'linalool and natural products known to be rich in linalool, such as bois de rose, coriander or ho wood oils, should only be used when the level of peroxides is kept to the lowest practical value. It is recommended to add antioxidants at the time of production of the raw material. The addition of 0.1% BHT or α-tocopherol demonstrates great efficiency. The maximum peroxide level for products in use should be 20™mmol/L' (IFRA 2009).

Linalool oxide

Synonyms: Linalyl oxide. Linalool monoxide. Linalool epoxide. Epoxylinalool
Systematic name: 5-Ethenyltetrahydro-α,α,5-trimethyl-2-furanmethanol
Chemical class: Monocyclic monoterpenoid alkene ether
Note: Different isomers of linalool oxide exist, and the following isomer-specific information has been published:

(E)-Linalool oxide

Synonyms: *trans*-Linalool oxide. (E)-(2R,5R)-Linalool oxide. Linalool A
CAS number: 34995-77-2

Sources >1.0%:

Osmanthus absolute	0.6–7.0%
Ho leaf (linalool CT)	0–2.8%
Mint (bergamot)	1.3–1.7%
Rosewood	~1.3%
Orange flower water absolute	1.1%
Linaloe wood	1.0%

(Z)-Linalool oxide

Synonyms: *cis*-Linalool oxide. (Z)-(2R,5S)-Linalool oxide. Linalool B
CAS number: 5989-33-3

Sources >1.0%:

Osmanthus absolute	0.7–5.6%
Champaca absolute (orange)	0.2–2.5%
Linaloe wood	2.0%
Orange flower water absolute	1.9%
Mint (bergamot)	1.2–1.6%
Rosewood	~1.5%
Thyme (lemon)	1.4%

Adverse skin reactions: Undiluted linalool oxide was moderately-to-severely irritating when applied to rabbit skin for 24 hours under occlusion. Tested at 8% on 28 volunteers linalool oxide was neither irritating nor sensitizing (Opdyke & Letizia 1983 p. 863–864).

Acute toxicity: Acute oral LD_{50} 1.15 g/kg in rats, acute dermal LD_{50} in rabbits 2.5 g/kg (Opdyke & Letizia 1983 p. 863–864).
Summary: Linalool oxide appears to be non-irritant and non-allergenic. It possesses 'slight' toxicity.

Linalyl acetate

Synonyms: Linalool acetate. Acetic acid linalyl ester. Bergamol
Systematic name: 2,6-Dimethyl-2,7-octadien-6-yl ethanoate
Chemical class: Aliphatic monoterpenoid alkene ester
Note: Different isomers of linalyl acetate exist, and the following isomer-specific information has been published:

(+)-Linalyl acetate

CAS number: 51685-40-6

(−)-Linalyl acetate

CAS number: 16509-46-9

Sources >5.0%:

Clary sage	45.3–73.6%
Orange leaf (bigarade)	51.0–71.0%
Clary sage absolute	66.5%
Orange leaf (Paraguayan)	47.4–58.0%
Mint (bergamot)	34.0–57.3%
Skimmia	55.6%
Orange leaf absolute	48.9%
Linaloe wood	47.0%
Lavender	25.0–46.0%
Lavender absolute	44.7%
Lavandin Super	38.6–44.3%
Snakeroot	28.0–41.4%
Bergamot (expressed)	17.1–40.4%
Lavandin Grosso	28.0–38.0%
Lavandin Abrialis	20.0–30.0%
Bergamot (FCF)	18.0–28.0%
Snowbush	18.0%
Orange flower absolute	7.0–16.8%
Chamomile (Cape)	14.1%
Marjoram (sweet)	7.4–10.5%
Neroli	0.6–10.0%
Thymus zygis (linalool CT)	3.4–8.6%
Cardamon	0.7–7.7%
Lemon leaf	tr–6.5%
Sage (Spanish)	0.1–5.8%

Pharmacokinetics: Linalyl acetate hydrolyses in gastric juice to yield linalool which, to some extent, is rapidly ring closed to yield α-terpineol (JECFA 1999a).
Adverse skin reactions: One irritation response occurred when 0.2% linalyl acetate was tested on 82 male and female dermatitis patients (Fujii et al 1972). Linalyl acetate was not irritating when tested at 5% on the upper arms of 12 male and 13 female

volunteers, nor when tested at 10% on the backs of 131 male and female volunteers (Letizia et al 2003b). It produced no irritation when tested at 20% on 40 volunteers (Fujii et al 1972) nor when tested at 32% on 50 male volunteers (Motoyoshi et al 1979).

Linalyl acetate was not sensitizing when tested at 12% in 25 volunteers (Greif 1967). A 20% concentration produced no adverse reactions in 25 volunteers. When five samples of the compound were tested at 10% in five groups of volunteers, there were 2/22, 0/26, 0/27, 1/26 and 0/30 sensitization reactions, totaling 3/131 (2.3%). The sensitizing samples were re-tested, or purified and re-tested, and then produced no reactions, suggesting that impurities may have been responsible for some of the reactions (Letizia et al 2003b).

There were no irritant or allergic reactions in a group of 100 consecutive dermatitis patients tested with 1% and 5% linalyl acetate (Frosch et al 1995a). None of 70 contact dermatitis patients reacted to 1% linalyl acetate (Nethercott et al 1989). No adverse effects were observed with 5% linalyl acetate in 7 patients with facial melanosis, 31 patients with cosmetic dermatitis, 27 patients with non-cosmetic eczema and dermatitis, or in 10 control subjects (Ishihara et al 1979, 1981). Of 119 eczema patients with contact allergy to cosmetics one (0.8%) was allergic to 3% linalyl acetate (De Groot et al 1988). There were no adverse reactions in 20 perfume-sensitive patients and 50 control patients tested with 5% linalyl acetate (Larsen 1977).

Linalyl acetate does not absorb UV light in the range of 290–400 nm and therefore would not have the potential to elicit photoirritation or photoallergy (Bickers et al 2003b).

Acute toxicity: Acute oral LD_{50} reported as 14.5 g/kg and >10 mL/kg in rats, and 13.36 g/kg and 13.5 g/kg in mice. Acute dermal LD_{50} >5 g/kg. Acute ip LD_{50} 2,778 mg/kg in male rats and 2,984 mg/kg in female rats (Letizia et al 2003b).

Inhalation toxicity: Two groups of 12 rats were exposed to an atmosphere saturated with steam at either 20°C or 100°C, the steam having been passed through a 5 cm layer of linalyl acetate. Animals were observed for 8 hours, and there were no mortalities at either exposure level. Slight mucous membrane irritation was seen at 100°C (Letizia et al 2003b).

Mutagenicity and genotoxicity: Linalyl acetate was not mutagenic in Ames tests with or without S9 activation (Heck et al 1989; Di Sotto et al 2008). Linalyl acetate was mutagenic in one of four assays, both with and without S9. The *E. coli* WP2*uvr*A assay detects a range of oxidative mutagens, free-radical generators and cross-linking agents (Di Sotto et al 2008). Linalyl acetate did not induce UDS in primary rat hepatocytes, and it was not clastogenic in cultured human lymphocytes (Heck et al 1989; Letizia et al 2003b).

Carcinogenic/anticarcinogenic potential: In male and female mice given 24 ip injections of linalyl acetate in tricaprylin in a total dose of 4.8 or 24.0 g/kg over 24 weeks the incidence of primary lung tumors was no higher than in the control group (Stoner et al 1973). Linalyl acetate was applied to the clipped backs of groups of mice three times a week for 460 days, either alone or with benzo[*a*]pyrene (B[*a*]P). No carcinogenic activity was observed when linalyl acetate was administered alone, or with 1 μg B[*a*]P. A weak cocarcinogenic activity was recorded when linalyl acetate was administered with 5 μg B[*a*]P (Van Duuren et al 1971).

Comments: The 'impurities' referred to by Letizia et al (2003b) were not investigated, so little can be deduced from this. However, it adds to the small and elusive body of evidence that synthetic compounds are sometimes more likely to elicit skin reactions than the same compounds as naturally present in essential oils.

Summary: Linalyl acetate is minimally skin reactive and is non-toxic. It was mutagenic in one of eight assays.

Regulatory guidelines: JECFA has set a group ADI of 0 to 0.5 mg/kg bw for citral, citronellol, geranyl acetate, linalool and linalyl acetate (JECFA 1999a).

Longifolene

Synonyms: Junipene. Kuromatsuene
Systematic name: [1S-(1α,3aβ,4α,8aβ)]-Decahydro-4,8,8-trimethyl-9-methylene-1,4-methanoazulene
Chemical class: Tricyclic sesquiterpenoid alkene
CAS number: 475-20-7

Sources >1.0%:

Black seed	1.2–10.2%
Cedarwood (Chinese)	4.2%
Pine (Scots)	0–3.5%
Grindelia	1.0–2.5%

Adverse skin reactions: Undiluted longifolene produced slight-to-moderate edema and erythema in rabbits patch-tested for 24 hours under occlusion. Tested at 10% on human volunteers, longifolene was neither irritant sensitizing (Ford et al 1992 p. 67S).

Acute toxicity: Acute oral LD_{50} in rats >5 g/kg; acute dermal LD_{50} in rabbits >5 g/kg (Ford et al 1992 p. 67S).

Summary: Longifolene is non-toxic, and there is no evidence of skin reactivity in humans.

Massoia lactone

Synonyms: (−)-Massoia lactone. 2-Decen-5-olide
Systematic name: (*R*)-(−)-6-Pentyl-5,6-dihydro-2*H*-pyran-2-one
Chemical class: Monoterpenoid alkene lactone
CAS number: 51154-96-2

Source >1.0%:

Massoia oil	68.2%
Sage (wild mountain)	1.4%

Adverse skin reactions: We could find no published safety data for massoia lactone. However, we were informed that, in private tests, 'massoia lactone was so irritating that the standard tests for sensitization and phototoxicity could not be conducted' (RIFM, private communication, 1994).

Comments: This compound merits further, more open investigation.

Summary: Massoia lactone may be highly irritant, but its irritancy has not been quantified.

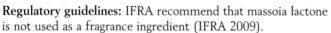

Regulatory guidelines: IFRA recommend that massoia lactone is not used as a fragrance ingredient (IFRA 2009).

Our safety advice: We recommend a maximum dermal use level of 0.01% for massoia lactone.

Menthofuran

Synonym: 3,9-Epoxy-*p*-mentha-3,8-diene
Systematic name: 3,6-Dimethyl-4,5,6,7-tetrahydrobenzo[*b*]furan
Chemical class: Bicyclic furanoid monoterpenoid alkene ether
Note: Different isomers of menthofuran exist, and the following isomer-specific information has been published:

(6*R*)-(+)-Menthofuran

CAS number: 17957-94-7

Sources >0.1%:

Palo santo	6.6–11.8%
Peppermint	tr–9.4%
Cornmint	0.4–0.6%
Pennyroyal (European)	tr–0.3%

(6*S*)-(−)-Menthofuran

CAS number: 80183-38-6

Pharmacokinetics: Various human CYP enzymes metabolize (6*R*)-(+)-menthofuran to 2-hydroxymenthofuran, which is an intermediate in the formation of mintlactone and isomintlactone (Khojasteh-Bakh et al 1999). It is also converted via an epoxide to a highly reactive metabolite, 8-pulegone aldehyde, which may be the ultimate toxicant (Thomassen et al 1990). Madyastha & Raj (1991, 1992) reported that *p*-cresol and benzoic acid can be formed from menthofuran, but Khojasteh et al (2010) failed to detect either substance as metabolites except at very low background levels, using rat or human liver microsomes, or rat liver slices. Other metabolites include diastereomeric keto acids and hydroxymintlactones (Khojasteh et al 2010). (*R*)-(+)-Menthofuran is a mechanism-based inhibitor of CYP2A6 (Di et al 2009). Inhibition of this enzyme may result in reduced metabolic oxidation, and hence, reduced production of toxic metabolites.

Acute toxicity: There are no reported LD_{50} values for menthofuran. Gordon et al (1982) recorded that 5/15 mice died within 24 hours from an ip dose of 200 mg/kg, and 10/16 mice died from 300 mg/kg, which suggests a mouse ip LD_{50} of about 250 mg/kg.

Subacute and subchronic toxicity: A toxicity screening test in rats was conducted on (6*R*)-(+)-menthofuran at dietary levels corresponding to an intake of 23 mg/kg for 14 days. No effects were seen on body weight gain or food consumption, nor on gross appearance or weight of liver and kidneys (Van Miller & Weaver 1987).

Hepatotoxicity: In rats, oral dosing with 250 mg/kg menthofuran once daily for three days caused hepatotoxicity, as demonstrated by changes in blood levels of enzyme markers for liver disease (Madyastha & Raj 1994). Menthofuran is reported to destroy CYP in rats (Thomassen et al 1990). However, while pulegone and pennyroyal oil caused marked depletion of hepatic glutathione, menthofuran caused only a very modest depletion. Menthofuran is at least twice as hepatotoxic as (1*R*)-(+)-β-pulegone, measured either as lethality or as degree of hepatic necrosis in male mice (Gordon et al 1982). Several potentially hepatotoxic metabolites are formed from menthofuran (Madyastha and Raj 1992, 2002), and at low doses hepatic glutathione protects the liver from these (Thomassen et al 1991). Menthofuran binds to various mouse tissues, with binding to protein in the liver exceeding that of the lungs and kidneys by approximately three times (McClanahan et al 1989; Thomassen et al 1992). Menthofuran is both activated by and destroys CYP (Thomassen et al 1990; Madyastha & Raj 1994).

Antioxidant/pro-oxidant activity: (6*R*)-(+)-Menthofuran scavenged singlet oxygen more effectively than (±)-α-tocopherol (Racine & Auffray 2005).

Mutagenicity and genotoxicity: (6*R*)-(+)-Menthofuran was not mutagenic in an Ames test with and without metabolic activation (Council of Europe 1999).

Summary: Menthofuran is hepatotoxic, possibly due to bioactivation to 8-pulegone aldehyde, a highly reactive metabolite. No toxicity was evident when rats ingested 23 mg/kg menthofuran for 14 days. Menthofuran is approximately twice as hepatotoxic as pulegone in male mice.

Regulatory guidelines: The CEFS of the Council of Europe have classed menthofuran as a hepatotoxic compound and consider it the proximate hepatotoxin of pulegone. They have set a group TDI for menthofuran and pulegone of 0.1 mg/kg bw based on the NOAEL of 20 mg/kg/day in a 28 day oral toxicity study of pulegone in rats (see Pulegone profile) with a safety factor of 200.

Our safety advice: Comparative toxicity testing shows menthofuran to be approximately twice as toxic as β-pulegone. We therefore propose a safety limit for menthofuran that is half that of β-pulegone, i.e. a maximum dose of 0.2 mg/kg/day. This is equivalent to 14 mg per adult oral dose, or to a dermal exposure of 0.5% (Table 14.1).

(−)-Menthol

Synonyms: (−)-*p*-Menthan-3-ol. (−)-3-Hydroxy-*p*-menthane. Levomenthol. Peppermint camphor
Systematic name: [1*R*-(1α,2β,5β)]-5-Methyl-2-(1-methylethyl)cyclohexanol
Chemical class: Monocyclic monoterpenoid alcohol
CAS number: 2216-51-5

Sources >1.0%:

Peppermint	19.0–54.2%
Cornmint	28.8–34.7%
Basil (lemon)	3.8–4.4%

Notes: Some safety information on (±)-menthol is included below. Where no isomer is specified, this could be naturally derived (−)-menthol, synthetic (−)-menthol, or synthetic (±)-menthol. Menthol is used in some topical preparations for the treatment of rheumatic conditions, and in aromatic inhalation mixtures for nasal decongestion. Menthol is an agonist of TRPM8 calcium channels, and these are found in the membranes of sensory neurons and cells of the blood vessels, respiratory tract, urinary system and the prostate. TRPM8 channels are cold receptors, but they also have other biological effects such as the regulation of vascular tone (Johnson CD et al 2009).

Pharmacokinetics: After oral administration of 800 mg/kg (−)-menthol to rats, the major urinary metabolites were p-menthane-3,8-diol and 3,8-dihydroxy-p-menthane-7-carboxylic acid (Madyastha & Srivastan 1988). In humans 50–79% of (−)-menthol was excreted in the urine as menthol glucuronide, and no unchanged menthol was detected. In rabbits high doses of (−)-menthol lead to lower glucuronide conjugation (20–48%) and in dogs only 5% was excreted as the glucuronide. In rats 38% was excreted in the urine, and 34% in the feces (Scheline 1991). Oral dosing of mice with 1.2, 2.0 or 9.3 mg/kg (−)-menthol resulted in an increase in hepatic glucuronidase activity compared to controls (Levvy et al 1948). When 500 mg of (−)-menthol was administered to 96 volunteers and 21 patients with confirmed liver disease, there was no significant difference between the two groups in the mean urinary excretion of (−)-menthol glucuronide (Bell et al 1981). The human systemic exposure to menthol from application in commercial skin patches was relatively low (Martin et al 2004).

Drug interactions: There have been two reported cases of menthol potentiating the anticoagulant effects of warfarin. In both cases the patient was concurrently taking menthol cough drops, and coagulation times reverted to normal after ceasing to take the cough drops (Kassebaum et al 2005; Coderre et al 2010).

Adverse skin and mucous membrane reactions: Undiluted (−)-menthol was not irritating to rabbit skin; tested at 8% on 24 human volunteers it was neither irritating nor sensitizing (Opdyke 1976 p. 471–472). (±)-Menthol was also not sensitizing when tested at 8% on 25 volunteers (Opdyke 1976 p. 473–474). In a modified Draize procedure on guinea pigs, menthol was sensitizing when used at 10% in the challenge phase (Sharp 1978). Patch testing with 5% menthol produced reactions in 9/877 dermatitis patients (1%) in central Europe (Rudzki & Kleniewska 1971). Tested at 1%, (−)-menthol produced reactions in 2/220 (0.9%) Japanese dermatitis patients (JCDRG 1981). Of 1,200 dermatitis patients patch tested, there were no irritant reactions and one allergic reaction (0.08%) to 5% (±)-menthol (Santucci et al 1987). In a retrospective multicenter study in Finland, there were no irritant or allergic reactions to menthol in 75 dermatitis patients (Kanerva et al 2001a). When 330 patients with either leg ulcers or eczematous dermatitis were patch tested with 1% menthol for 48 hours, adverse reactions were seen in 20 patients (6.1%) (Blondeel et al 1978).

A 31-year-old woman experienced strong allergic reactions both to dermal peppermint oil and to oral menthol (Papa & Shelly 1964). One report cites two cases of weak reactions to (−)-menthol and peppermint oil. One was an an eczema of the upper lip, the other a cheilitis (Wilkinson & Beck 1994). In two further cases a 26-year-old woman with recurrent oral ulceration tested positive to 2% menthol, and a 43-year-old man with orofacial granulomatosis tested positive to 2% menthol and 2% peppermint oil (Lewis et al 1995). There are further reports of oral mucous membrane sensitivity to menthol either on contact (Morton et al 1995) or after excessive prolonged use (Rogers & Pahor 1995; Fleming & Forsyth 1998). In each case, a burning sensation, ulceration and inflammation were the result.

In one case, hypersensitivity to menthol arose after prior sensitization to one or all of α-pinene, (+)-limonene and phellandrene (Dooms-Goosens et al 1977). Mentholated cigarettes have also caused hypersensitivity (Camarasa & Alomar 1978). Urticarial hypersensitivity has been reported in a young girl exposed to cigarettes, cough drops, aerosol room spray and topical medicaments all containing menthol. She tested positive to both oral and dermal challenges with menthol (McGowan 1966).

When tested on the skin of volunteers in an ethanol vehicle, menthol induced cold pain at 40%, but at 30% there was no cold pain, skin irritation or redness (Hatem et al 2006). (−)-Menthol was applied to the nasal passages of 16 volunteers at 0.1%, 0.2% and 0.5% in petrolatum or saline. Most found 0.5% irritating, 0.2% slightly or non-irritating, and 0.1% non-irritating (Bliss & Glass 1940). Menthol has been recommended as an agent which helps to soothe the skin in cases of dermatitis (Burkhart & Burkhart 2003).

In an in vitro assay, (−)-menthol was non-phototoxic (Placzek et al 2007).

Acute toxicity: (−)-Menthol acute oral LD_{50} reported as 3,300 mg/kg in rats and 900 mg/kg in cats; acute rabbit dermal LD_{50} >5 g/kg (Opdyke 1976 p. 471–472). For (±)-menthol, the rat LD_{50} has been reported as 3,180 mg/kg (Jenner et al 1964) and 940 mg/kg (Bhatia et al 2008g). In the latter study, severe irritation of the GI tract mucous membrane occurred. (±)-Menthol acute oral LD_{50} in mice reported as 4,400 mg/kg (Bhatia et al 2008g) and 6,600 mg/kg (Dmitrieva et al 1962).

Mice were given a single ip dose of 333 mg/kg (−)-menthol and observed for 14 days. There was significant liver damage after 24 hours, including fatty degeneration and necrosis around the central vein, and hypertrophy of the nuclei. Toxic signs persisted for 7 days, and repair was almost complete at 14 days. After 3 days some kidney damage was evident, and this resolved by day 14. Ip injection of 700 mg/kg (−)-menthol caused prolonged respiratory depression and unconsciousness (Levvy et al 1948).

Subacute and subchronic toxicity: In a 5.5 week gavage study, rats received 0, 100 or 200 mg/kg/day (−)-menthol. Body weight gain was not adversely affected, there was no interference with CNS reactions to stimulants, and urinary excretion of glucuronide, water and electrolytes were normal (Herken 1961, unpublished report cited in JECFA 1999b). A NOAEL of 200 mg/kg can be derived from these data.

Inhalation toxicity: In a 71–79 day study, rats inhaled air with 0.6, 1.0 or 1.7 mg/m^3 (0.087, 0.15 or 0.26 ppm) (−)-menthol. In the high dose group, histopathological changes suggesting irritation were observed (tracheitis and pulmonary congestion). In the low and mid-dose groups, no adverse effects were seen (Rakieten et al 1954). The calculated irritation threshold for menthol is 50 ppm.

Human toxicity: Instillation into the nose, or introducing by drops, results in a combination of oral ingestion and inhalation. There are reports of non-fatal, but serious toxicity in children who have had solutions containing menthol (4 cases) instilled into their noses (Melis et al 1989; Decocq et al 1996; Wyllie & Alexander 1994). The ages ranged from 1 month to 3 years and 9 months. The effects of poisoning included irritated mucous membranes, tachycardia, dyspnea, nausea, vomiting, vertigo, muscular weakness, drowsiness and coma (Melis et al 1989; Reynolds 1993). The most serious symptoms (including coma) were seen in a child of under 2 months, who had 1 mL of a menthol solution instilled into his nose. Some of the other cases suffered no more than mucous membrane irritation, but some of these were given gastric lavage.

In most cases the drops were given accidentally, in mistake for another, safer preparation. No details were given regarding the amounts of menthol administered, so it is difficult to extrapolate to essential oils. When menthol vapors were inhaled by 44 premature newborn infants, there was either a transient cessation of respiration, or a drop in the respiratory rate (Javorka et al 1980).

Cardiovascular effects: Inhalation of (−)-menthol dilates capillaries in the nasal mucosa, which correlates with the reported ability of (−)-menthol to dilate systemic blood vessels after iv administration (Rakieten & Rakieten 1957). In an ex vivo study, menthol caused small contractions in rat arteries, but dilated arteries that had been previously contracted (Johnson CD et al 2009). A balm containing 1.9% menthol reduced mean arterial pressure when applied to the skin adjacent to isometrically contracting muscles in cats (Ragan et al 2004).

Excessive daily consumption of peppermint confectionery has been anecdotally associated with auricular fibrillation in two patients prone to the condition who were being maintained on quinidine, a stabilizer of heart rhythm (Thomas 1962). Bradycardia (slowing of heartbeat), along with GI and neurological symptoms, were reported in a person smoking up to 80 mentholated cigarettes per day (Luke 1962). Mentholated cigarettes (more than non-mentholated) increased tricuspid valve deceleration time and right ventricular contraction time in 18 chronic smokers (Ciftçi et al 2008). When 20 otherwise healthy young smokers and 22 non-smokers smoked two mentholated cigarettes, mean heart rate increased from a baseline of 69 to 101, compared to 82 on smoking two non-mentholated cigarettes (Ciftçi et al 2009). However, in a retrospective 14 year study of 5,887 adult smokers of regular or mentholated cigarettes, there were no differences in hazard ratios for coronary heart disease, cardiovascular disease, lung cancer or death from any cause (Murray et al 2007). This study was sponsored by a division of the National Institutes of Health.

When nine healthy males cycled to exhaustion, swallowing 25 mL of a 0.01% (−)-menthol solution every 10 minutes, there was no difference in heart rate compared to controls (Mündel & Jones 2010). A 1.9% concentration of menthol had no effect on heart rate when applied to the skin of cats (Ragan et al 2004).

Reproductive toxicity: (−)-Menthol was not teratogenic when given by gavage to pregnant mice at up to 185 mg/kg, pregnant rats at up to 218 mg/kg, pregnant hamsters at up to 405 mg/kg, or pregnant rabbits at up to 425 mg/kg, on gestational days 6–15, 6–15, 6–10 and 6–18, respectively (Food & Drug Research Labs., Inc. 1973, cited in Nair 2001b).

Hepatotoxicity: When (−)-menthol was administered by gavage in soybean oil to rats at 200, 400 or 800 mg/kg/day for 28 days a significant increase in liver weights and vacuolization of hepatocytes was observed at all doses (Thorup et al 1983b). Rowachol enterically coated capsules contain 32 mg menthol, 17 mg pinene, 6 mg menthone, 5 mg camphene, 2 mg 1,8-cineole and 33 mg olive oil. One capsule per 10 kg of body weight per day was taken by 24 patients with gallstones. Twenty-three patients took the capsules for 6 months or longer, and every 6 weeks, tests were performed for liver function, ESR, erythrocytes, hemoglobin and platelets. There were no hematological abnormalities nor was there any biochemical evidence of hepatotoxicity (Bell & Doran 1979).

Menthol has been shown to provoke severe neonatal jaundice in babies with a deficiency of the enzyme G6PD (glucose-6-phosphate dehydrogenase). Usually, menthol is detoxified by a metabolic pathway involving G6PD. When babies deficient in this enzyme were given a menthol-containing dressing for their umbilical stumps, menthol was found to build up in their bodies (Olowe & Ransome-Kuti 1980). This is an enzyme deficiency inherited by 400 million people worldwide, though most are asymptomatic throughout their life. It primarily affects people in Africa, the Middle East, South-East Asia and Brazil (Cappellini & Fiorelli 2008). G6PD deficiency is also gender linked; 12% of male African Americans are G6PD deficient, but only 3% of females (Hardisty & Weatherall 1982).

Antioxidant/pro-oxidant activity: (−)-Menthol demonstrated an antioxidant action in human liver microsomes, producing reversible inhibition of nifedipine oxidation and showed moderate activity as an inhibitor of CYP3A4 (Dresser et al 2002).

Mutagenicity and genotoxicity: Neither (−)-menthol nor (±)-menthol was mutagenic in Ames tests, with or without metabolic activation (Andersen & Jensen 1984; Nohmi et al 1985; Zeiger et al 1988; Gomes-Carneiro et al 1998). (−)-Menthol was also non-mutagenic in a *Bacillus subtilis* rec assay (Oda 1978) and in *E. coli* strain WP2*uvr*A (Yoo 1986). Neither (−)-menthol nor (±)-menthol was genotoxic in Chinese hamster fibroblasts (Ishidate et al 1984; Sofuni et al 1985). (±)-Menthol showed no genotoxic effect in a mouse micronucleus test, an all cell comet assay, and a comet assay in Chinese hamster ovary cells (Shelby et al 1993; Kiffe et al 2003). (−)-Menthol was not mutagenic in a dominant lethal assay, and was not clastogenic in a bone marrow CA test (FDA 1975, cited in Belsito et al 2008).

Carcinogenic/anticarcinogenic potential: When (±)-menthol was given in feed to male and female rats at 3,750 or 7,500 ppm or to male and female mice at 2,000 or 4,000 ppm for 2 years, it was not carcinogenic, and there were no treatment-related histopathological changes. Tissues microscopically examined included the brain (frontal cortex, basal ganglia, parietal cortex, thalamus, cerebellum, pons), pituitary, spinal cord, eyes, esophagus, trachea, salivary gland, mandibular lymph node, thyroid, parathyroid, heart, thymus, lungs, mainstem bronchi, liver, gallbladder, pancreas, spleen, kidney, adrenal gland, stomach, small intestine, colon, bladder, prostate or uterus, testes or ovaries, sternebrae, femur or vertebrae and mammary gland (National Cancer Institute 1979). In male and female mice given 20 ip injections of menthol in impure tricaprylin in a total dose of 0.5 or 2.0 g/kg over 24 weeks the incidence of primary lung tumors was no higher than in the control group (Stoner et al 1973). (−)-Menthol dose-dependently inhibited the growth of mouse leukemia WEHI-3 cells, mouse ascites sarcoma BP8 cells and human gastric SNU-5 cancer cells (Bernson & Pettersson 1983; Lin et al 2005; Lu et al 2007). (−)-Menthol had a significant chemopreventive action during DMBA initiation of rat mammary tumors (Russin et al 1989).

Menthol activates TRPM8 channels, causing a cellular influx of calcium. Carcinogenesis might therefore be enhanced or inhibited by menthol in cells that express these channels, especially since some cancer cells depend on controlled calcium increases at certain stages of cell proliferation. Tatman & Huanbiao (2002) reported that the proliferation of mouse B16 melanoma cells was very weakly inhibited by (−)-menthol with an IC_{50} value of 250 mM (39 g/L). In human malignant melanoma cells, the presence of menthol caused a dose-dependent, sustainable intracellular calcium increase, with an EC_{50} value of 286 μM (44.6 mg/L), and a corresponding decrease in cell viability (Yamamura et al 2008). Similarly, (−)-menthol induced cell death associated with calcium production in both human leukemia HL60 cells and human bladder cancer T24 cells (Lu et al 2006; Li Q et al 2009). TRPM8 channels are highly expressed in T24 cells.

TRPM8 channels are also found in normal prostate epithelial cells, and they are highly expressed in prostate cancer cells, especially those that are androgen-sensitive (Zhang & Barritt 2006). Menthol does inhibit prostate cancer cell proliferation in androgen-sensitive LNCaP cells, but only at above millimolar concentrations. However, (+)- and (−)-menthol enhance the antiproliferative efficacy of vitamin D(3) at 0.8 mM (124 mg/L) (Park et al 2009). Menthol was similarly toxic to androgen-independent PC-3 prostate cancer cells at above millimolar concentrations, but the mechanism was independent of TRPM8 channels (Kim SH et al 2009). TRPM8 channels are also expressed by human gliobastoma (brain cancer) cells. In in vitro studies, the TRPM8-mediated action of menthol was associated with an increase in cellular migration, possibly through activation of BK ion channels (Wondergem et al 2008; Wondergem & Bartley 2009).

Comments: There are very few reports of menthol allergy in relation to the widespread use of peppermint- and menthol-infused products such as chewing gum, toothpaste and confectionary. The two year carcinogenesis study found no evidence of cancer in brain or spinal cord tissue, so menthol is not carcinogenic per se. However, the possibility that it may exacerbate the development of a type of brain cancer requires further study.

Summary: Nasal instillation of liquids containing menthol is hazardous in young children. Hypersensitivity to menthol may occur from dermal or oral contact, but such cases are relatively rare. Chronic smoking of mentholated cigarettes may affect heart rate and function, but does not increase morbidity or mortality. Taken orally in small doses or applied to the skin, menthol appears to have no effect on heart rate. Gavage dosing of menthol for four weeks at >200 mg/kg/day was hepatotoxic in rats.

However in humans, similar oral doses taken for six months in enterically coated capsules were not hepatotoxic. Menthol is not teratogenic or carcinogenic.

Regulatory guidelines: An ADI for menthol was set at 0.2 mg/kg bw by the Joint FAO/WHO Expert Committee on Food Additives (JECFA 1999b). Concentrations of menthol up to 16% have been approved for OTC topical use by the FDA (Patel et al 2007).

Our safety advice: Menthol should be avoided, at least in oral doses, by anyone with a G6PD deficiency. These people will characteristically have had abnormal blood reactions to at least one of the following drugs, or will have been advised to avoid them: antimalarials, sulfonamides, chloramphenicol, streptomycin, aspirin. Menthol-rich essential oils should possibly be avoided in cases of cardiac fibrillation, and great care should be taken in regard to infants inhaling menthol.

Menthone

Synonyms: 1-Methyl-4-isopropylcyclohexan-3-one. *p*-Menthan-3-one
Systematic name: 2-(1-Methylethyl)-5-methylcyclohexanone
Chemical class: Monocyclic monoterpenoid ketone
Note: Different isomers of menthone exist, and the following isomer-specific information has been published:

(−)-Menthone

Synonyms: (2*S*)-*trans*-Menthone. (2*S*,5*R*)-Menthone. *l*-Menthone
CAS number: 14073-97-3

(+)-Menthone

Synonyms: (2*R*)-*cis*-Menthone. (2*R*,5*R*)-Menthone. *d*-Menthone
CAS number: 1196-31-2

Sources >1.0%:

Calamint (lesser)	7.0–55.8%
Peppermint	8.0–31.6%
Cornmint	16.3–31.1%
Buchu (diosphenol CT)	2.5–25%
Pennyroyal (European)	1.5–16.0%
Buchu (pulegone CT)	1.3–7.0%
Pennyroyal (Turkish)	3.5%
Geranium	0.1–2.4%
Spearmint	0.1–1.7%
Pennyroyal (N. American)	0.6–1.4%

Pharmacokinetics: (−)-Menthone is excreted in rabbits as a glucuronide conjugate, 10–15% being metabolized to (+)-neomenthol (Scheline 1991).

Acute toxicity: Subcutaneous LD_{50} in mice 2.18 g/kg (Wenzel & Ross 1957).

Subacute and subchronic toxicity: Given orally to rats for 28 days, menthone produced cerebellar lesions at 400 and 800 mg/kg/day, but not at 200 mg/kg/day. There were dose-dependent increases in plasma content of creatinine and bilirubin, and in plasma activity of alkaline phosphatase; the relative weights of liver and spleen were increased (Madsen et al 1986). Menthone does not deplete hepatic microsomal CYP (Madyastha et al 1985).

Antioxidant/pro-oxidant activity: Menthone has demonstrated significant radical scavenging activity against DPPH and OH radicals (Mimica-Dukic et al 2003).

Mutagenicity and genotoxicity: Menthone is mutagenic in the Ames test (Andersen and Jensen 1984) and is genotoxic in fruit flies (Franzios et al 1997).

Carcinogenic/anticarcinogenic potential: In male and female mice given 19 ip injections of menthone in impure tricaprylin in a total dose of 1.9 or 4.75 g/kg over 24 weeks the incidence of primary lung tumors was no higher than in the control group (Stoner et al 1973).

Summary: Menthone is subchronically toxic in rats at doses of >200 mg/kg/day po, and there are reports of mutagenicity.

(−)-Menthyl acetate

Synonym: Acetic acid (−)-menthyl ester
Systematic name: (1α,2β,5α)-5-Methyl-2-(1-methylethyl) cyclohexan-1-yl ethanoate
Chemical class: Monocyclic monoterpenoid ester
CAS number: 89-48-5

Sources >1.0%:

Peppermint	2.1–10.6%
Cornmint	1.8–3.4%

Adverse skin reactions: Undiluted (−)-menthyl acetate was mildly irritating to rabbit skin; tested at 8% on 25 volunteers it was neither irritating nor sensitizing (Opdyke 1976 p. 477).

Acute toxicity: Acute oral LD_{50} in rats >5 g/kg; acute dermal LD_{50} in rabbits >5 g/kg (Opdyke 1976 p. 477).

Antioxidant/pro-oxidant activity: (−)-Menthyl acetate demonstrated an antioxidant action in human liver microsomes, producing reversible inhibition of nifedipine oxidation and showed moderate activity as an inhibitor of CYP3A4 (Dresser et al 2002).

Summary: (−)-Menthyl acetate is non-toxic, and there is no evidence of skin reactivity in humans.

Methoxsalen

Synonyms: 8-Methoxypsoralen. 8-MOP. Xanthotoxin. 8-Methoxy-4′,5′:6,7-furocoumarin. Ammoidin
Systematic name: 9-Methoxy-7H-furo[3,2-g][1]benzopyran-7-one
Chemical class: Furanocoumarin ether
CAS number: 298-81-7

Sources:

Rue	0.032%
Lime (expressed)	<0.0005%
Parsnip	Uncertain

Pharmacokinetics: There is extensive first-pass metabolism of methoxsalen in the liver before it reaches the general circulation (Department of Health 1998). The in vitro uptake of methoxsalen into human skin was proportional to concentration and time of application, and increased with increasing vehicle polarity. No metabolic changes to the compound were detected while present in the skin for up to 16.7 hours (Gazith et al 1978). Methoxsalen inhibits CYP1A1, CYP2B1 and CYP3A (Koenigs & Trager 1998; Guo et al 2000; Baumgart et al 2005). It inhibited CYP3A4, with IC_{50} values of 35 μM and 39 μM (7.6 and 8.4 mg/L) in two different human livers (Ho et al 2001).

Adverse skin reactions: Methoxsalen is phototoxic (Zaynoun et al 1977a, 1977b) and potentially photocarcinogenic (Grube 1977). There is a long-term risk of skin cancer in patients receiving PUVA (psoralen + UVA) therapy (see Immunotoxicity below) with methoxsalen (Department of Health 1988).

Subacute and subchronic toxicity: Methoxsalen was orally administered to rats once, or for 16 or 90 days in a variety of doses. Of ten rats that received a single dose of 1,000 mg/kg, four males and five females died. In the 16 day studies, all the rats receiving 800 mg/kg died within 5 days, and there were later fatalities at both 400 mg/kg and 200 mg/kg, in addition to reductions of body weight. In the 90 day studies, there was significant weight loss at 200 and 400 mg/kg. At doses of 50 mg/kg and higher there were signs of hepatotoxicity in both sexes, and in males there was atrophy of the testes, seminal vesicles and prostate. No toxicity was observed in the 90 day studies at 25 mg/kg (National Toxicology Program 1989b).

Methoxsalen was orally administered to male and female monkeys at 0, 2, 6 or 18 mg/kg three times a week for 26 weeks. Dose-dependent emesis was the most sensitive indicator of toxicity, and the lowest dose to elicit emesis was 3 x 6 mg/kg/week. Metabolic saturation occurred between 3 × 2 and 3 × 6 mg/kg/week (Rozman et al 1989).

Chronic toxicity: Methoxsalen was orally administered to rats five days per week for two years at 0, 37.5 or 75 mg/kg. In the dosed groups, both body weights and survival were lower than controls, and signs of toxicity were more prevalent in males than in females. These included various dose-dependant signs of nephrotoxicity in addition to hypertrophy of the thyroid, hyperplasia and ulcers of the forestomach, carcinomas, adenomas and adenocarcinomas (National Toxicology Program 1989b).

Reproductive toxicity: Dietary methoxsalen was orally administered to pregnant female rats at 0, 1,250 or 2,500 ppm (corresponding to 0, ~100 and ~200 mg/kg) for 39–49 days (until the day before expected parturition). Both total weight gain and the number of pups per female were significantly lower in the high dose group, and in both dosed groups there was a significant reduction in uterine weight and in the number of corporea lutea. Circulating 17β-estradiol levels were dose-dependently reduced, and liver mRNAs for CYP1A1 and UGT1A6 were significantly induced. Enhanced metabolism of estrogens may explain the reproductive toxicity of methoxsalen (Diawara et al 1999; Diawara & Kulkosky 2003).

In a developmental toxicity study, pregnant rats were given gavage doses of 20, 80, 120 or 160 mg/kg/day of methoxsalen on gestational days 6–15. The developmental toxicity NOAEL was 80 mg/kg, and the maternal toxicity NOAEL was 20 mg/kg (National Toxicology Program 1994a). In a similar study, pregnant rabbits were given gavage doses of 40, 80, or 105 mg/kg/day of methoxsalen on gestational days 6–19. The developmental toxicity NOAEL was greater than or equal to 105 mg/kg (National Toxicology Program 1994b)

When male rats were given dietary methoxsalen at 0, 1,250 or 2,500 ppm (corresponding to 0, ~75 or ~150 mg/kg) for eight weeks, treated males had smaller pituitary and prostate glands. Sperm counts were reduced in the high-dose group and more breeding attempts were required to impregnate females. Dosing significantly elevated levels of testosterone and relative liver weight was significantly increased (Diawara et al 2001).

Immunotoxicity: Some information on the toxic effects of methoxsalen comes from studies in patients undergoing treatment for severe psoriasis and other skin diseases (PUVA therapy). Treatment involves an oral dose of 0.6 mg/kg followed by UVA exposure. At therapeutic doses in psoriasis patients, PUVA with methoxsalen causes some signs of mild immunosuppression characterized by reduced delayed-type hypersensitivity, changes to immunocompetent cells in the skin, and small reductions in the number and function of circulating T lymphocytes. Reductions in T cell number were also found in volunteers receiving the same treatment (Department of Health 1988).

Hepatotoxicity: Methoxsalen was a potent inhibitor of CYP3A, as indicated by reduced microsomal testosterone 6β-hydroxylation, with an IC_{50} value of 2.9 μM (626 μg/L) (Guo et al 2000). Dietary administration of 1,000 ppm (equivalent to ~100 mg/kg) of methoxsalen for four weeks significantly reduced total CYP levels in female mice, but not in males. In both sexes there was hypertrophy of the centrilobular hepatocytes (Diawara et al 2000)

Mutagenicity and genotoxicity: Methoxsalen was mutagenic in some *S. typhimurium* strains and not in others. It was mutagenic in Chinese hamster ovary cells in the absence of metabolic activation (National Toxicology Program 1989b). Methoxsalen was photomutagenic in *S. typhimurium*, and in the presence of UVA it was genotoxic in human lymphocytes (Koch 1986; Abel 1987b). It was also photomutagenic in Chinese hamster V79 cells (Uwaifo et al 1983). The treatment of human blood cultures with methoxsalen, followed by UVA exposure, results in chromosome damage. The methoxsalen was at concentrations of 0.1 or 1.0 μg/mL, and was present for periods of up to 72 hours (Youssefi et al 1994). The formation of photoadducts in cellular DNA is similar after bergapten or methoxsalen treatment. The primary photoproducts are 4,5-monoadducts, which crosslink on subsequent exposure to UVA radiation (Amici & Gasparro 1995).

Carcinogenic/anticarcinogenic potential: There are several reports of nonmelanocytic skin cancer developing in patients treated with oral methoxsalen and UVA radiation for psoriasis or mycosis fungoides. These are summarized an IARC report (IARC 1986c). In a follow-up of 1,380 psoriasis patients, the incidence of squamous cell carcinoma rose from 4.1% for patients receiving low-dose PUVA therapy, to 22.3% for those receiving medium doses, and 56.8% at high doses (Stern et al 1984). The doses refer to UVA light exposure, not methoxsalen.

Methoxsalen significantly reduced NNK-induced lung tumorigenesis in female mice at daily oral doses of 12.5 or 50 mg/kg for three days prior to ip administration of NNK. Tumor incidence was reduced from 93.8% to 20.0% or 16.7%, probably due to CYP2A6 inhibition (Takeuchi et al 2003). Subsequent research suggests that the effect is due to inhibiting CYP2A5-mediated metabolic activation of NNK (Miyazaki et al 2005b).

Summary: Methoxsalen is phototoxic and photocarcinogenic to humans, and is photomutagenic. It is toxic to the reproductive and endocrine systems of rats. Some hepatotoxicity has been seen in mice, and some immunotoxicity has occurred in patients receiving PUVA therapy. The rat oral NOAEL was 25 mg/kg.

Regulatory guidelines: The IARC have determined that methoxsalen, in combination with UV radiation, is carcinogenic to humans (IARC 1986c). For tanning products, the SCCNFP set a maximum of 1 ppm for 'furocoumarin-like substances' in 1995, later reviewed and confirmed (SCCNFP 2003b). This has now been extended to apply to all cosmetic products (SCCP 2005b).

Methyl allyl disulfide

Synonyms: Allyl methyl disulfide. 4,5-Dithia-1-hexene
Systematic name: Methyl 2-propenyl disulfide
Chemical class: Aliphatic alkene disulfide
CAS number: 2179-58-0

Source:

Garlic   3.9–12.2%

Carcinogenic/anticarcinogenic potential: Methyl allyl disulfide significantly reduced NDEA-induced forestomach tumor and pulmonary adenoma formation in mice (Wattenberg et al 1989). The compound also inhibited benzo[a]pyrene-induced neoplasia of the forestomach and lung in female mice when given prior to the carcinogen challenge (Sparnins et al 1988).
Summary: We could find no dermal or toxicity data for methyl allyl disulfide. It has demonstrated in vivo antitumoral effects.

Methyl allyl trisulfide

Synonyms: Allyl methyl trisulfide. 4,5,6-Trithia-1-heptene
Systematic name: Methyl 2-propenyl trisulfide
Chemical class: Aliphatic alkene trisulfide
CAS number: 34135-85-8

Source:

Garlic   8.3–18.2%

Cardiovascular effects: Methyl allyl trisulfide inhibits platelet aggregation (Boullin, 1981; Fenwick & Hanley 1985).

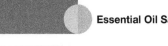

Carcinogenic/anticarcinogenic potential: Methyl allyl trisulfide induced glutathione *S*-transferase in mouse forestomach, small bowel, liver and lung. Two doses of 15.0 μmol (2.3 mg) inhibited benzo[*a*]pyrene-induced neoplasia of the forestomach but not the lung (Wattenberg et al 1985).
Summary: We could find no dermal or toxicity data for methyl allyl trisulfide. It inhibits platelet aggregation in vitro, and has demonstrated in vivo antitumoral effects.

Methyl anthranilate

Synonyms: Methyl 2-aminobenzoate. 2-Aminobenzoic acid methyl ester
Chemical class: Benzenoid amine ester
CAS number: 134-20-3

Sources >1.0%:

Orange flower absolute	3.0–15.0%
Champaca absolute (orange)	2.1–9.0%
Jasmine sambac absolute	5.5%
Orange flower water absolute	3.0%

Adverse skin reactions: Tested at 10% on 25 volunteers, methyl anthranilate was neither irritating nor sensitizing (Opdyke 1974 p. 935–936).
Acute toxicity: Acute oral LD_{50} in rats 2.91 g/kg, in mice 3.9 g/kg, and in guinea pigs 2.78 g/kg (Jenner et al 1964).
Subacute and subchronic toxicity: In a 90 day feed study in rats, no macroscopic effects were found from either 1,000 or 10,000 ppm methyl anthranilate (Hagan et al 1967). We estimate that the high dose used here is equivalent to within the range of 400–800 mg/kg body weight.
Mutagenicity and genotoxicity: Methyl anthranilate was not mutagenic in the Ames test (Kasamaki et al 1982; Mortelmans et al 1986). It was weakly genotoxic in Chinese hamster cells (Kasamaki et al 1982).
Carcinogenic/anticarcinogenic potential: In male and female mice given 24 ip injections of methyl anthranilate in impure tricaprylin in a total dose of 2.25 or 11.20 g/kg over 24 weeks the incidence of primary lung tumors was no higher than in the control group (Stoner et al 1973).
Summary: Methyl anthranilate appears to be non skin-reactive, and presents only a slight risk of acute or subchronic toxicity.

Methyl benzoate

Synonym: Benzoic acid methyl ester
Chemical class: Benzenoid ester
CAS number: 93-58-3

Sources >1.0%:

Jonquil absolute	23.4%
Tuberose absolute	7.8%
Ginger lily absolute	5.7%
Ylang-ylang	0.2–5.6%
Champaca absolute (orange)	1.0–5.0%
Bakul absolute	3.8%

Ylang-ylang absolute	3.5%
Jasmine sambac absolute	2.6%
Jasmine absolute	0.2–1.0%

Adverse skin reactions: Tested at 4% on human subjects methyl benzoate was not sensitizing (Opdyke 1974 p. 937). In an in vitro assay, methyl benzoate was non-phototoxic (Placzek et al 2007).
Acute toxicity: Acute oral LD_{50} has been reported as 1.35, 2.17, 3.42 and 3.5 g/kg in rats, 3.0 and 3.33 g/kg in mice, 4.1 g/kg in guinea pigs, and 2.17 g/kg in rabbits (Adams et al 2005b).
Mutagenicity and genotoxicity: Methyl benzoate was not mutagenic in the Ames test (Zeiger et al 1992).
Summary: Methyl benzoate appears to be minimally skin reactive, minimally toxic and non-mutagenic.

Methyl cinnamate

Synonyms: Cinnamic acid methyl ester. Methyl β-phenylacrylate
Systematic name: Methyl 3-phenyl-2-propenoate
Chemical class: Phenylpropenoid ester
Note: Different isomers of methyl cinnamate exist, and the following isomer-specific information has been published:

(2*E*)-Methyl cinnamate

Synonym: *trans*-Methyl cinnamate
CAS number: 1754-62-7

Sources >1.0%:

Narcissus absolute	1.1–15.8%
Sugandha	13.7%
Jonquil absolute	7.8%
Boronia absolute	6.7%
Galangal (greater)	2.6–5.3%
Bakul absolute	3.6%
Peru balsam	tr–1.7%

(2*Z*)-Methyl cinnamate

Synonym: *cis*-Methyl cinnamate
CAS number: 19713-73-6

Sources >1.0%:

Boronia absolute (+ *N*-tiglamide)	9.3%

Methyl cinnamate (isomer not specified)

Sources >1.0%:

Basil (methyl cinnamate CT)	58.0–63.1%
Tomar seed	12.2%
Finger root	3.0%

Note: Also found in a chemotype of *Ocimum basilicum* at 45-60%.
Pharmacokinetics: Methyl cinnamate is rapidly hydrolysed in rats and rabbits to cinnamic acid and methanol. Cinnamic acid

is subsequently converted mainly to hippuric acid in rats, rabbits, cats, dogs and man. In man, 50–75% of a 6 g oral dose was metabolized to hippuric acid in 4 hours, together with 3–6% of cinnamoyl glucuronide. In rat studies, several additional ring-hydroxylated compounds and their monomethyl ethers were also found (Scheline 1991 p. 150, 183).

Adverse skin reactions: Tested at 2% and 10% on 25 human volunteers, methyl cinnamate was neither irritating nor sensitizing (Opdyke 1975 p. 849). Methyl cinnamate was not sensitizing in tests on guinea pigs (Hausen et al 1992). Of 102 dermatitis patients sensitive to Peru balsam, three tested positive to 10% methyl cinnamate (Hausen 2001). Of 142 dermatitis patients sensitive to Peru balsam, six reacted to an unstated concentration of methyl cinnamate (Mitchell 1975; Mitchell et al 1976). In an in vitro assay, methyl cinnamate was non-phototoxic (Placzek et al 2007).

Mucous membrane irritation: In a private RIFM report, 15% methyl cinnamate was considered non-irritating to rabbit vaginal tissue, with observations made at periods ranging from 4.5 to 72 hours. In a similar private RIFM report, methyl cinnamate was non-irritant to the eyes of rabbits (Bhatia et al 2007b).

Acute toxicity: Acute oral LD_{50} in rats 2.61 g/kg, acute dermal LD_{50} in rabbits >5 g/kg (Opdyke 1975 p. 849).

Mutagenicity and genotoxicity: Methyl cinnamate was not mutagenic in a *Bacillus subtillis* rec assay (Oda et al 1978), but was genotoxic in Chinese hamster ovary cells (Sasaki et al 1989).

Summary: Methyl cinnamate appears to be minimally skin reactive, non-irritant to mucous membranes and minimally toxic. There are inconsistent mutagenicity data.

O-Methyleugenol

Synonyms: Eugenol methyl ether. 4-Allylveratrole
Systematic name: 3,4-Dimethoxy-(2-propenyl)benzene
Chemical class: Phenylpropenoid ether
CAS number: 93-15-2

Sources >0.05%:

Tea tree (black)	97.7%
Pine (huon)	95.0–97.0%
Snakeroot	36.1–44.5%
Cinnamomum rigidissimum	28.6%
Pimento berry	2.9–13.1%
Pteronia	7.2%
Basil (estragole CT)	0–4.2%
Laurel leaf	1.4–3.8%
Rose (Damask)	0.5–3.3%
Champaca absolute (white)	2.3%
Sassafras albidum	1.4–2.3%
Calamus (tetraploid form)	tr–2.0%
Ocotea odorifera	0–2.0%
Pimento leaf	tr–1.9%
Tuberose absolute	1.7%
Betel	0.3–1.7%
Citronella (Sri Lankan)	0–1.7%
Hyacinth absolute	1.5%
Tarragon	0.1–1.5%
Chaste tree seed	0–1.5%
Bay (West Indian)	0–1.4%
Nutmeg (East Indian)	0.1–1.2%
Myrtle	0.3–1.0%
Savory (winter)	0–0.9%
Rose absolute (Provencale)	0–0.8%
Sugandha	0.6%
Tejpat	0.5%
Ho leaf (camphor CT)	0–0.5%
Hyssop (pinocamphone CT)	0–0.5%
Basil (pungent)	0.4%
Ho leaf (linalool CT)	0.1–0.4%
Basil (holy)	0.2–0.3%
Elemi	0.2–0.3%
African bluegrass	0.2–0.3%
Mace (Indian)	0.2%
Mace (East Indian)	0.1–0.2%
Nutmeg (West Indian)	0.1–0.2%
Cascarilla (Bahamian)	0–0.2%
Clove bud	0–0.2%
Ho leaf (cineole CT, Chinese)	0.1%
Magnolia leaf	0.1%
Rose (Japanese)	0.1%
Cassia leaf	tr–0.1%
Basil (linalool CT)	tr–0.1%
Mastic	tr–0.1%
Citronella (Javanese)	0–0.1%
Cananga	0.07%
Tea tree	tr–0.06%

Notes: Methyleugenol has been anecdotally reported as a constituent of essential oils not listed above, but we could not find it in any reports of commercial essential oils of anise, black pepper, cardamon, carrot seed, cinnamon leaf, East Indian lemongrass or melissa at concentrations of 0.01% or higher. Rosemary oil can reportedly contain up to 0.01% of methyleugenol (Burfield, private communication, 2004).

Pharmacokinetics: The major metabolic routes for methyleugenol in rats involve modifications to the propenyl rather than to the methoxyl groups. The principal products are 2'-hydroxy-3,4-dimethoxyphenylpropanoic acid, 3,4-dimethoxycinnamic acid, 3,4-dimethoxybenzoic acid, and the glycine conjugates of the latter two compounds (Scheline 1991 p. 68). Epoxidation of the propenyl group yields methyleugenol 2'3'-epoxide which is rapidly detoxified and does not lead to genotoxicity (Burkey et al 2000; Luo and Guenthner 1995). Hydroxylation produces 1'-hydroxymethyleugenol, which can be further metabolized to 1'-sulfooxymethyleugenol, the likely ultimate carcinogen (Miller et al 1983). In rats, the formation of 1'-sulfooxymethyleugenol increased from 0.043% of the dose at 0.05 mg/kg, to 0.06% of the dose at 300 mg/kg (Al-Subeihi et al 2011).

In liver samples taken from 13 humans, the rate of 1'-hydroxylation of methyleugenol in vitro varied by up to 27-fold, with the highest activity being equal to that of liver microsomes from Fischer 344 rats. This implies that the toxicity of methyleugenol is subject to wide variability in the human population, but that rat data are equivalent to the worst-case scenario for humans (Gardner et al 1997). In a similar study of human liver microsomes in 15 individuals, variation of only 5-fold was noted (Jeurissen et al 2006). 1'-Hydroxylation of methyleugenol is catalyzed primarily by CYP1A2 (Jeurissen et al 2007).

Methyleugenol was detected in the serum of 98% of 206 samples taken from a cross-section of US adults, at a mean concentration of 24 pg/g (range <3.1– 390 pg/g). No demographic variable was a good predictor of exposure or dose (Barr et al 2000). After eating 12 gingersnaps containing a relatively high concentration of methyleugenol, the mean blood level of methyleugenol rose from a baseline of 16.2 pg/g to 53.9 pg/g in nine male and female volunteers. This was followed by a rapid decline, the mean half-life of elimination being 90 minutes (Schecter et al 2004). The average daily intake of methyleugenol from food and beverages by Europeans has been estimated to be 0.19 mg/kg (SCF 2001a).

Using data from Schmitt et al (2010) we calculate the human dermal absorption of methyleugenol to be within the range of 2–5% (see Ch. 4, p. 44).

Adverse skin reactions: Undiluted methyleugenol was irritating to rabbit skin; tested at 8% on 25 volunteers it was neither irritating nor sensitizing (Opdyke 1975 p. 857). Tested at 10% on 10 guinea pigs, methyleugenol was not sensitizing (Itoh 1982). In a worldwide multicenter study, four (1.8%) of 218 dermatitis patients with proven sensitization to fragrance materials, were sensitive to 5% methyleugenol (Larsen et al 2002).

Acute toxicity: The acute oral LD$_{50}$ in rats has been reported as 1,560 mg/kg (Jenner et al 1964) and 810 mg/kg; acute dermal LD$_{50}$ in rabbits >5 g/kg. The NOAEL of methyleugenol in rats and mice was estimated to be 10 mg/kg (Abdo et al 2001).

Subacute and subchronic toxicity: In 14-week gavage studies in rats and mice, methyleugenol was given in 0.5% methylcellulose at 10, 30, 100, 300 and 1,000 mg/kg. Changes observed included alterations in protein, carbohydrate or fat metabolism, increases in serum alanine aminotransferase and sorbitol dehydrogenase activities, and hepatocellular changes, signifying hepatic toxicity. Atrophic changes in the fundic region of the stomach were also noted. NOAEL values of 10 mg/kg applied to hematology and clinical chemistry data (only rats were tested) and to selected lesions (all tested organs/glands in both rats and mice). For body and organ weight changes, 10 mg/kg was the rat NAOEL and the mouse LOAEL. In further testing over 90 days at different doses, 75 mg/kg was the rat NOAEL and 300 mg/kg the mouse NOAEL for serum gastrin levels, and 37 mg/kg (rats) and 9 mg/kg (mice) were the LOAEL values for cell proliferation (Abdo et al 2001). Considering all endpoints at 90 days, 10 mg/kg is the rat NOAEL and 9 mg/kg is the mouse LOAEL.

Reproductive toxicity: Pregnant rats were given 80, 200 or 500 mg/kg/day methyleugenol by gavage on gestational days 6–19. In the mid and high dose groups, maternal weight gain was reduced, and there were minimal signs of hepatotoxicity. Increases in maternal liver weights (both absolute and relative) occurred in all three dosed groups. Prenatal mortality and live litter size were not affected at any dose, but in the high dose animals, average fetal body weight was reduced to 86% of controls, and one type of skeletal abnormality was increased (Price et al 2006).

Antioxidant/pro-oxidant activity: Methyleugenol was moderately effective in inhibiting the formation of hydroperoxides in methyl linoleate, and in this assay was approximately ten times less effective than eugenol (Park et al 2003). In a cerebral ischemia model, methyleugenol significantly reduced injury caused by oxidative stress, and elevated the activities of superoxide dismutase and catalase (Choi et al 2010).

Mutagenicity and genotoxicity: Methyleugenol was mutagenic in the *Bacillus subtilis* DNA repair test (Sekizawa & Shibamoto 1982), in *Saccharomyces cerevisiae* (Schiestl et al 1989), but not in the Ames test (Sekizawa & Shibamoto 1982; Mortelmans et al 1986). However, expression of human sulfotransferases in *S. typhimurium* TA100 causes methyleugenol to be metabolized to 1'-hydroxymethyleugenol, and leads to DNA adducts (Herrmann et al 2012). Methyleugenol was antimutagenic in the *S. typhimurium* TA135/pSK1002 umu test, due to inhibition of the metabolic activity of S9 (Miyazawa & Kohno 2005).

Methyleugenol is genotoxic in rat hepatocytes (Phillips et al 1984; Randerath et al 1984; Howes et al 1990; Chan and Caldwell 1992; Burkey et al 2000). It readily forms adducts with DNA and proteins in rats and mice (De Vincenzi et al 2000a), and can also form adducts with human cellular DNA (hepatoma cells) (Zhou et al 2007). The generation of protein adducts in the livers of rats fed with methyleugenol appears to require intact hepatocytes (Gardner 1996). In mice given 75 mg/kg/day of methyleugenol in the diet for four weeks, significant changes in the expression of genes related to tumor formation were noted, in some instances after only two weeks (Iida et al 2005).

Carcinogenic/anticarcinogenic potential: In a 2-year study, male and female Fischer 344 rats and B6C3F$_1$ mice received 37, 75 or 150 mg/kg/day methyleugenol by gavage five days a week. There was clear evidence of carcinogenesis in all groups at some dose level. There were significant increases in liver and glandular stomach tumors in male and female rats, and 2/10 male mice at 150 mg/kg developed malignant glandular stomach tumors. However, 37 mg/kg/day was the NOAEL for some types of tumor in both sexes of rat, and in male mice (National Toxicology Program 2000). In this study, the administration of high doses by gavage is likely to have caused significant hepatotoxicity, gastric damage and malnutrition in both rats and mice. The hepatotoxicity of high doses probably played a significant role in the formation of hepatic tumors (Smith et al 2002). The NOAEL for methyleugenol is below 37 mg/kg/day in rats and mice (Johnson et al 2000).

A RIFM evaluation of toxicological and exposure data for methyleugenol and estragole concluded: 'The currently available metabolic, biochemical and toxicological data found for methyleugenol in laboratory species provide clear evidence of nonlinearity in the dose–response relationships for methyleugenol and estragole with respect to metabolic activation and mechanisms associated with the carcinogenic effects. Consideration of this data indicates, that in all probability, a No-Observed-Effect-Level (NOEL) for methyleugenol in the rat exists in the dose-range of 1–10 mg/kg body weight/kg. If the combined exposure to methyleugenol from its use in fragrance products (added as such and from essential oils) is taken as the conservative estimate of 12.5 µg/kg body weight/day, then the margin of safety can be calculated to be in the range of 80–800, according to the NOEL.' The panel concluded that, based on the available data, 'neither methyleugenol nor estragole is likely to present a human cancer risk at current levels of exposure resulting from their addition to fragranced products (added as such or from essential oils)' (RIFM 2001). The panel commented that the NTP bioassays are hazard identifications, not safety assessments, although they 'may provide relevant data for safety assessment, if they are appropriately designed and conducted.'

Comments: Human epidemiological data for methyleugenol are lacking, and there are concerns about the relevance of high-dose carcinogenicity testing in rats. A comparision of both DNA adduct formation, and $BMDL_{10}$ values in rats suggests that there is no more than a three to fivefold difference between the carcinogenic potential of estragole, safrole and methyleugenol (Martati et al 2011). Therefore the 25-fold difference in the IFRA guideline for estragole and safrole (0.01%) and methyleugenol (0.0004%) seems excessive. In addition, the IFRA calculation allows for 40% dermal absorption, but permeability coefficient data suggest that this is in the range of 2–5% for methyleugenol (Ch. 4, p. 44). Very low methyleugenol-containing oils (such as rose) are being offered by some essential oil suppliers.

Summary: From the limited data available it appears that methyleugenol does not present a significant risk of skin irritation or sensitization. The developmental toxicity NOAEL in rats was 200 mg/kg. In rats and mice, the single dose NOAEL was estimated to be 10 mg/kg, and the long-term NOAEL 1–10 mg/kg/day. Methyleugenol is genotoxic, and is carcinogenic and hepatotoxic in rodents, when administered in sufficiently high doses.

Regulatory guidelines: The NTP class methyleugenol as being 'reasonably anticipated to be a human carcinogen based on sufficient evidence of its carcinogenicity in experimental animals.' The Council of Europe lists methyleugenol under 'substances which are suspected to be genotoxic carcinogens and therefore no MDI can be set' (Council of Europe 2003). Both IFRA and the SCCNFP have indicated that methyleugenol as such should not be added to cosmetic products, but that certain maximum concentrations are acceptable for methyleugenol-containing essential oils.

Taking the RIFM lower end NOAEL of 1 mg/kg/day arrived at by the RIFM working party, IFRA applied a safety factor of 1,000 to allow for systemic effects, leading to an acceptable dose of 1 µg/kg body weight/day. IFRA calculated that 40% dermal penetration of methyleugenol would result in an acceptable dose of 1.5 µg/kg body weight/day, corresponding to 150 µg/day of methyleugenol for a 60 kg person. Some further calculations, which take into account a theoretical total daily human exposure to methyleugenol from a variety of sources, result in the recommendation that the maximum concentration of methyleugenol in a body lotion should be 0.0004%. There are

other, higher levels for products only applied to a small area of skin, such as fragrancing cream (0.004%) and fine fragrance (0.02%) (IFRA 2009).

Most of the European Commission's SCCNFP exposure levels for methyleugenol are exactly half those recommended by IFRA. So the maximum for fine fragrance is 0.01%, the maximum for fragrancing cream is 0.002% and the maximum for other leave-on products (and oral hygiene products) is 0.0002%. Methyleugenol is not permitted as a fragrance ingredient added as such, but it is permitted as a constituent of natural essences (European Commission 2002). It should be remembered that the IFRA code is a voluntary one, but an EC directive is mandatory for member states. Health Canada has copied the EU guidelines.

It has been suggested that a limit of 0.05 mg/kg should be applied to the use of methyleugenol in food (De Vincenzi et al 2000a). The expert panel of the Flavor and Extract Manufacturer's Association (FEMA) determined that exposure to methyleugenol from the consumption of food and spices does not pose a significant cancer risk (Smith at al 2002). The European Commission's Scientific Committee on Food published a report on methyleugenol and concluded that, since it was genotoxic and carcinogenic, the existence of a threshold could not be assumed, and reductions in exposure and restrictions in use levels were indicated (SCF 2001a). In November 2001, under Proposition 65, the Office of Environmental Health Hazard Assessment of the California Environmental Protection Agency added methyleugenol to its list of chemicals known to the state to cause cancer (http://www.oehha.ca.gov/prop65/out_of_date/111601Not.html, accessed August 8th 2011)

Our safety advice: The metabolic data from Gardner et al (1997) suggests that rat metabolism of methyleugenol is equivalent to that of humans, even allowing for human interindividual variation. Taking the 90 day rat NOAEL of 10 mg/kg, this would typically be reduced by a factor of ten for lifetime exposure, giving 1 mg/kg/day. Although Al-Subeihi et al (2011) found that 1'-sulfooxymethyleugenol was being formed in rats, even with a methyleugenol dose of 0.05 mg/kg, this may be efficiently detoxified. In carcinogenesis studies, 37 mg/kg/day was the LOAEL, suggesting an NOAEL of approximately 3.7 mg/kg/day for carcinogenesis. There are insufficient data to calculate a true lifetime NOAEL for all types of toxicity. Therefore we have taken the 0.05 mg/kg level and applied a human variability of fivefold (as found by by Jeurissen et al 2006) to give 0.01 mg/kg/day, equivalent to a dermal maximum of 0.02% (Table 14.1).

Methyl heptenone

Synonyms: Methyl isohexenyl ketone. Sulcatone
Systematic name: 6-Methylhept-5-en-2-one
Chemical class: Aliphatic alkene ketone
CAS number: 409-02-9

Sources >1.0%:

Fenugreek	4.5%
May chang	0.5–4.4%

Lemongrass (West Indian)	0.1–2.6%
Myrtle (lemon)	0.1–2.5%
Melissa	0–2.5%
Basil (lemon)	1.0–1.9%
Lemongrass (East Indian)	0.3–1.4%
Verbena (lemon)	0.4–1.0%

Adverse skin reactions: In a modified Draize procedure on guinea pigs, methyl heptenone was non-sensitizing when used at 20% in the challenge phase (Sharp 1978). Methyl heptenone was irritating when applied full-strength to rabbit skin; it was neither irritating nor sensitizing when tested at 3% on 25 volunteers (Opdyke 1975 p. 859).
Acute toxicity: Acute oral LD_{50} in rats reported as 3.5 g/kg and 4.1 g/kg; acute dermal LD_{50} >5 g/kg (Opdyke 1975 p. 859).
Summary: Methyl heptenone appears to be minimally skin reactive and minimally toxic.

O-Methyl isoeugenol

Synonyms: Isoeugenol methyl ether. 4-Propenylveratrole
Systematic name: 3,4-Dimethoxy-(1-propenyl)benzene
Chemical class: Benzenoid alkene ether
Note: Different isomers of O-methyl isoeugenol exist, and the following isomer-specific information has been published:

(E)-O-Methyl isoeugenol

CAS number: 6379-72-2

Sources >1.0%:

Citronella (Sri Lankan)	0–10.7%

(Z)-O-Methyl isoeugenol

CAS number: 6380-24-1

Sources >1.0%:

Citronella (Sri Lankan)	0–1.2%

O-Methyl isoeugenol (isomer not specified)

Sources >1.0%:

Tuberose absolute	32.5%
Boswellia serrata	1.3–3.1%
Calamus (tetraploid form)	tr–2.8%
Narcissus absolute	0–1.6%

Pharmacokinetics: Metabolism is similar to O-methyleugenol, but 4-O-demethylation is more important. The principal metabolites are 3,4-dimethoxycinnamic acid and 3,4-dimethoxybenzoic acid as their glycine conjugates, and 3-methoxy-4-hydroxycinnamic acid (Scheline 1991 p. 68).
Adverse skin reactions: In a worldwide multicenter study, of 218 dermatitis patients with proven sensitization to fragrance materials, 16 (7.3%) were sensitive to 5% methyl isoeugenol (Larsen et al 2002).

Subacute and subchronic toxicity: Methyl isoeugenol was given to 16 male and 16 female rats in the diet for 28 consecutive days at 30, 100 and 300 mg/kg/day, with a similar group as a control. Although several minor variations were observed in the high dose group, such as differences in serum and urine chemical analyses, and increased liver weight and white blood cell counts, none of these were considered to be toxicologically significant (Purchase et al 1992).
Summary: Methyl heptenone appears to be minimally skin reactive and minimally toxic.

Methyl jasmonate

Synonym: Jasmonic acid methyl ester
Systematic name: Methyl 3-oxo-2-(2-pentenyl) cyclopentane ethanoate
Chemical class: Monocyclic monoterpenoid alkene ketone ester
Notes: Different isomers of methyl jasmonate exist. (1R,2R)-Methyl jasmonate and (1R,2S)-methyl epi-jasmonate predominate in jasmine (Tamogami et al 2001). The following isomer-specific information has been published:

[1R-(1α,2β(E))]-Methyl jasmonate

CAS number: 136233-36-8

[1R-(1α,2α (Z))]-Methyl jasmonate

CAS number: 95722-42-2

[1S-(1α,2β(Z))]-Methyl jasmonate

CAS number: 78609-06-0

Sources >1.0%

Ginger lily absolute	1.8%
Jasmine absolute	0.2–1.3%
Boronia absolute	1.2%
Tansy (blue)	tr–1.0%

Adverse skin reactions: In an in vitro assay, methyl cinnamate was non-phototoxic (Placzek et al 2007).
Carcinogenic/anticarcinogenic potential: Methyl jasmonate significantly inhibited the proliferation of two types of human prostate cancer cells in vitro (Samaila et al 2004). It similarly suppressed cell proliferation in human breast, melanoma and lymphoblastic leukemia cells (Fingrut & Flescher 2002). Methyl jasmonate induced cell death in leukemia cells isolated from the blood of leukemia patients, and increased the survival of lymphoma-bearing mice. A characteristic of jasmonates is that they selectively kill cancer cells while sparing normal cells (Flescher 2005). They act directly on mitochondria derived from cancer cells, by-passing premitochondrial apoptotic blocks, and inducing a non-apoptotic cell death (Fingrut et al 2005; Rotem et al 2005). Methyl jasmonate may also target cancer cells via apoptosis, such as in human lung cancer cells (Kim JH et al 2004). Methyl jasmonate suppressed metastasis of both normal and drug-resistant B16-F10 melanoma cells (Reischer et al 2007). Several more recent in vitro

studies showing cytotoxic effects by methyl jasmonate are cited in a review by Cohen & Flescher (2009).

Comments: Methyl jasmonate is produced widely in plants, notably as a 'stress hormone', a response to attack by insects, which deters feeding. Being volatile, it can also signal such attack to neighboring undamaged plants, which may then increase production of jasmonates.

Summary: We could find no acute toxicity or skin reaction data for methyl jasmonate. Significant in vitro anticancer effects have been reported.

Methyl salicylate

Synonym: 2-Hydroxybenzoic acid methyl ester
Systematic name: Methyl 2-hydroxybenzoate
Chemical class: Phenolic ester
CAS number: 119-36-8

Sources >1.0%:

Wintergreen	96.0–99.5%
Birch (sweet)	90.4%
Ylang-ylang	0–10.4%
Tuberose absolute	8.4%
Cassie absolute	<5.0%
Bakul absolute	1.9%

Notes: Widely used in topical preparations for treating skin infections, and as a counterirritant for rheumatic disorders. Some sources, especially older ones, use 'methyl salicylate' and 'wintergreen oil' as synonyms. Being a substituted phenol, methyl salicylate is a weak acid which may be corrosive to tissues.

Pharmacokinetics: After topical application, methyl salicylate is extensively metabolized to salicylic acid in human dermal and subcutaneous tissues (Cross et al 1997). Similarly, oral methyl salicylate is rapidly and extensively hydrolysed to salicylic acid in rats and dogs and also, to a lesser extent, in humans. Following oral ingestion of 0.42 mL methyl salicylate by six volunteers, a mean of 39% after 15 minutes, and 21% after 90 minutes of unchanged methyl salicylate was found in the blood. An appreciable proportion of salicylic acid is excreted unchanged in the urine of all species studied. The principal site of hydrolysis is the liver. In addition, significant amounts of the glycine acid conjugate and its phenolic O-glucuronide, and the phenolic and acid O-glucuronides of salicylic acid were found (Scheline 1991 p. 155, 183). It is conceivable that in man the relatively slow hydrolysis of methyl salicylate equates to higher toxicity (Davison et al 1961). In cases of human poisoning, methyl salicylate has been detected in saliva, bile, milk; spinal, synovial and peritoneal fluid (Adams et al 1957).

Human systemic exposure to methyl salicylate from application in commercial skin patches was reported as being relatively low (Martin et al 2004). With in vitro tests using human skin, the amount of methyl salicylate passing through the epidermis (0.3–0.4 mm) varied from 11.0–32.0%, with higher epidermal absorption from lower concentrations (Moody et al 2007). This compares with in vivo transcutaneous penetration, which was estimated to be 12.0–20.0%. This was calculated from total urinary excretion of salicylate after 10 hours dermal application of

one of five creams or salves, containing 12.0–50% methyl salicylate (Roberts et al 1982). Similarly, when volunteers applied 5 g of an ointment containing 12.5% methyl salicylate twice daily, salicylate recovered from urine was 15.5% on day one of application, and 22.0% on days two, three and four (Morra et al 1996). Uptake of methyl salicylate was similarly estimated at 22% from a 20 minute bath containing 0.03 g/L of methyl salicylate. This was calculated from urinary salicylate content over 48 hours in 10 volunteers (Pratzel et al 1990).

Drug interactions: Topically applied methyl salicylate can potentiate the anticoagulant effects of warfarin, causing internal hemorrhage (Le Bourhis & Soenen 1973; Chow et al 1989; Yip et al 1990). It is likely that either vitamin K metabolism is affected, or warfarin is displaced from protein binding sites. Even small doses topically applied can cause problems. In one case, a 22-year-old woman presented with an elevated INR (12.2) after applying a methyl salicylate-containing pain-relieving gel to her knees daily for eight days (Joss & LeBlond 2000). A similar interaction is possible, but by no means certain, with other anticoagulants such as aspirin and heparin.

Adverse skin reactions: Reported as severely irritating to guinea pig skin and eye; moderately irritating to rabbit skin when applied undiluted; tested at 8% on 25 volunteers, methyl salicylate was neither irritating nor sensitizing (Opdyke 1978 p. 821–825). Tested on nine human volunteers, methyl salicylate was irritating at 30% or 60% (Lapczynski et al 2007b). Tested at 50%, it was not sensitizing (Montelius et al 1998). One of 70 patients with contact dermatitis reacted to 1% methyl salicylate (Nethercott et al 1989). Of 276 health care employees with contact dermatitis, none were allergic to 2% methyl salicylate (Stingeni et al 1995). In patch tests on eczema or dermatitis patients using 2% methyl salicylate, results were as follows: 0/457 (0%) (Addo et al 1982), 6/3,109 (0.2%) (Romaguera & Grimalt 1980), 7/1,825 (0.4%) (De Groot et al 2000), 3/585 (0.5%) (Mitchell et al 1982), 3/241 (1.2%) (Ferguson & Sharma 1984) and 3/183 (1.6%) (Rudner 1977).

In a predictive endpoints assay for contact sensitizers, methyl salicylate was classed as a non-sensitizer (Ashikaga et al 2002). Based on literature published in German, methyl salicylate was classified as Category C, not significantly allergenic, by Schlede et al (2003). The compound is not phototoxic (Addo et al 1982).

Acute toxicity: The human adult oral LD_{50} has been estimated at 500 mg/kg, and human child LDlo as 170 mg/kg. Acute oral LD_{50} reported as 887 and 1,250 mg/kg in rats; 1,110 and 1,440 mg/kg in mice; 700 and 1,060 mg/kg in guinea pigs, 2,800 mg/kg in rabbits and 2,100 mg/kg in dogs (Jenner et al 1964; Opdyke 1978 p. 821–825; Clayton & Clayton 1981–1982 p. 2310; National Toxicology Program 1984a, 1984b). Acute dermal LD_{50} >5 g/kg (Opdyke 1978 p. 821–825). Convulsions were noted in guinea pigs, but not in rats.

Subacute, subchronic and chronic toxicity: Single oral doses of 700 mg/kg methyl salicylate in dogs damaged skeletal and cardiac muscle, possibly via salicylic acid-induced uncoupling of oxidative phosphorylation (Ojiambo 1971a). In dogs there was no observable effect from 500 mg/kg for nine days, 250 mg/kg for 52 days or 50 mg/kg for two years orally. Both 150 mg/kg/day and 350 mg/kg/day for two years resulted in macroscopic and microscopic liver toxicity, and both 800 mg/kg/day for four days and 1,200 mg/kg/day for three days were fatal. In rats, 1,000 ppm for 17 weeks and 1,000 ppm for two years (equivalent to 50 mg/kg) had no adverse effect; 10,000 ppm for 17 weeks and 10,000 ppm for 2 years caused growth retardation; and 20,000 ppm for 49 weeks was fatal (Webb & Hansen 1963; Hagan et al 1967). Doses of 4 mL/kg of methyl salicylate, applied to the skin of rabbits five days a week for up to 96 days, caused early deaths and kidney damage; lower doses (0.5, 1.0, or 2.0 mL/kg) caused a higher than normal incidence of 'spontaneous' nephritis (Webb & Hansen 1963).

Inhalation toxicity: There were no toxic signs or organ abnormalities in four female rats exposed to 700 mg/m^3 (120 ppm) of methyl salicylate for seven hours per day for 20 days (Gage 1970).

Human toxicity: Numerous cases of methyl salicylate poisoning in humans have been reported, with a 50–60% mortality rate. Signs of poisoning include nausea, vomiting, acidosis, convulsions, fever, tachycardia, rapid and labored breathing, pneumonia, pulmonary edema and respiratory alkalosis. There is often enlargement of the heart, congestion of the lungs, liver and kidneys and generalized lymphoid hyperplasia (Hughes 1932). Death results from cardiovascular collapse and respiratory failure, after a period of unconsciousness (Adams et al 1957). Ingestion of up to 85 mL of wintergreen oil resulted in mental confusion, severe respiratory distress, tachycardia and coma (Ojiambo 1971b). One of these subjects developed congestive heart failure and died, and myocardial muscle degeneration was identified at autopsy. Another subject died of a subendocardial hemorrhage after having been found to have a prolonged prothrombin time.

Cases of methyl salicylate poisoning have been notorious for their poor prognosis. In one report from 1937, 25 of 43 cases in the USA (59%) proved fatal (Rubin et al 1949). In British reports of accidental poisoning in the 1950s, wintergreen oil (36 deaths) featured far more frequently than camphor (12 deaths) citronella oil or eucalyptus oil (1 death each) (Craig 1953). Methyl salicylate has been a frequent cause of serious poisoning in children (Graham 1961). In the years 1926, 1928 and 1939–1943, 427 deaths were reported in the US from methyl salicylate poisoning after ingesting wintergreen oil, or products containing it (Davison et al 1961). The problem is also widespread in South East Asia, where inadequate labeling and inappropriate packaging has resulted in cases of poisoning (Malik et al 1994; Lee et al 1997).

Doses as small as 4 mL of of methyl salicylate have been fatal in infants (Reynolds 1993). The ingestion of 10 mL by an adult has been survived (Jacobziner & Raybin 1962b). One teaspoon (5 mL) of methyl salicylate is equivalent to approximately 7.0 g of salicylate, or 21.7 adult aspirin tablets (Botma et al 2001).

Methyl salicylate toxicity has been implicated as a cause of topical necrosis and kidney damage after application of a preparation containing it to the skin. In this case, a 62-year-old man presented with large blisters on his arms and thighs. He had been using an ointment containing methyl salicylate and menthol, and applied a heat pad on top of the ointment. The clinical picture was initially that of acute eczema, such as occurs in contact dermatitis. But over the following 3 days, it became clear that the full thickness of skin was necrotic and that the necrosis extended even into the muscle layers. The patient had a high temperature and complained of muscle weakness. His skin lesions were treated by grafting and he was hospitalized for almost a year. Residual kidney damage was still evident two years later (Heng 1987). In a second case a 40-year-old man became acutely unwell after using a methyl salicylate-containing cream for treating psoriasis. Transcutaneous absorption was enhanced due to his skin condition and to the use of an occlusive dressing. His symptoms included tinnitus, vomiting, tachypnea and acid/base disturbance typical of salicylate toxicity (Bell & Duggin 2002).

Cardiovascular effects: When 5 g of a 30% methyl salicylate preparation was applied to the anterior thigh of nine healthy males, statistically significant platelet inhibition was seen on blood and urine analysis six hours later, and this was equivalent to ingestion of 162 mg of aspirin. There was no effect on thromboxane levels (Tanen et al 2008).

Reproductive toxicity: Salicylates in general are known to dose-dependently inhibit growth and cause congenital abnormalities in experimental animals (Wilson 1973). Their teratogenic action is thought to involve free oxygen radicals, since superoxide dismutase, an antioxidant enzyme, reduced salicylate teratogenicity in rat embryos (Karabulut et al 2000). Salicylates do cross the placental barrier (Ellenhorn & Barceloux 1988, p.564).

When pregnant rats were given ip injections of methyl salicylate at 200 or 400 mg/kg on gestational days 9 and 10, there were dose-related reductions in the development of fetal brain, liver, lung and kidney (Kavlock et al 1982). In female rats administered 0.05 mL or 0.1 mL methyl salicylate ip on days 10 and 11 of pregnancy, fetal kidney development was retarded, without causing permanent abnormality; the higher dose females gained less weight, had fewer and smaller offspring, and there were more resorptions and malformed young than in the controls (Woo & Hoar 1972). Increased fetal deaths, decreased fetal body weight, and anomalies of cleft palate and tail in surviving fetuses were observed in the progeny of female rats given a single sc injection of methyl salicylate (1.5 mL/kg) on day 7, 9 or 11 of gestation (Pyun 1970). Given to pregnant rats at 200, 250 or 300 mg/kg/day ip, on gestation days 11–12, methyl salicylate was both teratogenic and embryotoxic (Daston et al 1988).

Pregnant rats weighing 170–200 g were given a single sc injection of methyl salicylate, doses ranging from 0.1–0.5 mL, on gestational day 9, 10 or 11. Of 116 animals, most lost some weight, 26 died and 47 resorbed their young. Of the 298 young produced, 45 were externally abnormal (compared to none of the 484 controls) and a total of 120 (40.3%) were abnormal in some way. Multiple abnormalities were found in the digestive tract, CNS, liver and skeleton of offspring (Warkany & Takacs 1959). A significant lowering of plasma calcium levels in pregnant rats and mice administered 400 mg/kg sc of methyl salicylate may be related to the compound's fetal toxicity (Saito et al 1982).

Whether topically or orally administered to pregnant hamsters, methyl salicylate produced the same defect in embryos, a failure of fusion of the neural tube. Oral dosing was by gavage at 1,750 mg/kg on gestational day seven. For dermal administration, an unmeasured quantity of undiluted methyl salicylate was applied to the shaved back on gestational day seven. Serum salicylate levels following both treatments were similar, demonstrating that teratogenic levels of salicylate can reach the maternal circulation after intensive topical exposure (Overman & White 1983). When undiluted methyl salicylate was topically applied to pregnant rats at 2,000 mg/kg/day on gestational days 6–15, 25% of the animals died, and in surviving animals, 100% of embryos were resorbed. However, when methyl salicylate was topically applied to pregnant rats at 3% in petrolatum at doses corresponding to 30, 60, 90 or 180 mg/kg/day methyl salicylate, there were no signs of maternal, developmental or embryo/fetotoxicity at any dose (Infurna et al 1990).

When methyl salicylate was administered to two generations of male and female mice at 25, 50 or 100 mg/kg/day by gavage, no adverse effects on body weight or reproductive indices in either the first or second generation were seen (National Toxicology Program 1984a). When similarly given to mated pairs at 100, 250 or 500 mg/kg/day for 18 weeks, body weight was not altered in either sex and there were no adverse clinical signs, but there were reductions in the number of litters and the number of pups per litter. The reproductive NOAEL was 100 mg/kg/day (National Toxicology Program 1984b). In a three generation study, dietary methyl salicylate was fed to rats of both sexes for 100 days at 500, 1,500, 3,000 and 5,000 ppm, and then animals were mated. Third generation pups were not given methyl salicylate. There was no effect on fertility at any dose in the first generation, but second generation fertility was reduced at 5,000 ppm. There was a dose-related reduction in litter size and number of live-born progeny at all doses except for the 500 ppm animals, although taken alone, the reductions at 1,500 were not statistically significant. There were no gross signs of teratogenicity, nor were there any histopathological signs of liver or kidney toxicity in any generation, at any dose (Collins et al 1971). The NOAEL in this study was 500 ppm, equivalent to 25 mg/kg/day.

Mutagenicity and genotoxicity: Methyl salicylate was not genotoxic in Chinese hamster fibroblasts (Ishidate et al 1984), was not mutagenic in the Ames test (Ishidate et al 1984; Mortelmans et al 1986), and was not mutagenic in the *B. subtilis* rec-assay (Oda et al 1978; Kuboyama & Fuji 1992).

Carcinogenic/anticarcinogenic potential: In male and female mice given 24 ip injections of methyl salicylate in tricaprylin in a total dose of 2.4 or 12.0 g/kg over 24 weeks the incidence of primary lung tumors was no higher than in the control group (Stoner et al 1973).

Comments: Fatalities following ingestion of large amounts of methyl salicylate or wintergreen oil have been mainly accidental, and adequate labeling and appropriate packaging is an obvious step in reducing this risk. The principal safety concern is reproductive toxicity.

Summary: At high doses, acute or chronic administration of methyl salicylate in animals causes damage to the liver, kidneys, heart and skeletal muscle, and may be fatal. However, moderate doses are well tolerated acutely and chronically. A comparison of animal and human acute toxicity data suggests that methyl salicylate is 1.5–4.5 times more toxic to humans than rodents (see Ch. 3, p. 32). In 2-year toxicity studies, the NOAEL was 50 mg/kg/day for both rats and dogs. In multi-generational reproductive toxicity studies, oral NOAEL doses were 100 mg/kg/day in mice, and 25 mg/kg/day in rats; the rat dermal NOAEL was 180 mg/kg/day. No evidence has been found to link methyl salicylate with mutagenicity or carcinogenicity, but there are few studies. There have been isolated reports of skin and internal damage following topical application. The average response to patch testing with methyl salicylate for allergy is 0.33% (22/6,676), which suggests an allergen of negligible risk. Methyl salicylate, applied topically or orally, can inhibit platelet aggregation, and potentiate the action of warfarin. It may similarly interact with other anticoagulant drugs. There is a comprehensive review of methyl salicylate toxicity by the Cosmetic Ingredient Review Expert Panel (2003).

Regulatory guidelines: In 1967, an ADI for methyl salicylate was set at 0.5 mg/kg bw by the Joint FAO/WHO Expert Committee on Food Additives (JECFA 2001b), based on a two year feeding study in dogs (NOAEL 50 mg/kg) and applying an uncertainty factor of 100. The same ADI, based on a two year rat study in 1963, was adopted by the Council of Europe Committee of Experts on Flavoring Substances. The Health Canada maximum for methyl salicylate is 1% in topical products (Health Canada Cosmetic Ingredient Hotlist, March 2011).

Our safety advice: We recommend a maximum oral dose of 2.5 mg/kg/day, based on the multi-generational rat reproductive toxicity NOAEL of 25 mg/kg, with an uncertainty factor of 10 (5 for inter-species, and 5 for inter-individual differences). This is equivalent to a dermal limit of 2.4% (Table 14.1). Internal use of methyl salicylate-rich essential oils should be avoided in gastroesophageal reflux disease, and salicylates are contraindicated in children due to the risk of developing Reye's syndrome. We advise that essential oils with a high methyl salicylate content be avoided by any route in pregnancy and lactation, by anyone concurrently taking anticoagulant drugs (due to possible potentiation) and by anyone with salicylate sensitivity, which applies to most children with ADD/ADHD. Caution is advised in people with dermatological conditions where the integrity of the skin is impaired.

β-Myrcene

Synonym: Myrcene
Systematic name: 7-Methyl-3-methylene-1,6-octadiene
Chemical class: Aliphatic monoterpenoid alkene
CAS number: 123-35-3

Sources >5.0%:

Rosemary (β-myrcene CT)	19.5–52.1%
Cape may	43.8%
Celery leaf	33.6%
Hemp	21.2–31.1%
Grindelia	14.0–26.0%
Hop	25.4%
Bay (West Indian)	6.4–25.0%
Parsley leaf	7.8–23.8%
Juniperberry	0–22.0%
Boswellia sacra (α-pinene CT)	0–20.7%
Pepper (pink)	5.0–20.4%

African bluegrass	15.4–20.2%
Lemongrass (West Indian)	5.6–19.2%
Pepper (Sichuanese)	16.4%
Lavender cotton	3.6–15.0%
Tansy (blue)	1.1–13.8%
Pine (white)	4.7–13.1%
Mastic	0.2–12.3%
Myrtle (honey)	10.9%
Pteronia	10.3%
Myrtle (bog)	9.5%
Goldenrod	9.4%
Verbena (honey)	4.7–8.3%
Ravensara leaf	5.0–7.3%
Yarrow (chamazulene CT)	7.0%
Pine (dwarf)	0.5–7.0%
Honey verbena	6.5%
Sage (blue mountain)	6.2%
Pine (grey)	4.1–6.1%
Rosemary (α-pinene CT)	1.1–6.0%
Boswellia frereana	0–6.0%
Chaste tree seed	0–5.6%
Angelica root	1.6–5.5%
Rosemary (verbenone CT)	0.5–5.4%
Spruce (Norwegian)	3.0–5.2%
Fern (sweet)	5.1%
Pine (red)	4.3–5.0%
Longoza	1.0–5.0%

Notes: Only the β-isomer of myrcene is found in essential oils. β-Myrcene has been identified in over 200 plant species, and is present in emissions from many trees (National Toxicology Program 2010b).

Pharmacokinetics: β-Myrcene, administered intragastrically for 20 days at 800 mg/kg/day in rats, and 670 mg/kg/day in rabbits, was mainly metabolized to a pair of glycols, presumably via epoxidation and hydration, followed by oxidation to a corresponding pair of hydroxycarboxylic acids. A cyclic neutral compound was also detected, but its structure remains inconclusive (Scheline 1991). In rats, orally administered β-myrcene was metabolized to 10-hydroxylinalool, 7-methyl-3-methylene-oct-6-ene-1,2-diol, 1-hydroxymethyl-4-isopropenyl cyclohexanol, 10-carboxylinalool and 2-hydroxy-7-methyl-3-methylene-oct-6-enoic acid (Madyastha & Srivatsan 1987). In female rats, oral administration of 1 g/kg body weight of β-myrcene resulted in a 60 minute blood level of 14.1 ± 3.0 μg/mL, with an elimination half-life of 285 minutes. The parent compound was detected in adipose tissue, brain, liver, kidney, and testis (Delgado et al 1993b).

β-Myrcene prolonged pentobarbital-induced sleeping time in rats, probably by inhibiting the barbiturate's metabolism by CYP (Freitas et al 1993). β-Myrcene is an inducer of isoenzymes belonging to the CYP2B subfamily (De-Oliveira et al 1997b).

Adverse skin reactions: β-Myrcene was moderately irritating when applied full-strength to rabbit skin, but was neither irritating nor sensitizing when tested at 4% on 25 volunteers (Opdyke 1976 p. 615). Tested at 5%, β-myrcene was sensitizing to two of eleven dermatitis patients sensitive to tea tree oil (Hausen et al

1999). In a multicenter study involving 1,511 consecutive dermatitis patients, only one (0.07%) tested positive to 3% oxidized β-myrcene, containing 30% β-myrcene (Matura et al 2005).

Acute toxicity: Acute oral LD_{50} in rats >5 g/kg; acute dermal LD_{50} in rabbits >5 g/kg (Opdyke 1976 p. 615). ALD 5.06 g/kg in mice, 11.39 g/kg in rats (Paumgartten et al 1990). The oral NOAEL of β-myrcene in rats has been estimated as 300 mg/kg (Paumgartten et al 1998).

Subacute and subchronic toxicity: In a 14-week gavage study, groups of male and female rats and mice were dosed with β-myrcene at 250, 500, 1,000, 2,000 or 4,000 mg/kg/day 5 days per week (a range equivalent to human daily doses of 17.5–280 g). Thirty-nine of the 40 high-dose rats and mice died in the first week. By the end of the study, renal tubule necrosis was significantly increased in all surviving rats. This was not tested for in mice. There were no adverse effects on hematology at 250 mg/kg in rats, and at 500 mg/kg in mice. The absolute and/or relative liver and kidney weights of most of the dosed rats and mice were significantly increased, and degenerative lesions in the olfactory epithelium were noted in rats on 2,000 mg/kg. However, no histopathological lesions of any kind were seen in mice (National Toxicology Program 2010b).

Reproductive toxicity: Gavage doses of β-myrcene up to 2 g/kg in rats and up to 1 g/kg in mice had no effect on the weight of reproductive organs, on sperm count in males, or on the estrus cycle of females (National Toxicology Program 2010b). No effect on peri- or post-natal development was observed at doses of up to 250 mg/kg of 90% pure β-myrcene given orally to pregnant rats from day 15 of pregnancy to postnatal day 21. Above 500 mg/kg, some adverse effect on birth weight, perinatal mortality and postnatal development was seen (Delgado et al 1993a, 1993b; Paumgartten et al 1998). This does not represent a level of fetotoxicity which would present any problems in essential oils as used in aromatherapy.

Mutagenicity and genotoxicity: β-Myrcene was not mutagenic in an Ames test using *Salmonella* strains TA97, TA98, TA100 and TA1535 with and without metabolic activation (Gomes-Carneiro et al 2005a; National Toxicology Program 2010b). It was similarly negative in *E. coli* strain WP2 *uvrA*/pKM101 with and without metabolic activation, and in a mouse micronucleus test (National Toxicology Program 2010b). β-Myrcene showed strong antimutagenic activity through concentration-dependent, competitive inhibition of PROD, with an IC_{50} of 0.14 μM (19.0 μg/L) (De-Oliveira et al 1997a). β-Myrcene is not genotoxic (Kauderer et al 1991; Zamith et al 1993) and may reduce the genotoxicity of toxic agents such as DMBA, benzo[a]pyrene and cyclophosphamide by inhibiting their oxidation to reactive metabolites (Röscheisen et al 1991). At nanomolar concentrations, β-myrcene suppressed *t*-butyl hydroperoxide induced genotoxicity, both in bacteria and cultured human cells. This was predominantly mediated by radical scavenging activity (Mitić-Culafić et al 2009).

Carcinogenic/anticarcinogenic potential: β-Myrcene inhibited the in vitro formation of the carcinogen NDMA by 88% (Sawamura et al 1999). β-Myrcene did not significantly increase or reduce the average number of tumors per rat or the median tumor latency period in a DMBA-induced rat mammary carcinogenesis model (Russin et al 1989). β-Myrcene inhibited proliferation of human breast cancer MCF-7 cells in vitro, with an IC$_{50}$ of 291 μM (39.6 mg/L), but was only mildly toxic to normal Chang liver cells, with an IC$_{50}$ of 9.5 mM (1,292 mg/L) (Chaouki et al 2009).

In gavage studies, groups of male and female rats and mice were given 250, 500 or 1,000 mg/kg/day of β-myrcene, 5 days per week for 2 years. However, so many high-dose rats and mice died before the end of the study period that these groups could not be included in the assessment. More than 30 types of gland or organ tissue were examined. In both groups of dosed male rats (but not female rats, or mice of either sex) there was an increased incidence of combined benign and malignant renal tubule tumors. In male mice, but not females, there was a dose-dependent increase in hepatocellular carcinomas, though this was not statistically significant in the 250 mg/kg group. In rats, no hepatic lesions of any kind were seen in either sex (National Toxicology Program 2010b).

Comments: The logic behind the massive doses used in the National Toxicology Program (2010b) study was that, since previous data suggested that β-myrcene was not very toxic, high doses would be needed to elicit toxic effects. This is unfortunate, since the results of the study have little relevance to actual human exposure to β-myrcene. The lowest dose used, 250 mg/kg, is equivalent to a 70 kg human ingesting 35 g of an essential oil consisting of 50% β-myrcene. This at least 35 times a therapeutic oral dose, and 100–1,000 times the amount that would be absorbed from a body oil or lotion. The standard grade of commercially available β-myrcene used in testing was only 90% pure. In the NTP study, impurities were reported as 5% ψ-limonene and 1.4% (±)-limonene. The remainder, presumably up to 3.6%, was tentatively identified as isomers and dimers of β-myrcene, and their presence could arguably invalidate all of the findings. The increase in liver weight (noted in the 14 week study) combined with a lack of genotoxicity and the sex/species differences, is a pattern typical in chemicals that are mildly or moderately carcinogenic in some rodents but not humans. The increased liver weight is a function of a higher metabolic rate (Monro 1992, 1993).

Summary: β-Myrcene can be regarded as non-irritant, non-allergenic, non-toxic and antimutagenic. The rat NOAEL for reproductive toxicity was 250 mg/kg. The renal tubule lesions seen in male rats on chronic dosing, are typical of the male rat-specific nephrotoxicity also seen with (+)-limonene and 1,8-cineole, and can be discounted as a human risk. Hepatic cancers were seen in male mice on chronic dosing, but these were not reflected by any toxicity in rats. This, combined with the massive doses applied, and the doubts about the purity of the β-myrcene used, make it impossible to extrapolate any meaningful human risk data.

Myristicin

Synonyms: Methoxysafrole. 3-Methoxy-4,5-(methylenedioxy) allylbenzene
Systematic name: 3-Methoxy-4,5-(methylenedioxy)-1-(2-propenyl)benzene
Chemical class: Phenylpropenoid ether
CAS number: 607-91-0

Sources >1.0%:

Parsnip	17.2–40.1%
Parsleyseed	0.7–37.9%
Nutmeg (East Indian)	3.3–13.5%
Parsley leaf	1.9–8.8%
Mace (Indian)	5.9%
Mace (East Indian)	1.3–3.8%
Sugandha	2.5%
Nutmeg (West Indian)	0.5–0.9%

Note: Non-alcoholic drinks, especially cola, are a major source of human myristicin intake (Yun et al 2003).

Pharmacokinetics: Experiments in rats showed that the methylenedioxy group of myristicin is particularly susceptible to cleavage, resulting in catechol derivatives (Peele 1976). Several alcohol and carboxylic acid oxidation products were also identified in rat urine, as well as nitrogen-containing aminopropiophenone derivatives analogous to the Mannich reaction products reported by Oswald et al (1971). Other workers have identified 3-methoxy-4,5-methylenedioxyamphetamine as a metabolite from in vitro experiments using isolated rat liver or rat liver homogenates, although its relevance is not known (Scheline 1991). Demethylenyl myristicin and dihydroxy myristicin were present in human urine after nutmeg ingestion (Beyer et al 2006). From in vitro and in vivo studies in rats, two metabolites were identified, 1'-hydroxymyristicin and 5-allyl-1-methoxy-2,3-dihydroxybenzene (Lee et al 1998). The latter compound was the major metabolite in human liver, and CYP3A4 and CYP1A2 were the enzymes primarily responsible for the oxidation of myristicin (Yun et al 2003).

Myristicin shows high activity (up to 14-fold increase) as an inducer of glutathione S-transferase (Zheng et al 1992b; Ahmad et al 1997) and is a potent inducer of cytochrome P448 (Ioannides et al 1985). At a dose of 500 μmol/kg (96 mg/kg) ip, myristicin induced several rat liver CYP enzymes (CYP1A1, CYP1A2, CYP2B1, CYP2B2 and CYP2E1) with increases ranging from 2–20-fold (Jeong & Yun 1995). This may have important implications for the efficacy of drugs and their toxicity.

Drug interactions: Myristicin is a moderate inhibitor of monoamine oxidase (MAO) in rodents (Truitt & Ebersberger 1962, Truitt et al 1963).

Acute toxicity: Cat oral LD$_{100}$ 570 mg/kg (Spector 1956). Myristicin is believed to be especially toxic to cats; the odor of nutmeg repels cats.

Subacute and subchronic toxicity: It is estimated that a typical daily intake of myristicin in essential oils and spices in food is unlikely to cause adverse effects in humans (Hällström & Thuvander 1997).

Neurotoxicity: Myristicin can reproduce many of the psychotropic characteristics of ground nutmeg, and increases the levels of the neurotransmitter serotonin in rat brain (Truitt 1967). If this occurs in humans, a psychotropic consequence is almost certain. A metabolic pathway has been proposed which could convert myristicin to 3,4,5-trimethoxyamphetamine (TMA) (Weil 1965, 1966) or 3-methoxy-4,5-methylenedioxyamphetamine (MMDA) (Weil 1965), both known hallucinogens. Further work has confirmed that myristicin is potentially convertible to chemicals similar to hallucinogens (Kalbhen 1971). Myristicin is itself very similar in structure to MMDA, an analogue of MDMA, or Ecstasy (Shulgin 1966). However, there is no evidence that myristicin is converted in vivo to either TMA or MMDA. Taken orally by humans in doses of 400 mg, myristicin appears to have no psychotropic effect (Truitt et al 1961) and is insufficiently potent to explain the psychotropic effects of nutmeg (Truitt 1967).

Hepatotoxicity: Myristicin was found to possess 'extraordinarily potent hepatoprotective activity' in rats, against liver damage caused by lipopolysaccharide (LPS) or d-galactosamine (D-GalN). Myristicin markedly suppressed LPS or D-GalN-induced enhancement of serum TNF-α concentrations and hepatic DNA fragmentation in mice (Morita et al 2003).

Antioxidant/pro-oxidant activity: Myristicin inhibited lipid peroxidation in liver homogenates, probably by scavenging free radicals or ROS directly (Hattori et al 1993).

Mutagenicity and genotoxicity: Myristicin was not genotoxic in either repair-proficient or repair-deficient Chinese hamster ovary cells (Martins et al 2011). Myristicin did not cause UDS in rat hepatocytes (Hasheminejad & Caldwell 1994). But in two ^{32}P post-labelling studies, a low but possibly significant level of DNA adduct formation was reported for myristicin in newborn male and adult female mice (Phillips et al 1984; Randerath et al 1984). Myristicin forms weak adducts in human cellular DNA (hepatoma cells) (Zhou et al 2007). Myristicin binding to hepatic DNA in mice is three to four times weaker than that of safrole (Randerath et al 1993). Myristicin produces only two DNA adducts in mouse liver (Phillips et al 1984) and a minimum of three adducts is thought to be required for cancerous cells to form (Williams et al 2005b).

Carcinogenic/anticarcinogenic potential: In a novel assay for carcinogens, groups of male rats were dosed for 2, 14 or 90 days with 0.2 or 2.0 mmol/kg/day (38 or 384 mg/kg/day) of myristicin, and then hepatic tissue was analyzed for precancerous changes in gene expression. The results suggest that myristicin is weakly hepatocarcinogenic in male rats (Auerbach et al 2010). Myristicin shows high activity as an inducer of glutathione S-transferase (Zheng et al 1992b). Myristicin was not carcinogenic in male mice when a total dose of 4.75 μmol (912 μg) was injected ip in increasing doses on days 1, 8, 15 and 22 prior to weaning (Miller et al 1983). Myristicin inhibits benzo[a]pyrene-induced tumors in mice, and induces cytotoxicity in human neuroblastoma SK-N-SH cells by an apoptotic mechanism (Zheng et al 1992a; Lee et al 2005a). It is cytotoxic to cells for myelogenous leukemia (K562, IC_{50} 18.5 μg/mL) non-small cell lung cancer (NCI-H460, IC_{50} 16.0 μg/mL) and breast cancer (MCF-7, IC_{50} 16.0 μg/mL) (Di Stefano et al 2011).

Comments: Under normal circumstances, the intake of myristicin from essential oils and spices is unlikely to pose any problems in humans. However, owing to its actions on MAO and CYP enzyme activity, myristicin-containing essential oils should be used cautiously or avoided altogether in patients taking prescription drugs, notably MAOIs and pethidine.

Summary: Myristicin is a moderate inhibitor of MAO, and an inducer of glutathione S-transferase and various CYP enzymes. Evidence indicates that myristicin is, at most, weakly psychotropic in man. It has been suggested that TMA, MMDA or similar substances may be formed during metabolism, but this remains speculative. Although myristicin is potentially genotoxic at high doses, there is no evidence for carcinogenicity, and mouse data suggests that it affords some protection against B[a]P-induced tumors.

Regulatory guidelines: The Council of Europe lists myristicin under 'substances which are suspected to be genotoxic carcinogens and therefore no MDI can be set' (Council of Europe 2003).

Our safety advice: Because of its MAO inhibiting action, essential oils high in myristicin should be used with caution in oral doses by anyone taking MAOIs, SSRIs, pethidine, and indirect sympathomimetics (see Table 4.10 for more detail).

Myrtenyl acetate

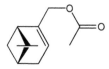

Synonym: 2-Pinen-10-yl acetate
Systematic name: (1R)-6,6-Dimethylbicyclo[3.1.1]hept-2-en-2-ylmethyl ethanoate
Chemical class: Bicyclic monoterpenoid alkene ester
CAS number: 36203-31-3

Sources >1.0%:

Myrtle	0.1–21.1%
Valerian (European)	tr–9.1%
Lavender (Spanish)	2.0–4.3%
Thyme (thujanol CT)	4.0%
Thyme (geraniol CT)	2.0%

Adverse skin reactions: Tested at 10% on 26 volunteers myrtenyl acetate was neither irritating nor sensitizing (Ford et al 1988a p. 297–298).

Acute toxicity: The acute oral LD_{50} in rats has been reported as between 1.0 and 2.5 g/kg and as 2.6 g/kg ; acute dermal LD_{50} in rabbits >5 g/kg (Ford et al 1988a p. 297–298).

Summary: Limited data suggest that myrtenyl acetate is non-irritant, non-allergenic and possesses only slight toxicity.

Nepetalactone

Synonym: 2-(2-Hydroxy-1-methylethenyl)-5-methylcyclopentanecarboxylic acid δ-lactone
Systematic name: 5,6,7,7a-Tetrahydro-4,7-dimethylcyclopenta[c]pyran-1(4aH)-one
Chemical class: Bicyclic monoterpenoid alkene lactone
Note: Different isomers of nepetalactone exist, and the following isomer-specific information has been published:

(Z,E)-Nepetalactone

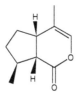

Synonyms: (4aα,7α,7aα)-Nepetalactone. *cis,trans*-Nepetalactone
CAS number: 21651-62-7

(E,Z)-Nepetalactone

Synonyms: (4aα,7α,7aβ)-Nepetalactone. *trans,cis*-Nepetalactone
CAS number: 17257-15-7

Source:

Catnip   12.7–84% (mixture of (Z,E)- and (E,Z)-isomers)

Pharmacokinetics: Following oral administration of ^{14}C-labelled (Z,E)-nepetalactone to domestic cats, 86–94% of the ^{14}C label was excreted in the urine, 1–2% in the feces, and 1–12% in the expelled air. The major metabolite (50–75%) was α-nepetalinic acid, which was excreted in the urine together with small amounts of dihydronepetalactone, unchanged nepetalactone, and several unidentified compounds (Waller et al 1969).
Acute toxicity: Mouse ip LD$_{50}$ 1.55 g/kg for nepetalactone, isomer not specified (Harney et al 1978).
Summary: Nothing useful can be deduced from the limited data available.

Nepetalic acid

Synonym: 2-Carboxy-α,3-dimethylcyclopentylethanal
Systematic name: 2-Methyl-5(1-methyl 2-oxoethyl)-cyclopentanecarboxylic acid
Chemical class: Monocyclic monoterpenoid aldehyde carboxylic acid
Note: Different isomers of nepetalic acid exist, and the following isomer-specific information has been published:

(R)-α-Nepetalic acid

CAS number: 21651-54-7

(S)-α-Nepetalic acid

CAS number: 32203-60-4

Source:

Catnip   1.2–43%

Acute toxicity: Mouse ip LD$_{50}$ 1.05 g/kg (isomer not specified) (Harney et al 1978).
Summary: Nothing useful can be deduced from the limited data available.

Neral

Synonyms: (Z)-Citral. *cis*-Citral. β-Citral. Citral b
Systematic name: (2Z)-3,7-Dimethyl-2,6-octadienal
Chemical class: Aliphatic monoterpenoid alkene aldehyde
CAS number: 106-26-3
Note: Neral is an isomer of geranial, and a component of citral.

Sources >1.0%:

Myrtle (lemon)	32.0–40.9%
Lemongrass (East Indian)	30.1–36.1%
Lemongrass (West Indian)	25.0–35.2%
May chang	25.5–33.8%
Tea tree (lemon-scented)	31.3%
Verbena (lemon)	22.9–29.6%
Myrtle (honey)	29.0%
Melissa	9.7–26.1%
Lemon leaf	6.5–25.3%
Basil (lemon)	16.0–17.1%
Lemon balm (Australian)	7.7%
Thyme (lemon)	7.1%
Bergamot (wild)	1.4–2.0%
Lemon (expressed)	0.4–2.0%
Lemon (distilled)	0.5–1.5%
Lime (expressed, Mexican)	1.4%
African bluegrass	0.1–1.4%
Orange (sweet)	<1.3%
Lime (expressed, Persian)	0.5–1.2%
Geranium	0–1.1%

Adverse skin reactions: In 20 eczema patients suspected of suffering from contact sensitization to cosmetics, there were no reactions to 1% neral on patch testing. Of 182 dermatitis patients suspected of contact allergy to cosmetics, 2.6% (presumably either four or five) tested positive to 1% neral (Malten et al 1984).
Summary: We could find no toxicity data for neral but see Citral, of which neral is a naturally-occurring constituent.

Nerol

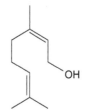

Synonyms: (Z)-Geraniol. *cis*-Geraniol
Systematic name: (2Z)-3,7-Dimethyl-2,6-octadien-1-ol
Chemical class: Aliphatic monoterpenoid alkene alcohol
CAS number: 106-25-2
Note: Isomeric with geraniol and linalool
Sources >1.0%:

Basil (lemon)	13.0–15.3%
Helichrysum italicum subsp. *microphyllum*	14.6%
Davana	10.0%
Rose (Damask)	0.8–8.7%
Lemon leaf	1.3–7.4%
Orange flower absolute	0.9–4.0%
Orange flower & leaf water absolute	3.7%
Helichrysum angustifolium	2.6–3.4%
Wormwood (sabinyl acetate CT)	3.2%
Orange flower water absolute	3.0%
Rose absolute (Provencale)	0–3.0%
Myrtle (honey)	2.8%
Lemon balm (Australian)	1.9%
Thyme (lemon)	1.9%
Ghandi root	1.4%
Bergamot (wild)	0.8–1.4%
Melissa	0.6–1.3%
Neroli	0.3–1.3%
Geranium	0–1.2%
Orange leaf (bigarade)	0.4–1.1%
May chang	0.2–1.1%
Wormwood ((Z)-epoxy ocimene CT)	0.5–1.0%

Pharmacokinetics: Approximately 25–30% of an oral dose of 17–55 g nerol (given to an unstated species in 2–10 g daily doses) was recovered as a pair of dicarboxylic acids. These were supposedly formed via an intermediate diol resulting from oxidation of one of the allylic methyl groups. Some nerol was also recovered as the glucuronide (Scheline 1991 p. 34).

Adverse skin reactions: Nerol was moderately irritating when applied undiluted to rabbit skin, but was neither irritating nor sensitizing when tested at 4% on 25 volunteers (Opdyke 1976 p. 623–624). In a worldwide multicenter study, of 218 dermatitis patients with proven sensitization to fragrance materials, 13 (6.0%) were sensitive to 5% nerol (Larsen et al 2002). In an in vitro assay, nerol was non-phototoxic (Placzek et al 2007).

Acute toxicity: Acute oral LD_{50} in rats 4.5 g/kg; acute dermal LD_{50} in rabbits >/kg (Opdyke 1976 p. 623–624).

Inhalation toxicity: When mice were exposed for one minute to nerol vapors, the dose causing a 25% reduction in respiratory rate (irritation) was 591 µg/L (Lapczynski et al 2008i).

Reproductive toxicity: Using chick embryos at 72 hours of incubation, Forschmidt (1979) determined that nerol had a teratogenic value of 11.9% relative to a control value of 7.9%. The implications of these data for humans are unknown. Since nerol is an isomer of linalool, their degree of reproductive toxicity may be very similar. When gavage doses of linalool were given to pregnant rats at 250, 500 or 1,000 mg/kg/day, on gestational days 7–17, no fetal toxicity or teratogenicity was seen at any dose. Since there was some maternal increase in relative body weight and feed consumption in the high dose group, the NOAEL for maternal toxicity was 500 mg/kg/day (Politano et al 2008).

Summary: Nerol possesses minimal irritancy, allergenicity and acute toxicity.

Nerolidol

Synonym: Peruviol
Systematic name: 3,7,11-Trimethyl-1,6,10-dodecatrien-3-ol
Chemical class: Aliphatic sesquiterpenoid alkene alcohol
Note: Different isomers of nerolidol exist, and the following isomer-specific information has been published:

(R,E)-Nerolidol
CAS number: 77551-75-8

(R,Z)-Nerolidol
CAS number: 132958-73-7

(S,E)-Nerolidol
CAS number: 1119-38-6

(S,Z)-Nerolidol
CAS number: 142-50-7

Sources >1.0%:

(E)-Nerolidol

Niaouli (nerolidol CT)	75.7–92.5%
Niaouli (linalool CT)	61.1%
Siam wood	35.5%
Cedrela	8.0%
Niaouli (viridiflorol CT)	3.0–6.0%
Balsam poplar	5.8%
Neroli	1.3–4.0%
Fern (sweet)	3.7%
Cardamon	0.1–2.7%
Chaste tree leaf	0–2.5%
Southernwood	2.2%
Sandalwood (W. Australian)	0–2.2%
Ambrette	0.1–2.0%
Spikenard	1.9%
Myrtle (bog)	1.5%
Amyris	0.4–1.1%

(Z)-Nerolidol

Cabreuva	65–80%

Nerolidol (isomer not specified)

Vassoura	20.0–30.0%
Orange flower absolute	0–7.6%
Cubeb	1.4–3.5%
Bakul absolute	3.2%

Ho leaf (linalool CT)	0.5–3.2%
Lantana	2.3%
Damiana	2.2%
Honeysuckle absolute	2.2%
Boswellia serrata	0–2.1%
Peru balsam	2.0%

Pharmacokinetics: In an uptake study using human skin, 39.6% of the nerolidol applied was found in the stratum corneum (Cornwell et al 1996).

Adverse skin reactions: In a modified Draize procedure on guinea pigs, nerolidol was non-sensitizing when used at 20% in the challenge phase (Sharp 1978). Undiluted nerolidol was not irritating when applied to rabbit skin, and was neither irritating nor sensitizing when tested at 4% on 25 volunteers (Opdyke 1975 p. 887). Of 102 dermatitis patients sensitive to Peru balsam, three tested positive to 1% nerolidol (Hausen 2001).

Acute toxicity: Acute oral LD_{50} in rats >5 g/kg; acute dermal LD_{50} in rabbits >5 g/kg (Opdyke 1975 p. 887).

Reproductive toxicity: In an ex vivo assay, nerolidol did not bind to estrogen receptors in female rat uterus tissue (Blair et al 2000).

Mutagenicity and genotoxicity: Neither (Z)-nerolidol nor mixed isomer nerolidol was mutagenic in *S. typhimurium* strains TA98 and TA100 with or without S9 (Gonçalves et al 2011). Nerolidol was weakly genotoxic in mouse peripheral blood leucocytes and hepatocytes, and was genotoxic in a mouse micronucleus test (Piculo et al 2011).

Carcinogenic/anticarcinogenic potential: The proliferation of mouse B16 melanoma cells was very weakly inhibited by nerolidol with an IC_{50} value of 65 mM (14.4 g/L) (Tatman & Huanbiao 2002). Nerolidol exhibited moderate in vitro cytotoxicity against two human carcinoma cell lines (Kubo & Morimitsu 1995) and significantly inhibited colon carcinogenesis induced by azoxymethane in male F344 rats (Wattenberg 1991). (Z)-Nerolidol was cytotoxic to human leukemia HL60 cells with an IC_{50} of 29.47 µg/mL (Nibret & Wink 2010).

Summary: Nerolidol is non-irritating, non-allergenic, non-toxic and non-estrogenic, and has demonstrated anticarcinogenic activity.

Neryl acetate

Synonym: Acetic acid neryl ester
Systematic name: (Z)-3,7-Dimethyl-2,6-octadien-1-yl ethanoate
Chemical class: Aliphatic monoterpenoid alkene ester
CAS number: 141-12-8

Sources >1.0%:

Helichrysum angustifolium	34.5–39.9%
Helichrysum italicum subsp. microphyllum	38.6%
Fenugreek	17.3%
Lemon leaf	3.7–7.4%
Helichrysum italicum	6.1%
Melissa	1.5–4.0%

Orange flower absolute	0.8–4.0%
Orange leaf (Paraguayan)	2.1–3.0%
Orange leaf (bigarade)	0–2.6%
Linaloe wood	2.5%
Neroli	0.3–2.1%
Wormwood (β-thujone / (Z)-epoxy ocimene CT)	0.4–2.1%
Lemon balm (Australian)	1.6%
Lemon (expressed)	0.1–1.5%
Bergamot (expressed)	0.1–1.2%
Skimmia	1.1%
Orange leaf absolute	1.0%

Adverse skin reactions: Not irritating when applied full-strength to rabbit skin. Neither irritating nor sensitizing when tested at 10% on 25 volunteers (Opdyke 1976 p. 625).

Acute toxicity: Acute oral LD_{50} in rats >5 g/kg; acute dermal LD_{50} in rabbits >5 g/kg (Opdyke 1976 p. 625).

Summary: Limited data suggest that neryl acetate is non-irritant, non-allergenic and non-toxic.

Neryl isobutyrate

Synonym: Isobutyric acid neryl ester
Systematic name: (2Z)-3,7-Dimethyl-2,6-octadien-1-yl 2-methylpropanoate
Chemical class: Aliphatic monoterpenoid alkene ester
CAS number: 2345-26-8

Sources >1.0%:

Wormwood (sabinyl acetate CT)	2.6%
Wormwood (β-thujone CT)	0–1.4%
Wormwood ((Z)-epoxy ocimene CT)	0.5–1.1%

Adverse skin reactions: Undiluted neryl isobutyrate produced slight irritant effects in rabbits patch-tested for 24 hours under occlusion. Tested at 5% on the skin of human subjects, it was neither irritating nor sensitizing (Ford et al 1988a p. 391).

Acute toxicity: Acute oral LD_{50} in rats >5 g/kg; acute dermal LD_{50} in rabbits >5 g/kg (Ford et al 1988a p. 391).

Summary: Limited data suggest that neryl isobutyrate is non-irritant, non-allergenic and non-toxic.

Neryl isovalerate

Synonym: Isovaleric acid neryl ester
Systematic name: (2Z)-3,7-Dimethyl-2,6-octadien-1-yl 3-methylbutanoate
Chemical class: Aliphatic monoterpenoid alkene ester
CAS number: 3915-83-1

Sources >1.0%:

Wormwood (sabinyl acetate CT)	9.1%
Wormwood ((Z)-epoxy ocimene CT)	1.6–2.2%
Wormwood (β-thujone/(Z)-epoxy ocimene CT)	1.0–1.1%

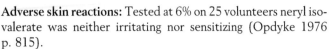

Adverse skin reactions: Tested at 6% on 25 volunteers neryl iso-valerate was neither irritating nor sensitizing (Opdyke 1976 p. 815).

Acute toxicity: Acute oral LD_{50} in rats >5 g/kg, acute dermal LD_{50} in rabbits >5 g/kg (Opdyke 1976 p. 815).

Summary: Limited data suggest that neryl isovalerate is non-irritant, non-allergenic and non-toxic.

Neryl propionate

Synonyms: Propionic acid neryl ester. Neryl propanoate
Systematic name: (2Z)-3,7-Dimethyl-2,6-octadien-1-yl propanoate
Chemical class: Aliphatic monoterpenoid alkene ester
CAS number: 105-91-9

Sources >1.0%:
Helichrysum angustifolium	4.8–6.7%
Helichrysum italicum subsp. microphyllum	1.8%

Adverse skin reactions: The undiluted material produced mild irritant effects in rabbits patch-tested for 24 hours under occlusion. Tested at 6% on the skin of human subjects, neryl propionate was neither irritant nor sensitizing (Opdyke 1976 p. 629).

Acute toxicity: Acute oral LD_{50} in rats >5 g/kg; acute dermal LD_{50} in rabbits >5 g/kg (Opdyke 1976 p. 629).

Summary: Limited data suggest that neryl propionate is non-irritant, non-allergenic and non-toxic.

2-Nonanone

Synonym: Methyl heptyl ketone
Chemical class: Aliphatic ketone
CAS number: 821-55-6

Sources >1.0%:
Rue	18.0–24.7%
Sugandha	1.9%

Pharmacokinetics: 2-Nonanone has been identified as a component of normal human urine (Ford et al 1988a p. 393).

Adverse skin reactions: Tested at 5% on human subjects 2-nonanone was neither irritating nor sensitizing (Ford et al 1988a p. 393).

Acute toxicity: Both the acute oral LD_{50} in rats and the acute dermal LD_{50} in rabbits exceeded 5 g/kg (Ford et al 1988a p. 393).

Summary: 2-Nonanone appears to possess minimal irritancy, allergenicity and acute toxicity.

Nootkatone

Synonym: 1(10),11-Eremophiladien-2-one
Systematic name: 1,2,3,5,6,7,8,8a-Octahydro-1,8a-dimethyl-7-(1-methylethenyl)-naphthalene-3-one
Chemical class: Bicyclic sesquiterpenoid alkene ketone
CAS number: 4674-50-4

Sources >0.1%:
Grapefruit	0.1–0.8%
Bergamot	0.01–0.1%

Pharmacokinetics: The metabolic pathway of nootkatone in rabbits is via epoxidation of the isopropenyl group followed by hydration. Six male rabbits with an average body weight of 2.5 kg were given 2 g nootkatone orally in suspension. Two urinary metabolites were identified, (+)-nootkatone-13,14-diol, the major metabolite, constituted ~35% of the neutral metabolites, and (+)-nootkatone-13,14-diol monoacetate (Asakawa et al 1986).

Adverse skin reactions: Nootkatone was not irritating when applied at a concentration of 10% to three groups of healthy human volunteers, 25, 25 and 28 in number. When tested on 25 healthy male and female volunteers a sample of 86% pure nootkatone elicited one sensitization reaction. A second sample of 86% pure nootkatone was tested at 10% on 28 male volunteers and elicited three sensitization reactions. A third sample, 98% pure, was not sensitizing at 10% in a group of 25 male and female volunteers (Letizia et al 2000 p. S165–167). Nootkatone with a purity of 86% is a potential skin sensitizer. However, this is counteracted when 1 part nootkatone is mixed with 4 parts limonene, and is not present when 98% pure nootkatone is used (IFRA 2009). Grapefruit oil consists of ~90% limonene and bergamot 27.4–52.0%.

Acute toxicity: Acute oral LD_{50} in rats >5 g/kg; acute dermal LD_{50} in rabbits >5 g/kg (Letizia et al 2000 p. S165–167).

Summary: Nootkatone of 86% purity was allergenic, while nootkatone of 98% purity was not. This might suggest that nootkatone, as it occurs in essential oils, is not allergenic. However, this conclusion is tentative since we do not know what the impurities are in each case.

β-Ocimene

Systematic name: 3,7-Dimethyl-1,3,6-octatriene
Chemical class: Aliphatic monoterpenoid polyalkene
Note: Different isomers of β-ocimene exist, and the following isomer-specific information has been published:

(3*E*)-β-Ocimene

Synonym: *trans*-β-Ocimene
CAS number: 3779-61-1

Sources >5.0%:
Jonquil absolute	35.3%
Opopanax	33.0%

Finger root	22.8%
Basil (pungent)	20.6%
Hemp	2.1–10.2%
Tarragon	tr–9.1%
Arina	7.0%
Neroli	4.6–7.0%
Lavandin Abrialis	3.0–7.0%
Blackcurrant bud absolute	0.6–6.7%
Basil (holy)	3.4–6.2%
Lavender	<5.0%

(3Z)-β-Ocimene

Synonym: *cis*-β-Ocimene
CAS number: 3338-55-4

Sources >5.0%:

Taget	16.6–69.8%
Celery leaf	14.1%
African bluegrass	10.3–11.5%
Tarragon	tr–9.5%
Lovage seed	9.2%
Lavender	<9.0%
Galangal (greater)	0–6.4%
Asafoetida	0–6.1%
Rhododendron	5.3%

β-Ocimene (isomer not specified)

Sources >5.0%:

| Jamrosa | 7.8% |

Adverse skin reactions: Undiluted mixed isomer ocimene was moderately irritating when applied to rabbit skin, but was neither irritating nor sensitizing when tested at 5% on 25 volunteers (Opdyke 1978 p. 829).
Acute toxicity: Mixed isomer ocimene acute oral LD_{50} in rats >5 g/kg; acute dermal LD_{50} in rabbits >5 g/kg (Opdyke 1978 p. 829).
Carcinogenic/anticarcinogenic potential: The proliferation of mouse B16 melanoma cells was very weakly inhibited by 'ocimene' with an IC_{50} value of 250 mM (34.0 g/L) (Tatman & Huanbiao 2002).
Summary: β-Ocimene appears to be non-irritant and non-allergenic. It is non-toxic.

3-Octanol

Synonyms: Octan-3-ol. Octanol-3. 3-*n*-Octanol. *n*-Octan-3-ol
Chemical class: Aliphatic alcohol
Note: Different isomers of 3-octanol exist, and the following isomer-specific information has been published:

(R)-3-Octanol

CAS number: 70492-66-9

(S)-3-Octanol

CAS number: 22658-92-0

Sources >1.0%:

Spearmint	0.6–2.6%
Cornmint	0.4–2.4%
Calamint (lesser)	1.0–2.1%
Pennyroyal (European)	0.6–2.0%
Bay (West Indian)	0.6–1.0%
Thyme (limonene CT)	1.0%

Note: Should not be confused with 1-octen-3-ol.
Adverse skin reactions: Tested at 12% on human volunteers, 3-octanol was neither irritant nor sensitizing. The undiluted material produced moderate irritant effects in rabbits patch-tested for 24 hours under occlusion (Opdyke 1979a p. 881).
Acute toxicity: Acute oral LD_{50} in rats >5 g/kg; acute dermal LD_{50} in rabbits >5 g/kg (Opdyke, 1979a p881).
Subacute and subchronic toxicity: Groups of ten male and ten female rats were administered 0, 25, 100 or 400 mg/kg of 3-octanol by gavage for 90 days. Relative liver weights of high-dose males were significantly elevated. Incidence of bile duct proliferation were increased in both males and females at the highest dosage level. Some degradation of kidney tissue occurred in males on 100 or 400 mg/kg doses. A NOAEL of 25 mg/kg in rats was established (Lindecrona et al 2003).
Comments: Increased hepatotoxicity from gavage dosing has been seen with other essential oil constituents, and the toxicity apparent here may be misleading.
Summary: 3-Octanol appears to be non-irritant and non-allergenic. It is non-toxic on acute dosing, and the rat 90 day NOAEL was 25 mg/kg.

1-Octen-3-yl acetate

Synonym: Acetic acid octenyl ester
Systematic name: 1-Octen-3-yl ethanoate
Chemical class: Aliphatic alkene ester
CAS number: 2442-10-6

Source:

| Lavender absolute | 1.1% |

Comments: We could find no record of skin sensitizing data in the public domain. The presence of 1-octen-3-yl acetate would appear to have negligible safety implications for essential oils, as far as skin sensitization goes.
Summary: 1-Octen-3-yl acetate may be skin allergenic (see Regulatory guidelines, below).
Regulatory guidelines: 1-Octen-3-yl acetate should not be used such that the level in finished cosmetic products exceeds 0.3% (SCCNFP 2001, IFRA 2009). IFRA further recommend that, for use in consumer products for which no skin contact is foreseeable under normal conditions of use, the level in the consumer product should not exceed 0.6%. This recommendation is based on test results of RIFM showing sensitization potential at 10% and no sensitization reaction when tested at 3% (private communication to IFRA; IFRA 2009).

Octyl acetate

Synonyms: *n*-Octyl acetate. *n*-Octanyl acetate. Acetic acid octyl ester
Systematic name: Octyl ethanoate
Chemical class: Aliphatic ester
CAS number: 112-14-1

Sources >1.0%:

Boswellia papyrifera	50.0–60.0%
Boswellia frereana	0–1.5%
Boswellia sacra (α-pinene CT)	0–1.5%

Adverse skin reactions: Octyl acetate was slightly irritating to rabbit skin when applied undiluted for 24 hours under occlusion. Tested at 8% on 24 volunteers the material was neither irritating nor sensitizing (Opdyke 1974 p. 815–816).
Acute toxicity: Acute oral LD_{50} in rats 3 g/kg; acute dermal LD_{50} in rabbits >5 g/kg (Opdyke 1974 p. 815–816).
Subacute and subchronic toxicity: In a gavage study, octyl acetate was administered to rats 5 days per week for 13 weeks at 100, 500 or 1,000 mg/kg/day. After 45 days of dosing several treatment-related effects were observed in the 1,000 mg/kg group. These included slight reductions in body weight and food consumption, increased liver and kidney weights, and evidence of hydrocarbon nephropathy in high-dose males only. With the exception of increased liver weights in the mid-dose group, no other significant treatment-related effects were observed in the mid- or low-dose groups. It is believed that the increases in liver weight were a compensatory response to an increased metabolic load, and not a reflection of true hepatotoxicity (Daughtrey et al 1989a).
Reproductive toxicity: Octyl acetate was administered via oral gavage to pregnant Sprague–Dawley rats on gestational days 6–15 at 0, 100, 500, and 1,000 mg/kg. The mid- and high-doses resulted in maternal toxicity as evidenced by reductions in body weight gain and food consumption. There were no statistically significant effects on embryo-fetal lethality or fetal growth for any treatment group. The number of litters with at least one malformed fetus and the mean percentage of the litter malformed were significantly elevated in the high-dose group only. Octyl acetate produced some evidence of developmental toxicity at a dose (1,000 mg/kg) that was maternally toxic. Developmental toxicity was not observed at the maternally toxic 500 mg/kg dose or the maternally non-toxic dose (100 mg/kg). It was determined that octyl acetate was not a selective developmental toxicant in rats (Daughtrey et al 1989b).
Comment: Both the subchronic and reproductive toxicity data point to a NOAEL of 100 mg/kg/day.
Summary: Octyl acetate appears to be non-irritant and non-allergenic, and it possesses minimal acute toxicity. The rat NOAEL for reproductive toxicity was 100 mg/kg.

Oxypeucedanin

Synonym: Prangolarin
Systematic name: 4-(2,3-Epoxy-3-methylbut-2-enoxy)-7*H*-furo[3,2-*g*][1]benzopyran-7-one
Chemical class: Tetracyclic furanocoumarin ether epoxide

Note: Different isomers of oxypeucedanin exist, and the following isomer-specific information has been published:

(*R*)-(+)-Oxypeucedanin

CAS number: 3173-02-2

(*S*)-(−)-Oxypeucedanin

CAS number: 26091-73-6

Sources >0.01%:

Lemon (expressed)	0.09–0.82%
Lime (expressed)	0.02–0.3%

Adverse skin reactions: Oxypeucedanin elicited photopigmentation on colored-guinea pig skin, and its phototoxic potency is about 25% of that of bergapten (Naganuma et al 1985). Oral oxypeucedanin was photosensitive to 2-week-old broiler chicks (Egyed & Williams 1977).
Hepatotoxicity: In rats receiving 100 mg/kg/day oxypeucedanin ip for 8 weeks, there were no hepatic lesions, changes in hepatic enzyme activity, reduced glutathione or DNA concentrations (Emerole et al 1981).
Mutagenicity and genotoxicity: Oxypeucedanin was not mutagenic in the Ames test (Uwaifo 1984).
Carcinogenic/anticarcinogenic potential: Oxypeucedanin dose-dependently inhibited in vitro proliferation of human cell lines for cancers of colon, lung, ovary, CNS and skin (melanoma) (Kim YK et al 2007).
Comments: Oxypeucedanin has not been studied for photomutagenicity or photocarcinogenicity.
Summary: Oxypeucedanin is phototoxic. It does not appear to be mutagenic, though it may be photomutagenic. It is not hepatotoxic in rats.
Regulatory guidelines: For tanning products, the SCCNFP set a maximum of 1 ppm for 'furocoumarin-like substances' in 1995, later reviewed and confirmed (SCCNFP 2003b). This has now been extended to apply to all cosmetic products, and specifically includes isopimpinellin (SCCP 2005b).

Pentadecanolide

Synonyms: 15-Pentadecanolide. Cyclopentadecanolide
Systematic name: 15-Hydroxypentadecanoic acid, ξ-lactone
Chemical class: Monocyclic sesquiterpenoid lactone
CAS number: 106-02-5

Source:

Angelica root	0.4–2.4%

Adverse skin reactions: Tested at 10% on human subjects pentadecanolide was neither irritating nor sensitizing. The compound is not phototoxic (Opdyke 1975 p. 787).
Acute toxicity: The acute oral LD_{50} in rats exceeded 5 g/kg (Opdyke 1975 p. 787).
Summary: Pentadecanolide appears to possess minimal irritancy, allergenicity and acute toxicity.

Perilla ketone

Synonym: β-Furyl isoamyl ketone
Systematic name: 1-(3-Furanyl)-4-methyl-1-pentanone
Chemical class: Furanoid monoterpenoid ketone
CAS number: 553-84-4

Sources: Found as the principal constituent of some perilla oils.
Acute toxicity: Intraperitoneal LD_{50} was 6 mg/kg in male mice, 10 mg/kg in male rats. A single iv injection of 19 mg/kg in a male sheep was followed by respiratory distress on day 3, and capillary congestion in the lungs (Wilson et al 1977). It is not clear whether perilla ketone (and hence perilla oil) represents a hazard to humans. Perilla ketone is a highly potent lung toxin to laboratory animals, and it often poisons grazing cattle that eat perilla leaves (Wilson et al 1977; Wilson 1979).
Comments: Perilla oil is used as a flavor ingredient in Japan, and no reports linking its use with pulmonary conditions in humans have as yet been noted (Wilson 1979).
Summary: Perilla ketone appears to possess considerable acute toxicity.

Perillaldehyde

Synonyms: Perilla aldehyde. Perillyl aldehyde. *p*-Mentha-1,8-dien-7-al
Systematic name: 4-(1-Methylethenyl)-1-cyclohexene-1-carboxaldehyde
Chemical class: Monocyclic monoterpenoid alkene aldehyde
Note: Different isomers of perillaldehyde exist, and the following isomer-specific information has been published:

(S)-(−)-Perillaldehyde

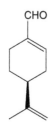

CAS number: 18031-40-8

Sources >1.0%:

Perilla   86.8%

(R)-(+)-Perillaldehyde

CAS number: 5503-12-8

Pharmacokinetics: The urine of rabbits orally dosed with 0.7–0.8 g/kg perillaldehyde contained mainly carboxylic acids including perillic acid, resulting from oxidation. Traces of aromatic acids, including cumic acid, were also detected, along with small amounts of alcoholic reduction products (Scheline 1991 p. 87).

Adverse skin reactions: Undiluted perillaldehyde was moderately irritating to guinea pig skin; tested at 1% and 4% it was not irritating to three separate panels of volunteers. In a maximation test at 4%, there were three questionable reactions; tested at 4% on a different panel, there were 2/29 sensitization reactions; tested at 1% on a further panel of 25, there were no reactions (Opdyke 1982 p. 799–800).
Acute toxicity: Acute oral LD_{50} in mice 1.72 g/kg; acute dermal LD_{50} in guinea pigs >5 g/kg (Opdyke 1982 p. 799–800).
Antioxidant/pro-oxidant activity: Perillaldehyde inhibits hydrogen peroxide-induced cytotoxicity and activates the antioxidant responsive element (ARE), which regulates important cellular antioxidants (Masutani et al 2009).
Mutagenicity and genotoxicity: (−)-Perillaldehyde was not mutagenic in the Ames test but produced CA in Chinese hamster fibroblasts (Ishidate et al 1984). In micronucleus tests in mice, (−)-perillaldehyde was not genotoxic (Hayashi et al 1988).
Carcinogenic/anticarcinogenic potential: The proliferation of mouse B16(F10) melanoma cells was inhibited by perillaldehyde with an IC_{50} value of 120 μM (18.0 mg/L) (He et al 1997b). Perillaldehyde dose- and time-dependently inhibited cell proliferation in human BroTo (head and neck cancer) and A549 lung cancer cells (Elegbede et al 2003). Perillaldehyde is capable of inducing apoptosis in cancer cells (Boon et al 2000).
Comments: (−)-Perillaldehyde is said to be 2,000 times sweeter than sucrose, and is used as a sweetening agent in Japan.
Summary: Perillaldehyde appears to be non-irritant, but possesses a degree of allergenicity and is restricted by IFRA. There are conflicting mutagenicity data for (−)-perillaldehyde. Perillaldehyde possesses antioxidant and anticarcinogenic activity.
Regulatory guidelines: IFRA recommends a maximum use level of 0.1% of perillaldehyde in most topical product types due to sensitization potential. This is based on an estimated maximum NOAEL of 700 μg/cm^2 (IFRA 2009).
Our safety advice: The IFRA NOAEL is equivalent to 7% for topical application. Exactly how IFRA derives 0.1% from 7% is not clear, but since there are no clinical data recording adverse effects from either perillaldehyde or perilla oil, we see no need to impose any restriction, especially one derived from multiple assumptions.

Perillyl alcohol

Synonyms: Perilla alcohol. Perillic alcohol. *p*-Mentha-1,8-dien-7-ol. Isocarveol
Systematic name: 4-(1-Methylethenyl)-1-cyclohexene-1-methanol
Chemical class: Monocyclic monoterpenoid alkene alcohol
Note: Different isomers of perillyl alcohol exist, and the following isomer-specific information has been published:

(R)-Perillyl alcohol

CAS number: 57717-97-2

(S)-Perillyl alcohol

CAS number: 18457-55-1

Sources >1.0%:

Perilla   5.4%

Pharmacokinetics: Perillyl alcohol, like limonene, is rapidly metabolized to perillic acid, dihydroperillic acid (DHPA), and lesser amounts of their methyl esters in both rats and humans (Crowell et al 1994a; Haag & Gould 1994). Both (Z)-DHPA and (E)-DHPA are found in equal amounts in rats and humans, as is a small amount of unchanged perillyl alcohol (Zhang et al 1999). Perillaldehyde is a major intermediary metabolite (Boon et al 2000).

Adverse skin reactions: On patch testing 25 volunteers, 4% perillyl alcohol was neither irritating nor sensitizing (RIFM 1977, cited in Bhatia et al 2008a). In a phase 1 trial for skin cancer, 0.76% w/w perillyl alcohol applied twice daily for 30 days produced no cutaneous or systemic toxicity in 25 subjects (Stratton et al 2008).

Acute toxicity: Perillyl alcohol acute oral LD_{50} in rats, 2.1 g/kg; acute dermal LD_{50} in rabbits, >5 g/kg (RIFM 1977, cited in Bhatia et al 2008a). Perillyl alcohol mouse ip MTD 75 mg/kg; 1 g/kg ip is lethal in mice (Lantry et al 1997).

Subacute and subchronic toxicity: In a six week assay, the dietary MTD for perillyl alcohol in rats was 2.5 g/kg (Reddy et al 1997).

Human toxicity: In five phase I clinical trials, perillyl alcohol was administered orally to a total of 92 cancer patients, in divided doses ranging from 1,200 to 8,400 mg/m^2 per day. (This refers to body surface area, which is often used to calculate doses for cancer drugs; these doses are equivalent to approximately 31–218 mg/kg po.) Treatment duration varied with each patient, but was generally between 2 and 9 months. Nausea is cited as a side effect in all five trials, vomiting or gastrointestinal distress in three, and fatigue in four. In three of the trials, the side effects were dose-limiting (Ripple et al 1998, 2000; Hudes et al 2000; Murren et al 2002; Bailey et al 2004). In four phase II clinical trials (colorectal, ovarian, breast and prostate cancers), oral doses of 1,200 mg/m^2 four times daily were not well tolerated, with fatigue and gastrointestinal symptoms often being dose-limiting. In all nine trials, clinical antitumor activity was only evident in a single patient, with metastatic colorectal cancer, possibly because therapeutic doses could not be acheived (Bailey et al 2002, 2008; Meadows et al 2002; Liu et al 2003). In a pilot study of pancreatic cancer patients, perillyl alcohol was administered orally at 1,200 mg/m^2 four times daily for 15 days. This shorter duration of therapy was tolerated slightly better than the above protocols, but gastrointestinal symptoms were still prevalent (Matos et al 2008).

Cardiovascular effects: In a clinical trial for the treatment of progessive brain cancer, 55 mg perillyl alcohol (0.3% v/v) was administered intranasally four times a day for 6 months or longer. Hematological and non-hematological parameters were monitored weekly. There were no clinical signs of toxicity, and laboratory tests remained normal (Da Fonseca et al 2008).

Mutagenicity and genotoxicity: Perillyl alcohol prevented DMBA-DNA binding in MCF-7 cells through inhibition of CYP1B1 activity (Chan et al 2006).

Carcinogenic/anticarcinogenic potential: Perillyl alcohol inhibits the activation of the tobacco-specific carcinogen NNK in mouse pulmonary and hepatic microsomes (Morse &

Toburen 1996) and demonstrates chemopreventive efficacy in a mouse lung assay (Lantry et al 1997), a rat colon assay (Reddy et al 1997), a mouse melanoma model (Lluria-Prevatt et al 2002) and a mouse photocarcinogenesis model (Barthelman et al 1998). The compound induced the regression of 81% of small rat mammary carcinomas and 75% of advanced mammary carcinomas initiated by DMBA (Haag & Gould 1994). Liver tumors in rats were significantly inhibited by perillyl alcohol, due to a 10-fold increase in apoptosis (Mills et al 1995). Hamster pancreatic tumors were reduced to less than half that of controls by perillyl alcohol administration, and 16% of tumors completely regressed (Stark et al 1995).

Perillyl alcohol inhibited the in vitro growth of four types of human breast cancer cells (KPL-1, MCF-7, MLK-F and MDS-MB-231), and suppressed cell growth and metastasis in vivo (Yuri et al 2004). It also inhibited the in vitro proliferation of the human head and neck cancer cells BroTo and SCC-25, and of the human lung carcinoma cells HTB-182 and CRL-5928 (Samaila et al 2004). Perillyl alcohol induced apoptosis in human BroTo and A549 (lung cancer) cells, inhibiting cell proliferation by 50% at concentrations of 1 and 2 mM (152 and 304 mg/L), respectively (Elegbede et al 2003). Apoptosis in human glioblastoma multiforme (brain tumor) cells was induced by perillyl alcohol (Fernandes et al 2005). A culture of LNCaP, a type of human prostate cancer cell, was treated with perillyl alcohol, which inhibited androgen-induced cell growth and androgen-stimulated secretion of prostate-specific antigen (Chung et al 2006).

The proliferation of mouse B16 melanoma cells was very weakly inhibited by perillyl alcohol with an IC_{50} value of 250 mM (38.0 g/L) (Tatman & Huanbiao 2002). Perillyl alcohol induced apoptosis and dose-dependently inhibited proliferation by 15% to 83% in the human lung cancer cells H322 and H838. It is suggested that the compound may be most useful in combination therapy for lung cancer, sensitizing cells to DNA damage by stimulating caspase-3 activity (Xu et al 2004). Perillyl alcohol inhibited colon cancer (HCT 116) cell proliferation, with an IC_{50} of 0.5 mM (76.0 mg/L), by regulating the expression of cell-cycle proteins (Bardon et al 2002).

Comments: Perillyl alcohol is a metabolite of limonene, and is thought to be a more potent anticarcinogenic agent. Because perillyl alcohol inhibited UVB-induced tumorigenesis in mice, it is being considered as a potential chemopreventive agent in skin cancer (Barthelman et al 1998; Stratton et al 2000). It is often cited anecdotally as a constituent of lavender oil, but we could find no analysis of lavender oil listing perillyl alcohol.

Summary: Perillyl alcohol appears to be non-irritant and non-allergenic. In a clinical trial, a total daily inhalation of 220 mg perillyl alcohol was non-toxic. In clinical trials, daily oral doses of 31 mg/kg or more often caused fatigue or gastrointestinal symptoms.

α-Phellandrene

Synonym: *p*-Mentha-1,5-diene
Systematic name: 2-Methyl-5-(1-methylethyl)-1,3-cyclo-hexadiene

Chemical class: Monocyclic monoterpenoid alkene
Note: Different isomers of α-phellandrene exist, and the following isomer-specific information has been published:

(5R)-(−)-α-Phellandrene

CAS number: 4221-98-1

(5S)-(+)-α-Phellandrene

CAS number: 2243-33-6

Sources >5.0%:

Turmeric leaf	53.4%
Boswellia sacra (α-pinene CT)	0–41.8%
Dill weed	18.2–30.2%
Angelica root	7.5–20.0%
Pepper (pink)	5.3–17.3%
Eucalyptus dives	16.9%
Elemi	4.3–15.1%
Turmeric rhizome	0.7–12.8%
Goldenrod	11.9%
Turpentine	0–8.0%
Lemon balm (Australian)	7.1%
Dill seed (Indian)	tr–6.5%
Boswellia frereana	0–5.9%
Nutmeg (E. Indian)	0.4–5.8%
Peta	5.5%

Pharmacokinetics: α-Phellandrene is metabolized in sheep along at least two pathways. One of these entails reduction and oxidation to give phellandric and phellanduric acids, and the other involves hydroxylation and glucuronide conjugation. Both *p*-cymene and carvotanacetone are found in the conjugate (Scheline 1991).

Adverse skin reactions: α-Phellandrene has been reported as a skin irritant (Budavari et al 1989). Undiluted α-phellandrene was moderately irritating to rabbit skin; tested at 4% and 8% on 25 volunteers it was not irritating. Tested at 8% it was not sensitizing; a 4% concentration produced one positive reaction in 25 volunteers, thought to be due to autoxidation of the compound (Opdyke 1978 p. 843–844). Tested at 5%, α-phellandrene was sensitizing to 4 of 11 dermatitis patients sensitized to tea tree oil (Hausen et al 1999).

Acute toxicity: Acute oral LD_{50} in rats 5.7 g/kg; acute dermal LD_{50} in rabbits >5 g/kg (Opdyke 1978 p. 843–844). Budavari et al (1989) report that ingestion of α-phellandrene can cause vomiting and diarrhea, but no details are given and this sounds like a reponse to an oral overdose.

Mutagenicity and genotoxicity: '*l*-Phellandrene' was not genotoxic in Chinese hamster ovary cells (Sasaki et al 1989).

Carcinogenic/anticarcinogenic potential: α-Phellandrene has been reported to promote tumor formation on the skin of mice treated with the primary carcinogen DMBA, but is not carcinogenic in its own right (Roe & Field 1965).

Summary: α-Phellandrene presents minimal risk of irritation sensitization or toxicity.

2-Phenylethanol

Synonyms: Phenyl ethanol. Phenethyl alcohol. β-Phenylethyl alcohol. Benzyl carbinol
Systematic name: 2-Phenylethanol
Chemical class: Benzenoid alcohol
CAS number: 60-12-8

Sources >1.0%:

Rose absolute (Provencale)	64.8–73.0%
Bakul absolute	38.8%
Orange flower absolute	4.5–35.0%
Champaca absolute (orange)	25.0–34.0%
Champaca absolute (white)	6.4%
Hyacinth absolute	3.7%
Jasmine sambac absolute	2.4%
Osmanthus absolute	tr–2.2%
Rose (Damask)	0.3–2.0%
Narcissus absolute	0–1.6%

Pharmacokinetics: In rabbits ~7% of the amount ingested was excreted combined with glucuronic acid, and ~3% is excreted as hippuric acid. Large amounts are oxidized to phenylacetic acid which is conjugated with glycine and excreted as phenaceturic acid (Scheline 1991). Toxicity data for phenylacetic acid may therefore also be relevant.

Adverse skin reactions: Undiluted 2-phenylethanol was slightly irritating to the skin of guinea pigs, but not to the skin of 25 volunteers; tested at 8% it was not sensitizing in 25 volunteers (Opdyke 1975 p. 903–904). There was one reaction (0.6%) to 25% 2-phenylethanol in 179 dermatitis patients suspected of allergy to cosmetics (De Groot et al 1985). There were no irritant or allergic reactions in a group of 100 consecutive dermatitis patients tested with 1% 2-phenylethanol (Frosch et al 1995a).

Acute toxicity: Acute oral LD_{50} 1.79 g/kg in rats (Jenner et al 1964), 1.15 g/kg in mice and 600 mg/kg in guinea pigs; acute dermal LD_{50} guinea pigs 5–10 mL/kg (Opdyke 1975 p. 903–904). Rat acute oral LD_{50} also cited as 1.5, 1.7 and 1.8 g/kg (Adams et al 2005b).

Subacute and subchronic toxicity: In a 90 day dermal toxicity study, 2-phenylethanol was applied to the skin of male and female rats at 0.25, 0.5, 1.0 or 2.0 mL/kg/day. Weight gain was suppressed at the two higher doses, and there were decreases in hemoglobin concentration and white blood cell count in high dose males. Otherwise, there were no changes in blood or urine chemistry, and no gross or microscopic changes were seen in tissues examined, including the eyes. The dermal NOAEL was therefore 0.5 mL/kg/day (Owston & Lough 1981). This is equivalent to 35 mL in a 70 kg human.

Reproductive toxicity: Pregnant rats were fed a diet containing microencapsulated 2-phenylethanol at 1,000, 3,000 or 10,000 ppm during gestational days 6–15. Consumption was equivalent to doses of 83, 266 and 799 mg/kg. Maternal effects were limited to transient reduction in food consumption during the first two days in the high dose group. In the offspring, there was an increased incidence of incomplete calcification in the high dose group. There were no significant differences between control and treated groups in terms of implants, embryolethality, live young, litter weight, mean fetal weight or sex ratio. The NOAEL in this study was 266 mg/kg (Bottomley et al 1987, cited in Adams et al 2005a).

2-Phenylethanol was applied to the skin of pregnant rats on gestational days 6–15, at 0.14, 0.43 or 1.40 mL/kg. An occlusive bandage was used to prevent oral ingestion of the test substance, though this will also have increased transcutaneous absorption. Fetuses were examined on day 20. In the high dose group there was clear evidence of toxicity assessed as increased lethality, weight depression, and a range of soft tissue and skeletal changes. In the mid-dose group there was no evidence of an effect on litter values, but there were some adverse fetal effects. In the 0.14 mL/kg group there were marginal skeletal irregularities, and this was considered the 'threshold for developmental toxicity' in rats from dermal exposure (Palmer et al 1986, cited in Adams et al 2005a). This dose is equivalent to an adult human dermal dose of 9.8 mL.

Mutagenicity and genotoxicity: 2-Phenylethanol was not mutagenic in the Ames test (Florin et al 1980) and did not induce SCE in human whole-blood lymphocyte cultures (Norppa & Vaino 1983). Phenylacetic acid, the major metabolite, did not increase UDS in rat hepatocytes (Heck et al 1989).

Comments: 2-Phenylethanol appears to be relatively safe for dermal application.

Summary: 2-Phenylethanol presents minimal risk of irritation sensitization or toxicity. The rat NOAEL for reproductive toxicity was 266 mg/kg po. For dermal application, 0.14 mL/kg was considered the threshold for developmental toxicity in rats. 2-Phenylethanol is not mutagenic.

Regulatory guidelines: The CIR recommended maximum for 2-phenylethanol in cosmetics is 1%.

Our safety advice: For reproductive toxicity, we propose an oral dose limit of 2.7 mg/kg/day for 2-phenylethanol, based on the rat oral NOAEL of 266 mg/kg/day and an uncertainty factor of 100.

2-Phenylethyl acetate

Synonyms: β-Phenylethyl acetate. Phenethyl acetate. Acetic acid 2-phenylethyl ester
Systematic name: 2-Phenylethyl ethanoate
Chemical class: Benzenoid ester
CAS number: 103-45-7

Sources >1.0%:

Kewda	2.8–3.5%
Bakul absolute	2.6%
Champaca absolute (orange)	0.4–2.0%

Adverse skin reactions: Undiluted 2-phenylethyl acetate was slightly irritating to the skin of rabbits, when applied for 24 hours under occlusion, but not to the skin of 20 human volunteers. Tested at 10% it was not sensitizing in 25 volunteers (Opdyke 1974 p. 957–958).

Acute toxicity: Acute oral LD_{50} in rats reported as 3.7, 5.2, >5.0 g/kg and 3.2 mL/kg (Adams et al 2005a). Acute dermal LD_{50} 6.21 g/kg in rabbits (Opdyke 1974 p. 957–958).

Carcinogenic/anticarcinogenic potential: In male and female mice given 24 ip injections of 2-phenylethyl acetate in impure tricaprylin in a total dose of 1.2 or 6.0 g/kg over 20 weeks the incidence of primary lung tumors was no higher than in the control group (Stoner et al 1973).

Summary: 2-Phenylethyl acetate appears to be non-irritant, non-allergenic and non-toxic.

Phenylethyl isothiocyanate

Synonyms: 2-Phenylethyl isothiocyanate. β-Phenylethyl isothiocyanate. Phenethyl isothiocyanate. PEITC
Systematic name: (2-Isothiocyanatoethyl)benzene
Chemical class: Benzenoid thiocarbonyl compound
CAS number: 2257-09-2

Sources >1.0%:

Horseradish	38.4–51.3%
Mustard	2.4–5.0%

Note: Only produced when the root is crushed.

Pharmacokinetics: PEITC is metabolized to mercaptopyruvic acid and the N-acetylcysteine conjugate (Eklind et al 1990). Metabolism differs in experimental animals according to their age (Borghoff & Birnbaum 1986).

Mutagenicity and genotoxicity: PEITC caused CA in an Indian Muntjac cell line at concentrations which may imply a risk to humans even at dietary levels (Musk & Johnson 1993). Using human hepatoma G2 cell gel electrophoresis, no evidence could be found for a protective effect of PEITC against DNA damage caused by benzo[a]pyrene and (±)-anti-benzo[a]pyrene-7,8-dihydrodiol-9,10-epoxide (BPDE), its ultimate genotoxic metabolite. On the contrary, at 5 μM (815 μg/L) and above, PEITC itself caused DNA damage (Kassie et al 2003). However, the compound reduced NMBA-induced UDS in vivo in hamster buccal pouch mucosa when painted on at 0.5, 5.0, or 50 mM (81.5, 815 and 8,150 mg/L) (Solt et al 2003).

Carcinogenic/anticarcinogenic potential: In a male rat study, oral doses of >0.01% PEITC enhanced urinary bladder carcinogenesis, while weakly promoting hepatocarcinogenesis. It is suggested that >0.05% PEITC has tumorigenic potential (Ogawa et al 2001). Other work confirms that PEITC is a carcinogen for male rat urinary bladder, with the potential to give rise to non-papillary carcinomas with frequent p53 mutations (Hirose et al 1998; Sugiura et al 2003). Epithelial cell inflammation, due to cytotoxicity and irritation, leads to continuous cell proliferation, and this seems to play an important role in the early stages of carcinogenesis (Akagi et al 2003).

PEITC induced apoptosis in the PC-3, p53-deficient human prostate cancer cell line (Xiao & Singh 2002). It induced apoptosis of human leukemia HL60 and human myeloblastic leukemia ML-1 cells (Xu & Thornalley 2001). It also potently induced apoptosis and cell cycle arrest in HepG2 cells (Rose et al 2003).

PEITC protected rodents against nitrosamine-induced carcinogenesis (Chung et al 1984, 1992; Smith et al 1990) and F-344 rats and A/J mice against NNK-induced lung tumors (Wattenberg 1990; Hecht 1995). Consequently, it was proposed that the presence of PEITC in the diet may inhibit the development of preneoplastic lesions while having little effect on normal cells (Musk et al 1995). PEITC had a significant anticarcinogenic action in azoxymethane-induced colonic aberrant crypt foci in rats (Chung et al 2000). PEITC, used at 50 mM (8,150 mg/L), reduced hamster buccal pouch tumor formation induced by NMBA by 94% (Solt et al 2003).

Given by gavage to A/J mice at 0.3, 1.0 or 3.0 μmol/g (49, 163 or 489 μg/g), PEITC effectively inhibited lung tumorigenesis induced by 3 μmol (756 μg) benzo[a]pyrene, 3 μmol (621 μg) NNK or a combination of the two (3 μmol each), but not when benzo[a]pyrene was used alone. Dosing was started one week before, and continued through to one week after eight weekly treatments with the carcinogen(s). PEITC was also effective when given in combination with benzyl isothiocyanate, although PEITC was the more potent compound. Daily dosing in the diet gave more effective protection than weekly dosing by gavage (Hecht et al 2000). Similar results were obtained using the N-acetylcysteine conjugate of PEITC (Yang et al 2002).

Summary: PEITC has demonstrated both mutagenicity and antimutagenicity. It is carcinogenic to male rat bladder, but anticarcinogenic in prostate, colon and lung cancers. It is considered a promising candidate for cancer treatment.

Phenylethyl methyl ether

Synonyms: 2-Phenylethyl methyl ether. Methyl 2-phenylethyl ether
Systematic name: 1-Methoxy-2-phenylethane
Chemical class: Benzenoid ether
CAS number: 3558-60-9

Source:

Kewda	65.6–75.4%

Adverse skin reactions: Phenylethyl methyl ether was mildly irritating when applied undiluted to rabbit skin for 24 hours under occlusion, and was neither irritating nor sensitizing when tested at 8% on 25 volunteers (Opdyke 1982 p. 807).
Acute toxicity: Acute oral LD_{50} in rats 4.1 g/kg; acute dermal LD_{50} in rabbits 3.97 g/kg (Opdyke 1982 p. 807).
Summary: Phenylethyl methyl ether appears to be non-irritant, non-allergenic and non-toxic.

(E)-Phenylpropyl cinnamate

Synonyms: trans-3-Phenylpropyl cinnamate. trans-Cinnamic acid phenylpropyl ester
Systematic name: (E)-3-Phenylpropyl 3-phenylpropenoate
Chemical class: Phenylpropenoid ester
CAS number: 122-68-9

Source:

Styrax (American)	32.3%

Adverse skin reactions: (E)-Phenylpropyl cinnamate was not irritating when applied undiluted to rabbit skin., and was neither irritating nor sensitizing when tested at 4% on 25 volunteers (Opdyke 1974 p. 969).
Acute toxicity: Acute oral LD_{50} in rats >5 g/kg; acute dermal LD_{50} in rabbits >5 g/kg (Opdyke 1974 p. 969).
Summary: (E)-Phenylpropyl cinnamate appears to be non-irritant, non-allergenic and non-toxic.

Phytol

Synonym: 2-Phyten-1-ol
Systematic name: 3,7,11,15-Tetramethyl-2-hexadecen-1-ol
Chemical class: Aliphatic diterpenoid alkene alcohol
Notes: Phytol is ubiquitous in plants as an esterified component and decomposition product of chlorophyll, but it is not frequently found in essential oils. Different isomers of phytol exist, and the following isomer-specific information has been published:

(R,E)-Phytol

CAS number: 99265-64-2

Sources >1.0%:

Jasmine absolute	7.0–12.5%
Mugwort (common)	1.2%

Pharmacokinetics: In man phytol is metabolized in part to CO_2, phytanic acid detected in plasma (Steinberg et al 1966). There are numerous other metabolites (Scheline 1991).
Adverse skin reactions: Moderately irritating when applied undiluted to rabbit skin; neither irritating nor sensitizing when tested at 10% on 25 volunteers (Opdyke 1982 p. 811–815).
Acute toxicity: Acute oral LD_{50} in rats >5 g/kg; acute dermal LD_{50} in rabbits >5 g/kg (Opdyke 1982 p. 811–815).
Hepatotoxicity: People with Refsum's disease have an impaired ability to metabolize phytanic acid, which tends to accumulate in the plasma and tissues (Steinberg et al 1966). Refsum's disease is a rare recessive familial disorder caused by a deficiency of phytanic acid hydroxylase. It is characterized clinically by peripheral neuropathy, cerebellar ataxia, retinitis pigmentosa and bone and skin changes (Berkow & Fletcher 1992).

Phytanic acid accumulated in the livers and serum of rats, mice, chinchillas and rabbits fed 2% or 5% phytol in the diet for ~3 weeks. At the 5% level growth was retarded, livers appeared to be mottled, and ~50% of the rats died. At the 2% level hepatotoxicity and growth retardation were reduced but observable in all four species. There was no evidence of growth retardation or toxicity in rats fed 0.5% phytol in the diet for 15 months (Steinberg et al 1966). There are many other reports of phytanic accumulation in animals fed phytol (Opdyke 1982 p. 811–815).
Comment: Phytol is a decomposition product of chlorophyll, so people with Refsum's disease need to avoid chrorophyll-containing foods.
Summary: Phytol is only found in amounts over 1.2% in jasmine absolute, and this in turn is used in such small amounts it would not lead to any hepatotoxicity. Jasmine absolute is only used in external preparations, generally at less than 1%, which would mean a maximum of 0.13% of phytol being present. In a whole body massage using 30 mL of oil with jasmine absolute at 1% this would entail a maximum of 0.04 mL of phytol being applied to the

skin, not all of which will be absorbed. This means that very much less phytol would be absorbed than the dietary 0.5% found to cause no adverse effect in rats over 15 months. However, some caution may be appropriate in people with Refsum's disease.

α-Pinene

Synonym: 2-Pinene
Systematic name: 2,6,6-Trimethylbicyclo[3.1.1]hept-2-ene
Chemical class: Bicyclic monoterpenoid alkene
Note: Different isomers of α-pinene exist, and the following isomer-specific information has been published:

(1*R*)-(+)-α-Pinene

Synonym: Australene
CAS number: 7785-70-8

(1*S*)-(−)-α-Pinene

CAS number: 7785-76-4

Sources > 10.0%:

Turpentine	44.1–94.3%
Boswellia frereana	41.7–80.0%
Ferula	79.5%
Mastic	58.8–78.6%
Myrtle	18.5–56.7%
Cistus	3.5–56.0%
Kanuka	55.5%
Juniperberry	24.1–55.4%
Camphor (Borneo)	54.3%
Juniper (Phoenician)	41.8–53.5%
Pine (red)	47.7–52.8%
Cypress	20.4–52.7%
Boswellia sacra (α-pinene CT)	10.3–51.3%
Pine (Scots)	20.3–45.8%
Sumach (Venetian)	44.0%
Labdanum	4.9–44.0%
Larch needle	38.5%
Rhododendron	37.4%
Pine (white)	30.8–36.8%
Rosemary (α-pinene CT)	19.1–35.8%
Pine (black)	11.5–35.1%
White cloud	33.2%
Pine (grey)	23.1–32.1%
Fir cone (silver)	18.0–31.7%
Pine (dwarf)	4.1–31.5%
St. John's Wort	31.4%
Rosemary (bornyl acetate CT)	24.0–28.5%

Fragonia	21.0–27.0%
Mace (East Indian)	16.3–26.7%
Nutmeg (East Indian)	18.0–26.5%
Rosemary (β-myrcene CT)	12.0–25.0%
Longoza	18.0–24.0%
Grindelia	17.0–24.0%
Angelica root	4.4–24.0%
Chaste tree seed	1.2–23.1%
Tana	16.0–23.0%
Rosemary (camphor CT)	4.4–22.0%
Helichrysum italicum	21.7%
Spruce (Norwegian)	14.2–21.5%
Hemp	7.6–19.4%
Fir needle (Himalayan)	19.1%
Pteronia	18.6%
Curry leaf	17.5%
Parsleyseed	8.3–16.9%
Boswellia neglecta	16.7%
Spruce (white)	16.6%
Vassoura	1.2–16.5%
Pepper (black)	1.1–16.2%
Laurel leaf	7.1–15.9%
Wormwood (annual)	0–15.7%
Spruce (red)	15.4%
Mace (Indian)	15.2%
Ormenis mixta	15.0%
Cascarilla (El Salvadorian)	14.7%
Eucalyptus globulus	3.7–14.7%
Eucalyptus camaldulensis	1.3–14.7%
Fir needle (Canadian)	6.2–14.3%
Chaste tree leaf	1.0–13.9%
Fir needle (Siberian)	13.7%
Spruce (black)	13.7%
Boswellia rivae	13.3%
Eucalyptus maidenii	13.1%
Fir (Douglas)	13.0%
Piri-piri	5.7–12.9%
Rosemary (cineole CT)	9.6–12.7%
Nutmeg (West Indian)	1.6–12.6%
Tea tree (lemon-scented)	12.3%
Fir needle (Japanese)	12.2%
Galbanum	12.0%
Niaouli (cineole CT)	7.0–12.0%
Sage (African wild)	11.5%
Carrot seed	0.9–11.2%
Boswellia serrata	0–11.2%
Sage (Spanish)	4.7–10.9%
Coriander seed	0.1–10.5%
Fennel (bitter)	tr–10.4%
Valerian (European)	0–10.1%
Rosalina	5.0–10.0%

Notes: α-Pinene occurs in over 400 essential oils. North American pine oils usually contain mainly (+)-α-pinene, whereas in European pine oils (−)-α-pinene generally predominates (Budavari 1989).

Pharmacokinetics: Following a dose of ~0.6 g/kg iv administered to humans, ~5% α-pinene was excreted in the expired air after two hours (Römmelt et al 1974). In rabbits, α-pinene undergoes hydroxylation and conjugation with glucuronic acid; a major urinary metabolite is verbenol (Ishida et al 1981; Scheline 1991). In humans 1–4% of inhaled (+)- and (−)-α-pinene was excreted as (Z)- and (E)-verbenol, most of which was eliminated 20 hours after a two hour exposure. The renal excretion of unchanged α-pinene was <0.001% (Levin et al 1992). It is suggested that the verbenols are formed from α-pinene by hydroxylation (Eriksson & Levin 1990). In a case of attempted suicide, a man ingested 400–500 mL of pine oil containing 57% α-pinene. The major urinary metabolite was bornyl acetate (Köppel et al 1981).

Adverse skin reactions: Twenty-eight dermatitis patients who were not sensitive to turpentine oil were patch tested with various dilutions of freshly distilled, unoxidized α-pinene. Concentrations of 70–80% were irritating in most patients, at 50% weak reactions were obtained 'in some cases' while no reactions were observed at 25–30% (Pirilä et al 1964). Of 1,200 dermatitis patients patch tested, there were no irritant reactions and no allergic reactions to 5% (presumably unoxidized) α-pinene (Santucci et al 1987). Undiluted α-pinene was moderately irritating to rabbit skin, but was not irritating to hairless mice or swine. Tested at 10% it was not irritating when tested in two panels of 25 volunteers (Opdyke 1978 p. 853–857).

Three sensitization reactions occurred when α-pinene was tested on 25 volunteers. In view of the autoxidation problems associated with α-pinene the maximation procedure was repeated using a freshly distilled sample of α-pinene processed under a blanket of nitrogen and containing added butylated hydroxyanisole as an antioxidant. The subsequent test on 25 volunteers produced no sensitization reactions (Opdyke 1978 p. 853–857). A concentration of 20% α-pinene in mineral oil produced a papulovesicular reaction in a 54 year-old man (Keil 1947). Four of 106 patients sensitized to turpentine oil reacted strongly to α-pinene (Pirilä et al 1969). Tested at 10%, α-pinene was not sensitizing to 11 dermatitis patients sensitized to tea tree oil (Hausen et al 1999).

α-Pinene was only eczematogenic after autoxidation in light and air, and potency corresponded to α-pinene peroxide content. The presence of antioxidants inhibited the formation of eczematogenic agents (Pirilä & Siltanen 1955). Autoxidation of α-pinene followed by concentration by vacuum distillation yielded peroxides which were eczematogenic in proportion to their concentrations. Purification of the α-pinene greatly reduced its eczematogenic activity (Pirilä & Siltanen 1956). It is believed that δ-3-carene, present as an impurity in α-pinene derived from wood oils, can significantly contribute to its eczematogenic activity, even at concentrations as low at 0.1–0.2% (Pirilä & Siltanen 1955, 1956, 1957). The principal degradation product of α-pinene, in reaction with hydroxyl radicals, is pinonaldehyde, with smaller amounts of acetone, formaldehyde, campholenealdehyde and acetaldehyde (Van den Bergh et al 2002).

It was reported that α-pinene could quench citral sensitization in volunteers in the ratio of four parts citral to one part α-pinene (Opdyke 1976 p. 197–198). The compound is not phototoxic (Opdyke 1978 p. 853–857). α-Pinene did not enhance the skin penetration of either chlorpromazine or haloperidol (Almirall et al 1996) but showed significant skin absorption in a human subject when present in a hot bath (inhalation was controlled for) (Römmelt et al 1974).

Acute toxicity: Acute oral LD_{50} in rats reported as 2.1, 3.2 and 3.7 g/kg; acute dermal LD_{50} in rabbits <5 g/kg (Opdyke 1978 p. 853–857).

Inhalation toxicity: In rats kept in an atmosphere saturated with α-pinene, glycogen levels rose sharply in the liver, to a lesser degree in muscle tissue, and in brain tissue normal levels were maintained. Blood sugar levels also remained normal (Epshtein & Khil'ko 1960). The brain respiration of rats exposed to α-pinene vapor was not affected directly, but brain glucokinase and ATP levels, as well as the activities of succinic dehydrogenase and lactic dehydrogenase, were lowered. Brain glucokinase levels returned to normal 40–45 days after exposure was terminated (Epshtein 1959). After male rats were exposed to 300 ppm turpentine vapor for 6 hours daily, five days per week for 8 weeks, α-pinene was found to accumulate in the perinephric fat and brain tissue (Savolainen & Pfäffli 1978). This suggests the possibility of a neurotoxic effect.

The LCt_{50} values (lethal concentrations for the shortest period causing death) for inhalation of saturated vapors (26.0 mg/L) of α-pinene from steam distillation of wood were 625 (rat), 572 (guinea pig) and 364 (mouse) mg/L/min. The vapors produced local eye, nose and lung irritation and affected the CNS (Opdyke 1978 p. 853–857).

Subjects exposed as a result of their work in sawmills to aerosol terpenes (including pinenes and δ-3-carene) have been found to have slightly reduced lung function that does not deteriorate upon further acute exposure (Hedenstierna 1983). Respiratory parameters were monitored in male mice for 60 minutes during inhalational exposure to oxidation products of ozone and the terpenes (+)-α-pinene, limonene and isoprene. Upper airway irritation was a prominent effect, as was the development of airflow limitation that persisted for at least 45 minutes after exposure. All effects from the terpene/ozone exposures were reversible within six hours, suggesting that they are not long-lasting (Rohr et al 2002).

Reproductive toxicity: When pregnant rats were given gavage doses of 3, 12, 56, or 260 mg/kg/day α-pinene on gestation days 6–15, there were no apparent adverse effects at any dose. Parameters measured included maternal and fetal survival, maternal and fetal body weight, implantations, resorptions, sex ratio and gross examination of the urogenital tract. In pups, there was no dose-related increase in skeletal abnormalities, or signs of toxicity in tissues examined (Environmental Protection Agency 1973).

Hepatotoxicity: α-Pinene is porphyrigenic and so especially hazardous to those with defects in hepatic heme synthesis (Bonkovsky et al 1992).

Mutagenicity and genotoxicity: α-Pinene was not mutagenic in the Ames test (Florin et al 1980; Connor et al 1985). Neither (+)-α-pinene nor (−)-α-pinene was mutagenic in an Ames test using *Salmonella* strains TA100, TA98, TA97a and TA1535 with and without metabolic activation (Gomes-Carneiro et al 2005a). α-Pinene shows strong antimutagenic activity through concentration-dependent, competitive inhibition of PROD, with IC_{50} values of 0.087 μM (11.8 μg/L) for (−)-α-pinene,

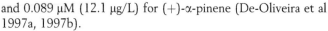

and 0.089 µM (12.1 µg/L) for (+)-α-pinene (De-Oliveira et al 1997a, 1997b).

Carcinogenic/anticarcinogenic potential: α-Pinene caused the appearance of benign skin tumors in mice following treatment with a single application of DMBA (Roe & Field 1965). (±)-α-Pinene did not significantly increase or reduce the average number of tumors per rat or the median tumor latency period in a DMBA-induced rat mammary carcinogenesis model. It was given for 20 weeks at 1% in the diet, and tumors began appearing after 11 weeks (Russin et al 1989). α-Pinene moderately inhibited the in vitro cell growth of myelogenous leukemia (K562) cells, with an IC_{50} of 117.3 µM (16.0 mg/L) (Lampronti et al 2006).

Comments: The fairly extensive inhalation toxicity data is related to the occupational exposure to α-pinene of workers in sawmills in Northern Europe.

Summary: Due to the formation of sensitizing peroxides on autoxidation, there is a risk of sensitization from old or poorly stored batches of essential oils rich in α-pinene. 'Rich' is not defined here, since the total content of oxidation-prone monoterpenes should be taken into account for each essential oil. α-Pinene appears to be neither carcinogenic nor anticarcinogenic. It has no detectable reproductive toxicity.

Regulatory guidelines: Based on literature published in German, α-pinene and its oxidation products were classified as category B, moderately allergenic, by Schlede et al (2003). The Swedish occupational exposure limit to inhaled terpenes such as α-pinene is 150 mg/m^3 (Eriksson et al 1997).

Our safety advice: In order to prevent oxidation the use of antioxidants in combination with α-pinene-rich essential oils is recommended. Such oils should be stored in a refrigerator in a closed container. Commercial products containing α-pinene will keep longer in light-proof packaging.

β-Pinene

Synonyms: Nopinene. Pseudopinene. Terebenthene
Systematic name: 6,6-Dimethyl-2-methylenebicyclo[3.1.1]heptane
Chemical class: Bicyclic monoterpenoid alkene
Note: Different isomers of β-pinene exist, and the following isomer-specific information has been published:

(+)-β-Pinene

CAS number: 19902-08-0

(−)-β-Pinene

CAS number: 18172-67-3
Note: β-Pinene usually occurs in plants together with α-pinene, but in smaller amounts.

Sources >10%:

Galbanum	45.1–58.8%
Fir needle (Canadian)	28.1–56.1%
Longoza	30.0–52.0%
Mace (Indian) (+ sabinene)	45.5%
Arina	39.7%

Pine (white)	31.1–33.3%
Pine (Scots)	1.9–33.3%
Pteronia	32.5%
Spruce (Norwegian)	4.8–31.9%
Combava fruit	25.9–31.5%
Pine (red)	29.4–29.9%
Turpentine	0.9–29.5%
Pine (ponderosa)	28.9%
Blackcurrant bud	0.2–24.0%
Spruce (white)	23.0%
Fir cone (silver)	3.0–22.5%
Vassoura	3.8–22.0%
Lime expressed (Mexican)	21.1%
Spruce (hemlock)	20.8%
Pine (dwarf)	1.3–20.7%
Mace (East Indian)	10.6–20.0%
Nutmeg (East Indian)	8.7–17.7%
Cumin	4.4–17.7%
Lemon (expressed)	6.0–17.0%
Lime expressed (Persian)	12.2–16.0%
Rhododendron	16.0%
Pine (grey)	11.1–15.4%
Fenugreek	15.1%
Pepper (black)	4.9–14.3%
Spruce (black)	14.2%
Lemon (distilled)	8.2–14.0%
Lemon leaf	3.5–13.6%
Neroli	3.5–13.0%
Galangal (greater)	12.9%
Ferula	12.7%
Nutmeg (West Indian)	7.8–12.1%
Spruce (red)	11.9%
Fir (Douglas)	11.6%
Sumach (Venetian)	11.4%
Bergamot (FCF)	4.0–11.0%
St. John's Wort	10.7%
Parsleyseed	5.4–10.7%
Larch needle	10.2%
Peta	10.2%

Pharmacokinetics: When β-pinene was administered to humans iv, ~3% was excreted in the expired air (Römmelt et al 1974). In rabbits β-pinene undergoes hydroxylation, giving rise to several alcohols, including (E)-pinocarveol, and acids, including myrtenic acid (Ishida et al 1977, 1981). (−)-β-Pinene was metabolized in rabbits to (−)-10-pinanol and (−)-1-p-menthene-7,8-diol (Ishida et al 1981).

Adverse skin reactions: Twenty-eight dermatitis patients who were not sensitive to turpentine oil were patch tested with various dilutions of freshly distilled, unoxidized β-pinene. Concentrations of 70–80% were irritating in most patients, at 50% weak reactions were obtained "in some cases" while no reactions were observed at 25–30% (Pirilä et al 1964). In one report, autoxidation of turpentine oil resulted in minimal amounts of eczematogen being formed from β-pinene. In another, β-pinene could not be oxidized to an agent eczematogenic to human skin (Opdyke 1978 p. 859–861). The principal degradation products of β-pinene, in reaction with hydroxyl radicals, are nopinone and formaldehyde, with smaller amounts of acetone and acetaldehyde (Van den Bergh et al 2002).

Undiluted β-Pinene was moderately irritating to rabbit skin. When tested at 12% it was neither irritating nor sensitizing in 25 volunteers. Of 1,200 dermatitis patients patch tested, there were no irritant reactions and two allergic reactions (0.17%) to 1% β-pinene (Santucci et al 1987). One case of hypersensitivity to gum turpentine was largely attributed to β-pinene (Keil 1947). β-Pinene showed significant skin absorption in a human subject when present in a hot bath (inhalation was controlled for) (Römmelt et al 1974).

Acute toxicity: Acute oral LD_{50} in rats >5 g/kg, acute dermal LD_{50} in rabbits >5 g/kg, subcutaneous LD_{50} in mice 1.42 g/kg. The LCt_{50} values (lethal concentrations for the shortest period causing death) for inhalation of saturated β-pinene vapor (19.6 mg/L) were 627 mg/L/min for rats, 627 mg/L/min for mice and 608 mg/L/min for guinea pigs. The vapor irritated eyes, nose and lungs and affected the CNS (Opdyke 1978 p. 859–861).

Reproductive toxicity: β-Pinene was administered by gavage to pregnant rats and mice on gestational days 6–15, and to pregnant hamsters on gestational days 6–10 at doses up to 43, 93 and 99 mg/kg/day, respectively. There were no adverse effects on nidation, reproduction, fetal development or maternal survival (Morgareidge 1973a, 1973b, 1973c, cited in FFHPVC 2006). β-Pinene was given as 15–18% of a mixture also including 20–25% α-pinene and 38–42% sabinene.

Mutagenicity and genotoxicity: β-Pinene was not mutagenic in an Ames test (Florin et al 1980), and was not genotoxic in Chinese hamster ovary cells (Sasaki et al 1989).

Carcinogenic/anticarcinogenic potential: (−)-β-Pinene showed moderate in vitro antiproliferative activity against human cancer cell lines MCF-7 (breast) A375 (malignant melanoma) and HepG2 (liver), while (+)-β-pinene was only weakly effective (Li et al 2008).

Comments: It would seem that β-pinene is less prone to give rise to potentially allergenic oxidation products than α-pinene.

Summary: β-Pinene is virtually non-irritant and non-sensitizing, but skin reactivity increases moderately as β-pinene oxidizes. β-Pinene is not mutagenic, and (−)-β-pinene demonstrates moderate in vitro antitumoral activity. The Swedish occupational exposure limit to inhaled β-pinene is 150 mg/m^3.

Regulatory guidelines: Based on literature published in German, β-pinene was classified as category B, moderately allergenic, by Schlede et al (2003). The Swedish occupational exposure limit to inhaled terpenes such as β-pinene is 150 mg/m^3 (Eriksson et al 1997).

Pinocamphone

Synonym: 3-Pinanone
Systematic name: 2,6,6-Trimethylbicyclo[3.1.1]heptan-3-one
Chemical class: Bicyclic monoterpenoid ketone
Note: Different isomers of pinocamphone exist, and the following isomer-specific information has been published:

(−)-Pinocamphone

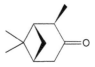

Synonyms: (1S,2R,5R)-3-Pinanone. (E)-Pinocamphone. *trans*-Pinocamphone
CAS number: 547-60-4

(+)-Pinocamphone

Synonym: (1R,2S,5S)-3-Pinanone
CAS number: 18492-59-6

Note: Isomeric with isopinocamphone.

Sources >1.0%:

Hyssop (pinocamphone CT)	31.2–42.7%
Labdanum	0–1.3%
Hyssop (linalool CT)	0.5–1.0%

Pharmacokinetics: Pinocamphone is metabolized in vitro and in vivo primarily by CYP enzymes to hydroxyl derivatives. This has been proposed as a probable detoxification pathway (Höld et al 2002).

Acute toxicity: Acute ip LD_{50} in mice >250 mg/kg (Höld et al 2002).

Neurotoxicity: Pinocamphone is largely responsible for the neurotoxicity of hyssop oil (Millet et al 1980). The lowest known convulsant dose of pinocamphone isomers in humans was ~210 mg (10 drops of hyssop oil containing ~70% pinocamphone and isopinocamphone); this is equivalent to 3 mg/kg (Millet 1981). Subcutaneous pinocamphone was convulsant but not lethal to mice at 585 mg/kg (Wenzel & Ross 1957) and it was convulsant and lethal to rats above 0.05 mL/kg ip (Millet et al 1981). In ip LD_{50} testing, mice exhibited neurological signs 1–2 minutes after injection and these progressed to generalized, unremitting convulsions, followed by either death or recovery. Pinocamphone acts as a GABA-gated chloride channel blocker, and its convulsant activity can be reversed by administration of diazepam (Höld et al 2002).

Comments: Thujone, a structurally similar cyclic monoterpenoid ketone, shares many of the properties of pinocamphone. Both are convulsant, both noncompetitively antagonize GABA$_A$ receptors, and both are metabolized by CYP enzymes to less harmful hydroxyl derivatives (Höld et al 2002). Both have similar convulsant dose thresholds in mice: 585 mg/kg sc for pinocamphone and 590 mg/kg for thujone isomers (Wenzel & Ross 1957). They also seem to have similar toxicities in humans, the lowest known convulsant dose of pinocamphone isomers being 3 mg/kg (Millet 1981), and the equivalent dose for thujone isomers being 2.2–2.9 mg/kg (Burkhard et al 1999).

Summary: Pinocamphone is neurotoxic, elevated doses causing convulsions in mice, rats and humans.

Regulatory guidelines: In France, pinocamphone is limited, in absinthe or similar alcoholic beverages, to 20 mg/L (Lachenmeier et al 2008).

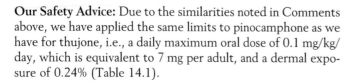

Our Safety Advice: Due to the similarities noted in Comments above, we have applied the same limits to pinocamphone as we have for thujone, i.e., a daily maximum oral dose of 0.1 mg/kg/day, which is equivalent to 7 mg per adult, and a dermal exposure of 0.24% (Table 14.1).

Piperitone

Synonyms: 3-Carvomenthenone. *p*-Menth-1-en-3-one
Systematic name: 3-Methyl-6-(1-methylethyl)-2-cyclohexen-1-one
Chemical class: Monocyclic monoterpenoid alkene ketone
Note: Different isomers of piperitone exist, and the following isomer-specific information has been published:

(6S)-(+)-Piperitone

CAS number: 6091-50-5

(6R)-(−)-Piperitone

CAS number: 4573-50-6

Sources >1.0%:

Eucalyptus dives	54.5%
Calamint (lesser)	0–7.4%
Eucalyptus radiata	0.4–4.7%
Cornmint	0.6–3.8%
Jamrosa	3.4%
Catnip	0–1.5%
Verbena (white)	0.7–1.4%
Peppermint	0–1.3%
Oregano (Mexican)	0.9–1.2%
Chaste tree seed	0–1.2%

Note: Piperitone is isomeric with pulegone, but is less toxic.
Pharmacokinetics: The metabolism of piperitone has received little attention. In sheep given 9.3 g piperitone orally, the presence of thymol, diosphenol, carvotanacetone and unchanged piperitone in the urine were proposed (Scheline 1991 p. 104).
Adverse skin reactions: Undiluted piperitone was moderately irritating to rabbit skin; tested at 10% on 25 volunteers it was neither irritating nor sensitizing (Opdyke 1978 p. 863–864).
Acute toxicity: Acute oral LD_{50} in rats 3.55 g/kg, acute dermal LD_{50} in rabbits >5 g/kg (Opdyke 1978 p. 863–864); subcutaneous LD_{50} in mice 1.42 g/kg (Wenzel & Ross 1957).
Neurotoxicity: High doses of subcutaneously injected piperitone reduced sleep duration in mice, but even lethal doses did not cause seizures (Wenzel & Ross 1957).
Mutagenicity and genotoxicity: Piperitone was not mutagenic in the Ames test (Florin et al 1980).
Comments: Wenzel & Ross (1957) describe piperitone as a CNS stimulant because it was 'lethal at the convulsant dose', on sc administration, but no further details are given. In the acute oral toxicity report, there is no mention of seizures (Opdyke 1978 p. 863–864).

Summary: Piperitone appears to be non-irritant and non-allergenic. It has caused convulsions in mice, but only on lethal sc dosing. Piperitone is not mutagenic.

Piperonal

Synonyms: Piperonaldehyde. Heliotropin. Geliotropin
Systematic name: 3,4-Methylenedioxybenzaldehyde
Chemical class: Benzenoid aldehyde
CAS number: 120-57-0

Source:

Vanilla

Pharmacokinetics: Following oral administration of piperonal to rabbits, ~28% of the dose was recovered in the urine as piperonylic acid. In mice 89% of an oral dose was recovered in the urine, the major metabolite being piperonylglycine. In rats 93% of an oral dose was recovered in 24 hours in the urine, 71% as piperonylglycine and 20% as piperonylic acid (Scheline 1991).
Adverse skin reactions: A patch test using undiluted piperonal for 24 hours resulted in one irritation reaction in 20 volunteers. Tested at 6%, piperonal produced no sensitization reactions in 25 volunteers (Opdyke 1974 p. 907–908). Tested at 5%, the compound induced six allergic reactions (0.4%) of 1,606 dermatitis patients. When tested at 1% in the same group there were two (0.1%) allergic reactions (Frosch et al 2002b).
Acute toxicity: The acute oral LD_{50} in rats was 2.7 g/kg (Hagan et al 1967).
Subacute, subchronic & chronic toxicity: In feeding studies, neither 1,000 ppm fed to rats for 28 weeks nor 10,000 ppm for 15 weeks had any adverse effects (Hagan et al 1967). Groups of 20 male and 20 female rats were fed diets containing 0.1% or 0.5% piperonal for two years with no adverse effects (Bär Vn & Griepentrog 1967).
Mutagenicity and genotoxicity: Piperonal was not mutagenic in the Ames test (White et al 1977; Sekizawa & Shibamoto 1982; Haworth et al 1983; Heck et al 1989). It was genotoxic in one *Bacillus subtilis* DNA rec assay (Sekizawa & Shibamoto 1982) and not in another (Oda et al 1978).
Summary: Piperonal is minimally irritant, allergenic and toxic.
Regulatory guidelines: Piperonal is listed under the FDA Controlled Substances Act as a 'List 1 chemical', one that can be used in the manufacture of illegal drugs (http://www.fda.gov/regulatoryinformation/legislation/ucm148726.htm#cntlsba accessed August 5th 2012).

Propyl allyl disulfide

Synonyms: Allyl propyl disulfide. 4,5-Dithia-1-octene
Systematic name: Propyl 2-propenyl disulfide
Chemical class: Aliphatic alkene disulfide
CAS number: 2179-59-1

Sources:

Leek	8.1%
Garlic	0.26–7.2%

Adverse skin reactions: Has been known to cause contact allergy in a garlic-sensitive individual (Papageorgiou et al 1983). **Mutagenicity and genotoxicity:** Propyl allyl disulfide was not mutagenic in the Ames test (Eder et al 1982). **Summary:** There are insufficient data to draw any conclusions.

Psoralen

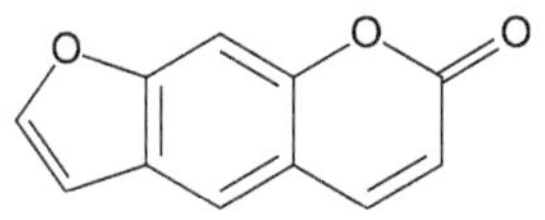

Synonyms: Ficusin. Furo[3,2-g]coumarin
Systematic name: 7H-Furo[3,2-g][1]benzopyran-7-one
Chemical class: Tricyclic benzofuranoid lactone
CAS number: 66-97-7

Sources:

Rue	0.015%
Angelica root	0.0112%
Taget	0.011%
Orange (bitter)	0.007%
Bergamot (expressed)	0–0.0026%
Grapefruit	Undetermined

Pharmacokinetics: Psoralen was a potent inhibitor of CYP3A, as indicated by reduced microsomal testosterone 6β-hydroxylation, with an IC_{50} value of 5.1 μM (949 μg/L) (Guo et al 2000). It inhibited CYP3A4 only weakly, with IC_{50} values of 116 μM and 257 μM (21.6 and 47.8 mg/L) in two different human livers (Ho et al 2001).
Adverse skin reactions: Psoralen is one of a group of furanocoumarins which have shown photosensitizing and phototoxic effects in both animals and humans (Anderson & Voorhees 1980; Parsons 1980).
Mutagenicity and genotoxicity: Psoralen was positive in the SOS chromotest (a modified *E. coli* PQ37 genotoxicity assay) with or without S9 activation (Kevekordes et al 1999). Psoralen was also genotoxic both in human lymphocytes and in the human hepatoma cell line Hep G2 (Kevekordes et al 2001). Psoralen is photomutagenic in the presence of UVA (Schimmer & Kühne 1990). Psoralen was mutagenic in an HPRT assay, and was photogenotoxic in a micronucleus assay at >5 μg/mL (Lohr et al 2010).
Summary: Psoralen is phototoxic, mutagenic, and photomutagenic.
Regulatory guidelines: For tanning products, the SCCNFP set a maximum of 1 ppm for 'furocoumarin-like substances' in 1995, later reviewed and confirmed (SCCNFP 2003b). This has now been extended to apply to all cosmetic products (SCCP 2005b).

α-Pulegone

Synonyms: *p*-Menth-8-en-3-one. Isopulegone
Systematic name: 5-Methyl-2-(1-methylethenyl)cyclohexanone

Chemical class: Monocyclic monoterpenoid alkene ketone
Note: Different isomers of α-pulegone exist, and the following isomer-specific information has been published:

(+)-(Z)-α-pulegone

Synonyms: (1R,4R)-α-pulegone. (+)-*cis*-α-Pulegone. Isoisopulegone
CAS number: 3391-89-7

Sources >1.0%:

Buchu (pulegone CT)	2.2–3.9%

(−)-(E)-α-Pulegone

Synonyms: (1R,4S)-α-Pulegone. (−)-*trans*-α-Pulegone
CAS number: 57129-09-6

Sources >1.0%:

Buchu (pulegone CT)	1.8–4.8%
Pennyroyal (European)	0.2–1.6%
Pennyroyal (Turkish)	1.5%

(+)-(Z)-α-Pulegone + (−)-(E)-α-pulegone

Buchu (diosphenol CT)	0.4–4.6%

Acute toxicity: In male mice given α-pulegone at 400, 500 or 600 mg/kg ip, there was dose-dependent hepatotoxicity measured as degree of necrosis, and there was dose-dependent lethality. At 400 mg/kg no animals died, and minimal hepatic necrosis was seen in five of 20 animals. At the same dose of (1R)-(+)-β-pulegone, nine of 16 mice died (Gordon et al 1982). Therefore, α-pulegone is significantly less toxic than (1R)-(+)-β-pulegone.
Summary: There are insufficient data to draw any conclusions, but the structural similarity to β-pulegone suggests a similar toxicity.

β-Pulegone

Synonym: *p*-Menth-4(8)-en-3-one
Systematic name: 5-Methyl-2-(1-methylethylidene)cyclohexanone
Chemical class: Monocyclic monoterpenoid alkene ketone
Note: Different isomers of β-pulegone exist, and the following isomer-specific information has been published:

(1R)-(+)-β-Pulegone

CAS number: 89-82-7

Sources >1.0%:

Pennyroyal (European)	67.6–86.7%
Pennyroyal (N. American)	61.3–82.3%
Calamint (lesser)	17.6–76.1%
Buchu (pulegone CT)	31.6–73.2%

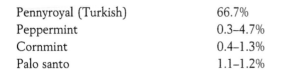

Pennyroyal (Turkish)	66.7%
Peppermint	0.3–4.7%
Cornmint	0.4–1.3%
Palo santo	1.1–1.2%

(1S)-(−)-β-Pulegone

CAS number: 3391-90-0

Sources >1.0%:

| Buchu (diosphenol CT) | 0.6–4.5% |

β-Pulegone (isomer not specified)

| Khella | 1.8% |

Pharmacokinetics: Oral doses of 0.8, 8.0 and 80 mg/kg (1R)-(+)-β-pulegone were well absorbed in rats and mice, with mice excreting 85–100% in 24 hours, and rats 59–81%, primarily in the urine and feces. There was accumulation in several tissues of both species on dosing 80 mg/kg once daily over four consecutive days. The accumulation in the liver was up to three times that of a single dose, that in the lungs was only slight, and there was no accumulation in the brain. In male rats only there was a substantial accumulation in the kidneys, suggesting male rat-specific toxicity (Chen LJ et al 2003).

Until 2001, the following was the conventional wisdom concerning metabolism. (1R)-(+)-β-Pulegone is extensively metabolized by hydroxylation in the 5- and 9-positions to form 5-hydroxypulegone and 9-hydroxypulegone, which then undergo further metabolism. The latter is the predominant pathway, and 9-hydroxypulegone undergoes cyclization to form (6R)-(+)-menthofuran. The 5-hydroxy metabolite dehydrates to form piperitenone (Moorthy et al 1989b; Madyastha & Raj 1993; Nelson et al 1992b). (1R)-(+)-β-Pulegone is also reduced to pulegol, and may isomerize reversibly to α-pulegone (Gordon et al 1987, McClanahan et al 1988). All these studies were performed in rats or mice. It was believed that the toxicity of pulegone was primarily due to its conversion to menthofuran, a major metabolite, and further conversion to a reactive intermediate, 8-pulegone aldehyde, the ultimate toxicant (Thomassen et al 1990).

At 250 mg/kg, (1S)-(−)-β-pulegone is metabolized qualitatively in a similar manner to (1R)-(+)-β-pulegone in male rats, but there are differences in the relative amounts of metabolites formed from the alternative metabolic pathways (Madyastha & Gaikwad 1998). Chen et al (2001) maintained that in most previous pharmacokinetic studies pulegone was used at close to lethal concentrations, and that lower concentrations do not lead to menthofuran formation. Fourteen metabolites were identified after oral administration of 0.8, 8.0 and 80 mg/kg (1R)-(+)-β-pulegone to male and female F344 rats. There were three major pathways: (1) hydroxylation to give monohydroxylated pulegones, followed by glucuronidation or further metabolism; (2) reduction of the carbon-carbon double bond to give diastereomeric menthone/isomenthone, followed by hydroxylation and glucuronidation; and (3) Michael addition of glutathione to pulegone, followed by further metabolism to give diastereomeric

8-(N-acetylcystein S-yl)menthone/isomenthone. All but one of the major metabolites are phase II metabolites.

The first human study was reported in 2003. When six volunteers ingested 1 mg/kg of (1S)-(−)-β-pulegone or 0.5 mg/kg of (1R)-(+)-β-pulegone, menthofuran was detected in the urine, but only in trace amounts as was mintlactone, a metabolite of menthofuran. These findings suggest substantial differences between rodent high-dose and human low-dose metabolism. Toxicity may not correlate linearly with dose, since high doses produce toxic metabolites that are produced only in traces, if at all, in low doses (Engel 2003).

Menthofuran has been found in the blood in cases of poisoning from pennyroyal oil, which may contain menthofuran in concentrations below 1%. Ten hours after ingestion of an unknown quantity of pennyroyal oil by a 22-month-old girl, 40 ng/mL (40 µg/L) of menthofuran was detected in the serum. Following medical intervention the girl made a full recovery (Mullen et al 1994). In a fatal case of poisoning from pennyroyal herbal extract in a 24-year-old female, plasma pulegone and menthofuran levels of 18 ng/mL and 1 ng/mL (18 µg/L and 1 µg/L) serum, respectively, were recorded 26 hours after death, and 72 hours after the final ingestion of the extract, which contained 293 times more pulegone than menthofuran (Anderson et al 1996).

Drug interactions: In rats, phenobarbitone (either 40 or 80 mg/kg/day for 4 days) potentiated the hepatotoxicity caused by pulegone given orally at 400 mg/kg once daily for five subsequent days. Because the activation of pulegone occurs via CYP, pretreatment with drugs that induce CYP greatly enhances pulegone's hepatotoxicity (Moorthy et al 1989a). Since such drugs are common, this makes pulegone-rich essential oils potentially hazardous, especially in oral doses.

Adverse skin reactions: Tested on 25 volunteers at 10%, pulegone was non-irritant and non-sensitizing (Opdyke 1978 p. 867–868).

Acute toxicity: Acute oral LD$_{50}$ 470 mg/kg in rats, approximate ip LD$_{50}$ in mice 150 mg/kg, acute dermal LD$_{50}$ in rabbits 3.09 g/kg (Opdyke 1978 p. 867–868). This work refers to 'd-pulegone', which is still sometimes used as a synonym for (1R)-(+)-β-pulegone. Subcutaneous LD$_{50}$ in mice 1.7 g/kg (Wenzel & Ross 1957). The rat acute oral LD$_{50}$ of 470 mg/kg cited by Opdyke (1978) seems low, considering that 400 mg/kg/day po caused no fatalities in rats, even when given daily for five consecutive days (Moorthy et al 1989a). The mouse ip LD$_{50}$ of 150 mg/kg also seems low, considering that Gordon et al (1982) recorded nine of 16 mice dying within 24 hours from an ip dose of 400 mg/kg (1R)-(+)-β-pulegone, which suggests an LD$_{50}$ of 355 mg/kg. The Opdyke citations are from a private report to RIFM, and no details are given. Comparison of the acute ip toxicity of pulegone in male mice indicates that the (1R)-(+)- isomer is about three times more toxic than the (1S)-(−)- isomer; the former caused hepatic necrosis at 200 mg/kg, and the latter at 600 mg/kg (Gordon et al 1982).

Subacute and subchronic toxicity: In a two week gavage study, 96% pure (1R)-(+)-β-pulegone was administered to rats at 37.5, 75, 150, 300 or 600 mg/kg/day. All male and most female rats on the two higher doses died before the end of the study period due to liver toxicity with increased incidences of hepatic necrosis and cytoplasmic vacuolization. When (1R)-(+)-β-pulegone was administered to mice at 18.75, 37.5, 75, 150 or 300 mg/kg/day, there were similar incidences of hepatotoxicity and death in the high dose group (National Toxicology Program 2009).

When pulegone was fed to rats in the diet at 20, 80 or 160 mg/kg/day for 28 days, cyst-like spaces were reported to develop in the white matter of the brain, especially in the cerebellum, at the higher two levels (Olsen & Thorup 1984). However, in later studies, no such effect was seen from 160 mg/kg pulegone (Mølck et al 1998) or from 500 mg/kg of peppermint oil (Mengs & Stotzem 1989). The cyst-like spaces reported by Olsen & Thorup (1984) may have arisen from inadequate tissue fixation procedures. In rats given 160 mg/kg/day po for 28 days there were decreases in food consumption and body weight, increased plasma glucose, alkaline phosphatase and S-alanine aminotransferase and decreased plasma creatinine (Mølck et al 1998). In rats given gavage doses of 20, 80 or 160 mg/kg/day po for 28 days, atonia, decreased plasma creatinine and lowered body weight were recorded at the two higher doses. At 20 mg/kg no adverse effects were seen (Thorup et al 1983b).

In a 14 week gavage study, groups of male and female rats were dosed with (1R)-(+)-β-pulegone at 9.375, 18.75, 37.5, 75 or 150 mg/kg/day 5 days per week. All males and most females on the two higher doses died before the end of the study period due to liver toxicity, with increased incidences of hepatic necrosis. Of 27 hematology and clinical chemistry parameters measured, there were no adverse effects in rats at 9.375 mg/kg except for an increase in bile acids in females. Also at this dose, the relative kidney weight of females was significantly greater than controls. There were no adverse effects on sperm parameters or estrous cyclicity at doses up to 75 mg/kg, and there were no lesions seen in the kidney, liver, heart, bone marrow, glandular stomach (or lungs and ovaries in females) at the two lower doses, or in the brain at any dose. Therefore, the NOAEL for male rats was 9.38 mg/kg (National Toxicology Program 2009).

When (1R)-(+)-β-pulegone was administered to mice at 18.75, 37.5, 75, 150 and 300 mg/kg/day, there were increased incidences of hepatotoxicity and death in the high dose group. The only adverse effect in mice at the 18.75 mg/kg dose was an increase in the absolute liver weight of females. Therefore, the NOAEL for male mice was 18.75 mg/kg (National Toxicology Program 2009).

Chronic toxicity: In the two-year gavage studies described below under Carcinogenic/anticarcinogenic potential, there were dose-dependent signs of hyaline glomerulopathy in both rats and mice. There was also inflammation and degeneration of the olfactory epithelium in both species. This was also seen in studies with cresol and is thought to be due to chronic irritation due to repeated inhalation of the test substance while feeding (National Toxicology Program 2009).

Hepatotoxicity: (1R)-(+)-β-Pulegone depleted glutathione in vitro, or when injected ip into rats at 150 mg/kg or mice at 300 mg/kg, but menthofuran caused only a very modest depletion (Gordon et al 1982; Thomassen et al 1990). On ip injection in rats at 300 mg/kg, (1R)-(+)-β-pulegone caused biochemical, histological and ultrastructural changes in the liver suggestive of severe damage to the endoplasmic reticulum that are likely to

cause cell death (Moorthy et al 1991). Pulegone destroys hepatic CYP in rats (Madyastha et al 1985; Madyastha & Moorthy 1989; Moorthy 1991). Pretreatment with a variety of CYP inhibitors decreased hepatotoxicity from pulegone, demonstrating its CYP-mediated activation (Gordon et al 1987; Mizutani et al 1987; Moorthy et al 1989a). Single oral doses of 200 or 300 mg/kg (1R)-(+)-β-pulegone in rats dose-dependently decreased both CYP and heme, but 100 mg/kg had no effect (Moorthy et al 1989a). When rats and mice of both sexes were given gavage doses of 37.5 or 75 mg/kg for two years, there were dose-dependent signs of hepatotoxicity in all groups. In male rats at 18.75 mg/kg, the only hepatotoxic sign of 24 parameters measured was fatty change (National Toxicology Program 2009).

(1R)-(+)-β-Pulegone is notably more hepatotoxic than (1S)-(−)-β-pulegone in male mice, and menthofuran at least twice as hepatotoxic as (1R)-(+)-β-pulegone, measured as degree of hepatic necrosis in mice. By the same measure piperitenone is also hepatotoxic, but considerably less so than (1R)-(+)-β-pulegone, and only in doses of >400 mg/kg ip (Gordon et al 1982).

Menthofuran is converted via an epoxide to a highly reactive metabolite, 8-pulegone aldehyde, which can irreversibly bind to components of liver cells in which metabolism takes place (Thomassen et al 1990). The degree of binding to liver protein parallels the hepatotoxicity of pulegone in vivo. Binding to mouse liver, lung and kidney proteins has been observed from administration of both pulegone and menthofuran (McClanahan et al 1989; Thomassen et al 1992).

Mutagenicity and genotoxicity: (1R)-(+)-β-Pulegone was not mutagenic in two Ames tests, both with and without metabolic activation (Andersen & Jensen 1984; Council of Europe 1999). Pulegone was marginally genotoxic in fruit flies (Franzios et al 1997). After three months of gavage dosing, (1R)-(+)-β-pulegone was not genotoxic in a mouse micronucleus test (National Toxicology Program 2009).

Carcinogenic/anticarcinogenic potential: In a two-year gavage study, groups of 50 rats were administered (1R)-(+)-β-pulegone at 37.5 or 75 mg/kg/day five days per week. In addition, males were dosed at 18.75 mg/kg, and females at 150 mg/kg. Due to excessive morbidity and mortality, 75 mg/kg males and 150 mg/kg females were given no further pulegone after week 60. A total of 42 glands, organs or tissues were examined. There were increased incidences only of urinary bladder papilloma or carcinoma in the 150 mg/kg females. When mice were dosed with 37.5, 75 or 150 mg/kg/day (1R)-(+)-β-pulegone in a similar study, there was an increased incidence of liver tumors. The highest doses causing no benign tumors were 150 mg/kg for male rats, 75 mg/kg for female rats and mice, while none could be established for male mice. The highest doses that did not cause malignant tumors were 37.5 mg/kg for male mice, and 75 mg/kg for male rats, female rats and mice (National Toxicology Program 2009).

Comments: Considering that menthofuran is twice as hepatotoxic as (1R)-(+)-β-pulegone, and that menthofuran is at best only a minor metabolite of (1R)-(+)-β-pulegone, it does not make sense to treat both compounds as if they presented equal risk (see Regulatory guidelines). Comparative ip LD_{50} values in mice also show greater toxicity for menthofuran. Neurological symptoms of varying severity have occurred in some cases of poisoning from pennyroyal oil, but the only sign of neurotoxicity from pulegone dosing in animals is the report of Olsen & Thorup (1984). However, their findings were not seen in subsequent testing, even at a higher dose. Species-specific bladder cancer caused by non-genotoxic substances is often seen in experimental animals (Swenberg et al 1992).

Summary: $(1R)$-$(+)$-β-Pulegone is hepatotoxic in both rodents and humans, and it is hepatocarcinogenic in mice at >75 mg/kg. Pharmacokinetic studies suggest that rats are more susceptible than mice to toxicity from repeated doses. In rats, the 28 day NOAEL was 20 mg/kg, and the 14 week NOAEL was 9.4 mg/kg for males, with female rats at that dose showing elevated bile acid levels. Over two years, 18.75 mg/kg was the LOAEL in male rats (females were not tested at this dose). Therefore, the long-term rat NOAEL for all endpoints can be estimated as 5 mg/kg/day.

$(1R)$-$(+)$-β-Pulegone is notably more hepatotoxic than $(1S)$-$(-)$-β-pulegone, and the metabolite menthofuran is more hepatotoxic than either compound. However, while menthofuran has been found in human blood after pennyroyal oil poisoning, it has not been detected in either rats or humans given low doses of $(1R)$-$(+)$-β-pulegone. One study found that menthofuran was not formed following doses of 80 mg/kg pulegone in rats, but in a subchronic toxicity study, toxicological signs were observed at this dose. Cases of poisoning in humans suggest that human pennyroyal oil acute toxicity and rodent β-pulegone acute toxicity are quantitively and qualitively similar at elevated doses, even though there are interspecies differences in metabolism.

Regulatory guidelines: The CEFS of the Council of Europe have classed pulegone as a hepatotoxic compound. They have set a group TDI for pulegone and menthofuran of 0.1 mg/kg bw based on the NOAEL of 20 mg/kg/day in the 28 day oral toxicity study in rats, with a safety factor of 200. In the EU, the maximum permitted amounts of pulegone are 25 mg/kg food, 100 mg/kg in beverages, 250 mg/kg in mint-flavored beverages, and 350 mg/kg in mint confectionery. For peppermint oil, the CIR recommendation (for cosmetics) states: 'safe as used, except that the concentration of pulegone should not exceed 1%.' Presumably this means the concentration in peppermint oil.

Our safety advice: In proposing a safety limit some allowance is needed for vulnerable groups, but there is no reason to believe that humans are more susceptible than rats to β-pulegone toxicity. Taking the estimated rat NOAEL of 5 mg/kg, we propose an uncertainty factor of ten for interindividual differences. Therefore, a maximum dose of 0.5 mg/kg/day has been applied in this text to essential oils containing pulegone. This is equivalent to 35 mg per adult oral dose, or to a dermal exposure of 1.2% (Table 14.1). The maximum oral dose is one that we know does not lead to toxification in humans, and is broadly within the safety limits set for foods and beverages.

Rose oxide

Systematic name: Tetrahydro-4-methyl-2-(2-methyl-1-propenyl)-2H-pyran
Chemical class: Monocyclic monoterpenoid alkene ether

Note: Different isomers of rose oxide exist, and the following isomer-specific information has been published:

(−)-(Z)-Rose oxide

Synonyms: $(2S,Z)$-Rose oxide. $(2S,4R)$-Rose oxide. $(−)$-*cis*-Rose oxide
CAS number: 3033-23-6

(+)-(Z)-Rose oxide

Synonyms: $(2R,Z)$-Rose oxide. $(2R,4S)$-Rose oxide. $(+)$-*cis*-Rose oxide
CAS number: 4610-11-1

(−)-(E)-Rose oxide

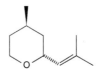

Synonyms: $(2R,E)$-Rose oxide. $(2R,4R)$-Rose oxide. $(−)$-*trans*-Rose oxide
CAS number: 5258-11-7

(+)-(E)-Rose oxide

Synonyms: $(2S,E)$-Rose oxide. $(2S,4S)$-Rose oxide. $(+)$-*trans*-Rose oxide
CAS number: Not found
Note: All four isomers are found in geranium oil, and $(2S,4R)$-rose oxide is a minor constituent ($\sim$0.5%) of rose oil.

Sources >1.0%:

Geranium	0.3–1.4%

Adverse skin reactions: Undiluted 'rose oxide levo' produced moderate irritant effects in rabbits patch-tested for 24 hours under occlusion. Tested at 2% on the skin of human subjects, this rose oxide was neither irritant nor sensitizing (Opdyke 1976 p. 855).
Acute toxicity: 'Rose oxide levo' oral LD_{50} in rats 4.3 g/kg; acute dermal LD_{50} in rabbits >5 g/kg (Opdyke 1976 p. 855).
Summary: Limited data suggest that 'rose oxide levo' is non-irritant, non-allergenic and possesses minimal toxicity.

Sabinene

Synonyms: Sabenene. Sabinane. β-Thujene. *d*-Thujane. Tanacetane
Systematic name: 1-(1-Methylethyl)-4-methylenebicyclo[3.1.0]hexane
Chemical class: Bicyclic monoterpenoid alkene
CAS number: 3387-41-5

Sources >10.0%:

Mullilam	66.3%
Nutmeg (W. Indian)	42.0–57.0%
Nutmeg (E. Indian)	14.0–44.1%

Chaste tree seed	7.1–44.1%
Savin	18.3–40.8%
Thorow-wax	39.7%
Juniperberry	0–28.8%
Cubeb	2.1–28.1%
Plai	27.0%
Yarrow (chamazulene CT)	26.2%
Boswellia frereana	0.5–21.0%
Combava fruit	15.6–20.4%
Goldenrod	18.8%
Chaste tree leaf	6.9–17.1%
Ravensara leaf	10.2–16.4%
Labrador tea	15.7%
Blackcurrant bud absolute	1.8–15.4%
Ho leaf (cineole CT, Madagascan)	11.4–14.0%
Black pepper	0.1–13.8%
Bergamot	0.8–12.8%

Reproductive toxicity: Sabinene was administered by gavage to pregnant rats and mice on gestational days 6–15, and to pregnant hamsters on gestational days 6–10 at doses up to 105, 224 and 240 mg/kg/day, respectively. There were no adverse effects on nidation, reproduction, fetal development or maternal survival (Morgareidge 1973a, 1973b, 1973c, cited in FFHPVC 2006). Sabinene was given as 38–42% of a mixture also including 20–25% α-pinene and 15–18% β-pinene.

(Z)-Sabinyl acetate

Synonyms: *cis*-Sabinyl acetate. *cis*-4-Thujanyl acetate
Systematic name: (Z)-4-Methylene-1-(1-methylethyl)bicyclo[3.1.0]hexan-3-yl ethanoate
Chemical class: Bicyclic monoterpenoid ester
CAS number: 3536-54-7

Sources >1.0%:

Plectranthus	>60.0%
Savin	19.1–53.1%
Wormwood (β-thujone CT)	18.1–32.8%
Wormwood (sabinyl acetate CT)	31.5%
Wormwood ((Z)-epoxy ocimene CT)	0.3–7.4%
Sage (Spanish)	0–6.6%
Yarrow (green)	3.7%
Boldo	2.4%

Notes: Sabinyl acetate is one of the very few toxic essential oil esters. Plectranthus oil is not commercially available.
Reproductive toxicity: A fraction of Spanish sage oil, containing 50% sabinyl acetate, was injected sc into pregnant mice on gestational days 6–15 at 15, 45 and 135 mg/kg. It was dose-dependently abortifacient in all groups (Pages et al 1992). Subcutaneously administered savin oil, containing 50% sabinyl acetate, prevented implantation in mice at 45 and 135 mg/kg, but not at 15 mg when given on gestational days 0–4. However, no antifertility effect was found when savin oil was given on gestational days 8–11, indicating that the abortifacient action

of sabinyl acetate is due to inhibition of implantation (Pages et al 1996). Plectranthus oil (~60% sabinyl acetate) dramatically increased both the rate of resorption and fetal toxicity in pregnant rats after oral administration of 0.5, 2.5 or 5.0 mg/kg on gestational days 6–15 (Pages et al 1988).
Comments: A dose of sabinyl acetate that would be safe in pregnancy cannot be determined from the data, but will be below 1 mg/kg oral. This suggests that sabinyl acetate presents significant reproductive toxicity risks.
Summary: In relation to reproductive toxicity, sabinyl acetate is both maternally toxic and abortifacient, and toxicity is seen on oral or sc dosing in rodents. The reproductive toxicity NOAEL is not known, but will be less than 1 mg/kg/day.

Safrole

Synonym: Shikimole
Systematic name: 1,2-Methylenedioxy-4-allylbenzene
Chemical class: Phenylpropenoid ether
CAS number: 94-59-7

Sources >0.1%:

Ocotea odorifera	71.2–92.9%
Cinnamomum porrectum	80.0–90.0%
Sassafras albidum	82.8–88.8%
Cinnamomum rigidissimum	61.7%
Camphor (brown)	50–60%
Betel	6.5–45.3%
Camphor (yellow)	20%
Ho leaf (camphor CT)	0.1–5.0%
Nutmeg (E. Indian)	0.3–3.3%
Mace (East Indian)	0.2–1.9%
Cinnamon leaf	0–1.0%
Ho leaf (linalool CT)	0.01–0.9%
Mace (Indian) (+ p-cymen-8-ol)	0.7%
Phoebe	0.5–0.7%
Cangerana	0.5%
Nutmeg (W. Indian)	0.1–0.5%
Ylang-ylang absolute	0.4%
Ho leaf (cineole CT, Chinese)	0.2%
Anise (star)	0–0.1%
Cubeb seed	0–0.1%
Cinnamon bark	0–0.04%

Pharmacokinetics: After oral administration of safrole, the principal metabolite was 1,2-dihydroxy-4-allylbenzene, which constituted 65.1% of the total urinary metabolites in man, and 45.1% in rats. 1′-Hydroxysafrole was found as a conjugate in rat urine, but could not be detected in human urine. Rats were given 600 mg/kg of safrole, while humans ingested 1.66 mg per person, some 25,000 times less. In humans, plasma levels were maximal after 30 minutes suggesting rapid absorption. Elimination was biphasic, with first and second half-lives of 2.5 hours and 15 hours, respectively, and 92% excreted in the urine by 24 hours. In rats given an oral dose of 0.63 mg/kg, 88% was excreted in the urine by 24 hours, but this reduced to 78% for a dose of 60 mg/kg (Benedetti et al 1977). In a percutaneous absorption study, 15% of applied safrole was absorbed by unoccluded excised human skin (Bronaugh et al 1985). However, acetone was used as a vehicle, and acetone disrupts barrier function, making the skin more permeable.

Both 1'-hydroxylation and 2',3'-epoxidation of safrole lead to potentially carcinogenic compounds (Wislocki et al 1976). Safrole and 1'-hydroxysafrole can both cause hepatic cell enlargement in experimental animals (Hagan et al 1965) but 1'-hydroxysafrole is the more potent hepatic carcinogen (Borchert et al 1973a, 1973b). 1'-Hydroxysafrole is further converted to 1'-sulfooxysafrole, and there is good evidence that this is the major carcinogenic metabolite (Boberg et al 1983, 1987; Burkey et al 2000). However, 1'-hydroxysafrole is also converted in rat and mouse liver enzyme systems in vitro to other electrophiles such as 1'-oxosafrole, safrole-1'-sulfate and 1'-hydroxysafrole-2',3'-oxide, which are also candidate ultimate carcinogens (Wislocki et al 1976, 1977; Ioannides et al 1981).

A prominent detoxification route in rodents and man is via oxidative opening of the heterocyclic ring to give catechol derivatives, which are then largely excreted as their conjugates. In rats, this may occur while the epoxide function remains intact (Delaforge et al 1980). These catechol products are potentially toxic as they can be oxidized to reactive o- and p-quinone methides that can bind covalently with DNA (Bolton et al 1994). In vitro tests using S. typhimurium lend support to the hypothesis that epoxides are the proximate carcinogens of safrole (Dorange et al 1977). However, although safrole 2',3'-oxide formed adducts with calf thymus DNA in vitro, no such adducts were detected in vivo, suggesting that 2',3'-oxidation is not relevant to in vivo genotoxicity (Qato & Guenthner 1995). Although the 2',3'-oxide is very reactive and therefore potentially genotoxic, its rate of metabolism is much greater than its rate of formation in rat liver.

Epoxide hydrolase activity in human liver varies by some 20-fold, but even those with the lowest hydrolase activity are equivalent to the mean value for rats. Therefore, epoxide hydrolyzation is more rapid in human liver than rat liver, allowing for a wide margin of safety in humans (Guenthner & Luo 2001). The epoxides are mainly further metabolized to 2',3'-diols and α-hydroxy acids (Stillwell et al 1974; Scheline 1991).

Adverse skin reactions: Tested at 8.0% in petrolatum, safrole produced no skin irritation in human subjects following a 48 hour closed-patch test, and no sensitization in 25 human subjects after a maximation test; it was also non-phototoxic (Opdyke 1974 p. 983–986).

Acute toxicity: Acute oral LD_{50} reported as 1.95 g/kg (Taylor et al 1964) and 1.95 g/kg in rat, and 2.35 g/kg in mouse (Jenner et al 1964). Subcutaneous LDLo 1.0 g/kg in rabbit

and 0.50 g/kg in cat; oral LDLo 1.0 g/kg in rabbit (Spector 1956). CNS depression has been reported after safrole was given to experimental animals in very high doses (Shipochliev 1968).

Subacute and subchronic toxicity: Oral administration of 750 mg/kg/day for 19 days was lethal to nine of ten rats; 500 mg/kg/day for 46 days was lethal to one of ten rats; 500 mg/kg/day for 34 days was not lethal to any rats. Safrole is non-toxic in the mouse pulmonary tumor response test (Stoner et al 1973).

Reproductive toxicity: When administered orally at 600 μmol/kg (97 mg/kg) to pregnant mice on day 18 of gestation, safrole formed adducts with maternal and fetal DNA in numerous organs, most notably the liver (Lu et al 1986a). After oral administration of safrole to pregnant mice at 120 mg/kg on four gestational days, kidney epithelial tumors occurred in 7% of offspring, compared to none of the control animals. When safrole was given to nursing mice at the same dose 12 times every second day following birth, 34% of male offspring developed hepatocellular tumors, compared to none of the females or controls. When safrole was administered directly to young mice, 48% of females and only 8% of males developed hepatocellular tumors. There were both benign and malignant tumors, with a higher incidence of carcinomas in females than males (Vesselinovitch et al 1979).

Hepatotoxicity: Administration of an unstated amount of safrole to rats resulted in liver hypertrophy and glycogen reduction; it induced hepatic reductase and hydroxylase enzymes as well as UDP-glucuronyltransferase and CYP (Parke & Rahman 1970). Microscopic liver lesions in rats were seen after oral administration of safrole at 650 mg/kg/day for four days (Taylor et al 1964). When single ip doses of safrole were given to rats at 250, 500 or 1,000 mg/kg, reversible lipid peroxidation and oxidative DNA damage occurred in the liver, as evidenced by dose-dependent increases in serum ALT and AST activities. This may contribute to the hepatocarcinogenic action of safrole (Liu et al 1999). Safrole caused liver enlargement and induced hepatic microsomal enzymes in rats after administration at 150 mg/kg/day for 32 weeks (Gray et al 1972).

Mutagenicity and genotoxicity: Safrole was not mutagenic using a dominant lethal assay (Epstein et al 1972). It was not mutagenic in a direct bacterial assay, or in an Ames test (Eder et al 1982) but was mutagenic in a microsomal mutagenesis assay (Green & Savage 1978). Neither safrole nor 1'-hydroxysafrole were mutagenic in an Ames test using Salmonella strains TA1535, TA100, TA1537, TA1538 or TA98 without S9, but safrole was mutagenic in TA1535 with S9. The corresponding epoxides were mutagenic in TA1535 and TA100. Mutagenesis appears to increase with electrophilic properties (Dorange et al 1977). Wislocki et al (1977) also found that neither safrole nor 1'-hydroxysafrole were mutagenic in TA1535 or TA100 without S9, but the four 2'-3'-oxides of safrole tested were mutagenic. In contrast, Swanson et al (1979) reported that 'highly purified' 1'-hydroxysafrole was mutagenic in TA100 without S9.

Safrole was neither genotoxic in the S. typhimurium TA135/pSK1002 umu test (Nakamura et al 1987) nor in the SOS chromotest with or without S9 activation (Kevekordes et al 1999). However, it was genotoxic in Saccharomyces cerevisiae (Schiestl et al 1989), Chinese hamster lung cells (Ishidate et al 1988),

Chinese hamster ovary cells (Tayama 1996), and in rat hepatocytes (Randerath et al 1984; Howes et al 1990). At <4,000 μM, safrole was genotoxic in a HepG2/single cell gel electrophoresis assay, thought to detect genotoxins that give false negative results in other assays (Uhl et al 2000). Safrole can form adducts with mouse liver DNA (Phillips et al 1984; Randerath et al 1984; Phillips 1990), and induces SCE and CA in rodents both in vitro and in vivo (Daimon et al 1997a, 1997b,8).

Carcinogenic metabolites of safrole bind to DNA, RNA and protein in the liver (Wislocki et al 1976). In mice, pregnancy led to a 2.3–3.5-fold increase in total binding to liver and kidney DNA after a single oral dose of 600 μmol/kg (97 mg/kg) of safrole or 400 μmol/kg (71 mg/kg) of 1'-hydroxysafrole administered on day 18 of gestation (Lu et al 1986b). Safrole preferentially binds to hepatic DNA. After a single oral dose of 2.47 mmol/kg (400 mg/kg), the number of adducts per ten million (10^7) nucelotides was 238 in mouse liver DNA, and only 5, 3, 5 and 0.6 in the DNA of the kidneys, lungs, white blood cells and spleen, respectively (Reddy & Randerath 1990). Although safrole also binds preferentially to human hepatic DNA (Liu et al 2000), it does so more weakly in humans than mice. In studies of three patients with hepatocellular carcinoma who were also habitual chewers of betel quid (which contains safrole), the number of safrole-DNA adducts per 10^7 nucleotides in hepatic DNA was 1.6, 2.3 and 9.7, compared to 110 in mice (Liu et al 2000; Chung et al 2008). Taken together, the above findings suggest that safrole–DNA binding in the liver is 10–150 times more potent in mice than humans.

In a ^{32}P-postlabelling assay, the dose and time dependence of hepatic safrole-DNA adducts was examined after ip administration of single doses of safrole to female mice at 0.001, 0.01, 0.1, 1.0 and 10.0 mg/mouse. Liver DNA was analyzed at 0.5, 1, 2, 3, 7, 15 and 30 days. Adduct formation was dose-dependent, with peak levels after two days (Gupta et al 1993). After single doses of 1, 10, 100, 250 and 500 mg/kg of safrole in rats, CA were not induced at any dose, but SCE increased at 100 mg/kg and higher. On multiple dosing (once a day for five days at 62.5, 125 and 250 mg/kg) CA increased at 125 and 250 mg/kg, and SCE increased at all doses (Daimon et al 1998). The rat data suggest that non-genotoxic levels exist for safrole, and that DNA adducts may be more closely associated with SCE than CA. In mice, hepatic safrole-DNA adducts can persist for up to 30 days after a dose of 0.001 mg/kg, and for up to 140 days after a dose of 10 mg/kg (Randerath et al 1984; Gupta et al 1993).

In Taiwan, the number of safrole-DNA adducts per 10^7 nucelotides varied from 0–7 in the peripheral blood leukocyte DNA of betel quid chewers (Liu et al 2004), and from 0.55 to 21.4 (a 39-fold variation) in the esophageal cells of six patients with esophageal cancers related to quid chewing (Lee JM et al 2005b). Depending on dose, safrole produces up to four adducts. The principal two adducts are N^2-((E)-isosafrol-3'-yl) deoxyguanosine 5'-monophosphate and N^2-(safrol-1'-yl) deoxyguanosine 5'-monophosphate (Gupta et al 1993).

Chronic toxicity and carcinogenic/anticarcinogenic potential: In male rats given safrole in the diet at 1,000 or 10,000 ppm for up to 370 days (rats were killed whenever they became moribund), significant hepatic changes occurred in animals on the higher dose, including fibrosis, fatty degeneration and hyperplasia. In the same group, body weights were reduced, and there were signs of testicular atrophy and bone marrow loss. One rat in the low-dose group developed a malignant kidney tumor, though this could not be definitively linked to safrole. Otherwise, lower dose animals were not adversely affected in any way (Homburger et al 1961). In a similar study but with female rats consuming 10,000 ppm safrole, similar signs of hepatotoxicity were seen, though no malignancies occurred in any organ (Homburger et al 1962). In both of these studies many of the animals were also on a riboflavin-deficient diet, which intensified the hepatotoxicity.

In a feeding study in rats of both sexes, 1,000, 2,500 or 5,000 ppm safrole was given over two years and 10,000 ppm was given over 62 weeks. Both 10,000 and 5,000 ppm were associated with benign and malignant tumors, with all rats in the high dose group dead at the end of the 62 weeks. At 2,500 and 1,000 ppm there was 'moderate' and 'slight' liver damage, respectively, but no tumors or increase in mortality. Growth retardation and slight kidney toxicity were seen at all doses (Hagan et al 1965, 1967). In another two year feeding study in the same species of rat, safrole was administered to both sexes at 100, 500, 1,000 or 5,000 ppm. Liver damage was 'very slight' at 100 ppm and 'slight' at 500 ppm; benign tumors developed in 8/46 (17%) at the 1,000 ppm level, while at 5,000 ppm, benign tumors were found in 5/47 (11%) and malignant tumors in 14/47 (30%) of animals (Long et al 1963). The lowest dose used in this study is equivalent to ~5 mg/kg/day.

Mice are also susceptible to hepatic tumors from safrole. After administration to males at 4,000 ppm, benign liver tumors were found in 4/10 and 7/10 mice at 36 and 52 weeks, respectively. At 75 weeks, they occurred in 5/5 mice. Hepatocellular carcinomas developed in 2/10 animals at 52 weeks and 3/5 at 75 weeks (Lipsky et al 1981). Malignant liver tumors also developed in 46/72 mice (two species, male and female, 18 mice per group) given safrole orally at 464 mg/kg/day from 7 to 28 days after birth, followed by 1,112 ppm in the diet for 78 weeks. In spite of the massive dose used during the first three weeks, no mice developed lymphomas or pulmonary tumors (Innes et al 1969).

Safrole dosing produced an increased incidence of hepatomas at 11–14 months, following four ip injections over 21 days totaling 9.45 μmol (1.3 mg) to preweanling male mice (Miller et al 1983). A similar increase in hepatoma incidence was found in mice one year after receiving four sc injections over 21 days totaling either 0.6 mg or 6.6 mg of safrole in infancy; the increases in the lower dose group were marginal (Epstein et al 1970). In both of these studies, there were minimal increases in lung tumor incidence. However, in male and female mature mice given 12 ip injections of safrole in a total dose of 0.9 or 4.5 g/kg over 24 weeks, the incidence of primary lung tumors was no higher than in the control group (Stoner et al 1973). This suggests a susceptibility of infant mice to lung tumors from safrole, and the virtual lack of DNA repair in infant mice for safrole and related substances has been noted (Gupta et al 1993).

In dogs fed daily doses of 20 mg/kg safrole over six years, 40 mg/kg over 91–116 days, or 80 mg/kg over 26–39 days, microscopic and macroscopic changes to the liver were observed at all doses, with emaciation and general weakness at 40 mg/kg, and marked weight loss and one death (of four dogs) at 80 mg/kg (Long et al 1963).

In a novel assay for carcinogens, groups of male rats were dosed for 2, 14 or 90 days with 0.2 or 2.0 mmol/kg/day (32 or 324 mg/kg/day) of safrole, and then hepatic tissue was analyzed for precancerous changes in gene expression. These were significant at 90 days on the higher dose, but not the lower dose. The changes in gene expression were more pronounced in younger animals, presumably due to their more rapid rate of growth (Auerbach et al 2010). Incubation of human oral cancer cells with 10–1,000 μM (1.6–162 mg/L) safrole increased cell proliferation by 50–70%. There was no effect from 1 μM (162 μg/L) (Huang et al 2005). This supports the idea of a zero-effect dose. Curiously, safrole induced apoptotic cell death in human tongue cancer (SCC-4) cells and human oral cancer (HSC-3) cells, due to changes in gene expression (Yu et al 2011, 2012).

Summary: Safrole is not irritating, sensitizing or phototoxic to human skin, and has low acute oral toxicity in rats, mice, rabbits and cats. In rats, hepatotoxicity is evident from short-term, high-dose administration, and long-term dosing causes hepatic fibrosis, fatty degeneration and hyperplasia. In rodent studies a progression is evident from hepatoxicity to benign tumors to malignant tumors, with toxicity dependent on dose and duration. There are mixed results in mutagenicity and genotoxicity tests, but safrole and its 2′,3′-epoxy, 1′-hydroxy and 1′-sulfate metabolites can form adducts with hepatic DNA, and are thus potentially carcinogenic. Metabolic studies suggest that humans are at no greater risk than rats from either 1′-hydroxylation or from epoxidation products. Although safrole-DNA adducts have been found in people with cancers epidemiologically associated with chronic exposure to safrole through betel quid chewing, the significance of these adducts is not known, and betel quid contains other carcinogenic substances.

The linear dose–response relationship of DNA adduct formation seen in mice may not predict a similar relationship for tumor induction, either in mice or humans. Mice, especially in infancy, are highly susceptible to safrole toxicity and carcinogenicity, probably due to inefficient DNA repair mechanisms. There is both in vitro and in vivo evidence of a theshold, non-toxic dose for safrole. In a gene expression study in rats, there were no pre-cancerous changes from 0.2 mmol/kg/day (32 mg/kg/day) of safrole for 90 days. Chronic toxicity studies in dogs suggest a safe dose of less than 20 mg/kg/day, and rat studies suggest that 5 mg/kg/day is approximately the lifetime minimal toxic dose. Even 50 mg/kg/day (1,000 ppm) causes no toxicity if only given for one year. There are insufficient data to firmly establish a NOAEL, although reducing the 5 mg/kg dose, effectively the LOEL, by five times suggests a NOAEL of 1 mg/kg/day.

Regulatory guidelines: Safrole was banned as a food additive in the USA in 1961. Both IFRA and the EU require that safrole as such is not used as a fragrance ingredient. When safrole-containing essential oils are used, both authorities recommend a maximum use level of 0.01% (IFRA 2009). In the EU, safrole is permitted at up to 50 ppm in adult dental hygiene products, but is prohibited in children's toothpaste. Both the UK and EU 'standard permitted proportion' of safrole in food flavorings is 1.0 mg/kg (1 ppm), except as a constituent of nutmeg or mace, when the limit is 15 ppm (Anon 1992b). Safrole is listed under substances 'reasonably anticipated to be human carcinogens' by the National Toxicology Program. In the absence of any pertinent human data, the carcinogenic potential of safrole in humans has been ranked as low (Environmental Protection Agency 1988). The Joint Expert Committee on Food Additives has not set an ADI for safrole, due to insufficient data (JECFA 2009). Safrole is prohibited in cosmetics in Canada, 'except when naturally occurring in plant extracts' (Health Canada Cosmetic Ingredient Hotlist, March 2011). Whether 'plant extracts' would include essential oils is not clear. Safrole is listed under the FDA Controlled Substances Act as a 'List 1 chemical', one that can be used in the manufacture of illegal drugs http://www.fda.gov/regulatoryinformation/legislation/ucm148726.htm#cntlsba accessed August 5th 2012.

Our safety advice: Since safrole-DNA binding is 10–150 times more prevalent in mouse liver than human liver, and safrole carcinogenicity is 8.6 times more potent in mouse liver than rat liver (Table 12.5), safrole is no more carcinogenic in humans than rats. Therefore, the rat NOAEL can be assumed to be a human NOAEL. Taking the approximate rat NOAEL of 1 mg/kg/day, we have applied an uncertainty factor of 40 to allow for inter-individual differences (based on safrole-DNA adducts in Taiwanese with esophageal cancer), giving 0.025 mg/kg as a safe human lifetime daily dose. This is equivalent to a dermal maximum of 0.05% (Table 14.1). The fact that 1′-hydroxysafrole could not be detected in human urine after an oral dose of 1.66 mg (equivalent to 0.024 mg/kg) would seem to confirm this as a non-carcinogenic dose. The dose of 0.025 mg/kg is 4,800 times less than the dose causing reproductive toxicity in mice.

Salicylaldehyde

Synonyms: Salicylic aldehyde. *o*-Hydroxybenzaldehyde. 2-Formylphenol
Systematic name: 2-Hydroxybenzaldehyde
Chemical class: Phenolic aldehyde
CAS number: 90-02-8

Sources >1.0%:

Cassia leaf	0.05–3.1%
Cassia bark	0.04–1.8%

Note: Being a substituted phenol, salicylaldehyde is a weak acid which may be corrosive to tissues.

Pharmacokinetics: Following oxidation, salicylic acid was the major metabolite in rabbits, cats and dogs (Scheline 1991 p. 90).
Adverse skin reactions: Salicylaldehyde was moderately-to-severely irritating to rabbit skin when applied undiluted for 24 hours under occlusion. Tested at 2% on 33 volunteers it was neither irritating nor sensitizing (Opdyke 1979a p. 903–905). One out of 747 dermatitis patients suspected of fragrance allergy (0.13%) reacted to 2% salicylaldehyde (Wöhrl et al 2001). There is one reported case of salicylaldehyde allergy (Aalto-Korte et al 2005).
Acute toxicity: In rats the acute oral LD_{50} was 520 mg/kg, the acute sc LD_{50} was 900 mg/kg and the minimum lethal dose was 1.0 g/kg. The acute dermal LD_{50} in rabbits was 3.0 g/kg (Opdyke 1979a p. 903–905).
Subacute and subchronic toxicity: Rats fed 2% dietary salicylaldehyde for 13 days showed a marked decrease in cytoplasmic basophilic bodies in liver cells and depletion of zymogen

granules from pancreatic acinar cells. A second group of rats fed 1% dietary salicylaldehyde for 13 days showed increases in the number, size and fibrillar material of hepatic and renal microbodies, and lipid droplets were observed in hepatocytes (Hruban et al 1966).

Reproductive toxicity: Salicylaldehyde, administered sc at 136 mg/kg to pregnant rats, caused significant increases in the number of fetal resorptions (17.9%), malformations (20.9%), toxicity (46.1%) and fatalities (7.8%). At the same time salicylaldehyde significantly lowered the maternal plasma calcium level. The induced hypocalcemia was believed to be related to the fetal toxicity observed (Saito et al 1982)

Hepatotoxicity: Salicylaldehyde inhibited hepatocyte respiration, depleted hepatocyte glutathione and has appreciable cytotoxicity. Its cytotoxicity may result from the formation of covalent bonds with amino groups of proteins involved in cell respiration (Niknahad et al 2003).

Mutagenicity and genotoxicity: Salicylaldehyde was nonmutagenic in the Ames test, with or without metabolic activation (Sasaki & Endo 1978; Florin et al 1980; Kono et al 1995). It did not induce SCE in lymphocytes taken from human blood (Jansson et al 1988) and was not genotoxic in the *S. typhimurium* TA135/pSK1002 umu test (Nakamura et al 1987).

Carcinogenic/anticarcinogenic potential: Salicylaldehyde inhibited the growth of cultured ascites sarcoma BP8 cells (a rat cell line) in concentrations of 1.0 mM (122 mg/L) (100% inhibition), 0.1 mM (12.2 mg/L) (79%) and 0.01 mM (1.22 mg/L) (1%) (Pilotti et al 1975). When 20% salicylaldehyde was applied to the skin of mice previously treated with DMBA there was no carcinoma or papilloma development (Boutwell & Bosch 1959; Wynder & Hoffman 1963).

Comments: Salicylaldehyde is not carcinogenic, but is moderately toxic, and this seems to be reflected in the (low) toxicity of cassia oil (see Cassia profile, Chapter 13).

Summary: Salicylaldehyde presents minimal risk of irritation or sensitization. It is 'moderately' toxic, is not mutagenic, and dermal application is not tumorigenic.

Santalol

Chemical class: Bicyclic sesquiterpenoid alkene alcohol
Note: Different isomers of santalol exist, and the following isomer-specific information has been published:

(Z)-α-Santalol

Synonyms: (+)-α-Santalol. *d*-α-Santalol. *cis*-α-Santalol. Santalol a. Sandal
Systematic name: (R,Z)-5-(2,3-dimethyltricyclo[2.2.1.0^{2,6}]hept-3-yl)-2-methyl-2-penten-1-ol
CAS number: 115-71-9

Sources >1.0%:

Sandalwood (East Indian)	46.2–59.9%
Sandalwood (New Caledonian)	42.3%
Sandalwood (West Australian distilled)	15.3–17.0%
Sandalwood (West Australian extracted)	13.3%

(Z)-β-Santalol

Synonyms: *cis*-β-Santalol. β-Santalol. Santalol b
Systematic name: (1S-(1α,2α(Z),4α)]-2-Methyl-5-(2-methyl-3-methylenebicyclo[2.2.1]hept-2-yl)-2-penten-1-ol
CAS number: 77-42-9

Sandalwood (East Indian)	20.5–29.0%
Sandalwood (New Caledonian)	17.5%
Sandalwood (West Australian extracted)	5.9%
Sandalwood (West Australian distilled)	4.6–4.8%

Adverse skin reactions: Using 20% santalol, there were no irritant reactions in five volunteers, nor allergic reactions in 25 volunteers (Belsito et al 2008). In a worldwide multicenter study of dermatitis patients with proven sensitization to fragrance materials, 2 of 178 (1.12%) were sensitive to 5% of a mixture of (Z)-α-santalol and (Z)-β-santalol (Larsen et al 2001).

Santalol was tested at 1%, 2% and 10%, producing reactions in 1/310, 2/305 and 5/306 patients with cosmetic dermatitis, respectively (0.32%, 0.65%, 1.63%) (Sugai 1980). In Japan, 47 of 3,123 patients with cosmetic dermatitis (1.5%), tested positive to 2% santalol (Utsumi et al 1992). In 141, 237 and 133 patients with cosmetic dermatitis there were one, three and two allergic reactions respectively (0.7%, 1.27%, 1.5%) to 2% santalol (Hashimoto et al 1990; Nagareda et al 1992, 1996). A mixture of (Z)-α- and (Z)-β-santalol, tested at 1%, 2% and 10%, caused allergic reactions in 2, 2, and 5 of 327 patients (0.6%, 0.6%, 1.5%) with cosmetic dermatitis (Mid-Japan Contact Dermatitis Research Group 1984). In a total of 511 patients with cosmetic dermatitis, there were no photoallergic responses to photopatch testing with 2% santalol (Hashimoto et al 1990; Nagareda et al 1992, 1996).

Acute toxicity: Santalol acute oral LD$_{50}$ 3.8 g/kg in rats, acute dermal LD$_{50}$ >5 g/kg in rabbits (Belsito et al 2008).

Carcinogenic/anticarcinogenic potential: (Z)-α-Santalol significantly decreased DMBA-induced and TPA-promoted skin papillomas in two strains of mice, reducing papilloma incidence from 100% to 40% and 23%, and reducing papilloma multiplicity approximately 10-fold. At the same time it reduced TPA-induced ODC activity (a marker of tumor promotion) by 60% and 89% (Dwivedi et al 2003). In a similar regime, (Z)-β-santalol inhibited skin cancer incidence in mice (Kim TH et al 2006). Whether applied to the skin at 1.2% or 2.5%, (Z)-α-santalol was equally effective in preventing skin cancers in mice, induced as above (Dwivedi et al 2005). Applied to mouse skin at 5%, (Z)-α-santalol significantly inhibited UVB-induced tumor development (Dwivedi et al 2006; Bommareddy et al 2007). (Z)-α-Santalol induced apoptosis in human epidermoid carcinoma A431 (skin cancer) cells in vitro (Kaur et al 2005). (Z)-α-Santalol is thought to prevent skin cancer development by inducing proapoptotic proteins via an extrinsic pathway and increasing p53 (Arasada et al 2008).

Summary: From a total of 4,266 Japanese people with cosmetic dermatitis, 57 (1.34%) reacted to 2% santalol, suggesting that lower concentrations should be used for people of Japanese origin. The number of fragrance-sensitive individuals reacting to 5% santalol (1.12%) is quite low for this sub-population, suggesting that santalol may not represent much risk of skin sensitization for Caucasians. Santalol is only minimally toxic. Both santalol isomers have shown in vivo chemopreventive effects in skin cancer.

Sclareol

Synonym: Labd-14-ene-8,13-diol
Systematic name: [1R-(1α(R*),2β,4aβ,8aα)]-Decahydro-α-ethenyl-α,2,5,5,8a-pentamethyl-2-hydroxy-1-naphthalenepropanol
Chemical class: Bicyclic diterpenoid alkene diol
CAS number: 515-03-7

Source:

Clary sage absolute	2.4%

Note: Because sclareol has an extremely low volatility it only shows up as a small percentage when analysed by gas chromatography. However, HPLC analysis reveals that clary sage absolute typically consists of 70–75% sclareol and 13-*epi*-sclareol (Burfield, private communication, 2003).

Adverse skin reactions: Undiluted sclareol was irritating to rabbit skin, but 3% sclareol was not; tested at 10% on 25 volunteers it was not irritating. Three samples of 10% sclareol were tested on four separate panels, totaling 106 individuals, with no irritation reactions. One sample produced 1/29 and 3/26 sensitization reactions, while the other two samples produced no reactions in 23 and 28 volunteers (Ford et al 1992 p. 115S). In human repeat insult patch tests, 3% sclareol in ethanol was not sensitizing in 35 volunteers, nor was 3% sclareol in petrolatum in 39 volunteers (Belsito et al 2008).

Acute toxicity: Acute oral LD_{50} in rats >5 g/kg, acute dermal LD_{50} in rabbits >5 g/kg (Ford et al 1992 p. 115S).

Subacute and subchronic toxicity: When 8.8 mg/kg/day sclareol was administered to rats by gavage for 30 days, only marginal toxic effects were observed, and this dose was determined to be the NOAEL (Bhatia et al 2008h).

Carcinogenic/anticarcinogenic potential: Sclareol exhibited strong cytotoxic activity against cell lines for mouse leukemia (P-388), human epidermal carcinoma (KB) and human lung cancer (NSCLC-N6) (Chinou et al 1994). Sclareol was cytotoxic to 13 of 14 human leukemia cell lines tested, with IC_{50} values ranging from 6.0–24.2 µg/mL, but was not cytotoxic to peripheral blood mononuclear leukocytes within the same dose range. Cytotoxicity was due to a phase-specific mechanism which induces apoptosis (Dimas et al 1999). Sclareol induced apoptosis and growth arrest in human breast cancer cells MN1 and MDD2 with IC_{50} values of 22.8 and 27.7 µM (7.0 and 8.6 mg/L), respectively. It also enhanced the in vitro activity of anticancer drugs (Dimas et al 2006). Sclareol showed in vitro activity against 10 human cancer cell lines whether free, or incorporated into microsomes. However, the latter form was less cytotoxic to peripheral blood mononuclear cells. Liposomal sclareol reduced the growth rate of human colon cancer tumors xenografted in mice (Hatziantoniou et al 2006). An isomer, 13-epi-sclareol, which is also present in clary sage, inhibits the growth of breast and uterine cancer cells in vitro, and was slightly more potent than Tamoxifen, but was not toxic to normal cells (Sashidhara et al 2007).

Summary: Naturally-occurring sclareol is non-irritant and non-sensitizing. It possesses minimal toxicity, and has demonstrated in vitro antitumoral activity. The rat NOAEL is 8.8 mg/kg/day.

Regulatory guidelines: IFRA recommends that sclareol, used as a fragrance ingredient, should have a minimum purity of 98% in order to avoid skin sensitization. This is based on RIFM test results showing a skin sensitizing potential for samples with a lower purity, but none for those with a minimum purity of 98% (IFRA 2009).

β-Sesquiphellandrene

Synonyms: (−)-β-Sesquiphellandrene. 1,3(15),10-Bisabolatriene
Systematic name: 3-(1,5-Dimethyl-4-hexenyl)-6-methylenecyclohexene
Chemical class: Monocyclic sequiterpenoid polyalkene
CAS number: 20307-83-9

Sources >1.0%:

Coleus	13.2%
Turmeric rhizome	8.8–9.5%
Amyris	1.5–8.6%
Ginger	7.2–7.3%
Pilocarpus microphyllus	0.5–3.4%
Calamus (diploid form)	0–3.0%
Tansy (blue)	0.2–1.8%

Antioxidant/pro-oxidant activity: β-Sesquiphellandrene has demonstrated marked DPPH scavenging activity (Zhao et al 2010).

Carcinogenic/anticarcinogenic potential: β-Sesquiphellandrene was active against the L1210 cell line (mouse, lymphocytic leukemia) and its cytotoxicity was potentiated fivefold by *ar*-turmerone (Ahn & Lee 1989).

Summary: β-Sesquiphellandrene has demonstrated in vitro antitumoral activity.

α-Terpinene

Synonyms: *p*-Mentha-1,3-diene. α-Terpine
Systematic name: 1-Methyl-4-(1-methylethyl)-1,3-cyclohexadiene
Chemical class: Monocyclic monoterpenoid alkene
CAS number: 99-86-5
Note: Isomeric with β- and γ-terpinenes.

Sources >1.0%:

Peta	14.9%
Tea tree	5.0–13.0%
Mace (East Indian)	4.8–7.5%
Ravensara leaf	1.8–7.1%
Marjoram (sweet)	3.0–5.9%
Nutmeg (East Indian)	0.1–5.2%
Pine (dwarf)	0.2–4.5%
Chamomile (Roman)	0–4.5%
Nutmeg (West Indian)	0.8–4.2%
Mace (Indian)	3.9%
Blackcurrant bud absolute	0.7–3.9%

Feverfew	2.2–3.8%
Mace (Indian) (+ *p*-cymene)	3.5%
Plai	3.5%
Savory (summer)	1.8–3.5%
Sage (African wild)	3.4%
Pine (Scots)	0.1–3.2%
Tana	1.0–3.0%
Curry leaf	2.8%
Juniperberry	0–2.6%
Thymus zygis (thymol CT)	0–2.2%
Lime Mexican (distilled)	tr–2.1%
Fir (Douglas)	2.0%
Labrador tea	1.5%
Boswellia frereana	0–1.5%
Savory (winter)	0–1.5%
Oregano (Mexican)	0.2–1.4%
Thymus serpyllum	tr–1.4%
Oregano	<1.4%
Thyme (spike)	1.3%
Thymus zygis (carvacrol CT)	1.3%
Marjoram wild (carvacrol CT)	1.2%
Tansy (blue)	0.1–1.2%
Hinoki leaf	1.1%
Atractylis	1.0%
Thyme (thujanol CT)	1.0%
Thymus vulgaris (carvacrol CT)	1.0%
Thymus vulgaris (thymol CT)	<1.0%

Adverse skin reactions: Tested at 5% on 25 volunteers α-terpinene was neither irritating nor sensitizing (Opdyke 1976 p. 873–874). Of seven dermatitis patients already sensitive to tea tree oil five were sensitive to α-terpinene tested at 1% (Knight & Hausen 1994). Tested at 5%, α-terpinene was sensitizing to 11 of 16 dermatitis patients sensitive to tea tree oil (Hausen et al 1999).

Acute toxicity: Acute oral LD$_{50}$ in rats 1.68 g/kg (Opdyke 1976 p. 873–874).

Hepatotoxicity: α-Terpinene hepatotoxicity is referred to in one paper, but this appears to be unsubstantiated (Bär Vn & Griepentrog 1967).

Reproductive toxicity: At doses of 30, 60, 125 and 250 mg/kg body weight, 89% pure α-terpinene in corn oil was given by gavage to female Wistar rats from day 6 to 15 of pregnancy. A reduction in body weight minus uterine weight at term indicated that the two highest doses tested were maternally toxic. No increase in the ratio of resorptions/implantations was observed over the dose range tested. Signs of delayed ossification and a higher incidence of minor skeletal malformations were observed at doses of 60 mg/kg or more (Araujo 1996). A NOAEL for embryofetotoxicity cannot be extrapolated, since the very low purity (89%) of the compound used in this study invalidates its findings.

Antioxidant/pro-oxidant activity: α-Terpinene is a scavenger of DPPH radicals (Kim HJ et al 2004; Li & Liu 2009).

Mutagenicity and genotoxicity: α-Terpinene was not mutagenic in an Ames test using *Salmonella* strains TA100, TA98, TA97a and TA1535 with and without metabolic activation (Gomes-Carneiro et al 2005a). α-Terpinene shows strong antimutagenic activity through concentration-dependent, competitive inhibition of PROD, with an IC$_{50}$ of 0.76 μM (103 μg/L) (De-Oliveira et al 1997a, 1997b).

Carcinogenic/anticarcinogenic potential: α-Terpinene inhibited the in vitro formation of the carcinogen NDMA by 82% (Sawamura et al 1999).

Summary: α-Terpinene was a cause of several cases of tea tree oil allergenicity. Thresholds of α-terpinene skin sensitization are not known. α-Terpinene is not mutagenic.

γ-Terpinene

Synonyms: *p*-Mentha-1,4-diene. Crithmene. Moslene
Systematic name: 1-Methyl-4-(1-methylethyl)-1,4-cyclohexadiene
Chemical class: Monocyclic monoterpenoid alkene
CAS number: 99-85-4
Note: Isomeric with α- and β-terpinenes.

Sources >5.0%:

Savory (summer)	19.5–42.8%
Ajowan	14.6–35.0%
Cumin	11.2–32.0%
Mandarin leaf	23.9–28.5%
Tea tree	10.0–28.0%
Narcissus absolute	10.3%–27.2%
Mandarin	16.4–22.7%
Tangelo	16.8%
Savory (winter)	1.8–15.1%
Lime expressed (Persian)	1.3–14.4%
Lemon (expressed)	3.0–13.3%
Yuzu	12.5%
Thymus serpyllum	4.4–12.3%
Bergamot (FCF)	3.0–12.0%
Thymus zygis (carvacrol CT)	11.9%
Lime distilled (Persian)	11.8%
Mace (East Indian)	4.9–11.6%
Bergamot (expressed)	5.0–11.4%
Rosemary (camphor CT)	0.5–10.8%
Thymus vulgaris (carvacrol CT)	10.7%
Lime distilled (Mexican)	9.5–10.7%
Lemon (distilled)	8.4–10.7%
Thymus zygis (thymol CT)	0.9–10.1%
Marjoram (sweet)	7.3–9.8%
Thyme (spike)	9.5%
Coriander seed	0.1–9.1%
Oregano	1.6–8.7%
Lime expressed (Mexican)	8.1%
Nutmeg (East Indian)	1.3–7.7%
Plai	6.5%

Thymus vulgaris (thymol CT)	5.2–6.4%	Marjoram (sweet)	16.4–31.6%
Thymus zygis (thymol/carvacrol CT)	6.3%	Basil (hairy)	7.5–26.8%
Juniperberry	0–5.8%	Kewda	0–21.0%
African bluegrass	0.1–5.7%	Ghandi root	17.2%
Bee balm	0.9–5.3%	Juniperberry	1.5–17.0%
Pine (dwarf)	0.1–5.0%	Mace (East Indian)	4.4–14.0%
		Boswellia neglecta	12.5%
		Nutmeg (East Indian)	1.0–10.9%
		Boswellia papyrifera	0–8.0%
		Labrador tea	7.6%
		Boswellia sacra (α-pinene CT)	0–6.9%
		Rosemary (β-myrcene CT)	1.8–6.8%
		Calamint (lesser)	0–6.8%
		Nutmeg (West Indian)	3.0–6.4%
		Blackcurrant bud absolute	0.5–6.3%
		Curry leaf	6.1%
		Lavender	<6.0%
		Pteronia	5.3%
		Saro	3.0–5.0%
		Peppermint	0–5.0%

Adverse skin reactions: Tested at 5% on 25 volunteers γ-terpinene was neither irritating nor sensitizing (Opdyke 1976 p. 875).

Acute toxicity: Acute oral LD_{50} in rats 3.65 g/kg; acute dermal LD_{50} in rabbits >5 g/kg (Opdyke 1976 p. 875).

Antioxidant/pro-oxidant activity: γ-Terpinene demonstrates considerable antioxidant activity, inhibiting oxidation of LDL and linoleic acid, and potently scavenges DPPH radicals (Choi et al 2000; Foti & Ingold 2003; Takahashi et al 2003; Li and Liu 2009).

Mutagenicity and genotoxicity: At low concentrations (0.00005–0.1 mM; 6.8–13,600 µg/L) γ-terpinene was not genotoxic in human lymphocytes, and in the same concentration range it protected them from DNA damage. However, at higher concentrations (0.2–1 mM; 27.2–136 mg/L) γ-terpinene was genotoxic, causing significant increases in DNA damage. At 0.2 mM (27.2 mg/L). γ-Terpinene on its own was genotoxic, but at this concentration also showed antigenotoxic activity (Aydin et al 2005).

Comments: Since antioxidant activity can become pro-oxidant at high doses, the dose-dependent genotoxic/antigenotoxic activity of γ-terpinene may be related to oxidative processes.

Summary: Limited data suggest that γ-terpinene is non-irritant and non-allergenic. It possesses minimal toxicity and may be mutagenic or non-mutagenic, depending on concentration.

Terpinen-4-ol

Synonyms: Terpin-4-ol. Terpinenol-4. 4-Terpineol. 4-Carvomenthol. *p*-Menth-1-en-4-ol

Systematic name: 4-Methyl-1-(1-methylethyl)-3-cyclohexen-1-ol

Chemical class: Monocyclic monoterpenoid alkene alcohol

Note: Different isomers of terpinen-4-ol exist, and the following isomer-specific information has been published:

(R)-(−)-Terpinen-4-ol

CAS number: 20126-76-5

Note: The (R)-(−)- form is found in eucalyptus and *Zanthoxylum* spp.

(S)-(+)-Terpinen-4-ol

CAS number: 2438-10-0

Note: The (S)-(+)- form is found in lavender and cypress spp.

Sources >5.0%:

Tea tree	30.0–48.0%
Plai	41.7%

Adverse skin reactions: Tested at 5% on 25 volunteers terpinen-4-ol was neither irritating nor sensitizing (Opdyke 1982 p. 833–834). Of seven dermatitis patients sensitive to tea tree oil, one was sensitive to terpinen-4-ol tested at 1% (Knight & Hausen 1994). Tested at 10%, terpinen-4-ol was not sensitizing to 11 dermatitis patients sensitive to tea tree oil (Hausen et al 1999). Terpinen-4-ol reduces the edema associated with contact hypersensitivity (Brand et al 2002b).

Acute toxicity: Acute oral LD_{50} in rats 1.3 g/kg; acute dermal LD_{50} in rabbits >2.5 g/kg (Opdyke 1982 p. 833–834). Terpinen-4-ol from juniperberry oil had a rat acute oral LD_{50} of 1.85 mL/kg (Schilcher & Leuschner 1997).

Subacute and subchronic toxicity: A dosage of 400 mg/kg of terpinen-4-ol administered orally to rats for 28 days produced no changes in function or morphology of the kidneys and was therefore not nephrotoxic (Schilcher & Leuschner 1997).

Chronic toxicity: After chronic administration to mice, terpinen-4-ol caused no discernable pathological changes (Janku et al 1960).

Mutagenicity and genotoxicity: Terpinen-4-ol was not mutagenic in *S. typhimurium* TA98, TA100 or TA102, with or without metabolic activation (Fletcher et al 2005).

Carcinogenic/anticarcinogenic potential: Terpinen-4-ol showed in vitro cytotoxic activity against five human cell lines: CTVR-1 (leukemia), Molt-4 (leukemia), K562 (myelogenous leukemia), HeLa (cervical adenocarcinoma) and HepG2 (hepatocellular carcinoma) with IC_{50} values ranging from 0.06–0.33 g/L after 24 hours incubation (Hayes et al 1997). Terpinen-4-ol inhibits the in vitro growth of human melanoma M14 WT cells and their drug-resistant counterparts, M14 adriamicin-resistant cells due to caspase-dependent apoptosis (Calcabrini et al 2004). Terpinen-4-ol significantly inhibited in vitro growth of mouse cancer cell lines AE17 mesothelioma and B16 melanoma. It was significantly less toxic to normal fibroblasts (Greay et al 2010a).

Summary: Terpinen-4-ol appears to be non-irritant and non-allergenic, and possesses 'slight' toxicity. It is not mutagenic, and has demonstrated in vitro antitumoral activity.

Terpineol

Chemical class: Monocyclic monoterpenoid alkene alcohol
Note: Different isomers of terpineol exist, and the following isomer-specific information has been published:

α-Terpineol

Synonyms: (*S*)-(−)-*p*-Menth-1-en-8-ol. (−)-α-Terpineol
Systematic name: (1*S*)-α,α,4-Trimethyl-3-cyclohexene-1-methanol
CAS number: 10482-56-1

Sources >5.0%:

Orange flower and leaf water absolute	23.5%
Orange flower water absolute	20%
Eucalyptus radiata	0–15.2%
Cedarwood (Port Orford)	14.3%
Ho leaf (cineole CT, Chinese)	14.3%
Lime distilled (Mexican)	5.4–12.7%
Palo santo	7.1–10.9%
Thyme (borneol CT)	10.0%
Niaouli (cineole CT)	4.0–10.0%
Galangal (greater)	2.3–9.3%
Chaste tree seed	0.2–9.3%
Chaste tree leaf	1.4–9.2%
Cajuput	6.5–8.7%
Linaloe wood	8.5%
Eucalyptus camaldulensis	0–8.4%
Ho leaf (cineole CT, Madagascan)	6.9–8.3%
Marjoram (sweet)	3.8–8.3%
Tea tree	1.5–8.0%
Lemon (expressed)	0.1–8.0%
Cardamon (black)	7.9%
Narcissus absolute	0.3–7.0%
Orange leaf (Paraguayan)	4.4–6.8%
Lime distilled (Persian)	6.6%
Sugandha	6.6%
Boswellia serrata	1.5–5.8%
Neroli	1.1–5.8%
Sage (African wild)	5.7%
Fragonia	5.6–5.7%
Rosewood	0.5–5.4%
Orange leaf (bigarade)	2.1–5.2%
Galangal (lesser)	5.0%

β-Terpineol

Synonym: *p*-Menth-8-en-1-ol
Systematic name: 1-Methyl-4-(1-methylethenyl)cyclohexanol
CAS number: 138-87-4

Sources >1.0%:

Cedarwood (Port Orford)	3.3%
Lime distilled (Mexican)	0.5–2.2%

γ-Terpineol

Synonym: *p*-Menth-4(8)-en-1-ol
Systematic name: 1-Methyl-4-(1-methylethylidene)cyclohexanol
CAS number: 586-81-2

Sources >1.0%:

Lime distilled (Mexican)	0.8–1.6%

δ-Terpineol

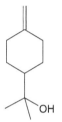

Synonym: *p*-Menth-1(7)-en-8-ol
Systematic name: α,α-Dimethyl-4-methylenecyclohexanemethanol
CAS number: 17023-62-0

Sources >1.0%:

Marjoram (Spanish)	1.0–2.0%
Cardamon (black)	1.6%

Notes: Found in a great many essential oils. A mixture of α, β and γ isomers was used in the RIFM toxicity testing.
Pharmacokinetics: α-Terpineol forms a glucuronide conjugate in rabbits and is excreted mainly unchanged in guinea pig urine. The major urinary metabolite in both rat and man is *p*-menthan-1,2,8-triol, which is excreted principally free and partly conjugated. Acidic metabolites have also been detected (Scheline 1991 p37).
Adverse skin reactions: Undiluted mixed isomer terpineol was moderately irritating to rabbit skin; tested at 12% on 25 human subjects it was not sensitizing (Opdyke 1974 p. 997–998). Tested at 5%, α-terpineol induced allergic responses in 1 (0.1%) of 1,606 consecutive dermatitis patients (Frosch et al 2002b). Of 1,200 dermatitis patients patch tested, there were no irritant reactions and two allergic reactions (0.17%) to 5% α-terpineol (Santucci et al 1987). There were no irritant or allergic reactions in a group of 100 consecutive dermatitis patients tested with 5% terpineol (isomer not specified) (Frosch et al 1995a). None of 70 patients with contact dermatitis reacted to 1% α-terpineol (Nethercott et al 1989). There were no reactions to 15% terpineol (mixed isomers) mixed with 10% terpinyl acetate in 179 dermatitis patients suspected of allergy to cosmetics. α-Terpineol can reduce the edema associated with contact

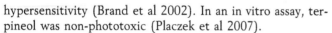

hypersensitivity (Brand et al 2002). In an in vitro assay, terpineol was non-phototoxic (Placzek et al 2007).

Acute toxicity: Acute oral LD_{50} in rats 4.3 g/kg, acute dermal LD_{50} in rabbits >3 g/kg for mixed isomer terpineol (Opdyke 1976 p. 877–878).

Reproductive toxicity: α-Terpineol demonstrated an anti-estrogenic effect in an in vitro assay using MCF-7 cells (Nielsen 2008).

Mutagenicity and genotoxicity: A slight but dose-related mutagenic effect was found for terpineol in the Ames test in one report (Gomes-Carneiro et al 1998). In two others, α-terpineol was not mutagenic (Florin et al 1980; Heck et al 1989). In a mouse lymphoma assay, α-terpineol was not mutagenic, with or without S9 (Heck et al 1989).

Carcinogenic/anticarcinogenic potential: α-Terpineol inhibited the in vitro cell growth of myelogenous leukemia (K562) cells, with an IC_{50} of 75 μM (11.6 mg/L) (Lampronti et al 2006). Hayes et al (1997) reported that α-terpineol was cytotoxic against five human cell lines: CTVR-1 (leukemia), Molt-4 (leukemia), K562 (myelogenous leukemia), HeLa (cervical adenocarcinoma) and HepG2 (hepatocellular carcinoma) with IC_{50} values ranging from 0.2 to 0.32 g/L after 24 hours incubation. Bicas et al (2011) also observed activity against K562 cells, and in addition found α-terpineol to be cytotoxic to cells for MCF-7 (breast cancer), NCI-ADR/RES (multidrug resistant breast adenocarcinoma), NIH:004FVCAR-3 (ovarian adenocarcinoma), PC-3 (prostate cancer) and NCI-H460 (non-small cell lung cancer). In male and female mice given 24 ip injections of α-terpineol or β-terpineol in tricaprylin in a total dose of 1.9 or 9.6 g/kg over 24 weeks, the incidence of primary lung tumors for either compound was no higher than in the control group (Stoner et al 1973).

Comments: α-Terpineol is the predominant isomer found in essential oils, and is virtually the only terpineol isomer that has been separately tested. Only Spanish marjoram oil contain more of another terpineol isomer.

Summary: There is a very low incidence of allergic skin reactions to α-terpineol (or unspecified isomer terpineol) in humans. Terpineol shows a low level of acute toxicity in experimental animals. α-Terpineol is not mutagenic.

Terpinolene

Synonyms: Isoterpinene. Methylcyclohexene. p-Mentha-1,4(8)-diene
Systematic name: 1-Methyl-4-(1-methylethylidene)cyclohexene
Chemical class: Monocyclic monoterpenoid alkene
CAS number: 586-62-9

Sources >5.0%:

Parsnip	40.3–69.0%
Pine (dwarf)	1.0–29.2%
Blackcurrant bud absolute	3.9–11.6%
Turmeric leaf	11.5%
Fir (Douglas)	9.1%
Hemp	1.6–9.1%
Blackcurrant bud	0–9.0%

Lime distilled (Mexican)	8.1–8.7%
Lemon balm (Australian)	6.6%
Parsley leaf	2.8–6.6%
Cypress	2.4–6.3%
Cajuput	0–5.9%
Lime distilled (Persian)	5.2%
Rosalina	2.0–5.0%
Tea tree	1.5–5.0%

Adverse skin reactions: Tested at 20% on human subjects terpinolene was neither irritating nor sensitizing (Opdyke 1976 p. 877–878). Tested at 10%, terpinolene was sensitizing to all of 16 dermatitis patients sensitive to tea tree oil (Hausen et al 1999).

Acute toxicity: Acute oral LD_{50} in both rats and mice 4.4 mL/kg (Opdyke 1976 p. 877–878).

Antioxidant/pro-oxidant activity: Terpinolene has demonstrated both marked DPPH scavenging activity (Choi et al 2000; Kim HJ et al 2004) and marked protection against LDL oxidation (Grassmann et al 2003, 2005).

Carcinogenic/anticarcinogenic potential: Terpinolene inhibited the in vitro formation of the carcinogen NDMA by 79% (Sawamura et al 1999).

Summary: Terpinolene was a cause of several cases of tea tree oil allergenicity. Thresholds of terpinolene skin sensitization are not known. Limited data suggests minimal toxicity. Terpinolene demonstrates radical scavenging activity.

Terpinyl acetate

Chemical class: Monocyclic monoterpenoid alkene ester
Notes: Mixed isomers were used in the toxicity testing. Different isomers of terpinyl acetate exist, and the following information has been published:

α-Terpinyl acetate

Synonyms: p-Menth-1-en-8-ol acetate. α-Terpineol acetate
Systematic name: α,α,4-Trimethylcyclohex-3-enylmethyl ethanoate
CAS number: 80-26-2

Sources >1.0%:

Lovage leaf	43.4–47.3%
Cardamon	29.2–39.7%
Sage (Spanish)	0–15.5%
Betel	6.8–11.0%
Hinoki leaf	9.1%
Hinoki root	9.1%
Lemon leaf	tr–7.3%
Laurel leaf	4.5–7.0%
Cypress	4.1–6.4%
Chaste tree seed	0.1–4.6%
Juniper (Phoenician)	0–4.6%
Myrtle	0–4.4%
Lovage seed	3.1%

| Thuja | 1.0–1.8% |
| *Thymus zygis* (thymol CT) | 0–1.2% |

β-Terpinyl acetate

Synonyms: *p*-Menth-8-en-1-ol acetate. β-Terpineol acetate
Systematic name: 1-Methyl-4-(1-methylethenyl) cyclohex-1-yl ethanoate
CAS number: 10198-23-9

Sources >1.0%:

| Blackcurrant bud absolute | 1.9% |

γ-Terpinyl acetate

Synonyms: *p*-Menth-4(8)-en-1-ol acetate. γ-Terpineol acetate
Systematic name: 1-Methyl-4-(1-methylethylidene)-cyclohexyl ethanoate
CAS number: 10235-63-9

Adverse skin reactions: Tested at 5% on 25 volunteers, terpinyl acetate was neither irritating nor sensitizing (Opdyke 1974 p. 999–1000). There were no reactions to 10% terpinyl acetate mixed with 15% terpineol (mixed isomers) in 179 dermatitis patients suspected of allergy to cosmetics (De Groot et al 1985). There were no irritant or allergic reactions in a group of 100 consecutive dermatitis patients tested with 5% terpinyl acetate (Frosch et al 1995a).

Acute toxicity: Terpinyl acetate acute oral LD_{50} in rats 5.1 g/kg (Jenner et al 1964).

Subacute and subchronic toxicity: No effect was observed from feeding terpinyl acetate to rats at 1,000, 2,500 or 10,000 ppm for 20 weeks (Hagan et al 1967).

Inhalation toxicity: In animals chronic inhalation of terpinyl acetate causes changes in the CNS, blood and liver. The minimum active concentration is 10 mg/m^3 (Rumiantsev et al 1993).

Summary: Terpinyl acetate is non-irritant and non-allergenic. It shows only minimal acute or subchronic toxicity. The maximum safe airborne concentration is 10 mg/m^3.

Thujaplicin

Chemical class: Monocyclic monoterpenoid polyalkene ketone alcohol
Note: Different isomers of thujaplicin exist, and the following isomer-specific information has been published:

α-Thujaplicin

Systematic name: 2-Hydroxy-3-(1-methylethyl)-2,4,6-cycloheptatrien-1-one
CAS number: 1946-74-3

Sources:

| Hibawood | Minor constituent |

β-Thujaplicin

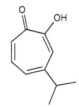

Synonyms: Hinokitiol. 4-Isopropyltropolone
Systematic name: 2-Hydroxy-4-(1-methylethyl)-2,4,6-cycloheptatrien-1-one
CAS number: 499-44-5

Sources:

| Hibawood | Major constituent |

γ-Thujaplicin

Systematic name: 2-Hydroxy-5-(1-methylethyl)-2,4,6-cycloheptatrien-1-one
CAS number: 672-76-4

Sources:

| Hibawood | Minor constituent |

Adverse skin reactions: β-Thujaplicin has been reported as a cause of ACD (Fujita & Aoki 1983).

Acute toxicity: β-Thujaplicin mouse acute oral LD_{50} 775 mg/kg (Ogata et al 1999); mouse ip LD_{50} values: 256 mg/kg for α-thujaplicin, 191 mg/kg for β-thujaplicin, 277 mg/kg for γ-thujaplicin (Matsumura et al 2001; Morita et al 2001, 2002).

Subacute and subchronic toxicity: Dietary β-thujaplicin was administered to male and female rats at 0.02%, 0.07% and 0.2% for 13 weeks. Significant body weight gain reduction was seen in 0.2% males and in 0.07% and 0.2% females, significant increases in relative liver weight was seen in 0.07% males and females, and increases in heart weight was seen in mid-dose and high-dose males. Various hematological parameters were adversely affected in 0.07% and/or 0.2% groups. The rat NOAEL was therefore 0.02%, equivalent to 12.7 mg/kg/day for males, and 14.8 mg/kg/day for females (Cho et al 2011).

Reproductive toxicity: A single dose of β-thujaplicin was administered orally to pregnant mice at 0, 420, 560, 750 or 1,000 mg/kg and was teratogenic at the three highest doses. At 560 mg/kg or greater it caused retardation in growth and developmental parameters in vitro and in vivo. The severity of the abnormalities was dose-dependent, and a 1% effective dose (ED_1) value of 190 mg/kg was derived for external malformations (Ogata et al 1999). Pregnant rats were given β-thujaplicin by gavage in doses of 15, 45 or 135 mg/kg on gestational days 6–15. There was a significant increase in postimplantation loss and in fetal malformations at 135 mg/kg. Based on decreases in maternal weight gain, and the weight of female fetuses at 45 mg/kg or higher, the NOAEL for both dams and fetuses was 15 mg/kg (Ema et al 2004).

Mutagenicity and genotoxicity: β-Thujaplicin was not mutagenic in an Ames test, but was mutagenic in a rec assay with

S9, and in a CA test. It was not genotoxic in a mouse micronucleus assay (Sofuni et al 1993, cited in Cho et al 2011).

Carcinogenic/anticarcinogenic potential: Groups of male and female rats received dietary β-thujaplicin at 0.015% or 0.05% for two years, equivalent to 7.8 and 25.9 mg/kg/day for females, and 6.4 and 20.9 mg/kg/day for males. Sixteen organs/tissues were examined, and no treatment-related increases in neoplastic lesions were seen. Hematological examination revealed no dose-related adverse effects (Imai et al 2006). α-Thujaplicin, β-thujaplicin and γ-thujaplicin were dose-dependently cytotoxic to both KATO-III (human stomach cancer) and Ehrlich's ascites carcinoma cell lines (Matsumura et al 2001; Morita et al 2001, 2002). γ-Thujaplicin was dose-dependently cytotoxic to mouse P388 lymphocytic leukemia cells (Morita et al 2004). β-Thujaplicin dose-dependently inhibited cell proliferation of human prostate cancer PC-3 and LNCaP cells, reduced intracellular and secreted PSA levels, and blocked the binding of a synthetic androgen to LNCaP cells (Liu & Yamauchi 2006). β-Thujaplicin inhibits ultraviolet B-induced apoptosis in keratinocytes and the inhibitory mechanism is thought to be due to the antioxidant activity of metallothionein induced by the agent (Baba et al 1998).

Comments: β-Thujaplicin has a relatively short half-life in the body, and is thought unlikely to represent a risk to humans (Ogata et al 1999). The compound has been permitted as a natural food preservative in Japan since 1996. There appear to be significant differences in reproductive toxicity tolerance levels between rats and mice.

Summary: β-Thujaplicin has moderate acute toxicity. The mouse reproductive toxicity NOAEL is 15 mg/kg. Similarly, the 13 week NOAEL in rats is 14.8 mg/kg/day for females and 12.7 mg/kg/day for males. β-Thujaplicin was not carcinogenic in rats at doses up to 25 mg/kg/day for 2 years. Thujaplicin isomers have shown in vitro antitumoral activity.

Thujone

Synonyms: Thujan-3-one. Absinthone. 3-Sabinone
Systematic name: 1-(1-Methylethyl)-4-methylbicyclo[3.1.0]hexan-3-one
Chemical class: Bicyclic monoterpenoid ketone
Notes: The α- and β- isomers are usually found together in nature. The following isomer-specific information has been published:

(−)-α-Thujone

Synonyms: [1S-(1α,4α,5α)]-Thujone. (1S,4R,5R)-Thujone. (−)-3-Isothujone
CAS number: 546-80-5

Sources >0.1:

Western red cedar	63.5–84.0%
Genipi	79.8%
Wormwood (sea)	63.3%
Thuja	48.7–51.5%
Sage (Dalmatian)	13.1–48.5%
Wormwood (white)	25.7–36.8%
Lanyana	22.5%

Boldo	14.3%
Mugwort (common, camphor/thujone CT)	11.4%
Wormwood (β-thujone CT)	2.3–3.4%
Artemisia vestita	1.8%
Boswellia frereana	0–1.2%
Tansy	1.1%
Yarrow (chamazulene CT)	1.1%
Balsamite	0.8%
Cistus	0–0.8%
Mugwort (common, chrysanthenyl acetate CT)	0.2–0.3%
Wormwood ((Z)-epoxy-ocimene CT)	0–0.2%
Wormwood (sabinyl acetate CT)	0.1%
Hyssop (pinocamphone CT)	0–0.1%

(+)-β-Thujone

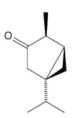

Synonyms: [1S-(1α,4β,5α)]-Thujone. (1S,4S,5R)-Thujone. (+)-3-Thujone. *cis*-Thujone
CAS number: 471-15-8

Sources >0.1%

Wormwood (β-thujone CT)	33.1–59.9%
Tansy	45.2%
Mugwort (great)	34.0%
Wormwood (β-thujone/(Z)-epoxy-ocimene CT)	20.9–21.7%
Sage (Dalmatian)	3.9–19.1%
Western red cedar	4.9–15.2%
Genipi	10.4%
Thuja	7.9–9.9%
Wormwood (white)	2.0–9.0%
Lanyana	8.9%
Boldo	7.2%
Mugwort (common, chrysanthenyl acetate CT)	2.1–2.3%
Boswellia neglecta	1.8%
Yarrow (chamazulene CT)	1.8%
Sage (Greek)	1.6%
Savin	0.2–1.5%
Wormwood ((Z)-epoxy-ocimene CT)	0.3–0.8%
Artemisia vestita	0.7%
Wormwood (sabinyl acetate CT)	0.6%
Hyssop (pinocamphone CT)	0–0.3%
Balsamite	0.2%

Pharmacokinetics: Both α- and β-thujone are rapidly detoxified by CYP-dependent oxidative metabolism (Höld et al 2001). In rabbits, thujone was hydroxylated to 4-*p*-menthanol-2-one and excreted in the urine as its glucuronide conjugate (Scheline 1991 p. 109). Following oral administration in rabbits of α- and β-thujone (ratio 9:2) two neutral urinary metabolites were identified as 3-hydroxy-α-thujane and 3-β-hydroxy-β-thujane (Ishida et al 1989). α-Thujone was metabolized by mouse liver microsomes to 7-hydroxy-α-thujone as the major product, plus five minor metabolites (Höld et al 2000). Hydroxylation at the 2-position of α-thujone was observed in mice, but not in rat or human liver microsomes (Höld et al 2001).

In humans, α-thujone is mainly metabolized to 4- and 7-hydroxythujone by CYP2A6. Minor metabolites include 2-hydroxythujone, resulting from CYP2B6 and CYP3A4-catalyzed reactions, and carvacrol. Interestingly, α-thujone inhibited CYP2A6 with an IC_{50} of 15.4 μM (2.34 mg/L), and CYP2B6 with an IC_{50} of 17.5 μM (2.66 mg/L) (Abass et al 2011). This is significant because it will prolong and augment α-thujone levels, and hence, α-thujone toxicity. Low doses of thujone have been shown to affect nervous tissue (Sampson & Fernandez 1939; Steinmetz et al 1985). This strongly suggests that it crosses the blood–brain barrier and enters the CNS after absorption into the bloodstream.

Using data from Schmitt et al (2010) we calculate the human dermal absorption of α-thujone to be within the range of 2–5% (see Ch. 4, p. 44).

Adverse skin reactions: Tested at 4% on volunteers α-thujone was neither irritating nor sensitizing (FEMA 1997).

Acute toxicity: The α-isomer is more toxic than the β-isomer. Subcutaneous mouse LD_{50} 87 mg/kg for α-thujone, 440 mg/kg for β-thujone, 134 mg/kg for α- + β-thujone (Rice and Wilson 1976). α-Thujone sc LD_{50} in rabbits 360 mg/kg (NLM 1997). For α- + β-thujone: mouse oral LD_{50} 230 mg/kg, rat oral LD_{50} reported as 190 mg/kg (Pinto-Scognamiglio 1967) and 500 mg/kg (NLM 1997); rat ip LD_{50} 1,250 mg/kg (Millet et al 1980). Dog oral LD_{Lo} for β-thujone 250 mg/kg (Opdyke et al 1976 p. 869). Rat ip LD_{50} for α + β-thujone 140 mg/kg (Sampson & Fernandez 1939). Rabbit iv LD_{50} 0.031 mg/kg (NLM 1997). Oral thujone is lethal, convulsive and psychotropic in mice at 250 mg/kg (Le Bourhis & Soenen 1973).

Subacute and subchronic toxicity: In a 16 day study, α-thujone was administered by gavage to B6C3F1 mice and to Fischer 344 rats at doses of 0, 1, 3, 10, 30 or 100 mg/kg. In mice, mortality was 4/5 males and 5/5 females in the highest dose group; mortality was no greater than controls in the lower dose groups. Histological changes, seen only at the highest dose, included mild renal tubular dilatation/focal degeneration, increased hematopoiesis in spleen, and bone marrow myeloid cell hyperplasia. There was no increased mortality in male rats but there was in females at the highest dose (3/5 animals). As in mice, the increased death rate was associated with seizures (National Toxicology Program 2011).

In a 16 day study using a mixture of 71% α-thujone, 12% β-thujone, 13% fenchone and 3% camphor, similar doses to those above were administered by gavage to mice and rats of the same strains. In mice on the highest dose there was increased mortality in males (5/5) and females (2/5) but this was not associated with any notable pathology. In rats, 1/5 males died in the highest dose group but gross and histological effects were minimal (National Toxicology Program 2011).

Thujone (isomer unspecified) was administered to rats by gavage at doses of 12.5, 25 or 50 mg/kg/day, five days per week for 13 weeks. There was an increased lethality in 60% of females and 37% of males at the high dose. The NOAEL for convulsions in the males was 12.5 mg/kg but no NOAEL for females could be established (Surber 1962). In a further gavage study, rats were given thujone at 5, 10 or 20 mg/kg/day on six days per week for 14 weeks. There were three deaths in females and one in males, associated with convulsions at the high dose. The NOAEL for convulsions was 10 mg/kg in males and 5 mg/kg in females. No changes were noted in hematologic parameters or histopathologic examinations (Margaria 1963). In a subsequent 14 week study, a mixture of 70% α-thujone, 11% β-thujone, 16% fenchone, 2% camphor was given to rats at 12.5, 25, 50, 75 or 100 mg/kg and to mice at 6.25, 12.5, 25, 50 or 75 mg/kg. The NOAEL for mice was 12.5 mg/kg. It would have been also for rats, except that all doses caused an increase in renal tubule mineralization in females (National Toxicology Program 2011).

Chronic toxicity: Data on non-neoplastic lesions from the two-year carcinogenicity gavage studies described below indicate a mouse NOAEL for all endpoints of 12 mg/kg. No NOAEL could be established for rats, since even at 12.5 mg/kg there was increased renal tubule mineralization in male rats, and some seizures in both sexes (National Toxicology Program 2011).

Neurotoxicity: Thujone can cause convulsions when taken by mouth (Budavari 1989) and is suspected of being particularly toxic to the CNS (Gerarde 1960). Administered sc to mice, α- + β-thujone was convulsant but not lethal in mice at 590 mg/kg (Wenzel & Ross 1957). Administered ip to rats, it was convulsant but not lethal at 36 mg/kg (Sampson & Fernandez 1939) but convulsant and lethal above 0.2 mL/kg (Millet et al 1981). Administered by gavage at 100 mg/kg/day for 16 days, α-thujone induced hyperactivity, tremors, tonic seizures, and was fatal, in a majority of male mice, female mice and female (but not male) rats (National Toxicology Program 2011).

However, in gavage studies using a mixture containing 70–71% α-thujone and 11–12% β-thujone, no rats or mice had seizures at doses up to 100 mg/kg for 16 days; in a 14 week study, there were no seizures at 12.5 mg/kg, but doses of 25 mg/kg or higher were convulsant in both species; in a two-year study, there were no seizures in mice at 12 mg/kg, but 3/50 female rats and 5/50 male rats on 12.5 mg/kg did have seizures, compared with 2/100 controls (National Toxicology Program 2011).

There are no recorded cases of thujone poisoning as such, but thujone-rich oils have caused seizures in humans when large doses were ingested. A 50-year-old woman took 20 drops of thuja oil twice a day for five days. Thirty minutes after her tenth dose she suffered a tonic seizure and fell, fracturing her skull (Millet et al 1981) (Table 14.7). This is evidence of a cumulative effect. Convulsions were induced in an adult who accidentally ingested one 'swallow' of sage oil (Arditti et al 1978) and in two other adults, who ingested 12 drops, and at least one 'swallow' (Burkhard et al 1999). Thujone may be the cause of tonic and clonic seizures and acute renal failure following wormwood oil intoxication (Weisbord et al 1997). Thujone neurotoxicity in rodents and humans in compared in Table 14.7.

There is much anecdotal belief, but little hard evidence, that absinthe toxicity is primarily due to thujone which derives from wormwood, one of the ingredients used to make the spirit. 'Absinthism', a syndrome of hallucinations, sleeplessness,

Table 14.7 Oral thujone neurotoxicity

A. Convulsant doses in humans

Essential oil	Convulsive dose	Equiv. dose of thujone	Dose per kg bw	Reference
Sage	12 drops (400 mg)	200 mg	2.86 mg/kg	Burkhard et al 1999
Thuja	20 drops[a] (666 mg)	400 mg	5.7 mg/kg	Millet et al 1981

B. Non-convulsant doses in rodents

Substance	Animal	Daily dose	Reference
α and β-Thujone	Rats and mice	30 mg/kg $\times$ 14 days	SCF 2003b
Not stated	Male rat	10 mg/kg $\times$ 1 day	Margaria 1963
Not stated	Female rat	5 mg/kg $\times$ 1 day	Margaria 1963

[a]Taken daily for five days

tremors, seizures and even paralysis, was associated with long-term ingestion of the liqueur (Bonkovsky et al 1992; Weisbord et al 1997). Absinthe is said to have originally contained 260 mg/kg of thujone, but there are doubts about the analytical methods available at the time. Some vintage absinthes were very low in thujone (less than 10 mg/L) but the thujone content may have degraded over time. However, absinthes produced according to historical recipes also turned out to be very low in thujone (0–4.3 mg/L) (Lachenmeier et al 2005).

Cognitive performance and mood can be affected by thujone. In a clinical trial with three groups, one drinking just alcohol, one drinking alcohol containing 10 mg/L of thujone, and the third drinking alcohol with 100 mg/L thujone, the high thujone group showed significant reductions in attention performance parameters, such as reaction times to visual stimuli. In addition, there was a relative increase in anxiety. The reactions observed are thought to be due to the antagonistic effect of thujone on GABA receptors (Dettling et al 2004).

α-Thujone is a non-competitive GABA antagonist at GABA$_A$ receptors, and modulates GABA-gated chloride channels. Although accumulating in the brain in higher concentrations, its metabolite, 7-hydroxy-α-thujone, binds to this receptor with much lower affinity (Höld et al 2000). β-Thujone is also a GABA$_A$ receptor antagonist (Hall et al 2004). When GABA$_A$ receptors are blocked, neurons fire too easily and their signaling goes out of control (Rietjens et al 2005b).

It has been suggested that thujone and δ-9-tetrahydrocannabinol, the most active ingredient in cannabis, interact with a common receptor in the CNS and so have similar psychotropic effects (Del Castillo et al 1975). However, subsequent studies showed that thujone binds with relatively low affinity to CB$_1$ and CB$_2$ receptors and fails to mimic δ-9-tetrahydrocannabinol at appropriate doses (Meschler & Howlett 1999).

Reproductive toxicity: In a three month gavage study in rats and mice of both sexes, there was no evidence of toxicity induced by a thujone-rich mixture (70% α-thujone, 11% β-thujone, 16% fenchone, 2% camphor) to the reproductive system of male rats; however, female rats in the highest dose group (50 mg/kg) were more likely to remain in extended diestrus than controls (National Toxicology Program 2011). No data could be found for thujone relating to possible toxicity in pregnancy.

Hepatotoxicity: Thujone was porphyrigenic in primary cultures of chick embryo hepatocytes and so may be especially hazardous to those with defects in hepatic heme synthesis (Bonkovsky et al 1992).

Mutagenicity and genotoxicity: Thujone was tested at 1.5% and 3.0% in DMSO for its effect on the mutagenicity of aflatoxin B$_1$ in *S. typhimurium* TA100. There was some evidence of colony damage which the researchers interpreted as moderate mutagenesis (Kim et al 1992). A mixture of α- and β-thujone (94.5%, 3.5%) was not mutagenic in *S. typhimurium* TA100, and inhibited UV-induced mutations in both *E. coli* and *S. cerevisiae* (Vuković-Gačić et al 2006). Similarly, mixed isomer thujone (composition as below) was not mutagenic in either *S. typhimurium* or *E. coli*, with or without S9. After three months of gavage dosing, mixed isomer thujone was not toxic to bone marrow in mice; in a micronucleus test it was not genotoxic to male mice, but was very slightly genotoxic to female mice (National Toxicology Program 2011). Thujone was not genotoxic in the wing somatic mutation and recombination test (SMART) of *Drosophila melanogaster* (Pavlidou et al 2004).

Carcinogenic/anticarcinogenic potential: In two-year gavage studies, rats and mice of both sexes were dosed with a mixture of 70% α-thujone, 11% β-thujone, 16% fenchone and 2% camphor. Rats were given 12.5, 25 or 50 mg/kg/day, mice were given 3, 6, 12 or 25 mg/kg/day. All the high-dose rats died before the end of the study, and survival was significantly reduced in all 25 mg/kg groups. In male rats, there was an increased incidence of preputial gland carcinoma, but this was not dose-dependent, and incidence in the 12.5 mg/kg group was 1/49 rats, compared to 3/49 in the control group. The existence of a preputial gland in humans is controversial. There was no evidence of carcinogenicity in any organ in female rats, or in mice of either sex. Therefore, a rodent NOAEL for carcinogenesis would be at least 12.5 mg/kg (National Toxicology Program 2011).

When mixed isomer thujone was administered ip to various mouse species at 1 mg/kg/day for five consecutive days, both humoral and cell-mediated immunity were significantly enhanced, and the development of solid tumors was inhibited (Siveen & Kuttan 2011). A thujone-rich fraction of *Thuja occidentalis* was cytotoxic to human melanoma (A375) cells. At

200 μg/mL it inhibited proliferation of 59% of cells and induced apoptosis, with only minimal cytotoxic effects on peripheral blood mononuclear cells (Biswas et al 2011).

Comments: It is curious that the increase in renal tubule mineralization seen in rats in the National Toxicology Program (2011) report was only in females in the 14 week study, yet only in males in the two year study. In neither case was the incidence dose-related. Taken together these observations cast doubt on the relevance of the renal toxicity data. In addition, the thujone mix used was only 81% pure. The authors explain that in most tests they used a mixture of thujone isomers because this reflects the occurrence of thujone in nature. However, they give no explanation for the presence of fenchone and camphor in the preparation used. Only one essential oil, thuja, contains significant quantities of both thujone and fenchone. In mice, subcutaneously injected fenchone was convulsant at 1,133 mg/kg but not at 500 mg/kg, while mixed isomer thujone was convulsant at 590 mg/kg (Wenzel & Ross 1957), suggesting that fenchone is significantly less neurotoxic than thujone.

The α-thujone used in the 16 day studies was 99% pure, the mixed isomer thujone used in the 16 day studies was 83% pure, and that used in the 14 week and two year studies was 81% pure. Historically, the relative proportions of α- and β-thujone used in testing are not always specified, and there is no standard mix that is universally used. In most essential oils that contain thujone, the α-isomer predominates, but there are exceptions. However, since α-thujone is the more toxic of the isomers, using a mixture containing more of it errs on the side of safety.

Summary: Thujone isomers are always found together in essential oils, though in relative proportions that vary greatly. In a mouse sc LD_{50} test, α-thujone was five times more toxic than β-thujone. α-Thujone, mixed isomer thujone, and thujone-rich oils are neurotoxic, causing convulsions in experimental animals and (in the case of essential oils) humans. The data suggest that humans are up to ten times more susceptible to thujone neurotoxicity than rats. When 30 mg/kg/day of an α-/β thujone mixture was administered to rats and mice for 16 days, no convulsions were seen (National Toxicology Program 2011), while in a human case, 12 drops (400 mg) of Dalmatian sage essential oil (containing an estimated 150–200 mg total thujone, equivalent to 2.2–2.9 mg/kg) did cause convulsions (Burkhard et al 1999). α-Thujone may be more neurotoxic than β-thujone. Current research does not support the hypothesis of a THC-like psychotropic effect for thujone, but it may adversely affect cognitive performance. Mixed isomer thujone is not carcinogenic in mice or in female rats. The relevance to humans of preputial gland carcinoma from thujone dosing seen in male rats is doubtful. There is evidence of marginal genotoxicity.

Regulatory guidelines: Thujone is banned as a food additive in the USA and its presence in foods and beverages is regulated in several countries; the limits for α- and/or β-thujone in Europe vary from 5–35 mg/kg depending on beverage type (Anon 1992b). Thujone is listed in the EPA's Toxic Substances Control Act inventory. In 1999 the Council of Europe allocated a TDI of 10 μg/kg of thujone, based on the NOAEL of 5 mg/kg in female rats and an uncertainty factor of 500 (Council of Europe 1999, cited in SCF 2003b). However, in a subsequent SCF report on thujone it was concluded that the available data were inadequate to establish a TDI/ADI (SCF 2003b). The

European Medicines Agency proposed an oral limit for thujone of 3 mg/adult, in 2009 (EMA 2009) and later revised this to 5 mg/kg (EMA 2010).

Our safety advice: Lachenmeier & Uebelacker (2010) have proposed an oral limit for thujone isomers of 0.11 mg/kg/day, based on benchmark dose modeling of the rodent data, including the NTP 2011 report. This is derived from a $BMDL_{10}$ value of 11 mg/kg/day for clonic sezures in male rats, and uncertainty factors of 10 for interspecies and 10 for interindividual differences. We recommend a rounded down value of 0.1 mg/kg/day. This is equivalent to 7 mg per adult, and a dermal exposure of 0.25% (Table 14.1).

Thymol

Synonyms: 2-Isopropyl-5-methylphenol. 2-(1-Methylethyl)-5-methylphenol. *p*-Cymen-3-ol. Thyme camphor
Systematic name: 1-Hydroxy-2-methylethyl-5-methylbenzene
Chemical class: Phenol
CAS number: 89-83-8

Sources >1.0%:

Thymus zygis (thymol CT)	30.9–74.0%
Thymus vulgaris (thymol CT)	48.3–62.5%
Oregano (Mexican)	0.2–60.6%
Ajowan	36.9–53.8%
Thyme (limonene CT)	27.6%
Thymus serpyllum	16.7–25.9%
Thymus zygis (thymol/carvacrol CT)	25.5%
Thyme (borneol CT)	10.0%
Savory (winter)	1.0–8.0%
Thymus vulgaris (carvacrol CT)	5.0%
Oregano	0.3–4.4%
Thyme (linalool CT)	1.0–3.8%
Fir needle (Canadian)	0–2.9%
Chaste tree seed	0–2.7%
Boswellia papyrifera	0–2.6%
Damiana	2.3%
Tansy (blue)	0.8–1.8%
Boswellia rivae	1.4%
Wormseed	1.0%
Chaste tree leaf	0–1.0%

Notes: Isomeric with carvacrol. Being a substituted phenol, thymol is a weak acid that may be corrosive to tissues. Thymol is used in aromatic inhalation mixtures for the relief of nasal congestion and colds, and in antiseptic mouthwashes for the treatment of oral ulcers.

Pharmacokinetics: Thymol is primarily excreted as glucuronide and ethereal sulfate conjugates in rabbits, dogs and man. A small amount of oxidation, giving thymoquinol, has also been observed. Following the ingestion of 0.6 g thymol by humans, thymol glucuronide, thymol sulfate, and small amounts of thymoquinol sulfate and of unchanged thymol were excreted in the urine (Scheline 1991). On human ingestion of 1.08 mg of thymol, thymol sulfate was detected in both plasma and urine, and thymol glucuronide was found in urine. No free thymol was detected in either plasma or urine, possibly due to the much smaller dose used in this study. Peak plasma concentrations were 93.1 ng/mL and were reached after 2.0 hours. The mean terminal elimination half-life was 10.2 hours. Thymol sulfate was detectable up to 41 hours after administration. The amount of both thymol sulfate and glucuronide excreted in 24-hour urine was 16.2% of the dose (Kohlert et al 2002).

Adverse skin reactions: Thymol is regarded as an irritant (Budavari 1989). In a CAM (chorioallantoic membrane of the fertile chicken egg) assay, an established model for detecting irritants, *Origanum onites* oil with 57.4% carvacrol and 11.6% thymol was strongly irritating. This irritation was due to thymol and not to carvacrol (Demirci et al 2004). However, *Lippia sidoides* leaf oil, consisting of 66.7% thymol, inhibited mouse ear inflammation by 45.9% when applied topically at 1 mg/ear (Monteiro et al 2007).

In a 48 hour occlusive patch test on 50 volunteers, the highest concentration of thymol producing no adverse reaction was 5%. Similarly tested at 1%, it produced no reactions in 290 eczema patients (Meneghini et al 1971). Of 1,200 dermatitis patients patch tested, there were no irritant or allergic reactions to 1% thymol (Santucci et al 1987). None of 70 patients with contact dermatitis reacted to patch tests with 1% thymol (Nethercott et al 1989). Two cases of ACD due to thymol have been reported (Fisher 1989; Lorenzi et al 1995).

Based on literature published in German, thymol was classified as category C, not significantly allergenic, by Schlede et al (2003).

Mucous membrane irritation: According to Reynolds (1993) thymol is irritant to the gastric mucosa; fats and alcohol increase its absorption and aggravate toxic symptoms. However, gastric irritation depends on dose and concentration. Monteiro et al (2007) reported that oral *Lippia sidoides* leaf oil, consisting of 66.7% thymol, dose-dependently inhibited alcohol-induced gastric lesions when given at 1, 5 and 10 mg/kg, but this effect reduced as the dose increased to 50 and 100 mg/kg.

Acute toxicity: Acute oral LD_{50} reported as 1,800 mg/kg in mice (Spector 1956), 980 mg/kg in rats, and 880 mg/kg in guinea pigs (Jenner et al 1964). Dog iv lethal dose 150 mg/kg (Caujolle and Franck 1944a). No toxicity was evident from the acute administration of up to 3 g/kg of *Lippia sidoides* oil (60% thymol) to mice (Fontenelle et al 2007).

Subacute and subchronic toxicity: Oral administration of 118 mg/kg/day of *Lippia sidoides* oil (60% thymol) to mice for 30 days was devoid of toxicity (Fontenelle et al 2007). No adverse effects were observed on gross pathology, hematology, body weight, food intake or organ weight from 1,000 ppm or 10,000 ppm thymol given to rats in the diet for 19 weeks (Hagan et al 1967).

Cardiovascular effects: Thymol inhibited arachidonic acid-induced platelet aggregation, and was over 30 times more potent than aspirin (Enomoto et al 2001).

Hepatotoxicity: A possible link has been proposed between thymol, used as an antioxidant in halothane, and a rare form of severe liver damage, in patients receiving anesthesia (Hutter & Laing 1993). In studies on isolated rat hepatocytes, leakage of glutamic oxaloacetic transaminase (GOT) was dose-dependently increased by 0.2–4.0 mM thymol (30–600 mg/L) (Manabe et al 1987). Thymol showed a considerable protection against carbon tetrachloride-induced hepatotoxicity in rats combined with a marked radical scavenger activity (Jiménez et al 1993). A similar protection was seen in mice, and it was noted that thymol acted as a free radical scavenger, inhibiting lipid peroxidation (Alam et al 1999).

Antioxidant/pro-oxidant activity: Thymol has considerable antioxidant activity (Aeschbach et al 1994; Lee and Shibamoto 2001; Vardar-Unlu et al 2003) and significant radical scavenging activity, even at concentrations less than 1 µg/mL (Braga et al 2005). Thymol dose-dependently inhibited LDL oxidation in human aortic endothelial cells at 1.25–10 µM (Pearson et al 1997).

Mutagenicity and genotoxicity: Thymol was not mutagenic in the Ames test (Florin et al 1980; Azizan & Blevins 1995). It was genotoxic in a CA test in the presence, but not in the absence, of metabolic activation (Hikiba et al 2005). Thymol was cytotoxic, but not genotoxic to human dental pulp fibroblasts (Chang et al 2000). When rats were injected ip with 40, 60, 80 or 100 mg/kg bw of thymol, it was dose-dependently genotoxic to their bone marrow cells (Azirak & Rencuzugullari 2008). Thymol protected K562 leukemic cells from DNA damage induced by hydrogen peroxide, with an IC_{50} of 450 µM (67.5 mg/L) (Horváthová et al 2007). At low concentrations (0.005–0.1 mM; 0.75–15 mg/L) thymol was not genotoxic in human lymphocytes, and also protected them from DNA damage. However, at higher concentrations (0.2–2 mM; 30–300 mg/L) thymol was genotoxic, causing significant increases in DNA damage. At 0.2 mM (30 mg/L), thymol was genotoxic, but at this concentration also showed antigenotoxic activity (Aydin et al 2005). However, this dose-dependency was not seen in another report, where genotoxicity occurred in human lymphocytes at all concentrations tested (Buyukleyla & Rencuzogullari 2009). In a comet assay, thymol was not genotoxic at 1 or 5 µM (150 or 750 µg/L), but was genotoxic at 25 µM (3.75 mg/L) (Ündeger et al 2009). The genotoxic potential of thymol is considered to be very weak, although the possibility of action at DNA level cannot be excluded (Stammati et al 1999; Nafisi et al 2004).

Carcinogenic/anticarcinogenic potential: In male and female mice given 24 ip injections of thymol in tricaprylin in a total dose of 1.2 or 6.0 g/kg over 24 weeks, the incidence of primary lung tumors was no higher than in the control group (Stoner et al 1973). A population of mouse B16(F10) melanoma cells were significantly inhibited by thymol with an IC_{50} value of 120 µM (18.0 mg/L) (He et al 1997b). Thymol completely inhibited the growth of ascites sarcoma BP8 cells (a rat cell line) at a concentration of 1.0 mM (150 mg/L) (Pilotti et al 1975). Thymol was dose-dependently cytotoxic to human leukemia (HL-60) cells at concentrations ranging from 25–100 µM

(3.75–15.0 mg/L), reducing cell viability at 24 hours to 5% at 100 µM, while having no cytotoxic effect on peripheral blood leukocytes. The selective antitumoral action of thymol was partly due to an induction of ROS, leading indirectly to apoptosis (Deb et al 2011). An essential oil of *Ocimum viride* containing 80.4% thymol was dose-dependently cytotoxic to human colon cancer (COLO 205) cells due to apoptosis induction (Sharma et al 2010).

Comments: As with eugenol, it is possible that the action of thymol is highly dependent on dose and concentration, with higher doses being toxic and lower doses being antitoxic. In justifying the CIR maximum of 0.5% for thymol (see below), Andersen (2006b) explains: 'It may be that…thymol…and carvacrol do not cause chemical leukoderma at concentrations higher than 0.5%, but data are not available to support that possibility.' However, the only reference given to suggest that thymol might cause skin depigmentation is Mathias (1988), and this report does not mention thymol or carvacrol. It states that common causes of toxic vitiligo (chemical leukoderma) 'include *para*-substituted phenols and catechols', and thymol is neither of these.

Summary: Patch tested at 1%, thymol caused no irritant or allergic reactions in a total of 1,560 dermatology patients, and is therefore safe to use at this concentration. Thymol is irritant to mucous membrane in high concentrations, but doses of 15 mg/kg bw counteract gastric irritation. The rodent acute toxicity of thymol is borderline 'slight'/'moderate', and thymol was non-toxic in mice at 71 mg/kg over 30 days. There are reports of both hepatotoxicity and hepatoprotection for thymol, and there are reports of it being genotoxic, non-genotoxic and antigenotoxic. These effects may be dose-dependent. Thymol inhibits platelet aggregation.

Regulatory guidelines: The CIR recommended maximum for thymol in cosmetics is 0.5% (Andersen et al 2006b).

Our safety advice: In order to avoid skin irritation, we recommend a maximum dermal use level of 1% for thymol. Because of its antiplatelet aggregation activity, oral dosing of essential oils high in thymol is cautioned in conjunction with anticoagulant drugs, major surgery, childbirth, peptic ulcer, hemophilia or other bleeding disorders (see Box 7.1 for more detail).

Thymoquinone

Synonyms: 2-Isopropyl-5-methyl-1,4-benzoquinone. Thymol. *p*-Mentha-3,6-dien-2,5-dione
Systematic name: 2-Methyl-5-(1-methylethyl)-2,5-cyclohexadien-1,4-dione
Chemical class: Bicyclic benzenoid ketone
CAS number: 490-91-5

Source:

Black seed	26.8–54.8%

Note: An inhaled thymoquinone aerosol dose-dependently protected guinea pigs against histamine-stimulated bronchospasm in the range of 2.5–10 mg/kg (Marozzi et al 1970).
Adverse skin reactions: Thymoquinone is a relatively potent contact allergen. Its action has been rationalized in terms of facile attack by nucleophiles such as amines and thiols (Cremer

et al 1987). Thymoquinone 1% in 96% ethanol was used as a skin irritant in patch testing of 600 allergic and non-allergic people with eczema and 33 healthy controls. There was a positive skin reaction (marked local erythema) in 53% to 63% of all three groups (Coenraads et al 1975).
Acute toxicity: Rat oral LD_{50} 794.3 mg/kg, rat ip LD_{50} 57.5 mg/kg, mouse oral LD_{50} 870.9 mg/kg (Al-Ali et al 2008). The mouse ip LD_{50} has been reported as 90.3 mg/kg and 104.7 mg/kg (Mansour et al 2001; Al-Ali et al 2008).
Subacute and subchronic toxicity: There were no incidents of mortality, toxicity or enzymatic changes in mice given thymoquinone in drinking water at concentrations of 0.01, 0.02, and 0.03% (equivalent to approximately 30, 60, or 90 mg/kg/day) for 90 days. Notably, there was no effect on hepatic glutathione levels (Badary et al 1998). Daily ip injections of rats with 8 mg/kg of thymoquinone resulted in the death of the majority of animals within a week. Surviving animals showed signs of severe peritonitis (Bamosa et al 2002).
Cardiovascular effects: Thymoquinone significantly inhibited VEGF-induced angiogenesis at 1 µM and almost completely abolished it at 10 µM in the matrigel plug assay. It inhibited micro-vessel growth in vitro at 50 nM-100 nM after 4 days incubation. At 6 mg/kg sc for 15 days, thymoquinone inhibited angiogenesis in prostate cancer tumors in mice (Yi et al 2008).
Nephrotoxicity: Thymoquinone protects the kidneys from the damaging effects of two anticancer drugs in rodents. At 5 mg/kg/day orally for five days before, during and after treatment with ifosfamide, thymoquinone significantly reduced ifosfamide-induced renal damage in rats (Badary 1999). Single injections of thymoquinone given iv at 5 mg/kg in rats, and ip at 7 or 14 mg/kg in mice, greatly ameliorated cisplatin nephrotoxicity (Badary et al 1997). When Rhesus monkey kidney epithelial cells were dosed with thymoquinone in vitro at 10, 50 or 100 µM (1.64, 8.20 or 16.4 mg/L), there was no evidence of a pro-oxidant effect, but at 72 hours, there was an increase in cellular glutathione, suggesting a protective effect (Vance et al 2008).
Reproductive toxicity: A single dose of thymoquinone was administered i.p. to pregnant rats on gestational days 11 or 14 at 15, 35 or 50 mg/kg. Dose-dependent fetal resorption and maternal toxicity were seen at the higher two doses, and 15 mg/kg was the NOAEL. At 50 mg/kg on gestational day 11, 100% of implants were resorbed (AbuKhader et al 2013). Diabetes during pregnancy is associated with free radical-mediated oxidative processes, raised levels of malondialdehyde, and teratogenicity or developmental toxicity in animals and humans. When thymoquinone was administered by gavage at 10 mg/kg/day on gestational days 1–19, to mice with induced diabetes, malondialdehyde formation was reduced, and hepatic glutathione was increased, compared to controls (Al-Enazi 2007).
Hepatotoxicity: Incubation of isolated rat hepatocytes with 1 mM (164 mg/L) thymoquinone prevented ALT and AST leakage and the depletion of intracellular glutathione induced by tert-butyl hydroperoxide (Daba et al 1998). Due to its antioxidant activity, thymoquinone protected mouse liver against chemically induced damage at doses of 12.5 mg/kg ip, or 100 mg/kg po (Nagi et al 1999; Mansour et al 2001). However, single ip doses of 25 or 50 mg/kg were not protective (Mansour et al 2001). When administered orally to mice at 1, 2 or 4 mg/kg/day for 5 days, thymoquinone dose-dependently induced

hepatic glutathione *S*-transferase and quinone reductase, demonstrating a protective effect (Nagi & Almakki 2009). The in vivo hepatoprotective action may be mediated through the combined antioxidant properties of thymoquinone and its metabolite, dihydrothymoquinone (Nagi et al 1999).

Antioxidant/pro-oxidant activity: In PC12 cells (an in vitro model for neurotoxicity) 2.34, 4.68 or 9.37 μM (384, 768 or 1,530 μg/L) thymoquinone protected against intracellular ROS and consequent cytotoxicity (Mousavi et al 2010). Thymoquinone appears to undergo reduction to dihydrothymoquinone, which, in an in vitro model, was a more potent antioxidant than thymoquinone or BHT (Nagi et al 1999). Both thymoquinone and dihydrothymoquinone acted as general free radical scavengers in mouse tissues, with IC_{50} values in the nanomolar and micromolar range, respectively (Mansour et al 2002). After rats with high serum cholesterol levels were fed thymoquinone at 20, 50 or 100 mg/kg for 8 weeks, there were dose-dependent increases in plasma hydroxyl radical scavenging activity, and in hepatic superoxide dismutase and glutathione peroxidase levels (Ismail et al 2009). In rats with gastric lesions induced by ischemia/reperfusion (linked with free radical damage), single oral doses 5 or 20 mg/kg thymoquinone inhibited lipid peroxidation, and increased mucosal reduced glutathione and superoxide dismutase after one hour. However, doses of 50 or 100 mg/kg greatly lowered glutathione levels (El-Abhar et al 2003).

Mutagenicity and genotoxicity: Thymoquinone demonstrated an antimutagenic action in protecting mouse cells against CA induced by schistosomiasis (Aboul-Ela 2002). In rat hepatocytes, concentrations of >1.25 mM (>205 mg/L) thymoquinone caused an increased incidence of CA and micronuclei (Khader et al 2009).

Carcinogenic/anticarcinogenic potential: Thymoquinone was cytotoxic to several parental and multi-drug resistant variant human tumor cell lines (Worthen et al 1998), and to cells for lung, larynx, pancreas and colon cancers (Rooney & Ryan 2005a). Cytotoxicity to laryngeal cancer cells was associated with depletion of glutathione (Rooney & Ryan 2005b). Thymoquinone inhibited the proliferation of five different human colon cancer cell lines through apoptosis, without being cytotoxic to normal human intestinal cells (El-Najjar et al 2010). Other studies have found anti-colorectal cancer effects for thymoquinone in vitro (Gali-Muhtasib et al 2004a, 2008a) and in vivo (Gali-Muhtasib et al 2008b). Thymoquinone was cytotoxic to cancerous mouse skin cells (papilloma and spindle cell melanoma), inducing apoptosis at concentrations not toxic to normal keratinocytes (Gali-Muhtasib et al 2004b). Thymoquinone induced oxidative damage and apoptosis in two human bone cancer cell lines (Roepke et al 2007), and inhibited proliferation of HL-60 human leukemia cells, inducing apoptosis (El-Mahdy et al 2005). In an in vitro study, thymoquinone dose-dependently decreased glutathione levels in Hep-2 human laryngeal carcinoma cells (Rooney & Ryan 2005b).

Thymoquinone inhibited the tumor growth of fibrosacrcoma (neoplasia in connective tissue) and squamous cell carcinoma in mice, after intratumoral injection at 5 mg/kg/day for 4 days. It was cytotoxic to the same cancers in vitro, but was less toxic to L929 mouse fibroblasts (Ivankovic et al 2006). Given at 0.01% in drinking water to mice, thymoquinone had a chemopreventive action against fibrosarcoma (Badary & Gamal El-Din

2001). Similarly administered, it also inhibited B[*a*]P-induced forestomach cancer in mice, possibly through an enhancement of antioxidant enzymes and detoxification processes (Badary et al 1999). At 40–100 μM (16.4 mg/L), thymoquinone inhibited the proliferation of three types of prostate cancer cells, but had no adverse effect on normal prostate epithelial cells. After 30 days sc administration at 20 mg/kg/day, thymoquinone reduced the growth of xenografted prostate tumors to half the size of the tumors in control mice (Kaseb et al 2007). Injected sc at 6 mg/kg/day for 15 days, thymoquinone inhibited the growth and angiogenesis of subcutaneous tumors in mice xenografted with human PC3 prostate cancer cells (Yi et al 2008). In both of these studies, thymoquinone had no adverse effect on body weight, suggesting low collateral toxicity.

Comments: Single oral doses of 50 or 100 mg/kg thymoquinone lowered levels of reduced glutathione in the gastric mucosa of rats with induced gastric lesions. However, hepatic glutathione was increased by oral doses of 10 mg/kg/day for 19 days in mice, or of 20–100 mg/kg/day in rats. Intraperitoneal administration of thymoquinone results in much higher toxicity than oral dosing. Taken together, these data suggest that the criteria for internal dosing need to be carefully considered.

Summary: Thymoquinone has a tendency to provoke skin reactions in humans. Rodent data indicates that daily oral doses of thymoquinone between 5 mg/kg and 90 mg/kg can be therapeutic and non-toxic. The ip NOAEL for reproductive toxicity is 15 mg/kg. This, and the strong antiangionenic activity, suggests that thymoquinone is unsafe in pregnancy.

ar-Turmerone

Synonym: Dehydroturmerone
Systematic name: 2-Methyl-6-(4-methylphenyl)-2-hepten-4-one
Chemical class: Benzenoid sesquiterpenoid alkene ketone
CAS number: 532-65-0
Note: The prefix '*ar*' denotes 'aromatic'. α-Turmerone and β-turmerone isomers also exist, both of which are major constituents of turmeric rhizome oil.

Source >1.0%:

Turmeric rhizome	15.5–27.5%

Cardiovascular effects: *ar*-Turmerone showed strong antiplatelet aggregation activity in vitro (Lee 2006). It also showed potent hypoglycemic activity with IC_{50} values against α-glucosidase and α-amylase of 0.28 μg and 24.5 μg respectively (Lekshmi et al 2012).

Mutagenicity and genotoxicity: A fraction of turmeric oil consisting of 44.5% *ar*-turmerone was antimutagenic (Jayaprakasha et al 2002).

Carcinogenic/anticarcinogenic potential: At 50 mg/kg *ar*-turmerone was active against sarcoma 180 ascites (connective tissue cancer) in mice (Itokawa et al 1985). In a 1:1 ratio, it potentiated the action of β-sesquiphellandrene against the muscine L1210 cell line fivefold at 5.2 μg/mL, and in the same ratio it potentiated the action of aurapten, a psoralen found in orange oil (at 1.6 μg/mL) of cyclophosphamide tenfold (at

1.81 µg/mL) and of MeCCNU tenfold (at 0.28 µg/mL) (Ahn & Lee 1989). *ar*-Turmerone, isolated from turmeric, exhibited potent, concentration-dependent apoptotic cytotoxicity towards cell lines for human, rat and mouse leukemia (K562, RBL-2H3 and L1210), and human lymphoma (U937) with IC_{50} values of 20–50 µg/mL (Ji et al 2004). The apoptotic action of *ar*-turmerone from turmeric oil on U937 lymphoma cells involves concentration-dependent caspase-3 activation, through induction of Bax and p53 proteins (Lee 2009). *ar*-Turmerone induced apoptosis in human myeloid leukemia cells (HL-60) through internucleosomal DNA fragmentation (Paek et al 1996). Selective, concentration- and time-dependent induction of apoptosis by *ar*-turmerone was observed in human leukemia HL-60 and Molt 4B cells, but not in human stomach cancer KATO III cells (Aratanechemuge 2002). *ar*-Turmerone showed a potent inhibition of both COX-2 (IC_{50} 5.2 µg/mL) and iNOS (IC_{50} 3.2 µg/mL) that correlates with a cancer chemopreventive action (Lee et al 2002).

Comments: We could find no acute toxicity or dermal data for *ar*-tumerone, but turmeric rhizome oil is non-toxic (see profile), suggesting that *ar*-tumerone probably is also. *ar*-Turmerone inhibits platelet aggregation in vitro.

Summary: *ar*-Turmerone inhibits platelet aggregation. It is anti-mutagenic, and demonstrates in vitro and in vivo antitumoral activity.

2-Undecanone

Synonym: Methylnonyl ketone
Chemical class: Aliphatic ketone
CAS number: 112-12-9

Sources >1.0%:

Rue	46.8–49.2%
Sugandha	3.6%
Ginger	<1.4%

Adverse skin reactions: In a modified Draize procedure on guinea pigs, 2-undecanone was non-sensitizing when used at 10% in the challenge phase (Sharp 1978). Full-strength 2-undecanone was not irritating to the skin of rabbits or hairless mice and swine when applied for 24 hours under occlusion. Tested at 5% on 25 volunteers the material was neither irritating nor sensitizing. No phototoxic effects were found in hairless mice and swine (Opdyke 1975 p. 869–870).

Acute toxicity: Acute oral LD_{50} reported as >5 g/kg in rats and 3.88 g/kg in mice; acute dermal LD_{50} reported as >5 g/kg in rabbits (Opdyke 1975 p. 869–870).

Summary: Limited data suggest that 2-undecanone is relatively non-skin reactive and non-toxic.

Valencene

Synonyms: (+)-Valencene. 1(10),11-Eremophiladiene
Systematic name: [1R-(1α,7β,8aα)]-1,2,3,5,6,7,8,8a-Octahydro-1,8a-dimethyl-7-(1-methylethenyl)naphthalene
Chemical class: Bicyclic sesquiterpenoid alkene
CAS number: 4630-07-3

Source >1.0%:

Tansy (blue)	0.5–1.6%

Adverse skin reactions: Acute dermal LD_{50} reported as >5 g/kg in rabbits. Full strength valencene was moderately to severely irritating to the skin of rabbits when applied for 24 hours under occlusion. Tested at 5% on 25 healthy male volunteers the material was neither irritating nor sensitizing (Letizia et al 2000 p. S235–S236).

Acute toxicity: Acute oral LD_{50} reported as >5 g/kg in rats (Letizia et al 2000 p. S235–S236).

Mutagenicity and genotoxicity: Valencene was not mutagenic in *S. typhimurium* strains TA98 and TA100 with or without S9 (Gonçalves et al 2011).

Summary: Limited data suggest that valencene is relatively non-skin reactive and non-toxic.

Vanillin

Synonyms: Vanillic aldehyde. Methylprotocatechuic aldehyde
Systematic name: 3-Methoxy-4-hydroxybenzaldehyde
Chemical class: Phenolic aldehyde ether
CAS number: 121-33-5

Sources >1.0%:

Vanilla	12.0–95.0%
Tolu balsam	1.4%

Notes: Widely used in food flavorings. Vanillin occurs as a glycoside in vanilla, and is liberated by enzymatic cleavage on curing. Being a substituted phenol, vanillin is a weak acid which may be corrosive to tissues.

Pharmacokinetics: Vanillin can be oxidized to vanillic acid or reduced to vanillyl alcohol. In rabbits, 69% of an oral dose was excreted as vanillic acid, either free (44%) or conjugated (25%). In rats, one study reported 17% (free) and 24% (conjugated) while another reported 47% for total urinary vanillic acid. In the latter study 8–9% of guaiacol and catechol, 7% of vanillin and 19% of vanillyl alcohol were also detected. In humans, 73% of vanillic acid was found in the urine, with 2% of unchanged vanillin (Scheline 1991).

Vanillin is a potent inhibitor of sulfotransferase enzymes which are involved in the metabolism of phenolic drugs, and it has been suggested that it might also be an inducer of microsomal drug metabolizing enzymes (Janbaz & Gilani 1999).

Adverse skin reactions: Vanillin was not irritating when applied to the skin of 30 volunteers at 2%, 29 volunteers at 20%, or 35 dermatitis patients at 0.4%. None of 70 patients with contact dermatitis reacted to 10% vanillin (Nethercott et al 1989). One out of 747 dermatitis patients suspected of fragrance allergy (0.13%) reacted to 10% vanillin (Wöhrl et al 2001). Tested at 2% or 5%, vanillin produced no sensitization reactions in groups of 25 volunteers. Vanillin was found not to be responsible for most cases of sensitivity to natural vanilla. Positive reactions to vanillin have been reported in 8/142 (5.7%) and 21/164 (13%) of people sensitive to Peru balsam (Opdyke 1977a p. 633–638). However, Hausen (2001) found that none of 102 dermatitis patients who were allergic to Peru balsam tested positive to 5% vanillin. In an in vitro assay, vanillin was non-phototoxic (Placzek et al 2007).

Acute toxicity: The acute oral LD_{50} has been reported as 2.0 g/kg, 2.8 g/kg (Opdyke 1977 p. 633–638) and 1.58 g/kg in rats and 1.4 g/kg in guinea pigs (Jenner et al 1964). The acute ip LD_{50} has been reported as 480 mg/kg and 780 mg/kg and in mice, 1.16 g/kg in rats and 1.19 g/kg in guinea pigs. The acute sc LD_{50} has been reported as 1.5 g/kg and 2.6 g/kg in rats (Opdyke 1977 p. 633–638).

Subacute and subchronic toxicity: There were no macroscopic liver lesions and no deaths following the administration of four daily oral doses of 530 mg/kg vanillin given to rats (Taylor et al 1964). No effects were observed in mice given vanillin for 91 days at 3,000 ppm in the diet while 10,000 ppm resulted in mild adverse effects, and at 50,000 ppm growth retardation and enlargement of liver, kidneys and spleen were reported (Opdyke 1977 p. 633–638). No effects were observed at any dose when vanillin was fed to rats at 1,000 ppm for 27–28 weeks, 5,000 ppm for two years, 10,000 ppm for 16 weeks, 10,000 ppm for two years, 20,000 ppm for one year, 20,000 ppm for two years, or 50,000 ppm for one year (Hagan et al 1967).

Reproductive toxicity: In an ex vivo assay, vanillin did not bind to estrogen receptors in female rat uterus tissue (Blair et al 2000).

Antioxidant/pro-oxidant activity: Both pro-oxidant and antioxidant activity have been reported for vanillin (Liu & Mori 1993).

Mutagenicity and genotoxicity: Vanillin was non-mutagenic in Ames tests (Florin et al 1980; Kasamaki et al 1982; Pool and Lin 1982; Ishidate et al 1984; Mortelmans et al 1986; Heck et al 1989). It was not mutagenic in a *B. subtilis* rec assay (Oda et al 1978) and was antimutagenic in mammalian cells, both in vitro and in vivo (Imanishi et al 1990). Vanillin was antimutagenic in TA104, but not in TA98 or TA100. Inhibition of mutagenesis occurred at GC sites, not AT sites. Vanillin is thought to reduce mutation through enhancing recombinational repair, and not through an antioxidant action (Shaughnessy et al 2001).

Vanillin was not genotoxic in *S. cerevisiae* (Rosin 1984), and did not induce UDS in rat hepatocytes (Heck et al 1989). It was not genotoxic in tests in Chinese hamster cells (Kasamaki et al 1982; Ishidate et al 1984), but it did induce SCE in human lymphocytes (Jansson et al 1988). Vanillin reduced CA induced by X-rays in bone marrow cells in mice (Sasaki et al 1990) and by methotrexate in Chinese hamster lung cells (Keshava et al 1997–1998). It was not mutagenic in a mouse lymphoma assay (Heck et al 1989). In human cell extracts, vanillin inhibited DNA end-joining, a potentially mutagenic process (Durant & Karran 2003). Vanillin was antigenotoxic in human hepatoma (HepG2) cells (Sanyal et al 1997). In mice, oral dosing with vanillin suppressed the formation of induced micronuclei in bone marrow cells (Inouye et al 1988). Vanillin may cause a type of genotoxicity that elicits recombinational repair, which fixes not only the damage caused by vanillin, but also other DNA damage. Antimutagenic effects have been seen in both *E. coli*

and human colon cancer cells (Shaughnessy et al 2006; King et al 2007).

Carcinogenic/anticarcinogenic potential: In male and female mice given 24 ip injections of vanillin in tricaprylin in a total dose of 3.6 or 18.0 g/kg over 24 weeks, the incidence of primary lung tumors was no higher than in the control group (Stoner et al 1973). Vanillin inhibited hepatic carcinogenesis in rats (Tsuda et al 1994), and inhibited the activation of carcinogenic nitrosamines in mouse hepatic and pulmonary microsomes (Morse et al 1995).

Summary: There is a low incidence of allergic skin reactions to vanillin in humans, and the compound has a low acute and subchronic toxicity in rodents. Vanillin appears to be non-carcinogenic.

Regulatory guidelines: In a preliminary report by an ECETOC taskforce, vanillin was classified as a weak allergen (on a scale of extreme, strong, moderate and weak) only likely to elicit a sensitization reaction if present at 3% or more (Kimber et al 2003). In 2009, IFRA set a limit of 0.5% for vanillin in leave-on products such as body lotions, but this standard was subsequently withdrawn pending a review of the data.

Verbenone

Synonym: 2-Pinen-4-one
Systematic name: 4,6,6-Trimethylbicyclo[3.1.1]hept-3-en-2-one
Chemical class: Bicyclic monoterpenoid alkene ketone
Note: Different isomers of verbenone exist, and the following isomer-specific information has been published:

(+)-Verbenone

Synonym: (1R,5R)-(+)-Verbenone
CAS number: 18309-32-5

(−)-Verbenone

Synonym: (1S,5S)-(−)-Verbenone
CAS number: 1196-01-6

Sources >1.0%:

Rosemary (verbenone CT)	7.6–12.3%
Rosemary (borneol CT)	8.4%
Boswellia frereana	0–6.5%
Boswellia sacra (α-pinene CT)	0–6.5%
Rosemary (camphor CT)	0–6.3%
Rosemary (α-pinene CT)	0.5–6.0%
Rosemary (bornyl acetate CT)	4.3–5.7%
Piri-piri	1.1–3.9%
Mastic	0–2.9%
Wormwood (annual)	0–2.6%
Hinoki root	2.4%
Cistus	0–2.0%
Rosemary (β-myrcene CT)	tr–1.8%
Labdanum	0–1.2%
Boswellia neglecta	1.0%

Pharmacokinetics: (−)-Verbenone is converted to (−)-10-hydroxyverbenone in both rats and humans, but this takes place primarily through CYP2A6 activity in humans, and through CYP2C11 activity in male rats (Miyazawa et al 2003).

Drug interactions: (−)-Verbenone alters the distribution of the antibiotics erythromycin and ampicillin in mice, increasing their concentration in the lungs, while not altering their hepatic concentration (Pintabona et al 1995).

Acute toxicity: Mouse ip LD_{50} 250 mg/kg (Harborne & Baxter 1993).

Cardiovascular effects: Verbenone shows strong antiplatelet aggregation activity in vitro (Chiariello et al 1986).

Summary: Verbenone inhibits platelet aggregation. It may interfere with the action of certain antibiotics.

Xanthorrhizol

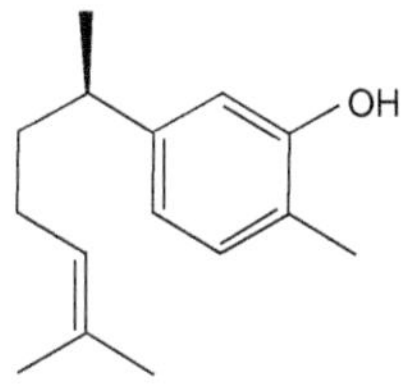

Synonym: 1,3,5,10-Bisabolatetraen-2-ol

Systematic name: 5-(1,5-Dimethyl-4-hexenyl)-2-methyl-phenol

Chemical class: Phenolic sesquiterpenoid alkene

CAS number: 30199-26-9

Sources >1.0%:

Turmeric (wild)   16.2–25.7%

Note: Being a substituted phenol, xanthorrhizol is a weak acid which may be corrosive to tissues.

Nephrotoxicity: Pretreatment with xanthorrhizol in mice, given orally at 200 mg/kg/day for 4 days, significantly attenuated the nephrotoxicity induced by cisplatin, a widely used anticancer drug (Kim et al 2005).

Carcinogenic/anticarcinogenic potential: Xanthorrhizol potently inhibited both COX-2 (IC_{50} 0.2 µg/mL) and iNOS (IC_{50} 1.0 µg/mL) which correlates with a cancer chemopreventive action (Lee et al 2002). Xanthorrhizol suppressed proliferation of both MCF-7 human breast cancer cells (EC_{50} 1.71 µg/mL) and HepG2 hepatoma cells (IC_{50} 4.17 µg/mL) via induction of apoptosis (Cheah et al 2006; Handayani et al 2007). At 50 mg/kg xanthorrhizol was active against sarcoma 180 ascites in mice (Itokawa et al 1985). In mice, ip doses of 0.1, 0.2, 0.5 and 1.0 mg/kg for 2 weeks inhibited the formation of lung tumor nodules by 36%, 63%, 61% and 52%, respectively (Choi et al 2005a).

Summary: Xanthorrhizol is antinephrotoxic and antitumoral.

General safety guidelines

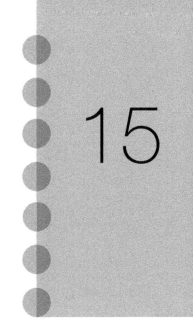

15

First aid

If you or someone you are with is suffering a serious adverse event, seek immediate help from your local poison center or hospital.

Most adverse reactions to essential oils are without any serious consequence, but if young children ingest any amount, medical attention should be sought urgently. After suspected ingestion of an essential oil, asymptomatic children are normally observed for six hours, and drinking of water is encouraged. Symptomatic children require hospital admission (Riordan et al 2002). Activated charcoal is regarded as ineffective for treating essential oil poisoning (Jepsen & Ryan 2005). A summary of first aid procedures for essential oil toxicity is given in Box 15.1.

Signs and symptoms of toxicity

Topical exposure to some essential oils may cause local skin reactions including irritation, allergic reaction, and photosensitization, especially if undiluted oils are used. If essential oils get into the eyes, reddening and lacrimation are likely to occur, and a child may rub their eyes. If essential oils have been instilled nasally, signs and symptoms of airway irritation are likely, ranging from nasal irritation through various degrees of respiratory edema and distress to respiratory arrest. If sufficient amounts are absorbed by this route, systemic poisoning may result, as for oral ingestion.

The advice given to doctors dealing with essential oil poisoning following oral ingestion is that the initial effects generally include mucosal irritation, epigastric pain, vomiting and diarrhea, and that convulsions, CNS depression and hepatic and renal failure may follow (Riordan et al 2002). Table 15.1 gives a summary of common signs and symptoms of poisoning by essential oils. Many published cases of poisoning are detailed in the appropriate essential oil profile in Chapter 13.

Reporting adverse events

In the US, consumers and health professionals can report adverse events from essential oils electronically by visiting the FDA's Medwatch site at https://www.accessdata.fda.gov/scripts/medwatch/medwatch-online.htm (accessed August 28th 2012).

In Canada, essential oil reactions can be reported to Health Canada, by visiting http://www.hc-sc.gc.ca/ahc-asc/media/advisories-avis/reaction-eng.php#Consumer (accessed August 28th 2012).

In the UK, the equivalent body is the MHRA, and their website can be accessed at http://www.mhra.gov.uk/index.htm (accessed August 28th 2012). However, there is no provision for reporting reactions to essential oils.

In Australia, adverse events can be reported to the Therapeutic Goods Administration http://www.tga.gov.au (accessed August 28th 2012).

http://dx.doi.org/10.1016/B978-0-443-06241-4.00015-1

Box 15.1

General first aid procedures in cases of adverse reactions following exposure to essential oils by different routes

Ingestion

- Do not induce vomiting (corrosive chemicals may destroy mucous membranes, and there is a risk of aspiration into the victim's lungs during vomiting)
- If the person is conscious and not convulsing, rinse mouth with water and immediately call a hospital or poison center. Avoid alcohol
- If the person is convulsing or unconscious do not give anything by mouth. Ensure their airway is open and lay them on their side with the head lower than the body
- Transport the person to a hospital as soon as possible

Inhalation

- Remove person to fresh air
- If not breathing, give artificial respiration, preferably mouth-to-mouth
- Seek medical attention

Eye contact

- Flush eye(s) with water for at least 15 minutes. If there are contact lenses, remove them after the first 5 minutes, then continue rinsing eye(s)

- Ensure adequate flushing of the eyes by separating the eyelids with fingers
- Seek medical advice if irritation persists

Skin contact

- Remove any contaminated clothing.
- Wash the skin gently with (preferably unperfumed) soap and water for at least 10 minutes
- Expose the skin to the air (but not to direct sunlight) to encourage evaporation of remaining essential oil.
- Lukewarm oatmeal baths may help soothe reactions spread over large areas of skin.
- Application of a simple barrier cream, or a mild corticosteroid cream is the normal medical approach (although ACD to topical corticosteroids is possible).
- Oral antihistamines may help reduce itching (topical antihistamines should be avoided because of the risk of ACD).
- Seek medical attention if irritation persists.

(Partly adapted from safety data sheets for essential oils.)

Table 15.1 Poisoning from specific essential oils after acute oral ingestion

Essential oil	Signs and symptoms
Camphor	Initially CNS stimulation (delirium, convulsions), followed by depression (ataxia, coma) Possibly nausea, vomiting, vertigo, confusion, respiratory failure
Cinnamon bark	A burning sensation in the mouth, chest and stomach, dizziness, double vision, nausea, vomiting, collapse
Citronella	Vomiting, shock, frothing at the mouth, fever, deep and rapid respiration, cyanosis, convulsions
Clove	Acidosis, deteriorating liver function, CNS depression, deep coma, convulsions, ketonuria, low blood glucose
Eucalyptus	CNS depression (drowsiness, coma), abnormal respiration (shallow or labored breathing), pinpoint pupils, ataxia, vertigo, epigastric pain, vomiting, weakness in the legs, cold sweats, headache
Hyssop	Convulsions
Parsley/apiole	Fever, severe abdominal pain, vaginal bleeding, vomiting, diarrhea
Pennyroyal	Fever, delirium, nausea, vomiting, dizziness, coma, tingling and numbness of the extremities, hemorrhage
Pine	Drowsiness, delirium, headache, nausea, ataxia, tachycardia, paresis, gastroenteritis, toxic nephritis, renal failure
Sage (Dalmatian)	Convulsions
Thuja	Convulsions, gastroenteritis, flatulence, hypotension
Sassafras	Principally shock, vomiting. CNS depression causing inadequacy of respiration and blood circulation. Similar clinical picture to that of eucalyptus, except for pinpoint pupils
Tea tree	Convulsions, ataxia, drowsiness
Wintergreen/methyl salicylate	Convulsions, vomiting, fever, rapid and labored breathing, cyanosis, tachycardia, respiratory alkalosis, tinnitus, deafness
Wormseed	Generalized edema, skin and mucous membrane irritation, headache, vertigo, tinnitus, double vision, nausea, vomiting, constipation, deafness, blindness

Safety in healthcare

The following are guidelines for preventing or managing adverse reactions.

Adverse skin reactions

- do not apply undiluted essential oils to any part of the body
- before applying to the skin, essential oils should be appropriately diluted, depending on the oils used
- adding undiluted essential oils to bathwater is inadvisable
- individuals with a personal or family history of atopic dermatitis, with a history of skin contact allergy or perfume allergy, or with a current skin condition, may be at greater risk of adverse skin reactions.

Child safety

- do not allow children to ingest essential oils
- do not add undiluted essential oils to the bathwater of children
- keep essential oils out of reach of children
- if possible, purchase bottles of essential oils with child-resistant caps
- do not apply essential oils to or near a child's face
- do not place essential oils or preparations containing them into the nose of a child
- do not expose children of five years or less to strong essential oil vapors.

Patient safety

- for general aromatherapy massage, it is recommended that essential oils are diluted to less than 3% by volume
- for children younger than 15 years, lower concentrations should be used (see Table 4.5)
- see Table 4.6 for how to calculate concentrations
- for pregnant women, certain essential oils should be avoided completely (Table 11.1)
- patch testing may be useful occasionally if there are doubts about the safety of a proposed treatment protocol. It is described on Ch. 5, p. 74
- if there is uncertainty about a possible reaction, a 1% concentration should be used initially for treatment, and increased in subsequent sessions if prudent
- we caution the direct inhalation of essential oil vapors by those with diagnosed asthma, or anyone reporting airway hyper-reactivity to fragrances, paint fumes or turpentine. A guideline maximum of 1% of essential oil for aromatherapy massage is recommended for this group
- a patient should not ingest essential oils unless advised to do so by a practitioner who is qualified/licensed to prescribe essential oils in this way

- practitioners should label clearly the contents and concentrations in every bottle of essential oil dispensed, including whether the oils are undiluted or diluted with an excipient and if so, by how much
- practitioners should be aware of safety issues concerning photosensitivity, pregnancy, contraindications, etc.

Practitioner safety

- the working space used by aromatherapists performing massage must have adequate ventilation, especially if it is small
- conditions of low relative humidity can exacerbate terpene airway irritation, which is an occupational risk in aromatherapy. In very dry climates, or where indoor heating is being used, a humidifier may be helpful
- ozone can exacerbate terpene airway irritation. Indoor concentrations of ozone in aromatherapy treatment rooms should therefore be minimized by removing sources of it such as photocopying machines, laser printers and ozone-generating air cleaners
- hand dermatitis is an occupational risk for aromatherapists who use massage. If you start to develop hand dermatitis, you should consider wearing thin plastic disposable gloves for massage until it subsides. In the meantime, visit a dermatologist to find out which essential oils may be causative
- individuals with a history of atopic dermatitis should be wary of a career involving regular skin contact with essential oils, as they are statistically more prone to adverse skin reactions
- frequent hand washing with detergents increases the risk of hand dermatitis, so their use should be minimized. Most liquid soaps are made with detergents
- the regular use of hand cream is recommended to counteract the increased roughness and dryness caused by frequent hand washing

General safety measures

The most toxic essential oils should not be sold (Table 15.2). Restrictions already apply in some regions to some of these.

Packaging

To minimize the risk of serious accidental poisoning from essential oils:

- undiluted essential oils should only be bought, sold and dispensed in bottles fitted with integral drop-dispensers
- child-resistant bottle closures (caps) should be used for the more toxic essential oils (Table 15.3).

The following or similar warnings should be included on the labels of all bottles of undiluted essential oils:

- keep away from children
- for external use only. Do not ingest

Table 15.2 Essential oils that present a high risk of acute toxicity or carcinogenicity

Essential oil[a]	Source	Botanical name
Almond oil (bitter, unrectified)	Kernels	*Prunus dulcis* (Mill.) var. *amara*
Boldo oil	Leaves	*Peumus boldus* Molina
Cade oil (unrectified)	Wood	*Juniperus oxycedrus* L.
Horseradish oil	Roots	*Armoracia rusticana* P. Gaertn. et al.
Mustard oil	Seeds	*Brassica nigra* L., *Brassica juncea* (L.) Czern.
Pine oil (huon)	Wood	*Dacrydium franklinii* J. D. Hook.
Sassafras oil	Roots	*Sassafras albidum* (Nutt.) Nees
Sassafras oil (Brazilian)	Roots	*Nectandra sanguinea* Rol. Ex Rottb., *Ocotea odorifera* (Vell.) Rohwer
Sassafras oil (Chinese)	Roots	*Cinnamomum porrectum* (Roxb.), *Cinnamomum rigidissimum* H.T. Chang
Snakeroot oil	Roots, rhizomes	*Asarum canadense* L.
Tea tree oil (black)	Leaves	*Melaleuca bracteata* F. von Müller
Wormseed oil	Seeds	*Chenopodium ambrosioides* L., *Chenopodium ambrosioides* L. var. *anthelminticum* L.

[a]These essential oils should not be sold in a retail environment, used by aromatherapists, or included in aromatherapy products

Table 15.3 Essential oils that present a known or probable risk of acute toxicity if ingested by children of 6 years or under

Essential oil[a]	Source	Botanical name
Ajowan oil	Seeds	*Trachyspermum ammi* L.
Basil oil	Leaves	*Ocimum gratissimum* L., *Ocimum tenuiflorum* L.
Birch oil (sweet)	Bark	*Betula lenta* L.
Birch tar oil	Bark & wood	*Betula lenta* L, *Betula pendula* Roth., *Betula pubescens* Ehrh.
Buchu oil (diosphenol CT)	Leaves	*Agathosma betulina* Bergius
Buchu oil (pulegone CT)	Leaves	*Agathosma crenulata* L.
Cajuput oil	Leaves & twigs	*Melaleuca cajuputi* Powell
Calamint (lesser)	Herb	*Calamintha nepeta* L. subsp. *glandulosa* Req.
Cassia oil	Bark or leaves	*Cinnamomum cassia* Blume
Cinnamon oil	Bark	*Cinnamomum verum* J. Presl.
Cinnamon oil	Leaves	*Cinnamomum verum* J. Presl.
Clove oil	Buds, leaves or stems	*Syzygium aromaticum* (L.) Merill et L.M. Perry
Cornmint oil	Leaves	*Mentha arvensis* L.
Eucalyptus oil	Leaves	Various *Eucalyptus* species
Feverfew oil	Leaves	*Tanacetum parthenium* L.
Garlic oil	Bulb	*Allium sativum* L.
Genipi	Herb	*Artemisia genepi* Weber syn.
Ho leaf (camphor CT)	Leaves	*Cinnamomum camphora* L.
Hyssop oil (pinocamphone CT)	Leaves & flowering tops	*Hyssopus officinalis* L.

Continued

Table 15.3 Essential oils that present a known or probable risk of acute toxicity if ingested by children of 6 years or under—Cont'd

Essential oil	Source	Botanical name
Lanyana oil	Leaves and stems	*Artemisia afra* von Jacquin
Lavender oil (Spanish)	Flowering tops	*Lavandula stoechas* L. ssp. *stoechas*
Leek oil	Herb	*Allium porrum* L.
Mugwort oil (great)	Herb	*Artemisia arborescens* L.
Niaouli oil (cineole CT)	Leaves	*Melaleuca quinquenervia* Cav.
Nutmeg oil	Kernels	*Myristica fragrans* Houtt.
Onion oil	Seeds	*Allium cepa* L.
Oregano oil	Leaves	*Lippia graveolens* HBK, *Origanum onites* L. *Origanum vulgare* L. subsp. *Hirtum* Link, *Thymbra capitata* L.
Parsley oil	Leaves or seeds	*Petroselinum crispum* Mill.
Pennyroyal oil	Leaves	*Hedeoma pulegioides* L., *Mentha pulegium* L.
Peppermint oil	Leaves	*Mentha* x *piperita* L.
Perilla oil	Leaves & flowering tops	*Perilla frutescens* L.
Pimento oil	Berries or leaves	*Pimenta dioica* L.
Rosemary oil	Leaves	*Rosmarinus officinalis* L.
Sage oil (Dalmatian)	Leaves	*Salvia officinalis* L.
Sage oil (Spanish)	Leaves	*Salvia lavandulifolia* Vahl.
Savory oil	Herb	*Satureia hortensis* L., *Satureia montana* L.
Southernwood oil	Herb	*Artemisia abrotanum* L.
Spike lavender oil	Flowering tops	*Lavandula latifolia* Medic.
Tansy oil	Herb	*Tanacetum vulgare* L.
Tea tree oil	Leaves	*Melaleuca alternifolia* Cheel
Tejpat oil	Leaves	*Cinnamomum tamala* Buch.-Ham.
Thuja oil	Leaves	*Thuja occidentalis* L.
Thyme oil	Leaves	*Thymbra spicata* L., *Thymus serpyllum* L., *Thymus vulgaris* L., *Thymus zygis* L.
Western red cedar	Leaves	*Thuja plicata* Donn ex D. Don
Wintergreen oil	Leaves	*Gaultheria fragrantissima* Wall., *Gaultheria procumbens* L.
Wormwood oil	Leaves & flowering tops	*Artemisia absinthium* L.
Wormwood oil (sea)	Leaves & flowering tops	*Artemisia maritima* L.
Wormwood oil (white)	Leaves & flowering tops	*Artemisia herba-alba* Asso

[a]We believe that these essential oils should only be sold in bottles with child-resistant closures if sold to consumers

- do not apply undiluted to any part of the body
- essential oils are flammable. Keep away from naked flames.

The label should also include:

- the botanical name of the plant source and the part of the plant used.
- appropriate 'use by' or 'sell by' dates or times.

Specific warnings should also be included for essential oils that are potentially phototoxic (Box 5.4), or that should be avoided in pregnancy (Table 11.1):

- this essential oil may burn the skin if applied in any dilution or amount up to 12 hours before exposure to UV light (sunbed or strong sunlight)
- do not use if pregnant.

The American Herbal Products Association trade guideline policy for essential oil labelling can be found here: http://www.ahpa.org/Default.aspx?tabid=224#section_undiluted_oils (accessed August 28th 2012).

Storage and quality control

The quality of essential oils changes with continual use and over time (see Chapter 2 for details of degradation). The following advice is therefore given to suppliers, retailers, health practitioners and others who use essential oils:

- keep essential oils cool, preferably in a refrigerator
- replace bottle caps immediately after use and return the bottle to a child-safe place
- observe 'use by' dates. If there are none, use within 12 months of purchase, or of first opening
- discard oxidation-prone essential oils that are more than 6 months old (after purchase or first opening) or when the bottle is about 90% empty (see Box 5.2 or individual oil profiles)

- keep essential oils away from sources of heat and direct sunlight
- keep essential oils away from naked flames, e.g., candles and vaporizers. Essential oils are flammable and many have flash points of 50–60°C.

Waste disposal

- essential oil waste is a fire hazard
- spills should be wiped up with a paper towel and placed in a closed metal waste container with a lid and a plastic liner
- used tissues, paper towels, empty bottles, etc., should be placed in a metal waste container
- waste containers should be emptied daily
- towels that have been used for aromatherapy massage have been known to self-combust in a tumble dryer. It is important to launder them at temperatures of at least 40°C in order to remove any oil residues http://www.wiltsfire.gov.uk/media/press_releases/2011/jul/media_press_releases_270711-2.html (accessed August 27th 2012).

Appendix A: Clinical Safety A–Z

Note: We advise checking the Safety Summary of individual essential oil profiles before using an essential oil.

Albinism

People with oculocutaneous albinism have reduced skin pigmentation, and are at an increased risk of photosensitivity and skin cancer. They should therefore avoid photosensitizing essential oils.

Allergic contact dermatitis (ACD)

This is defined as any skin allergy caused by dermal or airborne contact. Nickel is the most common cause of ACD, followed by fragrance materials. A person with a known allergic reaction to a particular essential oil or constituent should completely avoid contact with it. ACD may be acquired through repeated contact, and the most likely products to cause such a reaction are listed in Table 5.3. Also see: Atopic dermatitis; Skin: Asian; Skin diseases.

Anticoagulants

See Box 7.1 for essential oils that we contraindicate or caution orally.

Aspirin

See Box 7.1 for essential oils that we contraindicate or caution orally if taking aspirin regularly.

Asthma

Asthma is a chronic disease with acute episodes that can be triggered by viral infection, exercise, stress, irritants or allergens. Perfume is a known risk factor, and may act as an irritant or allergen. There is currently insufficient information to contraindicate specific essential oils, but great care should be taken in using aromatherapy to treat this condition. We caution the direct inhalation of essential oil vapors by those with diagnosed asthma, and anyone reporting airway hyper-reactivity to fragrances, paint fumes or turpentine. We recommend a maximum of 1% of essential oil for aromatherapy massage in the same group, and in atopic children.

Atopic dermatitis

Atopic dermatitis is a chronic skin condition. Its genesis is probably related to both genetic and environmental factors. Children or adults who are atopic are slightly more at risk for skin sensitization to essential oils and for inhaled allergy/asthma. See above comment.

Attention deficit disorder/attention deficit hyperactivity disorder (ADD/ADHD)

See Salicylate sensitivity.

Baths

Whenever essential oils are 'mixed' with water without a dispersing agent, there is a risk of irritation, since undiluted droplets of essential oil can attach to the skin, sometimes in sensitive areas. Therefore, essential oils should first be dispersed in a vegetable oil, or emulsified into an aqueous medium by use of an emulsifying agent. Full-fat milk helps to disperse essential oils in this way. However the dispersion is not complete, so this is not a perfect solution for anyone who might be sensitive, such as children or those with a skin disease.

Blood clotting deficiency/bleeding disorders

This group includes people with hemophilia, peptic ulcer, internal bleeding, severe hepatic or renal impairment, hypertensive or diabetic retinopathy, thrombocytopenia (decreased platelet count), vasculitis, breastfeeding mothers, people taking blood-thinning medication such as aspirin, heparin or warfarin, and up to one week before childbirth or any major surgery. See Box 7.1 for essential oils that we contraindicate or caution orally under these circumstances.

Blood-thinning drugs

See Blood clotting deficiency/bleeding disorders.

Breast cancer

See Estrogenic action.

Breastfeeding

Likely exposure in breast milk to most essential oil constituents is less than 1% of the maternal dose. This suggests that no particular caution is needed, except possibly from oral doses. See Tables 11.1 and 11.2, and Box 7.1 for essential oils to be avoided or restricted during breastfeeding.

Bronchial hyper-reactivity

See Asthma.

Bronchitis

See Chronic obstructive pulmonary disease.

Cancer treatment

Because of possible and unpredictable effects on immune mechanisms, we recommend that essential oils are avoided from one week before to one month following a course of chemotherapy or radiotherapy (see Possible adverse effects).

Cardiac fibrillation

As a cautionary measure, menthol-rich essential oils, i.e., peppermint and cornmint, are best avoided by people with cardiac fibrillation, because menthol has been associated with destabilization of heart rhythm. However, exposure to menthol is not associated with any increase in morbidity or mortality in this population.

Chemotherapy

See Cancer treatment.

Childbirth

There is no evidence that any essential oils have adverse effects when used to ease pain or anxiety during childbirth. See discussion on Ch. 11, p. 161. See Box 7.1 for essential oils that we contraindicate or caution orally up to one week before childbirth.

Children

Caution is advised for many essential oils in children under 2 years of age. Table 4.5 gives age-related maximum concentrations of essential oils for topical use in children. Essential oils high in 1,8-cineole or menthol can cause CNS and breathing problems in young children, and should not be applied to or near their faces. Sweet birch and wintergreen oils should not be used on or given to children in any amount due to the risk of developing Reye's syndrome.

Cholestasis (obstruction of bile flow)

Cholestasis can be caused by gallstones or tumors. Since they are known to or are likely to promote the secretion of bile, the following essential oils should not be taken orally in cases of cholestasis: cornmint, *Eucalyptus macarthurii*, jamrosa, peppermint, thyme (geraniol CT).

Chronic obstructive pulmonary disease (COPD)

We caution the direct inhalation of essential oil vapors by anyone with COPD.

Compresses

As with baths, there is a slight risk of irritation if essential oils are applied to the skin improperly dispersed.

Condoms

Latex condoms can be weakened by both vegetable oils and essential oils. Corn oil, for instance, has been shown to cause a loss of up to 77% of a condom's strength after only 15 minutes.

Cytochrome P450 inducers and inhibitors

Constituents of certain essential oils induce and/or inhibit cytochrome P450 (CYP450) enzymes (see Tables 4.10 and 4.11).

Dermatitis

See Skin diseases.

Diabetes

Because of their effects on blood sugar, some essential oils may interact with diabetic medication if taken in oral doses (see Table 4.10B).

Diabetic retinopathy

See Box 7.1 for essential oils that we contraindicate or caution orally.

Diuretics

Because of its antidiuretic action, anise oil may interact with diuretic medication if taken in oral doses.

Douching

Vaginal douching with essential oils is not recommended unless using a preparation made specifically for this purpose. It should be remembered that essential oils have an extremely low solubility in water, and that mucous membrane tissue is more sensitive to irritation than skin.

Driving (after aromatherapy massage)

It has been said that people should not drive after receiving aromatherapy massage with certain essential oils, such as clary sage. It might be more appropriate to recommend not driving if the person feels significantly disoriented or drowsy following aromatherapy massage with any essential oils. In the majority of cases these effects are both mild and transitory. Only in rare circumstances is driving proficiency likely to be affected.

Drug interactions

We caution the use of certain essential oils with specific drugs, either by any route (Table 4.10A) or only by oral administration (Table 4.10B). Also see Patches.

Ears

Undiluted essential oils should not be dripped into the ears, but diluted essential oils may be placed on a cotton wad for partial insertion.

Emphysema

See Chronic obstructive pulmonary disease.

Eczema

See Skin diseases.

Endometriosis

See Estrogenic action.

Epilepsy

Some essential oils, if taken orally, can cause convulsions in a vulnerable person. People with epilepsy who are taking suppressant medication may be no more vulnerable than non-epileptics. Epileptics who are not on medication are vulnerable, as are people who do not realize they are epileptics, and also infants and young children. Potentially convulsant essential oils are listed in Table 10.2. They should only be used at up to the recommended maximum amounts, which are intended to be safe for general use, including people who might be prone to seizures.

Estrogenic action

Because of their probable estrogenic action, essential oils high in (E)-anethole should be avoided in people with endometriosis or estrogen-dependent cancers. These include uterine cancers and some breast cancers. The essential oils to avoid are: anise, anise (star), fennel (bitter), fennel (sweet), myrtle (aniseed).

Eyes

Undiluted essential oils should not be applied to or very near the eyes. Great care should be taken, even with diluted essential oils. A 2009 report from an ophthalmologist in Bristol UK, describes partial loss of corneal tissue (ie erosion) when a 73-year-old man dripped Olbas Oil into his left eye because he thought he was using eye drops. He was "considerably incapacitated", but recovered after a week of treatment with topical antibiotics and lubricants. On checking, the author found that just his hospital, in the previous 18 months, had seen 12 patients who had mistakenly dripped Olbas Oil into one eye. He describes the result as a chemical burn. All 'Olbas Oil patients' recovered fully within one week following intensive treatment (Adams et al 2009). Olbas Oil is a mixture of essential oils and menthol.

Fever

Certain essential oils can precipitate convulsions in people with a fever, especially young children, who are more susceptible to convulsions when feverish. See Epilepsy.

Gastroesophageal reflux disease (GERD)

The following essential oils should be used with caution by the oral route in patients with GERD: birch (sweet), cornmint, peppermint, wintergreen.

G6PD deficiency

People who are G6PD deficient should avoid these essential oils altogether: cornmint, peppermint.

Heart disease

See Cardiac fibrillation.

Heme synthesis defects

See Porphyria.

Hemophilia

See Box 7.1 for essential oils that we contraindicate or caution orally.

Heparin

See Box 7.1 for essential oils that we contraindicate or caution orally if taking heparin.

Hormone replacement therapy (HRT)

It is unlikely that aromatherapy treatments could adversely affect hormone replacement therapy as any hormonal effect of the oil would be considerably weaker than that of the HRT.

Hypertension

There is currently no compelling evidence that any essential oils exacerbate hypertension. (see Ch. 7, p. 115).

Hypertensive retinopathy

See Box 7.1 for essential oils that we contraindicate or caution orally.

Hypotension

Many essential oils potentially lower blood pressure, including araucaria, pungent basil, blue cypress, emerald cypress and jade cypress. However, there is no evidence that any essential oils exacerbate hypotension.

Inhalation

A few drops of essential oil in a burner, vaporizer or in a steam inhalation is virtually risk-free. However, prolonged inhalation (more than about 30 minutes) of concentrated essential oil vapors (e.g., steam inhalation, or direct from a bottle) can lead to headaches, vertigo, nausea and lethargy. In certain instances more serious symptoms might be experienced, such as incoherence and double vision.

For children of 5 years old or less, direct inhalation should be avoided. Direct inhalation includes inhaling essential oils from the hands, a cotton ball, a nasal inhaler, a bowl of hot water or similar. Indirect, or ambient inhalation, is safe for young children, and includes any method that vaporizes essential oils into the air.

Interactions

See Drug interactions.

Kidney disease

See Box 7.1 for essential oils that we contraindicate or caution orally.

Leg ulcers

See Wounds.

Massage

Before being used in massage, essential oils should be diluted in a suitable vehicle, such as a vegetable oil. For massage over large areas of skin, it is not advisable to use a concentration greater than 3%. For concentrations suitable for children, see Table 4.5. See Table 4.6 for how to calculate concentrations of essential oil. Also see Undiluted oils.

Migraine

Migraine is the only disease known to be associated with a pronounced increase in olfactory sensitivity. Since odors can trigger migraine, great care is required in treating migraine sufferers with essential oils, and they should probably not be used at all during an attack.

Monoamine oxidase inhibitors (MAOIs)

Certain essential oil constituents may interact with MAOIs if taken in oral doses (see Table 4.10B)

Mucous membranes

Undiluted essential oils should not be applied to mucous membranes (eyes, mouth, nasal passages, vagina, rectum).

Do not use at all on mucous membranes: cinnamon bark, massoia, oakmoss absolute, treemoss absolute, verbena absolute.

Use with caution on mucous membranes: ajowan, anise (star), basil (pungent), cade (rectified), caraway, catnep, cinnamon leaf, citronella, clove bud, clove leaf, clove stem, combava leaf, cornmint, garlic, khella, leek, lemongrass, lemon myrtle, lemon-scented gum, may chang, melissa, onion, oregano, oregano (Mexican), peppermint, perilla, pimento leaf, savory, spearmint, thyme (thymol and/or carvacrol CTs).

Multiple chemical sensitivity

Inhaled fragrant molecules have been known to trigger attacks in people with multiple chemical sensitivity.

Oral dosing

Oral dosing is accompanied by an increased risk of toxic reactions because of the possibility of higher blood levels and the potential risk of overdosing. Oral dosing increases the risk of interactions with prescribed drugs or radiotherapy, and of adverse reactions in specific groups, such as those with porphyria, or in pregnant women.

In order to avoid gastric irritation, orally ingested essential oils should be diluted in a suitable vehicle. In order to be effective, enterically coated capsules are needed in some cases. It is not recommended that anyone self-prescribe essential oils orally. Only practitioners permitted to do so according to the laws of their country of residence should prescribe essential oils for oral ingestion.

For various safety reasons, the following essential oils should not be taken in oral doses: basil (estragole CT), basil (Madagascan), betel, birch tar, buchu (pulegone CT), cade (rectified), calamint (lesser), calamus (tetraploid/hexaploid), camphor (yellow), chervil, genipi, hyssop (pinocamphone CT), Mexican marigold, pennyroyal, pimento berry, pteronia, ravensara bark, sage (Dalmatian), tarragon, thuja, western red cedar, wormwood (β-thujone CT), wormwood (sea), wormwood (white).

Patches

Essential oils should not be applied to skin on which any medications or drug patches are being used, as the oils may dramatically increase the bioavailability of the drug.

Patch testing

This may be useful in identifying the cause of ACD in an individual. However, we do not recommend liberal use of precautionary patch testing. See Chapter 5 for a discussion and description of the procedure.

Peptic ulcer

See Box 7.1 for essential oils that we contraindicate or caution orally.

Photosensitivity/phototoxicity

See Sunlight/sunbeds.

Pigmented cosmetic dermatitis

This is a very rare skin condition that may be especially predominant in people of Asian ethnicity. See Skin: Asian.

Poisoning

If poisoning from essential oil ingestion is suspected, seek immediate help from your local poison center or hospital. If the person is showing severe signs of poisoning such as loss of consciousness, telephone the emergency service. Do not try to induce vomiting unless advised to by a health professional as this is not always useful, and can cause problems. See Box 15.1 for more detailed information.

Porphyria

An inherited or acquired disease resulting from a disorder of porphyrin metabolism. We caution the use of all essential oils orally in people with porphyria. See Porphyrin production in Chapter 9.

Pregnancy

It is likely that most essential oil constituents cross the placenta to the fetus after use by a pregnant woman. We therefore recommend that essential oils are only taken orally with great caution throughout pregnancy. Equal caution is recommended for rectal and vaginal administration, since the amount of essential oil reaching the fetus could be as high as from oral dosing. See Tables 11.1 and 11.2 for essential oils to be avoided or restricted during pregnancy.

Premature infants

Since premature newborns have very thin and sensitive skin, topical use of essential oils is inadvisable, unless there are very important benefits to be gained by the baby. Even vaporizing oils into the air might be best avoided, again unless there are important benefits to be gained.

Psoriasis

See Skin diseases.

Radiation

See Cancer treatment.

Renal impairment

See Box 7.1 for essential oils that we contraindicate or caution orally.

Salicylate sensitivity

People with salicylate sensitivity need to avoid certain foods, and they should also avoid the essential oils with high methyl salicylate content: sweet birch and wintergreen. Children with ADD/ADHD often have salicylate sensitivity.

Sensitive skin

See discussion of this on Ch. 5, p. 76.

Serotonin

Certain essential oils may interact with selective serotonin reuptake inhibitors (SSRIs) if taken in oral doses (see Table 4.10B).

Skin: Asian

Benzyl salicylate allergy is more common in Asia than in Europe or the US, although it is only a minor constituent of ylang-ylang, tuberose and carnation. Photoallergy to sandalwood oil may be more common in Asia. Asian races are more susceptible than those with white or black skin to a condition known as pigmented contact dermatitis (see Ch. 5, p. 79), and to similar conditions involving hyperpigmentation.

Skin: black

People with darker skin have some increased tolerability to phototoxicity and photocarcinogenesis, but are still susceptible to skin conditions caused by sunlight.

Skin: white

White races are more susceptible than Asians to the fragrance mix, and to isoeugenol and oakmoss. They are also more susceptible than those with ethnically darker skin to irritation, phototoxicity and photocarcinogenesis.

Skin diseases

Caution is needed when applying essential oils to diseased or damaged skin, because it is more prone to allergic reactions, as well as being more readily permeable to essential oils. See Patch testing.

Sunlight/sunbeds

Skin should not be exposed to sunlight or UV lamp irradiation for 12–18 hours, if any of the following are used at levels higher than those indicated. However, there is no risk of phototoxicity if the maximum levels are observed: angelica root (0.8%), bergamot (0.4%), cumin (0.4%), grapefruit (expressed) (4.0%), laurel leaf absolute 2.0%, lemon (expressed) (2.0%), lime (expressed) (0.7%), mandarin leaf (0.17%), orange (bitter, expressed) (1.25%), rue (0.15%), taget oil or absolute (0.01%).

There is reason to suspect the following materials of phototoxicity, but it is not known whether or not they are phototoxic, and if so at what level they could be safely used: angelica root absolute, angelica root CO_2 extract, celery leaf, celery seed absolute, clementine, combava (fruit), cumin seed absolute, cumin seed CO_2 extract, khella, lovage leaf, parsnip, skimmia.

Surgery: one week before or after

See Box 7.1 for essential oils that we contraindicate or caution orally.

Thrombocytopenia (decreased platelet count)

See Box 7.1 for essential oils that we contraindicate or caution orally.

Transplants

Due to the possible and unpredictable effects on immune mechanisms, we recommend that essential oils are avoided in patients undergoing organ or tissue transplants who are taking conventional immunosuppressant drugs.

Undiluted essential oils

Generally, undiluted essential oils are not used in massage, nor are they applied to eyes, mucous membranes, diseased or broken skin. This is to avoid causing irritation, inflammation and/or allergic reaction. However, there are instances in which benefits may outweigh risks. Such instances could include: bites and stings, burns, herpes simplex, herpes zoster, leg ulcers, malignant ulceration (fungating carcinomas), mouth ulcers, neutropenic ulceration, pressure sores, tinea, verrucae, warts, etc. In some of these instances medical supervision is advisable.

Uterine cancer

See Estrogenic action.

Vaporization

Devices that use a naked flame are a substantial fire risk, and it should be remembered that essential oils are flammable. Young children should not be left alone with any device that could catch fire or burn the child, and naked flame burners should never be left unattended.

Vasculitis

See Box 7.1 for essential oils to avoid orally.

Warfarin

See Box 7.1 for essential oils to avoid orally if taking warfarin. Warfarin is also known under the brand names Coumadin, Jantoven, Marevan, Lawarin, Waran, and Warfant.

Appendix B: Examples of drug substrates for CYP enzymes

Drug class	Generic name	CYP1A2	CYP1B1	CYP2B6	CYP2C9	CYP2D6	CYP2E1	CYP3A4
Acetylcholinesterase inhibitors	Donezepil					✓		✓
	Tacrine	✓						
Adrenaline α_2-receptor agonists	Tizanidine	✓						
Adrenaline β-receptor antagonists	Alprenolol					✓		
	Carvedilol					✓		✓
	Propranolol	✓				✓		✓
Analgesics, non-opioid	Acetaminophen (paracetamol)	✓					✓	
	Phenacetin	✓				✓		
Analgesics, opioid	Alfentanil			✓				✓
	Codeine					✓		✓
	Fentanyl							✓
	Methadone			✓				✓
Anesthetics	Halothane		✓				✓	
	Methoxyflurane		✓				✓	
	Propofol			✓				
Angiotensin II-receptor antagonists	Irbesartan				✓			
	Losartan				✓			✓
Antiandrogenic drugs	Flutamide	✓						
Antiarrhythmic drugs	Amiodarone (class III)							✓
	Lidocaine (class Ib)					✓		✓
	Mexiletine (class Ib)	✓				✓		
	Quinidine (class Ia)							✓
	Sparteine (class Ia)					✓		

Continued

Drug class	Generic name	CYP1A2	CYP1B1	CYP2B6	CYP2C9	CYP2D6	CYP2E1	CYP3A4
Anticoagulants	Warfarin	✓			✓			
Anticonvulsants	Losigamone		✓					
	Valproate			✓				
Antidepressants, tricyclic	Amitriptyline	✓			✓	✓		✓
	Clomipramine	✓				✓		✓
	Imipramine	✓				✓		✓
Antidepressants, other	Bupropion			✓				
	Mirtazapine	✓						✓
Antidiabetic drugs	Glibenclamide				✓			✓
	Nateglinide				✓			
	Rosiglitazone				✓			
	Tolbutamide				✓			
Antiepileptic drugs	Phenytoin				✓			
Antifungal drugs	Itraconazole							✓
	Ketoconazole							✓
	Terbinafine				✓			
Antipsychotic drugs	Clozapine	✓						
	Haloperidol	✓				✓		✓
	Pimozide							✓
	Thioridazine					✓		
Benzodiazepines	Diazepam	✓						✓
	Midazolam							✓
	Triazolam							✓
Bronchodilators	Theophylline	✓					✓	
Calcium channel blockers	Diltiazem							✓
	Felodipine							✓
	Nicardipine							✓
	Nifedipine							✓
	Nitrendipine							✓
	Verapamil	✓						✓
Chemotherapeutic drugs	Cyclophosphamide			✓				✓
	Doxorubicin							✓
	Vinblastine							✓
	Vincristine							✓
Diuretics	Torasemide				✓			
	Triamterene	✓						
Dopamine receptor agonists	Ropinirole	✓						
Dopamine receptor antagonists	Domperidone							✓
	Metoclopramide					✓		

Continued

Drug class	Generic name	CYP1A2	CYP1B1	CYP2B6	CYP2C9	CYP2D6	CYP2E1	CYP3A4
Estrogen receptor agonists	Estradiol	✓	✓					✓
	Ethinyl estradiol							✓
Estrogen receptor antagonists	Tamoxifen	✓		✓	✓	✓		✓
Glucocorticoids	Budenoside							✓
	Dexamethasone							✓
	Hydrocortisone							✓
	Prednisolone							✓
Histamine H_1-receptor antagonists	Astemizole							✓
	Chlorpheniramine					✓		✓
	Promethazine					✓		
	Terfenadine							✓
HMG Co-A reductase inhibitors	Atorvastatin							✓
	Fluvastatin				✓			
	Lovastatin							✓
	Simvastatin							✓
Hypnotic drugs	Zaleplon							✓
	Zopiclone							✓
Immunosuppressants	Cyclosporine							✓
	Tacrolimus							✓
5-Lipoxygenase inhibitors	Zileuton	✓						
Melatonin receptor agonists	Ramelteon	✓						
Monoamine oxidase inhibitors	Rasagiline	✓						
Nervous system stimulants	Amphetamine					✓		
	Caffeine	✓						✓
	Cocaine							✓
	Nicotine		✓	✓				
Non-steroidal anti-inflammatory drugs	Diclofenac				✓			
	Ibuprofen				✓			
	Naproxen	✓			✓			
	Piroxicam				✓			
Phosphodiesterase inhibitors	Cilostazol							✓
	Sildenafil				✓			✓
Platelet-activating factor antagonists	SM-12502		✓					
Reverse-transcriptase inhibitors	Efavirenz			✓				
	Nevirapine			✓				✓

Continued

Drug class	Generic name	CYP1A2	CYP1B1	CYP2B6	CYP2C9	CYP2D6	CYP2E1	CYP3A4
Serotonin receptor agonists	Buspirone (5-HT$_{1A}$)							✓
	Cisapride (5-HT$_4$)							✓
	Frovatriptan (5-HT$_{1B, D}$)	✓						
	Zolmitriptan (5-HT$_{1B, D}$)	✓						
Serotonin 5-HT$_3$-receptor antagonists	Alosetron	✓						
	Ondansetron	✓				✓		✓
	Tropisetron					✓		
Serotonin reuptake inhibitors (SSRIs)	Citalopram							✓
	Fluoxetine				✓	✓		
	Fluvoxamine	✓				✓		
	Paroxetine					✓		
	Sertraline							✓

The information above was derived from these sources

Flockhart, D.A., 2007. Drug interactions: cytochrome P$_{450}$ drug interaction table. Indiana University School of Medicine. http://medicine.iupui.edu/clinpharm/ddis/main-table/ accessed July 2012

Horn, J.R., Hansten, P.D., 2007. Get to know an enzyme: CYP1A2. http://www.pharmacytimes.com/publications/issue/2007/2007-11/2007-11-8279 accessed July 2012

[Swedish environmental classification of pharmaceuticals. Facts for prescribers.] http://www.fass.se/LIF/produktfakta/fakta_lakare_artikel.jsp?articleID=18352 accessed July 2012

Appendix C: Conversion tables for essential oils

Approximate conversions

1 mL of essential oil = approximately 0.9 g (depending on specific gravity)
1 g of essential oil = approximately 1.1 mL (depending on specific gravity)
1 fluid ounce of essential oil = 30 mL.

mg	mL
50	0.06
100	0.11
200	0.22
500	0.55
1,000	1.10
2,000	2.20
5,000	5.50

To convert mL to g: multiply by 0.9
To convert mL to mg: multiply by 900
To convert g to mL: multiply by 1.1
To convert mg to mL: multiply by 0.0011

mg	Drops
30	1
60	2
90	3
120	4
150	5
210	7
300	10
450	15
600	20
750	25
900	30

Drops	mL	Fluid oz
3	0.1	0.003
6	0.2	0.007
9	0.3	0.010
12	0.4	0.013
15	0.5	0.017
30	1	0.033
45	1.5	0.050
60	2	0.066
75	2.5	0.083
150	5	0.17
300	10	0.33
450	15	0.50
600	20	0.67
750	25	0.83
900	30	1.0

1 mL of essential oil = 20–40 drops (Svoboda et al 2001). We use the average of 30 drops.

Percent dilution	Drops per fluid oz	Drops per 10 mL
0.1%	1	0.3
0.2%	2	0.6
0.5%	5	1.5
1.0%	9	3
1.5%	14	4.5
2.0%	18	6
3.0%	27	9
4.0%	36	12
5.0%	45	15

For a more comprehensive dilution chart, see Table 4.6

Parts per million (ppm)	% in diet
1	0.0001%
5	0.0005%
10	0.001%
50	0.005%
100	0.01%
500	0.05%
1,000	0.1%
5,000	0.5%
10,000	1.0%
50,000	5.0%

mg/kg	mg per 70 kg (154 lb) human	Dermal %[a]
0.005	0.35	0.01%
0.01	0.7	0.02%
0.05	3.5	0.1%
0.1	7	0.2%
0.5	35	1.2%
1	70	2.3%
1.5	105	3.4%
2	140	4.5%
3	210	6.5%
5	350	10%
7.5	550	15%
10	700	19%
12.5	875	23%
15	1,050	26%

In this box we have assumed a specific gravity of 1.0, a dermal penetration of 10%, and dilution with 30 mL of carrier oil.

[a]The percentage of administered diluted oil $= (V_1) \times 100 / (V_1 + V_2)$, where $V_1 =$ volume of essential oil and $V_2 =$ volume of carrier oil, both in mL

$$V_1 = \frac{\text{oral dose (mg/kg)} \times \text{weight of a human adult (kg)}}{\text{fraction of constituent(s) absorbed} \times \text{specific gravity} \times 1000}$$

Glossary

Absolute An aromatic material extracted from a plant using solvent extraction. Unlike essential oils which are only produced by distillation or (in the case of citrus oils) cold pressing, absolutes tend to be more viscous than essential oils, and are more likely to be colored.

Adduct Used in the context of a 'DNA adduct', this is a product resulting from the reaction of a molecule with DNA, which leads to altered function.

Affinity The affinity of a molecule (ligand) for a binding site is a reflection of the strength of association between the two. Most ligands bind reversibly to their receptors.

Alcohol A compound possessing an –OH functional group. Terpenoid alcohols are commonly found in essential oils and are not noted for their toxicity.

Aldehyde A compound possessing a –CHO functional group. Terpenoid and phenylpropanoid aldehydes are commonly found in essential oils, and are implicated in some dermal sensitivity reactions.

Alkaloid A nitrogen-containing, usually basic, compound found in plants. Alkaloids are rarely found in essential oils, but include indole.

Alkene A compound containing one or more carbon-carbon double bonds, a common feature of many essential oil constituents.

Alkenylbenzene A class of essential oil constituent including safrole and estragole, some of which possess carcinogenic potential. Also known as phenyl alkenes, they contain both a benzene ring and an alkene functional group.

Alkylating agent A chemical which can react irreversibly with endogenous substrates, such as DNA, to attach an alkyl group. Alkylating agents are potential carcinogens.

Anophthalmia Absence of one or both eyes.

Anosmia Absence of the sense of smell.

Anthelmintic A remedy which expels or destroys intestinal worms.

Anticholinergic Antagonizing (counteracting) the actions of acetylcholine, an endogenous neurotransmitter.

Anxiolytic A remedy that prevents or reduces anxiety.

Ataxia Loss of control over voluntary movements, resulting in difficulty in walking or standing.

Atopy A genetic predisposition to developing immediate hypersensitivity to common environmental antigens such as pollen, animal dander and certain food items. Atopic reactions are mediated by immunoglobulin E (IgE), and commonly manifest as upper respiratory conditions such as asthma or hay fever, and as skin conditions such as urticaria.

Bioavailability The proportion of a substance that reaches the systemic circulation unchanged after administration. It is lower after dermal and oral dosing than after iv injection, which is, by definition, 100%.

Biocide A chemical agent, such as a bactericide, fungicide or pesticide that destroys micro-organisms.

Biotransformation The metabolic conversion of a chemical substance into another, which will usually possess a different pharmacological and toxicological profile.

Bradycardia Slow rate of beating of the heart.

Carboxylic acid A compound containing a –CO_2H functional group. Commonly found in foods, but relatively uncommon in essential oils. Examples from essential oils include valeric, cinnamic, anisic, citronellic and phenylacetic acids.

Cheilitis Inflammation of the lips.

Chemotype A variety of a plant species that may be virtually identical in appearance to another, but produces a different combination of major constituents. Chemotypes of aromatic plants produce essential oils with significant differences in chemical composition, and hence toxicity. See basil, oregano and thyme profiles for examples of chemotypes.

Chiral center A center of asymmetry in a molecule, usually a carbon atom, to which four different atoms or groups of atoms are attached.

Clastogenic Causing breaks in chromosomes.

Clinical relevance A positive patch test to a substance does not, in itself, demonstrate that the substance was the cause of an allergy. If a direct connection can be shown, then clinical relevance has been demonstrated.

Clonic Convulsions characterized by rapidly alternating muscular contraction and relaxation.

Conjugation In the context of phase II metabolism, this is the reaction of a substance with an endogenous water-soluble molecule such as glucuronic acid. Conjugation aids excretion into the urine.

Cultivar A plant variety produced from a naturally occurring species that has been developed and maintained by cultivation.

Cyanosis Bluish coloration of the skin and/or mucous membranes due to inadequate oxygenation of the blood.

Cytochrome P$_{450}$ A collective name for a group of metabolic enzymes found in many tissues, but most prevalent in the liver. They are responsible for the oxidation (phase I metabolism) of foreign molecules.

Cytotoxicity Toxicity to cells, leading to cell damage and death. Cytotoxic compounds are commonly reactive intermediates such as free radicals and epoxides. They interfere with the action of cytosolic enzymes, or with the metabolism and replication of DNA. They can do this in several ways, but all have the potential for great toxicity, as well as the ability to provoke malignant change, somewhat paradoxically, as anticancer drugs are, by definition, cytotoxic. Cytotoxic activity, which has been discovered in some essential oil constituents, is generally of a much lower order than that of anti-cancer drugs, and cytotoxic essential oils would not be expected to be toxic as used in aromatherapy.

Desquamation Shedding of outermost layer, usually of skin.

Diastereoisomer See Isomer, Optical isomers.

Diterpene A terpene hydrocarbon having the molecular formula $C_{20}H_{32}$.

Diterpenoid A compound containing a diterpene hydrocarbon skeleton and one or more functional groups such as aldehyde, ester or ketone. They are relatively uncommon in essential oils. Examples include geranyl linalool and phytol.

Ecchymosis Effusion of blood into tissue, giving the appearance of a bruise.

Electrophile An electron-deficient molecule or chemical group that is chemically reactive and has an affinity for electron-rich centers in macromolecules such as DNA and proteins. Metabolic electrophiles (e.g., epoxides) are very toxic, especially to the liver.

Enantiomer See Isomer, Optical isomers.

Endogenous Produced within the body.

Epoxidation An oxidation reaction leading to the formation of an epoxide.

Epoxide An organic compound produced by oxidation of an alkene. Epoxides are sometimes formed by metabolism of essential oil constituents in the liver, in which case they are frequently toxic to that organ. Epoxides tend to be highly reactive.

Ester A compound formed by reaction between a carboxylic acid and an alcohol. Esters may be converted back to these components on hydrolysis. Found in many essential oils, esters often have a sweet odor, and have relatively low toxicity.

Exchange transfusion The gradual removal of most or all of the recipient's blood with the simultaneous transfusion of an equal volume of exogenous blood.

Excoriation The stripping away of the surface layer of the skin, usually by mechanical means.

Exogenous Originating outside the body.

Ex vivo Literally, 'outside the living body'. A procedure for examining tissues or organs freshly removed from a living organism.

Fetotoxicity A general term for toxicity to the developing fetus, strictly speaking after the embryo stage.

Fraction In the context of distillation, a fraction is a mixture of constituents (e.g., of an essential oil), collected at a given boiling point. Splitting an essential oil into fractions is known as fractionation.

Functional group An atom or group of atoms that largely determine the chemical properties of any molecule containing it. In essential oils, they usually contain oxygen and are attached to a terpenoid or phenylpropanoid structure which contribute to the oils' chemical and physical characteristics. For example: alcohol, ester, ketone, aldehyde.

Furan A five-membered oxygen-containing aromatic ring compound. Furan derivatives are only found in a few essential oils.

Furanocoumarin Also known as furocoumarin or psoralen. A tricyclic aromatic compound containing oxygen, and most commonly found in cold-pressed citrus oils. Associated with phototoxicity on exposure to UV light.

Gastric lavage Washing out of the stomach, a procedure often used in cases of poisoning.

Gavage Feeding by a tube directly into the stomach.

Genotoxic Damaging to genes by interfering with the structure and/or function of cellular DNA. Genotoxicity may or may not lead to mutagenesis and carcinogenesis, since DNA damage can be repaired by endogenous mechanisms. It is possible to look for such abnormal cellular changes using cultures of human or animal cells.

Glutathione (reduced) (GSH) A sulfur-containing tripeptide (a thiol) in the liver responsible for detoxifying highly reactive metabolites. If endogenous glutathione levels are reduced, the toxicity of a reactive metabolite is often enhanced.

Hapten A small, reactive molecule which, when coupled with a protein, can cause the formation of antibodies, leading to an allergic reaction.

Hemolytic anemia A pathological condition resulting from destruction of red blood cells.

Hepatocarcinogen A chemical which can cause the development of liver cancer. Alkenylbenzenes, such as asarone, safrole and estragole are potential hepatocarcinogens.

Hepatocyte Liver cell.

Hepatotoxicity Toxicity to the liver in a general sense.

Histopathological Damaging to tissues.

Hydrophilic Literally, 'water-loving'. A substance that readily dissolves in water.

Hydrophobic Literally, 'water-hating'. A substance that dissolves sparingly in water.

Hydroxylation The addition of an –OH functional group to a carbon atom, often at a $C=C$ double bond.

Hyperkeratosis Thickening of the upper dead cell layer in the epidermis.

Hyperplasia An increase in the number of cells in an organ or tissue. Benign prostatic hyperplasia is common in older men, and results in enlargement of the prostate gland.

Hyperpyrexia A severely raised body temperature (over $41°C$).

Hypertrophy Enlargement or overgrowth of an organ or tissue.

Induction An increase in enzyme activity promoted by a substance.

In silico Using computer modelling or simulation of molecular structure and biological systems.

Intrinsic activity The ability of a molecule to trigger a physiological response when bound to a receptor. Also referred to as *efficacy*.

In vitro Literally, 'in glass'. A procedure for examining tissues (e.g., cultured cells) or organs in a controlled laboratory environment.

In vivo Literally, 'in a living organism', usually an animal.

Isomer One of two or more compounds that contain the same number of atoms of the same elements, but differ in the ways in which their atoms are arranged in the molecule. The properties of isomers are generally similar, but may occasionally be quite different. More on Ch. 2, p. 14 and Ch. 14, p. 483.

Ketone A compound possessing a $>C=O$ functional group, but lacking the hydrogen atom attached to the carbon, as found in aldehydes. Terpenoid ketones are commonly found in essential oils, and are often neurotoxic.

Lactone A cyclic ester formed by reaction of adjacent carboxylic acid and alcohol groups. Often skin sensitizing.

LD$_{50}$ Literally, the 'lethal dose 50%', this is the traditionally accepted index of acute toxicity, and represents the dose of a substance that kills 50% of a group of animals. Different doses of test substance are administered to groups of matched animals (one dose level per group) usually rats or mice. LD$_{50}$ values are expressed in grams of test substance per kilogram of body weight. This measure of toxicity is often used as a guide to toxicity in humans.

LD$_{Lo}$ The minimum amount of a chemical which tests have shown will be lethal to a specified type of animal.

Lipophilic Literally, 'lipid-loving'. A substance which dissolves in fatty solvents (often used as a synonym of hydrophobic).

Lymphoid hyperplasia Overgrowth of lymphatic tissue.

Maximation test Test for skin sensitization. The test substance is applied repeatedly to a patch of skin until a maximal response is obtained.

Metabolite Substance produced as a result of a biochemical reaction in the body, sometimes by way of detoxifying a chemical.

Microphthalmia Abnormally small, underdeveloped eyes.

Microsomal enzyme An enzyme, including the cytochrome P_{450}, which is located in sub-cellular structures called microsomes.

Mole The quantity of a substance expressed as its molecular or atomic weight, in grams.

Monoterpene A terpene hydrocarbon having the molecular formula $C_{10}H_{16}$.

Monoterpenoid An essential oil constituent containing a monoterpene hydrocarbon skeleton and one or more functional groups such as aldehyde, ester or ketone. Most essential oil constituents which are not monoterpene hydrocarbons are monoterpenoids.

Mutagenic Damaging to DNA, resulting in altered genetic codes being transcribed to mRNA, and consequently in the synthesis of mutant proteins. Mutagens can either act directly on DNA or on the replication of chromosomes, leading to the loss, addition or alteration of base pairs. Mutagenesis is often associated with the causation and progression of cancer. Mutagenic tests can be carried out in bacteria or fungi.

Myeloid Pertaining to the bone marrow.

Myelosuppression Suppressing the production of blood cells in the bone marrow.

Necrosis The death of living cells or tissues. It may be caused by such factors as infection, toxins, physical trauma, the direct action of a corrosive chemical, or insufficient flow of oxygenated blood.

Neoplasia/neoplastic Refers to abnormal, uncontrolled cell growth, which may be either benign or malignant.

Neurotoxic Having a damaging or toxic effect on nervous tissue.

Nidation Implantation: the embedding of the fertilized ovum in the uterine mucous membrane.

Normosmic A person with a normal sense of smell.

Occlusion The covering of the skin with an impermeable material which prevents evaporation of volatile substances from the skin, and enhances absorption.

Olfactory epithelium The small area of mucous membrane inside the top of the nose, into which the olfactory nerve endings project.

Oncogenesis A general term for malignant transformation leading to the formation of a cancer or tumor.

Orthostatic In the context of blood pressure, orthostatic hypotension occurs when a person stands up.

Oxidation The addition of oxygen to, or the removal of hydrogen or electrons from a molecule or atom.

Oxidative stress Adverse events occurring when the generation of reactive oxygen species in an organism exceeds its ability to neutralize and eliminate them through antioxidant systems. Oxidative stress can fatally damage a cell owing to the high reactivity of the free radicals, which contain an unpaired electron.

Patency The state or quality of being open, expanded or unblocked.

Pentoxyresorufin-O-dealkylase (PROD) A microsomal enzyme involved in the activation of genotoxic substances, and a selective marker for CYP2B1.

Percutaneous Through the skin. (In contrast to subcutaneous, which means beneath the skin).

Phenol A compound in which a hydroxyl group (–OH) is attached directly to a benzene ring. Simple phenols (like those often found in essential oils) are weak acids that are often irritant and moderately toxic. Many classes of plant substances are phenols.

Phenylpropanoid A plant secondary metabolite containing a propyl (3-carbon) chain joined to a benzene ring. Phenylpropanoids are biosynthesized via the shikimic acid pathway from plant sugars.

Photocarcinogenesis The initiation of cancer by UV light, or by a chemical in the presence of UV light.

Photochemical reaction A chemical reaction that is initiated by energy in the form of light.

Phototumorigenesis The initiation of tumors by UV light, or by a chemical in the presence of UV light.

Polar A term used to describe a molecule or functional group that has an affinity for polar solvents such as water. Polarity arises as a result of an uneven distribution of electrons in a molecule.

Polycyclic A molecular structure with several rings of atoms joined together.

Porphyria A metabolic disorder in which porphyrin is retained in the tissues. There is an excess of porphyrin in both blood and urine.

Porphyrigenic Inducing porphyria.

Porphyrin An organic compound commonly found in both plant and animal tissues that chelates atoms or ions.

Potentiate To give power to, or increase (the effect of). Methyl salicylate, for instance, potentiates the anticoagulant action of warfarin.

Proximate Used in the context of "proximate toxin" or "proximate carcinogen", this refers to the stage prior to the ultimate (final) toxin or carcinogen in the process of bioactivation.

Psoralen See Furanocoumarin.

Psychotropic Affecting the brain and influencing mood and behavior.

Radical A molecule containing one or more unpaired electrons. Radicals are normally generated in many metabolic pathways. Those that exist in free form may interact with somatic tissues causing dysfunction.

Reactive Likely to undergo a chemical reaction leading to a new product. Reactive compounds may have a pharmacological or toxicological action.

Reporter gene When attached to genes of interest in cultured cells, animals or plants, reporter genes act as markers and confer characteristics that allow them to be identified and measured.

Sesquiterpene A terpene hydrocarbon having the molecular formula $C_{15}H_{24}$.

Sesquiterpenoid An essential oil constituent containing a sesquiterpene hydrocarbon skeleton, $C_{15}H_{24}$, and one or more functional groups such as aldehyde, ester or ketone. They are relatively uncommon in essential oils. Examples include alantolactone and patchouli alcohol.

Spirometer An instrument used for measuring various parameters of pulmonary function.

Stomatitis Inflammation of the oral mucous membrane.

Subcutaneous Beneath the skin.

Substrate A compound which is chemically altered by an enzyme.

Sulfur compound These compounds are found in only a few essential oils, many of which are pungent, irritating and pharmacologically active. An example is diallyl disulfide in garlic.

Synergy A process whereby two or more compounds act together to produce an effect which is greater than the sum of their individual actions.

Teratogenic Causing developmental abnormalities in the fetus.

Teratology The study of the prediction of developmental abnormalities in fetuses caused by chemical agents.

Terpene A hydrocarbon plant secondary metabolite biosynthesized via the mevalonic acid pathway from combinations of isoprene (C_5H_8) units. Terpenes found in essential oils include monoterpenes, sesquiterpenes and diterpenes. Generally non-toxic.

Terpenoid An essential oil constituent containing a terpene hydrocarbon skeleton and one or more functional groups such as

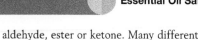

aldehyde, ester or ketone. Many different types are found in essential oils.

Toxicokinetics The absorption, distribution, metabolism and excretion of toxic substances.

Transcription The process by which genetic information is transferred from DNA to RNA.

Tumorigenic Tumor-inducing.

Xenobiotic A substance not normally found in the human body. Any chemical foreign to a biological system. Includes virtually all essential oil constituents.

Abbreviations

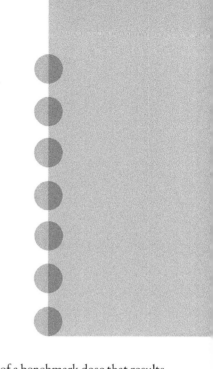

α	Alpha	BMDL₁₀	The lower bound of a benchmark dose that results in a 10% increase in toxicity over background level.

α   Alpha
β   Beta
γ   Gamma
δ   Delta
ε   Epsilon
ψ   Psi
ω   Omega
>   'More than', e.g. '>5 g/kg' means 'more than 5 g/kg'
<   'Less than', e.g. '<1 g/kg' means 'less than 1 g/kg'
~   Approximately
A375   A human malignant melanoma cell line
ABTS   2,2'-Azino-bis(3-ethylbenzthiazoline-6-sulfonic acid)
ACD   Allergic contact dermatitis
ACGIH   American Conference of Governmental Industrial Hygienists
ADI   Acceptable daily intake. The maximum dose of a substance that is anticipated to be without health risk to humans when taken daily over the course of a lifetime. ADIs are set by the EPA, and the term has now been replaced by Reference Dose (RfD).
ADP   Adenosine diphosphate
ADR   Adverse drug reaction
AE   Adverse event
AFB1   Aflatoxin B1
ALD   Approximate lethal dose
ALP   Alkaline phosphatase
ALT   Alanine transaminase (also known as alanine aminotransferase)
AST   Aspartate aminotransferase
B[a]P   Benzo[a]pyrene
BfR   Bundesinstitut für Risikobewertung (Federal Institute for Risk Assessment)
BHR   Bronchial hyper-reactivity
BHT   Butylated hydroxytoluene, an antioxidant
BMD   Benchmark dose

BMDL₁₀   The lower bound of a benchmark dose that results in a 10% increase in toxicity over background level.
bp   Boiling point
BP   Blood pressure
BPH   Benign prostatic hyperplasia
bw   Body weight
CA   Chromosomal aberrations, a type of mutagenicity
CCS   Common chemical sense
CEFS   Committee of Experts on Flavouring Substances
CIPEMC   International Commission for Protection Against Environmental Mutagens and Carcinogens
CIR   Cosmetic Ingredient Review
CITES   Convention on International Trade in Endangered Species of Wild Fauna and Flora
CNS   Central nervous system
COLIPA   European Cosmetic, Toiletry and Perfumery Association
COPD   Chronic obstructive pulmonary disease
COX-2   Cyclo-oxygenase 2
CSTEE   Scientific Committee on Toxicity, Ecotoxicity and the Environment
CT   Chemotype
CYP   Cytochrome P_{450}, a class of drug-metabolizing enzymes
DBP   Dibutyl phthalate
DEHP   Di-(2-ethylhexyl) phthalate
DHB   6,7-Dihydroxybergamottin
DIBP   Diisobutyl phthalate
DMBA   7,12-Dimethylbenz[a]anthracene
DMSO   Dimethyl sulfoxide
DPPH   1,1-Diphenyl-2-picrylhydrazyl
ECEAE   European Coalition to End Animal Experiments
ECETOC   European Centre for Ecotoxicology and Toxicology
ED   Effective dose
EFSA   European Food Safety Authority

EMA	European Medicines Agency	JECFA	Joint Expert Committee on Food Additives (a joint committee of the FAO and the WHO)
EPA	Environmental Protection Agency		
EPAA	The European Partnership for Alternative Approaches to Animal Testing	JMPR	Joint Meetings on Pesticide Residues (a joint committee of the FAO and the WHO)
EROD	Ethoxyresorufin-O-deethylase	K_i	The equilibrium dissociation constant of an enzyme/inhibitor (or enzyme/inhibitor/substrate) complex. It gives an indication of the potency of an inhibitor, and is expressed in concentration units, such as mM or mM.
ESS	Excited skin syndrome		
EU	European Union		
FAO	Food and Agriculture Organization of the United Nations		
FC	Furanocoumarin	LC_{50}	Median Lethal Concentration. The concentration of a substance that is lethal to 50% of a population.
FCF	Furanocoumarin-free		
FDA	Food and Drug Administration		
FEMA	Flavor and Extract Manufacturers Association	LD_{50}	Median Lethal Dose. The dose of a substance that is lethal to 50% of a population.
FFPA	Free from prussic acid		
FM	Fragrance mix	LDH	Lactate dehydrogenase
FRAME	Fund for the Replacement of Animals in Medical Experiments	LDLo	Lowest dose at which lethality occurs
		LH	Luteinizing hormone
FSH	Follicle-stimulating hormone	LLNA	Local lymph node assay
g	Grams	LOAEL	Lowest observed adverse effect level
GABA	Gamma-aminobutyric acid, the major inhibitory neurotransmitter of the central nervous system.	M	Molar (a concentration term; a 1 M solution contains 1 mole of solute in 1 liter of solvent)
GC	Gas chromatography	MAO	Monoamine oxidase
g/kg	Grams of administered substance per kilogram of body weight	MAOI	Monoamine oxidase inhibitor, a type of antidepressant drug
GI_{50}	The concentration of a substance that causes 50% growth inhibition in, for example, cancer cells. Similar to IC_{50}.	MCF-7	A human breast cancer cell line
		MCS	Multiple chemical sensitivity
		MDI	Maximum daily intake
GnRH	Gonadotropin-releasing hormone	MES	Maximal electroshock
GRAS	Generally recognized as safe	μg	Micrograms (millionths of a gram)
HepG2	A human hepatocellular (liver cancer) cell line	mg	Milligrams (thousandths of a gram)
HMG-CoA	3-Hydroxy-3-methylglutaryl coenzyme A	μL	Microliters (millionths of a liter)
HPRT	Hypoxanthine-guanine phosphoribosyltransferase (a mutagenicity test looks for mutations of the gene for this enzyme)	mL	Milliliters (thousandths of a liter)
		mL/kg	Milliliters of administered substance per kilogram of body weight
HRIPT	Human repeated insult patch test	mmol	Millimoles (thousandths of a mole)
IARC	International Agency for Research on Cancer	μmol	Micromoles (millionths of a mole)
IC	Inhibitory concentration	μM	Micromolar (a concentration term; a 1 μM solution contains 1 μmole of solute in 1 liter of solvent)
IC_{50}	The concentration of a substance required to inhibit 50% of a biological response. It is expressed in units such as mM or μM.	mM	Millimolar (a concentration term; a 1 mM solution contains 1 mmole of solute in 1 liter of solvent)
ICCVAM	Interagency Coordinating Committee on the Validation of Alternative Methods	MNU	N-methyl-N-nitrosourea (a mutagen and carcinogen)
ICD	Irritant contact dermatitis	Mole	An amount of a substance corresponding to its molecular weight in grams
IFRA	International Fragrance Association		
IIA	Irritant induced asthma	MROD	Methoxyresorufin O-dealkylase
im	Intramuscular	MRSA	Methicillin-resistant *Staphylococcus aureus*
iNOS	Nitric oxide synthase	MSDS	Material safety data sheet
INR	International normalized ratio (the ratio of the patient's clotting time to the lab's mean reference value)	MTD	Maximum tolerated dose
		NDEA	N-nitrosodiethylamine
		NDMA	N-nitrosodimethylamine
ip	Intraperitoneal (into the abdominal cavity)	NESIL	No expected sensitization induction level
ISO	International Organization for Standardization (ISO is not an acronym)	ng	Nanograms (thousand millionths of a gram)
		NGF	Nerve growth factor
iv	Intravenous	nL	Nanoliter (thousand millionths of a liter)
IVDK	Informationsverbund Dermatologischer Kliniken (Information Network of Departments of Dermatology)	NMBA	N-Nitrosomethylbenzylamine
		nmol	Nanomoles (thousand millionths of a mole)
		NNK	4-(Methylnitrosamino)-1-(3-pyridyl)-1-butanone

NOAEL	No observed adverse effect level (level at and below which no adverse effect is observed)
NOEL	No observed effect level (level at and below which no effect is observed)
NTP	National Toxicology Program
ODC	Ornithine decarboxylase (an enzyme associated with tumor promotion)
OECD	Organisation for Economic Co-operation & Development
OSHA	Occupational Safety & Health Administration
OTC	Over the counter
PAH	Polynuclear aromatic hydrocarbon
PCD	Pigmented contact dermatitis
pg	Picograms, trillionths of a gram
P-gp	P-glycoprotein
PIC	Picrotoxin, a convulsant
PMA	Phorbol myristate acetate
po	Per os, by mouth
ppb	Parts per billion
ppm	Parts per million
PROD	Pentoxyresorufin O-dealkylase
PTZ	Pentylenetetrazol, a convulsant
QRA	Quantitative risk assessment
QSAR	Quantitative structure–activity relationships
RADS	Reactive airways dysfunction syndrome
RCT	Randomized, controlled trial
RD$_{50}$	The dose or concentration of a substance that depresses the respiratory rate in a population by 50%.
REACH	Registration, Evaluation, Authorisation and Restriction of Chemical substances
RfC	Reference concentration, in mg/m^3, an EPA-determined maximum acceptable airborne concentration for continuous inhalation
RfD	Reference dose, an EPA-determined maximum acceptable oral dose. See ADI
RIFM	Research Institute for Fragrance Materials
ROS	Reactive oxygen species
sc	Subcutaneous

SCC	Squamous cell carcinoma
SCCNFP	Scientific Committee on Cosmetic Products and Non-Food Products Intended for Consumers (part of the EU)
SCCP	Scientific Committee on Consumer Products (replaced the SCCNFP in 2004) part of the EU
SCE	Sister-chromatid exchanges, a type of mutagenicity
SCF	Scientific Committee on Food (part of the EU)
SHR	Sensory hyper-reactivity
SI	Sensory irritation
SSO	Sorbitan sesquioleate
SSRI	Selective serotonin reuptake inhibitor, a type of antidepressant drug
TDI	Tolerable daily intake. (Intake quantity per 1 kg of human weight per day, that will not adversely affect a human over the course of a lifetime.)
TDS	Total DNA synthesis
TEWL	Trans-epidermal water loss, a sign of a compromised skin barrier function.
TI	Therapeutic index
TNBS	Trinitrobenzene sulfonic acid
TNF-α	Tumor necrosis factor *alpha*
TPA	12-O-Tetradecanoyl phorbol-13-acetate
tr	Trace (not a precise concentration, but usually less than either 0.05% or 0.01%)
TTC	Threshold of toxicological concern. It is based on the chemical structure and toxicity data of structurally-related chemicals
UDP	Uridine diphosphate
UDS	Unscheduled DNA synthesis (a measure of DNA damage)
UGT	UDP-glucuronosyltransferase
UNEP	United Nations Environment Programme
VEGF	Vascular endothelial growth factor
VEGF1	Vascular endothelial growth factor receptor 1
VOC	Volatile organic compound
WCMC	World Conservation Monitoring Centre
WHO	World Health Organization

Resources

Convention on International Trade in Endangered Species of Wild Fauna and Flora (CITES) http://www.cites.org/

Council of Europe http://www.coe.int/defaultEN.asp

Cosmetic Ingredient Review http://www.cir-safety.org/

Environmental Protection Agency (EPA) http://www.epa.gov

European Union Reference Laboratory for Alternatives to Animal Testing http://ihcp.jrc.ec.europa.eu/our_labs/eurl-ecvam

European Coalition to End Animal Experiments (ECEAE) http://www.eceae.org

Cosmetics Europe – The Personal Care Association (formerly COLIPA) http://www.cosmeticseurope.eu/

European Medicines Agency http://www.ema.europa.eu/ema

European Union (EU) http://www.europa.eu

The opinions of the European scientific committees may be found at: http://ec.europa.eu/health/scientific_committees/consumer_safety/opinions/

Federal Institute for Risk Assessment (BfR) (Germany) http://www.bfr.bund.de/cd/template/index_en

Fund for the Replacement of Animals in Medical Experiments (FRAME) http://www.frame.org.uk

Industrial Hygiene, Environmental, Occupational Health & Safety Resource (ACGIH) http://www.acgih.org/home.htm

Interagency Coordinating Committee on the Validation of Alternative Methods (ICCVAM) http://ntp-server.niehs.nih.gov

International Agency for Research on Cancer (IARC) http://www.iarc.fr/

International Fragrance Association (IFRA) http://www.ifraorg.org

International Organization for Standardization (ISO) http://www.iso.ch/iso/en/CatalogueListPage.CatalogueList For essential oils go to 71, then 100, then 60

IPCS INCHEM (Chemical safety information from intergovernmental organizations) http://www.inchem.org/

National Toxicology Program (NTP) http://iccvam.niehs.nih.gov

NTP carcinogenesis reports http://ntp.niehs.nih.gov/index.cfm?objectid=0847DDA0-F261-59BF-FAA04EB1EC032B61

Occupational Safety & Health Administration (OSHA) http://www.osha.gov

Personal Care Products Council (formerly CTFA) http://www.personalcarecouncil.org/

References

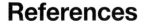

Note: Square brackets [] denote the English translation of the title of an article or book written in a different language.

Aalto-Korte, K., Välimaa, J., Henriks-Eckerman, M.L., et al., 2005. Allergic contact dermatitis from salicyl alcohol and salicylaldehyde in aspen bark (*Populus tremula*). Contact Dermatitis 52, 93–95.

Abanses, J.C., Arima, S., Rubin, B.K., 2009. Vicks VapoRub induces mucin secretion, decreases ciliary beat frequency, and increases tracheal mucus transport in the ferret trachea. Chest 135, 143–148.

Abass, K., Reponen, P., Mattila, S., et al., 2011. Metabolism of α-thujone in human hepatic preparations in vitro. Xenobiotica 41, 101–111.

Abaul, J., Bourgeois, P., 1995. Chemical composition of the essential oils of chemotypes of *Pimenta racemosa* var. *racemosa* (P. Miller) J.W. Moore (bois d'Inde) of Guadaloupe (F.W.I.). Flavour & Fragrance Journal 10, 319–321.

Abbott, D.D., Packman, E.W., Wagner, B.M., et al., 1961. Chronic oral toxicity of oil of sassafras and safrol. Pharmacologist 3, 62.

Abdel-Wahhab, M.A., Aly, S.E., 2005. Antioxidant property of *Nigella sativa* (black cumin) and *Syzygium aromaticum* (clove) in rats during aflatoxicosis. J. Appl. Toxicol. 25, 218–223.

Abdo, K.M., Huff, J.E., Haseman, J.K., et al., 1985. Benzyl acetate carcinogenicity, metabolism & disposition in Fischer 344 rats and B6C3F mice. Toxicology 37, 159–170.

Abdo, K.M., Wenk, M.L., Harry, G.J., et al., 1998. Glycine modulates the toxicity of benzyl acetate in F344 rats. Toxicol. Pathol. 26, 395–402.

Abdo, K.M., Cunningham, M.L., Snell, M.L., et al., 2001. 14-Week toxicity and cell proliferation of methyleugenol administered by gavage to F344 rats and B6C3F1 mice. Food Chem. Toxicol. 39, 303–316.

Abdollahi, M., Salehnia, A., Mortazavi, S.H., et al., 2003. Antioxidant, antidiabetic, antihyperlipidemic, reproduction stimulatory properties and safety of essential oil of *Satureja Khuzestanica* in rat *in vivo*: a toxicopharmacological study. Med. Sci. Monitor. 9, BR331–BR335.

Abdullaev, F.I., Espinosa-Aguirre, J.J., 2004. Biomedical properties of saffron and its potential use in cancer therapy and chemoprevention trials. Cancer Detect. Prev. 28, 426–432.

Abdullaev, J.F., Caballero-Ortega, H., Riveron-Negrete, L., et al., 2002. *In vitro* evaluation of the chemopreventive potential of saffron. Rev. Invest. Clin. 54, 430–436.

Abdullaev, F.I., Riveron-Negrete, L., Caballero-Ortega, H., et al., 2003. Use of *in vitro* assays to assess the potential antigenotoxic and cytotoxic effects of saffron (*Crocus sativus* L.). Toxicology In Vitro 17, 731–736.

Abdullah, D., Ping, Q.N., Liu, G.J., 1996. Enhancing effect of essential oils on the penetration of 5-fluorouracil through rat skin. Yao Xue Xue Bao 31, 214–221.

Abel, G., 1987a. Chromosome damaging effect of *beta*-asarone in human lymphocytes. Planta Med. 53, 251–253.

Abel, G., 1987b. Chromosome damage induced in human lymphocytes by 5-methoxypsoralen and 8-methoxypsoralen plus UV-A. Mutat. Res. 190, 63–68.

Aberchane, M., Fechtal, M., 2004. Analysis of Moroccan Atlas cedarwood oil (*Cedrus atlantica* Manetti). Journal of Essential Oil Research 16, 542–547.

Abernethy, M.K., Becker, L.B., 1992. Acute nutmeg intoxication. Am. J. Emerg. Med. 10, 429–430.

Aboul-Ela, E.I., 2002. Cytogenetic studies on *Nigella sativa* seeds extract and thymoquinone on mouse cells infected with schistosomiasis using karyotyping. Mutat. Res. 516, 11–17.

Aboutabl, E.A., El-Azzouny, A.A., Hammerschmidt, F.J., 1988. The essential oil of *Ruta graveolens* L. growing in Egypt. Scientica Pharmaceutica 56, 121–124.

Aboutabl, E.A., El Tohamy, S.F., De Pooter, H.L., et al., 1991. A comparative study of the essential oils from three *Melaleuca* species growing in Egypt. Flavour & Fragrance Journal 6, 139–141.

Abraham, M.H., Andonian-Haftvan, J., Cometto-Muñiz, J.E., et al., 1996. An analysis of nasal irritation thresholds using a new solvation equation. Fundam. Appl. Toxicol. 31, 71–76.

Abraham, S.K., 2001. Anti-genotoxicity of *trans*-anethole and eugenol in mice. Food Chem. Toxicol. 39, 493–498.

Abraham, M.H., Kumarsingh, R., Cometto-Muñiz, J.E., et al., 1998. An algorithm for nasal pungency thresholds in man. Arch. Toxicol. 72, 227–232.

Abraham, M.H., Gola, J.M., Cometto-Muñiz, J.E., et al., 2001. The correlation and prediction of VOC thresholds for nasal pungency, eye irritation and odour in humans. Indoor & Built Environment 10, 252–257.

Abramovici, A., 1972. The teratogenic effect of cosmetic constituents on the chick embryo. Adv. Exp. Med. Biol. 27, 161–174.

Abramovici, A., Sandbank, U., 1988. The mortician's mystery solved? N. Engl. J. Med. 319, 1157.

Abramovici, A., Kam, J., Liban, E., et al., 1978. Incipient histopathological lesions in citral-induced microphthalmos in chick embryos. Developments in Neuroscience 1, 177–185.

Abramovici, A., Rachmuth-Roizman, P., 1983. Molecular structure - teratogenicity relationships of some fragrance additives. Toxicology 29, 143–156.

Abramovici, A., Servadio, C., Sandbank, U., 1985. Benign hyperplasia of ventral prostate in rats induced by a monoterpene (preliminary report). Prostate 7, 389–394.

Abuhamdah, S., Huang, L., Elliott, M.S., et al., 2008. Pharmacological profile of an essential oil derived from *Melissa officinalis* with anti-agitation properties: focus on ligand-gated channels. J. Pharm. Phamacol. 60, 377–384.

AbuKhader, M.M., Khater, S.H., Al-Matubsi, H.Y., 2013. Acute effects of thymoquinone on the pregnant rat and embryo-fetal development. Drug Chem. Toxicol. 36, 27–34.

Acevedo, C., Opazo, J.L., Huidobro, C., et al., 2003. Positive correlation between single or combined genotypes of CYP1A1 and GSTM1 in relation to prostate cancer in Chilean people. Prostate 57, 111–117.

Achour, S., Abourazzak, S., Mokhtari, A., et al., 2011. Juniper tar (cade oil) poisoning in a new born after a cutaneous application. BMJ Case Reports doi: 10.1136/bcr.07.2011.4427.

Ackermann, L., Aalto-Korte, K., Jolanki, R., et al., 2009. Occupational allergic contact dermatitis from cinnamon including one case from airborne exposure. Contact Dermatitis 60, 96–99.

Adams, R.M., Maibach, H.I., 1985. A five-year study of cosmetic reactions. J. Am. Acad. Dermatol. 13, 1062–1069.

Adams, J.T., Bigler, J.A., Green, O.C., 1957. A case of methyl salicylate intoxication treated by exchange transfusion. J. Am. Med. Assoc. 165, 1563–1565.

Adams, R.P., Barrero, A.F., Lara, A., 1996. Comparisons of the leaf essential oils of Juniperus phoenicea, J. phoenicea subsp. eu-mediterranea Lebr. & Thiv. And J. phoenicea var. turbinata (Guss.) Parl. Journal of Essential Oil Research 8, 367–371.

Adams, T.B., Cohen, S.M., Doull, J., et al., 2004. The FEMA GRAS assessment of cinnamyl derivatives used as flavor ingredients. Food Chem. Toxicol. 42, 157–185.

Adams, T.B., Cohen, S.M., Doull, J., et al., 2005a. The FEMA GRAS assessment of phenethyl alcohol, aldehyde, acid, and related acetals and esters used as flavor ingredients. Food Chem. Toxicol. 43, 1179–1206.

Adams, T.B., Cohen, S.M., Doull, J., et al., 2005b. The FEMA GRAS assessment of benzyl derivatives used as flavor ingredients. Food Chem. Toxicol. 43, 1207–1240.

Adams, T.B., Cohen, S.M., Doull, J., et al., 2005c. The FEMA GRAS assessment of hydroxy- and alkoxy-substituted benzyl derivatives used as flavor ingredients. Food Chem. Toxicol. 43, 1241–1271.

Adams, M.K., Sparrow, J.M., Jim, S., et al., 2009. Inadvertent administration of Olbas oil into the eye: a surprisingly frequent presentation. Eye 23, 244.

Adcock, J.J., 2009. TRPV1 receptors in sensitisation of cough and pain reflexes. Pulm. Pharmacol. Ther. 22, 65–70.

Addo, H.A., Ferguson, J., Johnson, B.E., et al., 1982. The relationship between exposure to fragrance materials and persistent light reaction in the photosensitivity dermatitis with actinic reticuloid syndrome. Br. J. Dermatol. 107, 261–274.

Adebiyi, A., Adaikan, P.G., Prasad, R.N., 2004. Pregnancy outcomes following pre- and post-implantation exposure of Sprague-Dawley rats to benzyl isothiocyanate. Food Chem. Toxicol. 42, 715–720.

Adhikary, S.R., Tuladhar, B.S., Sheak, A., et al., 1992. Investigation of Nepalese essential oils. I. The oil of Cinnamomum glaucescens (Sugandha kokila). Journal of Essential Oil Research 4, 151–159.

Adisen, E., Onder, M., 2007. Allergic contact dermatitis from Laurus nobilis oil induced by massage. Contact Dermatitis 56, 360–361.

Aeschbach, R., Loliger, J., Scott, B.C., et al., 1994. Antioxidant actions of thymol, carvacrol, 6-gingerol, zingerone and hydroxytyrosol. Food Chem. Toxicol. 32, 31–36.

Afoulous, S., Ferhout, H., Raoelison, E.G., et al., 2011. Helichrysum gymnocephalum essential oil: chemical composition and cytotoxic, antimalarial and antioxidant activities, attribution of the activity origin by correlations. Molecules 16, 8273–8291.

Agarwal, M.K., 1993. Receptors for mammalian steroid hormones in microbes and plants. FEBS Lett. 322, 207–210.

Aggarwal, B.B., Shishodia, S., 2006. Molecular targets of dietary agents for prevention and therapy of cancer. Biochem. Pharmacol. 71, 1397–1421.

Agrawal, D., Durity, F.A., 2006. Seizure as a manifestation of intracranial hypotension in a shunted patient. Pediatr. Neurosurg. 42, 165–167.

Agrawal, O.P., Bharadwaj, S., Mathur, R., 1980. Antifertility effects of fruits of Juniperus communis. Planta Med. 39, 98–101.

Aguilar-Santamaría, L., Tortoriello, J., 1998. Anticonvulsant and sedative effects of crude extracts of Ternstroemia pringlei and Ruta chalepensis. Phytother. Res. 10, 531–533.

Aguirre, A., Oleaga, J.M., Zabala, R., et al., 1994. Allergic contact dermatitis from Reflex® spray. Contact Dermatitis 30, 52–53.

Ahmad, N., Mukhtar, H., 2004. Cytochrome p450: a target for drug development for skin diseases. J. Invest. Dermatol. 123, 417–425.

Ahmad, H., Tijerina, M.T., Tobola, A.S., 1997. Preferential overexpression of a class MU glutathione-S-transferase subunit in mouse liver by myristicin. Biochem. Biophys. Res. Commun. 236, 825–828.

Ahmed, M.M., Arif, M., Chikuma, T., et al., 2005. Pentylenetetrazol-induced seizures affect the levels of prolyl oligopeptidase, thimet oligopeptidase and glial proteins in rat brain regions, and attenuation by MK-801 pretreatment. Neurochem. Int. 47, 248–259.

Ahn, B.Z., Lee, J.H., 1989. Cytotoxic and cytotoxicity-potentiating effects of the Curcuma root on L1210 cell. Korean Journal of Pharmacognosy 20, 223–226.

Ait M'barek, L., Ait Mouse, H., Elabbadi, N., et al., 2007a. Anti-tumor properties of blackseed (Nigella sativa L.) extracts. Brazilian Journal of Medical & Biological Research 40, 839–847.

Ait M'barek, L., Ait Mouse, H., Jaafari, A., et al., 2007b. Cytotoxic effect of essential oil of thyme (Thymus broussonettii) on the IGR-OV1 tumor cells resistant to chemotherapy. Brazilian Journal of Medical & Biological Research 40, 1537–1544.

Akagi, K., Sano, M., Ogawa, K., et al., 2003. Involvement of toxicity as an early event in urinary bladder carcinogenesis induced by phenethyl isothiocyanate, benzyl isothiocyanate, and analogues in F344 rats. Toxicol. Pathol. 31, 388–396.

Åkesson, H.O., Wålinder, J., 1965. Nutmeg intoxication. Lancet 1, 1271–1272.

Akisue, G., 1977. Secreção de Myroxylon peruiferum L.F. IV Analise quantitativa de alguns components do balsamo e do oleo esencial apos separacão. An. Farm Quim. São Paulo 17, 25–41.

Al-Ali, A., Alkhawajah, A.A., Randhawa, M.A., et al., 2008. Oral and intraperitoneal LD50 of thymoquinone, an active principle of Nigella sativa, in mice and rats. J. Ayub Med. Coll. Abbottabad 20, 25–27.

Alam, K., Nagi, M.N., Badary, O.A., et al., 1999. The protective action of thymol against carbon tetrachloride hepatotoxicity in mice. Pharmacol. Res. 40, 159–163.

Alasalvar, C., Grigor, J.M., Quantick, P.C., 1999. Method for the static headspace analysis of carrot volatiles. Food Chem. 65, 391–397.

Albert-Puleo, M., 1980. Fennel and anise as estrogenic agents. J. Ethnopharmacol. 2, 337–344.

Alberts, W.M., Do Pico, G.A., 1996. Reactive airways dysfunction syndrome. Chest 109, 1618–1626.

Albery, W.J., Hadgraft, J., 1979. Percutaneous absorption: in vivo experiments. J. Pharm. Pharmacol. 31, 140–147.

Alcalay, J., Dall'Acqua, F., Kripke, M.L., 1990. Photocarcinogenesis in mice by 4,4',6 trimethylangelicin plus UVA radiation. Photodermatol. Photoimmunol. Photomed. 7, 116–118.

Aldridge, J.E., Meyer, A., Seidler, F.J., et al., 2005. Alterations in central nervous system serotonergic and dopaminergic synaptic activity in adulthood after prenatal or neonatal chlorpyrifos exposure. Environ. Health Perspect. 113, 1027–1031.

Al-Enazi, M.M., 2007. Effect of thymoquinone on malformations and oxidative stress-induced diabetic mice. Pakistan Journal of Biological Sciences 10, 3115–3119.

Alenmyr, L., Högestätt, E.D., Zygmunt, P.M., et al., 2009. TRPV1-mediated itch in seasonal allergic rhinitis. Allergy 64, 807–810.

Alexandrovich, I., Rakovitskaya, O., Kolmo, E., et al., 2003. The effect of fennel (Foeniculum vulgare) seed oil emulsion in infantile colic: a randomized, placebo-controlled study. Alternative Therapies 9, 58–61.

Al-Hader, A., Aqel, M., Hasan, Z., 1993. Hypoglycemic effects of the volatile oil of Nigella sativa seeds. International Journal of Pharmacognosy 31, 96–100.

Al-Hader, A., Hasan, Z.A., Aqel, M.B., 1994. Hyperglycemic and insulin release inhibitory effects of Rosmarinus officinalis. J. Ethnopharmacol. 43, 217–221.

Al-Harbi, M.M., Qureshi, S., Raza, M., et al., 1995. Influence of anethole treatment on the tumour induced by Ehrlich ascites carcinoma cells in paw of Swiss albino mice. Eur. J. Cancer Prev. 4, 307–318.

Al-Harrasi, A., Al-Saidi, S., 2008. Phytochemical analysis of the essential oil from botanically certified oleogum resin of Boswellia sacra (Omani Luban). Molecules 13, 2181–2189.

Alhusainy, W., Paini, A., Punt, A., et al., 2010. Identification of nevadensin as an important herb-based constituent inhibiting estragole bioactivation and physiology-based biokinetic modeling of its possible *in vivo* effect. Toxicol. Appl. Pharmacol. 245, 179–190.

Alkofahi, A., Al-Hamood, M.H., Elbetieha, A.M., 1996. Antifertility evaluation of some medicinal plants in male and female mice. Archives of STD/HIV Research 10, 189–196.

Allahverdiyev, A.M., Duran, N., Çetiner, S., 2001. Investigation of the anticancerogenic effect of the essential oil of *Melissa officinalis* L. Pharmaceutical & Pharmacological Letters 1, 26–29.

Allan, J., 1910. Poisoning by oil of eucalyptus. Br. Med. J. 1, 569.

Allavena, A., Martelli, A., Robbiano, L., et al., 1992. Evaluation in a battery of *in vivo* assays of four *in vitro* genotoxins proved to be noncarcinogens in rodents. Teratog. Carcinog. Mutagen. 12, 31–41.

Allen, W.T., 1897. Note on a case of supposed poisoning by pennyroyal. Lancet 1, 1022–1023.

Allen, C.M., Blozis, G.G., 1988. Oral mucosal reactions to cinnamon-flavored chewing gum. J. Am. Dent. Assoc. 116, 664–667.

Allenby, C.F., Goodwin, B.F.J., Safford, R.J., 1984. Diminution of immediate reactions to cinnamic aldehyde by eugenol. Contact Dermatitis 11, 322–323.

Almirall, L.M., Montana, J., Esribano, E., et al., 1996. Effect of *d*-limonene, *a*-pinene and cineole on *in vitro* transdermal human skin penetration of chlorpromazine and haloperidol. Arzneimittel-Forschung/Drug Research 46, 676–680.

Almora, K., Pino, J.A., Hernandez, M., et al., 2004. Evaluation of volatiles from ripening papaya (*Carica papaya* L., var. Maradol roja). Food Chem. 86, 127–130.

Al-Subeihi, A.A., Spenkelink, B., Rachmawati, N., et al., 2011. Physiologically based biokinetic model of bioactivation and detoxification of the alkenylbenzene methyleugenol in rat. Toxicology In Vitro 25, 267–285.

Altaei, D.T., 2012. Topical lavender oil for the treatment of recurrent aphthous ulceration. Am. J. Dent. 25, 39–43.

Altman, P.M., 1990. Summary of safety studies concerning Australian tea tree oil. In: Modern phytotherapy – the clinical significance of tea tree and other essential oils. Volume II. Proceedings of a conference on December 1–2, 1990 in Sydney, and a symposium on December 8 1990, in Surfers Paradise, 21–22.

Alvarez, M.S., Jacobs, S., Jiang, S.B., et al., 2003. Photocontact allergy to diallyl disulfide. Am. J. Contact Dermat. 14, 161–165.

Amantea, D., Fratto, V., Maida, S., et al., 2009. Prevention of glutamate accumulation and upregulation of phospho-Akt may account for neuroprotection afforded by bergamot essential oil against brain injury induced by focal cerebral ischemia in rat. Int. Rev. Neurobiol. 85, 389–405.

Amerio, A., De Benedictis, G., Leondeff, J., et al., 1968. La nefropatia da apiolo. Minerva Nefrol. 15 (1), 49–70.

Ames, B.N., Lee, F.D., Durston, W.E., 1973. An improved bacterial test system for the detection and classification of mutagens and carcinogens. Proc. Natl. Acad. Sci. U. S. A. 70, 782–786.

Ames, B.N., Magaw, R., Gold, L.S., 1987. Ranking possible carcinogenic hazards. Science 236, 271–280.

Amici, L.A., Gasparro, F.P., 1995. 5-Methoxypsoralen photoadduct formation: conversion of monoadducts to crosslinks. Photodermatol. Photoimmunol. Photomed. 11, 135–139.

Amini, A., Cheraghi, E., Safaee, M.R., et al., 2003. The role of eugenol in the reduction of teratogenic effects of retinoic acid on skeletal morphology of mice embryo. Yakhteh Medical Journal 4, 195–200.

Amonkar, A.J., Nagabhushan, M., D'Souza, A.V., et al., 1986. Hydroxychavicol: a new phenolic antimutagen from betel leaf. Food Chem. Toxicol. 24, 1321–1324.

An, Y.S., Sung, E., Xue, Y.G., et al., 1983. Experimental investigation of termination of early pregnancy by Chinese medicine - *Curcuma zedoaria* Rosc. Reproduction & Contraception 3, 57–58.

An, S., Lee, A.Y., Lee, C.H., 2005. Fragrance contact dermatitis in Korea: a joint study. Contact Dermatitis 320–323.

Analytical Methods Committee, 1988. Application of gas-liquid chromatography to the analysis of essential oils. Part XIV. Monograph of five essential oils. Analyst 113, 1125–1136.

Andersen, A., 2006a. Final report on the safety assessment of benzaldehyde. Int. J. Toxicol. 25 (Suppl. 1), 11–27.

Andersen, A., 2006b. Final report on the safety assessment of sodium *p*-chloro-*m*-cresol, *p*-chloro-*m*-cresol, chlorothymol, mixed cresols, *m*-cresol, *o*-cresol, *p*-cresol, isopropyl cresols, thymol, *o*-cymen-5-ol, and carvacrol. Int. J. Toxicol. 25 (Suppl. 1), 29–127.

Anderson, B.E., Zeiger, E., Shelby, M.D., et al., 1990. Chromosome aberration and sister chromatid exchange test results with 42 chemicals. Environ. Mol. Mutagen. 16 (Suppl. 18), 55–137.

Anderson, D., Styles, J.A., 1978. An evaluation of 6 short-term tests for detecting organic chemical carcinogens. Appendix II. The bacterial mutation test. Br. J. Cancer 37, 924–930.

Anderson, I.B., Mullen, W.H., Meeker, J.E., et al., 1996. Pennyroyal toxicity: measurement of toxic metabolite levels in two cases and review of the literature. Ann. Intern. Med. 124, 726–734.

Andersen, K.E., Johansen, J.D., Bruze, M., et al., 2001. The time-dose-response relationship for elicitation of contact dermatitis in isoeugenol allergic individuals. Toxicol. Appl. Pharmacol. 170, 166–171.

Andersson, L., Johansson, A., Millqvist, E., et al., 2008. Prevalence and risk factors for chemical sensitivity and sensory hyperreactivity in teenagers. Int. J. Hyg. Environ. Health 211, 690–697.

Andersen, P.H., Jensen, N.J., 1984. Mutagenic investigation of peppermint oil in the *Salmonella*/mammalian microsome test. Mutat. Res. 138, 17–20.

Anderson, R.C., Anderson, J.H., 1997a. Toxic effects of air freshener emissions. Arch. Environ. Health 52, 433–441.

Anderson, R.C., Anderson, J.H., 1997b. Neurotoxic effects of fragrance products. Advances in Occupational Medicine & Rehabilitation 3, 165–172.

Anderson, R.C., Anderson, J.H., 1998. Acute toxic effects of fragrance products. Archives of Environment Health 53, 138–146.

Anderson, T.F., Voorhees, J.J., 1980. Psoralen photochemotherapy of cutaneous disorders. Annu. Rev. Pharmacol. Toxicol. 20, 235–257.

Andrade-Neto, M., Cunha de., U.A., Mafezoli, J., et al., 2000. Volatile constituents of *Pilocarpus trachyllophus* Holmes and *Pilocarpus jaborandi* Holmes (Rutaceae) from Northeast Brazil. Journal of Essential Oil Research 12, 769–774.

Andrè, E., Campi, B., Materazzi, S., et al., 2008. Cigarette smoke-induced neurogenic inflammation is mediated by α, β-unsaturated aldehydes and the TRPA1 receptor in rodents. J. Clin. Invest. 118, 2574–2582.

Angelini, G., Vena, G.A., 1984. Allergic contact cheilitis to guaiazulene. Contact Dermatitis 10, 310–318.

Angelini, G., Vena, G.A., Foti, C., et al., 1997. Contact allergy to preservatives and perfumed compounds used in skin care products. Journal of Applied Cosmetology 15, 49–57.

Anigbogu, A.N., Williams, A.C., Barry, B.W., 1996. Permeation characteristics of 8-methoxypsoralen through human skin; relevance to clinical treatment. J. Pharm. Pharmacol. 48, 357–366.

Anjos, J.L., Neto, D.D., Alonso, A., 2007. Effects of 1,8-cineole on the dynamics of lipids and proteins of stratum corneum. Int. J. Pharm. 345, 81–87.

Anon, 1857. Medical Jurisprudence. Inquests and medical trials: poisoning by essential oil of bitter almonds. Lancet 69 (1741), 45–46.

Anon, 1934. The British pharmaceutical codex. The Pharmaceutical Press, London.

Anon, 1974. Oil of rue: proposed affirmation of GRAS status with specific limitations as direct human food ingredient. Fed. Regist. 39, 34215.

Anon, 1975. Safe and unsafe herbs in herbal teas. Department of Health Education & Welfare, Public Health Service Food & Drug Administration, Washington DC.

Anon, 1978. Fatality and illness associated with consumption of pennyroyal oil-Colorado. MMWR Morb. Mortal. Wkly. Rep. 27, 511–513.

Anon, 1982. Neonatal deaths associated with the use of benzyl alcohol - United States. MMWR Morb. Mortal. Wkly. Rep. 31, 290–291.

Anon, 1992a. Lemon burn warning. Int. J. Aromather. 4 (4), 4.

Anon, 1992b. The flavourings in food regulations 1992. Statutory Instruments No. 1971.

Anon, 1993. Condom concern. Int. J. Aromather. 5, 4.

Anon, 1999. Benzyl acetate. IARC Monogr. Eval. Carcinog. Risks Hum. 71, 1255–1264.

Anon, 2001a. Final report on the safety assessment of hydrogenated cottonseed oil, cottonseed (gossypium) oil, cottonseed acid, cottonseed glyceride, and hydrogenated cottonseed glyceride. Int. J. Toxicol. 20 (Suppl. 2), 21–29.

Anon, 2001b. Final report on the safety assessment of *Juniperus communis* extract, *Juniperus oxycedrus* extract, *Juniperus oxycedrus* tar, *Juniperus phoenicia* extracts, and *Juniperus virginiana* extract. Int. J. Toxicol. 20 (Suppl. 2), 41–56.

Anon, 2003a. Council directive of 27 July 1976 on the approximation of the laws of the member states relating to cosmetic products. Office for Official Publications of the European Communities. www.obelis.net/website/library/Directives/files/cos.pdf.

Anon, 2003b. Use of undiluted tea tree oil as a cosmetic. Opinion of the Federal Institute for Risk Assessment (BfR). 1st September 2003. http://www.bfr.bund.de/cm/257/use_of_undiluted_tea_tree_oil_as_a_cosmetic.pdf.

Anonis, D.P., 1993. Flower oils and floral compounds in perfumery. Allured, Carol Stream.

Anter, J., Romero-Jiménez, M., Fernández-Bedmar, Z., et al., 2011. Antigenotoxicity, cytotoxicity, and apoptosis induction by apigenin, bisabolol, and protocatechuic acid. J. Med. Food 14, 276–283.

Anthony, A., Caldwell, J., Hutt, A.J., et al., 1987. Metabolism of estragole in rat and mouse and influence of dose size on excretion of the proximate carcinogen 1'-hydroxyestragole. Food Chem. Toxicol. 25, 799–806.

Antunez-Solis, J., Hernández-Derramadero, F., Aquino-Vega, M., et al., 2009. 2,4,5-Trimethoxycinnamic acid: the major metabolite of α-asarone, retains most of the pharmacological properties of α-asarone. J. Enzyme Inhib. Med. Chem. 24, 903–909.

Aoshima, H., Hamamoto, K., 1999. Potentiation of GABAA receptors expressed in Xenopus oocytes by perfume and phytoncid. Biosci. Biotechnol. Biochem. 63, 743–748.

Aourell, M., Skoog, M., Carleson, J., 2005. Effects of Swedish massage on blood pressure. Complement. Ther. Clin. Pract. 11, 242–246.

Api, A.M., 2000. Quenching of citral, cinnamaldehyde and phenylacetaldehyde sensitization in human repeated insult patch tests. Contact Dermatitis 42 (Suppl. 2), Abstract 40.

Api, A.M., 2001a. Toxicological profile of diethyl phthalate: a vehicle for fragrance and cosmetic ingredients. Food Chem. Toxicol. 39, 97–108.

Api, A.M., 2001b. Lack of effect of coumarin on the formation of micronuclei in an *in vivo* mouse micronucleus assay. Food Chem. Toxicol. 39, 837–841.

Api, A.M., Isola, D., 2000. Quenching of citral sensitization demonstrated in a human repeated insult patch test. Contact Dermatitis 46 (Suppl. 4), 37.

Api, A.M., Vey, M., 2008. Implementation of the dermal sensitization Quantitative Risk Assessment (QRA) for fragrance ingredients. Regul. Toxicol. Pharmacol. 52, 53–61.

Api, A.M., Basketter, D.A., Cadby, P.A., et al., 2008. Dermal sensitization quantitative risk assessment (QRA) for fragrance ingredients. Regul. Toxicol. Pharmacol. 52, 3–23.

Apted, J.H., 1991. Contact dermatitis associated with the use of tea-tree oil. Australas. J. Dermatol. 32, 177.

Aqel, M., Shaheen, R., 1996. Effects of the volatile oil of *Nigella sativa* seeds on the uterine smooth muscle of rat and guinea pig. J. Ethnopharmacol. 52, 23–26.

Arasada, B.L., Bommareddy, A., Zhang, X., et al., 2008. Effects of α-santalol on proapoptotic caspases and p53 expression in UVB irradiated mouse skin. Anticancer Res. 28, 129–132.

Aratanechemuge, Y., Komiya, T., Moteki, H., et al., 2002. Selective induction of apoptosis by ar-turmerone isolated from turmeric (*Curcuma longa* L) in two human leukemia cell lines, but not in human stomach cancer cell line. Int. J. Mol. Med. 9, 481–484.

Araujo, I.B., Souza, C.A., De-Carvalho, R.R., 1996. Study of the embryofoetotoxicity of alpha-terpinene in the rat. Food Chem. Toxicol. 34, 477–482.

Arctander, S., 1960. Perfume and flavor materials of natural origin. Self-published, Elizabeth, New Jersey.

Arditti, J., Faizende, J.J., Bernard, J., et al., 1978. Trois observations d'intoxication par des essences végétales convulsivantes. Ann. Med. Nancy 17, 371–374.

Ariyoshi, T., Arakaki, M., Ideguchi, K., et al., 1975. Studies on the metabolism of *d*-limonene (*p*-mentha-1,8-diene). III. Effects of

d-limonene on the lipids and drug-metabolizing enzymes in rat livers. Xenobiotica 5 (1), 33–38.

Arnold, N., Bellomaria, B., Valentini, G., 1993. Comparative study of the essential oils from three species of *Origanum* growing wild in the Eastern Mediterranean region. Journal of Essential Oil Research 5, 71–77.

Aronow, R., 1976. Camphor poisoning. J. Am. Med. Assoc. 235, 1260.

Arora, R.B., Arora, C.K., 1963. Hypotensive and tranquillising activity of jatamansone (valeranone) a sesquiterpene from *Nardostachys jatamansi* DC. In: Chen, K.K., Mukerji, B. (Eds.), Pharmacology of oriental plants. Pergamon, Oxford, pp. 51–60.

Arora, C.K., Arora, R.B., Mesta, C.K., et al., 1967. Hypotensive activity of β-eudesmol and some related sesquiterpenes. Indian J. Med. Res. 55 (5), 463–472.

Arora, A., Siddiqui, I.A., Shukla, Y., 2004. Modulation of p53 in 7,12-dimethylbenz[a]anthracene-induced skin tumors by diallyl sulfide in Swiss albino mice. Mol. Cancer Ther. 3, 1459–1466.

Artuc, M., Stuettgen, G., Schalla, W., et al., 1979. Reversible binding of 5- and 8-methoxypsoralen to human serum proteins (albumin) and to epidermis *in vitro*. Br. J. Dermatol. 101, 669–677.

Aruna, K., Sivaramakrishnan, V.M., 1996. Anticarcinogenic effects of the essential oils from cumin, poppy and basil. Phytother. Res. 10, 577–580.

Arunasree, K.M., 2010. Anti-proliferative effects of carvacrol on a human metastatic breast cancer cell line, MDA-MB 231. Phytomedicine 17, 581–588.

Asakawa, Y., Ishida, T., Toyota, M., et al., 1986. Terpenoid biotransformation in mammals IV. Biotransformation of (+)-longifolene, (−)-caryophyllene, (−)-caryophyllene oxide, (−)-cyclocolorenone, (+)-nootkatone, (−)-elemol, (−)- abietic acid and (+)-dehydroabietic acid in rabbits. Xenobiotica 16, 753–767.

Asakawa, Y., Toyota, M., Ishida, T., 1988. Biotransformation of 1,4-cineole, a monoterpene ether. Xenobiotica 18, 1129–11340.

Asano, M., Yamakasa, T., 1950. The fate of branched chain fatty acids in animal body. I. A contribution to the problem of 'Hildebrandt Acid'. J. Biochem. (Tokyo) 37, 321–327.

Ashby, J., 1994. Benzyl acetate: from mutagenic carcinogen to non-mutagenic non-carcinogenic in 7 years? Mutat. Res. 306, 107–109.

Ashby, J., Lefevre, P.A., Odum, J., et al., 1997. Failure to confirm estrogenic activity for benzoic acid and clofibrate: Implications for lists of endocrine-disrupting agents. Regul. Toxicol. Pharmacol. 26, 96–101.

Ashikaga, T., Hoya, M., Itagaki, H., et al., 2002. Evaluation of CD86 expression and MHC class II molecule internalization in THP-1 human monocyte cells as predictive endpoints for contact sensitizers. Toxicol. In Vitro 16, 711–716.

Ashwood-Smith, M.J., Poulton, G.A., Liu, M., 1983. Photobiological activity of 5,7-dimethoxycoumarin. Experientia 39, 262–264.

Ashwood-Smith, M.J., Ceska, O., Warrington, P.J., et al., 1992. The photobiological activity of 5-geranoxypsoralen and its photoproducts. Photochem. Photobiol. 55, 529–532.

Aspres, N., Freeman, S., 2003. Predictive testing for irritancy and allergenicity of tea tree oil in normal human subjects. Exogenous Dermatology 2, 258–261.

Atanassova-Shopova, S., Roussinov, K., 1970a. Experimental studies on certain effects of the essential oil of *Salvia sclarea* L. on the central nervous system. Bulletin of the Institute of Physiology, Bulgarian Academy of Sciences 13, 89–95.

Atanassova-Shopova, S., Roussinov, K.S., 1970b. On certain central neurotropic effects of lavender essential oil. Bulletin of the Institute of Physiology, Bulgarian Academy of Sciences 13, 69–77.

Atanassova-Shopova, S., Roussinov, K.S., Boycheva, I., 1973. On certain central neurotropic effects of lavender essential oil. II communication: studies on the effects of linalool and of terpineol. Bulletin of the Institute of Physiology, Bulgarian Academy of Sciences 15, 149–156.

Athanasiadis, G.I., Pfab, F., Klein, A., et al., 2007. Erythema multiforme due to contact with laurel oil. Contact Dermatitis 57, 116–118.

Atkinson, H.C., Begg, E.J., Darlow, B.A., 1988. Drugs in human milk: clinical pharmacokinetic considerations. Clin. Pharmacokinet. 14, 217–240.

Atsumi, T., Tonosaki, K., 2007. Smelling lavender and rosemary increases free radical scavenging activity and decreases cortisol level in saliva. Psychiatry Res. 150, 89–96.

Aubin, F., Humbert, P.h., Agache, P., 1994. Effects of a new psoralen, 5-geranoxypsoralen, plus UVA radiation on murine ATPase positive Langerhans cells. J. Dermatol. Sci. 7, 176–184.

Audicana, M., Bernaola, G., 1994. Occupational contact dermatitis from citrus fuits: lemon essential oils. Contact Dermatitis 31, 183–185.

Auerbach, S.S., Shah, R.R., Mav, D., 2010. Predicting the hepatocarcinogenic potential of alkenylbenzene flavoring agents using toxicogenomics and machine learning. Toxicol. Appl. Pharmacol. 243, 300–314.

Auffray, B., 2007. Protection against singlet oxygen, the main actor of sebum squalene peroxidation during sun exposure, using Commiphora myrrha essential oil. Int. J. Cosmet. Sci. 29, 23–29.

Averbeck, D., Averbeck, S., Dubertret, L., et al., 1990. Genotoxicity of bergapten and bergamot oil in Saccharomyces cerevisiae. J. Photochem. Photobiol. 7, 209–229.

Aydelotte, M.B., 1963. The effects of vitamin A and citral on epithelial differentiation in vitro 2. The chick oesophageal and corneal epithelia and epidermis. J. Embryol. Exp. Morphol. 11, 621–635.

Aydin, S., Basaran, A.A., Basaran, N., 2005. The effects of thyme volatiles on the induction of DNA damage by the heterocyclic amine IQ and mitomycin C. Mutat. Res. 581, 43–53.

Aydin, Y., Kutlay, O., Ari, S., et al., 2007. Hypotensive effects of carvacrol on the blood pressure of normotensive rats. Planta Med. 73, 1365–1371.

Azirak, S., Rencuzogullari, E., 2008. The in vivo genotoxic effects of carvacrol and thymol in rat bone marrow cells. Environ. Toxicol. 23, 728–735.

Azizan, A., Blevins, R.D., 1995. Mutagenicity and antimutagenicity testing of six chemicals associated with the pungent properties of specific spices as revealed by the Ames Salmonella/microsomal assay. Arch. Environ. Contam. Toxicol. 28, 248–258.

Azuine, M.A., Amonkar, A.J., Bhide, S.V., 1991. Chemopreventive efficacy of betel leaf extract and its constituents on 7,12-dimethylbenz(a) anthracene induced carcinogenesis and their effect on drug detoxification system in mouse skin. Indian J. Exp. Biol. 29, 346–351.

Baba, T., Nakano, H., Tamai, K., et al., 1998. Inhibitory effect of beta-thujaplicin on ultraviolet B-induced apoptosis in mouse keratinocytes. J. Invest. Dermatol. 110, 24–28.

Babich, H., Stern, A., Borenfreund, E., 1993. Eugenol cytotoxicity evaluated with continuous cell lines. Toxicology In Vitro 7, 105–109.

Babu, P.S., Prabuseenivasan, S., Ignacimuthu, S., 2007. Cinnamaldehyde – a potential antidiabetic agent. Phytomedicine 14, 15–22.

Badary, O.A., 1999. Thymoquinone attenuates ifosfamide-induced Fanconi syndrome in rats and enhances its antitumor activity in mice. J. Ethnopharmacol. 67, 135–142.

Badary, O.A., Gamal El-Din, A.M., 2001. Inhibitory effects of thymoquinone against 20-methylcholanthrene-induced fibrosarcoma tumorigenesis. Cancer Detect. Prev. 25, 362–368.

Badary, O.A., Nagi, M.N., al-Shabanah, O.A., et al., 1997. Thymoquinone ameliorates the nephrotoxicity induced by cisplatin in rodents and potentiates its antitumor activity. Can. J. Physiol. Pharmacol 75, 1356–1361.

Badary, O.A., Alshabanah, O.A., Nagi, M.N., et al., 1998. Acute and subchronic toxicity of thymoquinone in mice. Drug Development Research 44, 56–61.

Badary, O.A., Al-Shabanah, O.A., Nagi, M.N., 1999. Inhibition of benzo(a) pyrene-induced forestomach carcinogenesis in mice by thymoquinone. Eur. J. Cancer Prev. 8, 435–440.

Badger, D.A., Smith, R.L., Bao, J., et al., 2002. Disposition and metabolism of isoeugenol in the male Fischer 344 rat. Food Chem. Toxicol. 40, 1757–1765.

Bailer, J., Witthöft, M., Rist, F., 2008. Modern health worries and idiopathic environmental intolerance. J. Psychosom. Res. 65, 425–433.

Bailey, H.H., Levy, D., Harris, L.S., et al., 2002. A phase II trial of daily perillyl alcohol in patients with advanced ovarian cancer: Eastern Cooperative Oncology Group Study E2E96. Gynecol. Oncol. 85, 464–468.

Bailey, D.G., Dresser, G.K., Bend, J.R., 2003. Bergamottin, lime juice, and red wine as inhibitors of cytochrome P450 3A4 activity: comparison with grapefruit juice. Clin. Pharmacol. Ther. 73, 529–537.

Bailey, H.H., Wilding, G., Tutsch, K.D., et al., 2004. A phase I trial of perillyl alcohol administered four times daily for 14 days out of 28 days. Cancer Chemother. Pharmacol. 54, 368–376.

Bailey, H.H., Attia, S., Love, R.R., et al., 2008. Phase II trial of daily oral perillyl alcohol (NSC 641066) in treatment-refractory metastatic breast cancer. Cancer Chemother. Pharmacol. 62, 149–157.

Baker, J.B.E., 1960. The effects of drugs on the foetus. Pharmacol. Rev. 12, 37–90.

Baker, R.B., 1999. Incidence of atopic dermatitis and eczema by ethnic group seen within a general pediatric practice. The Permanente Journal 3, 31–32.

Bakerink, J.A., Gospe, S.M., Dimand, R.J., et al., 1996. Multiple organ failure after ingestion of pennyroyal oil from herbal tea in two infants. Pediatrics 98, 944–947.

Bakkali, F., Averbeck, S., Averbeck, D., et al., 2005. Cytotoxicity and gene induction by some essential oils in the yeast Saccharomyces cerevisiae. Mutat. Res. 585, 1–13.

Bakkali, F., Averbeck, S., Averbeck, D., et al., 2006. Antigenotoxic effects of three essential oils in diploid yeast (Saccharomyces cerevisiae) after treatments with UVC radiation, 8-MOP plus UVA and MMS. Mutat. Res. 606, 27–38.

Bakkali, F., Averbeck, S., Averbeck, D., et al., 2008. Biological effects of essential oils – a review. Food Chem. Toxicol. 46, 446–475.

Bakker, C.V., Blömeke, B., Coenraads, P.J., et al., 2011. Ascaridole, a sensitizing component of tea tree oil, patch tested at 1% and 5% in two series of patients. Contact Dermatitis 65, 239–248.

Balachandran, B., Sivaswamy, S.N., Sivaramakrishnan, V.M., 1991. Genotoxic effects of some foods & food components in Swiss mice. Indian J. Med. Res. 94, 378–383.

Baldwin, C.M., Bell, I.R., O'Rourke, M.K., Lebowitz, M.D., 1997. The association of respiratory problems in a community sample with self-reported chemical intolerance. Eur. J. Epidemiol. 13, 547–552.

Baldwin, C.M., Bell, I.R., O'Rourke, M.K., 1999. Odor sensitivity and respiratory compaint profiles in a community-based sample with asthma, hay fever, and chemical odor intolerance. Toxicol. Ind. Health 15, 403–409.

Ball, J.C., Foxall-Van Aken, S., Jensen, T.E., 1984. Mutagenicity studies of p-substituted benzyl derivatives in the Ames Salmonella plate-incorporation assay. Mutat. Res. 138, 145–151.

Ballabeni, V., Tognolini, M., Chiavarini, M., et al., 2004. Novel antiplatelet and antithrombotic activities of essential oil from Lavandula hybrida Reverchon "grosso". Phytomedicine 11, 596–601.

Ballantyne, B., 1994. Acute percutaneous systemic toxicity of cyanides. Journal of Toxicology, Cutaneous & Ocular Toxicology 13, 249–262.

Ballantyne, M., 2002. Bergamottin: reverse mutation in five histidine-requiring strains of Salmonella typhimurium in the presence of ultraviolet light. Final Report. Cited in: SCCNFP 2003a.

Bamosa, A.O., Ali, B.A., al-Hawsawi, Z.A., 2002. The effect of thymoquinone on blood lipids in rats. Indian J. Physiol. Pharmacol. 46, 195–201.

Banerjee, S., Ecavade, A., Rao, A.R., 1993. Modulatory influence of sandalwood oil on mouse hepatic glutathione S-transferase activity and acid soluble sulphydryl level. Cancer Lett. 68, 105–109.

Banerjee, S., Sharma, R., Kale, R.K., et al., 1994. Influence of certain essential oils on carcinogen-metabolizing enzymes and acid-soluble sulfhydryls in mouse liver. Nutr. Cancer 21, 263–269.

Banerjee, S., Welsch, C.W., Rao, A.R., 1995. Modulatory influence of camphor on the activities of hepatic carcinogen metabolizing enzymes and the levels of hepatic and extrahepatic reduced glutathione in mice. Cancer Lett. 88, 163–169.

Banerjee, S., Kaseb, A.O., Wang, Z., et al., 2009. Antitumor activity of gemcitabine and oxaliplatin is augmented by thymoquinone in pancreatic cancer. Cancer Res. 69, 5575–5583.

Bang, J., Mortensen, O.S., Ebbehøj, N., 2008. Poisoning with anise oil. Ugeskr. Laeger 170, 461.

Bang Pedersen, N., Pla Arles, U.B., 1998. Phototoxic reaction to parsnip and UV-A sunbed. Contact Dermatitis 39, 97.

Bär Vn, F., Griepentrog, F., 1967. Die Situation in der gesundheitlichen Beurteilung der Aromatisierungsmittel für Lebensmittel. Medizin und Ernährung 8, 244–251.

Barany, E., Loden, M., 2000. Content of fragrance mix ingredients and customer complaints of cosmetic products. Am. J. Contact Dermat. 11, 74–79.

Barclay Dr., 1866. St. George's Hospital: case of poisoning by essential oil of bitter almonds; death; autopsy. Lancet 87 (2219), 255.

Bardon, S., Foussard, V., Fournel, S., et al., 2002. Monoterpenes inhibit proliferation of human colon cancer cells by modulating cell cycle-related protein expression. Cancer Lett. 181, 187–194.

Barja de Quiroga, G., López-Torres, M., Pérez-Campo, R., 1992. Relationships between antioxidants, lipid peroxidation and aging. In: Emerit, I., Chance, B. (Eds.), Free radicals and aging. Birkhauser Verlag, Basel, pp. 109–124.

Barker, N., Hadgraft, J., Rutter, N., 1987. Skin permeability in the newborn. J. Invest. Dermatol. 88, 409–411.

Barnes, K.C., 2010. An update on the genetics of atopic dermatitis: scratching the surface in 2009. J. Allergy Clin. Immunol. 126, 16–29.

Barnes, P.J., 1992. Neurogenic inflammation and asthma. J. Asthma 29, 165–180.

Barni, B., Barni, I., 1967. La intossicazione da apiolo. I. Rassegna casistica. Zacchia 3 (2), 197–221.

Barocelli, E., Calcina, F., Chiavarini, M., et al., 2004. Antinociceptive and gastroprotective effects of inhaled and orally administered Lavandula hybrida Reverchon "Grosso" essential oil. Life Sci. 76, 213–223.

Baron, J.M., Höller, D., Schiffer, R., et al., 2001. Expression of multiple cytochrome p450 enzymes and multidrug resistance-associated transport proteins in human skin keratinocytes. J. Invest. Dermatol. 116, 541–548.

Barr, D.B., Barr, J.R., Bailey, S.L., et al., 2000. Levels of methyleugenol in a subset of adults in the general U.S. population as determined by high resolution mass spectrometry. Environ. Health Perspect. 108, 323–328.

Barr, D.B., Bishop, A., Needham, L.L., 2007. Concentrations of xenobiotic chemicals in the maternal-fetal unit. Reprod. Toxicol. 23, 260–266.

Baratta, M.T., Dorman, H.J., Deans, S.G., et al., 1998. Antimicrobial and antioxidant properties of some commercial essential oils. Flavour & Fragrance Journal 13, 235–244.

Barrie, S.A., Wright, J.V., Pizzorno, J.E., 1987. Effects of garlic oil on platelet aggregation, serum lipids and blood pressure in humans. Journal of Orthomolecular Medicine 2 (1), 15–21.

Barros, M.A., Baptista, A., Correia, T.M., et al., 1991. Patch testing in children: a study of 562 schoolchildren. Contact Dermatitis 25, 156–159.

Barry, D.H., Chasseaud, L.F., Hunter, B., et al., 1972. The suppression of non-specific esterase activity in mouse skin sebaceous gland by "CS" gas. Nature 240, 560–561.

Bartek, M.J., LaBudde, J.A., Maibach, H.I., 1972. Skin permeability in vivo: comparison in rat, rabbit, pig and man. J. Invest. Dermatol. 58, 114–123.

Barthelman, M., Chen, W., Gensler, H.L., et al., 1998. Inhibitory effects of perillyl alcohol on UVB-induced murine skin cancer and AP-1 transactivation. Cancer Res. 58, 711–716.

Baser, K.H.C., Öztek, T., Tümen, G., et al., 1993. Composition of the essential oils of Turkish Origanum species with commercial importance. Journal of Essential Oil Research 5, 619–623.

Baser, K.H.C., Öztek, T., Kürkçüoglu, M., et al., 1994. The essential oil of Origanum vulgare subsp. hirtum of Turkish origin. Journal of Essential Oil Research 6, 31–36.

Baser, K.H.C., Demirci, B., Dekebo, A., Dagne, E., 2003. Essential oils of some Boswellia spp., myrrh and opopanax. Flavour & Fragrance Journal 18, 153–156.

Basketter, D.A., 1998. Chemistry of contact allergens and irritants. Am. J. Contact Dermat. 9 (2), 119–124.

Basketter, D., 2000. Quenching: fact or fiction? Contact Dermatitis 43, 253–258.

Basketter, D.A., Allenby, C.F., 1991. Studies of the quenching phenomenon in delayed contact hypersensitivity reactions. Contact Dermatitis 25, 160–171.

Basketter, D.A., Wilhelm, K.P., 1996. Studies on non-immune immediate contact reactions in an unselected population. Contact Dermatitis 35, 237–240.

Basketter, D., Dooms-Goossens, A., Karlberg, A.T., et al., 1995. The chemistry of contact allergy: why is a molecule allergenic? Contact Dermatitis 32, 65–73.

Basketter, D.A., Cookman, G., Gerberick, F., et al., 1997. Skin sensitization thresholds: determination in predictive models. Food Chem. Toxicol. 35, 417–425.

Basketter, D.A., Evans, P., Gerbick, G.F., et al., 2002a. Factors affecting thresholds in allergic contact dermatitis: safety and regulatory considerations. Contact Dermatitis 47, 1–6.

Basketter, D.A., Wright, Z.M., Colson, N.R., et al., 2002b. Investigation of the skin sensitizing activity of linalool. Contact Dermatitis 47, 161–164.

Basketter, D.A., York, M., McFadden, J.P., et al., 2004. Determination of skin irritation potential in the human 4-h patch test. Contact Dermatitis 51, 1–4.

Bassett, F., 1994. Journées de Digne. Le jasmin, la fleur le roi. Parfums Cosmétiques Arômes 119, 58–64.

Bassett, I.B., Pannowitz, D.L., Barnetson, R.S., 1990. A comparative study of tea-tree oil versus benzoylperoxide in the treatment of acne. Med. J. Aust. 153, 455–458.

Bassoli, A., Borgonovo, G., Caimi, S., et al., 2009. Taste-guided identification of high potency TRPA1 aginists from Perilla frutescens. Bioorg. Med. Chem. 17, 1636–1639.

Battaglia, S., 1997. The complete guide to aromatherapy. The Perfect Potion, Virginia, Queensland.

Battershill, J.M., Fielder, R.J., 1998. Mouse-specific carcinogens: an assessment of hazard and significance for validation of short-term carcinogenicity bioassays in transgenic mice. Hum. Exp. Toxicol. 17, 193–205.

Baumgart, A., Schmidt, M., Schmitz, H.J., et al., 2005. Natural furocoumarins as inducers and inhibitors of cytochrome P450 1A1 in rat hepatocytes. Biochem. Pharmacol. 69, 657–667.

Baur, X., Schneider, E.M., Wieners, D., et al., 1999. Occupational asthma to perfume. Allergy 54, 1334–1335.

Beamand, J.A., Barton, P.T., Price, R.J., Lake, B.G., 1998. Lack of effect of coumarin on unscheduled DNA synthesis in precision-cut human liver slices. Food Chem. Toxicol. 36, 647–653.

Beattie, K.D., Waterman, P.G., Forster, P.I., et al., 2011. Chemical composition and cytotoxicity of oils and eremophilanes derived from various parts of Eremophila mitchellii Benth. Myoporaceae. Phytochemistry 72, 400–408.

Beattie, R.T., 1968. Nutmeg as a psychoactive agent. Br. J. Addict. 63, 105–109.

Bechtel, D., Henderson, L., Proudlock, R., 1998. Lack of UDS activity in the livers of rats exposed to allyl isothiocyanate. Teratog. Carcinog. Mutagen. 18, 209–217.

Becker, K., Temesvari, E., Nemeth, I., 1994. Patch testing with fragrance mix and its constituents in a Hungarian population. Contact Dermatitis 30, 185–186.

Beckley-Kartey, S.A., Hotchkiss, S.A., Capel, M., 1997. Comparative in vitro skin absorption and metabolism of coumarin (1,2-benzopyrone) in human, rat and mouse. Toxicol. Appl. Pharmacol. 145, 34–42.

Bedford, P.G., Clarke, E.G., 1972. Experimental benzoic acid poisoning in the cat. Vet. Rec. 90, 53–58.

Behra, O., Rakotoarison, C., Harris, R., 2001. Ravintsara vs ravensara, a taxonomic classification. The International Journal of Aromatherapy 11, 4–7.

Belaiche, P., 1979. Traité de phytothérapie et d'aromathérapie. II. Les maladies infectieuses. Maloine S. A, Editeur, Paris.

Belanger, A., 1989. Residues of azinphos-methyl, cypermethrin, benomyl and chlorothalonil in monarda and peppermint oil. Acta Horticulturae 249, 67–73.

Bell, G.D., Doran, J., 1979. Gall stone dissolution in man using an essential oil preparation. Br. Med. J. 1, 24.

Bell, A.J., Duggin, G., 2002. Acute methyl salicylate toxicity complicating herbal skin treatment for psoriasis. Emerg. Med. (Fremantle) 14, 188–190.

Bell, G.D., Henry, D.A., Langman, M.J., et al., 1981. Glucuronidation of l-menthol in normal individuals and patients with liver disease. Br. J. Clin. Pharmacol. 12, 272–273.

Bell, I.R., Schwartz, G.E., Peterson, J.M., Amend, D., 1993. Self-reported illness from chemical odors in young adults without clinical syndromes or occupational exposures. Arch. Environ. Health 48, 6–13.

Bell, I.R., Schwartz, G.E., Baldwin, C.M., et al., 1997. Individual differences in neural sensitization and the role of context in illness from low-level environmental chemical exposures. Environ. Health Perspect. 105 (Suppl. 2), 457–466.

Bellman, M.H., 1973. Camphor poisoning in children. Br. Med. J. 2, 177.

Belloir, C., Singh, V., Daurat, C., et al., 2006. Protective effects of garlic sulfur compounds against DNA damage induced by direct- and indirect-acting genotoxic agents in HepG2 cells. Food Chem. Toxicol. 44, 827–834.

Belman, S., 1983. Onion and garlic oil inhibit tumour promotion. Carcinogenesis 4, 1063–1065.

Belova, L.F., Alibekov, S.D., Baginskaia, A.I., et al., 1985. Asarone and its biological properties. Farmakol. Toksikol. 48, 17–20.

Belsito, D.V., 1997. The rise and fall of allergic contact dermatitis. Am. J. Contact Dermat. 8, 193–201.

Belsito, D.V., Fowler, J.F., Sasseville, D., et al., 2006. Delayed-type hypersensitivity to fragrance materials in a select North American population. Dermatitis 17, 23–28.

Belsito, D., Bickers, D., Bruze, M., et al., 2007. A toxicologic and dermatologic assessment of related esters and alcohols of cinnamic acid and cinnamyl alcohol when used as fragrance ingredients. Food Chem. Toxicol. 45, S1–S23.

Belsito, D., Bickers, D., Bruze, M., et al., 2008. A toxicologic and dermatologic assessment of cylic and non-cyclic terpene alcohols when used as fragrance ingredients. Food Chem. Toxicol. 46, S1–S71.

Benda, G.I., Hiller, J.L., Reynolds, J.W., 1986. Benzyl alcohol toxicity: impact on neurologic handicaps among surviving very low weight birth infants. Pediatrics 77, 507–512.

Benedetti, M.S., Malnoe, A., Broillet, A.L., 1977. Absorption, metabolism and excretion of safrole in the rat and man. Toxicology 7, 69–83.

Bener, A., Abdulrazzaq, Y.M., Al-Mutawwa, J., et al., 1996. Genetic and environmental factors associated with asthma. Hum. Biol. 68, 405–414.

Bendaoud, H., Romdhane, M., Souchard, J.P., et al., 2010. Chemical composition and anticancer and antioxidant activities of Schinus molle L. and Schinus terebinthifolius Raddi berries essential oils. Journal of Food Science 75, C466–C472.

Benezra, C., 1990. Molecular recognition in allergic contact dermatitis to natural products. Pure Appl. Chem. 62, 1251–1258.

Benezra, C., Epstein, W.L., 1986. Molecular recognition patterns of sesquiterpene lactones in costus-sensitive patients. Contact Dermatitis 15, 223–230.

Benezra, C., Schlewer, G., Stampf, J.L., 1978. Lactones allergisantes naturelles et synthetiques. Rev. Fr. Allergol. 18, 31–33.

Benezra, C., Stampf, J.L., Barbier, P., et al., 1985. Enantiospecificity in allergic contact dermatitis. A review and new results in Frullania-sensitive patients. Contact Dermatitis 13, 110–114.

Benfeldt, E., Serup, J., Menné, T., 1999. Effect of barrier perturbation on cutaneous salicylic acid penetration in human skin: in vivo pharmacokinetics using microdialysis and non-invasive quantification of barrier function. Br. J. Dermatol. 140, 739–748.

Benham, F.L., 1905. Two cases of acute poisoning by oil of eucalyptus. Lancet 166 (4296), 1894.

Bénichou, C., 1990. Criteria of drug-induced liver disorders: report of an international consensus meeting. J. Hepatol. 11, 272–276.

Benjamin, J., 1906. Eucalyptus poisoning. Br. Med. J. 1, 1020.

Benjilali, B., Hammoumi, M., Richard, H., 1987. Polymorphisme chimique des huiles essentielles de thym de Maroc. Sci. Aliment 7, 77–91.

Benke, D., Barberis, A., Kopp, S., et al., 2009. GABA$_A$ receptors as in vivo substrate for the anxiolytic action of valerenic acid, a major constituent of valerian root extracts. Neuropharmacology 56, 174–181.

Benveniste, B., Azzo, N., 1992a. Geranium oil. Technical Bulletin & Newsletter, vol. II, July 1, Kato Worldwide Ltd, Mount Vernon, NY.

Berardesca, E., Fideli, D., Borroni, G., et al., 1990. In vivo hydration and water-retention capacity of stratum corneum in clinically uninvolved skin in atopic and psoriatic patients. Acta Derm. Venereol. 70, 400–404.

Berardesca, E., Fluhr, J.W., Maibach, H.I., 2006. Sensitive skin syndrome. Informa Health Care, London.

Berenbaum, M.R., Zangerl, A.R., Nitao, J.K., 1984. Furanocoumarins in seed of wild and cultivated parsnip. Phytochemistry 23, 1809–1810.

Berić, T., Nikolić, B., Stanojević, J., et al., 2007. Protective effect of basil (Ocimum basilicum L.) against oxidative DNA damage and mutagenesis. Food Chem. Toxicol. 46, 724–732.

Berggren, L., 1957. Lack of effect of citral on ocular tension. Acta Opthalmologica 35, 451–453.

Berkow, R., Fletcher, A.J., 1992. The Merck Manual. Merck Research Laboratories, Rahway N.J.

Berliocchi, L., Ciociaro, A., Russo, R., et al., 2011. Toxic profile of bergamot essential oil on survival and proliferation of SH-SY5Y neuroblastoma cells. Food Chem. Toxicol. 49, 2780–2792.

Bernard, G., Giménez-Arnau, E., Rastogi, S.C., 2003. Contact allergy to oak moss: search for sensitizing molecules using combined bioassay-guided chemical fractionation, GC-MS, and structure-activity relationship analysis. Arch. Dermatol. Res. 295, 229–235.

Berne, B., Tammela, M., Férm, G., et al., 2008. Can the reporting of adverse skin reactions to cosmetics be improved? A prospective clinical study using a structured protocol. Contact Dermatitis 58, 223–227.

Bernson, V.S., Pettersson, B., 1983. The toxicity of menthol in short-term bioassays. Chem. Biol. Interact. 46, 233–246.

Bertea, C.M., Azzolin, C.M., Bossi, S., et al., 2005. Identification of an EcoRI restriction site for a rapid and precise determination of beta-asarone-free Acorus calamus cytotypes. Phytochemistry 66, 507–514.

Bertrand, F., Basketter, D.A., Roberts, D.W., et al., 1997. Skin sensitization to eugenol and isoeugenol in mice: possible metabolic pathways involving ortho-quinone and quinone methide intermediates. Chem. Res. Toxicol. 10, 335–343.

Besaratinia, A., Pfeifer, G.P., 2004. Biological consequences of 8-methoxypsoralen-photoinduced lesions: sequence-specificity of mutations and preponderance of T to C and T to A mutations. J. Invest. Dermatol. 123, 1140–1146.

Bessac, B.F., Jordt, S.E., 2008. Breathtaking TRP channels: TRPA1 and TRPV1 in airway chemosensation and reflex control. Physiology 23, 360–370.

Bestmann, H.J., Classen, B., Kobold, U., et al., 1984. Pfanzliche Insektizide II (1.) Das ätherische Öle aus Blätteren des Balsamkrautes, Chrysanthemum balsamita L. Insektizide Wirkung und Zusammensetzung. Z. Naturforsch. 39C, 543–547.

Beyer, J., Ehlers, D., Maurer, H.H., 2006. Abuse of nutmeg (Myristica fragrans Houtt.): studies on the metabolism and the toxicologic detection of its ingredients elemicin, myristicin, and safrole in rat and human urine using gas chromatography/mass spectrometry. Ther. Drug Monit. 28, 568–575.

Bezard, M., Karlberg, A.T., Montelius, J., et al., 1997. Skin sensitization to linalyl hydroperoxide: support for radical intermediates. Chem. Res. Toxicol. 10, 987–993.

Bezerra, D.P., Marinho Filho, J.D., Alves, A.P., et al., 2009. Antitumor activity of the essential oil from the leaves of Croton regelianus and its component ascaridole. Chem. Biodivers. 6, 1224–1231.

Bhargava, A.K., Ali, S.M., Chauhan, C.S., 1967. Pharmacological investigation of the essential oil of Daucus carota. Indian J. Pharm. 28, 127–129.

Bhatia, S.P., Wellington, G.A., Cocchiaria, J., et al., 2007a. Fragrance material review on cinnamyl acetate. Food Chem. Toxicol. 45, S53–S57.

Bhatia, S.P., Wellington, G.A., Cocchiaria, J., et al., 2007b. Fragrance material review on methyl cinnamate. Food Chem. Toxicol. 46, S113–S119.

Bhatia, S.P., McGinty, D., Letizia, C.S., et al., 2008a. Fragrance material review on p-mentha-1,8-dien-7-ol. Food Chem. Toxicol. 46, S197–S200.

Bhatia, S.P., McGinty, D., Letizia, C.S., et al., 2008b. Fragrance material review on santalol. Food Chem. Toxicol. 46, S263–S266.

Bhatia, S.P., McGinty, D., Letizia, C.S., et al., 2008c. Fragrance material review on cedrol. Food Chem. Toxicol. 46, S100–S102.

Bhatia, S.P., McGinty, D., Letizia, C.S., et al., 2008d. Fragrance material review on α-santalol. Food Chem. Toxicol. 46, S267–S269.

Bhatia, S.P., McGinty, D., Letizia, C.S., et al., 2008e. Fragrance material review on isopulegol. Food Chem. Toxicol. 46, S185–S189.

Bhatia, S.P., McGinty, D., Letizia, C.S., et al., 2008f. Fragrance material review on l-borneol. Food Chem. Toxicol. 46, S81–S84.

Bhatia, S.P., McGinty, D., Letizia, C.S., et al., 2008g. Fragrance material review on menthol. Food Chem. Toxicol. 46, S209–S214.

Bhatia, S.P., McGinty, D., Letizia, C.S., et al., 2008h. Fragrance material review on sclareol. Food Chem. Toxicol. 46, S270–S274.

BHMA Scientific Committee, 1983. British herbal pharmacopoeia. British Herbal Medicine Association, Bournemouth.

Bhide, S.V., Shivapurkar, N.M., Gothoskar, S.V., et al., 1979. Carcinogenicity of betel quid ingredients: feeding mice with aqueous extract and the polyphenol fraction of betel nut. Br. J. Cancer 40, 922–926.

Bhide, S.V., Zariwala, M.B., Amonkar, A.J., et al., 1991a. Chemopreventive efficacy of a betel leaf extract against benzo[a]pyrene-induced forestomach tumors in mice. J. Ethnophamacol. 34, 207–213.

Bhide, S.V., Padma, P.R., Amonkar, A.J., 1991b. Antimutagenic and anticarcinogenic effects of betel leaf extract against the tobacco-specific nitrosamine 4-(N-nitrosomethylamino)-1-(3-pyridyl)-1-butanone (NNK). IARC Sci. Publ. 105, 520–524.

Bhide, S.V., Azuine, M.A., Lahiri, M., et al., 1994. Chemoprevention of mammary tumor virus-induced and chemical carcinogen-induced rodent mammary tumors by natural plant products. Breast Cancer Res. Treat. 30, 233–242.

Bhuiyan, N.I., Begum, J., Bhuiyan, N.H., 2009. Analysis of essential oil of eaglewood tree (Aquilaria agallocha Roxb.) by gas chromatography mass spectrometry. Bangladesh Journal of Pharmacology 4, 24–28.

Bhushan, M., Beck, M.H., 1997. Allergic contact dermatitis from tea tree oil in a wart paint. Contact Dermatitis 36, 117–118.

Bianchini, A., et al., 2001. Composition of Helichrysum italicum (Roth) G. Don fil. subsp. italicum essential oils from Corsica (France). Flavour & Fragrance Journal 16, 30–34.

Bicas, J.L., Neri-Numa, I.A., Ruiz, A.L., et al., 2011. Evaluation of the antioxidant and antiproliferative potential of bioflavors. Food Chem. Toxicol. 49, 1610–1615.

Bicchi, C., Fresia, M., Rubiolo, P., et al., 1997. Constituents of Tagetes lucida Cav. ssp. lucida essential oil. Flavour & Fragrance Journal 12, 47–52.

Bicchi, C., Rubiolo, P., Camargo, E.E.S., et al., 2003. Components of Turnera diffusa Willd. var. afrodisiaca (Ward) Urb. essential oil. Flavour & Fragrance Journal 18, 59–61.

Bickers, D.R., Miller, L., Kappas, A., 1975. Exacerbation of hereditary hepatic porphyria by surreptitious ingestion of an unusual provacative agent - a mouthwash preparation. N. Engl. J. Med. 292, 1115–1116.

Bickers, D., Calow, P., Greim, H., et al., 2003a. The safety assessment of fragrance materials. Regul. Toxicol. Pharmacol. 37, 218–273.

Bickers, D., Calow, P., Greim, H., et al., 2003b. A toxicologic and dermatologic assessment of linalool and related esters when used as fragrance ingredients. Food Chem. Toxicol. 41, 919–942.

Bidinotto, L.T., Costa, C.A., Salvadori, D.M., et al., 2010. Protective effects of lemongrass (Cymbopogon citratus STAPF) essential oil on DNA damage and carcinogenesis in female Balb/C mice. J. Appl. Toxicol doi: 10.1002/jat.1593.

Bidinotto, L.T., Costa, C.A., Costa, M., et al., 2012. Modifying effects of lemongrass essential oil on specific tissue response to the carcinogen N-methyl-N-nitrosurea in female BALB/c mice. J. Med. Food 15, 161–168.

Bignell, C.M., Dunlop, P.J., Brophy, J.J., 1998. Volatile leaf oils of some South-Western and Southern Australian species of the genus Eucalyptus (series 1) Part XIX. Flavour & Fragrance Journal 13, 131–139.

Biju, S.S., Ahuja, A., Khar, R.K., 2005. Tea tree oil concentration in follicular casts after topical delivery: determination by high-performance thin layer chromatography using a perfused bovine udder model. J. Pharm. Sci. 94, 240–245.

Bilia, A.R., Flamini, G., Taglioli, V., et al., 2002. GC-MS analysis of essential oil of some commercial Fennel teas. Food Chem. 76, 307–310.

Bilsland, D., Strong, A., 1990. Allergic contact dermatitis from the essential oil of French marigold (Tagetes patula) in an aromatherapist. Contact Dermatitis 23, 55–56.

Bischoff, K., Guale, F., 1998. Australian tea tree (Melaleuca alternifolia) oil poisoning in three purebred cats. J. Vet. Diagn. Invest. 10, 208–210.

Bissonnette, L., Arnason, J.T., Smith, M.L., 2008. Real-time fluorescence-based detection of furanocoumarin photoadducts of DNA. Photochemical Analysis 19, 342–347.

Biswas, R., Mandal, S.K., Dutta, S., et al., 2011. Thujone-rich fraction of Thuja occidentalis demonstrates major anti-cancer potentials: evidences

from in vitro studies on A375 cells. Evidence-Based Complementary & Alternative Medicine. http://www.ncbi.nlm.nih.gov/pmc/articles/PMC3106972.

Björnstad, K., Helander, A., Hultén, P., et al., 2009. Bioanalytical investigation of asarone in connection with Acorus calamus oil intoxications. J. Anal. Toxicol. 33, 604–609.

Black, H.S., Young, A.R., Gibbs, N.K., 1989. Effects of butylated hydroxytoluene upon PUVA-tumorigenesis and induction of ornithine decarboxylase activity in the mouse. J. Photochem. Photobiol. B. 3, 910–9100.

Blackmon, W.P., Curry, H.B., 1957. Camphor poisoning - report of a case occurring during pregnancy. J. Fla. Med. Assoc. 43 (10), 999–1000.

Blackwell, A.L., 1991. Tea tree oil and anaerobic (bacterial) vaginosis. Lancet 337, 300.

Blackwell, B., Mabbitt, L.A., 1965. Tyramine in cheese related to hypertensive crises after monoamine-oxidase inhibition. Lancet 1 (7392), 938–940.

Blair, R.M., Fang, H., Branham, W.S., et al., 2000. The estrogen receptor relative binding affinities of 188 natural and xenochemicals: structural diversity of ligands. Toxicol. Sci. 54, 138–153.

Blanchard, D.L., 1989. Sting Eze keratitis. Arch. Ophthal. 107, 791.

Blanco, M.M., Costa, C.A., Freire, A.O., et al., 2009. Neurobehavioral effect of essential oil of Cymbopogon citratus in mice. Phytomedicine 16, 265–270.

Blau, J.N., Solomon, F., 1985. Smell and other sensory disturbances in migraine. J. Neurol. 232, 275–276.

Bleasel, N., Tate, B., Rademaker, M., 2002. Allergic contact dermatitis following exposure to essential oils. Australas. J. Dermatol. 43, 211–213.

Bliss, J.A., Glass, H.B., 1940. A chemical and pharmacological comparison of the menthols. Pharmaceutical Abstracts 6, 171–175.

Blondeel, A., Oleffe, J., Achten, G., 1978. Contact allergy in 330 dermatological patients. Contact Dermatitis 4, 270–276.

Blumenthal, M., Busse, W.R., Goldberg, A., et al., 1998. The complete German Commission E monographs: therapeutic guide to herbal medicines. American Botanical Council, Austin, Texas.

Blumenthal, M., Goldberg, A., Brinckmann, J., 2000. Herbal medicine, expanded commission E monographs. Integrative Medicine Communications, Newton, MA.

Boberg, E.W., Miller, E.C., Miller, J.A., et al., 1983. Strong evidence from studies with brachymorphic mice and pentachlorophenol that 1′-sulfooxysafrole is the major ultimate electrophilic and carcinogenic metabolite of 1′-hydroxysafrole in mouse liver. Cancer Res. 43, 5163–5173.

Boberg, E.W., Liem, A., Miller, E.C., et al., 1987. Inhibition by pentachlorophenol of the initiating and promoting activities of 1′-hydroxysafrole for the formation of enzyme-altered foci and tumors in rat liver. Carcinogenesis 8, 531–539.

Bocca, C., Gabriel, L., Bozzo, F., 2004. A sesquiterpene lactone, costunolide, interacts with microtubule protein and inhibits the growth of MCF-7 cells. Chem. Biol. Interact. 147, 79–86.

Bodake, H.B., Panicker, K.N., Kailaje, V.V., et al., 2002. Chemopreventive effect of orange oil on the development of hepatic preneoplastic lesions induced by N-nitrosodiethylamine in rats: an ultrastructural study. Indian J. Exp. Biol. 40, 245–251.

Bode, C.W., Hansel, W., 2005. 5-(3-Phenylpropoxy)psoralen and 5-(4-phenylbutoxy)psoralen: mechanistic studies on phototoxicity. Pharmazie 60, 225–228.

Bode, C.W., Zager, A., Hansel, W., 2005. Photodynamic and photo-cross-linking potential of bergamottin. Pharmazie 60, 78–79.

Boelens, M., et al., 1971. Volatile flavour compounds from onion. J. Agric. Food Chem. 19, 984–991.

Boelens, M.H., 1985. The essential oils from Rosmarinus officinalis L. Perfumer & Flavorist 10, 21–37.

Boelens, M.H., 1994. Sensory and chemical evaluation of tropical grass oils. Perfumer & Flavorist 19, 29–45.

Boelens, M.H., Boelens, H., 1997. Differences in chemical and sensory properties of orange flower and rose oils obtained from hydrodistillation and from supercritical CO_2 extraction. Perfumer & Flavorist 22, 31–35.

Boissier, J.R., Simon, P., Le Bourhis, B., 1967. Action psychotrope expérimentale des anétholes isomères cis et trans. Therapie 22, 309–323.

Bollard, M., Stribbling, S., Mitchell, S., et al., 1997. The disposition of allyl isothiocyanate in the rat and mouse. Food Chem. Toxicol. 35, 933–943.

Bolton, J.L., Acay, N.M., Vukomanovic, V., 1994. Evidence that 4-allyl-o-quinones spontaneously rearrange to their more electrophilic quinone methides: potential bioactivation mechanism for the hepatocarcinogen safrole. Chem. Res. Toxicol. 7, 443–450.

Bommareddy, A., Hora, J., Cornish, B., et al., 2007. Chemoprevention by α-santalol on UVB radiation-induced skin tumor development in mice. Anticancer Res. 27, 2185–2188.

Bonamonte, D., Mundo, L., Daddabbo, M., et al., 2001. Allergic contact dermatitis from Mentha spicata (spearmint). Contact Dermatitis 45, 298.

Bonkovsky, H.L., Cable, E.E., Cable, J.W., et al., 1992. Porphyrogenic properties of the terpenes camphor, pinene, and thujone (with a note on historic implications for absinthe and the illness of Vincent van Gogh). Biochem. Pharmacol. 43, 2359–2368.

Bonnesen, C., Eggleston, I.M., Hayes, J.D., 2001. Dietary indoles and isothiocyanates that are generated from cruciferous vegetables can both stimulate apoptosis and confer protection against DNA damage in human colon cell lines. Cancer Res. 61, 6120–6130.

Bonneville, M., Chavagnac, C., Vocanson, M., et al., 2007. Skin contact irritation conditions the development and severity of allergic contact dermatitis. J. Invest. Dermatol. 127, 1430–1435.

Boon, P.J., van der Boon, D., Mulder, G.J., 2000. Cytotoxicity and biotransformation of the anticancer drug perillyl alcohol in PC12 cells and in the rat. Toxicol. Appl. Pharmacol. 167, 55–62.

Boonchai, W., Iamtharachai, P., Sunthonpalin, P., 2007. Occupational allergic contact dermatitis from essential oils in aromatherapists. Contact Dermatitis 56, 181–182.

Booth, A.N., Masri, M.S., Robbins, D.J., et al., 1959. Urinary metabolites of coumarin and o-coumaric acid. J. Biol. Chem. 234, 946–948.

Borchert, P., Wislocki, P.G., Miller, J.A., et al., 1973a. The metabolism of the naturally occurring hepatocarcinogen safrole to l-hydroxysafrole and the electrophilic reactivity of l-acetoxysafrole. Cancer Res. 33, 575–589.

Borchert, P., Miller, J.A., Miller, E.C., et al., 1973b. 1´-hydroxysafrole, a proximate carcinogenic metabolite of safrole in rat and mouse. Cancer Res. 33, 590–600.

Bordia, A., 1978. Effect of garlic on human platelet aggregation in vitro. Atherosclerosis 30, 355–360.

Bordia, A., Verma, S.K., Srivastava, K.C., 1998. Effect of garlic (Allium sativum) on blood lipids, blood sugar, fibrinogen and fibrinolytic activity in patients with coronary artery disease. Prostaglandins Leukot Essent Fatty Acids 58, 257–263.

Borghoff, S.J., Birnbaum, L.S., 1986. Age-related changes in the metabolism and excretion of allyl isothiocyanate. A model compound for glutathione conjugation. Drug Metab. Dispos. 14, 417–422.

Born, D., Barron, M.L., 2005. Herb use in pregnancy: what nurses should know. MCN Am. J. Matern. Child Nurs. 30, 201–206.

Born, S.L., Caudill, D., Smith, B.J., et al., 2000a. In vitro kinetics of coumarin 3,4-epoxidation: application to species differences in toxicity and carcinogenicity. Toxicol. Sci. 58, 23–31.

Born, S.L., Hu, J.K., Lehman-McKeeman, L.D., 2000b. o-Hydroxyphentlacetaldehyde is a hepatotoxic metabolite of coumarin. Drug Metab. Dispos. 28, 218–223.

Born, S.L., Caudill, D., Fliter, K.L., et al., 2002. Identification of the cytochromes P450 that catalyze coumarin 3,4-epoxidation and 3-hydroxylation. Drug Metab. Dispos. 30, 483–487.

Bosch, F.X., Ribes, J., Diaz, M., et al., 2004. Primary liver cancer: worldwide incidence and trends. Gastroenterology 127, S5–S16.

Boskabady, M.H., Jandaghi, P., 2003. Relaxant effects of carvacrol on guinea pig tracheal chains and its possible mechanisms. Pharmazie 58, 661–663.

Boskabady, M.H., Ramazani-Assari, M., 2001. Relaxant effect of Pimpinella anisum on isolated guinea pig tracheal chains and its possible mechanism (s). J. Ethnopharmacol. 74, 83–88.

Boskabady, M.H., Shaikhi, J., 2000. Inhibitory effect of Carum copticum on histamine (H1) receptors of isolated guinea-pig tracheal chains. J. Ethnopharmacol. 69, 217–227.

Boskabady, M.H., Khatami, A., Nazari, A., 2004. Possible mechanism(s) for relaxant effects of Foeniculum vulgare on guinea pig tracheal chains. Pharmazie 59, 561–564.

Boskabady, M.H., Kiani, S., Rakhshandah, H., 2006. Relaxant effects of Rosa damascena on guinea pig tracheal chains and its possible mechanism (s). J. Ethnopharmacol. 106, 377–382.

Botham, P.A., 2004a. The validation of in vitro methods for skin irritation. Toxicol. Lett. 149, 387–390.

Botham, P.A., 2004b. Acute systemic toxicity – prospects for tiered testing strategies. Toxicology In Vitro 18, 227–230.

Botma, M., Colquhoun-Flannery, W., Leighton, S., 2001. Laryngeal oedema caused by accidental ingestion of oil of wintergreen. International Journal of Pediatrics & Otorhinolaryngology 58, 229–232.

Bottone, F.G., Baek, S.J., Nixon, J.B., Eling, T.E., 2002. Diallyl disulfide (DADS) induces the antitumorigenic NSAID-activate gene (NAG-1) by a p53-dependent mechanism in human colorectal HCT 116 cells. J. Nutr. 132, 773–778.

Bouhlal, K., Meynadier, J.M., Peyron, J.L., et al., 1988a. Le cade en dermatologie. Parfums, Cosmetiques, Aromes 83, 73–82.

Bouhlal, K., Meynadier, J., Peyron, J.L., et al., 1988b. The cutaneous effects of the common concretes and absolutes used in the perfume industry. In: Lawrence, B.M. (Ed.), 2005. The antimicrobial/biological activity of essential oils. Allured, Carol Stream, Illinois, pp. 10–23.

Boukhman, M.P., Maibach, H.I., 2001. Thresholds in contact sensitisation: immunologic mechanisms and experimental evidence in humans – an overview. Food Chem. Toxicol. 39, 1125–1134.

Boukhris, M., Bouaziz, M., Feki, I., et al., 2012. Hypoglycemic and antioxidant effects of leaf essential oil of Pelargonium graveolens L'Her. in alloxan induced diabetic rats. Lipids Health Dis. 11, 81.

Boullin, D.J., 1981. Garlic as a platelet inhibitor. Lancet 1 (4 April), 776–777.

Bounds, S.V., Caldwell, J., 1996. Pathways of metabolism of [1'-14C]-trans-anethole in the rat and mouse. Drug Metab. Dispos. 24, 717–724.

Bourrel, C., Perineau, F., Michel, G., Bessiere, J.M., 1993a. Catnip (Nepeta cataria L.) essential oil: analysis of chemical constituents, bacteriostatic and fungistatic properties. Journal of Essential Oil Research 5, 159–167.

Bourrel, C., Vilarem, G., Perineau, F., 1993b. Chemical analysis, bacteriostatic and fungistatic properties of the essential oil of elecampane (Inula helenium L.). Journal of Essential Oil Research 5, 411–417.

Bourrel, C., Vilarem, G., Michel, G., et al., 1995. Etude des propriétés bacteriostatiques et fongistatiques en milieu solide de 24 huiles essentielles préamblement analysées. Rivista Italiana EPPOS 16, 3–12.

Boutwell, R.K., Bosch, D.K., 1959. The tumor promoting action of phenol and related compounds for mouse skin. Cancer Res. 19, 413.

Bowman, W.C., Rand, M.J., 1980. Textbook of pharmacology, second ed. Blackwell Scientific Publications, Oxford.

Bowman, W.C., Rand, M.J., 1982. Textbook of pharmacology, second ed. Blackwell Scientific Publications, Oxford (Chapter 40).

Boyer, C.S., Petersen, D.R., 1991. The metabolism of 3,7-dimethyl-2,6-octadienal (citral) in rat hepatic mitochondrial and cytosolic fractions. Interactions with aldehyde and alcohol dehydrogenases. Drug Metab. Dispos. 19, 81–86.

Boyland, E., 1940. Experiments on the chemotherapy of cancer. Further experiments with aldehydes and their derivatives. Biochem. J. 34, 1196–1201.

Boyland, E., Mawson, E.H., 1938. Experiments on the chemotherapy of cancer. II. The effect of aldehydes and glucosides. Biochem. J. 32, 1982–1987.

Boyland, E., Chasseaud, L.F., 1970. The effect of some carbonyl compounds on rat liver glutathione levels. Biochem. Pharmacol. 19, 1526–1528.

Bozin, B., Mimica-Dukic, N., Simin, N., et al., 2006. Characterization of the volatile composition of essential oils of some lamiaceae spices and the antimicrobial and antioxidant activities of the entire oils. J. Agric. Food Chem. 54, 1822–1828.

Bozin, B., Mimica-Dukic, N., Samojlik, I., Jovin, E., 2007. Antimicrobial and antioxidant properties of rosemary and sage (Rosmarinus officinalis L. and Salvia officinalis L., Lamiaceae) essential oils. J. Agric. Food Chem. 55, 7879–7885.

Bradley, P.R. (Ed.), 1992. British herbal compendium. British Herbal Medicine Association, Bournemouth.

Bradley, B.F., Brown, S.L., Chu, S., et al., 2009. Effects of orally administered lavender essential oil on responses to anxiety-provoking film clips. Hum. Psychopharmacol. 24, 319–330.

Braga, P.C., Dal Sasso, M., Culici, M., et al., 2005. Antioxidant potential of thymol determined by chemiluminescence inhibition in human neutrophils and cell-free systems. Pharmacology 76, 61–68.

Braithwaite, P.F., 1906. A case of poisoning by pennyroyal: recovery. Br. Med. J. 2, 865.

Brand, R.M., Jendrzejewski, J.L., 2008. Chronic ethanol ingestion alters xenobiotic absorption through the skin: potential role of oxidative stress. Food Chem. Toxicol. 46, 1940–1948.

Brand, C., Townley, S.L., Finlay-Jones, J.J., et al., 2002a. Tea tree oil reduces histamine-induced oedema in murine ears. Inflamm. Res. 51, 283–289.

Brand, C., Grimbaldeston, M.A., Gamble, J.R., et al., 2002b. Tea tree oil reduces the swelling associated with the efferent phase of a contact hypersensitivity response. Inflamm. Res. 51, 236–244.

Brandão, F.M., 1986. Occupational allergy to lavender oil. Contact Dermatitis 15, 249–250.

Brandenberger, A.W., Tee, M.K., Lee, J.Y., et al., 1997. Tissue distribution of estrogen receptors alpha (ER-alpha) and beta (ER-beta) mRNA in the midgestational human fetus. J. Clin. Endocrinol. Metab. 82, 3509–3512.

Brasch, J., Schnuch, A., Uter, W., et al., 2006. Strong allergic patch test reactions may indicate a general disposition for contact allergy. Allergy 61, 364–369.

Brenner, N., Frank, O.S., Knight, E., 1993. Chronic nutmeg psychosis. J. R. Soc. Med. 86, 179–180.

Brent, R.L., 2004. Utilization of animal studies to determine the effects and human risks of environmental toxicants (drugs, chemicals, and physical agents). Pediatrics 113 (Suppl.), 984–995.

Breuninger, H., Hildmann, A., Hildmann, H., 1970. Nasal application of volatile oils in infants and small children. Z. Laryngol. Rhinol. Otol. 40, 800–804.

Briganti, S., Picardo, M., 2003. Antioxidant activity, lipid peroxidation and skin diseases. What's new. J. Eur. Acad. Dermatol. Venereol. 17, 663–669.

Briggs, C.J., McLaughlin, L.D., 1974. Low-temperature thin-layer chromatograph for detection of polybutene contamination in volatile oils. J. Chromatogr. 101, 403–407.

Briggs, G.G., Freeman, R.K., Yaffe, S. (Eds.), 1998. Drugs in pregnancy and lactation: a reference guide to fetal and neonatal risk. fifth ed. Williams & Wilkins, Baltimore, pp. 577–578, 627–628.

Brock, M.P., McCarron, M.M., Mueller, J.A., 1989. Pine oil cleaner ingestion. Ann. Emerg. Med. 18, 391–395.

Broeckx, W., Blondeel, A., Dooms-Goossens, A., et al., 1987. Cosmetic Intolerance. Contact Dermatitis 16, 189–194.

Bronaugh, R.L., Stewart, R.F., Wester, R.C., et al., 1985. Comparison of percutaneous absorption of fragrances by humans and monkeys. Food Chem. Toxicol. 23, 111–114.

Bronaugh, R.L., Wester, R.C., Bucks, D., et al., 1990. In vivo percutaneous absorption of fragrance ingredients in rhesus monkeys and humans. Food Chem. Toxicol. 28, 369–373.

Broneck, W., Blondeel, A., Dooms-Goossens, A., et al., 1987. Cosmetic intolerance. Contact Dermatitis 16, 189–194.

Bronstein, A.C., Spyker, D.A., Cantilena, L.R., et al., 2007. 2006 Annual report of the American Association of Poison Control Centers National Poison Data System (NPDS). Clin. Toxicol. 45, 815–917.

Brophy, J.J., Davies, N.W., Southwell, I.A., et al., 1989. Gas chromatographic quality control for oil of Melaleuca terpinen-4-ol type (Australian tea tree). Journal of Agricultural & Food Chemistry 37, 1330–1335.

Brophy, J.J., Goldsack, R.J., Fookes, C.J.R., et al., 1995. Leaf oils of the genus Backhousia (Myrtaceae). Journal of Essential Oil Research 7, 237–254.

Brophy, J.J., Goldsack, R.J., Punruckvong, A., et al., 2000. Leaf essential oils of the genus Leptospermum (Myrtaceae) in Eastern Australia. Part 7. Leptospermum petersonii, L. liversidgei and allies. Flavour & Fragrance Journal 15, 342–351.

Brown, E.W., Scott, W.O., 1934. The absorption of methyl salicylate by the human skin. J. Pharmacol. Exp. Ther. 50, 32–50.

Brown, W.J., Buist, N.R., Gipson, H.T., et al., 1982. Fatal benzyl alcohol poisoning in a neonatal intensive care unit. Lancet 1, 1250.

Bruggeman, I.M., Temmink, J.H., van Bladeren, P.J., 1986. Glutathione- and cysteine-mediated cytotoxicity of allyl and benzyl isothiocyanate. Toxicol. Appl. Pharmacol. 83, 349–359.

Brun, R., 1982. Evolution of contact dermatitis factors in a population. Epidemiology 1975–1981. Dermatologica 165, 24–29.

Brunke, E.J., Hammerschmidt, F.J., Schmaus, G., 1992. Die Headspace-Analyse von Bluetendüften. Dragoco report 1/1992, 3–31.

Bruns, K., 1978. Ein Beitrag zur Untersuchung und Qualitätsbewertung von Patchouliöl. Parfümerie Kosmetik 59, 109–115.

Bruns, K., Meiertoberens, M., 1987. Volatile constituents of Pteronia incana (Compositae). Flavour & Fragrance Journal 2, 157–162.

Bruns, K., Heinrich, E., Pagel, I., 1981. Citronellaöl: Untersuchung von Handels- und Hybridölen Verschiedener Provinienz. In: Kubeczka, Vorkommen und Analytik ätherischer Öle, Band 2. Thieme Verlag, Stuttgart.

Bruns, K., Dolhaine, H., Weber, U., 1982. Über die Zusammensetzung des ätherischen Öls aus Atracylodes Lancea DC (Compositae). Parfümerie und Kosmetik 63, 237–239.

Bruynzeel, D.P., Maibach, H.I., 1986. Excited skin syndrome (angry back). AMA Arch. Derm. 122, 323–328.

Bruynzeel, D.P., van den Hoogenband, H.M., Koedijk, F., 1984. Purpuric vasculitis-like eruption in a patient sensitive to balsam of Peru. Contact Dermatitis 11, 207–209.

Bruynzeel, I., Bergman, W., Hartevelt, H.M., et al., 1991. 'High single-dose' European PUVA regimen also causes an excess of non-melanoma skin cancer. Br. J. Dermatol. 124, 49–55.

Buccellato, F., 1980. An anatomy of rose. Perfumer & Flavorist 5, 29–32.

Buccellato, F., 1982. Ylang survey. Perfumer & Flavorist 7, 9–12.

Buchbauer, G., Jirovetz, L., Jäger, W., et al., 1991. Aromatherapy: evidence for sedative effects of the essential oil of lavender after inhalation. Z. Naturforsch. 46C, 1067–1072.

Buchbauer, G., Jäger, W., Jirovetz, L., et al., 1992a. Effects of valerian root oil, borneol, isoborneol, bornyl acetate and isobornyl acetate on the motility of laboratory animals (mice) after inhalation. Pharmazie 47, 620–622.

Buchbauer, G., Jirovetz, L., Jäger, W., 1992b. Passiflora and lime-blossoms: motility effects after inhalation of the essential oils and of some of the main constituents in animal experiment. Arch. Pharm. (Weinheim) 325, 247–248.

Buchbauer, G., Jirovetz, L., Jäger, W., et al., 1993. Fragrance compounds and essential oils with sedative effects upon inhalation. J. Pharm. Sci. 82, 660–664.

Buchbauer, G., Jäger, W., Gruber, A., et al., 2005. R-(+)- and S-(-)-carvone: influence of chirality on locomotion activity in mice. Flavour & Fragrance Journal 20, 686–689.

Buck, D.S., Nidorf, D.M., Addino, J.G., 1994. Comparison of two topical preparations for the treatment of onychomycosis: Melaleuca alternifolia (tea tree) oil and clotrimazole. J. Fam. Pract. 38, 601–605.

Buckley, D.A., Wakelin, S.H., Seed, P.T., et al., 2000. The frequency of allergy in a patch-test population over a 17-year period. Br. J. Dermatol. 142, 279–283.

Buckley, D.A., Rycroft, R.J., White, I.R., et al., 2002. Contaminating resin acids have not caused the high rate of sensitivity to oakmoss. Contact Dermatitis 47, 19–20.

Buckley, D.A., Rycroft, R.J., White, I.R., et al., 2003. The frequency of fragrance allergy in patch-tested patients increases with their age. Br. J. Dermatol. 149, 986–989.

Budavari, S. (Ed.), 1989. The Merck Index, eleventh ed. Merck, New Jersey.

Buddhakala, N., Talubmook, C., Sriyotha, P., et al., 2008. Inhibitory effects of ginger essential oil on spontaneous and PGF2alpha-induced contraction of rat myometrium. Planta Med. 74, 385–391.

Buechel, D.W., Haverlah, C., Gardner, M.E., 1983. Pennyroyal oil ingestion: report of a case. J. Am. Osteopath. Assoc. 82, 793–794.

Bunge, A.L., Guy, R.H., Hadgraft, J., 1999. The determination of a diffusional path length through the stratum corneum. Int. J. Pharm. 188, 121–124.

Burfield, T., 2000. Natural aromatic materials - odours and origins, vols I & II. The Atlantic Institute of Aromatherapy, Tampa.

Burfield, T., 2003. The adulteration of essential oils – and the consequences to aromatherapy and natural perfumery practice. www.naha.org/articles/adulteration_1.htm (accessed 05.08.12.).

Burfield, T., 2004. Opinion document to the IFA: a brief safety guidance on essential oils. www.users.globalnet.co.uk/~nodice.

Burian, M., Freudenstein, J., Tegtmeier, M., et al., 2003. Single copy of variant CYP2A6 alleles does not confer susceptibility to liver dysfunction in patients treated with coumarin. Int. J. Clin. Pharmacol. Ther. 41, 141–147.

Burits, M., Bucar, F., 2000. Antioxidant activity of *Nigella sativa* essential oil. Phytother. Res. 14, 323–328.

Burits, M., Asres, K., Bucar, F., 2001. The antioxidant activity of the essential oils of *Artemisia afra*, *Artemisia abyssinica* and *Juniperus procera*. Phytother. Res. 15, 103–108.

Burke, Y.D., Ayoubi, A.S., Werner, S.R., et al., 2002. Effects of the isoprenoids perillyl alcohol and farnesol on apoptosis biomarkers in pancreatic cancer chemoprevention. Anticancer Res. 22, 3127–3134.

Burkey, J.L., Sauer, J.M., McQueen, C.A., et al., 2000. Cytotoxicity and genotoxicity of methyleugenol and related congeners – a mechanism of activation for methyleugenol. Mutat. Res. 453, 25–33.

Burke, B.E., Baillie, J.E., Olson, R.D., 2004. Essential oil of Australian lemon myrtle (*Backhousia citriodora*) in the treatment of molluscum contagiosum in children. Biomedicine & Pharmacology 58, 245–247.

Burkhard, P.R., Burkhard, K., Haenggeli, C.A., et al., 1999. Plant-induced seizures: reappearance of an old problem. J. Neurol. 246, 667–670.

Burkhart, C.G., Burkhart, H.R., 2003. Contact irritant dermatitis and anti-pruritic agents: the need to address the itch. J. Drugs. Dermatol. 2, 143–146.

Burns, E.E., Blamey, C., Ersser, S.J., et al., 2000. An investigation into the use of aromatherapy in intrapartum midwifery practice. J. Altern. Complement. Med. 6, 141–147.

Burns, E., Zobbi, V., Panzeri, D., et al., 2007. Aromatherapy in childbirth: a pilot randomised controlled trial. BJOG 114, 838–844.

Burt, S., 2004. Essential oils: their antibacterial properties and potential applications in foods - a review. Int. J. Food Microbiol. 94, 223–253.

Butani, L., Afshinnik, A., Johnson, J., et al., 2003. Amelioration of tacrolimus-induced nephrotoxicity in rats using juniper oil. Transplantation 76, 306–311.

Buyukleyla, M., Rencuzogullari, E., 2009. The effects of thymol on sister chromatid exchange, chromosome aberration and micronucleus in human lymphocytes. Ecotoxicol. Environ. Saf. 72, 943–947.

Cabello, C.M., Bair, W.B., Lamore, S.D., et al., 2009. The cinnamon-derived Michael acceptor cinnamic aldehyde impairs melanoma cell proliferation, invasiveness, and tumor growth. Free Radic. Biol. Med. 46, 220–231.

Caceres, A.I., Brackmann, M., Elia, M.D., et al., 2009. A sensory neuronal ion channel essential for airway inflammation and hyperreactivity in asthma. Proc. Natl. Acad. Sci. U. S. A. 106, 9099–9104.

Cachao, P., Menezes Brandao, F., Carmo, M., et al., 1986. Allergy to oil of turpentine in Portugal. Contact Dermatitis 14, 205–208.

Cadby, P.A., Troy, W.R., Vey, M.G., 2002. Consumer exposure to fragrance ingredients: providing estimates for safety evaluation. Regul. Toxicol. Pharmacol. 36, 246–252.

Cadéac, M., Meunier, A., 1891. Contribution à l'étude physiologique de l'intoxication par le vulnéraire. Nouvelles preuves des propriétés épileptisantes de l'essence d'hyssop. Bull. Acad. Natl. Med. 43, 261–264.

Caelli, M., Porteous, J., Carson, C.F., et al., 2000. Tea tree oil as an alternative topical decolonization agent for methicillin-resistant *Staphylococcus aureus*. J. Hosp. Infect. 46, 236–237.

Cai, Y., Baer-Dubowska, W., Ashwood-Smith, M., et al., 1997a. Inhibitory effects of naturally occurring coumarins on the metabolic activation of benzo[a]pyrene and 7,12-dimethylbenz[a]anthracene in cultured mouse keratinocytes. Carcinogenesis 18, 215–222.

Cai, Y., Kleiner, H., Johnston, D., 1997b. Effect of naturally occurring coumarins on the formation of epidermal DNA adducts and skin tumors induced by benzo[a]pyrene and 7,12-dimethylbenz[a]anthracene in SENCAR mice. Carcinogenesis 18, 1521–1527.

Cai, L., Yu, S.Z., Zhang, Z.F., 2001. Glutathione S-transferases M1, T1 genotypes and the risk of gastric cancer: a case-control study. World. J. Gastroenterol. 7, 506–509.

Caignard, A., Lagadec, P., Reisser, D., et al., 1985. Role of macrophage in the defense against intestinal cancers. Comp. Immunol. Microbiol. Infect. Dis. 8, 147–157.

Cal, K., 2006a. How does the type of vehicle influence the *in vitro* skin absorption and elimination kinetics of terpenes? Arch. Dermatol. Res. 297, 311–315.

Cal, K., 2006b. Skin penetration of terpenes from essential oils and topical vehicles. Planta Med. 72, 311–316.

Cal, K., 2006c. Aqueous solubility of liquid monoterpenes at 293 K and relationship with calculated Log P value. Yakugaku Zasshi 126, 307–309.

Cal, K., Sznitowska, M., 2003. Cutaneous absorption and elimination of three acyclic terpenes - *in vitro* studies. J. Control. Release 93, 369–376.

Cal, K., Kupiec, K., Sznitowska, M., 2006. Effect of physicochemical properties of cyclic terpenes on their *ex vivo* skin absorption and elimination kinetics. J. Dermatol. Sci. 41, 137–142.

Calabrese, E.J., 2002. Hormesis: changing view of the dose-response, a personal account of the history and current status. Mutat. Res. 511, 181–189.

Calabrese, E.J., Baldwin, L.A., 1998. Hormesis as a biological hypothesis. Environ. Health Perspect. 106 (Suppl. 1), 357–362.

Calabrese, E.J., Baldwin, L.A., 2003. Toxicology rethinks its central belief. Nature 421, 691–692.

Calcabrini, A., Stringaro, A., Toccacieli, L., et al., 2004. Terpinen-4-ol, the main component of *Melaleuca alternifolia* (tea tree) oil inhibits the *in vitro* growth of human melanoma cells. Journal of Investigative Dermatology 122, 349–360.

Caldwell, J., 1993. Perspective on the usefulness of the mouse lymphoma assay as an indicator of a genotoxic carcinogen: ten compounds which are positive in the mouse lymphoma assay but are not genotoxic carcinogens. Teratog. Carcinog. Mutagens. 13, 185–190.

Caldwell, J., Sutton, J.D., 1988. Influence of dose size on the disposition of *trans*-[methoxy-14C]anethole in human volunteers. Food Chem. Toxicol. 26, 87–91.

Caldwell, J., Farmer, P.B., Sangster, S.A., et al., 1983. Dose-dependent metabolism of trans-anethole in the rat. Br. J. Pharmacol. 79, 212P.

Caldefie-Chézet, F., Guerry, M., Chalchat, J.C., et al., 2004. Anti-inflammatory effects of *Melaleuca alternifolia* essential oil on human polymorphonuclear neutrophils and monocytes. Free Radic. Res. 38, 805–811.

Calnan, C.D., 1976. Cinnamon dermatitis from an ointment. Contact Dermatitis 2, 167–170.

Calnan, C.D., 1979. Perfume dermatitis from the cosmetic ingredients oakmoss and hydroxycitronellal. Contact Dermatitis 5, 194.

Calnan, C.D., Cronin, E., Rycroft, R.J., 1980. Allergy to perfume ingredients. Contact Dermatitis 6, 500–501.

Calogirou, A., Larsen, B.R., Kotzias, D., 1999. Gas-phase terpene oxidation products: a review. Atmos. Environ. 33, 1423–1439.

Camarasa, G., Alomar, A., 1978. Menthol dermatitis from cigarettes. Contact Dermatitis 4, 169–170.

Camarda, L., Dayton, T., Di Stefano, V., et al., 2007. Chemical composition and antimicrobial activity of some olegum resin essential oils from *Boswellia* spp. (Burseraceae). Ann. Chim. 97, 837–844.

Canbek, M., Uyanoglu, M., Bayramoglu, G., et al., 2008. Effects of carvacrol on defects of ischemia-reperfusion in the rat liver. Phytomedicine 15, 447–452.

Candan, F., Unlu, M., Tepe, B., et al., 2003. Antioxidant and antimicrobial activity of the essential oil and methanol extracts of *Achillea millefolium* subsp. *millefolium* Afan. (Asteraceae). J. Ethnopharmacol. 87, 215–220.

Canning, B.J., Farmer, D.G., Mori, N., 2006. Mechanistic studies of acid-evoked coughing in anesthetized guinea pigs. Am. J. Physiol. Regul. Integr. Comp. Physiol. 291, R454–R463.

Capasso, R., Pinto, L., Vuotto, M.L., Di Carlo, G., 2000. Preventive effect of eugenol on PAF and ethanol-induced gastric mucosal damage. Fitoterapia 71, S131–S137.

Cappellini, M.D., Fiorelli, G., 2008. Glucose-6-phosphate dehydrogenase deficiency. The Lancet 371, 64–74.

Cappello, G., Spezzaferro, M., Grossi, L., et al., 2007. Peppermint oil (Mintoil®) in the treatment of irritable bowel syndrome: a prospective double blind placebo-controlled randomized trial. Dig. Liver Dis. 39, 530–536.

Carder, K.R., 2005. Hypersensitivity reactions in neonates and infants. Dermatol. Ther. 18, 160–175.

Cardozo, M.T., De Conti, A., Ong, T.P., et al., 2011. Chemopreventive effects of β-ionone and geraniol during rat hepatocarcinogenesis promotion: distinct actions on cell proliferation, apoptosis, HMGCoA reductase, and RhoA. J. Nutr. Biochem. 22, 130–135.

Cardullo, A.C., Ruszkowski, A.M., DeLeo, V.A., 1989. Allergic contact dermatitis resulting from sensitivity to citrus peel, geraniol, and citral. J. Am. Acad. Dermatol. 21, 395–397.

Caress, S.M., Steinemann, A.C., Waddick, C., 2002. Symptomatology and etiology of multiple chemical sensitivities in the southeastern United States. Arch. Environ. Health 57, 429–436.

Caress, S.M., Steinemann, A.C., 2004. A national population study of the prevalence of multiple chemical sensitivity. Arch. Environ. Health 59, 300–305.

Cariddi, L., Escobar, F., Moser, M., et al., 2011. Monoterpenes isolated from *Minthostachys verticillata* (Griesb.) Epling essential oil modulates immediate-type hypersensitivity responses in vitro and in vivo. Planta Med. 77, 1687–1694.

Carlin, J.T., Kramer, S., Ho, C.T., 1988. Comparison of commercial citronella oils from various origins. In: Lawrence, B.M., Mookerjee, B.D., Willis, B.J. (Eds.), Flavor and fragrances: a world perspective. Elsevier Science, Amsterdam, pp. 495–504.

Carlsen, B.C., Andersen, K.E., Menné, T., et al., 2008. Patients with multiple contact allergies: a review. Contact Dermatitis 58, 1–8.

Carlsen, B.C., 2009. Patients with multiple contact allergies: population characteristics and clinical presentation. PhD Thesis. Faculty of Health Sciences, University of Copenhagen. www.videncenterforallergi.dk/Files/Filer/PHD/PhD-Carlsen.pdf

Carmichael, P.L., Crooks, N., Schenk, M., et al., 1999. A comparison of immunochemical and postlabelling methodologies for the detection of DNA adducts formed by methyleugenol. Hum. Exp. Toxicol. 18, 55.

Carnat, A.P., Lamaison, J.L., Rémery, A., 1991. Composition of leaf and flower essential oil from *Monarda didyma* L. cultivated in France. Flavour & Fragrance Journal 6, 79–80.

Carneiro Leite, V., Ferreira Santos, R., Chen, L., et al., 2004. Psoralen derivatives and longwave ultraviolet irradiation are active in vitro against human melanoma cell line. J. Photochem. Photobiol. B 76, 49–53.

Carnesecchi, S., Schneider, Y., Ceraline, J., et al., 2001. Geraniol, a component of plant essential oils, inhibits growth and polyamine biosynthesis in human colon cancer cells. J. Pharmacol. Exp. Ther. 298, 197–200.

Carnesecchi, S., Bras-Goncalves, R., Bradaia, A., et al., 2004. Geraniol, a component of plant essential oils, modulates DNA synthesis and potentiates 5-fluorouracil efficacy on human colon tumor xenografts. Cancer Lett. 215, 53–59.

Caron, E., 1986. D2-dopamine receptor: biochemical characterization. In: Ganong, W.F., Martini, L. (Eds.), Frontiers in neuroendocrinology. Raven Press, New York.

Carpenter, C.P., Smyth, H.F., Pozzani, U.C., 1949. The assay of acute vapor toxicity and the grading and interpretation of results on ninety-six compounds. J. Ind. Hyg. Toxicol. 31, 343–346.

Cartwright, L.E., Walter, J.F., 1983. Psoralen-containing sunscreen is tumorigenic in hairless mice. J. Am. Acad. Dermatol. 8, 830–836.

Carvalho-Freitas, M.I., Costa, M., 2002. Anxiolytic and sedative effects of extracts and essential oil from *Citrus aurantium*. Biological & Pharmacological Bulletin 25, 1629–1633.

Casetti, F., Bartelke, S., Biehler, K., et al., 2012. Antimicrobial activity against bacteria with dermatological relevance and skin tolerance of the essential oil from *Coriandrum sativum* L. fruits. Phytother. Res. 26, 420–424.

Caspary, W.J., Langenbach, R., Penman, B.W., et al., 1988. The mutagenic activity of selected compounds at the TK locus: rodent vs. human cells. Mutat. Res. 196, 61–81.

Casley-Smith, J.R., 1999. Benzo-pyrones in the treatment of lymphoedema. Int. Angiol. 18, 31–41.

Castilho, P.C., Do Ceu Costa, M., Rodrigues, A., et al., 2005. Characterization of laurel fruit oil from Madeira Island, Portugal. J. Am. Oil. Chem. Soc. 82, 863–868.

Caujolle, F., Franck, C., 1944a. Comparative toxicity of thymol and carvacrol. Bull. Soc. Chim. Biol. (Paris) 26, 334–342.

Caujolle, F., Franck, C., 1944b. On the pharmacodynamic action of lavender, lavandin and spike lavender oils. Ann. Pharm. Fr. 2, 147–148.

Caujolle, F., Franck, C., 1945a. Pharmacodynamic actions of clary sage and condiment sage. Comptes Rendues Société Biologique 139, 1109–1110.

Caujolle, F., Franck, C., 1945b. Sur l'action pharmacodynamique de l'essence d'hysope. Comptes Rendues Société Biologique 139, 1111.

Caujolle, F., Meunier, D., 1958. Toxicité de l'estragol et des anétholes (*cis* et *trans*). C. R. Hebd. Seances Acad. Sci. Paris 246, 1465–1468.

Cauthen, W.L., Hester, W.H., 1989. Accidental ingestion of oil of wintergreen. J. Fam. Pract. 29, 680–681.

Cavalieri, E., Mariotto, S., Fabrizi, C., et al., 2004. α-Bisabolol, a nontoxic natural compound, strongly induces apoptosis in glioma cells. Biochem. Biophys. Res. Commun. 315, 589–594.

Cavalieri, E., Bergamini, C., Mariotto, S., et al., 2009. Involvement of mitochondrial permeability transition pore opening in α-bisabolol induced apoptosis. FEBS J. 276, 3990–4000.

Cavalli, J.F., Tomi, F., Bernardini, A.F., et al., 2004. Combined analysis of the essential oil of Chenopodium ambrosioides by GC, GC-MS and 13C-NMR spectroscopy: quantitative determination of ascaridole, a heat-sensitive compound. Phytochem. Anal. 15, 275–279.

CEFS, 2000. Final version of the publication datasheet on estragole. Document RD 4/5/1–47 submitted by Italy for the 47th meeting in Strasbourg, 16–20 October, 2000.

Celik, S., Ozkaya, A., 2002. Effects of intraperitoneally administered lipoic acid, vitamin E, and linalool on the level of total lipid and fatty acids in guinea pig brain with oxidative stress induced by H2O2. J. Biochem. Mol. Biol. 35, 547–552.

Chadha, A., Madyastha, K.M., 1984. Metabolism of geraniol and linalool in the rat and effects on liver and lung microsomal enzymes. Xenobiotica 14, 365–374.

Chadwick, C.A., Potten, C.S., Cohen, A.J., et al., 1994. The time of onset and duration of 5-methoxypsoralen photochemoprotection from UVR-induced DNA damage in human skin. Br. J. Dermatol. 131, 483–494.

Chadwick, L.R., Pauli, G.F., Farnsworth, N.R., 2006. The pharmacognosy of *Humulus lupulus* L. (hops) with an emphasis on estrogenic properties. Phytomedicine 13, 119–131.

Chae, Y.H., Koenig, L.A., El-Bayoumy, K., 1997. Prenatal effect of *d*-limonene on the level of benzo[*a*]pyrene-(B[*a*]P)-DNA adducts in mouse fetuses exposed to B[*a*]P in utero. Proceedings of the American Association for Cancer Research 38, 363–364.

Chagonda, L.S., Makanda, C., 2000. Essential oils of cultivated *Cymbopogon winterianus* (Jowitt) and of C. *citratus* (DC) (Stapf) from Zimbabwe. Journal of Essential Oil Research 12, 478–480.

Chaieb, K., Zmantar, T., Ksouri, R., et al., 2007. Antioxidant properties of the essential oil of *Eugenia caryophyllata* and its antifungal activity against a large number of clinical Candida species. Mycoses 50, 403–406.

Chainy, G.B., Manna, S.K., Chaturvedi, M.M., et al., 2000. Anethole blocks both early and late cellular responses transduced by tumor necrosis factor: effect on NF-kappaB, AP-1, JNK, MAPKK and apoptosis. Oncogene 19, 2943–2950.

Chaiworapongsa, T., Romero, R., Kusanovic, J.P., et al., 2010. Unexplained fetal death is associated with increased concentrations of anti-angiogenic factors in amniotic fluid. J. Matern. Fetal. Neonatal Med. 23, 794–805.

Chalchat, J.C., Valade, I., 2000. Chemical composition of leaf oils of *Cinnamomum* from Madagascar: C. *zeylanicum* Blume, C. *camphora* L., C. fragrans Baillon and C. *angustifolium*. Journal of Essential Oil Research 12, 537–540.

Chalchat, J.C., Garry, R.P., Michet, A., Gorunovic, M., 1991. Essential oils of *Artemisia anuua* from Yugoslavia. Rivista Italiana EPPOS (Special Issue) 471–476.

Chalchat, J.C., Garry, R.P., Michet, A., et al., 1993. Essential oils of rosemary (*Rosmarinus officinalis* L.). The chemical composition of oils of various origins (Morocco, Spain, France). Journal of Essential Oil Research 5, 613–618.

Chalchat, J.C., Garry, R.P., Mathieu, J.P., 1994a. Composition of the volatile fraction from Honduras styrax, *Liquidambar styraciflua* L. Journal of Essential Oil Research 6, 73–75.

Chalchat, J.C., Garry, R.P., Lamy, J., 1994b. Influence of harvest time on yield and composition of *Artemisia annua* oil produced in France. Journal of Essential Oil Research 6, 261–268.

Chalchat, J.C., Garry, R.P., Michet, A., 1997. Variation of the chemical composition of essential oil of *Mentha piperita* L. during the growing time. Journal of Essential Oil Research 9, 463–465.

Chamorro, G., Salazar, M., Fournier, G., et al., 1990. The anti-implantation effects of various savine extracts on the pregnant rat. J. Toxicol. Clin. Exp. 10, 157–160.

Chamorro, G., Salazar, M., Salazar, S., et al., 1993. Pharmacology and toxicology of *Guatteria gaumeri* and alpha-asarone. Rev. Invest. Clin. 45, 597–604.

Chamorro, G., Garduño, L., Martínez, E., et al., 1998. Dominant lethal study of α-asarone in male mice. Toxicol. Lett. 99, 71–77.

Chamorro, G., Salazar, M., Tamariz, J., et al., 1999. Dominant lethal study of α-asarone in male and female mice after sub-chronic treatment. Phytother. Res. 13, 308–311.

Champagnat, P., Figueredo, G., Chalchat, J.C., 2006. A study on the composition of commercial *Vetiveria zizanoides* oils from different geographical origins. Journal of Essential Oil Research 18, 416–422.

Chan, T.Y., 1998. Drug interactions as a cause of overanticoagulation and bleedings in Chinese patients receiving warfarin. Int. J. Clin. Pharmacol. Ther. 36, 403–405.

Chan, V.S., Caldwell, J., 1992. Comparative induction of unscheduled DNA synthesis in cultured rat hepatocytes by allylbenzenes and their 1′-hydroxy metabolites. Food Chem. Toxicol. 30, 831–836.

Chan, K.C., Hsu, C.C., Yin, M.C., 2002. Protective effect of three diallyl sulphides against glucose-induced erythrocyte and platelet oxidation, and ADP-induced platelet aggregation. Thromb. Res. 108, 317–322.

Chan, N.L., Wang, H., Wang, Y., et al., 2006. Polycyclic aromatic hydrocarbon-induced CYP1B1 activity is suppressed by perillyl alcohol in MCF-7 cells. Toxicol. Appl. Pharmacol. 213, 98–104.

Chandhoke, N., Ghatak, B.J.R., 1969. Studies on *Tagetes minuta*:some pharmacological actions of the essential oil. Indian J. Med. Res. 57, 864–876.

Chandler, R.F., 1986. An inconspicuous but insidious drug. Can. Pharm. J. 119, 563–566.

Chandra, S., Prasad, M.C., Tandon, S.K., et al., 1989. Evaluation of a formulation of *Cedrus deodara* wood essential oil on blood urea nitrogen and blood glucose level and on skin irritation. Indian Vet. J. 66, 30–34.

Chang, Y.C., Karlberg, A.T., Maibach, H.I., 1997. Allergic contact dermatitis from oxidised *d*-limonene. Contact Dermatitis 37, 308–309.

Chang, Y.C., Tai, K.W., Huang, F.M., et al., 2000. Cytotoxic and nongenotoxic effects of phenolic compounds in human pulp cell cultures. J. Endod. 26, 440–443.

Chang, M.C., Uang, B.J., Wu, H.L., et al., 2002. Inducing the cell cycle arrest and apoptosis of oral KB carcinoma cells by hydroxychavicol: roles of glutathione and reactive oxygen species. Br. J. Pharmacol. 135, 619–630.

Chang, M.C., Wu, H.L., Lee, J.J., et al., 2004. The induction of prostaglandin E2 production, interleukin-6 production, cell cycle arrest, and cytotoxicity in primary oral keratinocytes and KB cancer cells by areca nut ingredients is differentially regulated by MEK/ERK activation. J. Biol. Chem. 279, 50676–50683.

Chao, L.K., Hua, K.F., Hsu, H.Y., et al., 2008. Cinnamaldehyde inhibits pro-inflammatory cytokines secretion from monocytes/macrophages through suppression of intracellular signaling. Food Chem. Toxicol. 46, 220–231.

Chaouki, W., Leger, D.Y., Liagre, B., 2009. Citral inhibits cell proliferation and induces apoptosis and cell cycle arrest in MCF-7 cells. Fundam. Clin. Pharmacol. 23, 549–556.

Charles, A.K., Darbre, P.D., 2009. Oestrogenic activity of benzyl salicylate, benzyl benzoate and butylphenylmethylpropional (Lilial) in MCF7 human breast cancer cells *in vitro*. J. Appl. Toxicol. 29, 422–434.

Chavasse, P.H., 1939. Poisoning by the essential oil of bitter almonds. Lancet 32 (838), 930–931.

Cheah, Y.H., Azimahtol, H.L., Abdullah, N.R., 2006. Xanthorrhizol exhibits antiproliferative activity on MCF-7 breast cancer cells via apoptosis induction. Anticancer Res. 26, 4527–4534.

Chen, W., Lu, Y., Gao, M., et al., 2011. Anti-angiogenesis effect of essential oil from *Curcuma zedoaria* in vitro and in vivo. J. Ethnopharmacol. 133, 220–226.

Cheminat, A., Stampf, J.L., Benezra, C., et al., 1981. Allergic contact dermatitis to costus: removal of haptens with polymers. Acta Derm. Venereol. (Stockholm) 61, 525–529.

Cheminat, A., Stampf, J.L., Benezra, C., 1984. Allergic contact dermatitis to laurel (*Laurus nobilis* L.): isolation and identification of haptens. Arch. Dermatol. Res. 276, 178–181.

Chen, I.S., Chang, C.T., Sheen, W.S., et al., 1996. Coumarins and antiplatelet aggregation constituents from Formosan *Peucedanum japonicum*. Phytochemistry 41, 525–530.

Chen, S.J., Wang, M.H., Chen, I.J., 1996. Antiplatelet and calcium inhibitory properties of eugenol and sodium eugenol acetate. General Pharmacology: The Vascular System 27, 629–633.

Chen, H., Chan, K.K., Budd, T., 1998. Pharmacokinetics of d-limonene in the rat by GC-MS assay. J. Pharm. Biomed. Anal. 17, 631–640.

Chen, C.L., Chi, C.W., Chang, K.W., et al., 1999. Safrole-like DNA adducts in oral tissue from oral cancer patients with a betel quid chewing history. Carcinogenesis 20, 2331–2334.

Chen, L.J., Lebetkin, E.H., Burka, L.T., 2001. Metabolism of (R)-(+)-pulegone in F344 rats. Drug Metab. Dispos. 29, 1567–1577.

Chen, L.J., Lebetkin, E.H., Burka, L.T., 2003. Comparative disposition of (R)-(+)-pulegone in B6C3F1 mice and F344 rats. DruNieg Metabolism & Disposition 31, 892–899.

Chen, Y.H., Dai, H.J., Chang, H.P., 2003. Suppression of inducible nitric oxide production by indole and isothiocyanate derivatives from Brassica plants in stimulated macrophages. Planta Med. 69, 696–700.

Chen, C.Y., Xu, K., Zhu, D.Y., et al., 2003. Treatment of secondary hepatocarcinoma by hepatic artery perfusion embolism of oleum Curcumae: a clinical observation of 28 cases. Xinzhongyi 35, 23–24.

Chen, R., Chen, J., Cheng, S., et al., 2010. Assessment of embryotoxicity of compounds in cosmetics by the embryonic stem cell test. Toxicology Mechanisms & Methods 20, 112–118.

Chen, W., Lu, Y., Gao, M., et al., 2011. Anti-angiogenesis effect of essential oil from *Curcuma zedoaria* in vitro and in vivo. J. Ethnopharmacol. 133, 220–226.

Cheng, J.H., Wu, W.Y., Liu, W.S., et al., 1999. Therapeutic effect of *Curcuma aromatica* oil infused via hepatic artery against primary liver neoplasms: 17 cases. Shijie Huaren Xiohua Zazhi 7, 92.

Cheng, J.H., Chang, G., Wu, W.Y., 2001. A controlled clinical study between hepatic arterial infusion with embolized *Curcuma aromatica* oil and chemical drugs in treating primary liver cancer. Zhingguo Zhingxiyi Jiehe Zazhi 21, 165–167.

Chericoni, S., Prieto, J.M., Iacopini, P., et al., 2005. *In vitro* activity of the essential oil of *Cinnamomum zeylanicum* and eugenol in peroxynitrite-induced oxidative processes. Journal of Agricultural & Food Chemistry 53, 4762–4765.

Cherng, J.M., Shieh, D.E., Chiang, W., 2007. Chemopreventive effects of minor dietary constituents in common foods on human cancer cells. Biosci. Biotechnol. Biochem. 71, 1500–1504.

Cheung, C., Hotchkiss, S.A., Pease, C.K., 2003. Cinnamic compound metabolism in human skin and the role metabolism may play in determining relative sensitisation potency. J. Dermatol. Sci. 31, 9–19.

Chhabra, S.K., Rao, A.R., 1993. Postnatal modulation of xenobiotic metabolizing enzymes in liver of mouse pups following translactational exposure to sandalwood oil. Nutrition Research 13, 1191–1202.

Chialva, F., Gabri, G., Liddle, P.A.P., et al., 1982. Qualitative evaluation of aromatic herbs by direct headspace GC analysis. Journal of HRC & CC 5, 182–188.

Chiang, A., Maibach, H.I., 2012. Towards a perfect vehicle(s) for diagnostic patch testing: an overview. Cutan. Ocul. Toxicol. doi: 10.3109/15569527.2012.684418.

Chiang, L.C., Chiang, W., Chang, M.Y., et al., 2003. Antileukemic activity of selected natural products in Taiwan. Am. J. Chin. Med. 31, 37–46.

Chiang, Y.H., Jen, L.N., Su, H.Y., et al., 2006. Effects of garlic oil and two of its major organosulfur compounds, diallyl disulfide and diallyl trisulfide, on intestinal damage in rats injected with endotoxin. Toxicol. Appl. Pharmacol. 213, 46–54.

Chiariello, M., Campana, G., Delfanti, G., et al., 1986. Platelet aggregation induced by arachidonic acid, ADP, thrombin. Study of the antiaggregation effects of verbenone and indomethacin. Boll. Chim. Farm. 125, 387–389.

Chidgey, M.A., Caldwell, J., 1986. Studies on benzyl acetate. I. Effect of dose size and vehicle on the plasma pharmacokinetics and metabolism of [methylene-14C]benzyl acetate in the rat. Food Chem. Toxicol. 24, 1257–1265.

Chidgey, M.A.J., Kennedy, J.F., Caldwell, J., et al., 1987. Studies on benzyl acetate III. The percutaneous absorption and disposition of methylene-C benzyl acetate in the rat. Food Chem. Toxicol. 25, 521–525.

Chinou, I., Demetzos, C., Harvala, C., et al., 1994. Cytotoxic and antibacterial labdane-type diterpenes from the aerial parts of *Cistus incanus* subsp. *creticus*. Planta Med. 60, 34–36.

Chiou, L.C., Ling, J.Y., Chang, C.C., 1995. *beta*-Eudesmol as an antidote for intoxication from organophosphorus anticholinesterase agents. Eur. J. Pharmacol. 292, 151–156.

Chiou, L.C., Ling, J.Y., Chang, C.C., 1997. Chinese herb constituent *beta*-eudesmol alleviated the electroshock seizures in mice and electrographic seizures in rat hippocampal slices. Neurosci. Lett. 231, 171–174.

Cho, Y.M., Hasumura, M., Takami, S., et al., 2011. A 13-week subchronic toxicity study of hinokitiol administered in the diet to F344 rats. Food Chem. Toxicol. 49, 1782–1786.

Chobanian, A.V., Bakris, G.L., Black, H.R., et al., 2003. The Seventh Report of the Joint National Committee on Prevention, Detection, Evaluation, and Treatment of High Blood Pressure (JNC 7). Hypertension 42, 1206–1252.

Choi, H.S., Song, H.S., Ukeda, H., et al., 2000. Radical-scavenging activities of citrus essential oils and their components: detection using 1,1-diphenyl-2-picrylhydrazyl. Journal of Agricultural & Food Chemistry 48, 4156–4161.

Choi, J., Lee, K.T., Ka, H., et al., 2001. Constituents of the essential oil of the *Cinnamomum cassia* stem bark and the biological properties. Archives of Pharmaceutical Research 24, 418–423.

Choi, J.H., Ha, J., Park, J.H., et al., 2002. Costunolide triggers apoptosis in human leukemia U937 cells by depleting intracellular thiols. Jpn. J Cancer Res. 93, 1327–1333.

Choi, M.A., Kim, S.H., Chung, W.Y., et al., 2005. Xanthorrhizol, a natural sesquiterpenoid from *Curcuma xanthorrhiza*, has an anti-metastatic potential in experimental mouse lung metastasis model. Biochem. Biophys. Res. Commun. 326, 210–217.

Choi, S.H., Im, E., Kang, H.K., et al., 2005. Inhibitory effects of costunolide on the telomerase activity in human breast carcinoma cells. Cancer Lett. 227, 153–162.

Choi, Y.K., Cho, G.S., Hwang, S., et al., 2010. Methyleugenol reduces cerebral ischemic injury by suppression of oxidative injury and inflammation. Free Radic. Res. 44, 925–935.

Choo, E.J., Rhee, Y.H., Jeong, S.J., et al., 2011. Anethole exerts antimetatstaic activity via inhibition of matrix metalloproteinase 2/9 and AKT/mitogen-activated kinase/nuclear factor kappa B signaling pathways. Biol. Pharm. Bull. 34, 41–46.

Choong, Y.M., Lin, H.J., 2001. A rapid and simple gas chromatographic method for direct determination of safrole in soft drinks. Journal of Food & Drug Analysis 9, 27–32.

Chopra, I.C., Jamwal, K.S., Khajuria, B.N., 1954. Pharmacological action of some common essential oil-bearing plants used in indigenous medicine. Indian J. Med. Res. 42, 381–384.

Choudhary, D., Kale, R.K., 2002. Antioxidant and non-toxic properties of Piper betle leaf extract: in vitro and in vivo studies. Phytother. Res. 16, 461–466.

Chow, W.H., Cheung, K.L., Ling, H.M., See, T., 1989. Potentiation of warfarin anticoagulation by topical methylsalicylate ointment. J. R. Soc. Med. 82, 501–502.

Christensen, B.V., Lynch, H.J., 1937. A comparative study of the pharmacological actions of natural and synthetic camphor. J. Am. Pharm. Assoc. 26, 786–796.

Christensson, J.B., Forsström, P., Wennberg, A.M., et al., 2009. Air oxidation increases skin irritation from fragrance terpenes. Contact Dermatitis 60, 32–40.

Christoph, G.R., Hansen, J.F., Leung, H.W., 2003. Subchronic inhalation neurotoxicity studies of ethyl acetate in rats. Neurotoxicology 24, 861–874.

Chuang, K.J., Chen, H.W., Liu, I.J., et al., 2012. The effect of essential oil on heart rate and blood pressure among solus por aqua workers. Eur. J. Prev. Cardiol. In Press.

Chu, Y.H., Zhou, M.H., Li, Q., et al., 1985. Antifertility effect of volatile oil of *Daucus carota* seeds. Reproduction & Contraception 5, 37–40.

Chung, F.L., Juchatz, A., Vitarius, J., et al., 1984. Effects of dietary compounds on α-hydroxylation of *N*-nitrosopyrrolidine and *N'*-nitrosonornicotine in rat target tissues. Cancer Res. 44, 2924–2928.

Chung, F.L., Morse, M.A., Eklind, K.I., 1992. New potential chemopreventive agents for lung carcinogenesis of tobacco-specific nitrosamine. Cancer Res. 52 (Suppl. 9), 2719S–2722S.

Chung, F.L., Conaway, C.C., Rao, C.V., et al., 2000. Chemoprevention of colonic aberrant crypt foci in Fischer rats by sulforaphane and phenethyl isothiocyanate. Carcinogenesis 21, 2287–2291.

Chung, B.H., Lee, H.Y., Lee, J.S., et al., 2006. Perillyl alcohol inhibits the expression and function of the androgen receptor in human prostate cancer cells. Cancer Lett. 236, 222–228.

Chung, Y.T., Chen, C.L., Wu, C.C., et al., 2008. Safrole-DNA adduct in hepatocellular carcinoma associated with betel quid chewing. Toxicol. Lett. 183, 21–27.

Chung, M.J., Cho, S.Y., Bhuiyan, M.J., et al., 2010. Anti-diabetic effects of lemon balm (*Melissa officinalis*) essential oil on glucose- and lipid-regulating enzymes in type 2 diabetic mice. Br. J. Nutr. 104, 180–188.

Cicció, J.F., 2004. A source of almost pure methyl chavicol: volatile oil from the aerial parts of *Tagetes lucida* (Asteraceae) cultivated in Costa Rica. Rev. Biol. Trop. 52, 853–857.

Ciftçi, O., Caliskan, M., Güllü, H., et al., 2008. Mentholated cigarette smoking induced alterations in left and right ventricular functions in chronic smokers. Anadolu Kardiyol. Derg. 8, 116–122.

Ciftçi, O., Güllü, H., Caliskan, M., et al., 2009. Mentholated cigarette smoking and brachial artery, carotid artery, and aortic vascular function. Türk Kardiyoloji Dernegi Arsivi 37, 234–240.

Ciftçi, O., Ozdemir, I., Tanyildizi, S., et al., 2011. Antioxidative effects of curcumin, β-myrcene and 1,8-cineole against 2,3,7,8-tetrachlorodibenzo-*p*-dioxin-induced oxidative stress in rats liver. Toxicol. Ind. Health 27, 447–453.

Ciganda, C., Laborde, A., 2003. Herbal infusions used for induced abortion. J. Toxicol. Clin. Toxicol. 41, 235–239.

CIR, 1999. Final report on the safety assessment of bisabolol. Int. J. Toxicol. 18 (Suppl. 3), 33–40.

Clark, G.C., 1988. Acute inhalation toxicity of eugenol in rats. Arch. Toxicol. 62, 381–386.

Clark, G.S., 1995. Coumarin. Perfumer & Flavorist 20, 23–34.

Clark, S.M., Wilkinson, S.M., 1998. Phototoxic contact dermatitis from 5-methoxypsoralen in aromatherapy oil. Contact Dermatitis 38, 289–290.

Clausen, P.A., Wilkins, C.K., Wolkoff, P., et al., 2001. Chemical and biological evaluation of a reaction mixture of R-(+)-limonene/ozone: formation of strong airways irritants. Environ. Int. 26, 511–522.

Clayton, D.G., Clayton, F.E., 1981–1982. Patty's industrial hygiene & toxicology: Vol 2A, 2B, 2C: Toxicology, third ed. John Wiley, New York.

Clayton, R., Orton, D., 2004. Contact allergy to spearmint oil in a patient with oral lichen planus. Contact Dermatitis 51, 314–315.

Clayton, R., Orton, D., 2005. Patch testing with tea tree oil: are we testing with the correct allergen? Br. J. Dermatol. 153 (Suppl. 1), 61.

Cleaver, J.E., Crowley, E., 2002. UV damage, DNA repair and skin carcinogenesis. Front. Biosci. 7, d1024–d1043.

Clerc, A., Sterne, J., Paris, R., 1934. Experiments on dogs with certain substances which lower the surface tension of the blood. C. R. Soc. Biol. 116, 864–867.

Clothier, R., Dierickx, P., Lakhanisky, T., et al., 2008. A database of IC50 values and principal component analysis of results from six basal cytotoxicity assays, for use in the modelling of the *in vivo* and *in vitro* data of the EU ACuteTox project. Altern. Lab. Anim. 36, 503–519.

Cockayne, S.E., Gawkrodger, D.J., 1997. Occupational contact dermatitis in an aromatherapist. Contact Dermatitis 37, 306–307.

Cocks, H., Wilson, D., 1998. Letter to the editor. Burns 24, 82.

Coderre, K., Faria, C., Dyer, E., 2010. Probable warfarin interaction with menthol cough drops. Pharmacotherapy 30, 110.

Coelho-de-Souza, L.N., Leal-Cardoso, J.H., De Abreu Matos, F.J., et al., 2005. Relaxant effects of the essential oil of *Eucalyptus tereticornis* and its main constituent 1,8-cineole on guinea-pig tracheal smooth muscle. Planta Med. 71, 1173–1175.

Coenraads, P.J., Bleumink, E., Nater, J.P., 1975. Susceptibility to primary irritants: age dependence and relation to contact allergic reactions. Contact Dermatitis 1, 377–381.

Cohen, A.J., 1979. Critical review of toxicology of coumarin with special reference to interspecies differences in metabolism and hepatotoxic response and their significance to man. Food Cosmet. Toxicol. 17, 277–289.

Cohen, D.M., Bhattacharyya, I., 2000. Cinnamon-induced oral erythema multiformelike sensitivity reaction. J Am Dent Assoc. 131, 929–934.

Cohen, B.M., Dressler, W.E., 1982. Acute aromatics inhalation modifies the airways. Effects of the common cold. Respiration 43, 285–293.

Cohen, S., Flescher, E., 2009. Methyl jasmonate: a plant stress hormone as an anti-cancer drug. Phytochemistry 70, 1600–1609.

Colalillo, R., 1974. Avvelenamento da apiolo in 7 donne e 2 bambini. Rivista di Tossicologia Sperimentale e Clinica 18 (2), 125–130.

Collins, F.W., Mitchell, J.C., 1975. Aroma chemicals: reference sources for perfume and flavour ingredients with special reference to cinnamic aldehyde. Contact Dermatitis 1, 43–47.

Collins, T.F.X., Hansen, W.H., Keeler, H.V., 1971. Effect of methyl salicylate on rat reproduction. Toxicol. Appl. Pharmacol. 18, 755–765.

Collins, N.F., Graven, E.H., van Beek, T.A., et al., 1996. Chemotaxonomy of commercial buchu species. (*Agathosma betulina* and *Agathosma crenulata*). Journal of Essential Oil Research 8, 229–235.

Colombo, G., Zucchi, A., Allegra, F., et al., 2003. *In vitro* and *in vivo* study of 5-methoxypsoralen skin concentration after topical application. Skin Pharmacol. Appl. Skin Physiol.

Cometto-Muñiz, J.E., Cain, W.S., 1991. Nasal pungency, odor, and eye irritation thresholds for homologous acetates. Pharmacol. Biochem. Behav. 39, 983–989.

Cometto-Muñiz, J.E., Cain, W.S., Abraham, M.H., et al., 1998a. Trigeminal and olfactory chemosensory impact of selected terpenes. Pharmacol. Biochem. Behav. 60, 765–770.

Cometto-Muñiz, J.E., Cain, W.S., Abraham, M.H., et al., 1998b. Sensory properties of selected terpenes. Thresholds for odor, nasal pungency, nasal localization, and eye irritation. Ann. N. Y. Acad. Sci. 855, 648–651.

Cometto-Muñiz, J.E., Cain, W.S., Abraham, M.H., 2005a. Determinants for nasal trigeminal detection of volatile organic compounds. Chem. Senses 30, 627–642.

Cometto-Muñiz, J.E., Cain, W.S., Abraham, M.H., 2005b. Molecular restrictions for human eye irritation by chemical vapors. Toxicol. Appl. Pharmacol. 207, 232–243.

Cometto-Muñiz, J.E., Cain, W.S., Abraham, M.H., et al., 2007. Cutoff in detection of eye irritation from vapors of homologous carboxylic acids and aliphatic aldehydes. Neuroscience 145, 1130–1137.

Committee for Veterinary Medicinal Products, 1999. Ruta graveolens, summary report. The European Agency for the Evaluation of Medicinal Products. www.emea.eu.int/pdfs/vet/mrls/054298en.pd.

Committee on Drugs, 1994. Camphor revisited: focus on toxicity (RE9422). Pediatrics 94, 127–128.

Concise International Chemical Assessment Document No 5. 1998 Limonene. World Health Organisation/Inter-Organization Programme for the Sound Management of Chemicals (IOMC).

Cone, J.E., Shusterman, D., 1991. Health effects of indoor odorants. Environ. Health Perspect. 95, 53–59.

Connor, M.J., 1991. Modulation of tumor promotion in mouse skin by the food additive citral (3,7-dimethyl-2,6-octadienal). Cancer Lett. 56, 25–28.

Connor, T.H., Theiss, J.C., Hanna, H.A., et al., 1985. Genotoxicity of organic chemicals frequently found in the air of mobile homes. Toxicol. Lett. 25, 33–40.

Conway, G.A., Slocumb, J.C., 1979. Plants used as abortifacients and emmenagogues by Spanish New Mexicans. J. Ethnopharmacol. 1, 241–261.

Coombs, H.C., Pike, F.H., 1931. Respiratory and cardio-vascular changes in the cat during convulsions of experimental origin. Am. J. Physiol. 97, 92–106.

Co-operative Group for Essential Oil of Garlic, 1986. The effect of essential oil of garlic on hyperlipemia and platelet aggregation – an analysis of 308 cases. J. Tradit. Chin. Med. 6, 117–120.

Corasaniti, M.T., Maiuolo, J., Maida, S., et al., 2007. Cell signaling pathways in the mechanisms of neuroprotection afforded by bergamot essential oil against NMDA-induced cell death *in vitro*. Br. J. Pharmacol. 151, 518–529.

Corazza, M., Mantovani, L., Maranini, C., Virgili, A., 1996. Allergic contact dermatitis from benzyl alcohol. Contact Dermatitis 34, 74–75.

Cornwell, P.A., Barry, B.W., Bootstrap, J.A., et al., 1996. Modes of action of terpene penetration enhancers in human skin; differential scanning calorimetry, small-angle X-ray diffraction and enhancer uptake studies. Int. J. Pharm. 127, 9–26.

Cornwell, C.P., Leach, D.N., Wyllie, S.G., 1999. The origin of terpinen-4-ol in the steam distillates of *Melaleuca argentea M. dissitiflora and M. linariifolia*. Journal of Essential Oil Research 11, 49–53.

Corthay, J., Medilanski, P., Benakis, A., 1977. Induction of hepatic microsomal enzymes by diuron, phenobenzuron, and metabolites in rats. Ecotoxicol. Environ. Saf. 1, 197–202.

Cortopassi, G.A., Wang, E., 1996. There is substantial agreement among interspecies estimates of DNA repair activity. Mech. Ageing Dev. 91, 211–218.

Cosmetic Ingredient Review Expert Panel, 2003. Safety assessment of salicylic acid, butyloctyl salicylate, calcium salicylate, C12–15 alkyl salicylate, capryloyl salicylic acid, hexyldodecyl salicylate, isocetyl salicylate, isodecyl salicylate, magnesium salicylate, MEA-salicylate, ethylhexyl salicylate, potassium salicylate, methyl salicylate, myristyl salicylate, sodium salicylate, TEA-salicylate, and tridecyl salicylate. Int. J. Toxicol. 22 (Suppl. 3), 1–108.

Cosmetic Ingredient Review Expert Panel, 2011. Tentative amended safety assessment of benzyl alcohol and benzoic acid and its salts and benzyl ester. CIR website: http://www.cir-safety.org/newreports.shtml (accessed 27.07.11.).

Costa, C.A., Bidinotto, L.T., Takahira, R.K., 2011. Cholesterol reduction and lack of genotoxic or toxic effects in mice after repeated 21-day oral intake of lemongrass (*Cymbopogon citratus*) essential oil. Food Chem. Toxicol. 49, 2268–2272.

Cotruvo, J.A., Simmon, V.F., Spanggord, R.J., 1977. Investigation of mutagenic effects of products of ozonation reactions in water. Ann. N. Y. Acad. Sci. 298, 124.

Coulson, I.H., Khan, A.S.A., 1999. Facial 'pillow' dermatitis due to lavender oil allergy. Contact Dermatitis 41, 111.

Council of Europe, 1992. Flavouring substances and natural sources of flavourings, Part 1, fourth ed. Maisonneuve, Strasbourg.

Council of Europe, 1999. Committee of Experts on Flavouring Substances 41st Meeting. RD 4.12/1–45. Datasheet on (R)-(+)-menthofuran.

Council of Europe, 2000. Committee of Experts on Flavouring Substances 47th Meeting. RD 4.6/1–47. Datasheet on eucalyptol.

Council of Europe, 2003. Committee of Experts on Flavouring Substances 51st Session RD 51 Rec. Strasbourg.

Coutts, I., Shaw, S., Orton, D., 2002. Patch testing with pure tea tree oil – 12 months experience. Br. J. Dermatol. 147 (Suppl. 62), 70.

Cox, D., O'Kennedy, R., Thornes, R.D., 1989. The rarity of liver toxicity in patients treated with coumarin (1,2-benzopyrone). Hum. Toxicol. 8, 501–506.

Coy, V., 2005. Genetics of essential hypertension. J. Am. Acad. Nurse. Pract. 17, 219–224.

Cragan, J.D., Friedman, J.M., Holmes, L.B., et al., 2006. Ensuring the safe and effective use of medications during pregnancy: planning and prevention through preconception care. Matern. Child Health J. 10, S129–S135.

Craig, J.O., 1953. Poisoning by the volatile oils in childhood. Arch. Dis. Child. 28, 475–483.

Craig, J.O., Fraser, M.S., 1953. Accidental poisoning in childhood. Arch. Dis. Child. 28, 259–267.

Craig, A.M., Karchesy, J.J., Blythe, L.L., et al., 2004. Toxicity studies on western juniper oil (*Juniperus occidentalis*) and Port-Orford-cedar oil (*Chamaecyparis lawsoniana*) extracts utilizing local lymph node and acute dermal irritation assays. Toxicol. Lett. 154, 217–224.

Craker, L.E., Simon, J.E., 1986. Herbs, spices, and medicinal plants: recent advances in botany, horticulture, & pharmacology, vol. 1. Oryx Press, Phoenix.

Craker, L.E., Simon, J.E., 1987. Herbs, spices, and medicinal plants: recent advances in botany, horticulture, and pharmacology, vol. 2. Oryx Press, Phoenix.

Crandon, K.L., Thompson, J.P., 2006. Olbas Oil and respiratory arrest in a child. Clin. Toxicol. 44, 568.

Craveiro, A.A., Andrade, C.H., Matos, F.J., et al., 1979. Essential oils from Brazilian *Rutaceae*. I. Genus *Pilocarpus*. J. Nat. Prod. 42, 669–671.

Crawford, G.H., Katz, K.A., Ellis, E., et al., 2004. Use of aromatherapy products and increased risk of hand dermatitis in massage therapists. Arch. Dermatol. 140, 991–996.

Crawford, M.J., Lehman, L., Slater, S., et al., 2009. Menstrual migraine in adolescents. Headache 49, 341–347.

Cremer, D., Hausen, B.M., Schmalle, H.W., 1987. Toward a rationalization of the sensitising potency of substituted *p*-benzoquinones: reaction of nucleophiles with *p*-benzoquinones. J. Med. Chem. 30, 1678–1681.

Crocker, T.T., Sanders, L.L., 1970. Influence of vitamin A and 3,7-dimethyl-2,6-octadienal (citral) on the effect of benzo(a)pyrene on hamster trachea in organ culture. Cancer Res. 30, 1312–1318.

Cronin, E., 1979. Oil of turpentine - a disappearing allergen. Contact Dermatitis 5, 308–311.

Cronin, M.T.D., Dearden, J.C., Moss, G.P., et al., 1999. Investigation of the mechanism of flux across human skin in vitro by quantitative structure-permeability relationships. Eur. J. Pharm. Sci. 7, 325–330.

Cross, S.E., Roberts, M., 2006. In-vitro human epidermal membrane penetration of tea tree oil components from pure oil and a 20% formulation. A report to RIRDC (Australian Rural Industry Research and Development Corporation).

Cross, S.E., Anderson, C., Thompson, M.J., et al., 1997. Is there tissue penetration after application of topical salicylate formulations? Lancet 350, 636.

Cross, S.E., Anderson, C., Roberts, M.S., 1998. Topical penetration of commercial salicylate esters and salts using human isolated skin and clinical microdialysis studies. Br. J. Clin. Pharmacol. 46, 29–35.

Cross, S.E., Megwa, S.A., Benson, H.A.E., et al., 1999. Self promotion of deep tissue penetration and distribution of methyl salicylate after topical application. Pharm. Res. 16, 427–433.

Cross, S.E., Russell, M., Southwell, I., et al., 2008. Human skin penetration of the major components of Australian tea tree oil applied in its pure form and as a 20% solution in vitro. Eur. J. Pharm. Biopharm. 69, 214–222.

Crowell, P.L., 1999. Prevention and therapy of cancer by dietary monoterpenes. J. Nutr. 129, 775S–778S.

Crowell, P.L., Lin, S., Vedejs, E., et al., 1992. Identification of metabolites of the antitumor agent *d*-limonene capable of inhibiting protein isoprenylation and cell growth. Cancer Chemother. Pharmacol. 31, 205–212.

Crowell, P.L., Elson, C.E., Bailey, H.H., et al., 1994a. Human metabolism of the experimental cancer therapeutic agent *d*-limonene. Cancer Chemother. Pharmacol. 35, 31–37.

Crowell, P.L., Ren, Z., Lin, S., et al., 1994b. Structure-activity relationships among monoterpene inhibitors of protein isoprenylation and cell proliferation. Biochem. Pharmacol. 47, 1405–1415.

Crowell, P.L., Siar Ayoubi, A., Burke, Y.D., 1996. Antitumorigenic effects of limonene and perillyl alcohol against pancreatic and breast cancer. Adv. Exp. Med. Biol. 401, 131–136.

CSTEE, 2001. Opinion on the results of the Risk Assessment of cyclohexane European Commission. Brussels,C2/JCD/csteeop/CycloHH09012002/D(02).http://ec.europa.eu/food/fs/sc/sct/out134_en.pdf

Culpeper, N., 1652. The English Physitian, or an Astro-physical discourse of the vulgar herbs of this nation. Being a compleat method of physick, whereby a man may preserve his body in health; or cure himself, being sick. Thomas Kelly, London.

Currie, G.P., Ayres, J.G., 2004. Assessment of bronchial responsiveness following exposure to inhaled occupational and environmental agents. Toxicol. Rev. 23, 75–81.

Cvetko, B., Vodopivec, S., Vatovec, S., 1973. Elektroencefalografske spremembe v epilepticnem statusu sprozenem z oljem morskega pelina. Neuropsihijatrija 21, 297–300.

Czygan, F.C., 1987. Warnung vor unkritischem Gebrauch von Wacholderbeeren. Zeitschrift für Phytotherapie 8, 10.

Daba, M.H., Abdel-Rahman, M.S., 1998. Hepatoprotective activity of thymoquinone in isolated rat hepatocytes. Toxicol. Lett. 95, 23–29.

Dadkhah, A., Allameh, A., Khalafi, H., et al., 2011. Inhibitory effects of dietary caraway essential oils on 1,2-dimethylhydrazine-induced colon carcinogenesis is mediated by liver xenobiotic metabolizing enzymes. Nutr. Cancer 63, 46–54.

Da Fonseca, C.O., Schwartsmann, G., Fischer, J., et al., 2008. Preliminary results from a phase I/II study of perillyl alcohol intranasal administration in adults with recurrent malignant gliomas. Surg. Neurol. 70, 259–266.

Dahl, A.R., Waruszewski, B.A., 1989. Metabolism of organonitriles to cyanide by rat nasal tissue enzymes. Xenobiotica 19, 1201–1205.

Daimon, H., Sawada, S., Asakura, S., et al., 1997a. Analysis of cytogenetic effects and DNA adduct formation induced by safrole in Chinese hamster lung cells. Teratog. Carcinog. Mutagen. 17, 7–18.

Daimon, H., Sawada, S., Asakura, S., et al., 1997. Inhibition of sulfotransferase affecting in vivo genotoxicity and DNA adducts induced by safrole in rat liver. Teratog. Carcinog. Mutagen 17, 327–337.

Daimon, H., Sawada, S., Asakura, S., et al., 1998. In vivo genotoxicity and DNA adduct levels in the liver of rats treated with safrole. Carcinogenesis 19, 141–146.

Dalle Carbonare, M., Pathak, M.A., 1992. Skin photosensitizing agents and the role of reactive oxygen species in photoaging. J. Photochem. Photobiol. B. 14, 105–124.

Dalton, P., 1999. Cognitive influences on health symptoms from acute chemical exposure. Health Psychol. 18, 579–590.

Dalton, P., 2003. Upper airway irritation, odor perception and health risk due to airborne chemicals. Toxicol. Lett. 140–141, 239–248.

Dalton, P., Doolittle, N., Breslin, P.A., 2002. Gender-specific induction of enhanced sensitivity to odors. Nat. Neurosci. 5, 199–200.

Damas, J., Deflandre, E., 1984. The mechanism of the anti-inflammatory effect of turpentine in the rat. Naunyn Schmiedebergs Arch. Pharmacol. 327, 143–147.

Damiani, C.E., Moreira, C.M., Zhang, H.T., et al., 2004. Effects of eugenol, an essential oil, on the mechanical and electrical activities of cardiac muscle. J. Cardiovasc. Pharmacol. 44, 688–695.

Dandiya, P.C., Menon, M.K., 1963. Effects of asarone and β-asarone on conditioned responses, fighting behaviour and convulsions. Br. J. Pharmacol. Chemother. 20, 436–442.

Dandiya, P.C., Sharma, J.D., 1962. Studies on *Acorus calamus*. Part V. Pharmacological actions of asarone and β-asarone on central nervous system. Indian J. Med. Res. 50, 46–60.

Danneman, P.J., Booman, K.A., Dorsky, J., et al., 1983. Cinnamic aldehyde: a survey of consumer patch-test sensitization. Food Chem. Toxicol. 21, 721–725.

D'Aprile, F., 1928. Studio clinico-sperimentale sull'intossicazione da apiolo. Annali di Ostetricia e Ginecologia 50, 1204–1227.

Darben, T., Cominos, B., Lee, C.T., 1998. Topical eucalyptus oil poisoning. Australian Journal of Dermatology 39, 265–267.

Darnall, B.D., Suarez, E.C., 2009. Sex and gender in psychoneuroimmunology research: past, present and future. Brain Behav. Immun. 23, 595–604.

Darra, E., Lenaz, G., Cavalieri, E., et al., 2007. *a*-Bisabolol: unexpected plant-derived weapon in the struggle against tumour survival? Ital. J. Biochem. 56, 323–328.

Darra, E., Abdel-Azeim, S., Manara, A., et al., 2008. Insight into the apoptosis-inducing action of *a*-bisabolol towards malignant tumor cells: involvement of lipid rafts and Bid. Arch. Biochem. Biophys. 476, 113–123.

Dasgupta, R., Saha, I., Pal, S., et al., 2006. Immunosuppression, hepatotoxicity and depression of antioxidant status by arecoline in albino mice. Toxicology 227, 94–104.

Da Silva, S.L., Figueiredo, P.M., Yano, T., 2007. Chemotherapeutic potential of the volatile oils from *Zanthoxylum rhoifolium* Lam leaves. Eur. J. Pharmacol. 576, 180–188.

Da Silva, S.L., Chaar, J.S., Figueiredo, P.M., et al., 2008. Cytotoxic evaluation of essential oil from *Casearia sylvestris* Sw on human cancer cells and erythrocytes. Acta Amazonica 38, 107–112.

Daston, G.P., Rehnberg, B.F., Carver, B., et al., 1988. Functional teratogens of the rat kidney. I. Colchicine, dinoseb, and methyl salicylate. Fundam. Appl. Toxicol. 11, 381–400.

Datnow, M.M., 1928. An experimental investigation concerning toxic abortion produced by chemical agents. J. Obstet. Gynaecol. 35, 693–724.

Daughtrey, W.C., Eutermoser, M., Thompson, S.W., et al., 1989a. A subchronic toxicity study of octyl acetate in rats. Fundam. Appl. Toxicol. 12, 313–320.

Daughtrey, W.C., Wier, P.J., Traul, K.A., et al., 1989b. Evaluation of the teratogenic potential of octyl acetate in rats. Fundam. Appl. Toxicol. 12, 303–309.

Davies, M.G., Hodgson, G.A., Evans, E., 1978. Contact dermatitis from an ostomy deodorant. Contact Dermatitis 4, 11–13.

Davis, C.A., 1970. Studies on identification of the causative agent in aspirin teratogenesis in the rat. Anat. Rec. 166, 295.

Davis, P., 1988. Aromatherapy an A–Z. CW Daniel, Saffron Walden.

Davis, P., 1999. Aromatherapy an A–Z. CW Daniel, Saffron Walden.

Davison, C., Zimmerman, E.F., Smith, P.K., 1961. On the metabolism and toxicity of methyl salicylate. J. Pharmacol. Exp. Ther. 132, 207–211.

Dawson, A.N., Walser, B., Jafarzadeh, M., et al., 2004. Topical analgesics and blood pressure during static contraction in humans. Med. Sci. Sports Exerc. 36, 632–638.

Day, L.M., Ozanne-Smith, J., 1997. Eucalyptus oil poisoning among young children: mechanisms of access and the potential for prevention. Aust. N. Z. J. Public Health 21, 297–302.

Dayawansa, S., Umeno, K., Takakura, H., et al., 2003. Autonomic responses during inhalation of natural fragrance of cedrol in humans. Auton. Neurosci. 108, 79–86.

Dayton, L., 1993. T-shirts find their place in the sun. New Sci. 139, 19.

Deans, S.G., Noble, R.C., Penzes, L., et al., 1993. Promotional effects of plant volatile oils on the polyunsaturated fatty acid status during aging. Age 16, 71–74.

Deans, S.G., Noble, R.C., Hiltunen, R., et al., 1995. Antimicrobial and antioxidant properties of Syzygium aromaticum (L.) Merr. & Perry: impact upon bacteria, fungi and fatty acid levels in ageing mice. Flavour & Fragrance Journal 10, 323–328.

Deb, D.D., Parimala, G., Saravana Devi, S., et al., 2011. Effect of thymol on peripheral blood mononuclear cell PBMC and acute promyelotic cancer cell line HL-60. Chem. Biol. Interact. 193, 97–106.

Debersac, P., Heydel, J.M., Amiot, M.J., et al., 2001. Induction of cytochrome P450 and/or detoxication enzymes by various extracts of rosemary: description of specific patterns. Food Chem. Toxicol. 39, 907–918.

Decapite, T.J., Anderson, B.E., 2004. Allergic contact dermatitis from cinnamic aldehyde found in an industrial odour-masking agent. Contact Dermatitis 51, 312–313.

Decocq, G., Dol, L., Leroy, D., et al., 1996. Lipid pneumonia after aerosol therapy with gomenol in a 4 month old child. Presse Méd. 25, 994–995.

De Feo, V., De Simone, F., Senatore, F., 2002. Potential allelochemicals from the essential oil of Ruta graveolens. Phytochemistry 61, 573–578.

De Freitas, T.G., Augusto, P.M., Montanari, T., 2005. Effect of Ruta graveolens L. on pregnant mice. Contraception 71, 74–77.

De Groot, A.C., 1987. Contact allergy to cosmetics: causative ingredients. Contact Dermatitis 17, 26–34.

De Groot, A.C., 1996. Airborne allergic contact dermatitis from tea tree oil. Contact Dermatitis 35, 304–305.

De Groot, A.C., Frosch, P.J., 1998. Fragrances as a cause of contact dermatitis in cosmetics: clinical aspects and epidemiological data. In: Frosch, P.J., Johansen, J.D., White, I.R. (Eds.), Fragrances, beneficial and adverse effects. Springer, Berlin.

De Groot, A.C., Liem, D.H., 1983. Facial psoriasis caused by contact allergy to linalool and hydroxycitronellal in an after-shave. Contact Dermatitis 9, 230–232.

De Groot, A.C., Weyland, J.W., 1992. Systemic contact dermatitis from tea tree oil. Contact Dermatitis 27, 279–280.

De Groot, A.C., Weyland, J.W., 1993. Contact allergy to tea tree oil. Contact Dermatitis 28, 309.

De Groot, A.C., Liem, D.H., Nater, J.P., et al., 1985. Patch tests with fragrance materials and preservatives. Contact Dermatitis 12, 87–92.

De Groot, A.C., Weyland, J.W., Bos, J.D., et al., 1986. Contact allergy to preservatives (I). Contact Dermatitis 14, 120–122.

De Groot, A.C., Bruynzeel, D.P., Bos, J.D., et al., 1988. The allergens in cosmetics. AMA Arch. Derm. 124, 1525–1529.

De Groot, A.C., van der Kley, A.M.J., Bruynzeel, D.P., et al., 1993. Frequency of false-negative reactions to the fragrance mix. Contact Dermatitis 28, 139–140.

De Groot, A.C., Coenraads, P.J., Bruynzeel, D.P., et al., 2000. Routine patch testing with fragrance chemicals in the Netherlands. Contact Dermatitis 42, 184–185.

Dekebo, A., Dagne, E., Sterner, O., 2002. Furanosesquiterpenes from Commiphora sphaerocarpa and related adulterants of true myrrh. Fitoterapia 73, 48–55.

Delaforge, M., Janiaud, P., Levi, P., et al., 1980. Biotransformation of allylbenzene analogues in vivo and in vitro through the epoxide-diol pathway. Xenobiotica 10, 737–744.

Delaney, T.A., Donnelly, A.M., 1996. Garlic dermatitis. Australas. J. Dermatol. 37, 109–110.

Del Beccaro, M.A., 1995. Melaleuca oil poisoning in a 17-month-old. Vet. Hum. Toxicol. 37, 557–558.

Del Castillo, J., Anderson, M., Rubottom, G.M., 1975. Marijuana, absinthe and the central nervous system. Nature 253, 365–366.

Deleo, V.A., Taylor, S.C., Belsito, D.V., 2002. The effect of race and ethnicity on patch test results. J. Am. Acad. Dermatol. 46, S107–S112.

Delgado, I.F., De Almeida Nogeira, A.C., Souza, C.A., et al., 1993a. Peri- and postnatal developmental toxicity of beta-myrcene in the rat. Food Chem. Toxicol. 31, 623–628.

Delgado, I.F., Carvalho, R.R., De Almeida Nogeira, A.C., et al., 1993b. Study on the embryo-foetotoxicity of β-myrcene in the rat. Food Chem. Toxicol. 31, 31–35.

Del Toro-Arreola, S., Flores-Torales, E., Torres-Lozano, 2005. Effect of d-limonene on immune response in BALB/c mice with lymphoma. Int. Immunopharmacol. 5, 829–838.

Demarquay, G., Royet, J.P., Mick, G., et al., 2008. Olfactory hypersensitivity in migraineurs: a H(2)(15)O-PET study. Cephalalgia 28, 1069–1080.

De Martino, L., De Feo, V., Nazzaro, F., 2009a. Chemical composition and in vitro antimicrobial and mutagenic activities of seven Lamiaciae essential oils. Molecules 14, 4213–4230.

De Martino, L., D'Arena, G., Minervini, M.M., et al., 2009b. Verbena officinalis essential oil and its component citral as apoptotic-inducing agent in chronic lymphocytic leukemia. Int. J. Immunopathol. Pharmacol. 22, 1097–1104.

De Medici, D., Pieretti, S., Salvatore, G., et al., 1992. Chemical analysis of essential oils of Malagasy medicinal plants by gas chromatography and NMR spectroscopy. Flavour & Fragrance Journal 7, 275–281.

Demeter, S.L., Cordasco, E.M., Guidotti, T.L., 2001. Permanent respiratory impairment and upper airway symptoms despite clinical improvement in patients with reactive airways dysfunction syndrome. Sci. Total Environ. 270, 49–55.

Demir, E., Kocaoglu, S., Kaya, B., 2008. Genotoxicity testing of four benzyl derivatives in the Drosophila wing spot test. Food Chem. Toxicol. 46, 1034–1041.

Demir, E., Kocaoglu, S., Kaya, B., 2010. Assessment of genotoxic effects of benzyl derivatives by the comet assay. Food Chem. Toxicol. 48, 1239–1242.

Demirci, F., Paper, D.H., Franz, G., et al., 2004. Investigation of the Origanum onites L. essential oil using the chorioallantoic membrane (CAM) assay. J Agric. Food Chem. 52, 251–254.

Denda, M., Tsuchiya, T., Elias, P.M., et al., 2000. Stress alters cutaneous permeability barrier homeostasis. Am. J. Physiol. Regul. Integr. Comp. Physiol. 278, R367–R372.

De-Oliveira, A.C., Ribeiro-Pinto, L.F., Paumgartten, F.J.R., 1997a. In vitro inhibition of CYP2B1 monooxygenase by β-myrcene and other monoterpenoid compounds. Toxicol. Lett. 92, 39–46.

De-Oliveira, A.C., Ribeiro-Pinto, L.F., Otto, S.S., et al., 1997b. Induction of liver monooxygenases by β-myrcene. Toxicology 124, 135–140.

De-Oliveira, A.C., Fidalgo-Neto, A.A., Paumgartten, F.J., 1999. In vitro inhibition of liver monooxygenases by β-ionone, 1,8-cineole, (−)-menthol and terpineol. Toxicology 135, 33–41.

Department of Health, 1998. 1996 Report of the committees on toxicity, mutagenicity, carcinogenicity of chemicals in food, consumer products and the environment. The Stationery Office, London.

De Pascual-T, J., Bellido, I.S., Torres, C., Pérez, M.A., 1980. Essential oil from Chenopodium ambroisioides. Rivista Italiana EPPOS 62, 123–125.

De Smet, P.A.G.M., Keller, K., Hänsel, R., Chandler, R.F. (Eds.), 1992. In: Adverse effects of herbal drugs, vol. 1. Springer-Verlag, Heidelberg.

De Smet, P.A.G.M., Keller, K., Hänsel, R., Chandler, R.F. (Eds.), 1993. In: Adverse effects of herbal drugs, vol. 2. Springer-Verlag, Heidelberg.

De Smet, R., Van Kaer, J., Van Vlem, B., et al., 2003. Toxicity of free p-cresol: a prospective and cross-sectional analysis. Clin. Chem. 49, 470–478.

De Sousa, A.C., Alviano, D.S., Blank, A.F., et al., 2004. Melissa officinalis L. essential oil: antitumoral and antioxidant activities. J. Pharm. Pharmacol. 56, 677–681.

De Sousa, D.P., Gonçalves, J.C., Quintans-Júnior, L., et al., 2006. Study of anticonvulsant effect of citronellol, a monoterpene alcohol, in rodents. Neurosci. Lett. 401, 231–235.

De Sousa, D.P., De Farias Nóbrega, F.F., De Almeida, R.N., 2007. Influence of the chirality of (R)-(−)- and (S)-(+)-carvone in the central nervous system: a comparative study. Chirality 19, 264–268.

De Sousa, D.P., Nóbrega, F.F., De Morais, L.C., et al., 2009. Evaluation of the anticonvulsant activity of terpinen-4-ol. Z. Naturforsch. B 64, 1–5.

Dettling, A., Grass, H., Schuff, A., et al., 2004. Absinthe: attention performance and mood under the influence of thujone. J. Stud. Alcohol. 65, 573–581.

De Vincenzi, M., Silano, M., Stacchini, P., et al., 2000a. Constituents of aromatic plants: I. Methyleugenol. Methyleugenol. Fitoterapia 71, 216–221.

De Vincenzi, M., Silano, M., Maialetti, F., et al., 2000b. Constituents of aromatic plants: II. Estragole. Fitoterapia 71, 725–729.

De Wolff, F.A., Thomas, T.V., 1986. Clinical pharmacokinetics of methoxsalen and other psoralens. Clin. Pharmacokinet. 11, 62–75.

DFG – Senate Commission on Food Safety, 2006. Toxicological assessment of furocoumarins in foodstuffs. http://www.dfg.de/download/pdf/dfg_im_profil/reden_stellungnahmen/2006/sklm_furocoumarine_en_2006.pdf.

Dhalla, N.S., Malhotra, C.L., Sastry, M.S., 1961. Effect of Acorus oil in vitro on the respiration of rat brain. J. Pharm. Sci. 50, 580–582.

Dhar, S.K., 1995. Anti-fertility activity and hormonal profile of trans-anethole in rats. Indian J. Physiol. Pharmacol. 391, 63–67.

Dhar, M.L., Dhar, M.M., Dhawan, B.N., et al., 1968. Screening of Indian plants for biological activity. Part I. Indian J. Exp. Biol. 6, 232.

Dharmagunawardena, B., Takwale, A., Sanders, K.J., et al., 2002. Gas chromatography: an investigative tool in multiple allergies to essential oils. Contact Dermatitis 47, 288–292.

Di, Y.M., Chow, V.D., Yang, L.P., et al., 2009. Structure, function, regulation and polymorphism of human cytochrome P450 2A6. Curr. Drug Metab. 10, 754–780.

Diamond, J., Dalton, P., Doolittle, N., et al., 2005. Gender-specific olfactory sensitization: hormonal and cognitive influences. Chem. Senses 30, i224–i225.

Diawara, M.M., Kulkosky, P.J., 2003. Reproductive toxicity of the psoralens. Pediatr. Pathol. Mol. Med. 22, 247–258.

Diawara, M.M., Chavez, K.J., Hoyer, P.B., et al., 1999. A novel group of ovarian toxicants: the psoralens. J. Biochem. Mol. Toxicol. 13, 195–203.

Diawara, M.M., Williams, D.E., Oganesian, A., et al., 2000. Dietary psoralens induce hepatotoxicity in C57 mice. J. Nat. Toxins 9, 179–195.

Diawara, M.M., Chavez, K.J., Simpleman, D., et al., 2001. The psoralens adversely affect reproductive function in male Wistar rats. Reprod. Toxicol. 15, 137–144.

Diba, V.C., Statham, B.N., 2003. Contact urticaria from cinnamal leading to anaphylaxis. Contact Dermatitis 46, 119.

Di Bella, G., Saitta, M., Pellegrino, M., et al., 1999. Contamination of Italian citrus essential oils: presence of phthalate esters. J. Agric. Food Chem. 47, 1009–1012.

Di Bella, G., Saitta, M., La Pera, L., et al., 2004. Pesticide and plasticizer residues in bergamot essential oils from Calabria (Italy). Chemosphere 56, 777–782.

Dickel, H., Taylor, J.S., Evey, P., et al., 2001. Comparison of patch test results with a standard series among white and black racial groups. Am. J. Contact Dermat. 12, 77–82.

Dickins, M., Bridges, J.W., Elcombe, C.R., et al., 1978. A novel haemoprotein induced by isosafrole pretreatment in the rat. Biochem. Biophys. Res. Commun. 80, 89–96.

Diego, M.A., Jones, N.A., Field, T., et al., 1998. Aromatherapy positively affects mood, EEG patterns of alertness and math computations. Int. J. Neurosci. 96, 217–224.

Diel, P., Smolnikar, K., Michna, H., 1999. In vitro test systems for the evaluation of the estrogenic activity of natural products. Planta Med. 65, 197–203.

Dieter, M.P., Goehl, T.J., Jameson, C.W., et al., 1993. Comparison of the toxicity of citral in F344 rats and B6C3F$_1$ mice when administered by microencapsulation in feed or by corn-oil gavage. Food Chem. Toxicol. 31, 463–474.

Dietrich, D.R., Swenberg, J.A., 1991. The presence of alpha 2u-globulin is necessary for d-limonene promotion of male rat kidney tumors. Cancer Res. 51, 3512–3521.

Dikshith, T.S., Kumar, S.N., Tandon, G.S., et al., 1989. Pesticide residues in edible oils and oil seeds. Bull. Environ. Contam. Toxicol. 42, 50–56.

Diliberto, J.J., Usha, G., Birnbaum, L.S., 1988a. Disposition of citral in male Fischer rats. Drug Metab. Dispos. 16, 721–727.

Diliberto, J.J., Usha, G., Burka, L.T., et al., 1988b. Biotransformation of citral in rats. Toxicologist 8, 208.

Dillon, D., Combes, R., Zeiger, E., 1998. The effectiveness of Salmonella strains TA100, TA102 and TA104 for detecting mutagenicity of some aldehydes and peroxides. Mutagenesis 13, 19–26.

Dimas, K., Kokkinopoulos, D., Demetzos, C., et al., 1999. The effect of sclareol on growth and cell cycle progression of human leukemic cell lines. Leuk. Res. 23, 217–234.

Dimas, K., Demetzos, C., Vaos, V., et al., 2001. Labdane type diterpenes down-regulate the expression of c-Myc protein, but not of Bcl-2, in human leukemia T-cells undergoing apoptosis. Leuk. Res. 25, 449–454.

Dimas, K., Papadaki, M., Tsimplouli, C., et al., 2006. Labd-14-ene-8,13-diol (sclareol) induces cell cycle arrest and apoptosis in human breast cancer cells and enhances the activity of anticancer drugs. Biomed. Pharmacother. 60, 127–133.

Din, J.K., 1983. The chemical composition of the Yunnan pine oil. Acta Botanica Yunnanica 5 (2), 250.

Dip, E.C., Pereira, N.A., Fernandes, P.D., 2004. Ability of eugenol to reduce tongue edema induced by Dieffenbachia picta Schott in mice. Toxicon 43, 729–735.

Dirsch, V.M., Stuppner, H., Vollmar, A.M., 2001. Cytotoxic sesquiterpene lactones mediate their death-inducing effect in leukemia T cells by triggering apoptosis. Planta Med. 67, 557–559.

Di Sotto, A., Evandri, M.G., Mazzanti, G., 2008. Antimutagenic and mutagenic activities of some terpenes in the bacterial reverse mutation assay. Mutat. Res. 653, 130–133.

Di Stefano, V., Pitonzo, R., Schillaci, D., 2011. Antimicrobial and antiproliferative activity of Athamanta sicula L. (Apiaceae). Pharmacognosy Magazine 7, 31–34.

Dixon, R.A., Ferreira, D., 2002. Genistein. Phytochemistry 60, 205–211.

Dixon, K., Kopras, E., 2004. Genetic alterations and DNA repair in human carcinogenesis. Semin. Cancer Biol. 14, 441–448.

Dmitrieva, N.M., Rubchinska, K.I., Svishchuk, A.A., 1962. Comparison of the effect of synthetic and natural menthol. Khimiko-Farmatsevticheskii Zhurnal 17, 53–57.

Dohare, P., Garg, P., Sharma, U., et al., 2008. Neuroprotective efficacy and therapeutic window of curcuma oil: in rat embolic stroke model. BMC. Complement. Altern. Med. 8, 55.

Doak, S.H., Jenkins, G.J., Johnson, G.E., 2007. Mechanistic influences for mutation induction curves after exposure to DNA-reactive carcinogens. Cancer. Res 67, 3904–3911.

Doimo, L., 2001. Azulenes, costols and γ-lactones from cypress-pines (Callitris columellaris, C. glaucophylla and C. intratropica) distilled oils and methanol extracts. Journal of Essential Oil Research 13, 25–29.

Domaracky, M., Rehak, P., Juhas, S., et al., 2007. Effects of selected plant essential oils on the growth and development of mouse preimplantation embryos in vivo. Physiol. Res. 56, 97–104.

Dong, J.Y., Xue, L.Q., Zhu, X.W., et al., 1981. Antifertility agents from seeds of Daucus carota. Zhongcaoyao 12, 61.

Dooms-Goossens, A., Deleu, H., 1991. Airborne contact dermatitis: an update. Contact Dermatitis 25, 211–217.

Dooms-Goossens, A., Degreef, H., Holvoet, C., et al., 1977. Turpentine-induced hypersensitivity to peppermint oil. Contact Dermatitis 3, 304–308.

Doppalapudi, R.S., Riccio, E.S., Rausch, L.L., et al., 2007. Evaluation of chemopreventive agents for genotoxic activity. Mutat. Res. 629, 148–160.

Dorai, T., Aggarwal, B.B., 2004. Role of chemopreventive agents in cancer therapy. Cancer Lett. 215, 129–140.

Dorange, J.L., Delaforge, M., Janiaud, P., et al., 1977. Mutagenicity of the metabolites of the epoxide-diol pathway of safrole and its analogs. Study on Salmonella typhimurium. Comptes Rendues Société Biologique Fil 171, 1041–1048.

Dorman, H.J.D., Deans, S.G., Noble, R.C., 1995. Evaluation in vitro of plant essential oils as natural antioxidants. Journal of Essential Oil Research 7, 645–651.

Dorne, J.L., 2004. Impact of inter-individual differences in drug metabolism and pharmacokinetics on safety evaluation. Fundam. Clin. Pharmacol. 18, 609–620.

Dorne, J.L., Renwick, A.G., 2005. The refinement of uncertainty/safety factors in risk assessment by the incorporation of data on toxicokinetic variability in humans. Toxicol. Sci. 86, 20–26.

Dorsch, W., Adam, O., Weber, J., et al., 1984. Antiasthmatic effects of onion extracts - detection of benzyl- and other isothiocyanates (mustard oils) as antiasthmatic compounds of plant origin. Eur. J. Pharmacol. 107, 17–24.

Dorsch, W., Ettl, M., Hein, G., et al., 1987. Antiasthmatic effects of onions. Inhibition of platelet-activating factor-induced bronchial obstruction by onion oils. Int. Arch. Allergy Appl. Immunol. 82, 535–536.

Dorsch, W., Wagner, H., Bayer, T., et al., 1988. Anti-asthmatic effects of onions. Alk(en)ylsulfinothioic acid alk(en)yl-esters inhibit histamine release, leukotriene and thromboxane biosynthesis in vitro and counteract PAF and allergen-induced bronchial obstruction in vivo. Biochem. Pharmacol. 37, 4479–4486.

Dos Santos, M.A., Santos Galvao, C.E., Morato Castro, F., 2001. Menthol-induced asthma: a case report. J. Investig. Allergol. Clin. Immunol. 11, 56–58.

Dotterud, L.K., Smith-Sivertsen, T., 2007. Allergic contact sensitization in the general adult population: a population-based study from Northen Norway. Contact Dermatitis 56, 10–15.

Doty, R.L., Cameron, E.L., 2009. Sex differences and reproductive hormone influences on human odor perception. Physiol. Behav. 97, 213–228.

Dourson, M.L., Felter, S.P., Robinson, D., 1996. Evolution of science-based uncertainty factors in noncancer risk assessment. Regul. Toxicol. Pharmacol. 24, 108–120.

Do Vale, T.G., Furtado, E.C., Santos, J.G., et al., 2002. Central effects of citral, myrcene and limonene, constituents of essential oil chemotypes from *Lippia alba* (Mill.) n.e. Brown. Phytomedicine 9, 709–714.

Downum, K.R., 1992. Light-activated plant defence. New Phytol. 122, 401–420.

Drake, T.E., Maibach, H.I., 1976. Allergic contact dermatitis and stomatitis caused by a cinnamic aldehyde-flavored toothpaste. Arch. Dermatol. 112, 202–203.

Dresser, G.K., Bailey, D.G., 2003. The effects of fruit juices on drug disposition: a new model for drug interactions. Eur. J. Clin. Invest. 33 (Suppl. 2), 10–16.

Dresser, G.K., Wacher, V., Wong, S., et al., 2002. Evaluation of peppermint oil and ascorbyl palmitate as inhibitors of cytochrome P4503A4 activity *in vitro* and *in vivo*. Clin. Pharmacol. Ther. 72, 247–255.

Drinkwater, N.R., Miller, E.C., Miller, J.A., et al., 1976. Hepatocarcinogenicity of estragole (1-allyl-4-methoxybenzene) and 1′-hydroxyestragole in the mouse and mutagenicity of 1′–-acetoxyestragole in bacteria. J. Natl. Cancer Inst. 57, 1323–1331.

Dryden, M.S., Dailly, S., Crouch, M., 2004. A randomized, controlled trial of tea tree topical preparations versus a standard topical regimen for the clearance of MRSA colonization. J. Hosp. Infect. 56, 283–286.

Du, J., Bai, B., Kuang, X., 2006a. Ligustilide inhibits spontaneous and agonists- or K⁺ depolarization-induced contraction of rat uterus. J. Ethnopharmacol. 108, 54–58.

Du, L., Neis, M.M., Ladd, P.A., et al., 2006b. Effects of the differentiated keratinocyte phenotype on expression levels of CYP1–4 family genes in human skin cells. Toxicol. Appl. Pharmacol. 213, 135–144.

Duarte, I., Lazzarini, R., Bedrikow, R., 2002a. Excited skin syndrome: study of 39 patients. Am. J. Contact Dermat. 12, 59–65.

Duarte, I., Lazzarini, R., Buense, R., 2002b. Interference of the position of substances in an epicutaneous patch test battery with the occurrence of false-positive results. Am. J. Contact Dermat. 13, 125–132.

Dubertret, L., Morliére, P., Averbeck, D., et al., 1990a. The photochemistry and photobiology of bergamot oil as a perfume ingredient: an overview. J. Photochem. Photobiol. B. 7, 362–365.

Dubertret, L., Serraf-Tircazes, D., Jeanmougin, M., et al., 1990b. Phototoxic properties of perfumes containing bergamot oil on human skin: photoprotective effect of UVA and UVB sunscreens. J. Photochem. Photobiol. B. 7, 251–259.

Ducombs, G., Benezra, C., Talaga, P., et al., 1990. Patch testing with the "sesquiterpene lactone mix": a marker for contact allergy to Compositae and other sesquiterpene-lactone-containing plants. A multicentre study of the EECDRG. Contact Dermatitis 22, 249–252.

Dudai, N., Weinstein, Y., Krup, M., et al., 2005. Citral is a new inducer of caspase-3 in tumor cell lines. Planta Med. 71, 484–488.

Dudek, W., Wittczak, T., Swierczynska-Machura, D., 2009. Occupational asthma due to turpentine in art painter – case report. Int. J. Occup. Med. Environ. Health 22, 293–295.

Duessel, S., Heuertz, R.M., Ezekiel, U.R., 2008. Growth inhibition of human colon cancer cells by plant compounds. Clin. Lab. Sci. 21, 151–157.

Dugo, G., 1994. The composition of the volatile fraction of the Italian citrus essential oils. Perfumer & Flavorist 19, 29–51.

Dugo, G., Cotroneo, A., Trozzi, A., et al., 1988. On the genuineness of citrus essential oils. Part XXV. The essential oil from 'Wenzhou honey' oranges. Flavour & Fragrance Journal 3, 161–166.

Dugo, G., Crotoneo, A., Verzera, A., Dugo, G., 1990. Mapo tangelo essential oil (3 samples). Flavour & Fragrance Journal 5, 205–210.

Dugo, G., Mondello, L., Cotroneo, A., et al., 1996. Characterization of Italian citrus petitgrain oils. Perfumer & Flavorist 21, 17–28.

Dugo, G., Saitta, M., Di Bella, G., et al., 1997. Organophosphorus and organochlorine pesticide residues in Italian citrus oils. Perfumer & Flavorist 22, 33–44.

Dugo, P., Mondello, L., Sebastiani, E., et al., 1999a. Identification of minor oxygen heterocyclic compounds of citrus essential oils by liquid chromatography-atmospheric pressure chemical ionisation mass spectrometry. Journal of Liquid Chromatography & Related Technologies 22, 2991–3005.

Dugo, P., Mondello, L., Proteggente, A.R., et al., 1999b. Oxygen heterocyclic compounds of bergamot essential oils. Rivista Italiana EPPOS 27, 31–41.

Duisken, M., Benz, D., Peiffer, T.H., et al., 2005. Metabolism of delta(3)-carene by human cytochrome p450 enzymes: Identification and characterization of two new metabolites. Curr. Drug Metab. 6, 593–601.

Duke, J.A., 1985. Handbook of medicinal herbs. CRC Press, Boca Raton.

Duncan, R.E., Lau, D., El-Sohemy, A., et al., 2004. Geraniol and β-ionone inhibit proliferation, cell cycle progression, and cyclin-dependent kinase 2 activity in MCF-7 breast cancer cells independent of effects on HMG-CoA reductase activity. Biochem. Pharmacol. 68, 1739–1747.

Dundar, E., Olgun, E.G., Isiksoy, S., et al., 2008. The effects of intra-rectal and intra-peritoneal application of *Origanum onites* L. essential oil on 2,4,6-trinitrobenzenesulfonic acid-induced colitis in the rat. Exp. Toxicol. Pathol. 59, 399–408.

Dunn, G.P., Old, L.J., Schreiber, R.D., 2004. The immunobiology of cancer immunosurveillance and immunoediting. Immunity 21, 137–148.

Dunn, G.P., Koebel, C.M., Schreiber, R.D., 2006. Interferons, immunity and cancer immunoediting. Nat. Rev. Immunol. 6, 836–848.

Dunnick, J.K., Prejean, J.D., Haseman, J., et al., 1982. Carcinogenesis bioassay of allyl isothiocyanate. Fundam. Appl. Toxicol. 2, 114–120.

Dunnick, J.K., Forbes, P.D., Eustis, S.L., et al., 1991. Tumors of the skin in the HRA/Skh mouse after treatment with 8-methoxypsoralen and UVA radiation. Fundam. Appl. Toxicol. 16, 92–102.

Dupuis, G., Brisson, J., 1976. Toxic effect of alantolactone and dihydroatlantolactone in *in vitro* cultures of leukocytes. Chem. Biol. Interact. 15, 205–217.

Durant, S., Karran, P., 2003. Vanillins - a novel family of DNA-PK inhibitors. Nucleic Acids Res. 31, 5501–5512.

D'Urben, J., 1998. Letters to the Editor. Int. J. Aromather. 9, 46.

Durnas, C., Cusack, B.J., 1992. Salicylate intoxication in the elderly. Recognition and recommendations on how to prevent it. Drugs Aging 2, 20–34.

Dutt, S., 1940. New Indian essential oils. Indian Soap Journal 6 (2), 248–255.

Duty, S.M., Silva, M.J., Barr, D.B., et al., 2003. Phthalate exposure and human semen parameters. Epidemiology 14, 269–277.

Duvoix, A., Delhalle, S., Blasius, R., et al., 2004. Effect of chemopreventive agents on glutathione S-transferase P1–1 gene expression mechanisms via activating protein 1 and nuclear factor kappaB inhibition. Biochem. Pharmacol. 68, 1101–1111.

Dwivedi, C., Abu-Ghazaleh, A., 1997. Chemopreventive effects of sandalwood oil on skin papillomas in mice. Eur. J. Cancer Prev. 6, 399–401.

Dwivedi, C., Zhang, Y., 1999. Sandalwood oil prevent skin tumour development in CD1 mice. Eur. J. Cancer Prev. 8, 449–455.

Dwivedi, C., Guan, X., Harmsen, W.L., et al., 2003. Chemopreventive effects of α-santalol on skin tumor development in CD-1 and SENCAR mice. Cancer Epidemiol. Biomarkers Prev. 12, 151–156.

Dwivedi, C., Maydew, E.R., Hora, J.J., et al., 2005. Chemopreventive effects of various concentrations of α-santalol on skin cancer development in CD-1 mice. Eur. J. Cancer Prev. 14, 473–476.

Dwivedi, C., Valluri, H.B., Guan, X., et al., 2006. Chemopreventive effects of a-santalol on ultraviolet B radiation-induced skin tumor development in SKH-1 hairless mice. Carcinogenesis 27, 1917–1922.

Dybing, E., Doe, J., Groten, J., et al., 2002. Hazard characterisation of chemicals in food and diet: dose response, mechanisms and extrapolation issues. Food Chem. Toxicol. 40, 237–282.

Early, D.F., 1961. Pennyroyal: a rare case of epilepsy. Lancet 281, 580–581.

Ebadi, M., 2001. Pharmacodynamic basis of herbal medicine. CRC Press, USA.

Edenharder, R., Tang, X., 1997. Inhibition of the mutagenicity of 2-nitrofluorene, 3-nitrofluoranthene and 1-nitropyrene by flavonoids, coumarins, quinones and other phenolic compounds. Food Chem. Toxicol. 35, 357–372.

Eder, E., Neudecker, T., Lutz, D., et al., 1980. Mutagenic potential of allyl and allylic compounds: structure-activity relationship as determined by alkylating and direct in vitro mutagenic properties. Biochem. Pharmacol. 29, 993–998.

Eder, E., Neudecker, T., Lutz, D., et al., 1982. Correlation of alkylating and mutagenic activities of allyl and allylic compounds: standard alkylation test vs. kinetic investigation. Chem. Biol. Interact. 38, 303–315.

Eder, E., Deininger, C., Muth, D., 1991. Genotoxicity of p-nitrocinnamaldehyde and related alpha, beta-unsaturated carbonyl compounds in two bacterial assays. Mutagenesis 6, 261–269.

Eder, E., Deininger, C., Neudecker, T., et al., 1992. Mutagenicity of β-alkyl substituted acrolein congeners in the Salmonella typhimurium strain TA100 and genotoxicity testing in the SOS chromotest. Environ. Mol. Mutagen. 19, 338–345.

Edris, A.E., 2007. Pharmaceutical and therapeutic potentials of essential oils and their individual volatile constituents: a review. Phytother. Res. 21, 308–323.

Edwards, A.J., Price, R.J., Renwick, A.B., Lake, B.G., 2000. Lack of effect of coumarin on unscheduled DNA synthesis in the in vivo rat hepatocyte DNA repair test. Food Chem. Toxicol. 38, 403–409.

EFFA, 2008. Allergens and essential oils. www.nhrorganicoils.com/uploads/Allegens%20essential%20oils.pdf.

Efferth, T., Davey, M., Olbrich, A., et al., 2002a. Activity of drugs from traditional Chinese medicine toward sensitive and MDR1- or MRP1-overexpressing multidrug-resistant human CCRF-CEM leukemia cells. Blood Cells Mol. Dis. 28, 160–168.

Efferth, T., Olbrich, A., Sauerbrey, A., et al., 2002b. Activity of ascaridol from the anthelmintic herb Chenopodium anthelminticum L. against sensitive and multidrug-resistant tumor cells. Anticancer Res. 22, 4221–4224.

EFSA, 2004. Opinion of the scientific panel on food additives, flavourings, processing aids and materials in contact with food (AFC) related to coumarin. http://www.efsa.europa.eu/en/efsajournal/pub/104.htm.

Egan, D., O'Kennedy, R., Moran, E., et al., 1990. The pharmacology, metabolism, analysis, and applications of coumarin and coumarin-related compounds. Drug Metab. Rev. 22, 503–529.

Egen-Schwind, C., Eckard, R., Kemper, F.H., 1992. Metabolism of garlic constituents in the isolated perfused rat liver. Planta Med. 58, 301–305.

Egyed, M.N., Williams, M.C., 1977. Photosensitizing effects of Cymopterus watsonii and Cymopterus longipes in chickens and turkey poults. Avian Dis. 21, 566–575.

Ehlers, D., Pfister, M., Bork, W.R., et al., 1995. HPLC analysis of tonka bean extracts. Z. Lebensm. Unters. Forsch. 201, 278–282.

Eickholt, T.H., Box, R.H., 1965. Toxicities of peppermint and Pycnanthemun albescens oils, Fam. Labiateae. J. Pharm. Sci. 54, 1071–1072.

Eidi, M., Eidi, A., Zamanizadeh, H., 2005. Effect of Salvia officinalis L. leaves on serum glucose and insulin in healthy and streptozotocin-induced diabetic rats. J. Ethnopharmacol. 100, 310–313.

Eiermann, H.J., Larsen, W., Maibach, H.I., et al., 1982. Prospective study of cosmetic reactions: 1977–1980. Journal of the American Acadmey of Dermatology 6, 909–917.

Eimas, A., 1938. Methyl salicylate poisoning in an infant. Report of a patient with partial necropsy. J. Pediatr. 13, 550–554.

Eklind, K.I., Morse, M.A., Chung, F.L., 1990. Distribution and metabolism of the natural anticarcinogen phenethyl isothiocyanate in A/J mice. Carcinogenesis 11, 2033–2036.

El-Abhar, H.S., Abdallah, D.M., Saleh, S., 2003. Gastroprotective activity of Nigella sativa oil and its constituent, thymoquinone, against gastric mucosal injury induced by ischaemia/reperfusion in rats. J. Ethnopharmacol. 84, 251–258.

Elahi, E.N., Wright, Z., Hinselwood, D., et al., 2004. Protein binding and metabolism influence the relative skin sensitization potential of cinnamic compounds. Chem. Res. Toxicol. 17, 301–310.

Elberling, J., Linneberg, A., Mosbech, H., et al., 2004. A link between skin and airways regarding sensitivity to fragrance products? Br. J. Dermatol. 151, 1197–1203.

Elberling, J., Linneberg, A., Dirksen, A., et al., 2005. Mucosal symptoms elicited by fragrance products in a population-based sample in relation to atopy and bronchial hyper-reactivity. Clin. Exp. Allergy 35, 75–81.

Elberling, J., Duus Johansen, J., Dirksen, A., et al., 2006. Exposure of eyes to perfume: a double-blind, placebo-controlled experiment. Indoor Air 16, 276–281.

Elcombe, C.R., Odum, J., Foster, J.R., et al., 2002. Prediction of rodent nongenotoxic carcinogenesis: evaluation of biochemical and tissue changes in rodents following exposure to nine nongenotoxic NTP carcinogens. Environ. Health Perspect. 110, 363–375.

Elegbede, J.A., Elson, C.E., Qureshi, A., et al., 1984. Inhibition of DMBA-induced mammary cancer by the monoterpene d-limonene. Carcinogenesis 5, 661–664.

Elegbede, J.A., Malzman, T.H., Verma, A.K., et al., 1986a. Mouse skin tumor promoting activity of orange peel oil and d-limonene: a re-evaluation. Carcinogenesis 7, 2047–2049.

Elegbede, J.A., Elson, C.E., Tanner, M.A., et al., 1986b. Regression of rat primary mammary tumours following dietary d-limonene. J. Natl. Cancer Inst. 76, 323–325.

Elegbede, J.A., Malzman, T.H., Elson, C.E., et al., 1993. Effects of anticarcinogenic monoterpenes on phase II hepatic metabolizing enzymes. Carcinogenesis 14, 1221–1223.

Elegbede, J.A., Flores, R., Wang, R.C., 2003. Perillyl alcohol and perillaldehyde induced cell cycle arrest and cell death in BroTo and A549 cells cultured in vitro. Life Sci. 73, 2831–2840.

Elias, P.M., Ghadially, R., 2002. The aged epidermal permeability barrier: basis for functional abnormalities. Clin. Geriatr. Med. 18, 103–120.

Elisabetsky, E., Coelho de Souza, G.P., Dos Santos, M.A.C., et al., 1995a. Sedative properties of linalool. Fitoterapia 66, 407–414.

Elisabetsky, E., Marschner, J., Souza, D.O., 1995b. Effects of linalool on glutamatergic system in the rat cerebral cortex. Neurochem. Res. 20, 461–465.

Elisabetsky, E., Brum, L.F., Souza, D.O., 1999. Anticonvulsant properties of linalool in glutamate-related seizure models. Phytomedicine 6, 107–113.

Ellahueñe, M.F., Pérez-Alzola, L.P., Orellana-Valdebenito, M., et al., 1994. Genotoxic evaluation of eugenol using the bone marrow micronucleus assay. Mutat. Res. 320, 175–180.

Ellenhorn, M.J., Barceloux, D.G., 1988. Medical toxicology: diagnosis and treatment of human poisoning. Elsevier Science, New York.

Elliott, C., 1993. Tea tree oil poisoning. Med. J. Aust. 159, 830–831.

Elliott, L., Longnecker, M.P., Kissling, G.E., et al., 2006. Volatile organic compounds and pulmonary function in the Third National Health and Nutrition Examination Survey, 1988–1994. Environ. Health Perspect. 114, 1210–1214.

Ellis, E., 1863. On a fatal case of poisoning by oil of bitter almonds. Lancet 82 (2094), 447.

El-Mahdy, M.A., Zhu, Q., Wang, Q.E., et al., 2005. Thymoquinone induces apoptosis through activation of caspase-8 and mitochondrial events in p53-null myeloblastic leukemia HL-60 cells. Int. J. Cancer 117, 409–417.

Elmann, A., Mordechay, S., Rindner, M., et al., 2009. Protective effects of the essential oil of Salvia fruticosa and its constituents on astrocytic susceptibility to hydrogen peroxide-induced cell death. J. Agric. Food Chem. 57, 6636–6641.

El-Najjar, N., Chatila, M., Moukadem, H., et al., 2010. Reactive oxygen species mediate thymoquinone-induced apoptosis and activate ERK and JNK signalling. Apoptosis 15, 183–195.

El-Rab, M.O., Al-Sheikh, O.A., 1995. Is the European standard series suitable for patch testing in Riyadh, Saudi Arabia? Contact Dermatitis 33, 310–314.

Elson, C.E., Maltzman, T.H., Boston, J.L., et al., 1988. Anti-carcinogenic activity of d-limonene during the initiation and promotion/progression stages of DMBA-induced rat mammary carcinogenesis. Carcinogenesis 9, 331–332.

El Tahir, K.E., Ashour, M.M., Al-Harbi, M.M., 1993. The cardiovascular actions of the volatile oil of the black seed (Nigella sativa) in rats: elucidation of the mechanism of action. Gen. Pharmacol. 24, 1123–1131.

EMA, 2009. Community herbal monograph on Artemisia absinthium L., herba. European Medicnes Agency, London.

EMA, 2010. Final community herbal monograph on Salvia officinalis L., folium. European Medicines Agency, London.

Ema, M., Harazono, A., Fujii, S., et al., 2004. Evaluation of developmental toxicity of β-thujaplicin (hinokitiol) following oral administration during organogenesis in rats. Food Chem. Toxicol. 42, 465–470.

Emamghoreishi, M., Bokaee, H.R., Keshavarz, M., et al., 2008. CYP2A6 allele frequencies in an Iranian population. Arch. Iran Med. 11, 613–617.

Emboden, W., 1979. Narcotic Plants. Macmillan, New York.

Emerole, G., Thabrew, M.I., Anosa, V., et al., 1981. Structure-activity relationship in the toxicity of some naturally occurring coumarins – chalepin, imperatorin and oxypeucedanine. Toxicology 20, 71–80.

Emmons, W.W., Marks, J.G., 1985. Immediate and delayed reactions to cosmetic ingredients. Contact Dermatitis 13, 258–265.

Enders, F., Przybilla, B., Ring, J., 1989. Patch testing with fragrance mix at 16% and 8%, and its individual constituents. Contact Dermatitis 20, 237–238.

Enders, F., Przybilla, B., Ring, J., 1991. Patch testing with fragrance-mix and its constituents: discrepancies are largely due to the presence or absence of sorbitan sesquioleate. Contact Dermatitis 24, 238–239.

Endo, H., Rees, T.D., 2007. Cinnamon products as a possible etiologic factor in orofacial granulomatosis. Med. Oral. Patol. Oral. Cir. Bucal. 12, E440–E444.

Engel, W., 2003. In vivo studies on the metabolism of the monoterpene pulegone in humans using the metabolism of ingestion-correlated amounts (MICA) approach: Explanation for the toxicity differences between (S)-(−)- and (R)-(+)-pulegone. J. Agric. Food Chem. 51, 6589–6597.

Engelstein, D., Shmueli, J., Bruhis, S., et al., 1996. Citral and testosterone interactions in inducing benign and atypical prostatic hyperplasia in rats. Comp. Biochem. Physiol. 115C, 169–177.

Enomoto, S., Asano, R., Iwahori, Y., et al., 2001. Hematological studies on black cumin oil from the seeds of Nigella sativa L. Biol. Pharm. Bull. 24, 307–310.

Enshaieh, S., Jooya, A., Siadat, A., et al., 2007. The efficacy of 5% topical tea tree oil gel in mild to moderate acne vulgaris: a randomized, double-blind placebo-controlled study. Indian J. Dermatol. Venereol. Leprol. 73, 22–25.

Environmental Health Research & Testing Inc, 1986. Screening of priority chemicals for reproductive hazards: benzyl alcohol, probenecid, trans-retinoic acid. NTIS Report No. PB89-139059.

Environmental Protection Agency, 1973. α-Pinene reproductive toxicity. iaspub.epa.gov/oppthpv/Public_Search.PublicEndPointReport?robust_summary_id=25253417&WhichButton=PrintTab&ep_name=Developmental+Toxicity/Teratogenicity&selchemid=101069 (accessed 21.08.11.).

Environmental Protection Agency, 1988. Evaluation of the potential carcinogenicity of safrole (94-59-7). Technical Report EPA/600/8-91/178.

Environmental Protection Agency, 1989. Health and environmental effects document for benzyl alcohol. NTIS Report No. PB91-213694.

Environmental Protection Agency, 1997. Reregistration Eligibility Decision (RED): Oil of citronella. http://www.epa.gov/oppsrrd1/REDs/3105red.pdf.

Environmental Protection Agency, 2006. Revised test plan for bicyclic terpene hydrocarbons. http://www.scribd.com/doc/1616281/Environmental-Protection-Agency-c13610rt (accessed 18.09.11.).

Epshtein, M.M., 1959. The effect of α-pinene on oxygen absorption and glycolytic activity in the rat brain in experiments in vivo. Ukr. Biokhim. Zh. 31, 751.

Epshtein, M.M., Khil'ko, O.K., 1960. Effect of 2-pinene on carbohydrate-phosphorus metabolism. Ukr. Biokhim. Zh. 32, 710–715.

Epstein, J.H., 1999. Phototoxicity and photoallergy. Semin. Cutan. Med. Surg. 18, 274–284.

Epstein, S.S., Fujii, K., Andrea, J., Mantel, N., 1970. Carcinogenicity testing of selected food additives by parenteral administration to infant Swiss mice. Toxicol. Appl. Pharmacol. 16, 321–334.

Epstein, S.S., Arnold, E., Andrea, J., et al., 1972. Detection of chemical mutagens by dominant lethal assay in the mouse. Toxicol. Appl. Pharmacol. 23, 288–325.

Eremenko, A.E., Nikolaevskii, V.V., Kostin, N.F., et al., 1987. Volatile fractions of essential oil-based phytoncides as a component of therapeutic-rehabilitative complexes in chronic bronchitis (article in Russian). Ter. Arkh. 59, 126–130.

Eriksson, K., Levin, J.O., 1990. Identification of cis- and trans-verbenol in human urine after occupational exposure to terpenes. Int. Arch. Occup. Environ. Health 62, 379–383.

Eriksson, K.A., Levin, J.O., Sandstrom, T., et al., 1997. Terpene exposure and respiratory effects among workers in Swedish joinery shops. Scand. J. Work Environ. Health 23, 114–120.

Eriksson, N.E., Löwhagen, O., Nilsson, J.E., et al., 1987. Flowers and other trigger factors in asthma and rhinitis - an inquiry study. Allergy 42, 374–381.

Escribano, J., Alonso, G.L., Coca-Prados, M., et al., 1996. Crocin, safranal and picrocrocin from saffron (Crocus sativus L.) inhibit the growth of human cancer cells in vitro. Cancer Lett. 100, 23–30.

Essential Science Publishing, 2004. Essential oils desk reference. Essential Science Publishing, Orem, Utah.

Essway, G.S., Sobbhy, H.M., El-Banna, H.A., 1995. The hypoglycaemic effect of volatile oils of some Egyptian plants. Veterinary Medical Journal, Giza 43, 167–172.

European Commission, 2002. Twenty-sixth commission directive 2002/34/EC of 15 April 2002. Official Journal of the European Communities L. 102, 19–31.

European Community Council, 1988. Maximum limits for certain undesirable substances present in foodstuffs as consumed as a result of the use of flavourings. Council directive, 15. 7. 88. Official Journal of the European Communities 1 (L), 184/61–184/65.

European Pharmacopoeia Commission, 2002. European Pharmacopoeia, fourth ed. Council of Europe, Strasbourg, France.

Evandri, M.G., Battinelli, L., Daniele, C., et al., 2005. The antimutagenic activity of Lavandula angustifolia (lavender) essential oil in the bacterial reverse mutation assay. Food Chem. Toxicol. 43, 1381–1387.

Evans, N.J., Rutter, N., 1986. Development of the epidermis in the newborn. Biol. Neonate 49, 74–80.

Evans, F.J., Schmidt, R.J., 1980. Plants and plant products that induce contact dermatitis. Planta Med. 38, 289–316.

Evans, J.G., Gaunt, I.F., Lake, B.G., 1979. Two-year toxicity study on coumarin in the baboon. Food Cosmet. Toxicol. 17, 187–193.

Fachini-Queiroz, F.C., Kummer, R., Estevão-Silva, C.F., et al., 2012. Effects of thymol and carvacrol, constituents of Thymus vulgaris L. essential oil, on the inflammatory response. Evid. Base. Compl. Alternative Med. http://dx.doi.org/10.1155/2012/657026.

Fahim, F.A., Esmat, A.Y., Fadel, H.M., Hassan, K.F.S., 1999. Allied studies on the effect of Rosmarinus officinalis L. on experimental hepatotoxicity and mutagenesis. Int. J. Food Sci. Nutr. 50, 413–427.

Fahrig, R., 1982. Effects of food additives in the mammalian spot test. Prog. Clin. Biol. Res. 109, 339–348.

Falk, A.A., Hagberg, M.T., Lof, A.E., et al., 1990. Uptake, distribution and elimination of alpha-pinene in man after exposure by inhalation. Scand. J. Work Environ. Health 16, 372–378.

Falk, A., Löf, A., Hagberg, M., et al., 1991a. Human exposure to 3-carene by inhalation: toxicokinetics, effects on pulmonary function and occurrence of irritative and CNS symptoms. Toxicol. Appl. Pharmacol. 110, 198–205.

Falk, A., Fischer, T., Hagberg, M., 1991b. Purpuric Rash caused by dermal exposure to d-limonene. Contact Dermatitis 25, 198–199.

Falk-Filipsson, A., 1996. Short term inhalation exposure to turpentine: toxicokinetics and acute effects in men. Occup. Environ. Med. 53, 100–105.

Falk-Filipsson, A., Löf, A., Hagberg, M., et al., 1993. *d*-Limonene exposure to humans by inhalation: uptake, distribution, elimination, and effects on the pulmonary function. J. Toxicol. Environ. Health 38, 77–88.

Fandohan, P., Gnonlonfin, B., Laleye, A., et al., 2008. Toxicity and gastric tolerance of essential oils from *Cymbopogon citratus*, *Ocimum gratissimum* and *Ocimum basilicum* in Wistar rats. Food Chem. Toxicol. 46, 2493–2497.

Fang, H.J., Su, X.L., Liu, H.Y., et al., 1989. Studies on the chemical components and anti-tumour action of the volatile oils from *Pelargonium graveolens*. Yao Xue Xue Bao 24, 366–371.

Farage, M.A., 2008. Perceptions of sensitive skin: changes in perceived severity and associations with environmental causes. Contact Dermatitis 59, 226–232.

Farage, M.A., Bjerke, D.L., Mahony, C., et al., 2003. Quantitative risk assessment for the induction of allergic contact dermatitis: uncertainty factor for mucosal exposures. Contact Dermatitis 49, 140–147.

Farage, M.A., Katsarou, A., Maibach, H.I., 2006. Sensory, clinical and physiological factors in sensitive skin: a review. Contact Dermatitis 55, 1–14.

Farhat, G.N., Affara, N.I., Gali-Muhtasib, H.U., 2001. Seasonal changes in the composition of the essential oil extract of East Mediterranean sage (*Salvia libanotica*) and its toxicity in mice. Toxicon 39, 1601–1605.

Farinola, N., Piller, N., 2005. Pharmacogenomics: its role in re-establishing coumarin as treatment for lymphedema. Lymphat. Res. Biol. 3, 81–86.

Farinola, N., Piller, N., 2007. CYP2A6 polymorphisms: is there a role for pharmacogenomics in preventing coumarin-induced hepatotoxicity in lymphedema patients? Pharmacogenomics 8, 151–158.

Farley, D.R., Howland, V., 1980. The natural variation of the pulegone content in various oils of peppermint. J. Sci. Food. Agric. 31, 1143–1151.

Farnsworth, N.R., Bingel, A.S., Cordell, G.A., et al., 1975. Potential value of plants as sources of new antifertility agents I. J. Pharm. Sci. 64, 535–598.

Farrow, A., Taylor, H., Northstone, K., et al., 2003. Symptoms of mothers and infants related to total volatile organic compounds in household products. Arch. Environ. Health 58, 633–641.

FASEB (Federation of American Societies for Experimental Biology), 1973. Evaluation of the health aspects of benzoic acid and sodium benzoate as food ingredients. NTIS Report No. PB-223-837.

Fassett, D.W., 1963. Organic acids and compounds. In: Patty, F.A. (Ed.), Industrial hygiene and toxicology, second ed., vol. II. Interscience Publishers, New York, p. 1838.

Fejes, S., Kery, A., Blazovics, A., et al., 1998. Investigation of the in vitro antioxidant effect of *Petroselinum crispum* (Mill.) Nym. ex A. W. Hill. Acta Pharm. Hung. 68, 150–156.

Felter, S.P., Ryan, C.A., Basketter, D.A., 2003. Application of the risk assessment paradigm to the induction of allergic contact dermatitis. Regul. Toxicol. Pharmacol. 37, 1–10.

Felter, S.P., Vassallo, J.D., Carlton, B.D., et al., 2006. A safety assessment of coumarin taking into account species-specificity of toxicokinetics. Food Chem. Toxicol. 44, 462–475.

FEMA, 1997. FEMA Database: Thujone. Flavor & Extract Manufacturers Association, Washington DC, 12pp.

Fenn, R.S., 1989. Aroma chemical usage trends in modern perfumery. Perfumer & Flavorist 14, 3–10.

Fenske, N.A., Lober, C.W., 1986. Structural and functional changes of normal aging skin. J. Am. Acad. Dermatol. 15 (4 pt 1), 571–585.

Fentem, J.H., Fry, J.R., 1993. Species differences in the metabolism and hepatotoxicity of coumarin. Comp. Biochem. Physiol. 104C, 1–8.

Fenwick, G.R., Hanley, A.B., 1985. The genus *Allium*-part 3. CRC Crit Rev Food Sci Nutr 23, 1–73.

Ferguson, J., Sharma, S., 1984. Cinnamic aldehyde test concentration. Contact Dermatitis 10, 191–192.

Ferguson, L.J., Lebetkin, E.H., Lih, F.B., et al., 2007. 14C-Labeled pulegone and metabolites binding to alpha2u-globulin in kidneys of male F-344 rats. J. Toxicol. Environ. Health A. 70, 1416–1423.

Ferley, J.P., Poutignat, N., Zmirou, D., et al., 1989. Prophylactic aromatherapy for supervening infections in patients with chronic bronchitis. Statistical evaluation conducted in clinics against a placebo. Phytother. Res. 3, 97–100.

Fernandes, J., da Fonseca, C.O., Teixeira, A., et al., 2005. Perillyl alcohol induces apoptosis in human glioblastoma multiforme cells. Oncol. Rep. 13, 943–947.

Fernández de Corres, L., 1986. Photosensitivity to oak moss. Contact Dermatitis 15, 118.

Fernández de Corres, L., Muñoz, D., Leaniz-Barrutia, I., et al., 1983. Photocontact dermatitis from oak moss. Contact Dermatitis 9, 528–529.

Fernandez-Vozmediano, J.M., Armario-Hita, J.C., Manrique-Plaza, A., 2000. Allergic contact dermatitis from diallyl disulfide. Contact Dermatitis 42, 108–109.

Feron, V.J., Til, H.P., De Vrijer, F., et al., 1991. Aldehydes: occurrence, carcinogenic potential, mechanism of action and risk assessment. Mutat. Res. 259, 363–385.

Ferracini, V.L., Paraiba, L.C., Leitão Filho, H.F., et al., 1995. Essential oils of seven Brazilian *Baccharis* species. Journal of Essential Oil Research 7, 355–367.

Ferrari, B., Castilho, P., Tomi, F., et al., 2005. Direct identification and quantitative determination of costunolide and dehydrocostuslactone in the fixed oil of Laurus novocanariensis by 13C-NMR spectroscopy. Phytochem. Anal. 16, 104–107.

Ferreira, A., Proenca, C., Serralheiro, M.L., et al., 2006. The in vitro screening for acetylcholinesterase inhibition and antioxidant activity of medicinal plants from Portugal. J. Ethnopharmacol. 108, 31–37.

Ferretti, J.J., Lu, W., Liu, M.B., 1977. Mutagenicity of benzidine and related compounds employed in the detection of hemoglobin. Am. J. Clin. Pathol. 67, 526.

Ferrini, A.M., Mannoni, V., Aureli, P., et al., 2006. *Melaleuca alternifolia* essential oil possesses potent anti-staphylococcal activity extended to strains resistant to antibiotics. Int. J. Immunopathol. Pharmacol. 19, 539–544.

Feuer, 1974. The metabolism and biological actions of coumarins. Prog. Med. Chem. 10, 85–158.

Feuer, G., Golberg, L., Le Pelley, J.R., 1965. Liver response tests. I. Exploratory studies on glucose 6-phosphatase and other liver enzymes. Food Cosmet. Toxicol. 3, 235–249.

Feuer, G., Golberg, L., Gibson, K.I., 1966. Liver response tests. VII. Coumarin metabolism in relation to the inhibition of rat liver glucose 6-phosphatase. Food Cosmet. Toxicol. 4, 157–167.

FFHPVC, 2006. Flavor & Fragrance High Production Volume Consortia. Revised test plan for bicyclic terpene hydrocarbons. http://www.scribd.com/doc/1616281/Environmental-Protection-Agency-c13610rt (accessed 29.01.12.).

Field, W.E., Roe, F.J., 1965. Tumor promotion in the forestomach epithelium of mice by oral administration of citrus oils. J. Natl. Cancer Inst. 35, 771–787.

Filipsson, A.F., 1996. Short term inhalation exposure to turpentine: toxicokinetics and acute effects in men. Occup. Environ. Med. 53, 100–105.

Fingrut, O., Flescher, E., 2002. Plant stress hormones suppress the proliferation and induce apoptosis in human cancer cells. Leukemia 16, 608–616.

Fingrut, O., Reischer, D., Rotem, R., et al., 2005. Jasmonates induce nonapoptotic death in high-resistance mutant p53-expressing B-lymphoma cells. Br. J. Pharmacol. 146, 800–808.

Fiorio, R., Bronzetti, G., 1994. Effects of cinnamaldehyde on survival and formation of HGPRT- mutants in V79 cells treated with methyl methanesulfonate, *N*-nitroso-*N*-methylurea, ethyl methanesulfonate and UV light. Mutat. Res. 324, 51–57.

Fischer, L., 1985. *In vitro* permeability of infant skin. In: Bronaugh, R.L., Maibach, H.I. (eds) Percutaneous absorption. Marcel Dekker, New York, p 213–222.

Fischer, I.U., von Unruh, G.E., Dengler, H.J., 1990. The metabolism of eugenol in man. Xenobiotica 20, 209–222.

Fisher, A.A., 1989. Allergic contact dermatitis due to thymol in Listerine for treatment of paronychia. Cutis 43, 531–532.

Fisher, A.A., Dooms-Goossens, A., 1976. The effect of perfume 'ageing' on the allergenicity of individual perfume ingredients. Contact Dermatitis 2, 155–159.

Fitzi, J., Furst-Jucker, J., Wegener, T., et al., 2002. Phytotherapy of chronic dermatitis and pruritus of dogs with a topical preparation containing tea tree oil (Bogaskin). Schweiz. Arch. Tierheilkd. 144, 223–231.

Fleming, C.J., Forsyth, A., 1998. D5 Patch test reactions to menthol and peppermint. Contact Dermatitis 38, 337.

Fleming, W.W., 2003. Mechanisms of drug action. In: Craig, C.R., Stitzel, R.E. (Eds.), Modern Pharmacology with Clinical Applications, sixth ed. Lippincott Williams & Wilkins, Philadelphia.

Flescher, E., 2005. Jasmonates - a new family of anti-cancer agents. Anticancer Drugs 16, 911–916.

Fletcher, J.P., Cassella, J.P., Hughes, D., et al., 2005. An evaluation of the mutagenic potential of commercially available tea tree oil in the United Kingdom. Int. J. Aromather. 15, 81–86.

Floch, F., Mauger, F., Desmurs, J.R., et al., 2002. Coumarin in plants and fruits: implication in perfumery. Perfumer & Flavorist 27 (2), 32–36.

Florence, A.T., Attwood, D., 1998. Physicochemical principles of pharmacy, third ed. Pharmaceutical Press, London.

Florey, H., Student, J.L., 1968. Observations on the action of the convulsant thujone. J. Pathol. Bacteriol. 28, 645–650.

Florin, I., Rutberg, L., Curvall, M., et al., 1980. Screening of tobacco smoke constituents for mutagenicity using the Ames test. Toxicology 15, 219–232.

Fluhr, J.W., Darlenski, R., Angelova-Fischer, I., et al., 2008. Skin irritation and sensitization: mechanisms and new approaches for risk assessment. 1. Skin irritation. Skin Pharmacol. Physiol. 21, 124–135.

Flury, F., Zernicke, F., 1931. Campher. In: Schädliche Gase Dämpfe, Nebel, Rauch- und Staubarten. FRG Julius Spinger, Berlin, pp. 451–452.

Flynn, E.F., 1893. Poisoning by essence of pennyroyal. Br. Med. J. 2, 1270.

Foggie, W.E., 1911. Eucalyptus oil poisoning. Br. Med. J. 1, 359–360.

Fontenelle, R.O., Morais, S.M., Brito, E.H., et al., 2007. Chemical composition, toxicological aspects and antifungal activity of essential oil from *Lippia sidoides* Cham. J. Antimicrob. Chemother. 59, 934–940.

Food and Drug Administration, 1983. Proposed rules: external analgesic drug products for over-the-counter human use; tentative final monograph. Fed. Regist. 48, 5852–5869.

Foray, L., Bertrand, C., Pinguet, F., et al., 1999. *In vitro* cytotoxic activity of three essential oils from *Salvia* species. In: Lawrence, B.M. (Ed.), 2005 The antimicrobial/biological activity of essential oils. Allured, Carol Stream, pp. 257–259.

Forbes, P.D., Urbach, F., Davies, R.E., 1977. Phototoxicity testing of fragrance raw materials. Food Cosmet. Toxicol. 15, 55–60.

Forbes, R.J., 1970. A short history of the art of distillation. E J Brill, Leiden.

Force, M., Sparks, W.S., Ronzio, R.A., 2000. Inhibition of enteric parasites by emulsified oil of oregano *in vivo*. Phytother. Res. 14, 213–214.

Ford, R.A., 1991. The toxicology and safety of fragrances. In: Müller, P.M., Lamparsky, D. (Eds.), Perfumes – art, science and technology. Elsevier, London.

Ford, R.A., Letizia, C., Api, A.M., 1988a. Monographs on fragrance raw materials. Food Chem. Toxicol. 26 (Suppl.).

Ford, R.A., Api, A.M., Suskind, R.R., 1988b. Allergic contact sensitization potential of hydroxycitronellal in humans. Food Chem. Toxicol. 26, 921–926.

Ford, R.A., Api, A.M., Letizia, C., 1992. Monographs on fragrance raw materials. Food Chem. Toxicol. 30 (Suppl.).

Ford, R.A., Domeyer, B., Easterday, O., et al., 2000. Criteria for development of a database for safety evaluation of fragrance ingredients. Regul. Toxicol. Pharmacol. 31, 166–181.

Ford, R.A., Hawkins, D.R., Mayo, B.C., Api, A.M., 2001. The *in vivo* dermal absorption and metabolism of [4-C^{14}]coumarin by rats and by human volunteers under simulated conditions of use in fragrances. Food Chem. Toxicol. 39, 153–162.

Formacek, K., Kubeczka, K.H., 1982. Essential oils analysis by capillary chromatography and carbon C-13 NMR spectroscopy. John Wiley, New York.

Forrest, J.E., Heacock, R.A., 1972. Nutmeg and mace, the psychotropic spices from *Myristica fragrans*. Lloydia 35, 440–449.

Forrest, J.E., Heacock, R.A., Forrest, T.P., 1972. Identification of the major components of the essential oil of mace. J. Chromatogr. 69, 115–121.

Forsbeck, M., Skog, E., 1977. Immediate reactions to patch tests with balsam of Peru. Contact Dermatitis 3, 201–205.

Forschmidt, P., 1979. Teratogenic activity of flavor additives. Teratology 19, 26A.

Fortini, P., Pascucci, B., Parlanti, E., et al., 2003. The base excision repair: mechanisms and its relevance for cancer susceptibility. Biochimie 85, 1053–1071.

Foti, M.C., Ingold, K.U., 2003. Mechanism of inhibition of lipid peroxidation by gamma-terpinene, an unusual and potentially useful hydrocarbon antioxidant. J. Agric. Food Chem. 51, 2758–2765.

Fotiades, J., Soter, N.A., Lim, H.W., 1995. Results of evaluation of 203 patients for photosensitivity in a 7.3-year period. J. Am. Acad. Dermatol. 33, 597–602.

Fournier, G., Pages, N., Dumitresco, S.M., et al., 1986. Contribution to the study of *Plectranthus fruticosus* essential oil. Planta Med. 53, 486–488.

Fournier, G., Pages, N., Baudron, V., et al., 1989. Étude d'échantillons commerciaux de sabine: rameaux, feuilles et huile essentielle. Plantes Medicinales et Phytothérapie 23, 169–179.

Fournier, G., Pages, N., Fournier, C., et al., 1990. Contribution à l'étude des huiles essentielles de différentes espèces de juniperus. J. Pharm. Belg. 45, 293–298.

Foussereau, M.J., 1963. L'allergie de contact à l'huile de laurier. Bull. Soc. Fr. Dermatol. Syphiligr. 70, 698–701.

Foussereau, J., Benezra, C., Ourisson, G., 1967a. Contact dermatitis from laurel I. Clinical aspects. Trans. St. Johns Hosp. Dermatol. Soc. 53, 141–146.

Foussereau, J., Benezra, C., Ourisson, G., 1967b. Contact dermatitis from laurel II. Chemical aspects. Trans. St. Johns Hosp. Dermatol. Soc. 53, 147–153.

Foussereau, J., Muller, J.C., Benezra, C., 1975. Contact allergy to *Frullania* and *Laurus nobilis*: cross-sensitization and chemical structure of the allergens. Contact Dermatitis 1, 223–230.

Francalanci, S., Sertoli, A., Giorgini, S., et al., 2000. Multicentre study of allergic contact cheilitis from toothpastes. Contact Dermatitis 43, 216–222.

Franchomme, P., Pénöel, D., 1990. L'aromathérapie exactement. Jollois, Limoges.

Frank, M.B., Yang, Q., Osban, J., et al., 2009. Frankincense oil derived from *Boswellia carteri* induces tumor cell specific cytotoxicity. BMC Complement. Altern. Med. doi: 10.1186/1472-6882-9-6.

Franz, T., 1975. Percutaneous absorption. On the relevance of in vitro data. J. Invest. Dermatol. 64, 190–195.

Franz, H., Frank, R., Rytter, M., et al., 1998. Allergic contact dermatitis due to cedarwood oil after dermatoscopy. Contact Dermatitis 38, 182–183.

Franzios, G., Mirotsou, M., Hatziapostolou, E., et al., 1997. Insecticidal and genotoxic activities of mint essential oils. J. Agric. Food Chem. 45, 2690–2694.

Freeman, R., 2006. Cardiovascular manifestations of autonomic epilepsy. Clin. Auton. Res. 16, 12–17.

Fregert, S., Hjorth, N., 1969. Results of standard patch tests with substances abandoned. Contact Dermatitis Newsletter 5, 85.

Freire, R.S., Morais, S.M., Catunda-Junior, F.E., et al., 2005. Synthesis and antioxidant, anti-inflammatory and gastroprotector activities of anethole and related compounds. Bioorg. Med. Chem. 13, 4353–4358.

Freire, C.M., Marques, M.O., Costa, M., 2006. Effects of seasonal variation on the central nervous system activity of *Ocimum gratissimum* L. essential oil. J. Ethnopharmacol. 105, 161–166.

Freitas, J.C., Presgrave, O.A., Fingola, F.F., et al., 1993. Effect of *beta*-myrcene on pentobarbital sleeping time. Braz. J. Med. Biol. Res. 26, 519–523.

Friedmann, P.S., 1990. The immunology of allergic contact dermatitis: the DNCB story. Advanced Dermatology 5, 175–195.

Friedmann, P.S., Moss, C., Shuster, S., et al., 1983a. Quantitative relationships between sensitizing dose of DNCB and reactivity in normal subjects. Clin. Exp. Immunol. 53, 709–715.

Friedmann, P.S., Moss, C., Shuster, S., et al., 1983b. Quantitation of sensitization and responsiveness to dinitrochlorobenzene in normal subjects. Br. J. Dermatol. 25, 86–88.

Friesen, M.S., Phillips, B., 2006. Status epilepticus following pediatric ingestion of thuja essential oil. Clin. Toxicol. 44, 557.

Frosch, P.J., 1992. Cutaneous irritation. In: Rycroft, R.J., Menné, T., Frosch, P.J. (Eds.), Textbook of contact dermatitis. Springer, Berlin.

Frosch, P.J., Pilz, B., Andersen, K.E., et al., 1995a. Patch testing with fragrances: results of a multicenter study of the European Environmental

& Contact Dermatitis Research Group with 48 frequently used constituents of perfumes. Contact Dermatitis 33, 333–342.

Frosch, P.J., Pilz, B., Burrows, D., et al., 1995b. Testing with fragrance mix. Is the addition of sorbitan sesquioleate to the constituents useful? Contact Dermatitis 32, 266–272.

Frosch, P.J., Johansen, J.D., Menné, T., et al., 2002a. Further important sensitizers in patients sensitive to fragrances. Contact Dermatitis 47, 78–85.

Frosch, P.J., Johansen, J.D., Menné, T., et al., 2002b. Further important sensitizers in patients sensitive to fragrances. Contact Dermatitis 47, 279–287.

Frosch, P., Pirker, C., Rastogi, S., 2004. The new fragrance mix II - test results of a multicentrre European study. Contact Dermatitis 50, 149.

Frosch, P.J., Rastogi, S.C., Pirker, C., 2005a. Patch testing with a new fragrance mix – reactivity to the individual constituents and chemical detection in relevant cosmetic products. Contact Dermatitis 52, 216–225.

Frosch, P.J., Pirker, C., Suresh, C., 2005b. Patch testing with a new fragrance mix detects additional patients sensitive to perfumes and missed by the current fragrance mix. Contact Dermatitis 52, 207–215.

Fuhr, U., 1998. Drug interactions with grapefruit juice. Extent, probable mechanism and clinical relevance. Drug Saf. 18, 251–272.

Fujii, T., Furukawa, S., Suzuki, S., 1972. Studies on compounded perfumes for toilet goods. On the non-irritative compounded perfumes for soaps. Yukagaku 21, 904–908.

Fujii, H., Yamamoto, M., Mogaki, M., et al., 1994. Glucagon responses in rabbits with obstructive jaundice and a low energy status in the liver. Surg. Today (Tokyo) 24, 982–986.

Fujisawa, S., Okada, N., Muraoka, E., 2001. Comparative effects of eugenol to bis-eugenol on oral mucous membranes. Dent. Mater. J. 20, 237–242.

Fujisawa, S., Atsumi, T., Kadoma, Y., et al., 2002. Antioxidant and prooxidant action of eugenol-related compounds and their cytotoxicity. Toxicology 177, 39–54.

Fujita, M., Aoki, T., 1983. Allergic contact dermatitis to pyridoxine ester and hinokitiol. Contact Dermatitis 9, 61–65.

Fujita, H., Sasaki, M., 1986. Mutagenicity test of food additives with Salmonella typhimurium TA97A and TA101. Kenku Nenpo-Tokyo-Toritsu Eisei Kenkyusho 37, 447–452.

Fukao, T., Hosono, T., Misawa, S., et al., 2004. The effects of allyl sulfides on the induction of phase II detoxification enzymes and liver injury by carbon tetrachloride. Food Chem. Toxicol. 42, 743–749.

Fukayama, M.Y., Easterday, O.D., Serafino, P.A., et al., 1999. Subchronic inhalation studies of complex fragrance mixtures in rats and hamsters. Toxicol. Lett. 111, 175–187.

Futami, T., 1984. Actions and mechanisms of counterirritants on the muscular circulation. Nippon Yakurigaku Zasshi 83, 219–226.

Fyhrquist-Vanni, N., Alenius, H., Lauerma, A., 2007. Contact Dermatitis. Dermatol. Clin. 25, 613–623.

Gabbanini, S., Lucchi, E., Carli, M., et al., 2009. In vitro evaluation of the permeation through reconstructed human epidermis of essentials oils from cosmetic formulations. J. Pharm. Biomed. Anal. 50, 370–376.

Gaddum, J.H., 1945. Lognormal distributions. Nature 156, 463–466.

Gafvert, E., Nilsson, J.L., Hagelthorn, G., et al., 2002. Free radicals in antigen formation: reduction of contact allergic response to hydroperoxides by epidermal treatment with antioxidants. Br. J. Dermatol. 146, 649–656.

Gage, J.C., 1970. The subacute inhalation toxicity of 109 industrial chemicals. Br. J. Ind. Med. 27, 1–18.

Gagnaire, F., Chalansonnet, M., Carabin, N., et al., 2006. Effects of subchronic exposure to styrene on the extracellular and tissue levels of dopamine, serotonin and their metabolites in rat brain. Arch. Toxicol. 80, 703–712.

Gaikwad, N.W., Bodell, W.J., 2003. Formation of DNA adducts in HL-60 cells treated with the toluene metabolite p-cresol: a potential biomarker for toluene exposure. Chem. Biol. Interact. 145, 149–158.

Gail, M.H., You, W.C., Chang, Y.S., et al., 1998. Factorial trial of three interventions to reduce the progression of precancerous gastric lesions in Shandong. China: design issues and initial data. Control Clin. Trials 19, 352–369.

Galfré, A., Martin, P., Petrzilka, M., 1993. Direct enantioselective separation and olfactory evaluation of all irone isomers. Journal of Essential Oil Research 5, 265–277.

Gali-Muhtasib, H., Affara, N.I., 2000. Chemopreventive effects of sage oil on skin papillomas in mice. Phytomedicine 7, 129–136.

Gali-Muhtasib, H., Diab-Assaf, M., Boltze, C., et al., 2004a. Thymoquinone extracted from black seed triggers apoptotic cell death in human colorectal cancer cells via a p53-dependent mechanism. Int. J. Oncol. 25, 857–866.

Gali-Muhtasib, H., Abou Kheir, W.G., Kheir, L.A., et al., 2004b. Molecular pathway for thymoquinone-induced cell-cycle arrest and apoptosis in neoplastic keratinocytes. Anticancer Drugs 15, 389–399.

Gali-Muhtasib, H., Kuester, D., Mawrin, C., et al., 2008a. Thymoquinone triggers inactivation of the stress response pathway sensor CHEK1 and contributes to apoptosis in colorectal cancer cells. Cancer Res. 68, 5609–5618.

Gali-Muhtasib, H., Ocker, M., Kuester, D., et al., 2008b. Thymoquinone reduces mouse colon tumor cell invasion and inhibits tumor growth in murine colon cancer models. J. Cell. Mol. Med. 12, 330–342.

Gallaway, S.M., Bloom, A.D., Resnick, M., et al., 1985. Development of a standard protocol for in vitro cytogenetic testing with Chinese hamster ovary cells: comparison of results for 22 compounds in two laboratories. Environ. Mutagen. 7, 1–51.

Galloway, S.M., Armstrong, M.J., Reuben, C., et al., 1987. Chromosome aberrations and sister chromatid exchanges in Chinese hamster ovary cells: evaluations of 108 chemicals. Environ. Mol. Mutagen. 10 (Suppl. 10), 1–175.

Gandhi, M., Lal, R., Sankaranarayanan, A., et al., 1991. Post-coital antifertility action of Ruta graveolens in female rats and hamsters. J. Ethnopharmacol. 34, 49–59.

Gangolli, S.D., Shilling, W.H., Grasso, P., et al., 1974. Studies on the metabolism and hepatotoxicity of coumarin in the baboon. Biochem. Soc. Trans. 2, 310–312.

Ganzera, M., Schneider, P., Stuppner, H., 2006. Inhibitory effects of the essential oil of chamomile (Matricaria recutita L.) and its major constituents on human cytochrome P450 enzymes. Life Sci. 78, 856–861.

Gao, Y.Y., Pascuale, M.A., Elizondo, A., et al., 2007. Clinical treatment for ocular demodecosis by lid scrub with tea tree oil. Cornea 26, 136–143.

Garcia, D.A., Bujons, J., Vale, C., et al., 2006. Allosteric positive interaction of thymol with the GABAA receptor in primary cultures of mouse cortical neurons. Neuropharmacology 50, 25–35.

García-Abujeta, J.L., De Larramendi, C.H., Berna, J.P., et al., 2005. Mud bath dermatitis due to cinnamon oil. Contact Dermatitis 52, 234.

Gardner, I., Bergin, P., Stening, P., et al., 1995. Protein adducts derived from methyleugenol. In: ISSX International Meeting, 4th 8, p. 208.

Gardner, I., Bergin, P., Stening, P., et al., 1996. Immunochemical detection of covalently modified protein adducts in livers of rats treated with methyleugenol. Chem. Res. Toxicol. 9, 713–721.

Gardner, I., Wakazono, H., Bergin, P., et al., 1997. Cytochrome P450 mediated bioactivation of methyleugenol to 1′-hydroxy methyleugenol in Fischer 344 rat and human liver microsomes. Carcinogenesis 18, 1775–1783.

Gardner, D.R., Panter, K.E., James, L.F., et al., 1998. Abortifacient effects of lodgepole pine (Pinus contorta) and common juniper (Juniperus communis) on cattle. Vet. Hum. Toxicol. 40, 260–263.

Garg, N., Misra, L.N., Siddiqui, M.S., Agarwal, S.K., 1989. Volatile constituents of the essential oil of Cyperus scariosus tubers. In: Proceedings 11th International Congress of Essential Oils. vol. 4. Fragrances & Flavours, New Delhi, pp. 161–165

Garg, A., Chren, M.M., Sands, L.P., et al., 2001. Psychological stress perturbs epidermal permeability barrier homeostasis: implications for the pathogenesis of stress-associated skin disorders. Arch. Dermatol. 137, 53–59.

Garland, S.M., Menary, R.C., Davies, N.W., 1999. Dissipation of propiconazole and tebuconazole in peppermint crops (Mentha piperita (Labiatae)) and their residues in distilled oils. J. Agric. Food Chem. 47, 294–298.

Garnero, J., Joulain, D., 1983. Massoia essential oil. In: Proceedings, 9th International Congress of Essential Oils, Singapore, 1983.

Garnett, A., Hotchkiss, S.A., Caldwell, J., 1994. Percutaneous absorption of benzyl acetate through rat skin in vitro. 3. A comparison with human skin. Food Chem. Toxicol. 32, 1061–1065.

Garty, B.Z., 1993. Garlic burns. Pediatrics 91, 658–659.

Gattefossé, R.M., 1936. article title unknown. Parfumerie Moderne 14, 511–529.

Gaunt, I.F., Agrelo, C.E., Colley, J., et al., 1971. Short-term toxicity of isobornyl acetate in rats. Food Cosmet. Toxicol. 9, 355–366.

Gaworski, C.L., Vollmuth, T.A., York, R.G., et al., 1992. Developmental toxicity evaluation of inhaled citral in Sprague-Dawley rats. Food Chem. Toxicol. 30, 269–277.

Gaworski, C.L., Vollmuth, T.A., Dozier, M.M., et al., 1994. An immunotoxicity assessment of food flavouring ingredients. Food Chem. Toxicol. 32, 409–415.

Gayathri, N.S., Dhanya, C.R., Indu, A.R., et al., 2004. Changes in some hormones by low doses of di (2-ethyl hexyl) phthalate (DEHP), a commonly used plasticizer in PVC blood storage bags and medical tubing. Indian J. Med. Res. 119, 139–144.

Gaydou, E.M., Randriamiharisoa, R.P., Bianchini, J.P., et al., 1988. Multidimensional data analysis of essential oils. Application to ylang-ylang (Cananga odorata Hook. Fil. et Thompson f. genuina) grades classification. J. Agric. Food Chem. 36, 574–579.

Gazith, J., Schalla, W., Bauer, E., Schaefer, H., 1978. 8-Methoxypsoralen (8-MOP) in human skin: penetration kinetics. J. Invest. Dermatol. 71, 126–130.

Gedeon, C., Koren, G., 2007. Designing pregnancy centered medications: Drugs which do not cross the human placenta. Placenta 27, 861–868.

Geier, J., Brasch, J., Schnuch, A., et al., 2002. Lyral has been included in the patch test standard series in Germany. Contact Dermatitis 46, 295–297.

Gelal, A., Jacob, P., Yu, L., et al., 1999. Disposition kinetics and effects of menthol. Clin. Pharmacol. Ther. 66, 128–135.

Galati, E.M., Miceli, M., Galluzzo, M.F., et al., 2004. Neuropharmacological effects of epinepetalactone from Nepeta sibthorpii behavioral and anticonvulsant activity. Pharmaceutical Biology 42, 391–395.

Geldof, A.A., Engel, C., Rao, B.R., 1992. Estrogenic action of commonly used fragrant agent citral induces prostatic hyperplasia. Urol. Res. 20, 139–144.

Geller, R.J., Spyker, D.A., Garrettson, L.K., et al., 1984. Camphor toxicity: development of a triage strategy. Vet. Hum. Toxicol. 26 (Suppl. 2), 8–10.

Gelot, P., Bara-Passot, C., Gimenez-Arnau, E., et al., 2012. Bullous drug eruption with Nigella sativa oil. Ann. Dermatol. Vénéréol. 139, 287–291.

Geng, Y., Li, C., Liu, J., et al., 2010. beta-Asarone improves cognitive function by suppressing neuronal apoptosis in the beta-amyloid hippocampus injection rats. Biol. Pharm. Bull. 33, 836–843.

George, J.D., Price, C.J., Marr, M.C., et al., 2001. Evaluation of the developmental toxicity of isoeugenol in Sprague-Dawley (CD) rats. Toxicol. Sci. 60, 112 120.

Gerarde, H.W., 1960. Toxicology and biochemistry of aromatic hydrocarbons. Elsevier, London, p. 59.

Gerberick, G.F., Robinson, M.K., Felter, S.P., et al., 2001a. Understanding fragrance allergy using an exposure-based risk assessment approach. Contact Dermatitis 45, 333–340.

Gerberick, G.F., Robinson, M.K., Ryan, C.A., et al., 2001b. Contact allergenic potency: correlation of human and local lymph node assay data. Am. J. Contact Dermat. 12, 156–161.

Gerberick, G.F., Ryan, C.A., Dearman, R.J., et al., 2007. Local lymph node assay (LLNA) for detection of sensitization capacity of chemicals. Methods 41, 54–60.

Gerhäuser, C., Klimo, K., Heiss, E., et al., 2003. Mechanism-based in vitro screening of potential cancer chemopreventive agents. Mutat. Res. 523-524, 163–172.

Gershanik, J.J., Beecher, B., George, W., et al., 1981. Gasping syndrome: benzyl alcohol poisoning. Clin. Res. 29, 895a.

Ghadially, R., 1998. Aging and the epidermal permeability barrier: implications for contact dermatitis. Am. J. Contact Dermat. 9, 162–169.

Ghadially, R., Brown, B.E., Sequeira-Martin, S.M., et al., 1995. The aged epidermal permeability barrier. Structural, functional, and lipid biochemical abnormalities in humans and a senescent murine model. J. Clin. Invest. 95, 2281–2290.

Ghannadi, A., Amree, S., 2002. Volatile oil constituents of Ferula gummosa Boiss. from Kashan, Iran. Journal of Essential Oil Research 14, 420–421.

Ghiringhelli, F., Menard, C., Martin, F., et al., 2006. The role of regulatory T cells in the control of natural killer cells: relevance during tumor progression. Immunol. Rev. 214, 229–238.

Ghosh, R., Nadiminty, N., Fitzpatrick, J.E., et al., 2005. Eugenol causes melanoma growth suppression through inhibition of E2F1 transcriptional activity. J. Biol. Chem. 280, 5812–5819.

Ghosh, R., Ganapathy, M., Alworth, W.L., et al., 2009. Combination of 2-methoxyestradiol (2-ME(2)) and eugenol for apoptosis induction synergistically in androgen independent prostate cancer cells. J. Steroid Biochem. Mol. Biol. 113, 25–35.

Gibbon, P., 1927. Poisoning by oil of eucalyptus. Br. Med. J. 1, 1005.

Gibson, P.R., Vogel, V.M., 2009. Sickness-related dysfunction in persons with self-reported multiple chemical sensitivity at four levels of severity. J. Clin. Nurs. 18, 72–81.

Gibson, D.E., Moore, G.P., Pfaff, J.A., 1989. Camphor ingestion. Am. J. Emerg. Med. 7, 41–43.

Gielen, M.H., Van der Zee, S.C., Van Wijnen, J.H., et al., 1997. Acute effects of summer air pollution on respiratory health of asthmatic children. Am. J. Respir. Crit. Care Med. 155, 2105–2108.

Gilani, A.H., Aziz, N., Khan, M.A., et al., 2000. Ethnopharmacological evaluation of the anticonvulsant, sedative and antispasmodic activities of Lavandula stoechas L. J. Ethnopharmacol. 71, 161–167.

Giles, A., Wamer, W., Kornhauser, A., 1985. In vivo protective effect of beta-carotene against psoralen phototoxicity. Photochem. Photobiol. 41, 661–666.

Gilman, A.G., Goodman, L.S., Gilman, A., 1980. The pharmacological basis of therapeutics, sixth ed. Baillière Tyndall, London, p. 31.

Gilpin, S., Maibach, H., 2010. Allergic contact dermatitis caused by farnesol: Clinical relevance. Cutan. Ocul. Toxicol. 29, 278–287.

Gilpin, S., Hui, X., Maibach, H., 2010. In vitro human skin penetration of geraniol and citronellol. Dermatitis 21, 41–48.

Giordano-Labadie, F., Rance, F., Pellegrin, F., et al., 1999. Frequency of contact allergy in children with atopic dermatitis: results of a prospective study of 137 cases. Contact Dermatitis 40, 192–195.

Girling, J., 1887. Poisoning by pennyroyal. Br. Med. J. 1, 1214.

Glaab, V., Collins, A.R., Eisenbrand, G., et al., 2001. DNA-damaging potential and glutathione depletion of 2-cyclohexene-1-one in mammalian cells, compared to food relevant 2-alkenals. Mutat. Res. 497, 185–197.

Gloxhuber, C., 1970. Prüfung von Kosmetik-Grundstoffen auf fototoxische Wirkung. J. Soc. Cosmet. Chem. 21, 825–833.

Gluck, S.J., Benko, M.H., Hallberg, R.K., et al., 1996. Indirect determination of octanol-water partition coefficients by microemulsion electrokinetic chromatography. J. Chromatogr. A 744, 141–146.

Gocke, E., 2001. Photochemical mutagenesis: examples and toxicological relevance. J. Environ. Pathol. Toxicol. Oncol. 20, 285–292.

Goeger, D.E., Anderson, K.E., Hsie, A.W., 1998. Coumarin chemoprotection against aflatoxin B_1-induced gene mutation in a mammalian cell system: a species difference in mutagen activation and protection with chick embryo and rat liver S9. Environ. Mol. Mutagen. 32, 64–74.

Goeger, D.E., Hsie, A.W., Anderson, K.E., 1999. Co-mutagenicity of coumarin (1,2-benzopyrone) with aflatoxin B_1 and human liver S9 in mammalian cells. Food Chem. Toxicol. 37, 581–589.

Goel, H.C., Singh, S., Singh, S.P., 1989. Radiomodifying influence of camphor on sister-chromatid exchange induction in mouse bone marrow. Mutat. Res. 224, 157–160.

Goel, N., Kim, H., Lao, R.P., 2005. An olfactory stimulus modifies nighttime sleep in young men and women. Chronobiol. Int. 22, 889–904.

Goetz, A.K., Ren, H., Schmid, J.E., et al., 2007. Disruption of testosterone homeostasis as a mode of action for the reproductive toxicity of triazole fungicides in the male rat. Toxicol. Sci. 95, 227–239.

Göggelmann, W., Schimmer, O., 1983. Mutagenicity testing of β-asarone and commercial calamus drugs with Salmonella typhimurium. Mutat. Res. 121, 191–194.

Goiriz, R., Delgado-Jimenez, Y., Sanchez-Perez, J., et al., 2007. Photoallergic contact dermatitis from lavender oil in topical ketoprofen. Contact Dermatitis 57, 381–382.

Golab, M., Skwarlo-Sonta, K., 2007. Mechanisms involved in the anti-inflammatory action of inhaled tea tree oil in mice. Exp. Biol. Med. 232, 420–426.

Golab, M., Burdzenia, O., Majewski, P., et al., 2005. Tea tree oil inhalations modify immunity in mice. Journal of Applied Biomedicine 3, 101–108.

Gold, J., Gates, W., 1980. Herbal abortifacients. J. Am. Med. Assoc. 243, 1365–1366.

Goldstein, D., Tate, S., 2005. Blunt Instrument. New Sci. 185, 23.

Gollhausen, R., Enders, F., Przybilla, B., et al., 1988. Trends in allergic contact sensitization. Contact Dermatitis 18, 147–154.

Gomes-Carneiro, M.R., Felzenszwalb, I., Paumgartten, F.J.R., 1998. Mutagenicity testing of (±)-camphor, 1,8-cineole, citral, citronellal, (-)-menthol and terpineol with the Salmonella/microsome assay. Mutat. Res. 416, 129–136.

Gomes-Carneiro, M.R., De-Oliveira, A.C.A.X., De-Carvalho, R.R., et al., 2003. Inhibition of cyclophosphamide-induced teratogenesis by β-ionone. Toxicol. Lett. 138, 205–213.

Gomes-Carneiro, M.R., Viana, M.E.S., Felzenszwalb, I., et al., 2005a. Evaluation of β-myrcene, α-terpinene and (+)- and (−)-α-pinene in the Salmonella/microsome assay. Food Chem. Toxicol. 43, 247–252.

Gomes-Carneiro, M.R., Dias, D.M., De-Oliveira, A.C.A.X., et al., 2005b. Evaluation of mutagenic and antimutagenic activities of α-bisabolol in the Salmonella/microsome assay. Mutat. Res. 585, 105–112.

Gomes-Carneiro, M.R., Dias, D.M., Paumgartten, F.J., 2006. Study on the mutagenicity and antimutagenicity of β-ionone in the Salmonella/microsome assay. Food Chem. Toxicol. 44, 522–527.

Gomes Do Espirito Santo, M.E., Marrama, L., Ndiaye, K., et al., 2002. Investigation of deaths in an area of groundnut plantations in Casamance, South of Senegal after exposure to Carbofuran, Thiram and Benomyl. J. Expo. Anal. Environ. Epidemiol. 12, 381–388.

Gómez, M.I., Azana, J.M., Arranz, I., et al., 1995. Plasma levels of 8-methoxypsoralen after bath-PUVA for psoriasis: relationship to disease severity. Br. J. Dermatol. 133, 37–40.

Gonçalves, O., Pereira, R., Gonçalves, F., et al., 2011. Evaluation of the mutagenicity of sesquiterpenic compounds and their influence on the susceptibility towards antibiotics of two clinically relevant bacterial strains. Mutat. Res. 723, 18–25.

Gonzalez-Trujano, M.E., Carrera, D., Ventura-Martinez, R., 2006. Neuropharmacological profile of an ethanol extract of Ruta chalepensis L. in mice. J. Ethnopharmacol. 106, 129–135.

Goossens, A., Merckx, L., 1997. Allergic contact dermatitis from farnesol in a deodorant. Contact Dermatitis 37, 179–180.

Gopalakrishnan, N., 1994. Studies on the storage quality of CO_2 extracted cardamom and clove bud oils. J. Agric. Food Chem. 42, 796–798.

Gordon, W.P., Forte, A.J., McMurtry, R.J., et al., 1982. Hepatotoxicity and pulmonary toxicity of pennyroyal oil and its constituent terpenes in the mouse. Toxicol. Appl. Pharmacol. 65, 413–424.

Gordon, W.P., Huitric, A.C., Seth, C.L., et al., 1987. The metabolism of the abortifacient terpene, (R)-(+)-pulegone to a proximate toxin, menthofuran. Drug Metab. Dispos. 15 (5), 589–594.

Gorelick, N.J., 1995. Genotoxicity of trans-anethole in vitro. Mutat. Res. 326, 199–209.

Gori, G.B., 2001. The costly illusion of regulating unknowable risks. Regul. Toxicol. Pharmacol. 34, 205–212.

Gorji, A., Khaleghi Ghadiri, M., 2001. History of epilepsy in Medieval Iranian medicine. Neurosci. Biobehav. Rev. 25, 455–461.

Gouin, S., Patel, H., 1996. Unusual cause of seizure. Pediatr. Emerg. Care 12, 298–300.

Gould, J.W., Mercurio, M.G., Elmets, C.A., 1995. Cutaneous photosensitivity diseases induced by exogenous agents. J. Am. Acad. Dermatol. 33, 551–573.

Gould, M.N., Malzman, T.H., Tanner, M.A., et al., 1987. Anticarcinogenic effects of terpenoids in orange peel oil. In: Proceedings of the 78th Annual Meeting of the American Association for Cancer Research, vol. 28, p. 153.

Goulden, V., Wilkinson, S.M., 1998. Patch testing for Compositae allergy. Br. J. Dermatol. 138, 1018–1021.

Gowder, S.J., Devaraj, H., 2008. Food flavor cinnamaldehyde-induced biochemical and histological changes in the kidney of male albino wistar rat. Environmental Toxicology & Pharmacology 26, 68–74.

Graham, J.R., 1943. One application of benzyl benzoate for scabies. Br. Med. J. 1 (4291), 413–414.

Graham, D.C., 1961. Methyl salicylate: a lethal hazard in the home. Can. Med. Assoc. J. 84, 960.

Gral, N., Beani, J.C., Bonnot, D., et al., 1993. Plasma levels of psoralens after celery ingestion. Ann. Dermatol. Vénéréol. 120, 599–603.

Gramosa, N.V., Silveira, E.R., 2005. Volatile constituents of Copaifera langsdorffii from the Brazilian Northeast. Journal of Essential Oil Research 17, 130–132.

Grande, G.A., Dannewitz, S.R., 1987. Symptomatic sassafras oil ingestion. Vet. Hum. Toxicol. 6, 447.

Grandjean, P., 1990. Skin penetration. Hazardous chemicals at work. Taylor & Francis, London, pp. 3–4.

Grandjean, P., Landrigan, P.J., 2006. Developmental neurotoxicity of industrial chemicals. Lancet 368, 2167–2178.

Granger, R.E., Campbell, E.L., Johnston, G.A., 2005. (+)- and (-)-borneol: efficacious positive modulators of GABA action at human recombinant $\alpha_1\beta_2\gamma_{2L}$ $GABA_A$ receptors. Biochem. Pharmacol. 69, 1101–1111.

Grassmann, J., Hippeli, S., Dornisch, K., et al., 2000. Antioxidant properties of essential oils. Possible explanations for their anti-inflammatory effects. Arzneimittelforschung 50, 135–139.

Grassmann, J., Hippeli, S., Vollmann, R., et al., 2003. Antioxidative properties of the essential oil from Pinus mugo. J. Agric. Food Chem. 51, 7576–7582.

Grassmann, J., Hippeli, S., Spitzenberger, R., et al., 2005. The monoterpene terpinolene from the oil of Pinus mugo L. in concert with alpha-tocopherol and beta-carotene effectively prevents oxidation of LDL. Phytomedicine 12, 416–423.

Gray, T.J.B., Parke, D.V., Grasso, P., et al., 1972. Biochemical and pathological differences in hepatic response to chronic feeding of safrole and butylated hydroxytoluene. Proceedings of the Biochemical Society 130, 91P–92P.

Greay, S.J., Ireland, D.J., Kissick, H.T., et al., 2010a. Induction of necrosis and cell cycle arrest in murine cancer cell lines by Melaleuca alternifolia (tea tree) oil and terpinen-4-ol. Cancer Chemother. Pharmacol. 65, 877–888.

Greay, S.J., Ireland, D.J., Kissick, H.T., et al., 2010b. Inhibition of established subcutaneous murine tumour growth with topical Melaleuca alternifolia (tea tree) oil. Cancer Chemother. Pharmacol. 66, 1095–1102.

Green, C.L., Espinosa, F., 1988. Jamaican and Central American pimento (allspice, Pimenta dioica): characterization of flavor differences and other distinguishing features. In: Lawrence, B.M., Mookherjee, B.D., Willis, B.J. (Eds.), Flavors & fragrances: a world perspective. Elsevier, Amsterdam, pp. 16–20.

Green Jr., R.C., 1959. Nutmeg poisoning. J. Am. Med. Assoc. 171, 1342–1344.

Green, C., Ferguson, J., 1994. Sesquiterpene lactone mix is not an adequate screen for Compositae allergy. Contact Dermatitis 31, 151–153.

Green, N.R., Savage, J.R., 1978. Screening of safrole, eugenol, their ninhydrin positive metabolites and selected secondary amines for potential mutagenicity. Mutat. Res. 57, 115–121.

Green, M., Newell, O., Aboyade-Cole, A., et al., 2007a. Diallyl sulfide induces the expression of estrogen metabolizing genes in the presence and/or absence of diethylstilbestrol in the breast of female ACI rats. Toxicol. Lett. 168, 7–12.

Green, M., Newell, O., Aboyade-Cole, A., et al., 2007b. Diallyl sulfide induces the expression of nucleotide excision repair enzymes in the breast of female ACI rats. Toxicol. Lett. 168, 40–44.

Greenblatt, D.J., von Moltke, L.L., Harmatz, J.S., et al., 2003. Time course of recovery of cytochrome P450 3A function after single doses of grapefruit juice. Clin. Pharmacol. Ther. 74, 121–129.

Greif, N., 1967. Cutaneous safety of fragrance materials as measured by the maximization test. American Perfumer & Cosmetics 82, 54–57.

Grieve, M., 1978. A modern herbal. Penguin Books, Harmondsworth.

Griffith, M., Zile, M.H., 2000. Retinoic acid, midkine, and defects of secondary neurulation. Teratology 62, 123–133.

Grigoleit, H.G., Grigoleit, P., 2005a. Peppermint oil in irritable bowel syndrome. Phytomedicine 12, 601–606.

Grigoleit, H.G., Grigoleit, P., 2005b. Pharmacology and preclinical pharmacokinetics of peppermint oil. Phytomedicine 12, 612–616.

Grisk, A., Fisher, W., 1969. Pulmonary elimination of cineole, menthol and thymol after rectal administration in rats. Zeitschrift Ärztliche Fortbildung 63, 233–236.

Grochulski Von, A., Borkowski, B., 1972. Effect of chamomile oil in experimental glomeronephritis in rabbits. Planta. Med. 21, 289–292.

Gronka, P.A., Bobkoskie, R.L., Tomchick, G.J., et al., 1969. Camphor exposures in a packaging plant. Am. Ind. Hyg. Assoc. J. 30, 276–279.

Grootendorst, D.C., Rabe, K.F., 2004. Mechanisms of bronchial hyperreactivity in asthma and chronic obstructive pulmonary disease. Proc. Am. Thorac. Soc. 1, 77–87.

Grossweiner, L.I., 1984. Mechanisms of photosensitization by furocoumarins. Nat. Cancer Inst. Monogr. 66, 47–54.

Grote, W., Schulz, L.C., Drommer, W., et al., 1977. Test of combination of the agents coumarin and troxerutin for embryotoxic and teratogenic side-effects in Gottingen miniature pigs. Arzneimittelforschung 27, 613–617.

Grube, D.D., 1977. Photosensitizing effects of 8-methoxypsoralen on the skin of hairless mice. II. Strain and spectral differences for tumorigenesis. Photochem. Photobiol. 25, 269–276.

Gu, Y., Ting, Z., Qiu, X., et al., 2010. Linalool preferentially induces robust apoptosis of a variety of leukemia cells via upregulating p53 and cyclin-dependent kinase inhibitors. Toxicology 268, 19–24.

Guarneri, F., Barbuzza, O., Vaccaro, M., et al., 2008. Allergic contact dermatitis and asthma caused by limonene in a labourer handling citrus fruits. Contact Dermatitis 58, 315–316.

Guba, R., 1998/1999. Wound healing: a pilot study using an essential oil-based cream to heal dermal wounds and ulcers. The International Journal of Aromatherapy 9, 67–74.

Guenther, E., 1949–1952. The essential oils. vols. 1–6. Van Nostrand, New York.

Guenthner, T.M., Luo, G., 2001. Investigation of the role of the 2′,3′-epoxidation pathway in the bioactivation and genotoxicity of dietary allylbenzene analogs. Toxicology 160, 47–58.

Guerra, M.O., Andrade, A.T., 1978. Contraceptive effects of native plants in rats. Contraception 18, 191–199.

Guerra, P., Aguilar, A., Urbina, F., et al., 1987. Contact dermatitis to geraniol in a leg ulcer. Contact Dermatitis 16, 298–299.

Guerrini, A., Sacchetti, G., Rossi, D., et al., 2009. Bioactivities of Piper aduncum L. and Piper obliquum Ruiz & Pavon (Piperaceae) essential oils from Eastern Ecuador. Environmental Toxicology & Pharmacology 27, 39–48.

Guerrini, A., Rossi, D., Paganetto, G., 2011. Chemical characterization (GC/MS and NMR fingerprinting) and bioactivities of South-African Pelargonium capitatum (L.) L' Her. (Geraniaceae) essential oil. Chem. Biodivers. 8, 624–642.

Guest, A., Jackson, J.R., James, S.P., 1982. Toxicity of benzyl cyanide in the rat. Toxicol. Lett. 10, 265–272.

Guillemain, J., Rousseau, A., Delaveau, P., 1989. Neurodepressive effects of essential oil of Lavandula angustifolia Mill. Ann. Pharm. Fr. 47, 337–343.

Guilliard, M., Delgado, W., Martinez, J.R., 2000. Determination of the enantiomeric purity of carvone, main component of Colombian Lippia alba (Mill) oil by means of bidimensional gas chromatography. In: 23rd International Symposium on Capillary Chromatography, June 5–10, www.richrom.com/assets/CD23PDF/i01.html.

Guillot, S., Peytavi, L., Bureau, S., et al., 2006. Aroma characterization of various apricot varieties using headspace–solid phase microextraction combined with gas chromatography–mass spectrometry and gas chromatography–olfactometry. Food Chem. 96, 147–155.

Guin, J.D., Jackson, D.B., 1988. Oakmoss photosensitivity in a ragweed-allergic patient. Contact Dermatitis 18, 240–242.

Guin, J.D., Meyer, B.N., Drake, R.D., et al., 1984. The effect of quenching agents on contact urticaria caused by cinnamic aldehyde. J. Am. Acad. Dermatol. 10, 45–51.

Güllüce, M., Sökmen, M., Daferera, D., et al., 2003. In vitro antibacterial, antifungal, and antioxidant activities of the essential oil and methanol extracts of herbal parts and callus cultures of Satureja hortensis L. J. Agric. Food Chem. 51, 3958–3965.

Gunby, P., 1979. Plant known for centuries still causes problems today. J. Am. Med. Assoc. 241, 2246–2247.

Gundert-Remy, U., Sonich-Mullin, C., 2002. The use of toxicokinetic and toxicodynamic data in risk assessment: an international perspective. Sci. Total Environ. 288, 3–11.

Gunn, J.W.C., 1921. The action of the 'emmenagogue' oils on the human uterus. J. Pharmacol. Exp. Ther. 16, 485–489.

Guo, L.Q., Taniguchi, M., Xiao, Y.Q., et al., 2000. Inhibitory effect of natural furanocoumarins on human microsomal cytochrome P450 3A activity. Jpn. J. Pharmacol. 82, 122–129.

Gupta, A., Myrdal, P.B., 2004. Development of a perillyl alcohol topical cream formulation. Int. J. Pharm. 269, 373–383.

Gupta, K.P., Van Golen, K.L., Putman, K.L., et al., 1993. Formation and persistence of safrole-DNA adducts over a 10,000-fold dose range in mouse liver. Carcinogenesis 14, 1517–1521.

Gurr, F.W., Scroggie, J.G., 1965. Eucalyptus oil poisoning treated by dialysis and mannitol infusion. Australas. Ann. Med. 14, 238–249.

Gurudut, K.N., Naik, J.P., Srinivas, P., et al., 1996. Volatile constituents of large cardamon (Amomum subulatum Roxb). Flavour & Fragrance Journal 11, 7–9.

Gutiérrez-Pajares, J.L., Lidia Zúñiga, J.P., 2003. Ruta graveolens aqueous extract retards mouse preimplantation embryo development. Reprod. Toxicol. 17, 667–672.

Guyonnet, D., Belloir, C., Suschetet, M., et al., 2001. Antimutagenic activity of organosulfur compounds from Allium is associated with phase II enzyme induction. Mutat. Res. 495, 135–145.

Guyonnet, D., Belloir, C., Suschetet, M., et al., 2002. Mechanisms of protection against aflatoxin B(1) genotoxicity in rats treated by organosulfur compounds from garlic. Carcinogenesis 23, 1335–1341.

Guyonnet, D., Berges, R., Siess, M.H., et al., 2004. Post-initiation modulating effects of allyl sulfides in rat hepatocarcinogenesis. Food Chem. Toxicol. 42, 1479–1485.

Gwak, H.S., Chun, I.K., 2002. Effect of vehicles and penetration enhancers on the in vitro percutaneous absorption of tenoxicam through hairless mouse skin. International Journal of Phamaceutics 236, 57–64.

Gyoubu, K., Miyazawa, M., 2007. In vitro metabolism of (−)-camphor using human liver microsomes and CYP2A6. Biol. Pharm. Bull. 30, 230–233.

Haag, J.D., Gould, M.N., 1994. Mammary carcinoma regression induced by perillyl alcohol, a hydroxylated analog of limonene. Cancer Chemother. Pharmacol. 34, 477–483.

Haag, J.D., Lindstrom, M.J., Gould, M.N., 1992. Limonene-induced regression of mammary carcinomas. Cancer Res. 52, 4021–4026.

Haber, D., Siess, M., Canivenc-Lavier, M., et al., 1995. Differential effects of dietary diallyl sulfide and diallyl disulfide on rat intestinal and hepatic drug-metabolizing enzymes. J. Toxicol. Environ. Health 44, 423–434.

Haber-Mignard, D., Suschetet, M., Berges, R., et al., 1996. Inhibition of aflatoxin B1- and N-nitrosodiethylamine-induced liver preneoplastic foci in rats fed naturally occurring allyl sulfides. Nutr. Cancer 25, 61–70.

Habersang, S., Leuschner, F., Isaac, O., et al., 1979. Pharmacological studies of chamomile constituents IV. Studies on the toxicity of (−)-α-bisabolol. Planta Med. 37, 115–123.

Hackzell-Bradley, M., Bradley, T., Fischer, T., 1997. Case report, Contact allergy caused by tea tree oil. Lakartidningen 94, 4359–4361.

Hadidi, H., Zahlsen, K., Idle, J.R., et al., 1997. A single amino acid substitution (Leu160His) in cytochrome P450 CYP2A6 causes switching from 7-hydroxylation to 3-hydroxylation of coumarin. Food Chem. Toxicol. 35, 903–907.

Hadidi, H., Irshaid, Y., Vågbø, C.B., et al., 1998. Variability of coumarin 7- and 3-hydroxylation in a Jordanian population is suggestive of a functional polymorphism in cytochrome P450 CYP2A6. Eur. J. Clin. Pharmacol. 54, 437–441.

Hafizoglu, H., 1982. Analytical studies on the balsam of Liquidambar orientalis Mill. by gas chromatography and mass spectrometry. Holforschung 36, 311–313.

Hagan, E.C., Jenner, P.M., Jones, W.I., et al., 1965. Toxic properties of compounds related to safrole. Toxicol. Appl. Pharmacol. 7, 18–24.

Hagan, E.C., Hansen, W.H., Fitzhugh, O.G., et al., 1967. Food flavorings and compounds of related structure II. Subacute and chronic toxicity. Food Cosmet. Toxicol. 5, 141–157.

Hagvall, L., Baron, J.M., Börje, A., et al., 2008. Cytochrome P450-mediated activation of the fragrance compound geraniol forms potent contact allergens. Toxicol. Appl. Pharmacol. 233, 308–313.

Hagvall, L., Karlberg, A.T., Christensson, J.B., 2012. Contact allergy to air-exposed geraniol: clinical obervations and report of 14 cases. Contact Dermatitis 67, 20–27.

Haider, F., Dwivedi, P.D., Naqvi, A.A., et al., 2003. Essential oil composition of Artemisia vulgaris harvested at different growth periods under Indo-Gangetic plain conditions. Journal of Essential Oil Research 15, 376–378.

Hakim, I.A., Harris, R.B., Ritenbaugh, C., 2000. Citrus peel use is associated with reduced risk of squamous cell carcinoma of the skin. Nutr. Cancer 37, 161–168.

Halicioglu, O., Astarcioglu, G., Yaprak, I., et al., 2011. Toxicity of *Salvia officinalis* in a newborn and a child: an alarming report. Pediatr. Neurol. 45, 259–260.

Hall, L., 2000. Chemotaxonomical investigation of frankincense producing Boswellia spp. from Somalia and a quest for quality standards. Thesis. University of Strathclyde.

Hall, A.C., Turcotte, C.M., Betts, B.A., et al., 2004. Modulation of human GABA$_A$ and glycine receptor currents by menthol and related monoterpenoids. Eur. J. Pharmacol. 506, 9–16.

Hällström, H., Thuvander, A., 1997. Toxicological evaluation of myristicin. Nat. Toxins 5, 186–192.

Hamada, M., Uezu, K., Matsushita, J., et al., 2002. Distribution and immune responses resulting from oral administration of *d*-limonene in rats. J. Nutr. Sci. Vitamino. (Tokyo) 48, 155–160.

Hamden, K., Keskes, H., Belhaj, S., et al., 2011. Inhibitory potential of omega-3 fatty and fenugreek essential oil on key enzymes of carbohydrate-digestion and hypertension in diabetes rats. Lipids Health Dis. 10, 226.

Hamaguchi, F., Tsutsui, T., 2000. Assessment of genotoxicity of dental antiseptics: ability of phenol, guaiacol, *p*-phenolsulfonic acid, sodium hypochlorite, *p*-chlorophenol, *m*-cresol or formaldehyde to induce unscheduled DNA synthesis in cultured Syrian hamster embryo cells. Jpn. J. Pharmacol. 83, 273–276.

Hammer, K.A., Carson, C.F., Riley, T.V., 2008. Frequencies of resistance to *Melaleuca alternifolia* (tea tree) oil and rifampicin in *Staphylococcus aureus*. *Staphylococcus epidermidis* and *Enterococcus faecalis*. Int. J. Antimicrob. Agents 32, 170–173.

Hammer, K.A., Carson, C.F., Riley, T.V., 2012. Effects of Melaleuca alternifolia (tea tree) essential oil and the major monoterpene component terpinen-4-ol on the development of single- and multistep antibiotic resistance and antimicrobial susceptibility. Antimicrob. Agents Chemother. 57, 909–915.

Hamond, P.W., 1906. Nutmeg poisoning. Br. Med. J. 2, 778.

Hanau, D., Grosshans, E., Barbier, P., et al., 1983. The influence of limonene on induced delayed hypersensitivity to citral in guinea pigs I. Histological study. Acta Derm. Venereol. 63, 1–7.

Hanausek, M., Walaszek, Z., Slaga, T.J., 2003. Detoxifying cancer causing agents to prevent cancer. Integr. Cancer Ther. 2, 139–144.

Hanawalt, P.C., 2001. Revisiting the rodent repairadox. Environ. Mol. Mutagen. 38, 89–96.

Handayani, T., Sakinah, S., Nallappan, M., 2007. Regulation of p53-, Bcl-2- and caspase-dependent signaling pathway in xanthorrhizol-induced apoptosis of HepG2 hepatoma cells. Anticancer Res. 27, 965–971.

Handjieva, N.V., Popov, S.S., 1996. Constituents of essential oils from *Nepeta cataria* L., *N. grandiflora* M.B. and *N. nuda* L. Journal of Essential Oil Research 8, 639–643.

Hannuksela-Svahn, A., Pukkala, E., Kuolu, L., et al., 1999. Cancer incidence among Finnish psoriasis patients treated with 8-methoxypsoralen bath PUVA. J. Am. Acad. Dermatol. 40, 694–696.

Hansch, C., Fujita, T., 1964. rho - delta - pi Analysis. A method for the correlation of biological activity and chemical structure. J. Am. Chem. Soc. 86, 1616–1626.

Hansson, S.O., Rudén, C., 2006. Evaluating the risk decision process. Toxicology 218, 100–111.

Hanus, L.O., Rezanka, T., Dembitsky, V.M., et al., 2005. Myrrh – *Commiphora* chemistry. Biomed. Pap. Med. Fac. Univ. Palacky Olomouc Czech. Repub. 149, 3–27.

Harada, M., Yano, S., 1975. Pharmacological studies on Chinese cinnamon. II. Effects of cinnamaldehyde on the cardiovascular and digestive systems. Chem. Pharm. Bull. (Tokyo) 23, 941–947.

Harbeson, A.E., 1936. A case of turpentine poisoning. Can. Med. Assoc. J. 549–550.

Harborne, J.B., Baxter, H. (Eds.), 1993. Phytochemical dictionary: a handbook of bioactive compounds from plants. Taylor & Francis, London.

Hard, G.C., Whysner, J., 1994. Risk assessment of *d*-limonene: an example of male rat-specific renal tumorigens. Crit. Rev. Toxicol. 24, 231–254.

Hard, G.C., Rodgers, I.S., Baetcke, K.P., et al., 1993. Hazard evaluation of chemicals that cause accumulation of alpha 2u-globulin, hyaline droplet nephropathy, and tubule neoplasia in the kidneys of male rats. Environ. Health Perspect. 99, 313–349.

Hardin, B.D., Schuler, R.L., Burg, J.R., et al., 1987. Evaluation of 60 chemicals in a preliminary developmental toxicity test. Teratog. Carcinog. Mutagen. 7, 29–48.

Hardisty, R.M., Weatherall, D.J., 1982. Blood and its disorders, second ed. Blackwell Scientific Publications, Oxford.

Hardy, M., 1991. Sweet scented dreams. Int. J. Aromather. 3, 12–13.

Harkenthal, M., Hausen, B.M., Reichling, J., 2000. 1,2,4-trihydroxymenthane, a contact allergen from oxidized Australian tea tree oil. Pharmazie 55, 153–154.

Harkiss, K.J., Linley, P.A., 1973. Evaluation of tolu balsam by gas-liquid chromatography. J. Pharm. Pharmacol 25 (Suppl.), 146.

Harney, J.W., Barofsky, I.M., Leary, J.D., 1978. Behavioral and toxicological studies of cyclopentanoid monoterpenes from *Nepeta cataria*. Lloydia 41, 367–374.

Harpin, V.A., Rutter, N., 1983. Barrier properties of the newborn infant's skin. Journal of Pediatrics 102, 419–425.

Harry, R.G., 1948. Cosmetic Materials, vol. II. Leonard Hill, London.

Hartiala, K.J., Pulkkinen, M., Ball, P., 1966. Inhibition of β-D-glucosiduronic acid conjugation by eugenol. Nature (London) 210, 739.

Hartman, D., Coetzee, J.C., 2002. Two US practitioners' experience of using essential oils for wound care. J. Wound Care 11, 317–320.

Hartnoll, G., Moore, D., Douek, D., 1993. Near fatal ingestion of oil of cloves. Arch. Dis. Child. 69, 392–393.

Hasani, A., Pavia, D., Toms, N., et al., 2003. Effect of aromatics on lung mucociliary clearance in patients with chronic airways obstruction. J. Altern. Complement. Med. 9, 243–249.

Haseman, J.K., Huff, J.E., Rao, G.N., 1985. Neoplasms observed in untreated and corn oil gavage control groups of F344/N rats and (C57BL/6 N X C3H/HeN)F1 (B6C3F1) mice. J. Natl. Cancer Inst. 75, 975–984.

Hasheminejad, G., Caldwell, J., 1994. Genotoxicity of the alkenylbenzenes *alpha*- and *beta*-asarone, myristicin and elemicin as determined by the UDS assay in cultured rat hepatocytes. Food Chem. Toxicol. 32, 223–232.

Hashim, S., Aboobaker, V.S., Madhubala, R., et al., 1994. Modulatory effects of essential oils from spices on the formation of DNA adduct by aflatoxin B$_1$ *in vitro*. Nutr. Cancer 21, 169–175.

Hashim, S., Banerjee, S., Madhubala, R., et al., 1998. Chemoprevention of DMBA-induced transplacental and translactational carcinogenesis in mice by oil from mustard seeds (*Brassica* spp.). Cancer Lett. 134, 217–226.

Hashimoto, M., Davis, D.C., Gillette, J.R., 1972. Effect of different routes of administration of cedrene on hepatic drug metabolism. Biochem. Pharmacol. 21, 1514–1517.

Hashimoto, Y., Sugai, T., Shoji, A., et al., 1990. Incidence of positive reactions in patch tests with ingredients of cosmetic products in 1989 and representative cases of cosmetic dermatitis. Skin Research 32 (Suppl. 9), 115–124.

Hashimoto, Y., Kawaguchi, M., Miyazaki, K., et al., 2003. Estrogenic activity of tissue conditioners in vitro. Dent. Mater. 19, 341–346.

Hassan, S.B., Gali-Muhtasib, H., Göransson, H., et al., 2010. Alpha terpineol: a potential anticancer agent which acts through suppressing NF-kappaB signalling. Anticancer Res. 30, 1911–1919.

Hata, T., Sakaguchi, I., Mori, M., et al., 2003. Induction of apoptosis by *Citrus paradisi* essential oil in human leukemic (HL-60) cells. In Vivo 17, 553–559.

Hatem, S., Attal, N., Willer, J.C., et al., 2006. Psychophysical study of the effects of topical application of menthol in healthy volunteers. Pain 122, 190–196.

Hattori, M., Yang, X.W., Miyashiro, H., et al., 1993. Inhibitory effects of monomeric and dimeric phenylpropanoids from mace on lipid peroxidation *in vivo* and *in vitro*. Phytotherapy Research 7, 395–401.

Hatziantoniou, S., Dimas, K., Georgopoulos, A., et al., 2006. Cytotoxic and antitumor activity of liposome-incorporated sclareol against cancer cell lines and human colon cancer xenografts. Pharmacol. Res. 53, 80–87.

Hau, K.M., Connell, D.W., Richardson, B.J., 1999. Quantitative structure-activity relationships for nasal pungency thresholds of volatile organic compounds. Toxicol. Sci. 47, 93–98.

Hausen, B.M., 2001. Contact allergy to balsam of Peru. II. Patch test results in 102 patients with selected balsam of Peru constituents. Am. J. Contact Dermat 12, 93–102.

Hausen, B.M., Evers, P., Stuwe, H.T., et al., 1992. Propolis allergy (IV). Studies with further sensitizers from propolis and constituents common to propolis, poplar buds and balsam of Peru. Contact Dermatitis 26, 34–44.

Hausen, B.M., Simatupang, T., Bruhn, G., et al., 1995. Identification of new allergenic constituents and proof of evidence for coniferyl benzoate in balsam of Peru. Am. J. Contact Dermat. 6, 199–208.

Hausen, B.M., Reichling, J., Harkenthal, M., 1999. Degradation products of monoterpenes are the sensitising agents of tea tree oil. Am. J. Contact Dermat. 10, 68–77.

Hausner, H., Bredie, W.L., Molgaard, C., et al., 2008. Differential transfer of dietary flavour compounds into human breast milk. Physiol. Behav. 95, 118–124.

Hawthorn, M., Ferrante, J., Luchowski, E., et al., 1988. The actions of peppermint oil and menthol on calcium channel dependent processes in intestinal, neuronal and cardiac preparations. Aliment. Pharmacol. Ther. 2, 101–118.

Haworth, S., Lawlor, T., Mortelmans, K., et al., 1983. Salmonella mutagenicity test results for 250 chemicals. Environ. Mutagen. 5, 3–38.

Hayashi, M., Kishi, M., Sofuni, T., et al., 1988. Micronucleus tests in mice on 39 food additives and eight miscellaneous chemicals. Food Chem. Toxicol. 26, 487–500.

Hayder, N., Kilani, S., Abdelwahed, A., 2003. Antimutagenic activity of aqueous extracts and essential oil isolated from Myrtus communis. Pharmazie 58, 523–524.

Hayder, N., Abdelwahed, A., Kilani, S., et al., 2004. Anti-genotoxic and free-radical scavenging activities of extracts from (Tunisian) Myrtus communis. Mutat. Res. 564, 89–95.

Hayes, A.J., Markovic, B., 2002. Toxicity of Australian essential oil Backhousia citriodora (Lemon myrtle). Part 1. Absorption and histopathology following application to human skin. Food Chem. Toxicol. 40, 535–543.

Hayes, A.J., Markovic, B., 2003. Toxicity of Australian essential oil Backhousia citriodora (Lemon myrtle). Part 2. Antimicrobial activity and in vitro cytotoxicity. Food Chem. Toxicol. 41, 1409–1416.

Hayes, A.J., Leach, D.N., Markham, J.L., 1997. In vitro cytotoxicity of Australian tea tree oil using human cell lines. Journal of Essential Oil Research 9, 575–582.

Haze, S., Sakai, K., Gozu, Y., 2002. Effects of fragrance inhalation on sympathetic activity in normal adults. Jpn. J. Pharmacol. 90, 247–253.

Hazleton, L.W., Tusing, T.W., Zeitlin, B.R., et al., 1956. Toxicity of coumarin. J. Pharmacol. Exp. Ther. 118, 348–358.

He, K., Zeng, L., Shi, G., et al., 1997a. Bioactive compounds from Taiwania cryptomerioides. J. Nat. Prod. 60, 38–40.

He, L., Mo, H., Hadisusilo, S., et al., 1997b. Isoprenoids suppress the growth of murine B16 melanomas in vitro and in vivo. J. Nutr. 127, 668–674.

Health Canada Cosmetic Ingredient Hotlist, March 2011. http://www.hc-sc.gc.ca/cps-spc/cosmet-person/indust/hot-list-critique/hotlist-liste-eng.php.

Heard, C.M., Gallagher, S.J., Congiatu, C., et al., 2005. Preferential pi-pi complexation between tamoxifen and borage oil/gamma linolenic acid: transcutaneous delivery and NMR spectral modulation. Int. J. Pharm. 302, 47–55.

Hébert, C.D., Yuan, J., Dieter, M.P., 1994. Comparison of the toxicity of cinnamaldehyde when administered by microencapsulation in feed or by corn oil gavage. Food Chem. Toxicol. 12, 1107–1115.

Hecht, S.S., 1995. Chemoprevention by isothiocyanates. Journal of Cell Biochemistry (Supplement) 22, 195–209.

Hecht, S.S., Kenney, P.M., Wang, M., et al., 2000. Effects of phenethyl isothiocyanate and benzyl isothiocyanate, individually and in combination, on lung tumorigenesis induced in A/J mice by benzo[a]pyrene and 4-(methylnitrosamino)-1-(3-pyridyl)-1-butanone. Cancer Lett. 150, 49–56.

Hecht, S.S., Kenney, P.M., Wang, M., et al., 2002. Benzyl isothiocyanate: an effective inhibitor of polycyclic aromatic hydrocarbon tumorigenesis in A/J mouse lung. Cancer Lett. 187, 87–94.

Heck, J.D., Vollmuth, T.A., Cifone, M.A., et al., 1989. An evaluation of food flavoring ingredients in a genetic toxicity screening battery. Toxicologist 9, 257.

Hedenstierna, G., Alexandersson, R., Wimander, K., et al., 1983. Exposure to terpenes: effects on pulmonary function. Int. Arch. Occup. Environ. Health 51, 191–198.

Heikkila, A., Renkonen, O.V., Erkkola, R., 1992. Pharmacokinetics and placental passage of imipenem during pregnancy. Antimicrob. Agents Chemother. 36, 2652–2655.

Heinemann, U., Louvel, J., 1983. Changes in $[Ca^{2+}]o$ and $[K^+]o$ during repetitive electrical stimulation and during pentetrazol induced seizure activity in the sensorimotor cortex of cats. Pflugers Archives 398, 310–317.

Heinonen, O.P., Slone, D., Shapiro, S., 1977. Birth defects and drugs in pregnancy. Publishing Science Group, Littleton.

Heinrichs, L., 2002. Linking olfaction with nausea and vomiting of pregnancy, recurrent abortion, hyperemesis gravidarum, and migraine headache. Am. J. Obstet. Gynecol. 186, S215–S219.

Heisterberg, M.V., Menné, T., Johansen, J.D., 2011. Contact allergy to the 26 specific fragrance ingredients to be declared on cosmetic products in accordance with the EU cosmetics directive. Contact Dermatitis 65, 266–275.

Held, J.L., Ruszkowski, A.M., DeLeo, V.A., 1988. Consort contact dermatitis due to oak moss. Arch. Dermatol. 124, 261–262.

Helen, A., Rajasree, C.R., Krishnakumar, K., et al., 1999. Antioxidant role of oils isolated from garlic (Allium sativum Linn.) and onion (Allium cepa Linn.) on nicotine-induced lipid peroxidation. Vet. Hum. Toxicol. 41, 316–319.

Hemmer, W., Focke, M., Leitner, B., et al., 2000. Axillary dermatitis from farnesol in a deodorant. Contact Dermatitis 42, 168–169.

Hendriks, H., Bos, R., Allersma, D.P., et al., 1981. Pharmacological screening of valerenal and some other components of the essential oil of Valeriana officinalis. Planta Med. 42, 62–68.

Hendriks, H., Bos, R., Woerdenbag, H.J., et al., 1985. Central nervous depressant activity of valerenic acid in the mouse. Planta Med. 51, 28–31.

Heng, M.C., 1987. Local necrosis and interstitial nephritis due to topical methyl salicylate and menthol. Cutis 39, 442–444.

Hendy, M.S., Beattie, B.E., Burge, P.S., 1985. Br. J. Ind. Med. 42, 51–54.

Henley, V., Lipson, N., Korach, K.S., Bloch, C.A., 2007. Prepubertal gynecomastia linked to lavender and tea tree oils. N. Engl. J. Med. 356, 479–485.

Herd, R.M., Tidman, M.J., Prescott, R.J., et al., 1996. Prevalence of atopic eczema in the community: the Lothian Atopic Dermatitis study. Br. J. Dermatol. 135, 18–19.

Herrman, J.L., Younes, M., 1999. Background to the ADI/TDI/PTWI. Regul. Toxicol. Pharmacol. 30, S109–S113.

Hermann, K., Le Roux, A., Fiddes, F.S., 1956. Death from apiol used as an abortifacient. Lancet 1, 937–939.

Hernandez-Ceruelos, A., Madrigal-Bujaidar, E., de la Cruz, C., 2002. Inhibitory effect of chamomile essential oil on the sister chromatid exchanges induced by daunorubicin and methyl menthanesulfonate in mouse bone marrow. Toxicol. Lett. 135, 103–110.

Herrmann, K., Engst, W., Appel, K.E., et al., 2012. Identification of human and murine sulfotransferases able to activate hydroxylated metabolites of methyleugenol to mutagens in Salmonella typhimurium and detection of associated DNA adducts using UPLC-MS/MS methods. Mutagenesis 27, 453–462.

Héthelyi, E.B., Cseko, I., Grósz, G.M., et al., 1995. Chemical composition of the Artemisia annua essential oils from Hungary. Journal of Essential Oil Research 7, 45–48.

Heuberger, E., Hongratanaworakit, T., Bohm, C., et al., 2001. Effects of chiral fragrances on human autonomic nervous system parameters and self-evaluation. Chem. Senses 26, 281–292.

Heydorn, S., Johansen, J.D., Andersen, K.E., et al., 2002. Identification of fragrances relevant to hand eczema. Contact Dermatitis 46, 21–22.

Heydorn, S., Menné, T., Andersen, K.E., et al., 2003a. Citral: a fragrance allergen and irritant. Contact Dermatitis 49, 32–36.

Heydorn, S., Johansen, J.D., Andersen, K.E., et al., 2003b. Fragrance allergy in patients with hand eczema - a clinical study. Contact Dermatitis 48, 317–323.

Heydorn, S., Menné, T., Andersen, K.E., et al., 2003c. The fragrance hand immersion study - an experimental model simulating real-life exposure for allergic contact dermatitis on the hands. Contact Dermatitis 48, 324–330.

Hibasami, H., Yamada, Y., Moteki, H., et al., 2003. Sesquiterpenes (costunolide and zaluzanin D) isolated from laurel (*Laurus nobilis* L.) induce cell death and morphological change indicative of apoptotic chromatin condensation in leukemia HL-60 cells. Int. J. Mol. Med. 12, 147–151.

Hiki, N., Kurosaka, H., Tatsutomi, Y., et al., 2003. Peppermint oil reduces gastric spasm during upper endoscopy: a randomized, double-blind, double-dummy controlled trial. Gastrointest. Endosc. 57, 475–482.

Hikiba, H., Watanabe, E., Barrett, J.C., et al., 2005. Ability of fourteen chemical agents used in dental practice to induce chromosome aberrations in Syrian hamster embryo cells. J. Pharmacol. Sci. 97, 146–152.

Hiller, J.L., Benda, G.I., Rahatzad, M., et al., 1986. Benzyl alcohol toxicity: impact on mortality and intraventricular hemorrhage among very low birth weight infants. Pediatrics 77, 500–506.

Hills, J.M., Aaronson, P.I., 1991. The mechanism of action of peppermint oil on gastrointestinal smooth muscle. Gastroenterology 101, 55–65.

Hilton, I., Dearman, R.J., Fielding, I., et al., 1996. Evaluation of the sensitizing potential of eugenol and isoeugenol in mice and guinea pigs. J. Appl. Toxicol. 16, 459–464.

Hindle, R.C., 1994. Eucalyptus oil ingestion. N. Z. Med. J. 107, 185–186.

Hiramatsu, N., Xiufen, W., Yakechi, R., et al., 2004. Antimutagenicity of Japanese traditional herbs, gennoshoko, yomogi, senburi and iwa-tobacco. Biofactors 22, 123–125.

Hiroi, T., Miyazaki, Y., Kobayashi, Y., et al., 1995. Induction of hepatic P450s in rat by essential wood and leaf oils. Xenobiotica 25, 457–467.

Hirose, O., Arima, Y., Hosokawa, K., et al., 1987. Patch test results of cosmetic allergens during recent 30 months. Skin Research 29, 95–100.

Hirose, M., Yamaguchi, T., Kimoto, N., et al., 1998. Strong promoting activity of phenylethyl isothiocyanate and benzyl isothiocyanate on urinary bladder carcinogenesis in F344 male rats. Int. J. Cancer 77, 773–777.

Hjorth, N., 1961. Eczematous allergy to balsams: allied perfumes and flavoring agents with special reference to Balsam of Peru. Munksgaard, Copenhagen.

Ho, P.C., Saville, D.J., Wanwimolruk, S., 2001. Inhibition of human CYP3A4 activity by grapefruit flavonoids, furanocoumarins and related compounds. J. Pharm. Pharm. Sci. 4, 217–227.

Ho, S., Calder, R.J., Thomas, C.P., et al., 2004. In-vitro transcutaneous delivery of tamoxifen and gamma-linolenic acid from borage oil containing ethanol and 1,8-cineole. J. Pharm. Pharmacol. 56, 1357–1364.

Hoberg, E., Sticher, O., Orjala, J.E., et al., 1999. Diterpene aus Agni-casti fructus und ihre Analytik. Zeitschrift für Phytotherapie 20, 149–150.

Hoberman, A.M., Vollmuth, T.A., Bennett, M.B., et al., 1989. An evaluation of food flavoring ingredients using an in vivo reproductive and developmental toxicity screening test. Private communication to FEMA, cited in www.epa.gov/hpv/pubs/summaries/monoterp/c13756tp.pdf (accessed 18.12.11.).

Hoeger, P.H., Enzmann, C.C., 2002. Skin physiology of the neonate and young infant: a prospective study of functional skin parameters during early infancy. Pediatr. Dermatol. 19, 256–262.

Hohenwallner, W., Klima, J., 1971. *In vivo* activation of glucuronyl transferase in rat liver by eucalyptol. Biochem. Pharmacol. 20, 3463–3472.

Holck, A.R., Estep, J.E., Hemeyer, R.D., 1991. Teratogenicity of *d*-limonene to *Xenopus* embryos. Journal of the American College of Toxicology 10, 624.

Höld, K.M., Sirisoma, N.S., Ikeda, T., et al., 2000. α-Thujone (the active component of absinthe): γ-aminobutyric acid type A receptor modulation and metabolic detoxification. Proc. Natl. Acad. Sci. U. S. A. 97, 3826–3831.

Höld, K.M., Sirisoma, N.S., Casida, J.E., 2001. Detoxification of alpha- and beta-thujones (the active ingredients of absinthe): site specificity and species differences in cytochrome P450 oxidation *in vitro* and *in vivo*. Chem. Res. Toxicol. 14, 589–595.

Höld, K.M., Sirisoma, N.S., Sparks, S.E., et al., 2002. Metabolism and mode of action of cis- and trans-3-pinanones (the active ingredients of hyssop oil). Xenobiotica 32, 251–265.

Holland, G.W., 1902. A case of poisoning from pennyroyal. Virginia Medical Semi-Monthly 7, 319.

Holland, B., Pokorny, M.E., 2001. Slow stroke back massage: its effect on patients in a rehabilitation setting. Rehabil. Nurs. 26, 182–186.

Holm, Y., Laakso, I., Hiltunen, R., 1994. The enantiometic composition of monoterpene hydrocarbons as a chemotaxonomic marker in A. sachalinensis & A. mayriana essential oils. Flavour & Fragrance Journal 9, 223–227.

Holmes, C., Hopkins, V., Hensford, C., et al., 2002. Lavender oil as a treatment for agitated behaviour in severe dementia: a placebo controlled study. Int. J. Geriatr. Psychiatry 17, 305–308.

Homburger, F., Boger, E., 1968. The carcinogenicity of essential oils, flavors and spices: a review. Cancer Res. 28, 2372–2374.

Homburger, F., Kelley, T., Friedler, G., et al., 1961. Toxic and possible carcinogenic effects of 4-allyl-1,2-methylenedioxy-benzene (safrole) in rats on deficient diets. Medicina Experimentalis 4, 1–11.

Homburger, F., Kelley, T., Baker, T.R., et al., 1962. Sex effect on hepatic pathology from deficient diet and safrole in rats. Arch. Pathol. 73, 118–125.

Homburger, F., Treger, A., Boger, E., 1971. Inhibition of murine subcutaneous and intravenous benzo(rst)pentaphene carcinogenesis by sweet orange oils and *d*-limonene. Oncology 25, 1–10.

Homer, L.E., Leach, D.N., Lea, D., et al., 2000. Natural variation in the essential oil content of *Melaleuca alternifolia* Cheel (Myrtaceae). Biochemical Systematics & Ecology 28, 367–382.

Hong, J.Y., Wang, Z.Y., Smith, T.J., et al., 1992. Inhibitory effects of diallyl sulfide on the metabolism and tumorigenicity of the tobacco-specific carcinogen 4-(methylnitrosamino)-1-(3-pyridyl)-1-butanone (NNK) in A/J mouse lung. Carcinogenesis 13, 901–904.

Hongratanaworakit, T., Buchbauer, G., 2004. Evaluation of the harmonizing effect of ylang-ylang oil on humans after inhalation. Planta Med. 70, 632–636.

Hongratanaworakit, T., Heuberger, E., Buchbauer, G., 2004. Evaluation of the effects of East Indian sandalwood oil and alpha-santalol on humans after transdermal absorption. Planta Med. 70, 3–7.

Hooth, M.J., Sills, R.C., Burka, L.T., et al., 2004. Toxicology and carcinogenesis studies of microencapsulated *trans*-cinnamaldehyde in rats and mice. Food Chem. Toxicol. 42, 1757–1768.

Horikawa, E., Okada, T., 1975. Expermental study on the acute toxicity of phenol camphor. Shikwa Gakuho 75, 934–939.

Horn, T.L., Long, L., Cwik, M.J., et al., 2005. Modulation of hepatic and renal drug metabolizing enzyme activities in rats by subchronic administration of farnesol. Chem. Biol. Interact. 152, 79–99.

Horning, M.G., Bell, L., Carman, M.J., et al., 1974. GC-MS studies of the metabolism of safrole, an hepatocarcinogen, in the rat and guinea pig. Toxicol. Appl. Pharmacol. 29, 89(Abstract).

Horst, K., Rychlik, M., 2010. Quantification of 1,8-cineole and of its metabolites in humans using stable isotope dilution assays. Mol. Nutr. Food Res. 54, 1515–1529.

Horváth, G., Szabó, L.G., Héthelyi, E., et al., 2006. Essential oil composition of three cultivated *Thymus* chemotypes from Hungary. Journal of Essential Oil Research 18, 315–317.

Horváthová, E., Sramková, M., Lábaj, J., et al., 2006. Study of cytotoxic, genotoxic and DNA-protective effects of selected plant essential oils on human cells cultured *in vitro*. Neuro. Endocrinol. Lett. 27 (Suppl. 2), 44–47.

Horváthová, E., Turcaniova, V., Slamenová, D., 2007. Comparative study of DNA-damaging and DNA-protective effects of selected components of essential plant oils in human leukemic cells K562. Neoplasma 54, 478–483.

Horváthová, E., Slamenová, D., Marsálková, L., et al., 2009. Effects of borneol on the level of DNA damage induced in primary rat hepatocytes and testicular cells by hydrogen peroxide. Food Chem. Toxicol. 47, 1318–1323.

Hoskyn, J., Guin, J.D., 2005. Contact allergy to cinnamal in a patient with oral lichen planus. Contact Dermatitis 52, 160–161.

Hosoi, J., Tsuchiya, T., 2000. Regulation of cutaneous allergic reaction by odorant inhalation. J. Invest. Dermatol. 114, 541–544.

Hosoi, J., Tanida, M., Tsuchiya, T., 2001. Mitigation of stress-induced suppression of contact hypersensitivity by odorant inhalation. Br. J. Dermatol. 145, 716–719.

Hosoi, J., Tanida, M., Tsuchiya, T., 2003. Regulation of plasma substance P and skin mast cells by odorants. J. Cutan. Med. Surg. 7, 287–291.

Hosomi, J., Kuroki, T., 1985. UV-induced unscheduled DNA synthesis in cultured human epidermal and dermal cells. Jpn. J. Cancer Res. 76, 1072–1077.

Hossain, S.J., Hamamoto, K., Aoshima, H., et al., 2002. Effects of tea components on the response of GABA(A) receptors expressed in Xenopus Oocytes. J. Agric. Food Chem. 50, 3954–3960.

Hossain, S.J., Aoshima, H., Koda, H., et al., 2004. Fragrances in oolong tea that enhance the response of GABAA receptors. Biosci. Biotechnol. Biochem. 68, 1842–1848.

Hosseinzadeh, H., Parvardeh, S., 2004. Anticonvulsant effects of thymoquinone, the major constituent of Nigella sativa seeds, in mice. Phytomedicine 11, 56–64.

Hosseinzadeh, H., Parvardeh, S., Asl, M.N., et al., 2007. Effect of thymoquinone and Nigella sativa seeds oil on lipid peroxidation level during global cerebral ischemia-reperfusion injury in rat hippocampus. Phytomedicine 14, 621–627.

Hostýnek, J.J., 1998. Exposure to fragrances: their absorption and potential toxicity. In: Roberts, M.S., Walters, K.A. (Eds.), Dermal absorption and toxicity assessment. Dekker, New York.

Hostýnek, J.J., Magee, P.S., 1997. Fragrance allergens: classification and ranking by QSAR. Toxicol. In Vitro 11, 377–384.

Hostýnek, J.J., Maibach, H.I., 2003a. Is there evidence that anisyl alcohol causes allergic contact dermatitis? Exogenous Dermatology 2, 230–233.

Hostýnek, J.J., Maibach, H.I., 2003b. Is there evidence that linalool causes allergic contact dermatitis? Exogenous Dermatology 2, 223–229.

Hostýnek, J.J., Maibach, H.I., 2004a. Thresholds of elicitation depend on induction conditions. Could low level exposure induce sub-clinical allergic states that are only elicited under the severe conditions of clinical diagnosis? Food Chem. Toxicol. 42, 1859–1865.

Hostýnek, J.J., Maibach, H.I., 2004b. Sensitization potential of citronellol. Exogenous Dermatology 3, 307–312.

Hostýnek, J.J., Maibach, H.I., 2004c. Is there evidence that geraniol causes allergic contact dermatitis? Exogenous Dermatology 3, 318–331.

Hostýnek, J.J., Maibach, H.I., 2008. Allergic contact dermatitis to linalool. Perfumer & Flavorist 33 (5), 52–56.

Hostýnek, J.J., Magee, P.S., Maibach, H.I., 1998. Identification of fragrance sensitizers by QSAR. In: Frosch, P.J., Johansen, J.D., White, I.R. (Eds.), Fragrances, beneficial and adverse effects. Springer, Berlin.

Hotchkiss, S.A., 1994. How thin is your skin? New Sci. 141 (1910), 24–27.

Hotchkiss, S.A., 1998. Absorption of fragrance ingredients using in vitro models with human skin. In: Frosch, P.J., Johansen, J.D., White, I.R. (Eds.), Fragrances: beneficial and adverse effects. Springer, Berlin.

Hotchkiss, S.A., Miller, J.M., Caldwell, J., 1992. Percutaneous absorption of benzyl acetate through rat skin in vitro 2. Effect of vehicle and occlusion. Food Chem. Toxicol. 30, 145–153.

Houghton, P.J., 1988. Biological activity of valerian and related plants. J. Ethnopharmacol. 22, 121–142.

Howes, A.J., Chan, V.S.W., Caldwell, J., 1990. Structure-specificity of the genotoxicity of some naturally occurring alkenylbenzenes determined by the unscheduled DNA synthesis assay in rat hepatocytes. Food Chem. Toxicol. 28, 537–542.

Howes, M.J., Houghton, P.J., Barlow, D.J., et al., 2002. Assessment of estrogenic activity in some common essential oil constituents. J. Pharm. Pharmacol. 54, 1521–1528.

Howes, M.J., Simmonds, M.S., Kite, G.C., 2004. Evaluation of the quality of sandalwood essential oils by gas chromatography-mass spectrometry. Journal of Chromatographic Analysis 1028, 307–312.

Howrie, D.L., Moriarty, R., Breit, R., 1985. Candy flavoring as a source of salicylate poisoning. Paediatrics 75, 869–871.

Hruban, Z., Swift, H., Slesers, A., 1966. Ultrastructural alterations of hepatic microbodies. Laboratory Investigations 15, 1884–1901.

Hsia, M.T.S., Adamovics, J.A., Kreamer, B.L., 1979. Microbial mutagenicity studies of insect growth regulators and other potential insecticidal compounds in Salmonella typhimurium. Chemosphere 8, 521–529.

Hsieh, T.J., Chang, F.R., Chia, Y.C., et al., 2001. Cytotoxic constituents of the fruits of Cananga odorata. J. Nat. Prod. 64, 616–619.

Hsu, B., 1980. The use of herbs as anticancer agents. Am. J. Chin. Med. 8, 301–306.

Hsu, H.C., Yang, W.C., Tsai, W.J., et al., 2006. Alpha-bulnesene, a novel PAF receptor antagonist isolated from Pogostemon cablin. Biochem. Biophys. Res. Commun. 345, 1033–1038.

Hu, L., Chen, D.Y., 2009. Application of headspace solid phase microextraction for study of noncovalent interaction of borneol with human serum albumin. Acta Pharmacol. Sin. 30, 1573–1576.

Hu, J.J., Yoo, J.S.H., Lin, M., et al., 1996. Protective effects of diallyl sulfide on acetaminophen-induced toxicities. Food Chem. Toxicol. 34, 963–969.

Huang, Y.B., Fang, J.Y., Hung, C.H., et al., 1999. Cyclic monoterpene extract from cardamom oil as a skin permeation enhancer for indomethacin: in vitro and in vivo studies. Biol. Pharm. Bull. 22, 642–646.

Huang, J.K., Huang, C.J., Chen, W.C., et al., 2005. Independent [Ca2+]i increases and cell proliferation induced by the carcinogen safrole in human oral cancer cells. Naunyn Schmiedeberg Arch. Pharmacol. 372, 88–94.

Huang, J., Wang, S., Luo, X., et al., 2007a. Cinnamaldehyde reduction of platelet aggregation and thrombosis in rodents. Thromb. Res. 119, 337–342.

Huang, T.C., Fu, H.Y., Ho, C.T., et al., 2007b. Induction of apoptosis by cinnamaldehyde from indigenous cinnamon Cinnamomum osmophloeum Kaneh through reactive oxygen species production, glutathione depletion, and caspase activation in human leukemia K562 cells. Food Chem. 103, 434–443.

Huberman, E., Sachs, L., Yang, S.K., 1976. Identification of mutagenic metabolites of benzo[a]pyrene in mammalian cells. Proc. Natl. Acad. Sci. U. S. A. 73, 607–611.

Hudes, G.R., Szarka, C.E., Adams, A., et al., 2000. Phase I pharmacokinetic trial of perillyl alcohol (NSC 641066) in patients with refractory solid malignancies. Clin. Cancer Res. 6, 3071–3080.

Hudson, J.B., 1989. Plant photosensitizers with antiviral properties. Antiviral Res. 12, 55–74.

Hudson, J.B., Miki, N., Towers, G.H., 1987. Isopimpinellin is not phototoxic to viruses and cells. Planta Med. 53, 306–307.

Huffman, J.L., Sundheim, O., Tainer, J.A., 2005. DNA base damage recognition and removal: new twists and grooves. Mutat. Res. 577, 55–76.

Hughes, C.L., 1988. Phytochemical mimicry of reproductive hormones and modulation of herbivore fertility by phytoestrogens. Environ. Health Perspect. 78, 171–174.

Hughes, R.F., 1932. A case of methyl salicylate poisoning. Can. Med. Assoc. J. 27, 417–418.

Hunter, M.V., Brophy, J.J., Ralph, B.J., et al., 1997. Composition of Polygonum odoratum Lour. from Southern Australia. Journal of Essential Oil Research 9, 603–604.

Huntose, Y., Pandey, K.K., Dwivedi, M., 1999. Response of herbal drug (kustha) on psychological and neurobehavior changes during labour. South-East Asian Seminar on Herbs & Herbal Medicines, Patna, India, January 16–19, pp. 63–68.

Huong, D.T.L., Jo, Y.S., Lee, M.K., et al., 2000. Monoamine oxidase inhibitors from Cinnamomi cortex. Natural Product Sciences 6, 16–19.

Huque, T., Ahmad, P., 1975. Effect of allyl isothiocyanate on blood and urine levels of uric acid and glucose in rats. Bangladesh Journal of Biological & Agricultrual Science 4, 12–13.

Hursting, S.D., Slaga, T.J., Fischer, S.M., et al., 1999. Mechanism-based cancer prevention approaches: targets, examples, and the use of transgenic mice. J. Natl. Cancer Inst. 91, 215–225.

Hutter, C., Laing, D., 1993. Possible role of thymol in the pathogenesis of 'halothane hepatitis'. Eur. J. Anaesthesiol. 10, 237–238.

Hwang, J.H., 2006. The effects of the inhalation method using essential oils on blood pressure and stress responses of clients with essential hypertension. Taehan Kanhoe Hakhoe Chi 36, 1123–1134.

Hyvönen, H., Torkkeli, H., Häkkinen, V.M.A., et al., 1991. Two-dimensional separation of the essential oil of chamomile oil by on-line HPLC-HRGC. Acta Pharmaceutica Fennica 100, 269–273.

IARC, 1986a. Furocoumarins. IARC Monogr. Eval. Carcinog. Risk Chem. Hum 40, 327. http://193.51.164.11/htdocs/monographs/vol40/5-methoxypsoralen.htm.

IARC, 1986b. Furocoumarins. IARC Monogr. Eval. Carcinog. Risk Chem. Hum. (Suppl. 7), 242.http://193.51.164.11/htdocs/monographs/suppl7/methoxypsoralen-5.html.

IARC, 1986c. Furocoumarins. IARC Monogr. Eval. Carcinog. Risk Chem. Hum. (Suppl. 7), 261.http://193.51.164.11/htdocs/monographs/suppl7/methoxypsoralen-8.html.

Ibrus-Määr, A., 1932. Fatal poisoning with oil of chenopodium. Dtsch. Z. Gesamte Gerichtl. Med. 20, 158–160.

Ichiyama, R.M., Ragan, B.G., Bell, G.W., et al., 2002. Effects of topical analgesics on the pressor response evoked by muscle afferents. Med. Sci. Sports Exerc. 34, 1440–1445.

Idaomar, M., El-Hamss, R., Bakkali, F., et al., 2002. Genotoxicity and antigenotoxicity of some essential oils evaluated by wing spot test of Drosophila melanogaster. Mutat. Res. 513, 61–68.

Ide, H., Toki, S., 1970. Metabolism of β-ionone. Biochem. J. 119, 281–287.

Idris, R., Ahmad, K., 1975. The effect of allylisothiocyanate and other antithyroid compounds on blood coagulation in rats. Biochemical Phamacology 24, 2003–2005.

IFRA, 2009. Standards, including amendments as of October 14th 2009. International Fragrance Association, Brussels. http://www.ifraorg.org.

Igimi, H., Nishimura, M., Kodama, R., et al., 1974. Studies on the metabolism of d-limonene (p-mentha-1,8-diene). I. The absorption, distribution and excretion of d-limonene in rats. Xenobiotica 4, 77–84.

Iida, M., Anna, C.H., Holliday, W.M., et al., 2005. Unique patterns of gene expression changes in liver after treatment of mice for 2 weeks with different known carcinogens and non-carcinogens. Carcinogenesis 26, 689–699.

Ikeda, R., Nagao, T., Okabe, H., et al., 1998. Antiproliferative constituents in umbelliferae plants. III. Constituents in the root and the ground part of Anthriscus sylvestris Hoffm. Chem. Pharm. Bull. (Tokyo) 46, 871–874.

Ilett, K.F., Kristensen, J.H., Begg, E.J., 1997. Drug distribution in human milk. Australian Prescriber 20, 35–40.

Imai, T., Yasuhara, K., Tamura, T., et al., 2002. Inhibitory effects of cinnamaldehyde on 4-(methylnitrosamino)-1-(3-pyridyl)-1-butanone-induced lung carcinogenesis in rasH2 mice. Cancer Lett. 175, 9–16.

Imai, N., Doi, Y., Nabae, K., et al., 2006. Lack of hinokitiol (beta-thujaplicin) carcinogenicity in F344.DuCrj rats. J. Toxicol. Sci. 31, 357–370.

Imaida, K., Hirose, M., Yamaguchi, S., et al., 1990. Effects of naturally occurring antioxidants on combined 1,2-dimethylhydrazine- and 1-methyl-1-nitrosourea-initiated carcinogenesis in F344 male rats. Cancer Lett. 55, 53–59.

Imaizumi, K., Hanada, K., Mawatari, K., et al., 1985. Effects of essential oils on concentration of serum lipids and apolipoproteins in rats. Agriculture Biology & Chemistry 49, 2796–2797.

Imanishi, H., Sasaki, Y.F., Matsumoto, K., et al., 1990. Suppression of 6-TG-resistant mutations in V79 cells and recessive spot formations in mice by vanillin. Mutat. Res. 243, 151–158.

Imokawa, G., Kawai, M., 1987. Differential hypermelanosis induced by allergic contact dermatitis. J. Invest. Dermatol. 89, 540–546.

Imumorin, I.G., Dong, Y., Zhu, H., et al., 2005. A gene-environment interaction model of stress-induced hypertension. Cardiovasc. Toxicol. 5, 109–132.

Infurna, R., Beyer, B., Twitty, L., et al., 1990. Evaluation of the dermal absorption and teratogenic potential of methyl salicylate in a petroleum based grease (Abstract). Teratology 41, 566.

Inman, R.D., Kiigemagi, U., Deinzer, M.L., 1981. Determination of chlorpyrifos and 3,5,6-trichloro-2-pyridinol residues in peppermint hay and peppermint oil. J. Agric. Food Chem. 29, 321–323.

Inman, R.D., Kiigemagi, U., Deinzer, M.L., 1983. Determination of carbofuran and 3-hydroxycarbofuran residues in peppermint hay and peppermint oil. J. Agric. Food Chem. 31, 918–919.

Innes, J.R., Ulland, B.M., Valerio, M.G., et al., 1969. Bioassay of pesticides and industrial chemicals for tumorigenicity in mice. J. Natl. Cancer Inst. 42, 1101–1114.

Innocenti, G., Dall'Acqua, S., Scialino, G., et al., 2010. Chemical composition and biological properties of Rhododendron anthopogon essential oil. Molecules 15, 2326–2338.

Inouye, T., Sasaki, Y.F., Imanishi, H., et al., 1988. Suppression of mitomycin C-induced micronuclei in mouse bone marrow cells by post-treatment with vanillin. Mutat. Res. 202, 93–95.

Interaminense, L.F., Leal-Cardoso, J.H., Magalhaes, P.J., et al., 2005. Enhanced hypotensive effects of the essential oil of Ocimum gratissimum leaves and its main constituent, eugenol, in DOCA-salt hypertensive conscious rats. Planta Med. 71, 376–378.

Inveresk Research International Ltd, 1983. Screening of priority chemicals for reproductive hazard. NTIS Report No. PB83-258616.

Ioannides, C., Delaforge, M., Parke, D.V., 1981. Safrole: its metabolism, carcinogenicity and interactions with cytochrome P450. Food Cosmet. Toxicol. 19, 657–666.

Ioannides, C., Delaforge, M., Parke, D.V., 1985. Interactions of safrole and isosafrole and their metabolites with cytochromes P-450. Chem. Biol. Interact. 53, 303–311.

Ioannou, Y.M., Burka, L.T., Matthews, H.B., 1984. Allyl isothiocyanate: comparative disposition in rats and mice. Toxicol. Appl. Pharmacol. 75, 173–181.

Ip, C., Lisk, D.J., Stoewsand, G.S., 1992. Mammary cancer prevention by regular garlic and selenium-enriched garlic. Nutr. Cancer 17, 279–286.

Ipek, E., Tüylü, B.A., Zeytinoglu, H., et al., 2003. Effects of carvacrol on sister chromatid exchanges in human lymphocyte cultures. Cytotechnology 43, 145–148.

Ipek, E., Zeytinoglu, H., Okay, S., et al., 2005. Genotoxicity and antigenotoxicity of Origanum oil and carvacrol evaluated by Ames Salmonella/microsomal test. Food Chem. 93, 551–556.

Iqbal, M., Athar, M., 1998. Attenuation of iron-nitrilotriacetate (Fe-NTA)-mediated renal oxidative stress, toxicity and hyperproliferative response by the prophylactic treatment of rats with garlic oil. Food Chem. Toxicol. 36, 485–495.

Isaacs, G., 1983. Permanent local anaesthesia and anhidrosis after clove oil spillage. Lancet 1 (April 16), 882.

Ishida, T., Asakawa, Y., Okano, M., et al., 1977. Biotransformation of terpenoids in mammals; biotransformation of 3-carene and related compounds in rabbits. Tetrahedron. Lett. 28, 2437–2440.

Ishida, T., Asakawa, Y., Takemoto, T., et al., 1981. Terpenoids biotransformation in mammals III. Biotransformation of α-pinene, β-pinene, pinane, γ-3-carene, carane, myrcene, and p-cymene in rabbits. J. Pharm. Sci. 70, 406–414.

Ishida, T., Toyota, M., Asakawa, Y., 1989. Terpenoid biotransformation in mammals V. Metabolism of (+)-citronellal, (±)-7-hydroxycitronellal, citral, (−)-perillaldehyde, (−)-myrtenal, cuminaldehyde, thujone, and (±)-carvone in rabbits. Xenobiotica 19, 843–855.

Ishidate, M., Sofuni, T., Yoshikawa, K., et al., 1984. Primary mutagenicity screening of food additives currently used in Japan. Food Chem. Toxicol. 22, 623–636.

Ishidate, M., Harnois, M.C., Sofuni, T., 1988. A comparative analysis of data on the clastogenicity of 951 chemical substances tested in mammalian cell cultures. Mutat. Res. 195, 151–213.

Ishiguro, S., Miyamoto, A., Obi, T., et al., 1993. Teratological studies on benzyl acetate in pregnant rats. Bulletin Faculty Agriculture Kagoshima University 43, 25–31.

Ishihara, M., 1978. The environment and the skin. Journal of the Medical Society of Toho University 25, 750–766.

Ishihara, M., Itoh, S., Hayashi, S., et al., 1979. Methods of diagnosis in cases of cosmetic dermatitis and facial melanosis in females. Nishinihon Journal of Dermatology 41, 426–439.

Ishihara, M., Itoh, M., Hosono, K., et al., 1981. Some problems with patch tests using fragrance materials. Skin Research 23, 808–817.

Ishizaki, M., Ueno, S., Oyamada, N., et al., 1985. The DNA-damaging activity of natural food additives (III). Journal of Food Hygiene Society, Japan 26, 523–527.

Islam, S.N., Begum, P., Ahsan, T., et al., 2004. Immunosuppressive and cytotoxic properties of Nigella sativa. Phytother. Res. 18, 395–398.

Ismail, M., Al-Naqeep, G., Chan, K.W., 2009. Nigella sativa thymoquinone-rich fraction greatly improves plasma antioxidant capacity and expression of antioxidant genes in hypercholesterolemic rats. Free Radic. Biol. Med. doi: 10.1016/j.freeradbiomed.2009.12.002.

ISO Technical Committee, 1996. Oil of *Melaleuca*, terpinen-4-ol type (tea tree oil). International Organization for Standardization 4730:1996 (E).

Itai, T., Amayasu, H., Kuribayashi, M., et al., 2000. Psychological effects of aromatherapy on chronic hemodialysis patients. Psychiatry Clin. Neurosci. 54, 393–397.

Itani, W.S., El-Banna, S.H., Hassan, S.B., et al., 2008. Anti colon cancer components from Lebanese sage (*Salvia libanotica*) essential oil: mechanistic basis. Cancer Biol. Ther. 7, 1765–1773.

Itoh, M., 1982. Sensitization potential of some phenolic compounds, with special emphasis on the relationship between chemical structure and allergenicity. J. Dermatol. 9, 223–233.

Itoh, M., Ishihara, M., Hosono, K., et al., 1986. Results of patch tests conducted between 1978 and 1985 using cosmetic ingredients. Skin Research 28 (Suppl.2), 110–119.

Itoh, M., Hosono, K., Kantoh, H., et al., 1988. Patch test results with cosmetic ingredients conducted between 1978 and 1986. Journal of the Society of Cosmetic Science 12, 27–41.

Itokawa, H., Fusayoshi, H., Funakoshi, K., et al., 1985. Studies on the antitumor bisabolane sesquiterpenoids isolated from *Curcuma xanthorriza*. Chem. Pharm. Bull. (Tokyo) 33, 3488–3492.

Ivankovic, S., Stojkovic, R., Jukic, M., et al., 2006. The antitumor activity of thymoquinone and thymohydroquinone in vitro and in vivo. Exp. Oncol. 28, 220–224.

Ivie, G.W., Beier, R.C., 1996. Isopimpinellin is not phototoxic in a chick skin assay. Photochem. Photobiol. 63, 306–307.

Ivie, G.W., Beier, R.C., Holt, D.L., 1982. Analysis of the garden carrot (*Daucus carota* L.) for linear furocoumarins (psoralens) at the sub parts per million level. J. Agric. Food Chem. 30, 413–416.

Iwasaki, Y., Tanabe, M., Kobata, K., et al., 2008. TRPA1 agonists - allyl isothiocyanate and cinnamaldehyde - induce adrenaline secretion. Biosci. Biotechnol. Biochem. 72, 2608–2614.

Iyer, L.V., Ho, M.N., Shinn, W.M., et al., 2003. Glucuronidation of 1'-hydroxyestragole (1'-HE) by human UDP-glucuronosyltransferases UGT2B7 and UGT1A9. Toxicol. Sci. 73, 36–43.

Izumi, T., Iwamoto, N., Kitaichi, Y., et al., 2006. Effects of co-administration of a selective serotonin reuptake inhibitor and monoamine oxidase inhibitors on 5-HT-related behavior in rats. Eur. J. Pharmacol. 532, 258–264.

Jackson, B., Reed, A., 1969. Catnip and the alteration of consciousness. J. Am. Med. Assoc. 207, 1349–1350.

Jacobs, M.R., Hornfeldt, C.S., 1994. Melaleuca oil poisoning. J. Toxicol. Clin. Toxicol. 32, 461–464.

Jacobziner, H., Raybin, H.W., 1962a. Camphor poisoning. Arch. Pediatr. 79, 28–30.

Jacobziner, H., Raybin, H.W., 1962b. Methyl salicylate poisoning. N. Y. State. J. Med. (Feb 1), 403–405.

Jäger, W., Buchbauer, G., Jirovetz, L., et al., 1992a. Percutaneous absorption of lavender oil from a massage oil. J. Soc. Cosmet. Chem. 43, 49–54.

Jäger, W., Nasel, B., Nasel, C., et al., 1996. Pharmacokinetic studies of the fragrance compound 1,8-cineol in humans during inhalation. Chem. Senses 21, 477–480.

Jäger, W., Mayer, M., Platzer, P., et al., 2000. Stereoselective metabolism of the monoterpene carvone by rat and human liver microsomes. J. Pharm. Pharmacol. 52, 191–197.

Jäger, W., Mayer, M., Reznicek, G., et al., 2001. Percutaneous absorption of the monoterpene carvone: implication of stereoselective metabolism on blood levels. J. Pharm. Pharmacol. 53, 637–642.

Jahangir, T., Sultana, S., 2008. Benzo[a]pyrene-induced genotoxicity: attenuation by farnesol in a mouse model. J. Enzyme Inhib. Med. Chem. 23, 888–894.

Jahangir, T., Khan, T.H., Prasad, L., et al., 2005. Alleviation of free radical mediated oxidative and genotoxic effects of cadmium by farnesol in Swiss albino mice. Redox Rep. 10, 303–310.

Jamal, A., Javed, K., Aslam, M., et al., 2006. Gastroprotective effect of cardamom. *Elettaria cardamomum* Maton. fruits in rats. J. Ethnopharmacol. 103, 149–153.

James, W.D., White, S.W., Yanklowitz, B., 1984. Allergic contact dermatitis to compound tincture of benzoin. J. Am. Acad. Dermatol. 11 (5, part 1), 847–850.

Janahmadi, M., Niazi, F., Danyali, S., et al., 2006. Effects of the fruit essential oil of *Cuminum cyminum* Linn. (Apiaceae) on pentylenetetrazol-induced epileptiform activity in F1 neurones of *Helix aspersa*. J. Ethnopharmacol. 104, 278–282.

Janbaz, K.H., Gilani, A.H., 1999. Potentiation of paracetamol and carbon tetrachloride-induced hepatotoxicity in rodents by the food additive vanillin. Food Chem. Toxicol. 37, 603–607.

Jandera, V., Hudson, D.A., De Wet, P.M., et al., 2000. Cooling the burn wound: evaluation of different modalites. Burns 26, 265–270.

Janes, S.E., Price, C.S., Thomas, D., 2005. Essential oil poisoning: N-acetylcysteine for eugenol-induced hepatic failure and analysis of a national database. Eur. J. Pediatr. 164, 520–522.

Janku, I., Hava, M., Kraus, R., et al., 1960. Das diuretische Prinzip des Wacholders. Naunyn Schmiedebergs Arch. Exp. Pathol. Pharmakol. 238, 112–113.

Jansen, L.A., Jongen, W.M., 1996. The use of initiated cells as a test system for the detection of inhibitors of gap junctional intercellular communication. Carcinogenesis 17, 333–339.

Janssens, J., Laekeman, G.M., Pieters, L.A.C., et al., 1990. Nutmeg oil: identification and quantification of its most active constituents as inhibitors of platelet aggregation. J. Ethnopharmacol. 29, 179–188.

Jansson, T., Curvall, M., Hedin, A., et al., 1988. In vitro studies of the biological effects of cigarette smoke condensate. III. Induction of SCE by some phenolic and related constituents derived from cigarette smoke. A study of structure-activity relationships. Mutat. Res. 206, 17–24.

Jantan, I.bin, Basni, I., Ahmad, A.S., et al., 2001. Constituents of the rhizome oils of *Boesenbergia pandurata* (Roxb.) Schlecht from Malaysia, Indonesia and Thailand. Flavour & Fragrance Journal 16, 110–112.

Jantan, I.bin, Ahmad, A.S., Ahmad, A.R., 2002. A comparative study of the oleoresins of three *Pinus* species from Malaysian pine plantations. Journal of Essential Oil Research 14, 327–332.

Janzowski, C., Glaab, V., Mueller, C., et al., 2003. α, β-Unsaturated carbonyl compounds: induction of oxidative DNA damage in mammalian cells. Mutagenesis 18, 465–470.

Jappe, U., Bonnekoh, B., Hausen, B.M., et al., 1999. Garlic-related dermatoses: case report and review of the literature. Am. J. Contact Dermat. 10, 37–39.

Jarabek, A.M., Pottenger, L.H., Andrews, L.S., et al., 2009. Creating context for the use of DNA adduct data in cancer risk assessment: I. Data organization. Crit. Rev. Toxicol. 39, 659–678.

Jardim, C.M., Jham, G.N., Dhingra, O.D., et al., 2008. Composition and antifungal activity of the essential oil of the Brazilian *Chenopodium ambroisioides* L. J. Chem. Ecol. 34, 1213–1218.

Jarry, H., Leonhardt, S., Wuttke, W., 1991. Agnus-castus als dopaminerges wirkprincip in mastodynon. Zeitschrift für Phytotherapy 12, 77–78.

Jarvis, J., Seed, M.J., Elton, R.A., et al., 2005. Relationship between chemical structure and the occupational asthma hazard of low molecular weight organic compounds. Occup. Environ. Med. 62, 243–250.

Javorka, K., Tomori, Z., Zavarska, L., 1980. Protective and defensive airway reflexes in premature infants. Physiol. Bohemoslav. 29, 29–35.

Jayaprakasha, G.K., Jena, B.S., Negi, P.S., et al., 2002. Evaluation of antioxidant activities and antimutagenicity of turmeric oil: a byproduct from curcumin production. Z. Naturforsch. 57, 828–835.

JCDRG, 1981. Japan Contact Dermatitis Research Group. Incidence of contact hypersensitivity in Japan: 1981. Skin Research 24, 514–525.

JECFA, 1974. Toxicological evaluation of some food additives including anticaking agents, antimicrobials, antioxidants, emulsifiers and thickening agents. Rome In: Food & Agriculture Organization Nutrition Meetings Report Series No. 53A, p. 34 WHO/Food Add./74.5.

JECFA, 1981. Joint FAO/WHO Expert Committee on Food Additives. Monograph on β-asarone. WHO Food Additive Series no 16 http://www.inchem.org/documents/jecfa/jecmono/v16je04.htm.

JECFA, 1982. Summary of evaluations performed by the Joint FAO/WHO Expert Committee on Food Additives: eugenol. http://www.inchem.org/documents/jecfa/jeceval/jec_841.htm.

JECFA, 1998. Summary of evaluations performed by the Joint FAO/WHO Expert Committee on Food Additives: trans-anethole. www.inchem.org/documents/jecfa/jeceval/jec_137.htm.

JECFA, 1999a. Summary of evaluations performed by the Joint FAO/WHO Expert Committee on Food Additives: linalool. http://www.inchem.org/documents/jecfa/jeceval/jec_1271.htm.

JECFA, 1999b. Safety evaluation of certain food additives. World Health Organization, Geneva. WHO food additives series 42. Prepared by the fifty-first meeting of the joint FAO/WHO Expert Committee on Food Additives (JECFA). http://www.inchem.org/documents/jecfa/jecmono/v042je04.htm.

JECFA, 2001a. Summary of evaluations performed by the Joint FAO/WHO Expert Committee on Food Additives: benzyl alcohol. http://www.inchem.org/documents/jecfa/jeceval/jec_194.htm.

JECFA, 2001b. Summary of evaluations performed by the Joint FAO/WHO Expert Committee on Food Additives: methyl salicylate. http://www.inchem.org/documents/jecfa/jeceval/jec_1599.htm.

JECFA, 2002. Summary of evaluations performed by the Joint FAO/WHO Expert Committee on Food Additives: octanal. http://www.inchem.org/documents/jecfa/jeceval/jec_1755.htm.

JECFA, 2009. Safety evaluation of certain food additives. WHO food additives series 60. Prepared by the sixty-ninth meeting of the joint FAO/WHO Expert Committee on Food Additives (JECFA). whqlibdoc.who.int/publications/2009/9789241660600_eng.pdf.

Jeena, K., Liju, V.B., Kuttan, R., 2011. A preliminary 13-week oral toxicity study of ginger oil in male and female Wistar rats. Int. J. Toxicol. 30, 662–670.

Jeng, J.H., Hahn, L.J., Lu, F.J., et al., 1994a. Eugenol triggers different pathobiological effects on human oral mucosal fibroblasts. J. Dent. Res. 73, 1050–1055.

Jeng, J.H., Kuo, M.L., Hahn, L.J., et al., 1994b. Genotoxic and non-genotoxic effects of betel quid ingredients on oral mucosal fibroblasts in vitro. J. Dent. Res. 73, 1043–1049.

Jeng, J.H., Hahn, L.J., Lin, B.R., et al., 1999a. Effects of areca nut, inflorescence piper betle extracts and arecoline on cytotoxicity, total and unscheduled DNA synthesis in cultured gingival keratinocytes. J. Oral Pathol. Med. 28, 64–71.

Jeng, J.H., Tsai, C.L., Hahn, L.J., et al., 1999b. Arecoline cytotoxicity on human oral mucosal fibroblasts related to cellular thiol and esterase activities. Food Chem. Toxicol. 37, 751–756.

Jenkins, G.J., Zaïr, Z., Johnson, G.E., et al., 2010. Genotoxic thresholds, DNA repair, and susceptiblility in human populations. Toxicology 278, 305–310.

Jenner, P.M., Hagan, E.C., Taylor, J.M., et al., 1964. Food flavorings and compounds of related structure I. Acute oral toxicity. Food Cosmet. Toxicol. 2, 327–343.

Jennings, W.G., Sevenants, M.R., 1964. Volatile components of peach. Journal of Food Science 29, 796–801.

Jensen, F.E., 1999. Acute and chronic effects of seizures in the developing brain: experimental models. Epilepsia 40, S51–S58.

Jeong, H.G., Yun, C.H., 1995. Induction of rat hepatic cytochrome P450 enzymes by myristicin. Biochem. Biophys. Res. Commun. 217, 966–971.

Jeong, H.G., Chun, Y.J., Yun, C.H., et al., 2002. Induction of cytochrome P450 1A and 2B by alpha- and beta-ionone in Sprague Dawley rats. Archives of Pharmaceutical Research 25, 197–201.

Jeong, S.J., Itokawa, T., Shibuya, M., et al., 2002. Costunolide, a sesquiterpene lactone from Saussurea lappa, inhibits the VEGFR KDR/Flk-1 signaling pathway. Cancer Lett. 187, 129–133.

Jepsen, F., Ryan, M., 2005. Poisoning in children. Current Paediatrics 15, 563–568.

Jeurissen, S.M., Bogaards, J.J., Awad, H.M., et al., 2004. Human cytochrome P450 enzyme specificity for bioactivation of safrole to the proximate carcinogen 1'-hydroxysafrole. Chem. Res. Toxicol. 17, 1245–1250.

Jeurissen, S.M., Bogaards, J.J., Boersma, M.G., et al., 2006. Human cytochrome P450 enzymes of importance for the bioactivation of methyleugenol to the proximate carcinogen 1'-hydroxymethyleugenol. Chem. Res. Toxicol. 19, 111–116.

Jeurissen, S.M., Punt, A., Boersma, M.G., et al., 2007. Human cytochrome P450 enzyme specificity for the bioactivation of estragole and related alkenylbenzenes. Chem. Res. Toxicol. 20, 798–806.

Jeurissen, S.M., Punt, A., Delatour, T., et al., 2008. Basil extract inhibits the sulfotransferase mediated formation of DNA adducts of the procarcinogen 1'-hydroxyestragole by rat and human liver S9 homogenates and in HepG2 human hepatoma cells. Food Chem. Toxicol. 46, 2296–2302.

Ji, M., Choi, J., Lee, J., et al., 2004. Induction of apoptosis by ar-turmerone on various cell lines. Int. J. Mol. Med. 14, 253–256.

Jiao, D., Ho, C.T., Foiles, P., et al., 1994. Identification and quantification of the N-acetylcysteine conjugate of allyl isothiocyanate in human urine after ingestion of mustard. Cancer Epidemiol. Biomarkers Prev. 3, 487–492.

Jimbo, Y., Ishihara, M., Osamura, H., et al., 1983. Influence of vehicles on penetration through human epidermis of benzyl alcohol, isoeugenol and methyl isoeugenol. J. Dermatol. 10, 241–250.

Jiménez, J., Navarro, M.C., Montilla, M.P., et al., 1993. Thymus zygis oil: its effects on CC1$_4$-induced hepatotoxicity and free radical scavenger activity. Journal of Essential Oil Research 5, 153–158.

Jirovetz, L., Jager, W., Buchbauer, G., et al., 1991. Investigations of animal blood samples after fragrance drug inhalation by gas chromatography/mass spectrometry with chemical ionization and selected ion monitoring. Biology & Mass Spectrometry 20, 801–803.

Jirovetz, L., Buchbauer, G., Jäger, W., et al., 1992. Analysis of fragrance compounds in blood samples of mice by gas chromatography, mass spectrometry, GC/FTIR and GC/AES after inhalation of sandalwood oil. Biochemical Chromatography 6, 133–134.

Jirovetz, L., Buchbauer, G., Shahabi, M., 2002. Comparative investigations of essential oils and their SPME headspace volatiles of Rosa damascena from Bulgaria and Rosa centifolia from Morocco using GC-FID, GC/MS and olfactometry. Journal of Essential Oil Bearing Plants 5, 111–121.

Jirovetz, L., Buchbauer, G., Stoilova, I., et al., 2006. Chemical composition and antioxidant properties of clove leaf essential oil. J. Agric. Food Chem. 54, 6303–6307.

Jirovetz, L., Buchbauer, G., Stoilova, I., et al., 2007. Spice plants: chemical composition and antioxidant properties of Pimenta Lindl. essential oils. Part 2: Pimenta racemosa (Mill.) J.W. Moore leaf oil from Jamaica. Ernaehrung (Vienna, Austria) 31 (7/8), 293–300.

Johansen, J.D., Menné, T., 1995. The fragrance mix and its constituents: a 14-year material. Contact Dermatitis 32, 18–23.

Johansen, J.D., Andersen, K.E., Rastogi, S.C., et al., 1996a. Threshold responses in cinnamic aldehyde-sensitive subjects: results and methodological aspects. Contact Dermatitis 34, 165–171.

Johansen, J.D., Andersen, K.E., Menné, T., 1996b. Quantitative aspects of isoeugenol contact allergy assessed by use and patch tests. Contact Dermatitis 34, 414–418.

Johansen, J.D., Andersen, T.F., Veien, N., et al., 1997. Patch testing with markers of fragrance contact allergy. Do clinical tests correspond to patients' self-reported problems? Acta Derm. Venereol. 77, 149–153.

Johansen, J.D., Skov, L., Volund, A., et al., 1998a. Allergens in combination have a synergistic effect on the elicitation response: a study of fragrance-sensitized individuals. Br. J. Dermatol. 139, 264s–270s.

Johansen, J.D., Andersen, T.F., Kjoller, M., et al., 1998b. Identification of risk products for fragrance contact allergy: a case-referent study based on patients' histories. Am. J. Contact Dermat. 9, 80–86.

Johansen, J.D., Menné, T., Christophersen, J., et al., 2000. Changes in the pattern of sensitisation to common contact allergens in Denmark between 1985–86 and 1997–98, with a special view to the effect of preventive strategies. Br. J. Dermatol. 142, 490–495.

Johansen, J.D., Heydorn, S., Menné, T., 2002. Oak moss extracts in the diagnosis of fragrance contact allergy. Contact Dermatitis 46, 157–161.

Johansen, J.D., Andersen, K.E., Svedman, C., et al., 2003a. Chloroatranol, an extremely potent allergen hidden in perfumes: a dose-response elicitation study. Contact Dermatitis 49, 180–184.

Johansen, J.D., Frosch, P.J., Svedman, C., 2003b. Hydroxyisohexyl 3-cyclohexene carboxaldehyde- known as Lyral: quantitative aspects and risk assessment of an important fragrance allergen. Contact Dermatitis 48, 310–316.

Johansson, A., Brämerson, A., Millqvist, E., 2005. Prevalence and risk factors for self-reported odour intolerance: the Skövde population-based study. Int. Arch. Occup. Environ. Health 78, 559–564.

Johansson, A., Millqvist, E., Nordin, S., et al., 2006. Relationship between self-reported odor intolerance and sensitivity to inhaled capsaicin: proposed definition of airway sensory hyperreactivity and estimation of its prevalence. Chest 129, 1623–1628.

Jøhnke, H., Norberg, L.A., Vach, W., et al., 2004. Reactivity to patch tests with nickel sulfate and fragrance mix in infants. Contact Dermatitis 51, 141–147.

Johnson, J.D., Ryan, M.J., Toft, J.D., et al., 2000. Two-year toxicity and carcinogenicity study of methyleugenol in F344/N rats and B6C3F₁ mice. J. Agric. Food Chem. 48, 3620–3632.

Johnson, A.D., Wang, D., Sadee, W., 2005. Polymorphisms affecting gene regulation and mRNA processing: broad implications for pharmacogenetics. Pharmacol. Ther. 106, 19–38.

Johnson, C.D., Melanaphy, D., Purse, A., et al., 2009. Transient receptor potential melastatin 8 channel involvement in the regulation of vascular tone. Am. J. Physiol. Heart Circ. Physiol. 296, H1868–H1877.

Johnson, G.E., Doak, S.H., Griffiths, S.M., et al., 2009. Non-linear dose-response of DNA-reactive genotoxins: recommendations for data analysis. Mutat. Res. 678, 95–100.

Joly, C., Bouillie, C., Hummel, M., 1980. Acute toxicity from camphor administered in an infant. Ann. Pédiatr. (Paris) 27, 395–396.

Jones, C.O., 1913. A case of poisoning by pennyroyal. Br. Med. J. 2, 746.

Jori, A., Briatico, G., 1973. Effect of eucalyptol on microsomal enzyme activity of foetal and newborn rats. Biochem. Pharmacol. 22, 543–544.

Jori, A., Bianchetti, A., Prestini, P.E., 1969. Effect of essential oils on drug metabolism. Biochem. Pharmacol. 18 (9), 2081–2085.

Jori, A., Bianchetti, A., Prestini, P.E., et al., 1970. Effect of eucalyptol (1,8-cineole) on the metabolism of other drugs in rats and in man. Eur. J. Pharmacol. 9, 362–366.

Jori, A., Di Salle, E., Pescador, R., 1972. On the inducing activity of eucalyptol. J. Pharm. Pharmacol. 24, 464–469.

Joshi, P.C., Pathak, M.A., 1983. Production of singlet oxygen and superoxide radicals by psoralens and their biological significance. Biochem. Biophys. Res. Commun. 112, 638–646.

Joshi, J., Ghaisas, S., Vaidya, A., et al., 2003. Early human safety study of turmeric oil (Curcuma longa oil) administered orally in healthy volunteers. Journal of Association of Physicians of India 51, 1055–1060.

Joss, J.D., LeBlond, R.F., 2000. Potentiation of warfarin anticoagulation associated with topical methyl salicylate. Ann. Pharmacother. 34, 729–733.

Joulain, D., 1986. Study of the fragrance given off by certain springtime flowers. In: Brunke, E.J. (Ed.), Progress in essential oil research. De Gruyter, Berlin, pp. 57–67.

Joulain, D., Laurent, R., 1986. Paper no. 50. Proceedings of the 10th International Congress of Essential Oils. Fragrances & Flavors, Washington DC.

Joulain, D., Tabacchi, R., 2009a. Lichen extracts as raw materials in perfumery. Part 1: oakmoss. Flavour & Fragrance Journal 24, 49–61.

Joulain, D., Tabacchi, R., 2009b. Lichen extracts as raw materials in perfumery. Part 2: treemoss. Flavour & Fragrance Journal 24, 105–116.

Juergens, U.R., Stober, M., Schmidt-Schilling, L., et al., 1998a. Antiinflammatory effects of eucalyptol (1,8-cineole) in bronchial asthma: inhibition of arachidonic acid metabolism in human blood monocytes ex vivo. Eur. J. Med. Res. 173, 407–412.

Juergens, U.R., Stober, M., Vetter, H., 1998b. Inhibition of cytokine production and arachidonic acid metabolism by eucalyptol (1,8-cineole) in human blood monocytes in vitro. Eur. J. Med. Res. 173, 508–510.

Juergens, U.R., Stober, M., Vetter, H., 1998c. The anti-inflammatory activity of L-menthol compared to mint oil in human monocytes in vitro: a novel perspective for its therapeutic use in inflammatory diseases. Eur. J. Med. Res. 3, 539–545.

Juergens, U.R., Dethlefsen, U., Steinkamp, G., et al., 2003. Anti-inflammatory activity of 1,8-cineole (eucalyptol) in bronchial asthma: a double-blind placebo-controlled trial. Respir. Med. 97, 250–256.

Juliani, H.R., Simon, J.E., 2002. Antioxidant activity of basil. In: Janick, J., Whipkey, A. (Eds.), Trends in new crops and new uses. ASHS Press, Alexandria, pp. 575–579.

Juliano, C., Mattana, A., Usai, M., 2000. Composition and in vitro antimicrobial activity of the essential oil of Thymus herba-barona Loisel growing wild in Sardinia. Journal of Essential Oil Research 12, 516–522.

Ka, H., Park, H.J., Jung, H.J., et al., 2003. Cinnamaldehyde induces apoptosis by ROS-mediated mitochondrial permeability transition in human promyelocytic leukemia HL-60 cells. Cancer Lett. 196, 143–152.

Kadir, R., Barry, B.W., 1991. α-Bisabolol, a possible safe penetration enhancer for dermal and transdermal therapeutics. Int. J. Pharm. 70, 87–94.

Kaddu, S., Kerl, H., Wolf, P., 2001. Accidental bullous phototoxic reactions to bergamot aromatherapy oil. J. Am. Acad. Dermatol. 45, 458–461.

Kagan, J., Gabriel, R., Reed, S.A., 1980. α-Terthienyl, a non-photodynamic phototoxic compound. Photochem. Photobiol. 31, 465–469.

Kagawa, D., Jokura, H., Ochiai, R., et al., 2003. The sedative effects and mechanism of action of cedrol inhalation with behavioral pharmacological evaluation. Planta Med. 69, 637–641.

Kaidbey, K.H., Kligman, A.M., 1980. Identification of contact photosensitizers by human assay. Current Concepts in Cutaneous Toxicity. Academic Press, New York, p. 55–68.

Kaidbey, K.H., Kligman, A.M., 1981. Photosensitization by coumarin derivatives. Arch. Dermatol. 17, 258–263.

Kaiser, R., 1988. New volatile constituents of Jasminum sambac (L.) Aiton. In: Lawrence, B.M., Mookherjee, B.D., Willis, B.J. (Eds.), Flavors & fragrances: a world perspective. Elsevier, Amsterdam, pp. 669–695.

Kaiser, R., 1991. New volatile constituents of the flower concrete of Michelia champaca L. Journal of Essential Oil Research 3, 129–146.

Kaji, I., Tatsuta, M., Iishi, H., et al., 2001. Inhibition by d-limonene of experimental hepatocarcinogenesis in Sprague-Dawley rats does not involve p21(ras) plasma membrane association. Int. J. Cancer 93, 441–444.

Kalantari, H., Salehi, M., 2001. The protective effect of garlic oil on hepatotoxicity induced by acetaminophen in mice and comparison with N-acetylcysteine. Saudi. Med. J. 22, 1080–1084.

Kalbhen, D.A., 1971. Nutmeg as a narcotic. A contribution to the chemistry and pharmacology of nutmeg (Myristica fragrans). Angewandte Chemie International Edition 10, 370–374.

Kaledin, V.I., Pakharukova, M.Y., Pivovarova, E.N., et al., 2009. Correlation between hepatocarcinogenic effect of estragole and its influence on glucocorticoid induction of liver-specific enzymes and activities of FOXA and HNF4 transcription factors in mouse and rat liver. Biochemistry (Moscow) 74, 377–384.

Kamienski, F.X., Casida, J.E., 1970. Importance of demethylenation in the metabolism in vivo and in vitro of methylenedioxyphenyl synergists and related compounds in mammals. Biochem. Pharmacol. 19, 91–112.

Kamin, W., Kieser, M., 2007. Pinimenthol ointment in patients suffering from upper respiratory tract infections - a post-marketing observational study. Phytomedicine 14, 787–791.

Kamo, A., Tominaga, M., Negi, O., et al., 2011. Topical application of emollients prevents dry skin-inducible intraepidermal nerve growth in acetone-treated mice. J. Dermatol. Sci. 62, 64–66.

Kampf, G., Ennen, J., 2006. Regular use of a hand cream can attenuate skin dryness and roughness caused by frequent hand washing. BMC Dermatol. 6, 1. doi: 10.1186/1471-5945-6-1.

Kan, W.L., Cho, C.H., Rudd, J.A., et al., 2008. Study of the anti-proliferative effects and synergy of phthalides from Angelica sinensis on colon cancer cells. J. Ethnopharmacol. 120, 36–43.

Kanakis, C.D., Tarantilis, P.A., Tajmir-Riahi, H.A., et al., 2007. Crocetin, dimethylcrocetin, and safranal bind human serum albumin: stability and antioxidative properties. J. Agric. Food Chem. 55, 970–977.

Kanerva, R.L., Alden, C.L., 1987. Review of kidney sections from a subchronic d-limonene oral dosing study conducted by the National Cancer Institute. Food Chem. Toxicol. 25, 355–358.

Kanerva, R.L., Ridder, G.M., Lefever, F.R., et al., 1987. Comparison of short-term renal effects due to oral administration of decalin or d-limonene in young adult male Fischer-344 rats. Food Chem. Toxicol. 25, 345–353.

Kanerva, L., Jolanki, R., Estlander, T., 1999. Hairdresser's dermatitis caused by oak moss in permanent waving solution. Contact Dermatitis 41, 55–56.

Kanerva, L., Rantanen, T., Aalto-Korte, K., et al., 2001a. A multicenter study of patch test reactions with dental screening series. Am. J. Contact Dermat. 12, 83–87.

Kanerva, L., Estlander, T., Alanko, K., et al., 2001b. Patch test sensitization to Compositae mix, sesquiterpene-lactone mix, Compositae extracts, laurel leaf, Chlorophorin, Mansonone A, and dimethoxydalbergione. Am. J. Contact Dermat. 12, 18–24.

Kang, J.S., Yoon, Y.D., Lee, K.H., et al., 2004. Costunolide inhibits interleukin-1beta expression by down-regulation of AP-1 and MAPK activity in LPS-stimulated RAW 264.7 cells. Biochem. Biophys. Res. Commun. 313, 171–177.

Kang, L., Yap, C.W., Lim, P.F., et al., 2007. Formulation development of transdermal dosage forms: Quantitative structure-activity relationship model for predicting activities of terpenes that enhance drug penetration through human skin. J. Control. Release 120, 211–219.

Kapur, R.D., 1948. Action of some indigenous drugs on uterus: a preliminary note. Indian J. Med. Res. 36, 47–55.

Karabulut, A.K., Ulger, H., Pratten, M.K., 2000. Protection by free oxygen radical scavenging enzymes against salicylate-induced embryonic malformations in vitro. Toxicol. In Vitro 14, 297–307.

Karia, C., Harwood, J.L., Morris, A.P., et al., 2004. Simultaneous permeation of tamoxifen and gamma linolenic acid across excised human skin. Further evidence of the permeation of solvated complexes. Int. J. Pharm. 271, 305–309.

Karimzadeh, F., Hosseini, M., Mangeng, D., et al., 2012. Anticonvulsant and neuroprotective effects of Pimpinella anisum in rat brain. BMC Complement. Altern. Med. 12, 76.

Karkabounas, S., Kostoula, O.K., Daskalou, T., et al., 2006. Anticarcinogenic and antiplatelet effects of carvacrol. Exp. Oncol. 28, 121–125.

Karlberg, A.T., Dooms-Goossens, A., 1997. Contact allergy to oxidized d-limonene among dermatitis patients. Contact Dermatitis 36, 201–206.

Karlberg, A.T., Bowman, A., Melin, B., 1991. Animal experiments on the allergenicity of d-limonene – the citrus solvent. Ann. Occup. Hyg. 35, 419–426.

Karlberg, A.T., Magnusson, K., Nilsson, U., 1992. Air oxidation of d-limonene (the citrus solvent) creates potent allergens. Contact Dermatitis 26, 332–340.

Karlberg, A.T., Shao, L.P., Nilsson, U., et al., 1994a. Hydroperoxides in oxidized d-limonene identified as potent contact allergens. Arch. Dermatol. Res. 286, 97–103.

Karlberg, A.T., Magnusson, K., Nilsson, U., 1994b. Influence of an antioxidant on the formation of allergenic compounds during auto-oxidation of d-limonene. Ann. Occup. Hyg. 38, 199–207.

Karlberg, A.T., Nilsson, A.M., Luthman, K., et al., 2001. Structural analogues inhibit the sensitizing capacity of carvone. Acta Derm. Venereol. 81, 398–402.

Karpouhtsis, I., Pardali, E., Feggou, E., et al., 1998. Insecticidal and genotoxic activities of oregano essential oils. J. Agric. Food Chem. 46, 1111–1115.

Karrow, N.A., Leffel, E.K., Guo, T.L., et al., 2001. Dermal exposure to cinnamaldehyde alters lymphocyte subpopulations, number of interferon-gamma-producing cells, and expression of B7 costimulatory molecules and cytokine messenger RNAs in auricular lymph nodes of B6C3F1 mice. Am. J. Contact Dermat. 12, 6–17.

Kasamaki, A., Takahashi, H., Tsumura, N., et al., 1982. Genotoxicity of flavoring agents. Mutat. Res. 105, 387–392.

Kasanen, J.P., Pasanen, A.L., Pasanen, P., et al., 1999. Evaluation of sensory irritation of Δ3-carene and turpentine, and acceptable levels of monoterpenes in occupational and indoor environment. J. Toxicol. Environ. Health 57, 89–114.

Kaseb, A.O., Chinnakannu, K., Chen, D., et al., 2007. Androgen receptor and E2F-1 targeted thymoquinone therapy for hormone-refractory prostate cancer. Cancer Res. 67, 7782–7788.

Kasper, S., Gastpar, M., Muller, W.E., et al., 2010. Silexan, an orally administered lavandula oil preparation, is effective in the treatment of 'subsyndromal' anxiety disorder: A randomized, double-blind, placebo controlled trial. Int. Clin. Psychopharmacol. 25, 277–287.

Kassebaum, P.J., Shaw, D.L., Tomich, D.J., 2005. Possible warfarin interaction with menthol cough drops. Ann. Pharmacother. 39, 365–367.

Kassie, F., Laky, B., Gminski, R., et al., 2003. Effects of garden and water cress juices and their constituents, benzyl and phenethyl isothiocyanates, towards benzo(a)pyrene-induced DNA damage: a model study with the single cell gel electrophoresis/Hep G2 assay. Chem. Biol. Interact. 142, 285–296.

Kato, M., Ohgami, N., Kawamoto, Y., et al., 2007. Protective effect of hyperpigmented skin on UV-mediated cutaneous cancer development. J. Invest. Dermatol. 127, 1244–1249.

Katsarou, A., Armenaka, M., Kalogeromitros, D., et al., 1999. Contact reactions to fragrances. Ann. Allergy Asthma Immunol. 82, 449–455.

Katz, A., 1946. Dermal irritating properties of essential oils and aromatic chemicals. Spice Mill 69, 46–51.

Kauderer, B., Zamith, H., Paumgartten, F.J., et al., 1991. Evaluation of the mutagenicity of β-myrcene in mammalian cells in vitro. Environ. Mol. Mutagen. 18, 28–34.

Kauffman, R.E., Banner, W., Berlin, C.M., 1994. Camphor revisited: focus on toxicity. Pediatrics 94, 127–128.

Kaul, P.N., Bhaskaruni, R., Rajeswara, R., et al., 1997. Changes in chemical composition of rose-scented geranium (Pelargonium sp.) oil during storage. Journal of Essential Oil Research 9, 115–117.

Kaul, I.P., Kapila, M., Agrawal, R., 2007. Role of novel delivery systems in developing topical antioxidants as therapeutics to combat photoageing. Ageing Res. Rev. 6, 271–288.

Kaur, P., Singh, R., 2007. In vivo interactive effect of garlic oil and vitamin E against stavudine induced genotoxicity in Mus musculus. Indian J. Exp. Biol. 45, 807–811.

Kaur, M., Agarwal, C., Singh, R.P., et al., 2005. Skin cancer chemopreventive agent, α-santalol, induces apoptotic death of human epidermoid carcinoma A431 cells via caspase activation together with dissipation of mitochondrial membrane potential and cytochrome c release. Carcinogenesis 26, 369–380.

Kaur, G., Athar, M., Alam, M.S., 2010. Eugenol precludes cutaneous chemical carcinogenesis in mouse by preventing oxidative stress and inflammation and by inducing apoptosis. Mol. Carcinog. 49, 290–301.

Kavli, G., Volden, G., 1984. Phytophotodermatitis. Photodermatology 1, 65–75.

Kavli, G., Raa, J., Johnson, B.E., et al., 1983. Furocoumarins of Heracleum laciniatum: isolation, phototoxicity, absorption and action spectra studies. Contact Dermatitis 9, 257–262.

Kavlock, R.J., Chernoff, N., Rogers, E., et al., 1982. An analysis of fetotoxicity using biochemical endpoints of organ differentiation. Teratology 26, 183–194.

Kawamori, T., Tanaka, T., Hara, A., et al., 1995. Modifying effects of naturally occurring products on the development of colonic aberrant crypt foci induced by azoxymethane in F344 rats. Cancer Res. 55, 1277–1282.

Kawana, S., Liang, Z., Nagano, M., et al., 2006. Role of substance P in stress-derived degranulation of dermal mast cells in mice. J. Dermatol. Sci. 42, 47.

Keane, F.M., Smith, H.R., White, I.R., et al., 2000. Occupational allergic contact dermatitis in two aromatherapists. Contact Dermatitis 43, 49–51.

Kehrl, W., Sonnemann, U., Dethlefsen, U., 2004. Therapy for acute nonpurulent rhinosinusitis with cineole: results of a double-blind, randomized, placebo-controlled trial. Laryngoscope 114, 738–742.

Keil, H., 1947. Contact dermatitis due to oil of citronella. J. Invest. Dermatol. 8, 327–334.

Keinan, E., Alt, A., Amir, G., et al., 2005. Natural ozone scavenger prevents asthma in sensitized rats. Bioorg. Med. Chem. 13, 557–562.

Kejlová, K., Jírová, D., Bendová, H., et al., 2007. Phototoxicity of bergamot oil assessed by in vitro techniques in combination with human patch tests. Toxicol. In Vitro 21, 1298–1303.

Kelm, M.A., Nair, M.G., Strasburg, G.M., et al., 2002. Antioxidant and cyclooxygenase inhibitory phenolic compounds from Ocimum sanctum Linn. Phytomedicine 7, 7–13.

Kelman, L., 2004. Osmophobia and taste abnormality in migraineurs: a tertiary care study. Headache 44, 1019–1023.

Kemp, C.J., Donehower, L.A., Bradley, A., et al., 1993. Reduction of p53 gene dosage does not increase initiation or promotion but enhances malignant progression of chemically induced skin tumors. Cell 74, 813–822.

Kenerva, L., Estlander, T., Jolanki, R., 1995. Occupational allergic contact dermatitis caused by ylang-ylang oil. Contact Dermatitis 33, 198–199.

Kerr, J., 2002. The use of essential oils in wound healing. The International Journal of Aromatherapy 12, 202–206.

Kerr, H.A., Lim, H.W., 2007. Photodermatoses in African Americans: a retrospective analysis of 135 patients over a 7-year period. J. Am. Acad. Dermatol. 57, 638–643.

Keshava, C., Keshava, N., Whong, W.Z., 1997. Inhibition of methotrexate-induced chromosomal damage by vanillin and chlorophyllin in V79 cells. Teratog. Carcinog. Mutagen. 17, 313–326.

Ketterer, B., 1988. Protective role of glutathione and glutathione transferases in mutagenesis and carcinogenesis. Mutat. Res. 202, 343–361.

Kevekordes, S., Mersch-Sundermann, V., Burghaus, C.M., et al., 1999. SOS induction of selected naturally occurring substances in Escherichia coli (SOS chromotest). Mutat. Res. 445, 81–91.

Kevekordes, S., Spielberger, J., Burghaus, C.M., et al., 2001. Micronucleus formation in human lymphocytes and in the metabolically competent human hepatoma cell line Hep-G2: results with 15 naturally occurring substances. Anticancer Res. 21, 461–469.

Khader, M., Bresgen, N., Eckl, P.M., 2009. In vitro toxicological properties of thymoquinone. Food Chem. Toxicol. 47, 129–133.

Khalil, Z., Pearce, A.L., Satkunanathan, N., et al., 2004. Regulation of wheal and flare by tea tree oil: complementary human and rodent studies. J. Invest. Dermatol. 123, 683–690.

Khan, F.D., Roychowdhury, S., Gaspari, A.A., et al., 2006. Immune response to xenobiotics in the skin: from contact sensitivity to drug allergy. Expert Opin. Drug. Metab. Toxicol. 2, 261–272.

Khanna, M., Qasem, K., Sasseville, D., 2000. Allergic contact dermatitis to tea tree oil with erythema multiforme-like id reaction. Am. J. Contact Dermat. 11, 238–242.

Khattab, M.M., Nagi, M.N., 2007. Thymoquinone supplementation attenuates hypertension and renal damage in nitric oxide deficient hypertensive rats. Phytother. Res. 21, 410–414.

Khojasteh, S.C., Oishi, S., Nelson, S.D., 2010. Metabolism and toxicity of menthofuran in rat liver slices and in rats. Chem. Res. Toxicol. 23, 1824–1832.

Khojasteh-Bakht, S.C., Koenigs, L.L., Peter, R.M., et al., 1998. (R)-(+)-Menthofuran is a potent, mechanism-based inactivator of human liver cytochrome P450 2A6. Drug Metab. Dispos. 26, 701–704.

Khojasteh-Bakht, S.C., Chen, W., Koenigs, L.L., et al., 1999. Metabolism of (R)-(+)-pulegone and (R)-(+)-menthofuran by human liver cytochrome P-450s: evidence for formation of a furan epoxide. Drug Metab. Dispos. 27, 574–580.

Khokhar, O., Monroe, J., Kachemoune, A., 2004. Skin & Aging. http://www.skinandaging.com/article/2757.

Kieckebusch, W., Lang, K., 1960. The tolerability of benzoic acid in chronic feeding experiments. Arzneimittelforschung 10, 1001–1003.

Kiffe, M., Christen, P., Arni, P., 2003. Characterization of cytotoxic and genotoxic effects of different compounds in CHO K5 cells with the comet assay (single-cell gel electrophoresis assay). Mutat. Res. 537, 151–168.

Kligemagi, U., Heatherbell, C.J., Deinzer, M.L., 1984. Determination of oxamyl residues in peppermint hay and oil using a radioisotope dilution technique. J. Agric. Food Chem. 32, 628–633.

Kilani, S., Abdelwahed, A., Chraief, I., et al., 2005. Chemical composition, antibacterial and antimutagenic activities of essential oil from (Tunisian) Cyperus rotundus. Journal of Essential Oil Research 17, 695–700.

Kilani, S., Ledauphin, J., Bouhlel, I., et al., 2008. Comparative study of Cyperus rotundus essential oil by a modified GC/MS analysis method. Evaluation of its antioxidant, cytotoxic, and apoptotic effects. Chem. Biodivers. 5, 729–742.

Kim, H.M., Cho, S.H., 1999. Lavender oil inhibits immediate-type allergic reaction in mice and rats. J. Pharm. Pharmacol. 51, 221–226.

Kim, J.O., Kim, Y.S., Lee, J.H., et al., 1992. Antimutagenic effect of the major volatile compounds identified from mugwort (Artemisia asiatica Nakai) leaves. Journal of the Korean Society of Food & Nutrition 21, 308–313.

Kim, H.M., Lee, E.H., Kim, C.Y., et al., 1997. Antianaphylactic properties of eugenol. Pharmacol. Res. 36, 475–480.

Kim, S.G., Liem, A., Stewart, B.C., et al., 1999. New studies on trans-anethole oxide and trans-asarone oxide. Carcinogenesis 20, 1303–1307.

Kim, M.H., Chung, W.T., Kim, Y.K., et al., 2001. The effect of the oil of Agastache rugosa O. Kuntze and three of its components on human cancer cell lines. Journal of Essential Oil Research 13, 214–218.

Kim, S.H., Kang, S.N., Kim, H.J., et al., 2002. Potentiation of 1,25-dihydroxyvitamin D(3)-induced differentiation of human promyelocytic leukemia cells into monocytes by costunolide, a germacranolide sesquiterpene lactone. Biochem. Pharmacol. 64, 1233–1242.

Kim, H.J., Chen, F., Wu, C., et al., 2004. Evaluation of antioxidant activity of Australian tea tree (Melaleuca alternifolia) oil and its components. J. Agric. Food Chem. 52, 2849–2854.

Kim, J.H., Lee, S.Y., Oh, S.Y., et al., 2004. Methyl jasmonate induces apoptosis through induction of Bax/Bcl-XS and activation of caspase-3 via ROS production in A549 cells. Oncol. Rep. 12, 1233–1238.

Kim, N.H., Hyun, S.H., Jin, C.H., et al., 2004. Pretreatment with 1,8-cineole potentiates thioacetamide-induced hepatotoxicity and immunosuppression. Archives of Pharmaceutical Research 27, 781–789.

Kim, S.H., Hong, K.O., Hwang, J.K., et al., 2005. Xanthorrhizol has a potential to attenuate the high dose cisplatin-induced nephrotoxicity in mice. Food Chem. Toxicol. 43, 117–122.

Kim, H.Y., Lee, S.B., Chung, Y.H., et al., 2006. Evaluation of subchronic inhalation toxicity of dimethyl disulfide in rats. Inhal. Toxicol. 18, 395–403.

Kim, T.H., Ito, H., Hatano, T., et al., 2006. New antitumor sesquiterpenoids from Santalum album of Indian origin. Tetrahedron 62, 6981–6989.

Kim, D.H., Kim, C.H., Kim, M.S., et al., 2007. Suppression of age-related inflammatory NF-κB activation by cinnamaldehyde. Biogerontology 8, 545–554.

Kim, Y.K., Kim, Y.S., Ryu, S.Y., 2007. Antiproliferative effect of furanocoumarins from the root of Angelica dahurica on cultured human tumor cell lines. Phytother. Res. 21, 288–290.

Kim, H., Kim, K.B., Ku, H.Y., et al., 2008. Identification and characterization of potent CYP2B6 inhibitors in woohwangcheongsimwon suspension, an herbal preparation used in the treatment and prevention of apoplexy in Korea and China. Drug Metab. Dispos. 36, 1010–1015.

Kim, S.H., Nam, J.H., Park, E.J., et al., 2009. Menthol regulates TRPM8-independent processes in PC-3 prostate cancer cells. Biochim. Biophys. Acta 1792, 33–38.

Kim, Y.K., Kim, M., Kim, H., et al., 2009. Effect of lavender oil on motor function and dopamine receptor expression in the olfactory bulb of mice. J. Ethnopharmacol. 125, 31–35.

Kimata, H., 2004. Effect of exposure to volatile organic compounds on plasma levels of neuropeptides, nerve growth factor and histamine in patients with self-reported multiple chemical sensitivity. Int. J. Hyg. Environ. Health 207, 159–163.

Kimball, H.W., 1898. A case of poisoning by oil of pennyroyal: recovery. Atlantic Medical Weekly 307–308.

Kimber, I., Gerberick, G.F., Basketter, D.A., 1999. Thresholds in contact sensitization: theoretical and practical considerations. Food Chem. Toxicol. 37, 553–560.

Kimber, I., Basketter, D.A., Gerberick, G.F., et al., 2002. Allergic contact dermatitis. Int. Immunopharmacol. 2, 201–211.

Kimber, I., Basketter, D.A., Butler, M., et al., 2003. Classification of contact allergens according to potency: proposals. Food Chem. Toxicol. 41, 1799–1809.

Kimber, I., Dearman, R.J., Basketter, D.A., et al., 2008. Dose metrics in the acquisition of skin sensitization: thresholds and importance of dose per unit area. Regul. Toxicol. Pharmacol. 52, 39–45.

Kimmel, C.A., Wilson, J.G., Schumacher, H.J., 1971. Studies on metabolism and identification of the causative agent in aspirin teratogenesis in rats. Teratology 4, 15–24.

Kimura, E.T., Darby, T.D., Krause, R.A., et al., 1971. Parenteral toxicity studies with benzyl alcohol. Toxicol. Appl. Pharmacol. 18, 60–68.

Kimura, Y., Okuda, H., 1997. Histamine-release effectors from Angelica dahurica var. dahurica root. J. Nat. Prod. 60, 249–251.

King, A.A., Shaughnessy, D.T., Mure, K., et al., 2007. Antimutagenicity of cinnamaldehyde and vanillin in human cells: global gene expression and possible role of DNA damage and repair. Mutat. Res. 616, 60–69.

Kirkland, D., Aardema, M., Henderson, L., et al., 2005. Evaluation of the ability of a battery of three in vitro genotoxicity tests to discriminate rodent carcinogens and non-carcinogens I. Sensitivity, specificity and relative predictivity. Mutat. Res. 584, 1–256.

Kirkness, W.R., 1910. Poisoning by oil of eucalyptus. Br. Med. J. 1, 261.

Kirov, M., Bainova, A., Spasovski, M., 1988a. Rose oil: acute and subacute oral toxicity. Medico Biologic Information, Sofia 3, 8–14.

Kirov, M., Burkova, T., Kapurdov, V., et al., 1988b. Rose oil: lipotropic effect in modelled fatty dystrophy of the liver (morphological and enzymohistochemical study). Medico Biologic Information, Sofia 3, 18–22.

Kirsch, C.M., Yenokida, G.G., Jensen, W.A., et al., 1990. Non-cardiogenic pulmonary oedema due to the intravenous administration of clove oil. Thorax 45, 235–236.

Kirschbaum, C., Kudielka, B.M., Gaab, J., et al., 1999. Impact of gender, menstrual cycle phase, and oral contraceptives on the activity of the hypothalamus-pituitary-adrenal axis. Psychosom. Med. 61, 154–162.

Kishore, N., Chansouria, J.P., Dubey, N.K., 1996. Antidermatophytic action of the essential oil of Chenopodium ambrosioides and an ointment prepared from it. Phytother. Res. 10, 453–455.

Kiso, Y., Tohkin, M., Hikino, H., 1983. Antihepatotoxic principles of Atractylodes rhizomes. J. Nat. Prod. 46, 651–654.

Kitahara, M., Ishiguro, F., Takayama, K., et al., 1993. Evaluation of skin damage of cyclic monoterpenes, percutaneous absorption enhancers, by using culture human skin cells. Biological & Pharmacological Bulletin 16, 912–916.

Kiyotani, K., Yamazaki, H., Fujieda, M., et al., 2003. Decreased coumarin 7-hydroxylase activities and CYP2A6 expression levels in humans caused by genetic polymorphism in CYP2A6 promoter region (CYP2A6*9). Pharmacogenetics 13, 689–695.

Klaunig, J.E., Kamendulis, L.M., 2004. The role of oxidative stress in carcinogenesis. Annu. Rev. Pharmacol. Toxicol. 44, 239–267.

Kleeberg, J., 1959. Pharmacological and clinical studies on almonds. Inhibition of peptic activity by benzaldehyde. Arch. Int. Pharmacodyn. Thér. 120, 152.

Kleiner, H.E., Vulimiri, S.V., Miller, L., 2001. Oral administration of naturally occurring coumarins leads to altered phase I and II enzyme activities and reduced DNA adduct formation by polycyclic aromatic hydrocarbons in various tissues of SENCAR mice. Carcinogenesis 22, 73–82.

Kleiner, H.E., Vulimiri, S.V., Starost, M.F., 2002. Oral administration of the citrus coumarin, isopimpinellin, blocks DNA adduct formation and skin tumor initiation by 7,12-dimethylbenz[a]anthracene in SENCAR mice. Carcinogenesis 23, 1667–1675.

Kleiner, H.E., Reed, M.J., DiGiovanni, J., 2003. Naturally occurring coumarins inhibit human cytochromes P450 and block benzo[a]pyrene and 7,12-dimethylbenz[a]anthracene DNA adduct formation in MCF-7 cells. Chem. Res. Toxicol. 16, 415–422.

Kleinsasser, N.H., Kastenbauer, E.R., Weissacher, H., 2000. Phthalates demonstrate genotoxicity on human mucosa of the upper aerodigestive tract. Environ. Mol. Mutagen. 35, 9–12.

Kleinsasser, N.H., Kastenbauer, E.R., Wallner, B.C., 2001. Genotoxicity of phthalates. On the discussion of plasticizers in children's toys. HNO 49, 378–381.

Kleinschmidt, J., Römmelt, H., Zuber, A., 1985. The pharmacokinetics of the bronchosecretolytic ozothin after intravenous injection. Int. J. Clin. Pharmacol. 23, 200–203.

Klesse, P., Lukoschek, P., 1955. Investigations of the bacteriostatic action of some mustard oils. Arzneimittelforschung 5, 505–507.

Kligman, A.M., 1966. The identification of contact allergens by human assay: III. The maximation test: a procedure for screening and rating contact sensitizers. J. Invest. Dermatol. 47, 393–409.

Kligman, A.M., 1979. Perspectives and problems in cutaneous gerontology. J. Invest. Dermatol. 73, 39–46.

Kligman, A.M., 1990. The spectrum of contact urticaria. Wheals, erythema, and pruritus. Dermatol. Clin. 8, 57–60.

Kligman, A.M., 1998. A reappraisal of the guinea pig maximation test. In: Frosch, P.J., Johansen, J.D., White, I.R. (Eds.), Fragrances, beneficial and adverse effects. Springer, Berlin.

Klimes, I., Lamparsky, D., 1976. Vanilla volatiles, a comprehensive analysis. International Flavour & Food Additives 7, 272–291.

Kline, R.M., Kline, J.J., Di Palma, J., et al., 2001. Enteric-coated, pH-dependent peppermint oil capsules for the treatment of irritable bowel syndrome in children. J. Pediatr. 138, 125–128.

Klingensmith, W.R., 1934. Poisoning by camphor. J. Am. Med. Assoc. 102, 2182–2183.

Klopell, F.C., Lemos, M., Sousa, J.P., et al., 2007. Nerolidol, an antiulcer constituent from the essential oil of Baccharis dracunculifolia DC (Asteraceae). Z. Naturforsch. [C] 62, 537–542.

Kloss, J.L., Boeckman, C.R., 1967. Methyl salicylate poisoning. Ohio State Med. J. 63, 1064–1065.

Kluwe, W.M., Montgomery, C.A., Giles, H.D., et al., 1983. Encephalopathy in rats and nephropathy in rats and mice after subchronic oral exposure to benzaldehyde. Food Chem. Toxicol. 21, 245–250.

Knežević-Vukčević, J., Vuković-Gacić, B., Stevic, T., et al., 2005. Antimutagenic effect of sage (Salvia officinalis L.) and its fractions against UV-induced mutations in bacterial and yeats cells. Archives of Biological Sciences Belgrade 57, 163–172.

Knight, T.E., Hausen, B.M., 1994. Melaleuca oil (tea tree oil) dermatitis. J. Am. Acad. Dermatol. 30, 423–427.

Knowles, L.M., Milner, J.A., 1998. Depressed p34cdc2 kinase activity and G2/M phase arrest induced by diallyl disulfide in HCT-15 cells. Nutr. Cancer 30, 169–174.

Ko, Y.C., Huang, Y.L., Lee, C.H., et al., 1995. Betel quid chewing, cigarette smoking and alcohol consumption related to oral cancer in Taiwan. J. Oral Pathol. Med. 24, 450–453.

Koch, W.H., 1986. Psoralen photomutagenic specificity in Salmonella typhimurium. Mutat. Res. 160, 195–205.

Koch, H.M., Drexler, H., Angerer, J., 2003. An estimation of the daily intake of di(2-ethylhexyl)phthalate (DEHP) and other phthalates in the general population. Int. J. Hyg. Environ. Health 206, 77–83.

Kochi, M., Takeuchi, S., Mizutani, T., et al., 1980. Antitumor activity of benzaldehyde. Cancer Treat. Rep. 64, 21–23.

Kodama, R., Noda, K., Ide, H., 1974. Studies on the metabolism of d-limonene II. The metabolic fate of d-limonene in rabbit. Xenobiotica 4, 85–95.

Kodama, R., Okubo, A., Araki, E., et al., 1977a. Studies on d-limonene as a gallstone solubilizer (VII). Effects on development of mouse fetuses and offspring. Oyo Yakuri 13, 863–873.

Kodama, R., Okubo, A., Sato, K., et al., 1977b. Studies on d-limonene as a gallstone solubilizer (IX). Effects on development of rabbit fetuses and offspring. Oyo Yakuri 13, 885–898.

Koenigs, L.L., Trager, W.F., 1998. Mechanism-based inactivation of cytochrome P450 2B1 by 8-methoxypsoralen and several other furanocoumarins. Biochemistry 37, 13184–13193.

Koenigs, L.L., Peter, R.M., Thompson, S.J., et al., 1997. Mechanism-based inactivation of human liver cytochrome P450 2A6 by 8-methoxypsoralen. Drug Metab. Dispos. 25, 1407–1415.

Koh, K.J., Pearce, A.L., Marshman, G., et al., 2002. Tea tree oil reduces histamine-induced skin inflammation. Br. J. Dermatol. 147, 1212–1217.

Kohl, L., Blondeel, A., Song, M., 2002. Allergic contact dermatitis from cosmetics: retrospective analysis of 819 patch-tested patients. Dermatology 204, 334–337.

Kohlert, C., van Rensen, I., März, R., et al., 2000. Bioavailability and pharmacokinetics of natural volatile terpenes in animals and humans. Planta Med. 66, 495–505.

Kohlert, C., Schindler, G., Marz, R.W., et al., 2002. Systemic availability and pharmacokinetics of thymol in humans. J. Clin. Pharmacol. 42, 731–737.

Kohrman, K.A., Booman, K.A., Dorsky, J., et al., 1983. Benzyl salicylate: a survey of consumer patch-test sensitization. Food Chem. Toxicol. 21, 741–744.

Koizumi, K., Iwasaki, Y., Narukawa, M., et al., 2009. Diallyl sulfides in garlic activate both TRPA1 and TRPV1. Biochem. Biophys. Res. Commun. 382, 545–548.

Kojima, H., Yanai, T., Toyota, A., 1998. Essential oil constituents from Japanese and Indian Curcuma aromatica rhizomes. Planta Med. 64, 380–381.

Komericki, P., Aberer, W., Kränke, B., 2004. An 8-year experience in airborne contact dermatitis. Wien. Klin. Wochenschr. 116, 322–325.

Komori, T., Matsumoto, T., Motomura, E., et al., 2006. The sleep-enhancing effect of valerian inhalation and sleep-shortening effect of lemon inhalation. Chem. Senses 31, 731–737.

Kong, Y.C., Xie, J.X., But, P.P.H., 1986. Fertility regulating agents from traditional Chinese medicines. J. Ethnopharmacol. 15, 1–44.

Kong, Y.C., Lau, C.P., Wat, K.H., et al., 1989. Antifertility principle of Ruta graveolens. Planta Med. 55, 176–178.

Konishi, T., Shimada, Y., Nagao, T., et al., 2002. Antiproliferative sesquiterpene lactones from the roots of *Inula helenium*. Biol. Pharm. Bull. 25, 1370–1372.

Kono, M., Yoshida, Y., Itaya, Y., et al., 1995. Antimicrobial activity and mutagenicity of allyl isothiocyanate and several essential oils from spices. Kinki Daigaku Nogakubu Kiyo 28, 11–19.

Koo, T.H., Lee, J.H., Park, Y.J., et al., 2001. A sesquiterpene lactone, costunolide, from *Magnolia grandiflora* inhibits NF-kappa B by targeting I kappa B phosphorylation. Planta Med. 67, 103–107.

Koo, B.S., Park, K.S., Ha, J.H., et al., 2003. Inhibitory effects of the fragrance inhalation of essential oil from *Acorus gramineus* on central nervous system. Biological & Pharmaceutical Bulletin 26, 978–982.

Koo, B.S., Lee, S.I., Ha, J.H., et al., 2004. Inhibitory effects of the essential oil from SuHeXiang Wan on the central nervous system after inhalation. Biol. Pharm. Bull. 27, 515–519.

Koparal, A.T., Zeytinoglu, M., 2003. Effects of carvacrol on a human non-small cell lung cancer (NSCLC) cell line, A549. Cytotechnology 43, 149–154.

Kopelman, R., Miller, S., Kelley, R., et al., 1979. Camphor intoxication treated by resin hemoperfusion. J. Am. Med. Assoc. 241, 727–728.

Köppel, C., Tenczer, J., Tönnesmann, U., et al., 1981. Acute poisoning with pine oil – metabolism of monoterpenes. Arch. Toxicol. 49, 73–78.

Köppel, C., Tenczer, J., Schirop, T., et al., 1982. Camphor poisoning. Abuse of camphor as a stimulant. Arch. Toxicol. 51, 101–106.

Kordali, S., Kotan, R., Mavi, A., et al., 2005a. Determination of the chemical composition and antioxidant activity of the essential oil of *Artemisia dracunculus* and of the antifungal and antibacterial activities of Turkish *Artemisia absinthium*, *A. dracunculus*, *Artemisia santonicum*, and *Artemisia spicigera* essential oils. J. Agric. Food Chem. 53, 9452–9458.

Kordali, S., Cakir, A., Mavi, A., et al., 2005b. Screening of chemical composition and antifungal and antioxidant activities of the essential oils from three Turkish artemisia species. J. Agric. Food Chem. 53, 1408–1416.

Koren, G. (Ed.), 1990. Maternal-fetal toxicology - a clinicians' guide. Marcel Dekker, New York.

Koren, H.S., Graham, D.E., Devlin, R.B., 1992. Exposure of humans to a volatile organic mixture. III. Inflammatory response. Arch. Environ. Health 47, 39–44.

Koruk, S.T., Ozyilkan, E., Kaya, P., et al., 2005. Juniper tar poisoning. Clin. Toxicol. (Phila) 43, 47–49.

Köse, E., Sarsilmaz, M., Meydan, S., et al., 2011. The effect of lavender oil on serum testosterone levels and epididymal sperm characteristics of formaldehyde treated male rats. Eur. Rev. Med. Pharmacol. Sci. 15, 538–542.

Köse, E., Sarsilmaz, M., Tag, U., et al., 2012. Rose oil protects against formaldehyde-induced testicular damage in rats. Andrologia 44 (Suppl. 1), 342–348.

Kothari, S.K., Battacharya, A.K., Ramesh, S., et al., 2005a. Volatile constituents in oil from different plants of methyl eugenol-rich *Ocimum tenuiflorum* L.f. (syn. *O. sanctum* L.) grown in South India. Journal of Essential Oil Research 17, 656–658.

Kothari, S.K., Battacharya, A.K., Ramesh, S., et al., 2005b. Pre-flowering harvesting of *Ocimum gratissimum* for higher essential oil and eugenol yields under semi-arid tropics. Journal of Essential Oil Research 17, 212–216.

Kourounakis, A.P., Rekka, E.A., Kourounakis, P.N., 1997a. Effect of guaiazulene on some cytochrome P450 activities. Implication in the metabolic activation and hepatotoxicity of paracetamol. Arch. Pharm. 330, 7–11.

Kourounakis, A.P., Rekka, E.A., Kourounakis, P.N., 1997b. Antioxidant activity of guaiazulene and protection against paracetamol hepatotoxicity in rats. J. Pharm. Pharmacol. 49, 938–942.

Koussoulakou, D.S., Margaritis, L.H., Koussoulakos, S.L., 2011. Antagonists of retinoic acid and BMP4 affect fetal mouse osteogenesis and odontoblast differentiation. Pathophysiology 18, 103–109.

Kovacs, R., Kardos, J., Heinemann, U., et al., 2005. Mitochondrial calcium ion and membrane potential transients follow the pattern of epileptiform discharges in hippocampal slice cultures. J. Neurosci. 25, 4260–4269.

Kovar, K.A., Gropper, B., Friess, D., et al., 1987. Blood levels of 1,8-cineole and locomotor activity of mice after inhalation and oral administration of rosemary oil. Planta Med. 53, 315–318.

Kovats, E., 1987. Composition of essential oils part 7. Bulgarian oil of rose (*Rosa damascena* Mill). J. Chromatogr. 406, 185–222.

Kozam, G., Mantell, G.M., 1978. The effect of eugenol on oral mucous membrane. J. Dent. Res. 57, 954–957.

Kraus, A., Hammerschmidt, F.J., 1980. An investigation of fennel oils. Dragoco Report 1 (2), 3–12.

Kreckmann, K.H., Baldwin, J.K., Roberts, L.G., et al., 2000. Inhalation developmental toxicity and reproduction studies with cyclohexane. Drug Chemistry & Toxicology 23, 555–573.

Kreipl, A.T.h., König, W.A., 2004. Sesquiterpenes from the east African sandalwood *Osyris tenuifolia*. Phytochemistry 65, 2045–2049.

Kresel, J.J., 1982. Camphor. Clinical & Toxicological Revue 4, 1.

Kreutzer, R., Neutra, R.R., Lashuay, N., 1999. Prevalence of people reporting sensitivities to chemicals in a population-based survey. Am. J. Epidemiol. 150, 1–12.

Kreydiyyeh, S.I., Usta, J., Knio, K., et al., 2003. Aniseed oil increases glucose absorption and reduces urine output in the rat. Life Sci. 74, 663–673.

Krishnaiah, Y.S., Al-Saidan, S.M., Chandrasekhar, D.V., et al., 2006. Controlled *in vivo* release of nicorandil from a carvone-based transdermal therapeutic system in human volunteers. Drug Deliv. 13, 69–77.

Kristiansen, E., Madsen, C., 1995. Induction of protein droplet (alpha 2 mu-globulin) nephropathy in male rats after short-term dosage with 1,8-cineole and l-limonene. Toxicol. Lett. 80, 147–152.

Krob, H.A., Fleischer, A.B., D'Agostino, R., et al., 2004. Prevalence and relevance of contact dermatitis allergens: a meta-analysis of 15 years of published T.R.U.E. Test data. J. Am. Acad. Dermatol. 51, 349–353.

Kröber, F., 1936. A case of severe poisoning with chenopodium oil following its therapeutic use. Dtsch. Med. Wochenschr. 62, 1759.

Kroes, R., Renwick, A.G., Feron, V., et al., 2007. Application of the threshold of toxicological concern (TTC) to the safety evaluation of cosmetic ingredients. Food Chem. Toxicol. 45, 2533–2562.

Kronmiller, J.E., Beeman, C.S., Nguyen, T., et al., 1995. Blockade of the initiation of murine odontogenesis in vitro by citral, an inhibitor of endogenous retinoic acid synthesis. Arch. Oral. Biol. 40, 645–652.

Krüger, H., Hammer, K., 1999. Chemotypes of fennel (*Foeniculum vulgare* Mill). Journal of Essential Oil Research 11, 79–82.

Kruhlak, N.L., Contrera, J.F., Benz, R.D., et al., 2007. Progress in QSAR toxicity screening of pharmaceutical impurities and other FDA regulated products. Adv. Drug Deliv. Rev. 59, 43–55.

Kubeczka, K.H., 2002. Essential oils analysis by capillary gas chromatography and carbon-13 NMR spectroscopy, second ed. John Wiley, Chichester.

Kubeczka, K.H., Schultze, W., 1987. Biology and chemistry of conifer oils. Flavour & Fragrance Journal 2, 137–148.

Kubeczka, K.H., Stahl, E., 1975. Über ätherische Öle der Apiaceae (Umbelliferae). I. Das Wurzelol von *Pastinaca sativa*. Planta Med. 27, 235–241.

Kubo, I., Morimitsu, Y., 1995. Cytotoxicity of green tea flavor compounds against two solid tumor cells. J. Agric. Food Chem. 43, 1626–1628.

Kubo, I., Chaudhuri, S.K., Kubo, Y., et al., 1996. Cytotoxic and antioxidative sesquiterpenoids from *Heterotheca inuloides*. Planta Med. 62, 427–430.

Kuboyama, N., Fuji, A., 1992. Mutagenicity of analgesics, their derivatives, and anti-inflammatory drugs with S-9 mix of several animal species. J. Nihon Univ. Sch. Dent. 34, 183–195.

Kudrzycka-Bieloszabska, F.W., Glowniak, K., 1966. Pharmacodynamic properties of oleum chamomillae and oleum millefolii. Dissertationes Pharmaceuticae et Pharmacologicae (Pol) 18 (5), 449–454.

Kuge, T., Shibata, T., Willett, M.S., et al., 2001. Lack of oncogenicity of wood creosote, the principal active ingredient of Seirogan, an herbal antidiarrheal medication, in Sprague-Dawley rats. Int. J. Toxicol. 20, 297–305.

Kuiper, G.G., Enmark, E., Pelto-Huikko, M., et al., 1996. Cloning of a novel receptor expressed in rat prostate and ovary. Proc. Natl. Acad. Sci. U. S. A. 93, 5925–5930.

Kulieva, Z.T., 1980. Analgesic, hypotensive and cardiotonic action of the essential oil of thyme growing in Azerbaijan. Vestn. Akad. Med. Nauk SSSR 9, 61–63.

Kumagai, H., Kashima, N., Seki, T., et al., 1994. Analysis of volatile components in essential oil of upland wasabi and their inhibitory effects on platelet aggregation. Biosci. Biotechnol. Biochem. 58, 2131–2135.

Kumar, P., Caradonna-Graham, V.M., Gupta, S., et al., 1995. Inhalation challenge effects of perfume scent strips in patients with asthma. Ann. Allergy Asthma Immunol. 75, 429–433.

Kumar, A., Nadda, G., Shanker, A., 2004. Determination of chlorpyrifos 20% EC (Dursban 20 EC) in scented rose and its products. J. Chromatogr. A 1050, 193–199.

Kumar, A., D'Souza, S.S., Tickoo, S., et al., 2009. Antiangiogenic and proapoptotic activities of allyl isothiocyanate inhibit ascites tumor growth in vivo. Integr. Cancer Ther. 8, 75–87.

Kumaravelu, P., Dakshinamoorthy, D.P., Subranamiam, S., et al., 1995. Effect of eugenol on drug-metabolizing enzymes of carbon tetrachloride-intoxicated rat liver. Biochem. Pharmacol. 49, 1703–1707.

Kumaravelu, P., Subramaniyam, S., Dakshinamoorthy, D.P., et al., 1996. The antioxidant effect of eugenol on CCl4-induced erythrocyte damage in rats. Nutritional Biochemistry 7, 23–28.

Kundu, R.V., Scheman, A.J., Gutmanovich, A., et al., 2004. Contact dermatitis to white petrolatum. Skinmed 3, 295–296.

Kunkeler, A.C.M., Weiland, J.W., Bruynzeel, D.P., 1998. The role of coumarin in patch testing. Contact Dermatitis 39, 327–328.

Kurishita, A., Ihara, T., 1990. Inhibitory effects of cobalt chloride and cinnamaldehyde on 5-azacytidine-induced digital malformations in rats. Teratology 41, 161–166.

Kurita, M., Kato, H., Yoshimura, K., 2009. A therapeutic strategy based on histological assessment of hyperpigmented skin lesions in Asians. J. Plast. Reconstr. Aesthet. Surg. 62, 955–963.

Kuroda, K., Yoo, Y.S., Ishibashi, T., 1984a. Antimutagenic activity of food additives. Mutat. Res. 130, 369.

Kuroda, K., Tanaka, S., Yoo, Y.S., et al., 1984b. Rec-assay of food additives. Nihon Koshu Eisei Zasshi (Japanese Journal of Public Health) 31, 277–281.

Kusilic, T., Radionic, A., Katalinic, V., et al., 2004. Use of different methods for testing antioxidative activity of oregano essential oil. Food Chem. 85, 633–640.

Kütting, B., Brehler, R., Traupe, H., 2004. Allergic contact dermatitis in children: strategies of prevention and risk management. Eur. J. Dermatol. 14, 80–85.

Kutzman, R.S., Meyer, G.J., Wolf, A.P., 1980. Biodistribution and excretion of [11C]benzaldehyde by the rat after two-minute inhalation exposures. Xenobiotica 10, 281–288.

Kuwabara, Y., Alexeeff, G.V., Broadwin, R., et al., 2007. Evaluation and application of the RD50 for determining acceptable exposure levels of airborne sensory irritants for the general public. Environ. Health Perspect. 115, 1609–1616.

Kwak, M.K., Kim, S.G., Kim, N.D., 1995. Effects of garlic oil on rat hepatic P4502E1 expression. Xenobiotica 25, 1021–1029.

Kwon, K.B., Yoo, S.J., Ryu, D.G., et al., 2002. Induction of apoptosis by diallyl disulfide through activation of caspase-3 in human leukaemia HL-60 cells. Biochem. Pharmacol. 63, 41–47.

Kwon, H.J., Shin, J.O., Lee, J.M., et al., 2011. Retinoic acid modulates chondrogenesis in the developing mouse cranial base. J. Exp. Zoology B Mol. Dev. Evol. 316, 574–583.

Lachenmeier, D.W., Uebelacker, M., 2010. Risk assessment of thujone in foods and medicines containing sage and wormwood - evidence for a need of regulatory changes? Regul. Toxicol. Pharmacol. 58, 437–443.

Lachenmeier, D.W., Nathan-Maister, D., Breaux, T.A., et al., 2008. Chemical composition of vintage preban absinthe with special reference to thujone, fenchone, pinocamphone, methanol, copper, and antimony concentrations. J. Agric. Food Chem. 56, 3073–3081.

Lachenmeier, D.W., Emmert, J., Kuballa, T., et al., 2005. Thujone - cause of absinthism? Forensic. Sci. Int. 158, 1–8.

Lacour, M., Zunder, T., Schmidtke, K., et al., 2005. Multiple chemical sensitivity syndrome (MCS) - suggestions for an extension of the US MCS-case definition. Int. J. Hyg. Environ. Health 208, 141–151.

Laederich, L., Mamou, H., Arager, 1932. Fatal intoxication from apiol. Bulletin Société Médicale des Hospitaux de Paris 48, 746–751.

Lagouri, V., Blekas, G., Tsimidou, M., et al., 1993. Composition and antioxidant activity of essential oils from oregano plants grown wild in Greece. Z. Lebensm. Unters. Forsch. 197, 20–23.

Lahlou, S., Figueiredo, A.F., Magalhães, P.J., et al., 2002a. Cardiovascular effects of 1,8-cineole, a terpenoid oxide present in many plant essential oils, in normotensive rats. Can. J. Physiol. Pharmacol. 80, 1125–1131.

Lahlou, S., Galindo, C.A., Leal-Cardoso, J.H., 2002b. Cardiovascular effects of the essential oil of Alpinia zerumbet leaves and its main constituent, terpinen-4-ol, in rats: role of the autonomic nervous system. Planta Med. 68, 1097–1102.

Lahlou, S., Interaminense, L.F., Magalhaes, P.J., et al., 2004. Cardiovascular effects of eugenol, a phenolic compound present in many plant essential oils, in normotensive rats. J. Cardiovasc. Pharmacol. 43, 250–257.

Lahlou, S., Magalhaes, P.J., de Siqueira, R.J., et al., 2005. Cardiovascular effects of the essential oil of Aniba canelilla bark in normotensive rats. J. Cardiovasc. Pharmacol. 46, 412–421.

Lahti, A., 1980. Non-immunologic contact urticaria. Acta Dermatologica Venereologica (Stockh.) 60 (Suppl. 91), 1–49.

Lahti, A., Hannuksela, M., 1981. Is benzoic acid really harmful in cases of atopy and urticaria? Lancet 318 (8254), 1055.

Lai, E.C., Chyau, C.C., Mau, J.L., et al., 2004. Antimicrobial activity and cytotoxicity of the essential oil of Curcuma zedoaria. Am. J. Chin. Med. 32, 281–290.

Lai, M.W., Klein-Schwartz, W., Rodgers, G.C., et al., 2006. 2005 Annual report of the American Association of Poison Control Centers National Poisoning & Exposure Database. Clin. Toxicol. 44, 803–932.

Lake, B.G., 1984. Investigations into the mechanism of coumarin-induced hepatotoxicity in the rat. Arch. Toxicol. Suppl. 7, 16–29.

Lake, B.G., 1999. Coumarin metabolism, toxicity and carcinogenicity: relevance for human risk assessment. Food Cosmet. Toxicol. 37, 423–453.

Laleye, A., Gbenou, J., Edorh, P., et al., 2004. Evaluation de l'embryotoxicité de l'huile essentielle de Melaleuca quinquenervia (Cav) S.T. Black (niaouli) chez le rat Wistar. Journal de la Société Ouest-Africaine de Chimie 18, 149–164.

Lalko, J., Api, A.M., 2006. Investigation of the dermal sensitization potential of various essential oils in the local lymph node assay. Food Chem. Toxicol. 44, 739–746.

Lalko, J., Api, A.M., 2008. Citral: identifying a threshold for induction of dermal sensitization. Regul. Toxicol. Pharmacol. 52, 62–73.

Lalko, J., Lapczynski, A., Politano, V.T., et al., 2007a. Fragrance Material Review on α-ionone. Food Chem. Toxicol. 45, S235–S240.

Lalko, J., Lapczynski, A., McGinty, D., et al., 2007b. Fragrance Material Review on β-ionone. Food Chem. Toxicol. 45, S241–S247.

Lalko, J., Lapczynski, A., McGinty, D., et al., 2007c. Fragrance Material Review on α-irone. Food Chem. Toxicol. 45, S272–S275.

Lam, L.K., Zheng, B., 1991. Effects of essential oils on glutathione-S-transferase activity in mice. J. Agric. Food Chem. 39, 660–662.

Lamarti, A., Badoc, A., Bouriquet, R., 1991. A chemotaxonomic evaluation of Petroselinum crispum (Mill.) A.W. Hill (parsley) marketed in France. Journal of Essential Oil Research 3, 425–433.

Lammintausta, K., Maibach, H.I., Wilson, D., 1988. Mechanisms of subjective (sensory) irritation. Propensity to non-immunologic contact urticaria and objective irritation in stingers. Derm. Beruf Umwelt 36, 45–49.

Lamorena, R.B., Jung, S.G., Bae, G.N., et al., 2007. The formation of ultra-fine particles during ozone-initiated oxidations with terpenes emitted from natural paint. J. Hazard. Mater. 141, 245–251.

Lampronti, I., Saab, A.M., Gambari, R., 2006. Antiproliferative activity of essential oils derived from plants belonging to the Magnoliophyta division. Int. J. Oncol. 29, 989–995.

Lane, C.G., 1922. Dermatitis caused by oil of citronella. Arch. Derm. Syphilol. 5, 589–590.

Lane, B.W., Ellenhorn, M.J., Hulbert, T.V., et al., 1991. Clove oil ingestion in an infant. Hum. Exp. Toxicol. 10, 291–294.

Langer, P., Stolc, V., 1965. Goitrogenic activity of allylisothiocyanate – a widespread natural mustard oil. Endocrinology 76, 151–155.

Langley, G., 2005. Acute toxicity testing without animals. ECAE, London. http://www.eceae.org/downloads/pdf/ECEAE_Acute_Toxicity.pdf.

Lantry, L.E., Zhang, Z., Gao, F., et al., 1997. Chemopreventive effect of perillyl alcohol on 4-(methylnitrosamino)-1-(3-pyridyl)-1-butanone induced tumorigenesis in (C3H/HeJ X A/J)F1 mouse lung. J. Cell. Biochem. Suppl. 27, 20–25.

Lapczynski, A., Isola, D.A., Christian, M.S., et al., 2006. Evaluation of the developmental toxicity of acetyl cedrene. Int. J. Toxicol. 25, 423–428.

Lapczynski, A., McGinty, D., Jones, L., et al., 2007a. Fragrance material review on benzyl salicylate. Food Chem. Toxicol. 45, S362–S380.

Lapczynski, A., Jones, L., McGinty, D., et al., 2007b. Fragrance material review on methyl salicylate. Food Chem. Toxicol. 45, S428–S452.

Lapczynski, A., Bhatia, S.P., Letizia, C.S., et al., 2008b. Fragrance material review on l-citronellol. Food Chem. Toxicol. 46 (Suppl. 1), S110–S113.

Lapczynski, A., Letizia, C.S., Api, A.M., 2008c. Fragrance material review on (+)-(R)-citronellol. Food Chem. Toxicol. 46 (Suppl. 1), S114–S116.

Lapczynski, A., Bhatia, S.P., Letizia, C.S., et al., 2008d. Fragrance material review on farnesol. Food Chem. Toxicol. 46 (Suppl. 1), S149–S156.

Lapczynski, A., Letizia, C.S., Api, A.M., 2008e. Fragrance material review on d-linalool. Food Chem. Toxicol. 46 (Suppl. 1), S193–S194.

Lapczynski, A., Letizia, C.S., Api, A.M., 2008f. Fragrance material review on l-linalool. Food Chem. Toxicol. 46 (Suppl. 1), S195–S196.

Lapczynski, A., Letizia, C.S., Api, A.M., 2008g. Addendum to fragrance material review on linalool. Food Chem. Toxicol. 46 (Suppl. 11), S190–S192.

Lapczynski, A., Bhatia, S.P., Letizia, C.S., et al., 2008h. Fragrance material review on nerolidol. Food Chem. Toxicol. 46 (Suppl. 1), S247–S250.

Lapczynski, A., Foxenberg, R.J., Bhatia, S.P., et al., 2008i. Fragrance material review on nerol. Food Chem. Toxicol. 46 (Suppl. 1), S241–S244.

Larsen, W.G., 1977. Perfume dermatitis: a study of 20 patients. Arch. Dermatol. 113, 623–626.

Larsen, W., Nakayama, H., Fischer, T., et al., 1996a. A study of new fragrance mixtures. Am. J. Contact Dermat. 9, 202–206.

Larsen, W., Nakayama, H., Lindberg, M., et al., 1996b. Fragrance contact dermatitis: a worldwide multicenter investigation (Part I). Am. J. Contact Dermat. 7, 77–83.

Larsen, W., Nakayama, H., Fischer, T., et al., 1998. A study of new fragrance mixtures. American Dermatology 113, 623–626.

Larsen, S.T., Hougaard, K.S., Hammer, M., et al., 2000. Effects of R-(+)- and S-(-)-limonene on the respiratory tract in mice. Hum. Exp. Toxicol. 19, 457–466.

Larsen, W., Nakayama, H., Fischer, T., et al., 2001. Fragrance contact dermatitis: a worldwide multicentre investigation (part II). Contact Dermatitis 44, 344–346.

Larsen, W., Nakayama, H., Fischer, T., et al., 2002. Fragrance contact dermatitis: a worldwide multicentre investigation (part III). Contact Dermatitis 46, 141–144.

Lassak, E.V., McCarthy, T., 1983. Australian Medicinal Plants. Methuen, Sydney.

Låstbom, L., Boman, A., Camner, P., et al., 1998. Does airway responsiveness increase after skin sensitisation to 3-carene: a study in isolated guinea pig lungs. Toxicology 125, 59–66.

Låstbom, L., Boman, A., Camner, P., et al., 2000. Increased airway responsiveness after skin sensitisation to 3-carene, studied in isolated guinea pig lungs. Toxicology 147, 209–214.

Låstbom, L., Boman, A., Johnsson, S., et al., 2003. Increased airway responsiveness of a common fragrance component, 3-carene, after skin sensitisation – a study in isolated guinea pig lungs. Toxicol. Lett. 145, 189–196.

Latini, G., Verrotti, A., De Felice, C., 2004. Di-2-ethylhexyl phthalate and endocrine disruption: a review. Curr. Drug Targets Immune Endocr. Metabol. Disord. 4, 37–40.

Laude, E.A., Morice, A.H., Grattan, T.J., 1994. The antitussive effects of menthol, camphor and cineole in conscious guinea-pigs. Pulm. Pharmacol. 7, 179–184.

Lewith, G.T., Godfrey, A.D., Prescott, P., 2005. A single-blinded, randomized pilot study evaluating the aroma of Lavandula augustifolia as a treatment for mild insomnia. J. Altern. Complement. Med. 11, 631–637.

Lavker, R.M., Zheng, P.S., Dong, G., 1986. Morphology of aged skin. Dermatology Clinic 4, 379–389.

Lavy, G., 1987. Nutmeg intoxication in pregnancy: a case report. J. Reprod. Med. 32, 63–64.

Lawrence, B.M., 1979. Essential oils 1976–1978. Allured Publishing, Wheaton.

Lawrence, B.M., 1981. Essential oils 1979–1980. Allured Publishing, Wheaton.

Lawrence, B.M., 1989. Essential oils 1981–1987. Allured Publishing, Wheaton.

Lawrence, B.M., 1993. Essential oils 1988–1991. Allured Publishing, Wheaton.

Lawrence, B.M., 1995. Progress in essential oils. Perfumer & Flavorist 20. 1995a (no 1); 1995b (no 2); 1995c (no 3); 1995d (no 4); 1995e (no 5); 1995f (no 6).

Lawrence, B.M., 1995g. Essential oils 1988–1991. Allured Publishing, Wheaton.

Lawrence, B.M., 1996. Progress in essential oils. Perfumer & Flavorist 21. 1996a (no 1); 1996b (no 2); 1996c (no 3); 1996d (no 4); 1996e (no 5); 1996f (no 6).

Lawrence, B.M., 1997. Progress in essential oils. Perfumer & Flavorist 22. 1997a (no 1); 1997b (no 2); 1997c (no 3); 1997d (no 4); 1997e (no 5); 1997f (no 6).

Lawrence, B.M., 1998. Progress in essential oils. Perfumer & Flavorist 23. 1998a (no 1); 1998b (no 2); 1998c (no 3); 1998d (no 4); 1998e (no 5); 1998f (no 6).

Lawrence, B.M., 1999. Progress in essential oils. Perfumer & Flavorist 24. 1999a (no 1); 1999b (no 2); 1999c (no 3); 1999d (no 4); 1999e (no 5); 1999f (no 6).

Lawrence, B.M., 2000. Progress in essential oils, Numbers 1–6. Perfumer & Flavorist 25, 2000a (no 1); 2000b (no 2); 2000c (no 3); 2000d (no 4); 2000e (no 5); 2000f (no 6).

Lawrence, B.M., 2001. Progress in essential oils. Perfumer & Flavorist 26. 2001a (no 1); 2001b (no 2); 2001c (no 3); 2001d (no 4); 2001e (no 5); 2001f (no 6).

Lawrence, B.M., 2002. Progress in essential oils. Perfumer & Flavorist 27. 2002a (no 1); 2002b (no 2); 2002c (no 3); 2002d (no 4); 2002e (no 5); 2002f (no 6).

Lawrence, B.M., 2003. Progress in essential oils. Perfumer & Flavorist 28, 84–86.

Lawrence, B.M., 2005. Progress in essential oils. Perfumer & Flavorist 30, 52–57.

Lawrence, B.M., 2008. Progress in essential oils. Perfumer & Flavorist 33, 38–41.

Lawrence, B.M., 2009. Progress in essential oils. Perfumer & Flavorist 34, 54–56.

Lawrence, B.M., 2012. Progress in essential oils. Perfumer & Flavorist 37, 42–43.

Lawrence, N.J., McGowan, A.T., Nduka, J., et al., 2001. Cytotoxic Michael-type amine adducts of α-methylene lactones alantolactone and isoalantolactone. Bioorg. Med. Chem. Lett. 11, 429–431.

Lawson, L.D., Wang, Z.Y.J., Hughes, B.G., 1991. Identification and HPLC quantitation of the sulfides and dialk(en)yl thiosulfinates in commercial garlic products. Planta Med. 57, 363–370.

Lawson, L.D., Ransom, D.K., Hughes, B.G., 1992. Inhibition of whole blood platelet-aggregation by compounds in garlic clove extracts and commercial garlic products. Thromb. Res. 65, 141–156.

Lazarou, J., Pomeranz, B.H., Corey, P.N., 1998. Incidence of adverse drug reactions in hospitalized patients: a meta-analysis of prospective studies. J. Am. Med. Assoc. 279, 1200–1205.

Lazutka, J.R., Mierauskien, J., Slapyt, G., et al., 2001. Genotoxicity of dill (Anethum graveolens L.), peppermint (Mentha x piperita L.) and pine (Pinus sylvestris L.) essential oils in human lymphocytes and Drosophila melanogaster. Food Chem. Toxicol. 39, 485–492.

Leach, E.H., Lloyd, J.P.F., 1956a. Citral poisoning. Proc. Nutr. Soc. 15, xv–xvi.

Leach, E.H., Lloyd, J.P.F., 1956b. Experimental ocular hypertension in animals. Trans. Ophthalmol. Soc. U. K. 76, 453–460.

Lear, J.T., Heagerty, A.H., Tan, B.B., et al., 1996. Transient re-emergence of oil of turpentine allergy in the pottery industry. Contact Dermatitis 35, 169–172.

LeBel, M., Ferron, L., Masson, M., et al., 1988. Benzyl alcohol metabolism and elimination in neonates. Developments in Pharmacology & Therapy 11, 347–356.

Le Bouffant, R., Guerquin, M.J., Duquenne, C., et al., 2010. Meiosis initiation in the human ovary requires intrinsic retinoic acid synthesis. Hum. Reprod. 25, 2579–2590.

Le Bourhis, B., 1968. Recherches préliminaires sur le métabolisme du trans-anéthole. Ann. Biol. Clin. (Paris) 26, 711–715.

Le Bourhis, B., 1970. Identification de quelques métabolites du trans-anéthole chez l'homme, le lapin et le rat. Ann. Pharm. Fr. 28, 355–361.

Le Bourhis, B., Soenen, A.M., 1973. Recherches sur l'action psychotrope de quelques substances aromatiques utilisées en alimentation. Food Cosmet. Toxicol. 11, 1–9.

Lee, W.M., 2003. Drug-induced hepatotoxicity. N. Engl. J. Med. 349, 474–485.

Lee, H.S., 2006. Antiplatelet property of *Curcuma longa* L. rhizome-derived *ar*-turmerone. Bioresour. Technol. 97, 1372–1376.

Lee, Y., 2009. Activation of apoptotic protein in U937 cells by a component of turmeric oil. BMB Reports 42, 96–100.

Lee, K.G., Shibamoto, T., 2001. Inhibition of malonaldehyde formation from blood plasma oxidation by aroma extracts and aroma components isolated from clove and eucalyptus. Food Chem. Toxicol. 39, 1199–1204.

Lee, K.G., Shibamoto, T., 2002. Determination of antioxidant potential of volatile extracts isolated from various herbs and spices. J. Agric. Food Chem. 50, 4947–4952.

Lee, K.K., Chan, T.Y., Lee, C.W., 1997. Improvements are needed in the existing packaging of medicated oils containing methyl salicylate. J. Clin. Pharm. Ther. 22, 279–281.

Lee, H.S., Jeong, T.C., Kim, J.H., 1998. *In vitro* and *in vivo* metabolism of myristicin in the rat. J. Chromatogr. B Biomed. Sci. Appl. 705, 367–372.

Lee, K.G., Mitchell, A., Shibamoto, T., 2000. Antioxidative activities of aroma extracts isolated from natural plants. Biofactors 13, 173–178.

Lee, M.G., Lee, K.T., Chi, S.G., et al., 2001. Costunolide induces apoptosis by ROS-mediated mitochondrial permeability transition and cytochrome C release. Biol. Pharm. Bull. 24, 303–306.

Lee, S.K., Hong, C.H., Huh, S.K., et al., 2002. Suppressive effect of natural sesquiterpenoids on inducible cyclooxygenase (COX-2) and nitric oxide synthase (iNOS) activity in mouse macrophage cells. J. Environ. Pathol. Toxicol. Oncol. 21, 141–148.

Lee, Y.M., Wu, T.H., Chen, S.F., et al., 2003. Effect of 5-methoxypsoralen (5-MOP) on cell apoptosis and cell cycle in human hepatocellular carcinoma cell line. Toxicol. In Vitro 17, 279–287.

Lee, E.H., Faulhaber, D., Hanson, K.M., et al., 2004. Dietary lutein reduces ultraviolet radiation-induced inflammation and immunosuppression. J. Invest. Dermatol. 122, 510–517.

Lee, B.K., Kim, J.H., Jung, J.W., et al., 2005a. Myristicin-induced neurotoxicity in human neuroblastoma SK-N-SH cells. Toxicol. Lett. 157, 49–56.

Lee, J.M., Liu, T.Y., Wu, D.C., et al., 2005b. Safrole-DNA adducts in tissues from esophageal cancer patients: clues to areca-related esophageal carcinogenesis. Mutat. Res. 565, 121–128.

Lee, S.J., Umano, K., Shibamoto, T., et al., 2005c. Identification of volatile components in basil (Ocimum basilicum L.) and thyme leaves (Thymus vulgaris L.) and their antioxidant properties. Food Chem. 91, 131–137.

Lee, S.P., Buber, M.T., Yang, Q., et al., 2008. Thymol and related alkyl phenols activate the hTRPA1 channel. Br. J. Pharmacol. 153, 1739–1749.

Legault, J., Pichette, A., 2007. Potentiating effect of beta-caryophyllene on anticancer activity of alpha-humulene, isocaryophyllene and paclitaxel. J. Pharm. Pharmacol. 59, 1643–1647.

Legault, J., Dahl, W., Debiton, E., et al., 2003. Antitumor activity of balsam fir oil: production of reactive oxygen species induced by alpha-humulene as possible mechanism of action. Planta Med. 69, 402–407.

Le Goff-Klein, N., Klein, L., Hérin, M., et al., 2004. Inhibition of in-vitro simvastatin metabolism in rat liver microsomes by bergamottin, a component of grapefruit juice. J. Pharm. Pharmacol. 56, 1007–1014.

Lehman-McKeeman, L.D., Rodriguez, P.A., Takigiku, R., et al., 1989. *d*-Limonene-induced male-rat-specific nephrotoxicity: evaluation of the association between *d*-limonene and alpha$_{2u}$-globulin. Toxicol. Appl. Pharmacol. 99, 250–259.

Lehrner, J., Eckersberger, C., Walla, P., et al., 2000. Ambient odor of orange in a dental office reduces anxiety and improves mood in female patients. Physiol. Behav. 71, 83–86.

Lehrner, J., Marwinski, G., Lehr, S., et al., 2005. Ambient odors of orange and lavender reduce anxiety and improve mood in a dental office. Physiol. Behav. 86, 92–95.

Leibman, K.C., Ortiz, E., 1973. Mammalian metabolism of terpenoids I. Reduction and hydroxylation of camphor and related compounds. Drug Metab. Dispos. 1, 543–551.

Lekshmi, P.C., Arimboor, R., Indulekha, P.S., et al., 2012. Turmeric (*Curcuma longa* L.) volatile oil inhibits key enzymes linked to type 2 diabetes. Int. J. Food Sci. Nutr. 63, 832–834.

LeMasters, G.K., Genaidy, A.M., Succop, P., et al., 2006. Cancer risk among firefighters: a review and meta-analysis of 32 Studies. J. Occup. Environ. Med. 48, 1189–1202.

Lepoittevin, J.P., Mutterer, V., 1998. Molecular aspects of fragrance sensitisation. In: Frosch, P.J., Johansen, J.D., White, I.R. (Eds.), Fragrances, beneficial and adverse effects. Springer, Berlin.

Lepoittevin, J.P., Meschkat, E., 2000. Presence of resin acids in "oakmoss" patch test material: a source of misdiagnosis? J. Invest. Dermatol. 114, 129–130.

Lerbaek, A., Rastogi, S.C., Menné, T., 2004. Allergic contact dermatitis from allyl isothiocyanate in a Danish cohort of 259 selected patients. Contact Dermatitis 51, 79–83.

Lertsatitthanakorn, P., Taweechaisupapong, S., Aromdee, C., et al., 2006. In vitro bioactivities of essential oils used for acne control. Int. J. Aromather. 16, 43–49.

Lesaffer, G., De Smet, R., D'Heuvaert, T., et al., 2001. Kinetics of the protein-bound, lipophilic, uremic toxin *p*-cresol in healthy rats. Life Sci. 69, 2237–2248.

Leseche, B., Levisalles, J., Rudler, H., 1984. L'essence de terebenthine du pin maritime (*Pinus pinaster* de Portugal). Parfumes, Cosmetiques et Aromes 58, 53–58.

Lessenger, J.E., 2001. Occupational acute anaphylactic reaction to assault by perfume spray in the face. J. Am. Board Fam. Pract. 14, 137–140.

Lesueur, D., Ban, N.K., Bighelli, A., et al., 2005. Analysis of the root oil of *Fokienia hodginsii* (Dunn) Henry et Thomas (Cupressaceae) by GC, GC-MS and 13C-NMR. Flavour & Fragrance Journal 21, 171–174.

Letizia, C.S., Api, A.M., 2000. A dermal safety evaluation of extracts from *Tagetes* plants used in fragrances. Toxicologist 54, 397.

Letizia, C.S., Cocchiara, G.A., Wellington, G.A., et al., 2000. Monographs on fragrance raw materials. Food Chem. Toxicol. 38 (Suppl. 3).

Letizia, C.S., Cocchiara, J., Lalko, J., et al., 2003a. Fragrance material review on linalool. Food Chem. Toxicol. 41, 943–964.

Letizia, C.S., Cocchiara, J., Lalko, J., et al., 2003b. Fragrance material review on linalyl acetate. Food Chem. Toxicol. 41, 965–976.

Letizia, C.S., Cocchiara, J., Lalko, J., et al., 2005. Fragrance material review on cinnamyl alcohol. Food Chem. Toxicol. 43, 837–866.

Leung, A.Y., Foster, S., 2003. Encyclopedia of common natural ingredients used in food, drugs and cosmetics, second ed. John Wiley, New Jersey.

Leuschner, J., 1997. Reproductive toxicity studies of *d*-camphor in rats and rabbits. Arzneimittel-Forschung/Drug Research 47, 124–128.

Levin, J.O., Eriksson, K., Falk, A., et al., 1992. Renal elimination of verbenols in man following experimental alpha-pinene inhalation exposure. Int. Arch. Environ. Health 63, 571–573.

Levy, R.L., 1914. Oil of chenopodium in the treatment of hookworm infections. J. Am. Med. Assoc. 63, 1946–1949.

Levvy, G.A., Kerr, L.M., Campbell, J.G., 1948. β-Glucuronidase and cell proliferation. Biochem. J. 42, 462–468.

Lewerenz, H.J., Plass, R., Bleyl, D.W., et al., 1988. Short-term toxicity study of allyl isothiocyanate in rats. Nahrung 32, 723–728.

Lewis, R.J. (Ed.), 1992. Sax's Dangerous Properties of Industrial Materials. eighth ed. John Wiley. New York.

Lewis, R.J. (Ed.), 2000. Sax's dangerous properties of industrial materials. tenth ed. John Wiley. New York.

Lewis, D.F., Ioannides, C., Walker, R., et al., 1994. Safety evaluations of food chemicals by "COMPACT". 1. A study of some acyclic terpenes. Food Chem. Toxicol. 32, 1053–1059.

Lewis, F.M., Shah, M., Gawkrodger, D.J., 1995. Contact sensitivity to food additives can cause oral and perioral symptoms. Contact Dermatitis 33, 429–430.

Leyden, J.J., Kligman, A.M., 1977. Contact sensitization to benzoyl peroxide. Contact Dermatitis 3, 273–275.

Li, M., Gow, E., 1995. Benzyl alcohol allergy. Australas. J. Dermatol. 36, 219–220.

Li, G.X., Liu, Z.Q., 2009. Unusual antioxidant behavior of alpha- and gamma-terpinene in protecting methyl linoleate, DNA, and erythrocyte. J. Agric. Food Chem. 57, 3943–3948.

Li, Y., Lu, Y.Y., 2002. Isolation of diallyl trisulfide inducible differentially expressed genes in human gastric cancer cells by modified cDNA representational difference analysis. DNA Cell Biology 21, 771–780.

Li, C., Li, L., Luo, J., et al., 1998. Effect of turmeric volatile oil on the respiratory tract. Zhongguo Zhong Yao Za Zhi 23, 624–625.

Li, Z., Wang, K., Chen, Y.R., et al., 2000. Studies on metabolite of beta-elemene in rat bile. Yao Xue Xue Bao 35, 829–831.

Li, Y., Li, M.Y., Wang, L., et al., 2004. Induction of apoptosis of cultured hepatocarcinoma cell by essential oil of Artemisia Annua L. Sichuan Da Xue Xue Bao Yi Xue Ban 35, 337–339.

Li, X., Wang, G., Zhao, J., et al., 2005. Antiproliferative effect of beta-elemene in chemoresistant ovarian carcinoma cells is mediated through arrest of the cell cycle at the G2-M phase. Cell. Mol. Life Sci. 62, 894–904.

Li, Q., Nakadai, A., Matsushima, H., 2006. Phytoncides (wood essential oils) induce human natural killer cell activity. Immunopharmacol. Immunotoxicol. 28, 319–333.

Li, P., Callery, P.S., Gan, L.S., et al., 2007. Esterase inhibition by grapefruit juice flavonoids leading to a new drug interaction. Drug Metab. Dispos. 35, 1203–1208.

Li, Y.L., Yeung, C.M., Chiu, L.C., et al., 2008. Chemical composition and antiproliferative activity of essential oil from the leaves of a medicinal herb, Schefflera heptaphylla. Phytother. Res. 23, 140–142.

Li, Q., Wang, X., Yang, Z., et al., 2009. Menthol induces cell death via the TRPM8 channel in the human bladder cancer cell line T24. Oncology 77, 335–341.

Li, Y., Wo, J.M., Liu, Q., et al., 2009. Chemoprotective effects of Curcuma aromatica on esophageal carcinogenesis. Ann. Surg. Oncol. 16, 515–523.

Li, Q.Q., Wang, G., Huang, F., et al., 2010. Antineoplastic effect of beta-elemene on prostate cancer cells and other types of solid tumour cells. J. Pharm. Pharmacol. 62, 1018–1027.

Lijinsky, W., Andrews, A.W., 1980. Mutagenicity of vinyl compounds in Salmonella typhimurium. Teratogens Carcinogens & Mutagens 1, 259–267.

Lilly, G.E., Cutcher, J.L., Jendresen, M.D., 1972. Reaction of oral mucous membranes to selected dental materials. J. Biomed. Mater. Res. 6, 545–551.

Lima, S.R., Junior, V.F., Christo, H.B., et al., 2003. In vivo and in vitro studies on the anticancer activity of Copaifera multijuga Hayne and its fractions. Phytother. Res. 17, 1048–1053.

Lima, C.F., Carvalho, F., Fernandes, E., et al., 2004. Evaluation of toxic/protective effects of the essential oil of Salvia officinalis on freshly isolated rat hepatocytes. Toxicol. In Vitro 18, 457–465.

Lima, C.S., De Medeiros, B.J., Favacho, H.A., et al., 2011. Pre-clinical validation of a vaginal cream containing copaiba oil (reproductive toxicity study). Phytomedicine 18, 1013–1023.

Limón, I.D., Medieta, L., Díaz, A., et al., 2009. Neuroprotective effect of alpha-asarone on spatial memory and nitric oxide levels in rats injected with amyloid-beta$_{(25-35)}$. Neurosci. Lett. 453, 98–103.

Lin, J.P., Lu, H.F., Lee, J.H., et al., 2005. (-)-Menthol inhibits DNA topoisomerases I, II alpha and beta and promotes NF-kappaB expression in human gastric cancer SNU-5 cells. Anticancer. Res. 25, 2069–2074.

Lin, C.T., Chen, C.J., Lin, T.Y., et al., 2008. Anti-inflammation activity of fruit essential oil from Cinnamomum insularimontanum Hayata. Bioresour. Technol. 99, 8783–8787.

Linck de, V.M., Da Silva, A.L., Figueiro, M., et al., 2009. Inhaled linalool-induced sedation in mice. Phytomedicine 16, 303–307.

Lindecrona, R.H., Mølk, A.M., Gry, J., et al., 2003. Subchronic oral toxicity study on the three flavouring substances: octan-3-ol, 2-methylcrotonic acid and oct-3-yl 2-methylcrotonate in Wistar rats. Food Chem. Toxicol. 41, 647–654.

Linden, W., Moseley, J.V., 2006. The efficacy of behavioral treatments for hypertension. Appl. Psychophysiol. Biofeedback 31, 51–63.

Lipsky, M.M., Hinton, D.E., Klaunig, J.E., et al., 1981. Biology of hepatocellular neoplasia in the mouse. 1. Histogenesis of safrole-induced hepatocellular carcinoma. J. Natl. Cancer Inst. 67, 365–376.

Lis-Balchin, M., Hart, S., 1999. Studies on the mode of action of the essential oil of lavender (Lavandula angustifolia P. Miller). Phytother. Res. 13, 540–542.

Lis-Balchin, M., Hart, S.L., Deans, S.G., 2000. Pharmacological and antimicrobial studies on different tea-tree oils (Melaleuca alternifolia, Leptospermum scoparium or Manuka and Kunzea ericoides or Kanuka), originating in Australia and New Zealand. Phytother. Res. 14, 623–629.

Lisi, P., Meligeni, L., Pigatto, P., et al., 2000. The prevalence of sensitivity to Melaleuca essential oil. Italian Annals of Clinical & Experimental Allergological Dermatology 54, 141–144.

List, P.H., Hörhammer, L., 1976. Hager's Handbuch der Pharmazeutischen Praxis, vols. 2–6. Springer-Verlag, Berlin.

Litovitz, T.L., Klein-Schwartz, W., Dyer, K.S., et al., 1998. 1997 Annual report of the American Association of Poison Control Centers Toxic Exposure Surveillance System. Am. J. Emerg. Med. 16, 443–497.

Litovitz, T.L., Klein-Schwartz, W., Caravati, E.M., et al., 1999. 1998 Annual report of the American Association of Poison Control Centers Toxic Exposure Surveillance System. Am. J. Emerg. Med. 17, 435–487.

Litovitz, T.L., Klein-Schwartz, W., White, S., et al., 2000. 1999 Annual report of the American Association of Poison Control Centers Toxic Exposure Surveillance System. Am. J. Emerg. Med. 18, 517–574.

Litovitz, T.L., Klein-Schwartz, W., White, S., et al., 2001. 2000 Annual report of the American Association of Poison Control Centers Toxic Exposure Surveillance System. Am. J. Emerg. Med. 19, 337–395.

Litovitz, T.L., Klein-Schwartz, W., Rodgers, G.C., et al., 2002. 2001 Annual report of the American Association of Poison Control Centers Toxic Exposure Surveillance System. Am. J. Emerg. Med. 20, 391–452.

Litton Bionetics Inc, 1975. Mutagenic evaluation of compound FDA 73–70, benzoic acid, certified A.C.S. U.S. Food & Drug Administration Report. NTIS Report No. PB-245-500.

Liu, K.H., Kim, J.H., 2003. In vitro dermal penetration study of carbofuran, carbosulfan, and furathiocarb. Arch. Toxicol. 77, 255–260.

Liu, Y., Kulesz-Martin, M., 2001. p53 Protein at the hub of cellular DNA damage response pathways through sequence-specific and non-sequence-specific DNA binding. Carcinogenesis 22, 851–860.

Liu, J., Mori, A., 1993. Antioxidant and pro-oxidant activities of p-hydroxybenzyl alcohol and vanillin: effects on free radicals, brain peroxidation and degradation of benzoate, deoxyribose, amino acids and DNA. Neuropharmacology 32, 659–669.

Liu, S., Yamauchi, H., 2006. Hinokitiol, a metal chelator derived from natural plants, suppresses cell growth and disrupts androgen receptor signaling in prostate carcinoma cell lines. Biochem. Biophys. Res. Commun. 351, 26–32.

Liu, J.H., Chen, G.H., Yeh, H.Z., 1997. Enteric-coated peppermint oil capsules in the treatment of irritable bowel syndrome: a prospective, randomized trial. J. Gastroenterol. 32, 765–768.

Liu, T.Y., Chen, C.C., Chen, C.L., et al., 1999. Safrole-induced oxidative damage in the liver of Sprague-Dawley rats. Food Chem. Toxicol. 37, 697–702.

Liu, C.J., Chen, C.L., Chang, K.W., et al., 2000. Safrole in betel quid may be a risk factor for hepatocellular carcinoma: case report. Can. Med. Assoc. J. 162, 359–360.

Liu, G., Oettel, K., Bailey, H., et al., 2003. Phase II trial of perillyl alcohol (NSC 641066) administered daily in patients with metastatic androgen independent prostate cancer. Invest. New Drugs 21, 367–372.

Liu, T.Y., Chung, Y.T., Wang, P.F., et al., 2004. Safrole-DNA adducts in human peripheral blood - an association with areca quid chewing and CYP2E1 polymorphisms. Mutat. Res. 559, 59–66.

Liu, J., Li, C., Xing, G., et al., 2010. beta-Asarone attenuates neuronal apoptosis induced by beta amyloid in rat hippocampus. Yakugaku Zasshi 130, 737–746.

Liu, W.X., Jia, F.L., He, Y.Y., et al., 2012. Protective effects of 5-methoxypsoralen against acetaminophen-induced hepatotoxicity in mice. World J. Gastroenterol. 18, 2197–2202.

Liu, L., Wang, J., Shi, L., et al., 2013. β-Asarone induces senescence in colorectal cancer cells by inducing lamin B1 expression. Phytomedicine 20, 512–520.

Livingston, A.E., 1922. Oil of chenopodium and its components. Journal of Pharmacology 19, 266–267.

Llano, J., Raber, J., Eriksson, L.A., 2003. Theoretical study of phototoxic reactions of psoralens. Journal of Photochemistry & Photobiology A: Chemistry 154, 235–243.

Lluria-Prevatt, M., Morreale, J., Gregus, J., et al., 2002. Effects of perillyl alcohol on melanoma in the TPras mouse model. Cancer Epidemiol. Biomarkers Prev. 11, 573–579.

Lohr, C., Raquet, N., Schrenk, D., 2010. Application of the concept of relative photomutagenic potencies to selected furocoumarins in V79 cells. Toxicol. In Vitro 24, 558–566.

Loizzo, M.R., Tundis, R., Menichini, F., et al., 2007. Cytotoxic activity of essential oils from labiatae and lauraceae families against in vitro human tumor models. Anticancer. Res. 27, 3293–3299.

Loizzo, M.R., Tundis, R., Menichini, F., et al., 2008. Antiproliferative effects of essential oils and their major constituents in human renal adenocarcinoma and amelanotic melanoma cells. Cell Prolif. 41, 1002–1012.

Long, E.L., Nelson, A.A., Fitzhugh, O.G., et al., 1963. Liver tumors produced in rats by feeding safrole. Arch. Pathol. 75, 595–604.

Longnecker, D.S., Roebuck, B.D., Curphey, T.J., et al., 1986. Effects of corn oil and benzyl acetate on number and size of azaserine-induced foci in the pancreas of LEW and F344 rats. Environ. Health Perspect. 68, 197–201.

Longnecker, D.S., Roebuck, B.D., Curphey, T.J., et al., 1990. Evaluation of promotion of pancreatic carcinogenesis in rats by benzyl acetate. Food Chem. Toxicol. 28, 665–668.

Lopes-Lutz, D., Alviano, D.S., Alviano, C.S., et al., 2008. Screening of chemical composition, antimicrobial and antioxidant activities of Artemisia essential oils. Phytochemistry 1732–1738.

López, M.L., Hernandez, A., Chamorro, G., et al., 1993. α-Asarone toxicity in long-term cultures of adult rat hepatocytes. Planta Med 59, 115–120.

López, P., Sánchez, C., Batlle, R., Nerín, C., 2007. Vapor-phase activities of cinnamon, thyme, and oregano essential oils and key constituents against foodborne microorganisms. J. Agric. Food Chem. 55, 4348–4356.

López, M.A., Stashenko, E.E., Fuentes, J.L., 2011. Chemical composition and antigenotoxic properties of Lippia alba essential oils. Genetics & Molecular Biology 34, 479–488.

Loprinzi, C.L., Kugler, J.W., Sloan, J.A., et al., 1999. Lack of effect of coumarin in women with lymphedema after treatment for breast cancer. N. Engl. J. Med. 340, 346–350.

Lorente, I., Ocete, M.A., Zarzuelo, A., et al., 1989. Bioactivity of the essential oil of Bupleurum fruticosum. J. Nat. Prod. 52, 267–272.

Lorenzi, S., Placucci, F., Vincenzi, C., et al., 1995. Allergic contact dermatitis due to thymol. Contact Dermatitis 33, 439–440.

Lou, H.C., Friis-Hansen, B., 1979. Arterial blood pressure elevations during motor activity and epileptic seizures in the newborn. Acta Paediatr. Scand. 68, 803–806.

Loughlin, R., Gilmore, B.F., McCarron, P.A., et al., 2008. Comparison of the cidal activity of tea tree oil and terpinen-4-ol against clinical bacterial skin isolates and human fibroblast cells. Lett. Appl. Microbiol. 46, 428–433.

Loutrari, H., Hatziapostolou, M., Skouridou, V., et al., 2004. Perillyl alcohol is an angiogenesis inhibitor. J. Pharmacol. Exp. Ther. 311, 568–575.

Loutrari, H., Magkouta, S., Pyriochou, A., et al., 2006. Mastic oil from Pistacia lentiscus var. chia inhibits growth and survival of human K562 leukemia cells and attenuates angiogenesis. Nutr. Cancer 55, 86–93.

Love, J.N., Sammon, M., Smereck, J., 2004. Are one or two dangerous? Camphor exposure in toddlers. J. Emerg. Med. 27, 49–54.

Lowenstein, L., Ballew, D.H., 1958. Fatal acute haemolytic anaemia, thrombocytopenic purpura, nephrosis and hepatitis resulting from ingestion of a compound containing apiol. Can. Med. Assoc. J. 78, 195–198.

Lu, L.J., Disher, R.M., Reddy, M.V., et al., 1986a. ^{32}P-Postlabeling assay in mice of transplacental DNA damage induced by the environmental carcinogens safrole, 4-aminobiphenyl, and benzo[a]pyrene. Cancer Res. 46, 3046–3054.

Lu, L.J., Disher, R.M., Randerath, K., 1986b. Differences in the covalent binding of benzo[a]pyrene, safrole, 1'-hydroxysafrole, and 4-aminobiphenyl to DNA of pregnant and non-pregnant mice. Cancer Lett. 31, 43–52.

Lu, X.G., Feng, B.A., Zhan, L.B., et al., 2003. d-Limonene induces apoptosis of gastric cancer cells. Zhonghua Zhong Liu Za Zhi 25, 325–327.

Lu, X.G., Zhan, L.B., Feng, B.A., et al., 2004. Inhibition of growth and metastasis of human gastric cancer implanted in nude mice by d-limonene. World J. Gastroenterol. 10, 2140–2144.

Lu, H.F., Sue, C.C., Yu, C.S., et al., 2004. Diallyl disulfide (DADS) induced apoptosis undergo caspase-3 activity in human bladder cancer T24 cells. Food Chem. Toxicol. 42, 1543–1552.

Lu, H.F., Hsueh, S.C., Yu, F.S., et al., 2006. The role of Ca^{2+} in (−)-menthol-induced human promyelocytic leukemia HL-60 cell death. In Vivo 20, 69–75.

Lu, H.F., Liu, J.Y., Hsueh, S.C., 2007. (−)-Menthol inhibits WEHI-3 leukemia cells in vitro and in vivo. In Vivo 21, 285–289.

Luan, F., Ma, W., Zhang, X., et al., 2006. Quantitative structure-activity relationship models for prediction of sensory irritants (logRD50) of volatile organic chemicals. Chemosphere 63, 1142–1153.

Lucks, B.C., 2002. Vitex agnus castus essential oil and menopausal balance: a self-care survey. Complement Ther. Nurs. Midwifery 8, 148–154.

Lucks, B.C., 2003. Vitex agnus castus essential oil and menopausal balance: a research update. Complement Ther. Nurs. Midwifery 9, 157–160.

Luke, E., 1962. Addiction to mentholated cigarettes. Lancet 279 (7220), 110–111.

Lund, C., Kuller, J., Lane, A., et al., 1999. Neonatal skin care: the scientific basis for practice. J. Obstet. Gynecol. Neonatal Nurs. 28, 241–254.

Lunder, T., Kansky, A., 2000. Increase in contact allergy to fragrances: patch-test results 1989–1998. Contact Dermatitis 43, 107–109.

Luo, G., Guenthner, T.M., 1995. Metabolism of allylbenzene 2',3'-oxide and estragole 2',3'-oxide in the isolated perfused rat liver. J. Pharmacol. Exp. Ther. 272, 588–596.

Luo, G., Guenthner, T.M., 1996. Covalent binding to DNA in vitro of 2',3'-oxides derived from allylbenzene analogs. Drug Metab. Dispos. 24, 1020–1027.

Luo, M., Jiang, L.K., Zou, G.L., 2005. Acute and genetic toxicity of essential oil extracted from Litsea cubeba (Lour.) Pers. J. Food Prot. 68, 581–588.

Lupidi, G., Scire, A., Camaioni, E., et al., 2010. Thymoquinone, a potential therapeutic agent of Nigella sativa, binds to site I of human serum albumin. Phytomedicine 17, 714–720.

Lutz, D., Eder, E., Neudecker, T., et al., 1982. Structure-mutagenicity relationship in α, β-unsaturated carbonylic compounds and their corresponding allylic alcohols. Mutat. Res. 93, 305–315.

Lutz, W., Tarkowski, M., Nowakowska, E., 2001. Genetic polymorphism of glutathione S-transferase as a factor predisposing to allergic dermatitis. Med. Pr. 52, 45–51.

Lysenko, L.V., 1962. Pharmacological study of geraniol, carvone, linalool and thymol (Russian). Tr. Khar'kovsk. Farmatsevt. Inst. 2, 176–178.

Ma, W., Wlaschek, M., Hommel, C., et al., 2002. Psoralen plus UVA (PUVA) induced premature senescence as a model for stress-induced premature senescence. Exp. Gerontol. 37, 1197–1201.

Ma, E.L., Li, Y.C., Tsuneki, H., et al., 2008. beta-Eudesmol suppresses tumour growth through inhibition of tumour neovascularisation and tumour cell proliferation. J. Asian Nat. Prod. Res. 10, 159–167.

MacDonald, D., VanCrey, K., Harrison, P., et al., 2004. Ascaridole-less infusions of Chenopodium ambrosioides contain a nematocide(s) that is (are) not toxic to mammalian smooth muscle. J. Ethnopharmacol. 92, 215–221.

MacEwen, E.G., 1986. Anti-tumor evaluation of benzaldehyde in the dog and cat. Am. J. Vet. Res. 47, 451–452.

Macht, D.I., 1913. The action of so-called emmenagogue oils on the isolated uterine strip. J. Pharm. Exp. Ther. 4, 547–553.

Macht, D., 1921. The action of so-called emmenagogue oils on the isolated uterus. J. Am. Med. Assoc. 61, 105–107.

Macht, D.I., Ting, G.C., 1921. Experimental inquiry into the sedative properties of some aromatic drugs and fumes. J. Pharm. Exp. Ther. 18, 361–372.

Mack, R.B., 1982. Toxic encounters of the dangerous kind. The nutmeg connection. N. C. Med. J. 43, 439.

Mack, R.B., 1988. Fair dinkum koala kuisine – eucalyptus oil poisoning. N. C. Med. J. 49, 599–600.

Maddocks-Jennings, W., 2004. Critical incident: idiosyncratic allergic reactions to essential oils. Complement. Ther. Nurs. Midwifery 10, 58–60.

Madische, A., Heydenreich, C.J., Wieland, V., et al., 1999. Treatment of functional dyspepsia with a fixed peppermint oil and caraway oil combination preparation as compared to Cisparide. A multicenter, reference-controlled, double-blind equivalence study. Arzneimittelforschung 49, 925–932.

Madison, K.C., 2003. Barrier function of the skin: "la raison d'etre" of the epidermis. J. Invest. Dermatol. 121, 231–241.

Madsen, C., Würtzen, G., Carstensen, J., 1986. Short-term toxicity study in rats dosed with menthone. Toxicol. Lett. 32 (1–2), 147–152.

Madyastha, K.M., Chadha, A., 1986. Metabolism of 1,8-cineole in rat: its effects on liver and lung microsomal cytochrome P_{450} systems. Bull. Environ. Contam. Toxicol. 37, 759–766.

Madyastha, K.M., Gaikwad, N.W., 1998. Metabolic fate of S-(-)-pulegone in rat. Xenobiotica 28, 723–734.

Madyastha, K.M., Moorthy, B., 1989. Pulegone mediated hepatotoxicity: evidence for covalent binding of R(+)-(14C)pulegone to microsomal proteins in vitro. Chem. Biol. Interact. 72, 325–333.

Madyastha, K.M., Raj, C.P., 1990. Biotransformations of R-(+)-pulegone and menthofuran in vitro: chemical basis for toxicity. Biochem. Biophys. Res. Commun. 173, 1086–1092.

Madyastha, K.M., Raj, C.P., 1991. Evidence for the formation of a known toxin, p-cresol, from menthofuran. Biochem. Biophys. Res. Commun. 177, 140–146.

Madyastha, K.M., Raj, C.P., 1992. Metabolic fate of menthofuran in rats: novel oxidative pathways. Drug Metab. Dispos. 20, 295–301.

Madyastha, P., Raj, C.P., 1993. Studies on the metabolism of a monoterpene ketone, (R)-(+)-pulegone – a hepatotoxin in rat: isolation and characterization of new metabolites. Xenobiotica 23, 509–518.

Madyastha, K.M., Raj, C.P., 1994. Effects of menthofuran, a monoterpene furan on rat liver microsomal enzymes, in vivo. Toxicology 89, 119–125.

Madyastha, K.M., Raj, C.P., 2002. Stereoselective hydroxylation of 4-methyl-2-cyclohexenone in rats: its relevance to R-(+)-pulegone-mediated hepatotoxicity. Biochem. Biophys. Res. Commun. 297, 202–205.

Madyastha, K.M., Srivastan, V., 1987. Metabolism of β-myrcene in vivo and in vitro: its effects on rat liver microsomal enzymes. Xenobiotica 17, 539–549.

Madyastha, K.M., Srivastan, V., 1988. Studies on the metabolism of l-menthol in rats. Drug Metab. Dispos. 16, 765–772.

Madyastha, P., Moorthy, B., Vaidyanathan, C.S., et al., 1985. In vivo and in vitro destruction of rat liver cytochrome P-450 by a monoterpene ketone, pulegone. Biochem. Biophys. Res. Commun. 128, 921–927.

Magiatis, P., Melliou, E., Skaltsounis, A.L., et al., 1999. Chemical composition and antimicrobial activity of the essential oils of Pistacia lentiscus var. chia. Planta Med. 65, 749–754.

Magnusson, B.M., Runn, P., Koskinen, L.O.D., 1997. Terpene-enhanced transdermal permeation of water and ethanol in human epidermis. Acta Derm. Venereol. 77, 264–267.

Magyar, J., Szentandrassy, N., Banyasz, T., et al., 2004. Effects of terpenoid phenol derivatives on calcium current in canine and human ventricular cardiomyocytes. Eur. J. Pharmacol. 487, 29–36.

Mahalwal, V.S., Ali, M., 2002. Volatile constituents of the rhizomes of Nardostachys jatamansi DC. Journal of Essential Oil Bearing Plants 5, 83–89.

Mahavorasirikul, W., Tassaneeyakul, W., Satarug, S., et al., 2009. CYP2A6 genotypes and coumarin-oxidation phenotypes in a Thai population and their relationship to tobacco smoking. Eur. J. Clin. Pharmacol. 65, 377–384.

Maheshwari, M.L., 1995. Composition of essential oil from flowers of keora (Pandanus odoratissimus Linn.) by capillary gas chromatography. Indian Perfumer 39, 45–48.

Mahindru, S.N., 1992. Indian plant perfumes. Metropolitan, New Delhi.

Maibach, H.I., 1986. Cheilitis: occult allergy to cinnamic aldehyde. Contact Dermatitis 15, 106–107.

Maibach, H., Johnson, H.L., 1975. Contact urticaria syndrome. Contact urticaria to diethyltoluenamide (immediate-type hypersensitivity). Arch. Dermatol. 111, 726–730.

Maibach, H.I., Lammintausta, K., Berardesca, E., et al., 1989. Tendency to irritation: sensitive skin. J. Am. Acad. Dermatol. 21, 833–835.

Maickel, R.P., Snodgrass, W.R., 1973. Physicochemical factors in maternal-fetal distribution of drugs. Toxicol. Appl. Pharmacol. 26, 218–230.

Maistro, E.L., Mota, S.F., Lima, E.B., et al., 2010. Genotoxicity and mutagenicity of Rosmarinus officinalis (Labiatae) essential oil in mammalian cells in vivo. Genet. Mol. Res. 9, 2113–2122.

Majeti, V.A., Suskind, R.R., 1977. Mechanism of cinnamaldehyde sensitization. Contact Dermatitis 3, 16–18.

Makki, S., Treffel, P., Humbert, P., et al., 1991. High-performance liquid chromatographic determination of citropten and bergapten in suction blister fluid after solar product application in humans. J. Chromatogr. B Biomed. Sci. Appl. 563, 407–413.

Males, Z., Blazevic, N., Antolic, A., 1998. The essential oil composition of Vitex agnus-castus f. rosea leaves and flowers. Planta Med. 64, 286–287.

Malik, A.S., Zabidi, M.H., Noor, A.R., 1994. Acute salicylism due to accidental ingestion of a traditional medicine. Singapore Med. J. 35, 215–216.

Malingré, T.M., Hendriks, H., Batterman, S., et al., 1973. The presence of cannabinoid components in the essential oil of Cannabis sativa L. Pharm. Weekbl. 108, 549–552.

Malingré, T.M., Hendriks, H., Batterman, S., et al., 1975. The essential oil of Cannabis sativa. Planta Med. 28, 56–61.

Malizia, R.A., Molli, J.S., Cardell, D.A., et al., 1996. Volatile constituents of the essential oil of Nepeta cataria L. grown in Cordoba province (Argentina). Journal of Essential Oil Research 8, 565–567.

Malizia, R.A., Molli, J.S., Cardell, D.A., et al., 1999. Essential oil of hop cones (Humulus lupulus L.). Journal of Essential Oil Research 11, 13–15.

Malki, A., El-Saadani, M., Sultan, A.S., 2009. Garlic constituent diallyl trisulfide induced apoptosis in MCF7 human breast cancer cells. Cancer Biol. Ther. 8, 2174–2184.

Mallavarapu, G.R., Rao, L., Ramesh, S., et al., 2002. Composition of the volatile oils of Alpinia galanga rhizomes and leaves from India. Journal of Essential Oil Research 14, 397–399.

Malley, L.A., Bamberger, J.R., Stadler, J.C., et al., 2000. Subchronic toxicity of cyclohexane in rats and mice by inhalation exposure. Drug Chem. Toxicol. 23, 513–537.

Malten, K.E., Van Ketel, W.G., Nater, J.P., et al., 1984. Reactions in selected patients to 22 fragrance materials. Contact Dermatitis 11, 1–10.

Maltzman, T.H., Hurt, L.M., Elson, C.E., et al., 1989. The prevention of nitrosomethylurea-induced mammary tumors by d-limonene and orange oil. Carcinogenesis 10, 781–783.

Maltzman, T.H., Christou, M., Gould, M.N., et al., 1991. Effects of monoterpenoids on in vivo DMBA-DNA adduct formation and on phase I hepatic metabolizing enzymes. Carcinogenesis 12, 2081–2087.

Manabe, A., Nakayama, S., Sakamoto, K., 1987. Effects of essential oils on erythrocytes and hepatocytes from rats and dipalmitoyl phosphatidylcholine-liposomes. Jpn. J. Pharmacol. 44, 77–84.

Manceau, P., Revol, L., Vernet, A.M., 1936. Les essences de sabine du commerce. Étude d'essences authentiques de Juniperus Sabina L. et de Juniperus phoenicea L. Bulletin de la Société de Pharmacologie 43, 14–24.

Mandadi, S., Nakanishi, S.T., Takashima, Y., et al., 2009. Locomotor networks are targets of modulation by sensory transient receptor potential vanilloid 1 and transient receptor potential melastatin 8 channels. Neuroscience 162, 1377–1397.

Manesh, C., Kuttan, G., 2003. Effect of naturally occurring allyl and phenyl isothiocyanates in the inhibition of experimental pulmonary metastasis induced by B16F-10 melanoma cells. Fitoterapia 74, 355–363.

Mangelsdorf, H.C., Fleischer, A.B., Sherertz, E.F., 1996. Patch testing in an aged population without dermatitis: high prevalence of patch test positivity. Am. J. Contact Dermat. 7, 155–157.

Manikandan, S., Devi, R.S., 2005. Antioxidant property of a-asarone against noise-stress-induced changes in different regions of rat brain. Pharmacol. Res. 52, 467–474.

Manikandan, P., Murugan, R.S., Priyadarsini, R.V., et al., 2010. Eugenol induces apoptosis and inhibits invasion and angiogenesis in a rat model of gastric carcinogenesis induced by MNNG. Life Sci. 86, 936–941.

Manikandan, P., Vinothini, G., Vidya Priyadarsini, R., et al., 2011. Eugenol inhibits cell proliferation via NF-kappaB suppression in a rat model of gastric carcinogenesis induced by MNNG. Invest. New Drugs 29, 110–117.

Mann, J., 1992. Murder magic and medicine. Oxford University Press, Oxford.

Manoguerra, A.S., Erdman, A.R., Wax, P.M., et al., 2006. Camphor poisoning: an evidence-based practice guideline for out-of-hospital management. Clin. Toxicol. (Phila) 44, 357–370.

Manosroi, J., Dhumtanom, P., Manosroi, A., 2005. Anti-proliferative activity of essential oil extracted from Thai medicinal plants on KB and P388 cell lines. Cancer Lett. 235, 114–120.

Mansour, M.A., Ginawi, O.T., El-Hadiyah, T., et al., 2001. Effects of volatile oil constituents of Nigella sativa on carbon tetrachloride-induced hepatotoxicity in mice: evidence for antioxidant effects of thymoquinone. Res. Commun. Mol. Pathol. Pharmacol. 110, 239–251.

Mansour, M.A., Nagi, M.N., El-Khatib, A.S., et al., 2002. Effects of thymoquinone on antioxidant enzyme activities, lipid peroxidation and DT-diaphorase in different tissues of mice: a possible mechanism of action. Cell Biochem. Funct. 20, 143–151.

Mant, A.K., 1961. A case of poisoning by oil of citronella. Medicine. Science & the Law-Association Proceeding VI 1–2, 170–171.

Mantovani, A., Stazi, A.V., Macri, C., et al., 1989. Pre-natal (segment II) toxicity study of cinnamic aldehyde in the Sprague-Dawley rat. Food Chem. Toxicol. 27, 781–786.

Manuele, M.G., Ferraro, G., Anesini, C., 2008. Effect of *Tilia x viridis* flower extract on the proliferation of a lymphoma cell line and on normal murine lymphocytes: contribution of monoterpenes, especially limonene. Phytother. Res. 22, 1520–1526.

Manunta, A., Tirillini, B., Fraternale, D., 1992. Secretory tissues and essential oil composition of *Bupleurum fruticosum* L. Journal of Essential Oil Research 4, 461–466.

Manzini, B.M., Ferdani, G., Simonetti, V., et al., 1998. Contact sensitization in children. Pediatr. Dermatol. 15, 12–17.

Manzur, F., El Sayed, F., Bazex, J., 1995. Conatct allergy to cinnamic aldehyde and cinnamic alcohol in Oléophytal®. Contact Dermatitis 32, 55.

Maralhas, A., Monteiro, A., Martins, C., et al., 2006. Genotoxicity and endoreduplication inducing activity of the food flavouring eugenol. Mutagenesis 21, 199–204.

Marchant, C.A., 1996. Prediction of rodent carcinogenicity using the DEREK system for 30 chemicals currently being tested by the National Toxicology Program. Environ. Health Perspect. 104S, 1065–1073.

Marcus, C., Lichtenstein, E.P., 1982. Interactions of naturally occurring food plant components with insecticides and pentobarbital in rats and mice. J. Agric. Food Chem. 30, 563–568.

Marcus, D.M., Snodgrass, W.R., 2005. Do no harm: avoidance of herbal medicines during pregnancy. Obstet. Gynecol. 105, 1119–1122.

Margaria, R., 1963. Acute and sub-acute toxicity study on thujone. Unpublished report of the Istituto Fisiologica. Università di Milano (cited in SCF 2003b, from Council of Europe Datasheet RD4.2/14–44, 1999).

Marincola, F.M., Drucker, B.J., Siao, D.Y., et al., 1987. Inhibition of activation of lymphokine-activated killer cells in vitro by the heparin preservative benzyl alcohol. Lancet 2 (8555), 399.

Markowitz, K., Moynihan, M., Liu, M., et al., 1992. Biologic properties of eugenol and zinc oxide-eugenol. A clinically oriented review. Oral Surg. Oral Med. Oral Pathol. 73, 729–737.

Marks, J.G., Belsito, D.V., DeLeo, V.A., et al., 1995. North American Contact Dermatitis Group standard tray patch test results (1992 to 1994). Am. J. Contact Dermat. 6, 160–165.

Marks, J.G., Belsito, D.V., DeLeo, V.A., et al., 1998. North American Contact Dermatitis Group patch test results for the detection of delayed-type hypersensitivity to topical allergens. J. Am. Acad. Dermatol. 38, 911–918.

Marnett, L.J., 2000. Oxyradicals and DNA damage. Carcinogenesis 21, 361–370.

Marnett, L.J., Hurd, H.K., Hollstein, M.C., et al., 1985. Naturally occurring carbonyl compounds are mutagens in *Salmonella* tester strain TA104. Mutat. Res. 148, 25–34.

Marotti, M., Piccaglia, R., Biavati, B., et al., 2004. Characterization and yield evaluation of essential oils from different *Tagetes* species. Journal of Essential Oil Research 16, 440–444.

Marozzi, E., Farneti, A., 1968. Recente esperienza in tema di avvelenamento da apiolo e sostanze correlate. Zacchia 4, 563–580.

Marozzi, F.J., Kocialski, A.B., Malone, M.H., 1970. Studies on the antihistaminic effects of thymoquinone, thymohydroquinone and quercetin. Arzneimittelforschung 20, 1574–1577.

Marquardt, P., 1960. On the tolerability of benzoic acid. Arzneimittelforschung 10, 1033.

Marshall, A.D., Caldwell, J., 1992. Influence of modulators of epoxide metabolism on the cytotoxicity of *trans*-anethole in freshly isolated rat hepatocytes. Food Chem. Toxicol. 30, 467–473.

Marshall, A.D., Caldwell, J., 1993. The cytotoxicity and genotoxicity of anethole 1,2-epoxide, a primary metabolite of the food flavour *trans*-anethole. Hum. Exp. Toxicol. 12, 427–428.

Marshall, A.D., Caldwell, J., 1996. Lack of influence of modulators of epoxide metabolism on the genotoxicity of *trans*-anethole in freshly isolated rat hepatocytes assessed with the unscheduled DNA synthesis assay. Food Chem. Toxicol. 34, 337–345.

Martati, E., Boersma, M.G., Spenkelink, A., et al., 2011. Physiologically based biokinetic (PBBK) model for safrole bioactivation and detoxification in rats. Chem. Res. Toxicol. 24, 818–834.

Martin, D., Valdez, J., Boren, J., et al., 2004. Dermal absorption of camphor, menthol, and methyl salicylate in humans. J. Clin. Pharmacol. 44, 1151–1157.

Martin, M.T., Brennan, R., Hu, W., et al., 2007. Toxicogenomic study of triazole fungicides and perfluoroalkyl acids in rat livers predicts toxicity and categorizes chemicals based on mechanisms of toxicity. Toxicol. Sci. 97, 595–613.

Martinkova, J., Rydlova, I., Subrtova, D., et al., 1990. Liver damage induced by intrabiliary turpentine in rats. J. Pharm. Pharmacol. 42, 108–114.

Martins, C., Doran, C., Laires, A., et al., 2011. Genotoxic and apoptotic activities of the food flavourings myristicin and eugenol in AA8 and XRCC1 deficient EM9 cells. Food Chem. Toxicol. 49, 385–392.

Maruyama, N., Takizawa, T., Ishibashi, H., et al., 2008. Protective activity of geranium oil and its component, geraniol, in combination with vaginal washing against vaginal candidiasis in mice. Biol. Pharm. Bull. 31, 1501–1506.

Marzouki, H., Piras, A., Marongiu, B., et al., 2008. Extraction and separation of volatile and fixed oils from berries of *Laurus nobilis* L. by supercritical CO2. Molecules 13, 1702–1711.

Marzulli, F.N., Maibach, H.I., 1970. Perfume phototoxicity. J. Soc. Cosmet. Chem. 21, 695–715.

Marzulli, F.N., Maibach, H.I., 1980. Contact allergy: predictive testing of fragrance ingredients in humans by draize and maximation methods. J. Environ. Pathol. Toxicol. 3, 235–245.

Masamoto, Y., Kawabata, F., Fushiki, T., 2009. Intragastric administration of TRPV1, TRPV3, TRPM8, and TRPA1 agonists modulates autonomic thermoregulation in different manners in mice. Biosci. Biotechnol. Biochem. 73, 1021–1027.

Mascher, H., Kikuta, C., Schiel, H., 2001. Pharmacokinetics of menthol and carvone after administration of an enteric coated formulation containing peppermint oil and caraway oil. Arzneimittelforschung 51, 465–469.

Massoco, C.O., Silva, M.R., Gorniak, S.L., et al., 1995. Behavioural effects of acute and long-term administration of catnip (*Nepeta cataria*) in mice. Vet. Hum. Toxicol. 37, 530–533.

Masutani, H., Otsuki, R., Yamaguchi, Y., et al., 2009. Fragrant unsaturated aldehydes elicit activation of the Keap1/Nrf2 system leading to the up-regulation of thioredoxin expression and protection against oxidative stress. Antioxidants & Redox Signalling 11, 949–962.

Masutomi, N., Toyoda, K., Shibutani, M., et al., 2001. Toxic effects of benzyl and allyl isothiocyanates and benzyl-isoform specific metabolites in the urinary bladder after a single intravesical application to rats. Toxicol. Pathol. 29, 617–622.

Masuyama, K., Ochiai, H., Niwayama, S., et al., 1987. Inhibition of experimental and spontaneous pulmonary metastasis of murine RCT (+) sarcoma by *beta*-cyclodextrin-benzaldehyde. Jpn. J. Cancer Res. 78, 705–711.

Masuyama, K., Ochiai, H., Ishizawa, S., et al., 1988. Inhibition of pulmonary metastases in mice by *beta*-cyclodextrin-benzaldehyde. Gan To Kagaku Ryoho 15, 443–447.

Materazzi, S., Nassini, R., Gatti, R., et al., 2009. Cough sensors. II. Transient receptor potential membrane receptors on cough sensors. Handb. Exp. Pharmacol. 187, 49–61.

Mathela, C.S., Melkani, A.B., Pant, A.K., 1992. Reinvestigation of *Skimmia laureola* essential oil. Indian Perfumer 36, 217–222.

Mathela, C.S., Kharkwal, H., Shah, G.C., 1994. Essential oil composition of some Himalayan *Artemisia* species. Journal of Essential Oil Research 6, 345–348.

Mathela, C.S., Tiwari, M., Subhash, S., et al., 2005. *Valeriana wallichii* DC, a new chemotype from Northwestern Himalaya. Journal of Essential Oil Research 17, 672–675.

Mathias, C.G., 1988. Occupational dermatoses. J. Am. Acad. Dermatol. 19, 1107–1114.

Mathias, C.G., Chappler, R.R., Maibach, H.I., 1980. Contact urticaria from cinnamic aldehyde. Arch. Dermatol. 116, 74–76.

Matos, F.J., Machado, M.I., Alencar, J.W., et al., 1993. Constituents of Brazilian chamomile oil. Journal of Essential Oil Research 5, 337–339.

Matos, J.M., Schmidt, C.M., Thomas, H.J., et al., 2008. A pilot study of perillyl alcohol in pancreatic cancer. J. Surg. Res. 147, 194–199.

Matsuda, H., Toguchida, I., Ninomiya, K., et al., 2003. Effects of sesquiterpenes and amino acid-sesquiterpene conjugates from the roots of Saussurea lappa on inducible nitric oxide synthase and heat shock protein in lipopolysaccharide-activated macrophages. Bioorganic & Medicial Chemistry 11, 709–715.

Matsumoto, T., Ishida, T., Yoshida, T., et al., 1992. The enantioselective metabolism of p-cymene in rabbits. Chem. Pharm. Bull. (Tokyo) 40, 1721–1726.

Matsumoto, F., Idetsuki, H., Harada, K., et al., 1993. Volatile components of Hedychium coronarium Koenig flowers. Journal of Essential Oil Research 5, 123–133.

Matsumura, E., Morita, Y., Date, T., et al., 2001. Cytotoxicity of the hinokitiol-related compounds, gamma-thujaplicin and beta-dolabrin. Biol. Pharm. Bull. 24, 299–302.

Matsuoka, A., Yamakage, K., Kusakabe, H., et al., 1996. Re-evaluation of chromosomal aberration induction on nine mouse lymphoma assay 'unique positive' NTP carcinogens. Mutat. Res. 369, 243–252.

Matthys, H., de Mey, C., Carls, C., et al., 2000. Efficacy and tolerability of myrtol standardized in acute bronchitis. A multi-centre, randomised, double-blind, placebo-controlled parallel group clinical trial vs. cefuroxime and ambroxol. Arzneimittelforschung 50, 700–711.

Mattia, C.J., Adams, J.D., Bondy, S.C., 1993. Free radical induction in the brain and liver by products of toluene catabolism. Biochem. Pharmacol. 46, 103–110.

Matura, M., Goossens, A., Bordalo, O., et al., 2002. Oxidized citrus oil (R-limonene): a frequent skin sensitizer in Europe. J. Am. Acad. Dermatol. 47, 709–714.

Matura, M., Goossens, A., Bordalo, O., et al., 2003. Patch testing with oxidized R-(+)-limonene and its hydroperoxide fraction. Contact Dermatitis 49, 15–21.

Matura, M., Skold, M., Borje, A., et al., 2005. Selected oxidized fragrance terpenes are common contact allergens. Contact Dermatitis 52, 320–328.

Mau, J.L., Lai, E.Y., Wang, N.P., et al., 2003. Composition and antioxidant activity of the essential oil from Curcuma zedoaria. Food Chem. 82, 583–591.

Maudsley, F., Kerr, K.G., 1999. Microbiological safety of essential oils used in complementary therapies and the activity of these compounds against bacterial and fungal pathogens. Suppor. Care Cancer 7, 100–102.

Maura, A., Pino, A., Ricci, R., 1989. Negative evidence in vivo of DNA-damaging, mutagenic and chromosomal effects of eugenol. Mutat. Res. 227, 125–129.

May, B., Köhler, S., Schneider, B., 2000. Efficacy and tolerability of a fixed combination of peppermint oil and caraway oil in patients suffering from functional dyspepsia. Aliment. Pharmacol. Ther. 14, 1671–1677.

Mazza, G., Chubey, B.B., Kiehn, F., 1987. Essential oil of Monarda fistulosa L. var. menthaefolia, a potential source of geraniol. Flavour & Fragrance Journal 2, 129–132.

Mazzoni, V., Tomi, F., Casanova, J., 1999. A daucene-type sesquiterpene from Daucus carota seed oil. Flavour & Fragrance Journal 14, 268–272.

McAdam, B., Keimowitz, R.M., Maher, M., et al., 1996. Transdermal modification of platelet function: an aspirin patch system results in marked suppression of platelet cyclooxygenase. J. Pharm. Exp. Ther. 277, 559–564.

McCann, J., Choi, E., Yamasaki, E., et al., 1975. Detection of carcinogens as mutagens in the Salmonella/microsome test: assay of 300 chemicals. Proc. Natl. Acad. Sci. U. S. A. 72, 5135–5139.

McClanahan, R.H., Huitric, A.C., Pearson, P.G., et al., 1988. Evidence for a cytochrome P-450 catalysed allylic rearrangement with double-bond topomerization. J. Am. Chem. Soc. 110, 1979–1981.

McClanahan, R.H., Thomassen, D., Slattery, J.T., et al., 1989. Metabolic activation of (R)-(+)-pulegone to a reactive enonal that covalently binds to mouse liver proteins. Chem. Res. Toxicol. 2, 349–355.

McConnell, R., Hruska, A.J., 1993. An epidemic of pesticide poisoning in Nicaragua: implications for prevention in developing countries. Am. J Public Health 83, 1559–1562.

McCord, J.A., Jervey, L.P., 1962. Nutmeg (myristicin) poisoning: case report. South Carolina Medical Journal 58, 436–439.

McCormick, M.A., Manoguerra, A.S., 1988. Toxicity of pennyroyal oil: a case report and review. Vet. Hum. Toxicol. 30, 347.

McDonald, T.A., 1999. Evidence on the carcinogenicity of estragole. Office of Environmental Health Hazard Assessment California Environmental Protection Agency Final Report, November 1999.

McGowan, E.M., 1966. Menthol urticaria. Arch. Dermatol. 94, 62–63.

McGregor, D.B., Brown, A., Cattanach, P., et al., 1988. Responses of the L5178Y tk+/tk- mouse lymphoma cell forward mutation assay: III. 72 coded chemicals. Environ. Mol. Mutagen. 12, 85–154.

McGregor, D.B., Brown, A., Howgate, S., et al., 1991. Responses of the L5178Y mouse lymphoma cell forward mutation assay. V: 27 coded chemicals. Environ. Mol. Mutagen. 17, 196–219.

McGuigan, M.A., 1987. A two-year review of salicylate deaths in Ontario. Arch. Intern. Med. 147, 510–512.

McHale, D., Sheridan, J.B., 1989. The oxygen heterocyclic compounds of citrus peel oils. Journal of Essential Oil Research 1, 139–149.

McHale, D., Laurie, W.A., Woof, M.A., 1977. Composition of West Indian bay oils. Food Chem. 2, 19–25.

McKenna, K.E., Patterson, C.C., Handley, J., et al., 1996. Cutaneous neoplasia following PUVA therapy for psoriasis. Br. J. Dermatol. 134, 639–642.

McMahon, M.A., Blair, I.S., Moore, J.E., et al., 2007. Habituation to sub-lethal concentrations of tea tree oil (Melaleuca alternifolia) is associated with reduced susceptibility to antibiotics in human pathogens. J. Antimicrob. Chemother. 59, 125–127.

McMahon, M.A., Tunney, M.M., Moore, J.E., et al., 2008. Changes in antibiotic susceptibity in staphylococci habituated to sub-lethal concentrations of tea tree oil (Melaleuca alternifolia). Lett. Appl. Microbiol. 47, 263–268.

McNamara, M.E., Burnham, D.C., Smith, C., et al., 2003. The effects of back massage before diagnostic cardiac catheterization. Altern. Ther. Health Med. 9, 50–57.

McNeely, W., Goa, K.L., 1998. 5-Methoxypsoralen: a review of its effects in psoriasis and vitiligo. Drugs 56, 667–690.

McPherson, J., 1925. The toxicology of eucalyptus oil. Med. J. Aust. 2, 108–110.

Meadows, S.M., Mulkerin, D., Berlin, J., et al., 2002. Phase II trial of perillyl alcohol in patients with metastatic colorectal cancer. Int. J. Gastrointest. Cancer 32, 125–128.

Mediavilla, V., Steinmann, S., 1997. Essential oil of cannabis sativa L. strains. Journal of the International Hemp Association 4, 82–84.

Meding, B., 1990. Epidemiology of hand eczema in an industrial city. Acta Derm. Venereol. 153, 1–43.

Meehan, T., Bond, D.M., 1984. Hydrolysis of benzo[a]pyrene diol epoxide and its covalent binding to DNA proceed through similar rate-determining steps. Proc. Natl. Acad. Sci. U. S. A. 81, 2635–2639.

Meeker, J.D., Ryan, L., Barr, D.B., et al., 2006. Exposure to nonpersistent insecticides and male reproductive hormones. Epidemiology 17, 61–68.

Meewes, C., Brenneisen, P., Wenk, J., et al., 2001. Adaptive antioxidant response protects dermal fibroblasts from UVA-induced phototoxicity. Free Radic. Biol. Med. 30, 238–247.

Meggs, W.J., 1993. Neurogenic inflammation and sensitivity to environmental chemicals. Environ. Health Perspect. 101, 234–238.

Meidan, V.M., Bonner, M.C., Michniak, B.B., 2005. Transfollicular drug delivery - is it a reality? Int. J. Pharm. 306, 1–14.

Meier, C., Mediavilla, V., 1998. Factors influencing the yield and the quality of hemp (Cannabis sativa L.) essential oil. Journal of the International Hemp Association 5, 16–20.

Mele, A., 1952. Acute fatal poisoning with chenopodium oil. Folia Medica 35, 955–963.

Melis, K., Bochner, A., Janssens, G., 1989. Accidental nasal eucalyptol and menthol instillation. Eur. J. Pediatr. 148, 786–788.

Melnick, R.L., 2001. Is peroxisome proliferation an obligatory precursor step in the carcinogenicity of di(2-ethylhexyl)phthalate (DEHP)? Environ. Health Perspect. 109, 437–442.

Melzig, M.F., Moller, I., Jarry, H., 2003. New investigations of the *in vitro* pharmacological activity of essential oils from the Apiaceae. Zeitschrift für Phytotherapie 24, 112–116.

Mendelsohn, H.V., 1944. Dermatitis from lemon grass oil (*Cymbopogon citratus* or *Andropogon citratus*). Arch. Dermatol. Syphilol. 50, 34–35.

Meneghini, C.L., Rantuccio, F., Lomuto, M., 1971. Additives, vehicles and active drugs of topical medicaments as causes of delayed-type allergic dermatitis. Dermatologica 143, 137–147.

Mennella, J.A., Beauchamp, G.K., 1993. The effects of repeated exposure to garlic-flavored milk on the nursling's behavior. Pediatr. Res. 34, 805–808.

Mennella, J.A., Johnson, A., Beauchamp, G.K., 1995. Garlic ingestion by pregnant women alters the odor of amniotic fluid. Chem. Senses 20, 207–210.

Menezes, I.A., Marques, M.S., Santos, T.C., et al., 2007. Antinociceptive effect and acute toxicity of the essential oil of *Hyptis fruticosa* in mice. Fitoterapia 78, 192–195.

Mengs, U., Stotzem, C.D., 1989. Toxicological evaluation of peppermint oil in rodents and dogs. Medical Science Research 17, 499–500.

Menichini, F., Tundis, R., Loizzo, M.R., et al., 2010. In vitro photo-induced cytotoxic activity of Citrus bergamia and C. medica L. cv. Diamante peel essential oils and identified active coumarins. Pharmaceutical Biology 48, 1059–1065.

Mennicke, W.H., Gorler, K., Krumbiegel, G., 1983. Metabolism of some naturally occurring isothiocyanates in the rat. Xenobiotica 13, 203–207.

Menon, P.A., Thach, B.T., Smith, C.H., et al., 1984. Benzyl alcohol toxicity in a neonatal intensive care unit. Incidence, symptomatology, and mortality. Am. J. Perinatol. 1, 288–292.

Mereto, E., Brambilla-Campart, G., Ghia, M., et al., 1994. Cinnamaldehyde-induced micronuclei in rodent liver. Mutat. Res. 322, 1–8.

Merkulova, O.S., 1957. Reflex mechanism of camphor and pyramidone experimental epilepsy. Doklady Akademii Nauk USSR 112, 968–971.

Meschler, J.P., Howlett, A.C., 1999. Thujone exhibits low affinity for cannabinoid receptors but fails to evoke cannabimimetic responses. Pharmacol. Biochem. Behav. 62, 473–480.

Messer, A., Raquet, N., Lohr, C., et al., 2012. Major furocoumarins in grapefruit juice II: phototoxicity, photogenotoxicity, and inhibitory potency vs. cytochrome P450 3A4 activity. Food Chem. Toxicol. 50, 756–760.

Meuling, W.J., Ravensberg, L.C., Roza, L., et al., 2005. Dermal absorption of chlorpyrifos in human volunteers. Int. Arch. Occup. Environ. Health 78, 44–50.

Meyer, J., 1970. Accidents dus à un cosmétique de bronzage à base d'essence de bergamote. Bulletin du Société Française de Dermatologie et de Syphiligraphie 77, 881–884.

Mezzoug, N., Elhadri, A., Dallouh, A., et al., 2007. Investigation of the mutagenic and antimutagenic effects of *Origanum compactum* essential oil and some of its constituents. Mutat. Res. 629, 100–110.

Michaels, A.S., Chandrasekaran, S.K., Shaw, J.E., 1975. Drug permeation through human skin: theory and *in vitro* experimental measurement. AIChE Journal 21, 985–996.

Mid-Japan Contact Dermatitis Research Group, 1984. Determination of suitable concentrations for patch testing of various fragrance materials. A summary of group study conducted over a 6-year period. J. Dermatol. 11, 31–35.

Miguel, M.G., Guerrero, H., Rodrigues, J., et al., 2003a. Essential oils of Portuguese *Thymus mastichina* (L.) L. ssp. *mastichina* grown on different substrates and harvested on different dates. Journal of Horticultural Science & Biotechnology 78, 355–358.

Miguel, M.G., Figueiredo, A.C., Costa, M.M., et al., 2003b. Effect of the volatile constituents isolated from *Thymus albicans, Th. mastichina, Th. carnosus* and *Thymbra capitata* in sunflower oil. Nahrung 47, 397–402.

Milchard, M.J., Clery, R., DaCosta, N., et al., 2004. Application of gas-liquid chromatography to the analysis of essential oils. Perfumer & Flavorist 29, 28–36.

Miller, C.S., 1996. Chemical sensitivity: symptom, syndrome or mechanism for disease? Toxicology 111, 69–86.

Miller, J.S., 2001. The biology of natural killer cells in cancer, infection, and pregnancy. Exp. Hematol. 29, 1157–1168.

Miller, J.A., Miller, E.C., 1983. The metabolic activation of nucleic acid adducts of naturally-occurring carcinogens: recent studies with ethyl

carbamate and the spice flavours safrole and estragole. Br. J. Cancer 48, 1–15.

Miller, E.C., 1979. The metabolic activation of safrole and related naturally occurring alkylbenzenes in relation to carcinogenesis by these agents. In: Naturally occurring carcinogens-mutagens and modulators of carcinogenesis. Proceedings of the 9th International Symposium of the Princess Takamatsu Cancer Research Fund, Tokyo University. Park Press, Baltimore.

Miller, E.C., Swanson, A.B., Phillips, D.H., et al., 1983. Structure-activity studies of the carcinogenicities in the mouse and rat of some naturally occurring and synthetic alkenylbenzene derivatives related to safrole and estragole. Cancer Res. 43, 1124–1134.

Miller, R.L., Gould, A.R., Bernstein, M.L., 1992. Cinnamon-induced stomatitis venenata, clinical and characterisitic histopathological features. Oral Surg. Oral Med. Oral Pathol. 73, 708–716.

Millet, Y., Tognetti, P., Lavaire-Pierlovisi, M., et al., 1979. Étude expérimentale des propriétés toxiques convulsivantes des essences de sauge et d'hysope du commerce. Rev. Electroencéphalogr. Neurophysiol. Clin. 1, 12–18.

Millet, Y., Tognetti, P., Steinmetz, M.D., et al., 1980. Étude de la toxicité d'huiles essentielles végétales du commerce: essence d'hysope et de sauge. Médecine Légale, Toxicologie 23, 9–21.

Millet, Y., Jouglard, J., Steinmetz, M.D., et al., 1981. Toxicity of some essential plant oils: clinical and experimental study. Clin. Toxicol. 18, 1485–1498.

Millqvist, E., 2000. Cough provocation with capsaicin is an objective way to test sensory hyperreactivity in patients with asthma-like symptoms. Allergy 55, 546–550.

Millqvist, E., 2006. Rhinitis as a part of sensory hyperreactivity characterized by increased capsaicin cough sensitivity. In: Baraniuk, J.N., Shusterman, D.J. (Eds.), Nonallergic rhinitis: clinical allergy and immunology. Infroma Healthcare USA, New York.

Millqvist, E., Löwhagen, O., 1996. Placebo-controlled challenges with perfume in patients with asthma-like symptoms. Allergy 51, 434–439.

Millqvist, E., Bende, M., Löwhagen, O., 1998. Sensory hyperreactivity - a possible mechanism underlying cough and asthma-like symptoms. Allergy 53, 1208–1212.

Millqvist, E., Bengtsson, U., Lowhagen, O., 1999. Provocations with perfume in the eyes induce airways symptoms in patients with sensory hyperreactivity. Allergy 54, 495–499.

Millqvist, E., Ternesten-Hasséus, E., Ståhl, A., et al., 2005. Changes in levels of nerve growth factor in nasal secretions after capsaicin inhalation in patients with airway symptoms from scents and chemicals. Environ. Health Perspect. 113, 849–852.

Mills, S., Bone, K., 2000. Principles & practice of phytotherapy. Churchill Livingstone, London.

Mills, S., Bone, K., 2005. The essential guide to herbal safety. Churchill Livingstone, London.

Mills, J.J., Chari, R.S., Boyer, I.J., et al., 1995. Induction of apoptosis in liver tumors by the monoterpene perillyl alcohol. Cancer Res. 55, 979–983.

Mimica-Dukic, N., Bozin, B., Sokovic, M., et al., 2003. Antimicrobial and antioxidant activities of three *Mentha* species essential oils. Planta Med. 69, 413–419.

Mimica-Dukic, N., Bozin, B., Sokovic, M., et al., 2004. Antimicrobial and antioxidant activities of *Melissa officinalis* L. (Lamiaceae) essential oil. J. Agric. Food Chem. 52, 2485–2489.

Mimica-Dukic, N., Bugarin, D., Grbovic, S., et al., 2010. Essential oil of *Myrtus communis* L. as a potential antioxidant and antimutagenic agent. Molecules 15, 2759–2770.

Mio, M., Yabuta, M., Kamei, C., 1999. Ultraviolet B (UVB) light-induced histamine release from rat peritoneal mast cells and its augmentation by certain phenothiazine compounds. Immunopharmacology 41, 55–63.

Miraldi, E., Ferri, S., Franchi, G.G., Giorgi, G., 1996. *Peumus boldus* essential oil: new constituents and comparison of oils from leaves of different origin. Fitoterapia 67, 227–230.

Mirsalis, J., Tyson, K., Beck, J., et al., 1983. Induction of unschedules DNA synthesis (UDS) in hepatocytes following in vitro and in vivo treatment. Environ. Mutagen. 5, 482.

Misharina, T.A., Polshkov, A.N., 2005. Antioxidant properties of essential oils: autoxidation of essential oils from laurel and fennel and effects of mixing with essential oil from coriander. article in RussianPrikladnaia Biokhimiia Mikrobiologiia 41, 693–702.

Mishra, A.K., Kishore, N., Dubey, N.K., et al., 1991. An evaluation of the toxicity of the oils of *Cymbopogon citratus* and *Citrus medica* in rats. Phytother. Res. 6, 279–281.

Misra, L.N., Tyagi, B.R., Ahmad, A., et al., 1994. Variability in the chemical composition of the essential oil of *Coleus forskohlii* genotypes. Journal of Essential Oil Research 6, 243–247.

Misra, R., Dash, P.K., Rao, Y.R., 2000. Chemical composition of the essential oils of kewda and ketaki. Journal of Essential Oil Research 12, 175–178.

Mitchell, J.C., 1975. Contact hypersensitivity to some perfume materials. Contact Dermatitis 1, 196–199.

Mitchell, J.C., Calnan, C.D., Clendenning, W.E., et al., 1976. Patch testing with some components of Balsam of Peru. Contact Dermatitis 2, 57–58.

Mitchell, J.C., Adams, R.M., Glendenning, W.E., et al., 1982. Results of standard patch tests with substances abandoned. Contact Dermatitis 8, 336–337.

Mitić-Culafić, D., Zegura, B., Nikolić, B., et al., 2009. Protective effect of linalool, myrcene and eucalyptol against *t*-butyl hydroperoxide induced genotoxicity in bacteria and cultured human cells. Food Chem. Toxicol. 47, 260–266.

Miyachi, T., Tsutsui, T., 2005. Ability of 13 chemical agents used in dental practice to induce sister-chromatid exchanges in Syrian hamster embryo cells. Odontology 93, 24–29.

Miyake, Y., Murakami, A., Sugiyama, Y., et al., 1999. Identification of coumarins from lemon fruit (*Citrus limon*) as inhibitors of *in vitro* tumor promotion and superoxide and nitric oxide generation. J. Agric. Food Chem. 47, 3151–3157.

Miyazaki, M., Sugawara, E., Yoshimura, T., et al., 2005a. Mutagenic activation of betel quid-specific *N*-nitrosamines catalyzed by human cytochrome P450 coexpressed with NADPH-cytochrome P450 reductase in *Salmonella typhimurium* YG7108. Mutat. Res. 581, 165–171.

Miyazaki, M., Yamazaki, H., Takeuchi, H., et al., 2005b. Mechanisms of chemopreventive effects of 8-methoxypsoralen against 4-(methylnitrosamino)-1-(3-pyridyl)-1-butanone-induced mouse lung adenomas. Carcinogenesis 26, 1947–1955.

Miyazawa, M., Kohno, G., 2005. Suppression of chemical mutagen-induced SOS response by allylbenzen from *Asiasarum heterotropoides* in the *Salmonella typhimurium* TA1535/PSK1002 umu test. Nat. Prod. Res. 19, 29–36.

Miyazawa, M., Shindo, M., Shimada, T., 2001a. Roles of cytochrome P450 3A enzymes in the 2-hydroxylation of 1,4-cineole, a monoterpene cyclic ether, by rat and human liver microsomes. Xenobiotica 31, 713–723.

Miyazawa, M., Shindo, M., Shimada, T., 2001b. Oxidation of 1,8-cineole, the monoterpene cyclic ether originated from *Eucalyptus polybractea*, by cytochrome P450 3A enzymes in rat and human liver microsomes. Drug Metab. Dispos. 29, 200–205.

Miyazawa, M., Sugie, A., Shimada, T., 2003. Roles of human CYP2A6 and 2B6 and rat CYP2C11 and 2B1 in the 10-hydroxylation of (−)-verbenone by liver microsomes. Drug Metab. Dispos. 31, 1049–1053.

Mizutani, T., Nomura, H., Nakanishi, K., et al., 1987. Effects of drug metabolism modifiers on pulegone-induced hepatotoxicity in mice. Res. Commun. Chem. Pathol. Pharmacol. 58, 75–83.

Mizutani, T., Satoh, K., Nomura, H., 1991. Hepatotoxicity of eugenol and related compounds in mice depleted of glutathione: structural requirements for toxic potency. Res. Commun. Chem. Pathol. Pharmacol. 73, 87–95.

MMWR, 1982. Neonatal deaths associated with use of benzyl alcohol - United States. Morbidity & Mortality Weekly Report 31, 290–291.

Modak, T., Mukhopadhaya, A., 2011. Effects of citral, a naturally occurring antiadipogenic molecule, on an energy-intense diet model of obesity. Indian J. Pharm. 43, 300–305.

Modarai, M., Suter, A., Kortenkamp, A., et al., 2011. The interaction potential of herbal medicinal products: a luminescence-based screening platform assessing effects on cytochrome P450 and its use with devil's claw (Harpagophyti radix) preparations. J. Pharm. Pharmacol. 63, 429–438.

Modjtahedi, B.S., Modjtahedi, S.P., Maibach, H.I., 2004. The sex of the individual as a factor in allergic contact dermatitis. Contact Dermatitis 50, 53–59.

Mølck, A.M., Poulsen, M., Lauridsen, S.T., et al., 1998. Lack of histological cerebellar changes in Wistar rats given pulegone for 28 days. Comparison of immersion and perfusion tissue fixation. Toxicol. Lett. 95, 117–122.

Molhave, L., Kjaergaard, S.K., Hempel-Jorgensen, A., et al., 2000. The eye irritation and odor potencies of four terpenes which are major constituents of the emissions of VOCs from Nordic soft woods. Indoor Air 10, 315–318.

Molina-Jasso, D., Álvarez-González, I., Madrigal-Bujaidar, E., 2009. Clastogenicity of beta-caryophyllene in mouse. Biol. Pharm. Bull. 32, 520–522.

Möllenbeck, S., König, T., Schreier, P., et al., 1997. Chemical composition and analyses of enantiomers of essential oils of Madagascar. Flavour & Fragrance Journal 12, 63–69.

Moller, P., Loft, S., 2004. Interventions with antioxidants and nutrients in relation to oxidative DNA damage and repair. Mutat. Res. 551, 79–89.

Momtaz, K., Fitzpatrick, T.B., 1998. The benefits and risks of long-term PUVA photochemotherapy. Dermatol. Ther. 16, 227–234.

Mondello, F., De Bernardis, F., Girolamo, A., et al., 2006. *In vivo* activity of terpinen-4-ol, the main bioactive component of *Melaleuca alternifolia* Cheel (tea tree) oil against azole-susceptible and -resistant human pathogenic Candida species. BMC Infect. Dis. 6, 158.

Monma-Ohtaki, J., Maeno, Y., Nagao, M., et al., 2002. An autopsy case of poisoning by massive absorption of cresol a short time before death. Forensic Sci. Int. 126, 77–81.

Monro, A., 1992. Contemporary issues in toxicology. Toxicol. Appl. Pharmacol. 112, 171–181.

Monro, A., 1993. The paradoxical lack of interspecies correlation between plasma concentrations and chemical carcinogenicity. Regul. Toxicol. Pharmacol. 18, 115–135.

Montaguti, P., Melloni, E., Cavalletti, E., 1994. Acute intravenous toxicity of dimethyl sulfoxide, polyethylene glycol 400, dimethylformamide, absolute ethanol, and benzyl alcohol in inbred mouse strains. Arzneimittelforschung 44, 566–570.

Monteiro, M.V., De Melo Leite, A.K., Bertini, L.M., et al., 2007. Topical anti-inflammatory, gastroprotective and antioxidant effects of the essential oil of *Lippia sidoides* Cham. leaves. J. Ethnopharmacol. 111, 378–382.

Montelius, J., Wahlkvist, H., Boman, A., Wahlberg, J.E., 1998. Murine local lymph node assay for predictive testing of allergenicity: two irritants caused significant proliferation. Acta Derm. Venereol. 78, 433–437.

Monzote, L., Montalvo, A.M., Scull, R., et al., 2007. Activity, toxicity and analysis of resistance of essential oil from *Chenopodium ambrosioides* after intraperitoneal, oral and intralesional administration in BALB/c mice infected with *Leishmania amazonensis*: a preliminary study. Biomedicine & Pharmacotherapy 61, 148–153.

Moody, R.P., Akram, M., Dickson, E., et al., 2007. *In vitro* dermal absorption of methyl salicylate, ethyl parathion, and malathion: first responder safety. J. Toxicol. Environ. Health A 70, 985–999.

Moon, K.H., Pack, M.Y., 1983. Cytotoxicity of cinnamic aldehyde on leukaemia L1210 cells. Drug Chem. Toxicol. 6, 521–535.

Moorthy, B., 1991. Toxicity and metabolism of R-(+)- pulegone in rats: its effects on hepatic cytochrome P450 *in vivo* and *in vitro*. Journal of the Indian Institute of Science 71, 76–78.

Moorthy, B., Madyastha, P., Madyastha, K.M., 1989a. Hepatotoxicity of pulegone in rats: its effects on microsomal enzymes, in vivo. Toxicology 55, 327–337.

Moorthy, B., Madyastha, P., Madyastha, K.M., 1989b. Metabolism of a monoterpene ketone, R-(+)-pulegone - a hepatotoxin in rat. Xenobiotica 19, 217–224.

Moorthy, B., Vijayasarathi, S.K., Basu, A., et al., 1991. Biochemical, histopathological and ultrastructural changes in rat liver induced by R-(+)-pulegone, a monoterpene ketone. Toxicol. Environ. Chem. 33, 121–131.

Morales-Ramírez, P., Madrigal-Bujaidar, E., Mercader-Martínez, J., et al., 1992. Sister-chromatid exchange induction produced by in vivo and in vitro exposure to alpha-asarone. Mutat. Res. 279, 269–273.

Mori, H., Kawamori, T., Tanaka, T., et al., 1994. Chemopreventive effect of costunolide, a constituent of oriental medicine, on azoxymethane-induced intestinal carcinogenesis in rats. Cancer Lett. 83, 171–175.

Morice, A.H., Marshall, A.E., Higgins, K.S., 1994. Effect of inhaled menthol on citric acid induced cough in normal subjects. Thorax 49, 1024–1026.

725

Morikawa, T., Matsuda, H., Ninomiya, K., et al., 2002. Medicinal foodstuffs. XXIX. Potent protective effects of sesquiterpenes and curcumin from Zedoariae Rhizoma on liver injury induced by D-galactosamine/lipopolysaccharide or tumor necrosis factor-alpha. Biol. Pharm. Bull. 25, 627–631.

Morita, Y., Matsumura, E., Tsujibo, H., et al., 2001. Biological activity of a-thujaplicin, the minor component of Thujopsis dolabrata Sieb. et Zucc. var. hondai Makino. Biol. Pharm. Bull. 24, 607–611.

Morita, Y., Matsumura, E., Tsujibo, H., et al., 2002. Biological activity of 4-acetyltropolone, the minor component of Thujopsis dolabrata Sieb. et Zucc. hondai Mak. Biological & Pharmacological Bulletin 25, 981–985.

Morita, T., Jinno, K., Kawagishi, H., et al., 2003. Hepatoprotective effect of myristicin from nutmeg (Myristica fragrans) on lipopolysaccharide/d-galactosamine-induced liver injury. J. Agric. Food Chem. 51, 1560–1565.

Morita, Y., Matsumura, E., Okabe, T., et al., 2004. Biological activity of β-dolabrin, γ-thujaplicin, and 4-acetyltropolone, hinokitiol-related compounds. Biological & Pharmacological Bulletin 27, 1666–1669.

Morlière, P., Bazin, M., Dubertret, L., et al., 1991. Photoreactivity of 5-geranoxypsoralen and lack of photoreaction with DNA. Photochem. Photobiol. 53, 13–19.

Morra, P., Bartle, W.R., Walker, S.E., et al., 1996. Serum concentrations of salicylic acid following topically applied salicylate derivatives. Ann. Pharmacother. 30, 935–940.

Morris, M.C., Donoghue, A., Markowitz, J.A., et al., 2003. Ingestion of tea tree oil (Melaleuca oil) by a 4-year-old boy. Pediatr. Emerg. Care 19, 169–171.

Morrone, L.A., Rombolà, L., Pelle, C., et al., 2007. The essential oil of bergamot enhances the levels of amino acid neurotransmitters in the hippocampus of rat: implication of monoterpene hydrocarbons. Pharmacol. Res. 55, 255–262.

Morrow, J.W., 1960. Chemotherapy of carcinoma of the bladder: Preliminary report of forty-four cases treated with citral. Br. J. Urol. 32, 69–78.

Morse, M.A., Stoner, G.D., 1993. Cancer chemoprevention: principles and prospects. Carcinogenesis 15, 1737–1746.

Morse, M.A., Toburen, A.L., 1996. Inhibition of metabolic activation of 4-(methylnitrosamino)-1-(3-pyridyl)-1-butanone by limonene. Cancer Lett. 104, 211–217.

Morse, M.A., Kresty, L.A., Toburen, A.L., 1995. Inhibition of metabolism of 4-(methylnitrosamino)-1-(3-pyridyl)-1-butanone by dietary benzaldehydes. Cancer Lett. 97, 255–261.

Mortelmans, K., Haworth, S., Lawlor, T., et al., 1986. Salmonella mutagenicity tests: II. Results from the testing of 270 chemicals. Environmental Mutagens 8 (Suppl. 7), 1–119.

Mortelmans, K., Zeiger, E., 2000. The Ames Salmonella/microsome mutagenicity assay. Mutat. Res. 455, 29–60.

Morteza-Semnani, K., Saeedi, M., 2003. Constituents of the essential oil of Commiphora myrrha (Nees) Engl. var. molmol. Journal of Essential Oil Research 15, 50–51.

Morton, C.A., Garioch, J., Todd, P., et al., 1995. Contact sensitivity to menthol and peppermint in patients with intra-oral symptoms. Contact Dermatitis 32, 281–284.

Mortz, C.G., Andersen, K.E., 2010. Fragrance mix I patch test reactions in 5006 consecutive dermatitis patients tested simultaneously with TRUE Test® and Torlab® test material. Contact Dermatitis 63, 248–253.

Mortz, C.G., Lauritsen, J.M., Bindslev-Jensen, C., et al., 2001. Prevalence of atopic dermatitis, asthma, allergic rhinitis and hand and contact dermatitis in adolescents. The Odense Adolescence Cohort Study on Atopic Diseases and Dermatitis. Br. J. Dermatol. 144, 523–532.

Mortz, C.G., Lauritsen, J.M., Bindslev-Jensen, C., et al., 2002. Contact allergy and allergic contact dermatitis in adolescents: prevalence measures and associations. The Odense Adolescence Cohort Study on Atopic Diseases and Dermatitis (TOACS). Acta Derm. Venereol. 82, 352–358.

Mosaffa, F., Behravan, J., Karimi, G., et al., 2006. Antigenotoxic effects of Satureja hortensis L. on rat lymphocytes exposed to oxidative stress. Archives of Pharmaceutical Research 29, 159–164.

Moseley, H., Davison, M., MacKie, R.M., 1983. Measurement of daylight UVA in Glasgow. Phys. Med. Biol. 28, 589–597.

Mossa, A.T., Nawwar, G.A., 2011. Free radical scavenging and antiacetylcholinesterase activities of Origanum majorana L. essential oil. Hum. Exp. Toxicol. 30, 1501–1513.

Mosselman, S., Polman, J., Dijkema, R., 1996. ER–beta: identification and characterization of a novel human estrogen receptor. FEBS Lett. 392, 49–53.

Moteki, H., Hibasami, H., Yamada, Y., et al., 2002. Specific induction of apoptosis by 1,8-cineole in two human leukemia cell lines, but not a in human stomach cancer cell line. Oncol. Rep. 9, 757–760.

Motl, O., Hodacova, J., Ubik, K., 1990. Composition of Vietnamese cajuput essential oil. Flavour & Fragrance Journal 5, 39–42.

Motohashi, N., Ashihara, Y., Yamagami, C., et al., 2001. Structure-antimutagenic activity relationships of benzalacetone derivatives against UV-induced mutagenesis in E. coli WP2uvrA and gamma-induced mutagenesis in Salmonella typhimurium TA2638. Mutat. Res. 474, 113–120.

Motoyoshi, K., Toyoshima, Y., Sato, M., et al., 1979. Comparative studies on the irritancy of oils and synthetic perfumes to the skin of rabbit, guinea pig, rat, miniature swine and man. Cosmetics & Toiletries 94, 41–48.

Moudachirou, M., Gbénou, J.D., 1999. Chemical composition of essential oils of eucalyptus from Bénin: Eucalyptus citriodora and E. camaldulensis: influence of location, harvest time, storage of plants and time of steam distillation. Journal of Essential Oil Research 11, 109–118.

Moura Rocha, N.F., Venâncio, E.T., Moura, B.A., et al., 2010. Gastroprotection of (-)-alpha-bisabolol on acute gastric mucosal lesions in mice: the possible involved pharmacological mechanisms. Fundam. Clin. Pharmacol. 24, 63–71.

Mousavi, S.H., Tayarani-Najaran, Z., Asghari, M., et al., 2010. Protective effect of Nigella sativa extract and thymoquinone on serum/glucose deprivation-induced PC12 cells death. Cell. Mol. Neurobiol. 30, 591–598.

Moyler, D.A., 1998. The flavour gum resins, their chemistry and uses. Rivista Italiana EPPOS (Numero Speciale) 351–360.

Moysan, A., Morliere, P., Averbeck, D., et al., 1993. Evaluation of phototoxic and photogenotoxic risk associated with the use of photosensitizers in suntan preparations: application to tanning preparations containing bergamot oil. Skin Pharmacol. 6, 282–291.

Mozaffari, F.S., Ghorbanli, M., Babai, A., et al., 2000. The effect of water stress on the seed oil of Nigella sativa L. Journal of Essential Oil Research 12, 36–38.

Mozelsio, N.B., Harris, K.E., McGrath, K.G., et al., 2003. Immediate systemic hypersensitivity reaction associated with topical application of Australian tea tree oil. Allergy Asthma Proc. 24, 73–75.

Mucciarelli, M., Caramiello, R., Maffei, M., et al., 1995. Essential oils from some Artemisia species growing spontaneously in North-West Italy. Flavour & Fragrance Journal 10, 25–32.

Muchtaridi, Subarnas, A., Apriyantono, A., et al., 2010. Identification of compounds in the essential oil of nutmeg seeds (Myristica fragrans Houtt.) that inhibit locomotor activity in mice. Int. J. Mol. Sci 11, 4771–4781.

Mullen, M.P., Pathak, M.A., West, J.D., et al., 1984. Carcinogenic effects of monofunctional and bifunctional furocoumarins. National Cancer Institute Monographs 66, 205–210.

Mullen, W., et al., 1994. Accidental pennyroyal oil ingestion in a toddler with the first human serum metabolite detection. Vet. Hum. Toxicol. 36, 342.

Müller, L., Kasper, P., Müller-Tegethoff, K., et al., 1994. The genotoxic potential in vitro and in vivo of the allyl benzene etheric oils estragole, basil oil and trans-anethole. Mutat. Res. 325, 129–136.

Müller, M., Byres, M., Jaspars, M., et al., 2004. 2D NMR spectroscopic analyses of archangelicin from the seeds of Angelica archangelica. Acta Pharm. 54, 277–285.

Mumcuoglu, K.Y., Miller, J., Zamir, C., et al., 2002. The in vivo pediculicidal efficacy of a natural remedy. Isr. Med. Assoc. J. 4, 790–793.

Mumcuoglu, K.Y., Magdassi, S., Miller, J., et al., 2004. Repellency of citronella for head lice: double-blind randomized trial of efficacy and safety. Isr. Med. Assoc. J. 6, 756–759.

Munday, R., Munday, C.M., 2001. Relative activities of organosulfur compounds derived from onions and garlic in increasing tissue activities of quinone reductase and glutathione transferase in rat tissues. Nutr. Cancer 40, 205–210.

Mündel, T., Jones, D.A., 2010. The effects of swilling an L: (−)-menthol solution during exercise in the heat. Eur. J. Appl. Physiol. 109, 59–65.

Munerato, M.C., Sinigaglia, M., Reguly, M.L., et al., 2005. Genotoxic effects of eugenol, isoeugenol and safrole in the wing spot test of *Drosophila melanogaster*. Mutat. Res. 582, 87–94.

Murase, J.E., Lee, E.E., Koo, J., 2005. Effect of ethnicity on the risk of developing nonmelanoma skin cancer following long-term PUVA therapy. Int. J. Dermatol. 44, 1016–1021.

Murayama, M., Kumaroo, K.K., 1986. Inhibitors of *ex vivo* aggregation of human platelets induced by decompression, during reduced barometric pressure. Thromb. Res. 42, 511–516.

Murray, R.P., Connett, J.E., Skeans, M.A., et al., 2007. Menthol cigarettes and health risks in Lung Health Study data. Nicotine Tob. Res. 9, 101–107.

Murren, J.R., Pizzorno, G., DiStasio, S.A., et al., 2002. Phase I study of perillyl alcohol in patients with refractory malignancies. Cancer Biol. Ther. 1, 130–135.

Musajo, L., Rodighiero, G., Caporale, G., 1953. L'attività fotodinamica delle cumarine naturali. La Chimica e L'Industria 35, 13–15.

Musajo, L., Rodighiero, G., Caporale, G., 1954. L'activité photodynamique des coumarines naturelles. Bull. Soc. Chim. Biol. 36, 1213–1224.

Musajo, L., Rodighiero, G., Breccia, A., et al., 1966. Skin-photosensitising furocoumarins: photochemical interaction between DNA and -O14CH3 bergapten (5-methoxy-psoralen). Photochem. Photobiol. 5, 739–745.

Musk, S.R., Johnson, I.T., 1993. The clastogenic effects of isothiocyanates. Mutat. Res. 300, 111–117.

Musk, S.R., Stephenson, P., Smith, T.K., et al., 1995. Selective toxicity of compounds naturally present in food toward the transformed phenotype of human colorectal cell line HT29. Nutr. Cancer 24, 289–298.

Musk, S.R., Clapham, P., Johnson, I.T., 1997. Cytotoxicity and genotoxicity of diallyl sulfide and diallyl disulfide towards Chinese hamster ovary cells. Food Chem. Toxicol. 35, 379–385.

Mustafa, A., Ali, M., Khan, N.Z., 2005. Volatile oil constituents of the fresh rhizomes of *Curcuma amada* Roxb. Journal of Essential Oil Research 17, 490–491.

Muztar, A.J., Ahmad, P., Huque, T., et al., 1979a. A study of the chemical binding of allyl isothiocyanate with thyroxine and of the effect of allyl isothiocyanate on lipid metabolism in the rat. Can. J. Physiol. Pharmacol. 57, 385–389.

Muztar, A.J., Huque, T., Ahmad, P., et al., 1979b. Effect of allyl isothiocyanate on plasma and urinary concentrations of some biochemical entities in the rat. Can. J. Physiol. Pharmacol. 57, 504–509.

Myhr, B., McGregor, D., Bowers, L., et al., 1990. L5178Y Mouse lymphoma cell mutation assay results with 41 compounds. Environ. Mol. Mutagen. 16 (Suppl. 18), 138–167.

Myllynen, P., Pasanen, M., Vähäkangas, K., 2007. The fate and effects of xenobiotics in human placenta. Expert Opin. Drug Metab. Toxicol. 3, 331–346.

Myott, E.C., 1906. Case of eucalyptus poisoning. Br. Med. J. 1, 558.

Mytton, O.T., McGready, R., Lee, S.J., et al., 2007. Safety of benzyl benzoate lotion and permethrin in pregnancy: a retrospective matched cohort study. BJOG 114, 582–587.

Nacak, M., Erbagci, Z., Aynacioglu, A.S., 2006. Human arylamine N-acetyltransferase 2 polymorphism and susceptibility to allergic contact dermatitis. International Journal of Dermatitis 45, 323–326.

Naef, R., Morris, A.F., 1992. Lavender and lavandin – a comparative analysis. Rivista Italiana EPPOS (Numero Speciale), 364–377.

Näf, R., et al., 1995. Agarwood oil (*Aquilaria agallocha* Roxb.). Its composition and eight new valencane-, eremophilane- and vetispirane-derivatives. Flavour & Fragrance Journal 10, 147–152.

Nafisi, S.h, Hajiakhoondi, A., Yektadoost, A., 2004. Thymol and carvacrol binding to DNA: model for drug-DNA interaction. Biopolymers 74, 345–351.

Nagababu, E., Lakshmaiah, N., 1994. Inhibition of microsomal lipid peroxidation and monooxygenase activities by eugenol. Free Radic. Res. 20, 253–266.

Nagababu, E., Sesikeran, B., Lakshmaiah, N., 1995. The protective effects of eugenol on carbon tetrachloride induced hepatotoxicity in rats. Free Radic. Res. 23, 617–627.

Naganuma, M., Hirose, S., Nakayama, Y., et al., 1985. A study of the phototoxicity of lemon oil. Arch. Dermatol. Res. 278, 31–36.

Nagappan, T., Ramasamy, P., Wahid, M.E., et al., 2011. Biological activity of carbazole alkaloids and essential oil of *Murraya koenigii* against antibiotic resistant microbes and cancer cell lines. Molecules 16, 9651–9664.

Nagareda, T., Sugai, T., Shouji, A., et al., 1992. Incidence of positive reactions to cosmetic products and their ingredients in patch tests and representative cases with cosmetic dermatitis in 1991. Skin Research 34, 176–182.

Nagareda, T., Sugai, T., Shouji, A., et al., 1996. Incidence of positive reactions to cosmetic products and their ingredients in patch tests and a representative case of cosmetic dermatitis in 1993. Environmental Dermatology 3, 16–24.

Nagi, M.N., Almakki, H.A., 2009. Thymoquinone supplementation induces quinone reductase and glutathione transferase in mice liver: possible role in protection against chemical carcinogenesis and toxicity. Phytother. Res. 23, 1295–1298.

Nagi, M.N., Alam, K., Badary, O.A., et al., 1999. Thymoquinone protects against carbon tetrachloride hepatotoxicity in mice via an antioxidant mechanism. Biochemical Molecular & Biological Interactions 47, 153–159.

Nair, B., 2001a. Final report on the safety assessment of benzyl alcohol, benzoic acid, and sodium benzoate. Int. J. Toxicol. 20 (Suppl. 3), 23–50.

Nair, B., 2001b. Final report on the safety assessment of *Mentha piperita* (peppermint) oil, *Mentha piperita* (peppermint) leaf extract, *Mentha piperita* (peppermint) leaf, and *Mentha piperita* (peppermint) leaf water. Int. J. Toxicol. 20 (Suppl. 3), 61–73.

Nair, J., Nair, U.J., Ohshima, H., et al., 1987. Endogenous nitrosation in the oral cavity of chewers while chewing betel quid with or without tobacco. IARC Sci. Publ. 84, 465–469.

Nair, S.C., Pannikar, B., Panikkar, K.R., 1991. Antitumour activity of saffron (*Crocus sativus*). Cancer Lett. 57, 109–114.

Nakagawa, Y., Suzuki, T., 2003. Cytotoxic and xenoestrogenic effects via biotransformation of trans-anethole on isolated rat hepatocytes and cultured MCF-7 human breast cancer cells. Biochem. Pharmacol. 66, 63–73.

Nakagawa, H., Tsuta, K., Kiuchi, K., et al., 2001. Growth inhibitory effects of diallyl disulfide on human breast cancer cell lines. Carcinogenesis 22, 891–897.

Nakaizumi, A., Baba, M., Uehara, H., et al., 1997. *d*-Limonene inhibits N-nitrosobis(2-oxopropyl)amine induced hamster pancreatic carcinogenesis. Cancer Lett. 117, 99–103.

Nakamura, S.I., Oda, Y., Shimada, T., et al., 1987. SOS-inducing activity of chemical carcinogens and mutagens in *Salmonella typhimurium* TA1535/pSK1002: examination with 151 chemicals. Mutat. Res. 192, 239–246.

Nakamura, Y., Kawakami, M., Yoshihiro, A., et al., 2002. Involvement of the mitochondrial death pathway in chemopreventive benzyl isothiocyanate-induced apoptosis. J. Biol. Chem. 277, 8492–8499.

Nakamura, Y., Miyamoto, M., Murakami, A., et al., 2003. A phase II detoxification enzyme inducer from lemongrass: identification of citral and involvement of electrophilic reaction in the enzyme induction. Biochem. Biophys. Res. Commun. 320, 593–600.

Nakano, Y., 2007. Effect of chronic topical exposure to low-dose noxious chemicals and stress on skin sensitivity in mice. J. Occup. Health 49, 431–442.

Nakayama, H., 1998. Fragrance hypersensitivity and its control. In: Frosch, P.J., Johansen, J.D., White, I.R. (Eds.), Fragrances: beneficial and adverse effects. Springer, Berlin.

Nakayama, H., Matsuo, S., Hayakawa, K., et al., 1984. Pigmented cosmetic dermatitis. Int. J. Dermatol. 23, 299–305.

Naldi, L., 2002. The epidemiology of fragrance allergy: questions and needs. Dermatology 205, 89–97.

Nanayakkara, G.R., Bartlett, A., Forbes, B., et al., 2005. The effect of unsaturated fatty acids in benzyl alcohol on the percutaneous permeation of three model penetrants. Int. J. Pharm. 301, 129–139.

Naqvi, A.A., Mandal, S., 1995. Detection of adulteration in sandalwood oil by GLC. Indian Perfumer 39, 62–63.

Nardelli, A., Degreef, H., Goossens, A., 2004. Contact allergic reactions of the vulva: a 14-year review. Dermatitis 15, 131–136.

Nasseri-Sina, P., Hotchkiss, S.A., Caldwell, J., 1997. Cutaneous xenobiotic metabolism: glycine conjugation in human and rat keratinocytes. Food Chem. Toxicol. 35, 409–416.

Nater, J.P., De Jong, M.C., Baar, A.J., et al., 1977. Contact urticarial skin responses to cinnamaldehyde. Contact Dermatitis 3, 151–154.

Nath, S., Aldridge, D., Green, C.E., 2001. Determination of urinary metabolites of Fischer 344 rats following single oral administration of estragole-UL-phenyl-[14C]. Toxicol. Sci. 60, 341 Abstract.

National Cancer Institute, 1979. Bioassay of DL-menthol for possible carcinogenicity. Cacinogenesis Technical Report 98, 125 p. http://ntp.niehs.nih.gov/ntp/htdocs/LT_rpts/tr098.pdf.

National Toxicology Program, 1980. Bioassay of benzoin for possible carcinogenicity (CAS no. 119-53-9). Technical Report 204. http://ntp-server.niehs.nih.gov.

National Toxicology Program, 1982. Carcinogenesis bioassay of allyl isothiocynate (CAS No: 57-06-7) in F344/N rats and B6C3F1 mice (gavage study). Technical Report 234 ntp.niehs.nih.gov/ntp/htdocs/LT_rpts/tr234.pdf.

National Toxicology Program, 1983. Carcinogenesis studies of eugenol (CAS No 97-53-0) in F344/N rats and B6C3F1 mice (feed studies). Technical Report 223. http://ntp-server.niehs.nih.gov.

National Toxicology Program, 1984a. Methyl Salicylate, CAS #119-36-8): Reproduction and Fertility Assessment in CD-1 Mice When Administered by Gavage. Technical Report RACB82104. http://ntp-server.niehs.nih.gov.

National Toxicology Program, 1984b. Methyl Salicylate (CAS 119-36-8): Reproduction and Fertility Assessment in CD-1 Mice When Administered by Gavage. RACB85061. http://ntp-server.niehs.nih.gov.

National Toxicology Program, 1986. Carcinogenesis studies of benzyl acetate in F344/N rats and B6C3F1 mice (gavage studies). Technical Report 250. http://ntp-server.niehs.nih.gov.

National Toxicology Program, 1987. Carcinogenesis studies of food grade geranyl acetate (71% geranyl acetate, 29% citronellyl acetate) (CAS No 105-87-3) in F344/N rats and B6C3F1 mice (gavage study). Technical Report 252. http://ntp-server.niehs.nih.gov.

National Toxicology Program, 1989a. NTP Toxicology and carcinogenesis studies of benzyl alcohol (CAS No. 100-51-6) in F344/N rats and B6C3F1 mice (gavage studies). Technical Report 343. http://ntp-server.niehs.nih.gov.

National Toxicology Program, 1989b. toxicology and carcinogenesis studies of 8-methoxypsoralen (CAS No. 298-81-7) in F344/N rats (gavage studies). Technical Report 359. http://ntp-server.niehs.nih.gov.

National Toxicology Program, 1990a. Toxicology and carcinogenesis studies of d-limonene in F344/N rats and B6C3F1 mice (gavage studies). Technical Report 347. http://ntp-server.niehs.nih.gov.

National Toxicology Program, 1990b. Toxicology and carcinogenesis studies of benzaldehyde in F344/N rats and B6C3F1 mice (gavage studies). Technical Report 378. http://ntp-server.niehs.nih.gov.

National Toxicology Program, 1990c. Toxicology and carcinogenesis studies of d-carvone in B6C3F1 mice (gavage studies). Technical Report 381. http://ntp-server.niehs.nih.gov.

National Toxicology Program, 1991. Toxicity studies of cresols (CAS nos. 95-48-7, 108-39-4, 106-44-5) in F344/N rats and B6C3F1 mice (feed studies). Toxicity Report 9. http://ntp-server.niehs.nih.gov.

National Toxicology Program, 1992a. Developmental toxicity of d-camphor (CAS no. 464-49-3) in Sprague Dawley (CD®) rats. Technical Report 91018. http://ntp-server.niehs.nih.gov.

National Toxicology Program, 1992b. Developmental toxicity of d-camphor (CAS no. 464-49-3) in New Zealand white (NZW) rabbits. Technical Report 91019. http://ntp-server.niehs.nih.gov.

National Toxicology Program, 1993a. NTP Toxicology and carcinogenesis studies of coumarin (CAS No. 91-64-5) in F344/N rats and B6C3F1 mice (gavage studies). Technical Report 422. http://ntp-server.niehs.nih.gov.

National Toxicology Program, 1993b. Toxicology and carcinogenesis studies of benzyl acetate in F344/N rats and B6C3F1 mice (feed studies). Technical Report 431. http://ntp-server.niehs.nih.gov.

National Toxicology Program, 1994a. Developmental toxicity evaluation of 8-methoxypsoralen (CAS No. 298-81-7) administered by gavage to Sprague-Dawley (CD®) rats on gestational days 6 through 15. Technical Report 91017. http://ntp-server.niehs.nih.gov.

National Toxicology Program, 1994b. Developmental toxicity of 8-methoxypsoralen (CAS No. 298-81-7) in New Zealand white (NZW) rabbits. Technical Report 91016. http://ntp-server.niehs.nih.gov.

National Toxicology Program, 1995. NTP Toxicology and carcinogenesis studies of diethylphthalate (CAS No. 84-66-2) in F344/N rats and B6C3F1 mice (dermal studies) with dermal initiation/promotion study of diethylphthalate and dimethylphthalate (CAS No. 131-11-3) in male swiss (CD-1(R)) mice. Technical Report 429. http://ntp-server.niehs.nih.gov.

National Toxicology Program, 2000. Toxicology and carcinogenesis studies of methyleugenol (CAS No 93-15-2) in F344/N rats and B6C3F1 mice (gavage studies). Technical Report 491. http://ntp-server.niehs.nih.gov.

National Toxicology Program, 2003. NTP toxicology and carcinogenesis studies of citral (microencapsulated) (CAS No. 5392-40-5) in F344/N rats and B6C3F1 mice (feed studies). Technical Report 505. http://ntp-server.niehs.nih.gov.

National Toxicology Program, 2004. Toxicology and carcinogenesis studies of trans-cinnamaldehyde (CAS No. 14371-10-9) in F344/N rats and B6C3F1 mice (feed studies). Technical Report 514. http://ntp-server.niehs.nih.gov.

National Toxicology Program, 2005. Report on Carcinogens, eleventh ed. U.S. Department of Health and Human Services.http://ntp.niehs.nih.gov/ntp/roc/eleventh/profiles/s150pah.pdf.

National Toxicology Program, 2008a. NTP technical report on the 3-month toxicity studies of estragole (CAS No. 140-67-0) administered by gavage to F344/N rats and B6C3F1 mice. Toxicity Report 82. http://ntp-server.niehs.nih.gov.

National Toxicology Program, 2008b. NTP technical report on the toxicology and carcinogenesis studies of cresols (CAS No. 1319-77-3) in male F344/N rats and female B6C3F1 mice (feed studies). Technical Report 550. http://ntp-server.niehs.nih.gov.

National Toxicology Program, 2009. NTP technical report on the toxicology and carcinogenesis studies of pulegone (CAS No. 89-82-7) in F344/N rats and B6C3F1 mice (gavage studies). Technical Report 563. http://ntp-server.niehs.nih.gov.

National Toxicology Program, 2010a. NTP technical report on the toxicology and carcinogenesis studies of isoeugenol (CAS No. 97-54-1) in F344/N rats and B6C3F1 mice (gavage studies). Technical Report 551. http://ntp-server.niehs.nih.gov.

National Toxicology Program, 2010b. NTP technical report on the toxicology and carcinogenesis studies of β-myrcene (CAS No. 123-35-3) in F344/N rats and B6C3F1 mice (gavage studies). Technical Report 557. http://ntp-server.niehs.nih.gov.

National Toxicology Program, 2011. NTP technical report on the toxicology and carcinogenesis studies of α,β-thujone (CAS No. 76231-76-0) in F344/N rats and B6C3F1 mice (gavage studies). Technical Report 570. http://ntp-server.niehs.nih.gov.

Neale, A., 1893. Case of death following blue gum (Eucalyptus globulus) oil. The Australasian Medical Gazette 12, 115–116.

Nedbal, J., 1967. The effect of olfactory stimuli on seizure disposition in epilepsy. Zeitschrift Ärzneimittel Fortbild 61, 21–23.

Nelson, S.D., Gordon, W.P., 1983. Mammalian drug metabolism. J. Nat. Prod. 46, 71–78.

Nelson, S.D., McClanahan, R.H., Thomassen, D., et al., 1992a. Investigations of mechanisms of reactive metabolite formation from R-(+)-pulegone. Xenobiotica 22, 1157–1164.

Nelson, S.D., McClanahan, R.H., Knebel, N., et al., 1992b. The metabolism of (R)-(+)-pulegone, a toxic monoterpene. Environmental Science Research 44, 287–296.

Nesnow, S., 1990. International Commission for Protection Against Environmental Mutagens and Carcinogens. ICPEMC Working Paper 1/2. A multi-factor ranking scheme for comparing the carcinogenic activity of chemicals. Mutat. Res. 239, 83–115.

Nesslany, F., Marzin, D., 1999. A micromethod for the in vitro micronucleus assay. Mutagenesis 14, 403–410.

Nestmann, E.R., Lee, E.G., 1983. Mutagenicity of constituents of pulp and paper mill effluent in growing cells of Saccharomyces cerevisiae. Mutat. Res. 119, 273–280.

Nethercott, J.R., Nield, G., Holness, D.L., 1989. A review of 79 cases of eyelid dermatitis. J. Am. Acad. Dermatol. 21, 223–230.

Nethercott, J.R., Holness, D.L., Adams, R.M., et al., 1991. Patch testing with a routine screening tray in North America, 1985 through 1989: I. Frequency of response. Am. J. Contact Dermat. 2, 122–129.

Neto, M.A., Alencar, J.W., Cunha, A.N., et al., 1994. Volatile constituents of *Psidium pohlianum* Berg. and *Psidium guyanensis* Pers. Journal of Essential Oil Research 6, 299–300.

Nettelblad, H., Vahlqvist, C., Krysander, L., et al., 1996. Psoralens used for cosmetic sun tanning: an unusual cause of extensive burn injury. Burns 22, 633–635.

Neubert, D., Chahoud, I., Platzek, T., et al., 1987. Principles and problems in assessing prenatal toxicity. Arch. Toxicol. 60, 238–245.

Neudecker, T., Henschler, D., 1985. Allyl isothiocyanate is mutagenic in *Salmonella typhimurium*. Mutat. Res. 156, 33–37.

Neudecker, T., Öhrlein, K., Eder, E., et al., 1983. Effect of methyl and halogen substitutions in the αC position on the mutagenicity of cinnamaldehyde. Mutat. Res. 110, 1–8.

Neustaedter, R., 2007. http://www.cure-guide.com/Natural_Health_Newsletter/Lavender_Dangers/lavender_dangers.html.

Neves, A., Rosa, S., Gonçalves, J., et al., 2010. Screening of Five essential oils for identification of potential inhibitors of IL-1-induced Nf-kappaB activation and NO production in human chondrocytes: characterization of the inhibitory activity of alpha-pinene. Planta Med. 76, 303–308.

Newberne, P.M., Carlton, W.W., Brown, W.R., 1989. Histopathological evaluation of proliferative liver lesions in rats fed *trans*-anethole in chronic studies. Food Chem. Toxicol. 27, 21–26.

Newberne, P., Smith, R.L., Doull, J., et al., 1999. The FEMA GRAS assessment of *trans*-anethole used as a flavouring substance. Food Chem. Toxicol. 37, 789–811.

Newsham, J., Rai, S., Williams, J.D., 2011. Two cases of allergic contact dermatitis to neroli oil. Br. J. Dermatol. 165 (Suppl. 1), 76.

Ngassoum, M.B., Yonkeu, S., Jirovetz, L., et al., 1999. Chemical composition of essential oils of *Lantana camara* leaves and flowers from Cameroon and Madagascar. Flavour & Fragrance Journal 14, 245–250.

Nguyen, S.H., Dang, T.P., MacPherson, C., et al., 2008. Prevalence of patch test results from 1970 to 2002 in a multi-centre population in North America (NACDG). Contact Dermatitis 58, 101–106.

Nibret, E., Wink, M., 2010. Trypanocidal and antileukaemic effects of the essential oils of *Hagenia abyssinica*, *Leonotis ocymifolia*, *Moringa stenopetala*, and their main individual constituents. Phytomedicine 17, 911–920.

Nielsen, J.B., 2006. Natural oils affect the human skin integrity and the percutaneous penetration of benzoic acid dose-dependently. Basic Clin. Pharmaol. Toxicol. 98, 575–581.

Nielsen, J.B., 2008. What you see may not always be what you get - bioavailability and extrapolation from in vitro tests. Toxicol. In Vitro 22, 1038–1042.

Nielsen, N.H., Menné, T., 1992. Allergic contact sensitization in an unselected Danish population: The Glostrup Allergy Study, Denmark. Acta Derm. Venereol. 72, 456–460.

Nielsen, J.B., Nielsen, F., 2006. Topical use of tea tree oil reduces the dermal absorption of benzoic acid and methiocarb. Arch. Dermatol. Res. 297, 395–402.

Nielsen, G.D., Hougaard, K.S., Larsen, S.T., 1999. Acute airway effects of formaldehyde and ozone in BALB/c mice. Hum. Exp. Toxicol. 18, 400–409.

Nielsen, J.B., Nielsen, F., Sørensen, J.A., 2004. *In vitro* percutaneous penetration of five pesticides - effects of molecular weight and solubility characteristics. Ann. Occup. Hyg. 48, 697–705.

Nielsen, G.D., Larsen, S.T., Hougaard, K.S., et al., 2005. Mechanisms of acute inhalation effects of (+) and (-)-alpha-pinene in BALB/c mice. Basic Clin. Pharmacol. Toxicol. 96, 420–428.

Nielsen, G.D., Wolkoff, P., Alarie, Y., 2007a. Sensory irritation: risk assessment approaches. Regul. Toxicol. Pharmacol. 48, 6–18.

Nielsen, G.D., Larsen, S.T., Olsen, O., et al., 2007b. Do indoor chemicals promote development of airway allergy? Indoor Air 17, 236–255.

Niesink, R.J.M., de Vries, J., Hollinger, M.A. (Eds.), 1996. Toxicology: principles and practice. CRC Press, Boca Raton.

Nigg, H.N., Nordby, H.E., Beier, R.C., et al., 1993. Phototoxic coumarins in limes. Food Chem. Toxicol. 31, 331–335.

Niknahad, H., Shuhendler, A., Galati, G., et al., 2003. Modulating carbonyl cytotoxicity in intact rat hepatocytes by inhibiting carbonyl metabolizing enzymes. II. Aromatic aldehydes. Chem. Biol. Interact. 143–144, 119–128.

Nilsson, U., Bergh, M., Shao, L.P., et al., 1996. Analysis of contact allergenic compounds in oxidized *d*-limonene. Chromatographia 42, 199–205.

Nilsson, A.M., Jonsson, C., Luthman, K., et al., 2004. Inhibition of the sensitizing effect of carvone by the addition of non-allergenic compounds. Acta Derm. Venereol. 84, 99–105.

NIOSH (National Institute for Occupational Safety & Health), 1977. Registry of toxic effects of chemical substances, vol. 2 179. Fairchild, E. J., Lewis, R.J., Tatken, R.L. (Eds.). NIOSH, Cincinnati.

Nishie, K., Daxenbichler, M.E., 1980. Toxicology of glucosinolates, related compounds (nitriles, R-goitrin, isothiocyanates) and vitamin U found in cruciferal. Food Cosmet. Toxicol. 18, 159–172.

Nishihara, T., Nishikawa, J., Kanayama, T., et al., 2000. Estrogenic activities of 517 chemicals by yeast two-hybrid assay. J. Health Sci. 46, 282–298.

Nishikawa, Y., Okabe, M., Yoshimoto, K., et al., 1976. Chemical and biochemical studies on carbohydrate esters. II. Antitumor activity of saturated fatty acids and their ester derivatives against Ehrlich ascites carcinoma. Chem. Pharm. Bull. (Tokyo) 24, 387–393.

Nishimura, M., Ishihara, M., Itoh, M., et al., 1984. Results of patch tests on cosmetic ingredients conducted between 1979 and 1982. Skin Research 26, 945–954.

Nissen, L., Zatta, A., Stefanini, I., et al., 2010. Characterization and antimicrobial activity of essential oils of industrial hemp varieties (*Cannabis sativa*). Fitoterapia 81, 413–419.

Nivsarkar, M., Kumar, G.P., Laloraya, M., 1996. Metal binding and resultant loss of phototoxicity of alpha-terthienyl: metal detoxification versus alpha-terthienyl inactivation. Bulletin of Enviromental Contamination Toxicology 56, 183–189.

NLM, 1997. Registry of toxic effects of chemical substances. National Library of Medicine, Bethesda.

Nogueira, A.C., Carvalho, R.R., Souza, C.A., et al., 1995. Study on the embryofeto-toxicity of citral in the rat. Toxicology 96, 105–112.

Nohmi, T., Miyata, R., Yoshikawa, K., et al., 1985. Mutagenicity tests on organic chemical contaminants in city water and related compounds I. Bacterial mutagenicity tests. Eisei Shikenjo Hokoku 103, 60–64.

Nøjgaard, J.K., Christensen, K.B., Wolkoff, P., 2005. The effect on human eye blink frequency of exposure to limonene oxidation products and methacrolein. Toxicol. Lett. 156, 241–251.

Noleau, I., Richard, H., Peyroux, A.S., 1991. Volatile compounds in leek and asafoetida. Journal of Essential Oil Research 3, 241–256.

Nolte, D.L., Provenza, F.D., Callan, R., et al., 1992. Garlic in the ovine fetal environment. Physiol. Behav. 52, 1091–1093.

Nomura, Y, Mitsui, N., Bhawal, U.K., et al., 2006. Estrogenic activity of phthalate esters by in vitro VTG assay using primary-cultured *Xenopus* hepatocytes. Dent. Mater. J. 25, 533–537.

Norbäck, D., Bjornsson, E., Janson, C., et al., 1995. Asthmatic symptoms and volatile organic compounds, formaldehyde, and carbon dioxide in dwellings. Occup. Environ. Med. 52, 388–395.

Norppa, H., Vaino, H., 1983. Induction of sister-chromatid exchanges by styrene analogues in cultured human lymphocytes. Mutat. Res. 116, 379–387.

Northover, B.J., Verghese, J., 1962. The pharmacology of certain terpene alcohols and oxides. Journal of Scientific & Industrial Research 21C, 342–345.

Nosbaum, A., Ben Said, B., Halpern, S.J., et al., 2011. Systemic allergic contact dermatitis due to black cumin essential oil expressing as generalized erythema multiforme. Eur. J. Dermatol. 21, 447–448.

Novak, E., Stubbs, S.S., Sanborn, E.C., et al., 1972. The tolerance and safety of intravenously administered benzyl alcohol in methylprednisolone sodium succinate formulations in normal human subjects. Toxicol. Appl. Pharmacol. 23, 54–61.

Nozaki, Y., 2001. Clinical studies of essential oil of *Pelargonium graveolens*. Aroma Research 2, 61–65.

NTIS, 1976. Teratologic evaluation of FDA 71-28 (oil of nutmeg). Food & Drug Research Labs Inc. National Technical Information Service.

Nutley, B.P., Farmer, P., Caldwell, J., 1994. Metabolism of *trans*-cinnamic acid in the rat and mouse and its variation with dose. Food Cosmet. Toxicol. 32, 877–886.

Nutrition International, 1990. First world congress on the health significance of garlic and garlic constituents. Nutrition International, Washington.

Nuwayser, E.S., Gay, M.H., DeRoo, D.J., et al., 1988. Proceedings of the 15th international symposium on controlled release of bioactive materials. August 15–19, Chicago, Illinois, pp. 213–214.

Oberly, T.J., Michaelis, K.C., Rexroat, M.A., et al., 1993. A comparison of the CHO/HGPRT+ and the L5178Y/TK+/- mutation assays using suspension treatment and soft agar cloning: results for 10 chemicals. Cell Biol. Toxicol. 9, 243–257.

Ocete, M.A., Risco, S., Zarzuelo, A., et al., 1989. Pharmacological activity of the essential oil of *Bupleurum gibraltaricum*: anti-inflammatory activity and effects on isolated rat uteri. J. Ethnopharmacol. 25, 305–313.

Ochiai, H., Niwayama, S., Masuyama, K., 1986. Inhibition of experimental pulmonary metastasis in mice by *beta*-cyclodextrin-benzaldehyde. J. Cancer Res. Clin. Oncol. 112, 216–220.

Oda, Y., Hamano, Y., Inoue, K., et al., 1978. Mutagenicity of food flavours in bacteria (1st report). Osaka-furitsu Koshu Eisei Kenkyu Hokoku Shokuhin Eisei Hen 9, 177–181.

Odeyemi, O.O., Yakubu, M.T., Masika, P.J., et al., 2008. Effect of administration of the essential oil from *Tagetes minuta* L. leaves in Wistar rats. J. Biol. Sci. 8, 1067–1071.

OECD, 2001. OECD guideline for the testing of chemicals: proposal for updating guideline 414. Prenatal developmental toxicity study. www.oecd.org/dataoecd/18/15/1948482.pdf.

Oesch, F., Fabian, E., Oesch-Bartlomowicz, B., et al., 2007. Drug-metabolizing enzymes in the skin of man, rat and pig. Drug Metab. Rev. 39, 659–698.

Ogata, A., Ando, H., Kubo, Y., et al., 1999. Teratogenicity of thujaplicin in ICR mice. Food Chem. Toxicol. 37, 1097–1104.

Ogawa, K., Hirose, M., Sugiura, S., et al., 2001. Dose-dependent promotion by phenylethyl isothiocyanate, a known chemopreventer, of two-stage rat urinary bladder and liver carcinogenesis. Nutr. Cancer 40, 134–139.

Ogawa, Y., Akamatsu, M., Hotta, Y., et al., 2010. Effect of essential oils, such as raspberry ketone and its derivatives, on antiandrogenic activity based on in vitro reporter gene assay. Bioorg. Med. Chem. Lett. 20, 2111–2114.

Oh, H.J., Oh, Y.K., Kim, C.K., 2001. Effects of vehicles and enhancers on transdermal delivery of melatonin. Int. J. Pharm. 212, 63–71.

Ohnishi, M., Yoshimi, N., Kawamori, T., et al., 1997. Inhibitory effects of dietary protocatechuic acid and costunolide on 7,12-dimethylbenz[a]anthracene-induced hamster cheek pouch carcinogenesis. Jpn. J. Cancer Res. 88, 111–119.

Ohno, Y., Sekigawa, S., Yamamoto, H., et al., 1978. Additive toxicity test of sorbic acid and benzoic acid in rats. Journal of Nara Medical Association 29, 695–708.

Ohsumi, T., Higashi, S., Ozumi, K., et al., 1996. Study on allergic contact dermatitis of eugenol in guinea pig. Oral Therapeutics & Pharmacology 15, 63–68.

Ohta, T., 1995. Mechanisms of antimutagenic action of flavorings. Kankyo Hen'igen Kenkyu [Environmental Mutagen Research Communications] 17, 23–33.

Ohta, T., Watanabe, K., Moriya, M., et al., 1983a. Antimutagenic effects of cinnamaldehyde on chemical mutagenesis in *Escherichia coli*. Mutat. Res. 107, 219–227.

Ohta, T., Watanabe, K., Moriya, M., et al., 1983b. Analysis of the antimutagenic effect of cinnamaldehyde on chemically induced mutagenesis in *Escherichia coli*. Mol. Gen. Genet. 192, 309–315.

Ohta, T., Watanabe, M., Watanabe, K., et al., 1986. Inhibitory effects of flavourings on mutagenesis induced by chemicals in bacteria. Food Chem. Toxicol. 24, 51–54.

Ohta, T., Imagawa, T., Ito, S., 2007. Novel agonistic action of mustard oil on recombinant and endogenous porcine transient receptor potential V1 (pTRPV1) channels. Biochem. Pharmacol. 73, 1646–1656.

Oikawa, A., Tohda, H., Kanai, M., et al., 1980. Inhibitors of poly(adenosine diphosphate ribose) polymerase induce sister chromatid exchanges. Biochem. Biophys. Res. Commun. 97, 1311–1316.

Ojala, T., Vuorela, P., Kiviranta, J., et al., 1999. A bioassay using *Artemia salina* for detecting phototoxicity of plant coumarins. Planta. Med. 65, 715–718.

Ojiambo, H.P., 1971a. Certain aspects of metabolism in myopathies induced by methyl salicylate intoxication in the dog. East. Afr. Med. J. 48 (6), 243–246.

Ojiambo, H.P., 1971b. Methyl salicylate myopathy in man. East. Afr. Med. J. 48 (12), 735–740.

Ojima, M., Tonori, H., Sato, T., et al., 2002. Odor perception in patients with multiple chemical sensitivity. Tohoku J. Exp. Med. 198, 163–173.

Okabe, H., Takayama, K., Ogura, A., et al., 1989. Effect of limonene and related compounds on the percutaneous absorption of indomethacin. Drug Des. Deliv. 4, 313–321.

Okada, N., Hirata, A., Murakami, Y., et al., 2005. Induction of cytotoxicity and apoptosis and inhibition of cyclooxygenase-2 gene expression by eugenol-related compounds. Anticancer Res. 25, 3263–3269.

Okazaki, K., Yamagishi, M., Son, H.Y., et al., 2002. Simultaneous treatment with benzyl isothiocyanate, a strong bladder promoter, inhibits rat urinary bladder carcinogenesis by N-butyl-N-(4-hydroxybutyl)nitrosamine. Nutr. Cancer 42, 211–216.

Okuyama, E., Umeyama, K., Saito, Y., et al., 1993. Ascaridole as a pharmacologically active principle of "Paico", a medicinal Peruvian plant. Chemical & Pharmaceutical Bulletin (Tokyo) 41, 1309–1311.

O'Mullane, N.M., Joyce, P., Kamath, S.V., et al., 1982. Adverse CNS effects of menthol-containing Olbas Oil. Lancet 1, 1121.

Olney, J.W., 2002. New insights and new issues in developmental neurotoxicology. Neurotoxicology 23, 659–668.

Olowe, S.A., Ransome-Kuti, O., 1980. The risk of jaundice in glucose-6-phosphate dehydrogenase deficient babies exposed to menthol. Acta Paediatr. Scand. 69, 341–345.

Olsen, P., Thorup, I., 1984. Neurotoxicity in rats dosed with peppermint oil and pulegone. Arch. Toxicol. Suppl. 7, 408–409.

Onder, M., Adisen, E., 2008. Patch test results in a Turkish paediatric population. Contact Dermatitis 58, 63–65.

Ong, T.P., Heidor, R., de Conti, A., et al., 2006. Farnesol and geraniol chemopreventive activities during the initial phases of hepatocarcinogenesis involve similar actions on cell proliferation and DNA damage, but distinct actions on apoptosis, plasma cholesterol and HMGCoA reductase. Carcinogenesis 27, 1194–1203.

Opdyke, D.L.J., 1973. Monographs on fragrance raw materials. Food Cosmet. Toxicol. 11 (Suppl).

Opdyke, D.L.J., 1974. Monographs on fragrance raw materials. Food Cosmet. Toxicol. 12 (Suppl).

Opdyke, D.L.J., 1975. Monographs on fragrance raw materials. Food Cosmet. Toxicol. 13 (Suppl).

Opdyke, D.L.J., 1976. Monographs on fragrance raw materials. Food Cosmet. Toxicol. 14 (Suppl).

Opdyke, D.L.J., 1977a. Monographs on fragrance raw materials. Food Cosmet. Toxicol. 15 (Suppl).

Opdyke, D.L.J., 1977b. Safety testing of fragrances: problems and implications. Clin. Toxicol. 10 (1), 61–77.

Opdyke, D.L.J., 1978. Monographs on fragrance raw materials. Food Cosmet. Toxicol. 16 (Suppl).

Opdyke, D.L.J., 1979a. Monographs on fragrance raw materials. Food Cosmet. Toxicol. 17 (Suppl).

Opdyke, D.L.J., 1979b. Monographs on fragrance raw materials. Food Cosmet. Toxicol. 17, 325–433.

Opdyke, D.L.J., Letizia, C., 1982. Monographs on fragrance raw materials. Food Cosmet. Toxicol. 20 (Suppl).

Opdyke, D.L.J., Letizia, C., 1983. Monographs on fragrance raw materials. Food Cosmet. Toxicol. 21, .

Opiekun, R.E., Smeets, M., Sulewski, M., et al., 2003. Assessment of ocular and nasal irritation in asthmatics resulting from fragrance exposure. Clin. Exp. Allergy 33, 1256–1265.

Orafidiya, L.O., 1993. The effect of autoxidation of lemongrass oil on its antibacterial activity. Phytother. Res. 7, 269–271.

Orani, G.P., Anderson, J.W., Sant'Ambrogio, G., et al., 1991. Upper airway cooling and l-menthol reduce ventilation in the guinea pig. J. Appl. Physiol. 70, 2080–2086.

Orav, A., Kuningas, K., Kailas, T., 1995. Computerized capillary gas chromatographic identification and determination of Siberian fir oil constituents. J. Chromatogr. 697, 495–499.

Orav, A., Kalias, T., Liiv, M., 1996. Analysis of terpenoic composition of conifer needle oils by steam distillation/extraction gas chromatography and gas chromatography-mass spectrometry. Chromatographia 43, 215–219.

Orr, J., Edin, S., 1906. Eucalyptus poisoning. Br. Med. J. 1, 1085.

Ortel, B., Maytum, D.J., Gange, R.W., 1991. Long persistence of monofunctional 8-methoxypsoralen-DNA adducts in human skin *in vivo*. Photochem. Photobiol. 54, 645–650.

Orton, D.I., Shaw, S., 2001. Sorbitan sesquioleate as an allergen. Contact Dermatitis 44, 190–191.

Osato, S., 1965. Chemotherapy of human carcinoma with citronellal and citral and their action on carcinoma tissue in its histological aspects up to healing. Tohoku J. Exp. Med. 86, 102–147.

Osato, S., Mori, H., Morita, M., 1961. Electron microscopy of cancer cells under the action of the chemotherapeutic agents. Tohoku J. Exp. Med. 75, 17.

Oser, B.L., Carson, S., Oser, M., 1965. Toxicological tests on flavouring matters. Food Cosmet. Toxicol. 3, 563–569.

Oshiro, Y., Balwierz, P.S., Eurell, T.E., et al., 1998. Exploration of the transformation potential of a unique male rat protein alpha2u-globulin using hamster embryonic cells. Toxicol. Pathol. 26, 381–387.

Osmundsen, P.E., 1970. Pigmented contact dermatitis. Br. J. Dermatol. 83, 296–301.

Ososki, A.L., Kennelly, E.J., 2003. Phytoestrogens: a review of the present state of research. Phytother. Res. 17, 845–869.

Ostad, S.N., Soodi, M., Shariffzadeh, M., et al., 2001. The effect of fennel essential oil on uterine contraction as a model for dysmenorrhea: pharmacology & toxicology study. J. Ethnopharmacol. 76, 299–304.

Ostad, S.N., Khakinegad, B., Sabzevari, O., 2004. Evaluation of the teratogenicity of fennel essential oil (FEO) on the rat embryo limb buds culture. Toxicol. In Vitro 18, 623–627.

Osterhoudt, K.C., Lee, S.K., Callahan, J.M., et al., 1997. Catnip and the alteration of human consciousness. Vet. Hum. Toxicol. 39, 373–375.

Oswald, E.O., Fishbein, L., Corbett, B.J., 1969. Metabolism of naturally occurring propenylbenzene derivatives. I. Chromatographic separation of ninhydrin-positive materials of rat urine. J. Chromatogr 45, 437–445.

Oswald, E.O., Fishbein, L., Corbett, B.J., 1971. Urinary excretion of tertiary aminomethoxy methylenedioxy propiophenones as metabolites of myristicin in the rat and guinea pig. Biochim. Biophys. Acta 244, 322–328.

Otto, D., Molhave, L., Rose, G., et al., 1990. Neurobehavioral and sensory irritant effects of controlled exposure to a complex mixture of volatile organic compounds. Neurotoxicol. Teratol. 12, 649–652.

Ou, C.N., Tsai, C.H., Tapley, K.J., et al., 1978. Photobinding of 8-methoxypsoralen and 5,7-dimethoxycoumarin to DNA and its effect on template activity. Biochemistry 17, 1047–1053.

Overman, D.O., White, J.A., 1983. Comparative teratogenic effects of methyl salicylate applied orally or topically to hamsters. Teratology 421–426.

Owlia, P., Rasooli, I., Saderi, H., 2007. Antistreptococcal and antioxidant activity of essential oil from *Matricaria chamomilla* L. Research Journal of Biological Sciences 2, 155–160.

Owston, E., Lough, R., 1981. A 90-day toxicity study of phenylethyl alcohol in the rat. Food Cosmet. Toxicol. 19, 713–715.

Oyen, L.P., Dung, N.X. (Eds.), 1999. Plant resources of South-East Asia. Backhuys, Leiden.

Özbek, H., Ugras, S., Dülger, H., et al., 2003. Hepatoprotective effect of *Foeniculum vulgare* essential oil. Fitoterapia 74, 317–319.

Özden, M.G., Oztas, P., Oztas, M.O., et al., 2001. Allergic contact dermatitis from *Laurus nobilis* (laurel) oil. Contact Dermatitis 45, 178.

Özgüven, M., Tansi, S., 1998. Drug yield and essential oil of *Thymus vulgaris* L. as influenced by ecological and ontogenetical variation. Turkish Journal of Agriculture & Forestry 22, 537–542.

Packman, E.W., Abbott, D.D., Wagner, B.M., et al., 1961. Chronic oral toxicity of oil sweet birch (methyl salicylate). Pharmacologist 3, 62.

Padma, P.R., Amonkar, A.J., Bhide, S.V., 1989a. Antimutagenic effects of betel leaf extract against the mutagenicity of two tobacco-specific N-nitrosamines. Mutagenesis 4, 154–156.

Padma, P.R., Lalitha, V.S., Amonkar, A.J., et al., 1989b. Anticarcinogenic effect of betel leaf extract against tobacco carcinogens. Cancer Lett. 45, 195–202.

Padmakumari, K.P., Sasidharan, I., Sreekumar, M.M., 2011. Composition and antioxidant activity of essential oil of pimento (*Pimenta dioica* (L) Merr.) from Jamaica. Nat. Prod. Res. 25, 152–160.

Paek, S.H., Kim, G.J., Jeong, H.S., et al., 1996. ar Turmerone and β-atlantone induce internucleosomal DNA fragmentation associated with programmed cell death in human myeloid leukaemia HL-60 cells. Arch. Pharm. Res. 19, 91–94.

Pages, N., Salazar, M., Chamorro, G., et al., 1988. Teratological evaluation of *Plectranthus fruticosus* leaf essential oil. Planta Med. 54, 296–298.

Pages, N., Fournier, G., Le Luyer, F., et al., 1989a. Les échantillons commerciaux de 'sabine' (rameaux feuilles et huile essentielle) sont-ils tératogènes? Étude chez la souris. Plantes Medicinales et Phytothérapie 23 (3), 186–192.

Pages, N., Fournier, G., Chamorro, G., et al., 1989b. Teratological evaluation of *Juniperus sabina* essential oil in mice. Planta Med. 55, 144–146.

Pages, N., Fournier, G., Le Luyer, F., et al., 1990. Les huiles essentielles et leurs propriétés tératogènes potentielles: example de l'huile essentielle d'eucalyptus étude préliminaire chez la souris. Plantes Medicinales et Phytothérapie 24, 21–26.

Pages, N., Fournier, G., Chamorro, G., et al., 1991. Teratogenic effects of *Plectranthus fruticosus* essential oil in mice. Phytother. Res. 5, 94–96.

Pages, N., Fournier, G., Velut, V., et al., 1992. Potential teratogenicity in mice of the essential oil of *Salvia lavandulifolia* Vahl. Study of a fraction rich in sabinyl acetate. Phytother. Res. 6, 80–83.

Pages, N., Fournier, G., Baduel, C., et al., 1996. Sabinyl acetate, the main component of *Juniperus Sabina* L'Hérit. essential oil, is responsible for antiimplantation effect. Phytother. Res. 10, 438–440.

Pages, N., Maurois, P., Delplanque, B., et al., 2010. Activities of α-asarone in various animal seizure models and in biochemical assays might be essentially accounted for by antioxidant properties. Neurosci. Res. 68, 337–344.

Paine, M.F., Criss, A.B., Watkins, P.B., 2005. Two major grapefruit juice components differ in time to onset of intestinal CYP3A4 inhibition. J. Pharm. Exp. Ther. 1151–1160.

Paini, A., Punt, A., Viton, F., et al., 2010. A physiologically based biodynamic (PBBD) model for estragole DNA binding in rat liver based on in vitro kinetic data and estragole DNA adduct formation in primary hepatocytes. Toxicol. Appl. Pharmacol. 245, 57–66.

Pal, D., Banerjee, S., Mukherjee, S., et al., 2010. Eugenol restricts DMBA croton oil induced skin carcinogenesis in mice: downregulation of c-Myc and H-ras, and activation of p53 dependent apoptotic pathway. J. Dermatol. Sci. 59, 31–39.

Palkin, S., Wells, P.A., 1933. Composition of the non-phenol portion of bay oil. J. Am. Chem. Soc. 55, 1549–1556.

Panayotopoulos, D.J., Chisholm, D.D., 1970. Hallucinogenic effect of nutmeg. Br. Med. J. 1, 754.

Pandey, B.N., Mishra, K.P., 2004. Modification of thymocytes membrane radiooxidative damage and apoptosis by eugenol. J. Environ. Pathol. Toxicol. Oncol. 23, 117 122.

Panigrahi, G.B., Rao, A.R., 1984. Induction of *in vivo* sister chromatid exchanges by arecaidine, a betel nut alkaloid, in mouse bone-marrow cells. Cancer Lett. 23, 189–192.

Papa, C.M., Shelly, W.B., 1964. Menthol hypersensitivity. J. Am. Med. Assoc. 189, 546–548.

Papageorgiou, C., Corbet, J.P., Menezes-Brandao, F., et al., 1983. Allergic contact dermatitis to garlic (*Allium sativum* L.). Identification of the allergens: the role of mono-, di-, and trisulfides present in garlic. Arch. Dermatol. Res. 275, 229–234.

Papavassiliou, M.J., 1935. Sur deux cas d'intoxication par la sabine la perméabilité placentaire a l'essence de sabine. Société de Médecine Légale 15, 778–781.

Papavassiliou, M.J., Eliakis, C., 1937. Rue as an abortifacient and poison. Ann. Méd. Lég. Criminol. Police Sci. Toxicol. 17, 993–999.

Parejo, I., Viladomat, F., Bastida, J., et al., 2002. Comparison between the radical scavenging activity and antioxidant activity of six distilled and nondistilled mediterranean herbs and aromatic plants. J. Agric. Food Chem. 50, 6882–6890.

Parish, R.A., McIntire, S., Heimbach, D.M., 1987. Garlic burns: a naturopathic remedy gone awry. Pediatr. Emerg. Care 3, 258–259.

Park, H.J., Kwon, S.H., Han, Y.N., et al., 2001. Apoptosis-Inducing costunolide and a novel acyclic monoterpene from the stem bark of *Magnolia sieboldii*. Archives of Pharmaceutical Research 24, 342–348.

Park, B.S., Lee, K.G., Shibamoto, T., et al., 2003. Antioxidant activity and characterization of volatile constituents of Taheebo (*Tabebuia impetiginosa* Martius ex DC). J. Agric. Food Chem. 51, 295–300.

Park, E.J., Kim, S.H., Kim, B.J., et al., 2009. Menthol enhances an antiproliferative activity of 1alpha,25-dihydroxyvitamin D(3) in LNCaP Cells. Journal of Clinical Biochemistry & Nutrition 44, 125–130.

Park, K.R., Lee, J.H., Choi, C., et al., 2007. Suppression of interleukin-2 gene expression by isoeugenol is mediated through down-regulation of NF-AT and NF-kappaB. Int. Immunopharmacol. 7, 1251–1258.

Parke, D.V., Rahman, H., 1969. The effects of some terpenoids and other dietary anutrients on hepatic drug-metabolizing enzymes. Proceedings of the Biochemical Society 113, 12P.

Parke, D.V., Rahman, H., 1970. The induction of hepatic microsomal enzymes by safrole. Proceedings of the Biochemical Society 119, 53P–54P.

Parke, D.V., Rahman, K.H., Walker, R., 1974a. Effect of linalool on hepatic drug-metabolizing enzymes in rhe rat. Biochem. Soc. Trans. 2, 615–618.

Parke, D.V., Rahman, K.H., Walker, R., 1974b. The absorption, distribution and excretion of linalool in the rat. Biochem. Soc. Trans. 2, 612–615.

Parry, E.J., 1922. The chemistry of essential oils and artificial perfumes, vols. 1 and 2. Scott, Greenwood, London.

Parsons, B.J., 1980. Psoralen photochemistry. Photochem. Photobiol. 32, 813–821.

Parys, B.T., 1983. Chemical burns resulting from contact with peppermint oil mar: a case report. Burns 9, 374–375.

Passos, G.F., Fernandes, E.S., Da Cunha, F.M., et al., 2006. Anti-inflammatory and anti-allergic properties of the essential oil and active compounds from *Cordia verbenacea*. J. Ethnopharmacol. 110, 323–333.

Patel, S., Wiggins, J., 1980. Eucalyptus oil poisoning. Arch. Dis. Child. 5, 405–406.

Patel, T., Ishiuji, Y., Yosipovitch, G., 2007. Menthol: A refreshing look at this ancient compound. J. Am. Acad. Dermatol. 57, 873–878.

Patel, B., Groom, L., Prasad, V., et al., 2008. Parental poison prevention practices and their relationship with perceived toxicity: cross-sectional study. Inj. Prev. 14, 389–395.

Pathak, M.A., Fitzpatrick, T.B., 1959. Bioassay of natural and synthetic furocoumarins (psoralens). J. Invest. Dermatol. 32, 509–518.

Pathak, M.A., Fitzpatrick, T.B., 1992. The evolution of photochemotherapy with psoralens and UVA (PUVA): 2000 BC to 1992 AD. J. Photochem. Photobiol. B 14, 3–22.

Pathak, M.A., Zarebska, Z., Mihm, M.C., et al., 1986. Detection of DNA-psoralen photoadducts in mammalian skin. J. Invest. Dermatol. 86, 308–315.

Pathak, S., Wanjari, M.M., Jain, S.K., et al., 2010. Evaluation of antiseizure activity of essential oil from the roots of *Angelica archangelica* Linn. in mice. Indian Journal of Pharmaceutical Sciences 72, 371–375.

Patlewicz, G., Basketter, D.A., Smith, C.K., et al., 2001. Skin-sensitization structure-activity relationships for aldehydes. Contact Dermatitis 44, 331–336.

Patlewicz, G.Y., Basketter, D.A., Smith Pease, C.K., et al., 2004. Further evaluation of quantitative structure-activity relationship models for the prediction of the skin sensitization potency of selected fragrance allergens. Contact Dermatitis 50, 91–97.

Patoir, A., Patoir, G., Bédrine, H., 1936. Le rôle abortif de l'apiol. Paris Méd. 3, 442–446.

Patoir, A., et al., 1938a. Action toxique de l'essence de sabine et de l'armoise sur l'organisme. Comptes Rendues Société Biologique 127, 1325–1326.

Patoir, A., Patoir, G., Bédrine, H., 1938b. Note sur l'action de l'essence de rue sur l'organisme animal. Comptes Rendues Société Biologique 127, 1324–1325.

Patton, D.W., Ferguson, M.M., Forsyth, A., et al., 1985. Oro-facial granulomatosis: a possible allergic basis. Br. J. Oral Maxillofac. Surg. 23, 235–242.

Paulsen, E., Andersen, K.E., Carlsen, L., et al., 1993a. Carvone: an overlooked contact allergen cross-reacting with sesquiterpene lactones? Contact Dermatitis 29, 138–143.

Paulsen, E., Andersen, K.E., Hausen, B.M., 1993b. Compositae dermatitis in a Danish dermatology department in one year (I). Results of routine patch testing with the sesquiterpene lactone mix supplemented with aimed patch testing with extracts and sesquiterpene lactones of Compositae plants. Contact Dermatitis 29, 6–10.

Paulsen, E., Sogaard, J., Andersen, K.E., 1998. Occupational dermatitis in Danish gardeners and greenhouse workers (III). Compositae-related symptoms. Contact Dermatitis 38, 140–146.

Paulsen, E., Andersen, K.E., 2005. Colophonium and Compositae mix as markers of fragrance allergy: cross-reactivity between fragrance terpenes, colophonium and compositae plant extracts. 53, 285–291.

Paumgartten, F.J., Delgado, I.F., Alves, E.N., et al., 1990. Single dose toxicity study of β-myrcene, a natural analgesic substance. Braz. J. Med. Biol. Res. 23, 873–877.

Paumgartten, F.J., De-Carvalho, R.R., Souza, C.A., et al., 1998. Study of the effects of β-myrcene on rat fertility and general reproductive performance. Braz. J. Med. Biol. Res. 31, 955–965.

Pavlidou, V., Karpouhtsis, I., Franzios, G., et al., 2004. Insecticidal and genotoxic effects of essential oils of Greek sage, *Salvia fruticosa*, and mint, *Mentha pulegium*, on *Drosophila melanogaster* and *Bactrocera oleae* (Diptera: Tephritidae). J. Agric. Urban Entomol. 21, 39–49.

Payne, R.B., 1963. Nutmeg intoxication. N. Engl. J. Med. 269, 36–38.

Peamkrasatam, S., Sriwatanakul, K., Kiyotani, K., et al., 2006. *In vivo* evaluation of coumarin and nicotine as probe drugs to predict the metabolic capacity of CYP2A6 due to genetic polymorphism in Thais. Drug Metab. Pharmacokinet. 21, 475–484.

Pearce, A.L., Finlay-Jones, J.J., Hart, P.H., 2005. Reduction of nickel-induced contact hypersensitivity reactions by topical tea tree oil in humans. Inflamm. Res. 54, 22–30.

Pearson, D.A., Frankel, E.N., Aeschbach, R., et al., 1997. Inhibition of endothelial cell-mediated oxidation of low-density lipoprotein by rosemary and plant phenolics. J. Agric. Food Chem. 45, 578–582.

Pecevski, J., Savkovic, N., Radivojevic, D., et al., 1981. Effect of oil of nutmeg on the fertility and induction of meiotic chromosome rearrangements in mice and their first generation. Toxicol. Lett. 7, 239–244.

Peele, J.D., 1976. Investigations on the metabolism of myristicin and the mechanism of formation of basic metabolites of allylbenzene in the rat. Dissertation Abstracts International 37B, 1234.

Peirce, W.E., 1961. Tumor-promotion by lime oil in the mouse forestomach. Nature 189, 497–498.

Pélissier, Y., Marion, C., Prunac, S., et al., 1995. Volatile components of leaves, stems and bark of *Cinnamomum camphora* Ness et Ebermaier. Journal of Essential Oil Research 7, 313–315.

Pelkonen, O., Raunio, H., Rautio, A., et al., 1993. Coumarin 7-hydroxylase: characteristics and regulation in mouse and man. J. Ir. Coll. Physicians Surg. 22, 24–28.

Peltonen, L., Wickström, G., Vaahtoranta, M., 1985. Occupational dermatoses in the food industry. Dermatosen 33, 166–169.

Pendlington, R.U., Barratt, M.D., 1990. Molecular basis of photocontact allergy. Int. J. Cosmet. Sci. 12, 91–103.

Perchellet, J.P., Perchellet, E.M., Abney, N.L., et al., 1986. Effects of garlic and onion oils on glutathione peroxidase activity, the ratio of reduced/oxidized glutathione and ornithine decarboxylase induction in isolated mouse epidermal cells treated with tumor promoters. Cancer Biochem. Biophys. 8, 299–312.

Pereira, F., Hatia, M., Cardoso, J., 2002. Systemic contact dermatitis from diallyl disulfide. Contact Dermatitis 46, 125.

Perera, F.P., Mooney, L.A., Stampfer, M., et al., 2002. Associations between carcinogen-DNA damage, glutathione S-transferase genotypes, and risk of lung cancer in the prospective Physicians' Health Cohort Study. Carcinogenesis 23, 1641–1646.

Perillo, M.A., Garcia, D.A., Marin, R.H., et al., 1999. Tagetone modulates the coupling of flunitrazepam and GABA binding sites at GABAA receptor from chick brain membranes. Mol. Membr. Biol. 16, 189–194.

Perrett, C.M., Evans, A.V., Russell-Jones, R., 2003. Tea tree oil dermatitis associated with linear IgA disease. Clin. Exp. Dermatol. 28, 167–170.

Perriot, R., Breme, K., Meierhenrich, U.J., et al., 2010. Chemical composition of French mimosa absolute. J. Agric. Food Chem. 58, 1844–1849.

Perry, P.A., Dean, B.S., Krenzelok, E.P., 1990. Cinnamon oil abuse by adolescents. Vet. Hum. Toxicol. 32, 162–164.

Perry, N.B., Anderson, R.E., Brennan, N.J., et al., 1999. Essential oils from dalmatian sage (*Salvia officinalis* L.): variations among individuals, plant parts, seasons, and sites. J. Agric. Food Chem. 47, 2048–2054.

Perry, N.S., Houghton, P.J., Sampson, J., et al., 2001. *In-vitro activity of S. lavandulaefolia* (Spanish sage) relevant to treatment of Alzheimer's disease. J. Pharm. Pharmacol. 53, 1347–1356.

Perry, N.S., Bollen, C., Perry, E.K., et al., 2003. Salvia for dementia therapy: review of pharmacological activity and pilot tolerability clinical trial. Pharmacol. Biochem. Behav. 75, 651–659.

Persson, E., Larsson, P., Tjalve, H., 2002. Cellular activation and neuronal transport of intranasally instilled benzo[*a*]pyrene in the olfactory system of rats. Toxicol. Lett. 133, 211–219.

Pettersen, E.O., Nome, O., Ronning, O.W., et al., 1983. Effects of benzaldehyde on survival and cell-cycle kinetics of human cells cultivated *in vitro*. Eur. J. Cancer Clin. Oncol. 19, 507–514.

Phelan III., W.J., 1976. Camphor poisoning: over-the-counter dangers. Pediatrics 57, 428–431.

Phillips, D.H., 1990. Further evidence that eugenol does not bind to DNA *in vivo*. Mutat. Res. 245, 23–26.

Phillips, J.C., Kingsnorth, J., Gangolli, S.D., et al., 1976. Studies on the absorption, distribution and excretion of citral in the rat and mouse. Food Cosmet. Toxicol. 14, 537–540.

Phillips, D.H., Miller, J.A., Miller, E.C., et al., 1981a. Structures of the DNA adducts formed in mouse liver after administration of the proximate hepatocarcinogen 1′-hydroxyestragole. Cancer Res. 41, 176–186.

Phillips, D.H., Miller, J.A., Miller, E.C., et al., 1981b. N2 atom of guanine and N6 atom of adenine residues as sites for covalent binding of metabolically activated 1′-hydroxysafrole to mouse liver DNA in vivo. Cancer Res. 41, 2664–2671.

Phillips, D.H., Reddy, M.V., Randerath, K., 1984. ^{32}P-post-labelling analysis of DNA adducts formed in the livers of animals treated with safrole, estragole and other naturally-occurring alkenylbenzenes II. Newborn male B6C3F1 mice. Carcinogenesis 5, 1623–1628.

Phillips, D.H., Schoket, B., Hewer, A., et al., 1990. DNA adduct formation in human and mouse skin by mixtures of polycyclic aromatic hydrocarbons. IARC Sci. Publ. 104, 223–229.

Pho, D.T., Nguyen, T.T.H., Vu, N.L., 1993. Toxicity of two types of *Eucalyptus* essential oils. Tap Chi Duoc Hoc 4, 19–20.

Phongpaichit, S., Kummee, S., Nilrat, L., et al., 2007. Antimicrobial activity of oil from the root of *Cinnamomum porrectum*. J. Sci. Technol. 29 (Suppl. 1), 11–16.

Phukan, R.K., Ali, M.S., Chetia, C.K., et al., 2001. Betel nut and tobacco chewing: potential risk factors of cancer of oesophagus in Assam. India. Br. J. Cancer 85, 661–667.

Piccaglia, R., Marotti, M., 1993. Characterization of several aromatic plants grown in northern Italy. Flavour & Fragrance Journal 8, 115–122.

Piccaglia, R., Marotti, M., Dellacecca, V., 1997. Effect of planting density and harvest date on yield and chemical composition of sage oil. Journal of Essential Oil Research 9, 187–191.

Piculo, F., Guiraldeli Macedo, G., De Andrade, S.F., et al., 2011. *In vivo* genotoxicity assessment of nerolidol. J. Appl. Toxicol. 31, 633–639.

Pienta, R.J., 1980. Evaluation and relevance of the Syrian hamster embryo cell system. Applied Methods in Oncology 3, 149–169.

Pigatto, P.D., Legori, A., Bigardi, A.S., et al., 1996. Gruppo Italiano Ricerca Dermatiti da Contatto ed ambientali italian multicenter study of allergic contact photodermatitis: epidemiological aspects. Am. J. Contact Dermat. 7, 158–163.

Pike, F.H., Elsberg, C.A., McCulloch, W.S., et al., 1929. Some observations on experimentally produced convulsions: the localization of the motor mechanisms from which the typical clonic movements of epilepsy arise. Am. J. Psychiatry 86, 259–283.

Pilapil, V.R., 1989. Toxic manifestations of cinnamon oil ingestion in a child. Clin. Pediatr. (Phila) 28, 276.

Piller, N.B., 1977. Tissue levels of (3-14C) coumarin in the rat: distribution and excretion. Br. J. Exp. Pathol. 58, 28–34.

Pilotti, A., Ancker, K., Arrhenius, E., et al., 1975. Effects of tobacco and tobacco smoke constituents on cell multiplication *in vitro*. Toxicology 5, 49–62.

Ping, H., Zhang, G., Ren, G., 2010. Antidiabetic effects of cinnamon oil in diabetic KK-Ay mice. Food Chem. Toxicol. 48, 2344–2349.

Pino, J.A., Rosado, A., 2001. Comparative. investigation of the distilled lime oils (*Citrus aurantifolia* Swingle and *Citrus latifolia* Tanaka) from Cuba. Journal of Essential Oil Research 13, 179–180.

Pintabona, A., Bianchi, G., Cappellini, V., 1995. Modification of the pharmacokinetics of some antibiotics after oral administration of an *l* (-) verbenone/beta-cyclodextrin complex. Boll. Chim. Farm. 134, 156–160.

Pintao, A.M., Pais, M.S., Coley, H., et al., 1995. *In vitro* and *in vivo* antitumor activity of benzyl isothiocyanate: a natural product from *Tropaeolum majus*. Planta Med. 61, 233–236.

Pinto-Scognamiglio, W., 1967. Current knowledge on the pharmacodynamic activity of the prolonged administration of thujone, a natural flavoring agent. Bolletino Chimico Farmaceutico 106, 292–300.

Pirilä, V., Pirilä, L., 1964. Turpentine allergy: eczematogenic effect of 2- and 3-carenes. Berufsdermatosen 12, 163–167.

Pirilä, V., Siltanen, E., 1955. On the chemical nature of the eczematogenic agent in oil of turpentine. I. Dermatologica 110, 144–155.

Pirilä, V., Siltanen, E., 1956. On the chemical nature of the eczematogenic agent in oil of turpentine II. Dermatologica 113, 1–13.

Pirilä, V., Siltanen, E., 1957. On the eczematous agent in oil of turpentine. Proceedings of the International Congress on Occupational Health-Helsinki (January 6) 3, 400–402.

Pirilä, V., Siltanen, E., 1958. On the chemical nature of the eczematogenic agent in oil of turpentine III. Dermatologica 117, 1–8.

Pirilä, V., Siltanen, E., Pirilä, L., 1964. On the chemical nature of the eczematogenic agent in oil of turpentine. IV. The primary irritant effect of terpenes. Dermatologica 128, 16–21.

Pirilä, V., Kilpio, O., Olkkonen, A., et al., 1969. On the chemical nature of the eczematogenic agent in oil of turpentine. V. Dermatologica 139, 183–194.

Pirker, C., Hausen, B.M., Uter, W., et al., 2003. Sensitization to tea tree oil in Germany and Austria. A multicenter study of the German Contact Dermatitis Group. J. Dtsch. Dermatol. Ges. 1, 629–634.

Pitman, V., 2004. Aromatherapy: a practical approach. Nelson Thornes, Cheltenham.

Placzek, M., Frömel, W., Eberlein, B., et al., 2007. Evaluation of phototoxic properties of fragrances. Acta Derm. Venereol. 87, 312–316.

Politano, V.T., Lewis, E.M., Hoberman, A.M., et al., 2008. Evaluation of the developmental toxicity of linalool in rats. Int. J. Toxicol. 27, 183–188.

Politano, V.T., McGinty, D., Lewis, E.M., et al., 2013. Uterotrophic assay of percutaneous lavender oil in immature female rats. Int. J. Toxicol. 32, 123–129.

Ponce-Monter, H., Campos, M.G., Perez, S., et al., 2008. Chemical composition and antispasmodic effect of *Casimiroa pringlei* essential oil on rat uterus. Fitoterapia 79, 446–450.

Pons-Guiraud, A., 2004. Sensitive skin: a complex and multifactorial syndrome. J. Cosmet. Dermatol. 3, 145–148.

Pool, B.L., Lin, P.Z., 1982. Mutagenicity testing in the *Salmonella typhimurium* assay of phenolic compounds and phenolic fractions obtained from smokehouse smoke condensates. Food Chem. Toxicol. 20, 383–391.

Poon, T.S., Freeman, S., 2006. Cheilitis caused by contact allergy to anethole in spearmint flavoured toothpaste. Australas J. Dermatol. 47, 300–301.

Porter, N.G., Wilkins, A.L., 1998. Chemical, physical and antimicrobial properties of essential oils of *Leptospermum scoparium* and *Kunzea ericoides*. Phytochemistry 50, 407–415.

Posadzki, P., Alotaibi, A., Ernst, E., 2012. Adverse effects of aromatherapy: a systematic review of case reports and case series. International Journal of Risk & Safety in Medicine 24, 147–161.

Posthumus, M.A., Van Beek, T.A., Collins, N.F., et al., 1996. Chemical composition of the essential oils of *Agathosma betulina*. *A. crenulata* and an *A. betulina* x *crenulata* hybrid (buchu). Journal of Essential Oil Research 8, 223–228.

Potten, C.S., Chadwick, C.A., Cohen, A.J., et al., 1993. DNA damage in UV-irradiated human skin *in vivo*: automated direct measurement by image analysis (thymine dimers) compared with indirect measurement (unscheduled DNA synthesis) and protection by 5-methoxypsoralen. Int. J. Radiat. Biol. 63, 313–324.

Potter, J., Smith, R.L., Api, A.M., 2001a. Urinary thiocyanate levels as a biomarker for the generation of inorganic cyanide from benzyl cyanide in the rat. Food Chem. Toxicol. 39, 141–146.

Potter, J., Smith, R.L., Api, A.M., 2001b. An assessment of the release of inorganic cyanide from the fragrance materials benzyl cyanide, geranyl nitrile and citronellyl nitrile applied dermally to the rat. Food Chem. Toxicol. 39, 147–151.

Potts, R.O., Francoeur, M.L., 1991. The influence of stratum corneum morphology on water permeability. J. Invest. Dermatol. 96, 495–499.

Pourgholami, M.H., Majzoob, S., Javadi, M., et al., 1999. The fruit essential oil of *Pimpinella anisum* exerts anticonvulsant effects in mice. J. Ethnopharmacol. 66, 211–215.

Powers, K.A., Beasley, V.R., 1985. Toxicological aspects of linalool: a review. Vet. Hum. Toxicol. 27, 484–486.

Power, F.B., Salway, A.H., 1908. Chemical examination and physiological action of nutmeg. American Journal of Pharmacy 80, 563–580.

Powers, M.F., Darby, T.D., Scheuler, F.W., 1961. A study of the toxic effects of cinnamon oil. Pharmacologist 3, 62.

Powolny, A.A., Singh, S.V., 2008. Multitargeted prevention and therapy of cancer by diallyl trisulfide and related *Allium* vegetable-derived organosulfur compounds. Cancer Lett. 269, 305–314.

Prakash, A.O., Saxena, V., Shukla, S., et al., 1985. Anti-implantation activity of some indigenous plants in rats. Acta Eur. Fertil. 16, 441–448.

Prashar, A., Locke, I.C., Evans, C.S., 2004. Cytotoxicity of lavender oil and its major components to human skin cells. Cell Prolif. 37, 221–229.

Prashar, A., Locke, I.C., Evans, C.S., 2006. Cytotoxicity of clove (*Syzygium aromaticum*) oil and its major components to human skin cells. Cell Prolif. 39, 241–248.

Pratt, M.D., Belsito, D.V., DeLeo, V.A., et al., 2004. North American Contact Dermatitis Group patch-test results, 2001–2002 study period. Dermatitis 15, 176–183.

Pratzel, H.G., Schubert, E., Muhanna, N., 1990. Pharmacokinetic study of percutaneous absorption of salicylic acid from baths with salicylate methyl ester and salicylic acid. Z. Rheumatol. 49, 185–191.

Price, C.J., George, J.D., Marr, M.C., et al., 2006. Developmental toxicity evaluation of methyleugenol (MEUG) administered to Sprague-Dawley rats on gestational days (gd) 6 through 19. Birth Defects Res. A Clin. Mol. Teratol. 76, 395.

Priestley, C.M., Williamson, E.M., Wafford, K.A., et al., 2003. Thymol, a constituent of thyme essential oil, is a positive allosteric modulator of human GABA(A) receptors and a homo-oligomeric GABA receptor from *Drosophila melanogaster*. Br. J. Pharmacol. 140, 1363–1372.

Prince, M., Campbell, C.T., Robertson, T.A., et al., 2006. Naturally occurring coumarins inhibit 7,12-dimethylbenz[a]anthracene DNA adduct formation in mouse mammary gland. Carcinogenesis 27, 1204–1213.

Prival, M.J., Sheldon, A.T., Popkin, D., 1982. Evaluation, using *Salmonella typhimurium*, of the mutagenicity of seven chemicals found in cosmetics. Food Chem. Toxicol. 20, 427–432.

Prudent, D., Perineau, F., Bravo, R., et al., 1991. Preparation et caracterisation d'extraits volatils de bois de Gaiac (*Bulnesia sarmienti* Lor.). Rivista Italiana EPPOS 5, 35–43.

Pultrini A de, M., Galindo, L.A., Costa, M., 2006. Effects of the essential oil from *Citrus aurantium* L. in experimental anxiety models in mice. Life Sci. 78, 1720–1725.

Punt, A., Delatour, T., Scholz, G., et al., 2007. Tandem mass spectrometry analysis of N2-(trans-Isoestragol-3'-yl)-2'-deoxyguanosine as a strategy to study species differences in sulfotransferase conversion of the proximate carcinogen 1'-hydroxyestragole. Chem. Res. Toxicol. 20, 991–998.

Punt, A., Freidig, A.P., Delatour, T., et al., 2008. A physiologically based biokinetic (PBBK) model for estragole bioactivation and detoxification in rat. Toxicol. Appl. Pharmacol. 231, 248–259.

Purchase, R., Ford, G.P., Creasy, D.M., et al., 1992. A 28-day feeding study with methyl isoeugenol in rats. Food Chem. Toxicol. 30, 475–481.

Purkayastha, J., Nath, S.C., Klinkby, N., 2006. Essential oil of the rhizome of *Curcuma zedoaria* (Christm.) Rosc. native to Northeast India. Journal of Essential Oil Research 18, 154–155.

Pybus, D.H., Sell, C.S., 1999. The chemistry of fragrances. Royal Society of Chemistry, Letchworth.

Pyun, J.S., 1970. Effect of methyl salicylate on developing rat embryos. Ch'oesin Uihak 13, 63–72.

Qadri, S.M., Mahmud, H., Föller, M., et al., 2009. Thymoquinone-induced suicidal erythrocyte death. Food Chem. Toxicol. 47, 1545–1549.

Qato, M.K., Guenthner, T.M., 1995. ^{32}P-Postlabeling analysis of adducts formed between DNA and safrole 2',3'-epoxide: absence of adduct formation *in vivo*. Toxicol. Lett. 75, 201–207.

Qian, B.C., Gong, W.G., Chen, J., et al., 1980. Pharmacological studies on the anti-asthmatic and anti-anaphylactic activities of the essential oil of Litsea cubeba (Lour.) Pers.]. Yao Xue Xue Bao 15, 584–589.

Quertermous, J., Fowler, J.F., 2010. Allergic contact dermatitis from carvone in hair conditioners. Dermatitis 21, 116–117.

Quintans-Júnior, L.J., Souza, T.T., Leite, B.S., 2007. Phythochemical screening and anticonvulsant activity of *Cymbopogon winterianus* Jowitt (Poaceae) leaf essential oil in rodents. Phytomedicine 15, 619–624.

Qureshi, A.A., Mangels, W.R., Din, Z.Z., 1988. Inhibition of hepatic mevalonate biosynthesis by the monoterpene *d*-limonene. J. Agric. Food Chem. 36, 1220–1224.

Rabbani, S.I., Devi, K., Khanam, S., et al., 2006. Citral, a component of lemongrass oil, inhibits the clastogenic effect of nickel chloride in mouse micronucleus test system. Pak. J. Pharm. Sci. 19, 108–113.

Rabl, W., Katzgraber, F., Steinlechner, M., 1997. Camphor ingestion for abortion (case report). Forensic. Sci. Int. 89, 137–140.

Racine, P., Auffray, B., 2005. Quenching of singlet molecular oxygen by *Commiphora myrrha* extracts and menthofuran. Fitoterapia 76, 316–323.

Rademaker, M., 1995. Allergic contact dermatitis from lavender fragrance in Difflam® gel. Contact Dermatis 31, 58–59.

Radonic, A., Milos, M., 2003. Chemical composition and *in vitro* evaluation of antioxidant effect of free volatile compounds from *Satureja montana* L. Free Radic. Res. 37, 673–679.

Radulović, N.S., Dekić, M.S., Stojanović-Radić, Z.Z., et al., 2010. *Geranium macrorrhizum* L. Geraniaceae essential oil: a potent agent against *Bacillus subtilis*. Chem. Biodivers 7, 2783–2800.

Radulović, N.S., Randjelović, P.J., Stojanović, N.M., et al., 2013. Toxic essential oils. Part II: Chemical, toxicological, pharmacological and microbiological profiles of *Artemisia annua* L. volatiles. Food Chem. Toxicol. 58C, 37–49.

Ragan, B.G., Nelson, A.J., Foreman, J.H., et al., 2004. Effects of a menthol-based analgesic balm on pressor responses evoked from muscle afferents in cats. Am. J. Vet. Res. 65, 1204–1210.

Raharivelomanana, P., Cambon, A., Azzaro, M., et al., 1993. Volatile constituents of *Neocallitropsis pancheri* (Carrière) de Laubenfels heartwood extracts (Cupressaceae). Journal of Essential Oil Research 5, 587–595.

Rahmani, H., Leonhardt, S., Beladdale, D., et al., 2004. Severe acute lung oedema after rectal enema with cade oil. Journal of Clinical Toxicology 42, 487.

Rai, L., Ahujarai, P.L., 1990. Effect of pure garlic oil (*Allium sativum*) on the protection against 3-methylcholanthrene-induced uterine cervical tumorigenesis. Journal of Research & Education in Indian Medicine 9, 20–26.

Raina, V.K., Srivastava, S.K., Syamsundar, K.V., 2005. Rhizome and leaf oil composition of *Curcuma longa* from the lower Himalayan region of Northern India. Journal of Essential Oil Research 17, 556–559.

Rakieten, N., Rakieten, M.L., 1957. The effect of *l*-menthol on the systemic blood pressure. J. Am. Pharm. Assoc. 46 (2), 82–84.

Rakieten, N., Rakieten, M., Boykin, M., 1954. Effects of menthol vapor on the intact animal with special reference to the upper respiratory tract. J. Am. Pharm. Assoc. 43, 390–392.

Rali, T., Wossa, S.W., Leach, D.N., 2007. Comparative chemical analysis of the essential oil constituents in the bark, heartwood and fruits of *Cryptocarya massoy* (Oken) Kosterm. (Lauraceae) from Papua New Guinea. Molecules 12, 149–154.

Ramachandraiah, O.S., Azeemoddin, G., Charyulu, J.K., 1998. Turmeric (*Curcuma longa* L.) leaf oil, a new essential oil for perfumery industry. Indian Perfumer 42, 124–127.

Ramadan, W., Mourad, B., Ibrahim, S., et al., 1996. Oil of bitter orange: new topical antifungal agent. Int. J. Dermatol. 35, 448–449.

Ramanoelina, P.A.R., Rasoarahona, J.R.E., 2006. Chemical composition of *Ravensara aromatica* Sonn. leaf essential oils from Madagascar. Journal of Essential Oil Research 18, 215–217.

Ramanoelina, P.A.R., Viano, J., Bianchini, J.P., Gaydou, E.M., 1994a. Occurrence of various chemotypes in niaouli (*Melaleuca quinquenervia*) essential oils from Madagascar using multivariate statistical analysis. J. Agric. Food Chem. 42, 1177–1182.

Ramanoelina, P.A.R., Rasoarahona, R.E., Masotti, V., et al., 1994b. Chemical composition of the leaf oil of *Psiadia altissima* (Compositae). Journal of Essential Oil Research 6, 565–570.

Ramezani, R., Moghimi, A., Rakhshandeh, H., et al., 2008. The effect of *Rosa damascena* essential oil on the amygdala electrical kindling seizures in rat. Pakistan Journal of Biological Sciences 11, 746–751.

Ramos, A., Visozo, A., Piloto, J., et al., 2003. Screening of antimutagenicity via antioxidant activity in Cuban medicinal plants. J. Ethnopharmacol. 87, 241–246.

Ramos-Ocampo, V.E., 1988. Mutagenicity and DNA-damaging activity of calamus oil, asarone isomers, and dimethoxypropenylbenzene analogues. The Philippine Entomologist 7 (3), 275–291.

Ramos-Ocampo, V.E., Hsia, M.T., 1987. Effects of acute treatments of calamus oil, β-asarone and dimethoxypropenylbenzenes in laboratory rats. Phillip. Ent. 7, 129–158.

Rampone, W.M., McCullough, J.L., Weinstein, G.D., et al., 1986. Characterization of cutaneous phototoxicity induced by topical alpha-terthienyl and ultraviolet A radiation. J. Invest. Dermatol. 87, 354–357.

Raña-Martínez, N., 2008. Migraines in women. Rev. Neurol. 46, 373–378.

Randerath, K., Haglund, R.E., Phillips, D.H., et al., 1984. ^{32}P-post-labelling analysis of DNA adducts formed in the livers of animals treated with safrole, estragole and other naturally-occurring alkenylbenzenes. I. Adult female CD-1 mice. Carcinogenesis 5, 1613–1622.

Randerath, K., Putman, K.L., Randerath, E., 1993. Flavor constituents in cola drinks induce hepatic DNA adducts in adult and fetal mice. Biochem. Biophys. Res. Commun. 192, 61–68.

Rao, A.R., 1984. Modifying influences of betel quid ingredients on B(a)P-induced carcinogenesis in the buccal pouch of hamster. Int. J. Cancer 33, 581–586.

Rao, Y.R., Rout, P.K., 2003. Geographical location and harvest time dependent variation in the composition of essential oils of *Jasminum sambac* (L.) Aiton. Journal of Essential Oil Research 15, 398–401.

Rao, A.R., Sinha, A., Selvan, R.S., 1985. Inhibitory action of *Piper betle* on the initiation of 7,12-dimethylbenz[*a*]anthracene-induced mammary carcinogenesis in rats. Cancer Lett. 26, 207–214.

Rao, B.R., Kaul, P.N., Bhattacharya, A.K., 1998. Java citronella (*Cymbopogon winterianus* Jowitt) cultivation in a tribal area of Andhra Pradesh. Journal of Essential Oil Bearing Plants 1, 114–118.

Rao, M., Kumar, M.M., Rao, M.A., 1999. *In vitro* and *in vivo* effects of phenolic antioxidants against cisplatin-induced nephrotoxicity. J. Biochem. (Tokyo) 125, 383–390.

Rao, P.G.P., Rao, L.J., Raghavan, B., 1999. Chemical composition of essential oils of garlic (*Allium sativum* L.). Journal of Spices & Aromatic Crops 8, 41–47.

Raphael, T.J., Kuttan, G., 2003a. Effect of naturally occurring monoterpenes carvone, limonene and perillic acid in the inhibition of experimental lung metastasis induced by B16F-10 melanoma cells. J. Exp. Clin. Cancer Res. 22, 419–424.

Raphael, T.J., Kuttan, G., 2003b. Immunomodulatory activity of naturally occurring monoterpenes carvone, limonene, and perillic acid. Immunopharmacol. 25, 285–294.

Rasheed, A., Laekeman, G.M., Vlietinck, A.J., et al., 1984. Pharmacological influence of nutmeg and nutmeg constituents on rabbit platelet function. Planta Med. 50, 222–226.

Rasoanaivo, P., De La Gorce, P., 1998. Essential oils of economical value in Madagascar: present state of knowledge. HerbalGram 43 (31–39), 58–59.

Rastogi, S.C., Johansen, J.D., Frosch, P., et al., 1998. Deodorants on the European market: quantitative chemical analysis of 21 fragrances. Contact Dermatitis 38, 29–35.

Rastogi, S.C., Heydorn, S., Johansen, J.D., et al., 2001. Fragrance chemicals in domestic and occupational products. Contact Dermatitis 45, 221–225.

Rastogi, S.C., Bossi, R., Johansen, J.D., et al., 2004. Content of oak moss allergens atranol and chloroatranol in perfumes and similar products. Contact Dermatitis 50, 367–370.

Rathee, J.S., Patro, B.S., Mula, S., et al., 2006. Antioxidant activity of *Piper betel* leaf extract and its constituents. J. Agric. Food Chem. 54, 9046–9054.

Rathore, P., Dohare, P., Varma, S., et al., 2008. Curcuma oil: reduces early accumulation of oxidative product and is anti-apoptogenic in transient focal ischemia in rat brain. Neurochem. Res. 33, 1672–1682.

Rauscher, F.M., Sanders, R.A., Watkins, J.B., 2001. Effects of isoeugenol on oxidative stress pathways in normal and streptozotocin-induced diabetic rats. J. Biochem. Mol. Toxicol. 15, 159–164.

Rautio, A., Kraul, H., Kojo, A., et al., 1992. Interindividual variability of coumarin 7-hydroxylation in healthy volunteers. Pharmacogenetics 2, 227–233.

Re, L., Barocci, S., Sonnino, S., et al., 2000. Linalool modifies the nicotinic receptor–ion channel kinetics at the mouse neuromuscular junction. Pharmacol. Res. 42, 177–181.

Recsan, Z., Pagliuca, G., Piretti, M.V., et al., 1997. Effect of essential oils on the lipids of the retina in the ageing rat: a possible therapeutic use. Journal of Essential Oil Research 9, 53–56.

Reddy, A.C., Lokesh, B.R., 1996. Effect of curcumin and eugenol on iron-induced hepatic toxicity in rats. Toxicology 107, 39–45.

Reddy, M.V., Randerath, K., 1990. A comparison of DNA adduct formation in white blood cells and internal organs of mice exposed to benzo[a]pyrene, dibenzo[c, g]carbazole, safrole and cigarette smoke condensate. Mutat. Res. 241, 37–48.

Reddy, B.S., Wang, C.X., Samaha, H., et al., 1997. Chemoprevention of colon carcinogenesis by dietary perillyl alcohol. Cancer Res. 57, 420–425.

Reed, P.M., Caldwell, J., 1992. Induction of cytochrome P450 and related enzyme activities following dietary administration of *trans*-anethole to Sprague-Dawley CD rats. Hum. Exp. Toxicol. 11, 580–581.

Reed, J.T., Ghadially, R., Elias, P.M., 1995. Skin type, but neither race nor gender, influence epidermal permeability barrier function. Arch. Dermatol. 131, 1134–1138.

Reekie, J.S., 1909. Nutmeg poisoning. J. Am. Med. Assoc. 52, 62.

Regan, J.W., Bjeldanes, L.F., 1976. Metabolism of (+)-limonene in rats. J. Agric. Food Chem. 24, 377–380.

Régimbal, J.M., Collin, G., 1994. Essential oil analysis of balsam fir *Abies balsamea* (L.) Mill. Journal of Essential Oil Research 6, 229–238.

Reich, K., Westphal, G., Konig, I.R., et al., 2003. Association of allergic contact dermatitis with a promoter polymorphism in the IL16 gene. J. Allergy Clin. Immunol. 112, 1191–1194.

Reichling, J., Fitzi, J., Hellmann, K., et al., 2004. Topical tea tree oil effective in canine localised pruritic dermatitis - a multi-centre randomised double-blind controlled clinical trial in the veterinary practice. Deutsche Tierarztliche Wochenschrifte 111, 408–414.

Reicks, M.M., Crankshaw, D., 1993. Effects of *d*-limonene on hepatic microsomal monooxygenase activity and paracetamol-induced glutathione depletion in mouse. Xenobiotica 23, 809–819.

Reid, F.M., 1979. Accidental camphor ingestion. Journal of the American College of Emergency Physicians 8, 339–340.

Reischer, D., Heyfets, A., Shimony, S., et al., 2007. Effects of natural and novel synthetic jasmonates in experimental metastatic melanoma. Br. J. Pharmacol. 150, 738–749.

Rekka, E.A., Kourounakis, A.P., Kourounakis, P.N., 1996. Investigation of the effect of chamazulene on lipid peroxidation and free radical processes. Res. Commun. Mol. Pathol. Pharmacol. 92, 361–364.

Remaut, K., 1992. Contact dermatitis due to cosmetic ingredients. J. Appl. Cosmetol. 10, 73–80.

Remberg, P., Björk, L., Hedner, T., et al., 2004. Characteristics, clinical effect profile and tolerability of a nasal spray preparation of *Artemisia abrotanum* L. for allergic rhinitis. Phytomedicine 11, 36–42.

Renaux, J., La Barre, J., 1941. Les effets ocytociques de rue et de sabine. Acta Biol. Belg. 1, 334–335.

Ress, N.B., Hailey, J.R., Maronpot, R.R., et al., 2003. Toxicology and carcinogenesis studies of microencapsulated citral in rats and mice. Toxicol. Sci. 71, 198–206.

Reverchon, E., Senatore, F., 1992. Isolation of rosemary oil: comparison between hydrodistilled and supercritical fluid CO2 extraction. Flavour & Fragrance Journal 7, 227–230.

Reynolds, J.E.F. (Ed.), 1993. Martindale: The extra pharmacopoeia. The Pharmaceutical Press, London.

Reznik, M., Sharif, I., Ozuah, P.O., 2004. Rubbing ointments and asthma morbidity in adolescents. J. Altern. Complement. Med. 10, 1097–1099.

Rice, K.C., Wilson, R.S., 1976. (−)-3-Isothujone, a small nonnitrogenous molecule with antinociceptive activity in mice. J. Med. Chem. 19, 1054–1057.

Reiter, M., Brandt, W., 1985. Relaxant effects on tracheal and ileal smooth muscles of the guinea pig. Arzneimittelforschung 35 (1A), 408–414.

Rietjens, I.M., Boersma, M.G., van der Woude, H., et al., 2005a. Flavonoids and alkenylbenzenes: mechanisms of mutagenic action and carcinogenic risk. Mutat. Res. 574, 124–138.

Rietjens, I.M., Martena, M.J., Boersma, M.G., et al., 2005b. Molecular mechanisms of toxicity of important food-borne phytotoxins. Mol. Nutr. Food Res. 49, 131–158.

Rietjens, I.M., Boersma, M.G., Zaleska, M., et al., 2008. Differences in simulated liver concentrations of toxic coumarin metabolites in rats and different human populations evaluated through physiologically based biokinetic (PBBK) modeling. Toxicol. In Vitro 22, 1890–1901.

RIFM, 2001. Position statement on methyl eugenol and estragole: safety with respect to use as fragrance ingredients (added as such and as components of natural oils). IFRA website:www.ifraorg.org/GuideLines.asp.

Riggs, J., Hamilton, R., Homel, S., et al., 1965. Camphorated oil intoxication in pregnancy. Obstetrics & Gynaecology 25, 255–258.

Rimini, E., 1901. Biological oxidation of fenchone. Accademia Nazionale dei Lincei 10, 244–249.

Rioja, A., Pizzey, A.R., Marson, C.M., et al., 2000. Preferential induction of apoptosis of leukaemic cells by farnesol. FEBS Lett. 467, 291–295.

Riordan, M., Rylance, G., Berry, K., 2002. Poisoning in children 4: household products, plants, and mushrooms. Arch. Dis. Child. 87, 403–406.

Rios Scherrer, M.A., 2006. Allergic contact dermatitis to petrolatum. Contact Dermatitis 54, 300–301.

Ripple, G.H., Gould, M.N., Stewart, J.A., et al., 1998. Phase I clinical trial of perillyl alcohol administered daily. Clin. Cancer Res. 4, 1159–1164.

Ripple, G.H., Gould, M.N., Arzoomanian, R.Z., et al., 2000. Phase I clinical and pharmacokinetic study of perillyl alcohol administered four times a day. Clin. Cancer Res. 6, 390–396.

Rissmann, R., Oudshoorn, M.H., Hennink, W.E., et al., 2009. Skin barrier disruption by acetone: observations in a hairless mouse skin model. Arch. Dermatol. Res. 301, 609–613.

Ristorcelli, D., Tomi, F., Casanova, J., 1996. Essential oils of *Calamintha nepeta* subsp. *nepeta* and subsp. *glandulosa* from Corsica (France). Journal of Essential Oil Research 8, 363–366.

Ristorcelli, D., Tomi, F., Casanova, J., 1998. ^{13}C-NMR as a tool for identification and enantiomeric differentiation of major terpenes exemplified by the essential oil of *Lavandula stoechas* L. ssp. *stoechas*. Flavour & Fragrance Journal 13, 154–158.

Ritschel, W.A., Brady, M.E., Tan, H.S.I., et al., 1977. Pharmacokinetics of coumarin and its 7-hydroxy-metabolites upon intravenous and peroral administration of coumarin in man. Eur. J. Clin. Pharmacol. 12, 457–461.

Ritschel, W.A., Brady, M.E., Tan, H.I.S., 1979. First-pass effect of coumarin in man. Int. J. Clin. Pharmacol. Biopharm. 17, 99–103.

Ritschel, W.A., Sabouni, A., Hussain, A.S., 1989. Percutaneous absorption of coumarin, griseofulvin and propranolol across human scalp and abdominal skin. Methods Find. Exp. Clin. Pharmacol. 11, 643–646.

Robbiano, L., Baroni, D., Carrozzino, R., et al., 2004. DNA damage and micronuclei induced in rat and human kidney cells by six chemicals carcinogenic to the rat kidney. Toxicology 204, 187–195.

Roberts, M.S., Favretto, W.A., Meyer, A., et al., 1982. Topical bioavailability of methyl salicylate. Aust. N. Z. J. Med. 12, 303–305.

Robertson, J.S., Hussain, M., 1969. Metabolism of camphors and related compounds. Biochem. J. 113, 57–65.

Robinson, M.K., Gerberick, G.F., Ryan, C.A., et al., 2000. The importance of exposure estimation in the assessment of skin sensitization risk. Contact Dermatitis 42, 251–259.

Robinson, S., Delongeas, J.L., Donald, E., et al., 2008. A European pharmaceutical company initiative challenging the regulatory requirement for acute toxicity studies in pharmaceutical drug development. Regul. Toxicol. Pharmacol. 50, 345–352.

Rockwell, P., Raw, I., 1979. A mutagenic screening of various herbs, spices and food additives. Nutr. Cancer 1, 10–15.

Roe, F.J.C., 1959. Oil of sweet orange: a possible role in carcinogenesis. Br. J. Cancer 13, 92–93.

Roe, F.J.C., Field, W.E.H., 1965. Chronic toxicity of essential oils and certain other products of natural origin. Food Cosmet. Toxicol. 3, 311–324.

Roe, F.J.C., Peirce, W.E.H., 1960. Tumor promotion by citrus oils: tumors of the skin and urethral orifice in mice. J. Natl. Cancer Inst. 24, 1389–1403.

Roebuck, B.D., Longnecker, D.S., Baumgartner, K.J., et al., 1985. Carcinogen-induced lesions in the rat pancreas: effects of varying levels of essential fatty acid. Cancer Res. 45, 5252–5256.

Roedel, W., Petrzika, M., 1991. Analysis of the volatile components of saffron. Journal of High Resolution Chromatography 14, 771–774.

Roepke, M., Diestel, A., BajBouj, K., et al., 2007. Lack of p53 augments thymoquinone-induced apoptosis and caspase activation in human osteosarcoma cells. Cancer Biol. Ther. 6, 160–169.

Roffey, S.J., Walker, R., Gibson, G.G., 1990. Hepatic peroxisomal and microsomal induction by citral and linalool in rats. Food Chem. Toxicol. 28, 403–408.

Rogan, E.G., Cavalieri, E.L., Walker, B.A., et al., 1986. Mutagenicity of benzylic acetates, sulfates and bromides of polycyclic aromatic hydrocarbons. Chem. Biol. Interact. 58, 253–275.

Rogers, S.N., Pahor, A.L., 1995. A form of stomatitis induced by excessive peppermint consumption. Dent. Update 22, 36–37.

Rohr, A.C., Wilkins, C.K., Clausen, P.A., et al., 2002. Upper airway and pulmonary effects of oxidation products of (+)-alpha-pinene, *d*-limonene, and isoprene in BALB/c mice. Inhal. Toxicol. 14, 663–684.

Roll, R., Bär, F., 1967. Die Wirkung von Cumarin (o-Hydroxyzimtsäure-lacton) auf trächtige Mäuseweibchen. Arzneimittel-Forschung/Drug Research 17, 97–100.

Rolseth, V., Djurhuus, R., Svardal, A.M., 2002. Additive toxicity of limonene and 50% oxygen and the role of glutathione in detoxification in human lung cells. Toxicology 170, 75–88.

Rolsted, K., Kissmeyer, A.M., Rist, G.M., et al., 2008. Evaluation of cytochrome P450 activity *in vitro*, using dermal and hepatic microsomes from four species and two keratinocyte cell lines in culture. Arch. Dermatol. Res. 300, 11–18.

Romaguera, C., Grimalt, F., 1980. Statistical and comparative study of 4600 patients tested in Barcelona (1973–1977). Contact Dermatitis 6, 309–315.

Romaguera, C., Vilaplana, J., 2000. Occupational contact dermatitis from ylang-ylang oil. Contact Dermatitis 43, 251.

Romano, L., Battaglia, F., Masucci, L., et al., 2005. *In vitro* activity of bergamot natural essence and furocoumarin-free and distilled extracts, and their associations with boric acid, against clinical yeast isolates. J. Antimicrob. Chemother. 55, 110–114.

Römmelt, H., Zuber, A., Dirnagl, K., et al., 1974. Zur Resorption von Terpenen aus Badezusätzen. München Medizin Wochenschrift 116, 537–540.

Römmelt, H., Schnizer, W., Swoboda, M., et al., 1987. Pharmakokinetik ätherische Öle nach Inhalation mit einer terpenhaltigen Salbe. Zeitschrift für Phytotherapie 9, 14–16.

Rompelberg, C.J., Verhagen, H., Van Bladeren, P.J., 1993. Effects of the naturally occurring alkenylbenzenes eugenol and *trans*-anethole on drug-metabolising enzymes in the rat liver. Food Chem. Toxicol. 31, 637–645.

Rompelberg, C.J., Stenhuis, W.H., de Vogel, N., et al., 1995. Antimutagenicity of eugenol in the rodent bone marrow micronucleus test. Mutat. Res. 346, 69–75.

Rompelberg, C.J., Steenwinkel, M.J., van Asten, J.G., et al., 1996b. Effect of eugenol on the mutagenicity of benzo[*a*]pyrene and the formation of benzo[*a*]pyrene-DNA adducts in the λ-*lacZ*-transgenic mouse. Mutat. Res. 369, 87–96.

Rompelberg, C.J., Vogels, J.T., de Vogel, N., et al., 1996c. Effect of short-term dietary administration of eugenol in humans. Hum. Exp. Toxicol. 25, 129–135.

Rooney, S., Ryan, M.F., 2005a. Effects of α-hederin and thymoquinone, constituents of *Nigella sativa*, on human cancer cell lines. Anticancer Res. 25, 2199–2204.

Rooney, S., Ryan, M.F., 2005b. Modes of action of α-hederin and thymoquinone, active constituents of *Nigella sativa*, against HEp-2 cancer cells. Anticancer Res. 25, 4255–4259.

Roots, I., Gerloff, T., Meisel, C., et al., 2004. Pharmacogenetics-based new therapeutic concepts. Drug Metab. Rev. 36, 617–638.

Röscheisen, C., Zamith, H., Paumgartten, F.J., et al., 1991. Influence of β-myrcene on sister-chromatid exchanges induced by mutagens in V79 and HTC cells. Mutat. Res. 264, 43–49.

Rose, P., Whiteman, M., Huang, S.H., et al., 2003. beta-Phenylethyl isothiocyanate-mediated apoptosis in hepatoma HepG2 cells. Cell. Mol. Life Sci. 60, 1489–1503.

Rosenhall, L., Zetterström, O., 1974. Asthma induced by analgesics and commonly used food and drug additives. Scand. J. Respir. Dis. 88 (Suppl.), 60.

Rosenhall, L., Zetterström, O., 1975. Asthmatic patients with hypersensitivity to aspirin, benzoic acid and tartrazine. Tubercle 56, 168.

Rosin, M.P., 1984. The influene of pH on the convertogenic activity of plant phenolics. Mutat. Res. 135, 109–113.

Roskos, K.V., Maibach, H.I., 1992. Percutaneous absorption and age. Implications for therapy. Drugs & Aging 2, 432–449.

Ross, J.S., du Peloux Menage, H., Hawk, J.L., et al., 1993. Sesquiterpene lactone contact sensitivity: clinical patterns of Compositae dermatitis and relationship to chronic actinic dermatitis. Contact Dermatitis 29, 84–87.

Ross, P.M., Whysner, J., Covello, V.T., et al., 1999. Olfaction and symptoms in the multiple chemical sensitivities syndrome. Prev. Med. 28, 467–480.

Rossi, T., Melegari, M., Bianchi, A., et al., 1988. Sedative, anti-inflammatory and anti-diuretic effects induced in rats by essential oils of varieties of *Anthemis nobilis*: a comparative study. Pharmacol. Res. Commun. 20, 71–74.

Rotem, R., Heyfets, A., Fingrut, O., et al., 2005. Jasmonates: novel anticancer agents acting directly and selectively on human cancer cell mitochondria. Cancer Res. 65, 1984–1993.

Rothenborg, H.W., Menné, T., Sjolin, K.E., 1977. Temperature dependent primary irritant dermatitis fom lemon perfume. Contact Dermatitis 3, 37–48.

Rothenstein, A.S., Booman, K.A., Dorsky, J., et al., 1983. Eugenol and clove leaf oil: a survey of consumer patch-test sensitization. Food Chem. Toxicol. 21, 727–733.

Rozman, T., Leuschner, F., Brickl, R., et al., 1989. Toxicity of 8-methoxypsoralen in cynomolgous monkeys (*Macaca fascicularis*). Drug Chem. Toxicol. 12, 21–37.

Rozman, K.K., Kerecsen, L., Viluksela, M.K., 1996. A toxicologist's view of cancer risk assessment. Drug Metab. Rev. 28, 29–52.

Rubel, D.M., Freeman, S., Southwell, I.A., 1998. Tea tree oil allergy: what is the offending agent? Report of three cases of tea tree oil allergy and review of the literature. Aust. J. Dermatol. 39, 244–247.

Ruberto, G., Biondi, D., Piattelli, M., et al., 1994. Essential oil of the new citrus hybrid, *Citrus clementina* x *C. limon*. Journal of Essential Oil Research 6, 1–8.

Ruberto, G., Baratta, M.T., Deans, S.G., et al., 2000. Antioxidant and antimicrobial activity of *Foeniculum vulgare* and *Crithmum maritimum* essential oils. Planta Med. 66, 687–693.

Rubin, M.B., Recinos, A., Washington, J.A., et al., 1949. Ingestion of poisons - survey of 250 children. Clinical Proceedings Childrens Hospital 5, 57–73.

Rücker, G., Tautges, J., Sieck, A., et al., 1978. Untersuchungen zur Isolierung und pharmakodynamischen Aktivität des Sesquiterpens Valeranon aus *Nardostachys jatamansi* DC. Arzneimittelforschung 28, 7–13.

Rudner, E.J., 1977. North American group results. Contact Dermatitis 3, 208–209.

Rudzki, E., Grzywa, Z., 1976. Sensitizing and irritating properties of star anise oil. Contact Dermatitis 2, 305–308.

Rudzki, E., Grzywa, Z., 1985. The value of a mixture of cassia and citronella oils for the detection of hypersensitivity to essential oils. Derm. Beruf Umwelt 33 (2), 59–62.

Rudzki, E., Kleniewska, D., 1971. Kontaktallergie auf einige Lokaltherapeutika und Konservierungsmittel. Dermatologica 143, 36–42.

Rudzki, E., Grzywa, Z., Brud, W.S., 1976. Sensitivity to 35 essential oils. Contact Dermatitis 2, 196–200.

Ruediger, H.W., 2006. Antagonistic combinations of occupational carcinogens. Int. Arch. Occup. Environ. Health 79, 343–348.

Rumchev, K.B., Spickett, J.T., Bulsara, M.K., et al., 2002. Domestic exposure to formaldehyde significantly increases the risk of asthma in young children. Eur. Respir. J. 20, 403–408.

Rumchev, K.B., Spickett, J.T., Bulsara, M.K., et al., 2004. Association of domestic exposure to volatile organic compounds with asthma in young children. Thorax 59, 746–751.

Rumiantsev, G.I., Novikov, S.M., Melnikova, N.N., et al., 1993. Experimental study of terpinyl acetate toxicity and its hygienic standards in the air at the workplace. Gig. Sanit. 10, 27–30.

Rupa, D.S., Riccio, E.S., Rausch, L.L., et al., 2003. Genetic toxicology testing of cancer chemopreventive agents. Environ. Mol. Mutagen. 41, 201.

Russin, W.A., Hoesly, J.D., Elson, C.E., et al., 1989. Inhibition of rat mammary carcinogenesis by monoterpenoids. Carcinogenesis 10, 2161–2164.

Rutherford, T., Nixon, R., Tam, M., et al., 2007. Allergy to tea tree oil: retrospective review of 41 cases with positive patch tests over 4.5 years. Australas. J. Dermatol. 48, 83–87.

Saab, A.M., Lampronti, I., Borgatti, M., et al., 2012a. In vitro evaluation of the anti-proliferative activities of the wood essential oils of three Cedrus species against K562 human chronic myelogenous leukaemia cells. Nat. Prod. Res. 26, 2227–2231.

Saab, A.M., Tundis, R., Loizzo, M.R., et al., 2012b. Antioxidant and antiproliferative activity of *Laurus nobilis* L. (Lauraceae) leaves and seeds essential oils against K562 human chronic myelogenous leukaemia cells. Nat. Prod. Res. 26, 1741–1745.

Sabulal, B., George, V., Dan, M., et al., 2007. Chemical composition and antimicrobial activities of the essential oils from the rhizomes of four *Hedychium* species from South India. Journal of Essential Oil Research 19, 93–97.

Sacchetti, G., Maietti, S., Muzzoli, M., et al., 2005. Comparative evaluation of 11 essential oils of different origin as functional antioxidants, antiradicals and antimicrobials in foods. Food Chem. 91, 621–632.

Sadhana, A.S., Rao, A.R., Kucheria, K., et al., 1988. Inhibitory action of garlic oil on the initiation of benzo[*a*]pyrene-induced skin carcinogenesis in mice. Cancer Lett. 40, 193–197.

Sadraei, H., Ghannadi, A., Takei-Bavani, M., 2003. Effects of *Zataria multiflora* and *Carum carvi* essential oils and hydroalcoholic extracts of *Passiflora incarnata*, *Berberis integerrima* and *Crocus sativus* on rat isolated uterus contractions. Int. J. Aromather. 13, 121–127.

Saeed, M.A., Sabir, A.W., 2004. Irritant potential of some constituents from oleo-gum-resin of *Commiphora myrrha*. Fitoterapia 75, 81–84.

Safayhi, H., Sabieraj, J., Sailer, E.R., et al., 1994. Chamazulene: an antioxidant-type inhibitor of leukotriene B4 formation. Planta Med. 60, 410–413.

Safford, R.J., Basketter, D.A., Allenby, C.F., 1990. Immediate contact reactions to chemicals in the fragrance mix and a study of the quenching action of eugenol. Br. J. Dermatol. 123, 595–606.

Sahraei, H., Ghoshooni, H., Hossein Salimi, S., et al., 2002. The effects of fruit essential oil of *Pimpinella anisum* on acquisition and expression of morphine induced conditioned place preference in mice. J. Ethnopharmacol. 80, 43–47.

Saïd, A., Makki, S., Muret, P., et al., 1997. Psoralens percutaneous permeation across the human whole skin and the epidermis in respect to their polarity (*in vitro* study). J. Dermatol. Sci. 14, 136–144.

Saint-Mezard, P., Krasteva, M., Chavagnac, C., et al., 2003a. Afferent and efferent phases of allergic contact dermatitis (ACD) can be induced after a single skin contact with haptens: evidence using a mouse model of primary ACD. J. Invest. Dermatol. 120, 641–647.

Saint-Mezard, P., Chavagnac, C., Bosset, S., et al., 2003b. Psychological stress exerts an adjuvant effect on skin dendritic cell functions in vivo. J. Immun. 171, 4073–4080.

Saint-Mezard, P., Rosières, A., Krasteva, M., et al., 2004. Allergic contact dermatitis. Eur. J. Dermatol. 14, 284–295.

Saito, H., Yokoyama, A., Takeno, S., et al., 1982. Fetal toxicity and hyopglycemia induced by acetylsalicylic acid analogues. Res. Commun. Chem. Pathol. Pharmacol. 38, 209–220.

Saito, K., Uwagawa, S., Kaneko, H., et al., 1991. Behavior of α-2u-globulin accumulating in kidneys of male rats treated with *d*-limonene: kidney-type α-2u-globulin in the urine as a marker of *d*-limonene nephropathy. Toxicology 79, 173–183.

Saito, Y., Shiga, A., Yoshida, Y., et al., 2004. Effects of a novel gaseous antioxidative system containing a rosemary extract on the oxidation induced by nitrogen dioxide and ultraviolet radiation. Biosci. Biotechnol. Biochem. 68, 781–786.

Saitta, M., Di Bella, G., Salvo, F., et al., 2000. Organochloride pesticide residues in Italian citrus essential oils, 1991–1996. J. Agric. Food Chem. 48, 797–801.

Sakai, H., Tsukamoto, T., Yamamoto, M., et al., 2002. Distinction of carcinogens from mutagens by induction of liver cell foci in a model for detection of initiation activity. Cancer Lett. 188, 33–38.

Sakurai, H., Yasui, H., Yamada, Y., et al., 2005. Detection of reactive oxygen species in the skin of live mice and rats exposed to UVA light: a research review on chemiluminescence and trials for UVA protection. Photochem. Photobiol. Sci. 4, 715–720.

Salam, T.N., Fowler, J.F., 2001. Balsam-related systemic contact dermatitis. J. Am. Acad. Dermatol. 45, 377–381.

Salant, W., Nelson, E.K., 1915. Toxicity of oil of chenopodium. Am. J. Physiol. 36, 440–463.

Salant, W.F., 1917. The pharmacology of the oil of chenopodium. JAMA 69, 2016–2017.

Salazar, M., Salazar, S., Ulloa, V., et al., 1992. Teratogenic action of α-asarone in the mouse. J. Toxicol. Clin. Exp. 12, 149–154.

Salido, S., Altarejos, J., Nogueras, M., et al., 2004. Chemical composition and seasonal variation of spike lavender oil from southern Spain. Journal of Essential Oil Research 16, 206–210.

Salim, E.I., Fukushima, S., 2003. Chemopreventive potential of volatile oil from black cumin (*Nigella sativa* L.) seeds against rat colon carcinogenesis. Nutr. Cancer 45, 195–202.

Salles Trevisan, M.T., Vasconcelos Silva, M.G., Pfundstein, B., et al., 2006. Characterization of the volatile patterns and antioxidant capacity of essential oils from different species of the genus *Ocimum*. J. Agric. Food Chem. 54, 4378–4382.

Salvatore, G., D'Andrea, A., Nicoletti, M., 1998. A pinocamphone poor oil of *Hyssopus officinalis* L. var. *decumbens* from France (Banon). Journal of Essential Oil Research 10, 563–567.

Samaila, D., Ezekwudo, D.E., Yimam, K.K., et al., 2004. Bioactive plant compounds inhibited the proliferation and induced apoptosis in human cancer cell lines. Transactions of the Integrated Biomedical Informatics & Enabling Technologies Symposium Journal 1, 34–42.

Sambuco, C.P., Forbes, P.D., Davies, R.E., et al., 1987. Protective value of skin tanning induced by ultraviolet radiation plus a sunscreen containing bergamot oil. J. Soc. Cosmet. Chem. 38, 11–19.

Samiec, P.S., Drews-Botsch, C., Flagg, E.W., et al., 1998. Glutathione in human plasma: decline in association with aging, age-related macular degeneration, and diabetes. Free Radic. Biol. Med. 24, 699–704.

Samojlik, I., Petkovic, S., Mimica-Dukic, N., et al., 2012. Acute and chronic pretreatment with essential oil of peppermint (Mentha × piperita L., Lamiaceae) influences drug effects. Phytother. Res. 26, 820–825.

Sampson, W.K., Fernandez, G., 1939. Experimental convulsions in the rat. J. Pharmacol. Exp. Ther. 65, 275–280.

Sams, W.M., 1941. Photodynamic action of lime oil (*Citrus aurantifolia*). Arch. Derm. Syphilol. 44, 571–587.

Sánchez-Pérez, J., García-Díez, A., 1999. Occupational allergic contact dermatitis from eugenol, oil of cinnamon and oil of cloves in a physiotherapist. Contact Dermatitis 41, 346–347.

Sandbank, M., Abramovici, A., Wolf, R., et al., 1988. Sebaceous gland hyperplasia following topical application of citral: an ultrastructural study. Am. J. Dermatopathol. 10, 415–418.

Sanders, J.M., Bucher, J.R., Peckham, J.C., et al., 2009. Carcinogenesis studies of cresols in rats and mice. Toxicology 257, 33–39.

Sangster, S.A., Caldwell, J., Smith, R.L., 1984a. Metabolism of anethole I. Pathways of metabolism in the rat and in the mouse. Food Chem. Toxicol. 22, 695–706.

Sangster, S.A., Caldwell, J., Smith, R.L., 1984b. Metabolism of anethole II. Influence of dose size on the route of *trans*-anethole in the rat and mouse. Food Chem. Toxicol. 22, 707–713.

Sangster, S.A., Caldwell, J., Hutt, A.J., et al., 1987. The metabolic disposition of (methoxy-C)-labelled *trans*-anethole, estragole and *p*-propylanisole in human volunteers. Xenobiotica 17, 1223–1232.

Sant'Ambrogio, F.B., Anderson, J.W., Sant'Ambrogio, G., 1992. Menthol in the upper airway depresses ventilation in newborn dogs. Respir. Physiol. 89, 299–307.

Sant'anna, J.R., Franco, C.C., Miyamoto, C.T., et al., 2009. Genotoxicity of *Achillea millefolium* essential oil in diploid cells of *Aspergillus nidulans*. Phytother. Res. 23, 231–235.

Santos, F.A., Rao, V.S.N., 1997. Mast cell involvement in the rat paw oedema response to 1,8-cineole, the main constituent of eucalyptus and rosemary oils. Eur. J. Pharmacol. 331, 253–258.

Santos, F.A., Rao, V.S., 2000. Antiinflammatory and antinociceptive effects of 1,8-cineole a terpenoid oxide present in many plant essential oils. Phytother. Res. 14, 240–244.

Santos, F.A., Rao, V.S., 2001. 1,8-cineole, a food flavoring agent, prevents ethanol-induced gastric injury in rats. Dig. Dis. Sci. 46, 331–337.

Santos, F.A., Rao, V.S., 2002. Possible role of mast cells in cineole-induced scratching behavior in mice. Food Chem. Toxicol. 40, 1453–1457.

Santos, F.A., Rao, V.S., Silveira, E.R., 1997. The leaf essential oil of *Psidium guyanensis* offers protection against pentylenetetrazole-induced seizures. Planta Med. 63, 133–135.

Santos, F.A., Silva, R.M., Tomé, A.R., et al., 2001. 1,8-cineole protects against liver failure in an in-vivo murine model of endotoxemic shock. J. Pharm. Pharmacol. 53, 505–511.

Santos, F.A., Silva, R.M., Campos, A.R., et al., 2004. 1,8-cineole (eucalyptol), a monoterpene oxide attenuates the colonic damage in rats on acute TNBS-colitis. Food Chem. Toxicol. 42, 579–584.

Santos, M.R., Carvalho, A.A., Medeiros, I.A., et al., 2007. Cardiovascular effects of Hyptis fruticosa essential oil in rats. Fitoterapia 78, 186–191.

Santos-Gomes, P.C., Fernandes-Ferreira, M., 2005. Composition of the essential oils from flowers and leaves of vervain [*Aloysia tryphylla* (L'Herit.) Britton] grown in Portugal. Journal of Essential Oil Research 17, 73–78.

Santucci, B., Cristaudo, A., Cannistraci, C., et al., 1987. Contact dermatitis to fragrances. Contact Dermatitis 16, 93–95.

Sanyal, R., Darroudi, F., Parzefall, W., et al., 1997. Inhibition of the genotoxic effects of heterocyclic amines in human derived hepatoma cells by dietary bioantimutagens. Mutagenesis 12, 297–303.

Sapienza, P.P., Ikeda, G.J., Warr, P.I., et al., 1993. Tissue distribution and excretion of 14C-labelled cinnamic aldehyde following single and multiple oral administration in male Fischer 344 rats. Food Chem. Toxicol. 31, 253–261.

Saratikov, A.S., Tarasova, E.N., Khomiakova, A.F., 1957. Camphor-adrenaline synergism. (Russian). Farmakol. Toksikol 20, 84–90.

Sarici, S.U., Kul, M., Candemir, G., et al., 2004. Neonatal convulsion after accidental ingestion of sage oil: a case report. Gulhane Tip Dergisi 46, 161–162.

Sasaki, Y., Endo, R., 1978. Mutagenicity of aldehydes in *Salmonella*. Mutat. Res. 54, 251–252.

Sasaki, Y.F., Imanishi, H., Ohta, T., et al., 1989. Modifying effects of components of plant essence on the induction of sister-chromatid exchanges in cultured Chinese hamster ovary cells. Mutat. Res. 226, 103–110.

Sasaki, Y.F., Ohta, T., Imanishi, H., et al., 1990. Suppressing effects of vanillin, cinnamaldehyde, and anisaldehyde on chromosome aberrations induced by X-rays in mice. Mutat. Res. 243, 299–302.

Sashidhara, K.V., Rosaiah, J.N., Kumar, A., et al., 2007. Cell growth inhibitory action of an unusual labdane diterpene, 13-*epi*-sclareol in breast and uterine cancers *in vitro*. Phytother. Res. 21, 1105–1108.

Satchell, A.C., Saurajen, A., Bell, C., et al., 2002a. Treatment of interdigital tinea pedis with 25% and 50% tea tree oil solution: a randomized, placebo-controlled, blinded study. Australas. J. Dermatol. 43, 175–178.

Satchell, A.C., Saurajen, A., Bell, C., et al., 2002b. Treatment of dandruff with 5% tea tree oil shampoo. J. Am. Acad. Dermatol. 47, 852–855.

Sato, A., Asano, K., Sato, T., 1990. The chemical composition of *Citrus hystrix* DC (Swangi peel oil). Journal of Essential Oil Research 2, 179–183.

Saunders, N.R., Knott, G.W., Dziegielewska, K.M., 2000. Barriers in the immature brain. Cell. Mol. Neurobiol. 20, 29–40.

Savolainen, H., Pfäffli, P., 1978. Effects of long-term turpentine inhalation on rat brain protein metabolism. Chem. Biol. Interact. 21, 271–276.

Sawamura, M., 2009. Development of eco-conscious technology for essential oil extraction from and treatment of Yuzu peel waste. Project Report of the Promoting Research Fund of Japan Science and Technology Agency, pp. 1–98.

Sawamura, M., 2010. Citrus essential oils: flavor and fragrance. Wiley, Hoboken.

Sawamura, M., Sun, S.H., Ozaki, K., et al., 1999. Inhibitory effects of citrus essential oils and their components on the formation of *N*-nitrosodimethylamine. J. Agric. Food Chem. 47, 4868–4872.

Sawamura, M., Son, U.S., Choi, H.S., et al., 2004. Compositional changes in commercial lemon essential oil for aromatherapy. The International Journal of Aromatherapy 14, 27–36.

Sawamura, M., Wu, Y., Fujiwara, C., et al., 2005. Inhibitory effect of yuzu essential oil on the formation of *N*-nitrosodimethylamine in vegetables. J. Agric. Food Chem. 53, 4281–4287.

Sawamura, M., Hasegawa, K., Kashiwagi, T., et al., 2009. Determination of bergapten in Japanese citrus essential oils. Japanese Journal of Aromatherapy 9, 30–37.

Sawyer, C., Peto, R., Bernstein, L., et al., 1984. Calculation of carcinogenic potency from long-term animal carcinogenesis experiments. Biometrics 40, 27–40.

Saygili, E.I., Akcay, T., Konukoglu, D., et al., 2003. Glutathione and glutathione-related enzymes in colorectal cancer patients. J. Toxicol. Environ. Health 66, 411–415.

Sayyah, M., Valizadeh, J., Kamalinejad, M., 2002a. Anticonvulsant activity of the leaf essential oil of *Laurus nobilis* against pentylenetetrazole- and maximal electroshock-induced seizures. Phytomedicine 9, 212–216.

Sayyah, M., Mahboubi, A., Kamalinejad, M., 2002b. Anticonvulsant effect of the fruit essential oil of *Cuminum cyminum* in mice. Pharmaceutical Biology 40, 478–480.

Sayyah, M., Nadjafnia, L., Kamalinejad, M., 2004. Anticonvulsant activity and chemical composition of *Artemisia dracunculus* L. essential oil. J. Ethnopharmacol. 94, 283–287.

Scardamaglia, L., Nixon, R., Fewings, J., 2003. Compound tincture of benzoin: a common contact allergen? Australas. J. Dermatol. 44, 180–184.

SCCNFP, 1999. Opinion concerning fragrance allergy in consumers: a review of the problem. SCCNFP/0017/98 Final.

SCCNFP, 2000. Opinion concerning the 1st update of the inventory of ingredients employed in cosmetic products section II: perfume and aromatic raw materials. SCCNFP /0389/00 Final.

SCCNFP, 2001a. Opinion of the scientific committee on cosmetic products and non-food products intended for consumers concerning an initial list of perfumery materials which must not form part of cosmetic products except subject to the restrictions and conditions laid down. 25th September 2001. SCCNFP/0392/00.

SCCNFP, 2001b. Opinion of the scientific committee on cosmetic products and non-food products intended for consumers concerning diethyl phthalate. 4th June 2002. SCCNFP/0411/01.

SCCNFP, 2003a. Opinion of the scientific committee on cosmetic products and non-food products intended for consumers concerning bergamottin. 20th October 2003. SCCNFP/0740/03.

SCCNFP, 2003b. Opinion of the scientific committee on cosmetic products and non-food products intended for consumers concerning furocoumarins in sun protection and bronzing products. 9th December 2003. SCCNFP/0765/03.

SCCNFP, 2003c. Opinion of the scientific committee on cosmetic products and non-food products intended for consumers concerning diethyl phthalate. 9th December 2003. SCCNFP/0767/03.

SCCNFP, 2003d. Opinion of the scientific committee on cosmetic products and non-food products intended for consumers concerning linalool. 9th December 2003. SCCNFP/0760/03.

SCCNFP, 2003e. Opinion of the scientific committee on cosmetic products and non-food products intended for consumers concerning essential oils. 24–25 June 2003. SCCNFP/0673/03 Final.

SCCP, 2004a. Opinion on tea tree oil. Scientific Committee on Consumer products. 7th December 2004. SCCP/0843/04.

SCCP, 2004b. Opinion on atranol and chloroatranol present in natural extracts (e.g. oak moss and tree moss extract). 7th December 2004. SCCP/00847/04. http://europa.eu.int/comm/health/ph_risk/committees/04_sccp/docs/sccp_o_006.pdf

SCCP, 2005a. Opinion on Tagetes erecta, T. minuta and T. patula extracts and oils (phototoxicity only). Scientific Committee on Consumer products. 21 June 2005. SCCP/0869/05.

SCCP, 2005b. Opinion on furocoumarins in cosmetic products. Scientific Committee on Consumer products. 13 December 2005. SCCP/0942/05.

SCCP, 2005c. Opinion on Commiphora glabrescens gum extract and oil (opoponax). Sensitization only. Scientific Committee on Consumer products. 15 March 2005. SCCP/0871/05.

SCCP, 2005d. Opinion on Liquidambar spp. balsam extracts and oils (storax). Sensitization only. Scientific Committee on Consumer products 15 March 2005. SCCP/0872/05.

SCCP, 2006. Opinion on methyl-n-methylanthranilate (photo-toxicity only). European Commission Health & Consumer Protection Directorate-General. SCCP/1068/06.

SCCP, 2008. Opinion on dermal sensitization quantitative risk assessment (citral, farnesol and phenylacetaldehyde). European Commission Health & Consumer Protection Directorate-General. SCCP/1153/08.

SCF, 2001a. Opinion of the Scientific Committee on Food on methyleugenol (4-allyl-1,2-dimethoxybenzene). European Commission. SCF/CS/FLAV/FLAVOUR/4 ADD1 Final. http://europa.eu.int/comm/food/fs/sc/scf/out102_en.pdf

SCF, 2001b. Opinion of the Scientific Committee on Food on estragole (1-allyl-4-methoxybenzene). European Commission. 26th September 2001. http://europa.eu.int/comm/food/fs/sc/scf/out104_en.pdf

SCF, 2002a. Opinion of the Scientific Committee on Food on the presence of β-asarone in flavourings and other food ingredients with flavouring properties. SCF/CS/FLAV/FLAVOUR/9 ADD1 Final 8 January 2002. http://ec.europa.eu/food/fs/sc/scf/out131_en.pdf

SCF, 2002b. Opinion of the Scientific Committee on Food on benzyl alcohol. European Commission. ec.europa.eu/food/fs/sc/scf/out138_en.pdf.

SCF, 2003a. Opinion of the Scientific Committee on Food on isosafrole. European Commission 9th April 2003. SCF/CS/FLAV/FLAVOUR/30.

SCF, 2003b. Opinion of the Scientific Committee on Food on thujone. European Commission. SCF/CS/FLAV/FLAVOUR/23 ADD2 Final. http://ec.europa.eu/food/fs/sc/scf/out162_en.pdf

Schafer, E.W., Bowles, W.A., 1985. Acute oral toxicity and repellency of 933 chemicals to house and deer mice. Arch. Environ. Contam. Toxicol. 14, 111–129.

Schafer, L., Kragballe, K., 1991. Abnormalities in epidermal lipid metabolism in patients with atopic dermatitis. J. Invest. Dermatol. 96, 10–15.

Schäfer, D., Schäfer, W., 1981. Pharmacological studies with an ointment containing menthol, camphene and essential oils for broncholytic and secretolytic effects. Arzneimittelforschung 31, 82–86.

Schafer, K., Braun, H.A., Isenberg, C., 1986. Effect of menthol on cold receptor activity. J. Gen. Physiol. 88, 757–776.

Schafer, T., Bohler, E., Ruhdorfer, S., et al., 2001. Epidemiology of contact allergy in adults. Allergy 56, 1192s–1196s.

Schaller, M., Korting, H.C., 1995. Allergic airborne contact dermatitis from essential oils used in aromatherapy. Clin. Exp. Dermatol. 20, 143–145.

Schaper, M., 1993. Development of a database for sensory irritants and its use in establishing occupational exposure. Am. Ind. Hyg. Assoc. J. 54, 488–544.

Schecter, A., Lucier, G.W., Cunningham, M.L., et al., 2004. Human consumption of methyleugenol and its elimination from serum. Environ. Health Perspect. 112, 678–680.

Scheinman, P.L., 1996. Allergic contact dermatitis to fragrance: a review. Am. J. Contact Dermat. 7, 65–76.

Scheline, R.R., 1991. CRC Handbook of mammalian metabolism of plant compounds. CRC Press, Boca Raton.

Scheman, A., 2000. Adverse reactions to cosmetic ingredients. Dermatol. Clin. 18, 685–698.

Scheman, A., Gupta, S., 2001. Photoallergic contact dermatitis from diallyl disulfide. Contact Dermatitis 45, 179.

Schempp, C.M., Schopf, E., Simon, J.C., 1999. Bullous phototoxic contact dermatitis caused by *Ruta graveolens* L. (garden rue), Rutaceae. Case report and review of literature. Hautzart 50, 432–434.

Scheper, M.A., Shirtliff, M.E., Meiller, T.F., et al., 2008. Farnesol, a fungal quorum-sensing molecule triggers apoptosis in human oral squamous carcinoma cells. Neoplasia 10, 954–963.

Scheuplein, R.J., Blank, I.H., 1971. Permeability of the skin. Physiol. Rev. 51, 702–747.

Schiestl, R.H., Chan, W.S., Gietz, R.D., et al., 1989. Safrole, eugenol and methyleugenol induce intrachromosomal recombination in yeast. Mutat. Res. 224, 427–436.

Schilcher, H., Leuschner, F., 1997. The potential nephrotoxic effects of juniper essential oil. Arzneimittelforschung 47, 855–858.

Schilcher, H., Emmrich, D., Koehler, C., 1993. Gas Chromatographischer Verleich von ätherischen Wacholderölen und deren toxikologische Bewertung. Pharmazeutische Zeitung 138, 85–91.

Schimmer, O., Kühne, I., 1990. Mutagenic compounds in an extract from Rutae Herba (*Ruta graveolens* L.). II. UV-A mediated mutagenicity in the green alga *Chlamydomonas reinhardtii* by furoquinoline alkaloids and furocoumarins present in a commercial tincture from Rutae Herba. Mutat. Res. 243, 57–62.

Schlatter, J., Zimmerli, B., Dick, R., et al., 1991. Dietary intake and risk assessment of phototoxic furocoumarins in humans. Food Chem. Toxicol. 29, 523–530.

Schlede, E., Aberer, W., Fuchs, T., et al., 2003. Chemical substances and contact allergy – 244 substances ranked according to allergenic potency. Toxicology 193, 219–259.

Schmeck-Lindenau, H.J., Naser-Hijazi, B., Becker, E.W., et al., 2003. Safety aspects of a coumarin-troxerutin combination regarding liver function in a double-blind placebo-controlled study. Int. J. Clin. Pharmacol. Ther. 41, 193–199.

Schmidt, E., 2003. The characteristics of lavender oils from Eastern Europe. Perfumer & Flavorist 28, 48–60.

Schmiedlin-Ren, P., Edwards, D.J., Fitzsimmons, M.E., et al., 1997. Mechanisms of enhanced oral availability of CYP3A4 substrates by grapefruit constituents: decreased enterocyte CYP3A4 concentration and mechanism-based inactivation by furanocoumarins. Drug Metab. Dispos. 25, 1228–1233.

Schmitt, S., Schäfer, U.F., Döbler, L., et al., 2009. Cooperative interaction of monoterpenes and phenylpropanoids on the in vitro human skin permeation of complex composed essential oils. Planta Med. 75, 1381–1385.

Schmitt, S., Schäfer, U.F., Döbler, L., et al., 2010. Variation of in vitro human skin permeation of rose oil between different application sites. Forsch. Komplementärmed. 17, 126–131.

Schnaubelt, K., 1995. Advanced aromatherapy: the science of essential oil therapy. Healing Arts Press, Rochester, p. 54.

Schnuch, A., Geier, J., Uter, W., et al., 1997. National rates and regional differences in sensitization to allergens of the standard series. Population-adjusted frequencies of sensitization (PAFS) in 40,000 patients from a multicenter study (IVDK). Contact Dermatitis 37, 200–209.

Schnuch, A., Uter, W., Geier, J., et al., 2002a. Epidemiology of contact allergy: an estimation of morbidity employing the clinical epidemiology and drug-utilization research (CE-DUR) approach. Contact Dermatitis 47, 32–39.

Schnuch, A., Geier, J., Uter, W., et al., 2002b. Another look at allergies to fragrances: frequencies of sensitisation to the fragrance mix and its constituents. Exogenous Dermatology 1, 231–237.

Schnuch, A., Lessmann, H., Geier, J., et al., 2004a. Contact allergy to fragrances: frequencies of sensitization from 1996 to 2002. Results of the IVDK. Contact Dermatitis 50, 65–76.

Schnuch, A., Uter, W., Geier, J., et al., 2004b. Contact allergy to farnesol in 2021 consecutively patch tested patients. Results of the IVDK. Contact Dermatitis 50, 117–121.

Schnuch, A., Lessmann, H., Geier, J., et al., 2006. White petrolatum (Ph. Eur.) is virtually non-sensitizing. Analysis of IVDK data on 80 000 patients tested between 1992 and 2004 and short discussion of identification and designation of allergens. Contact Dermatitis 54, 338–343.

Schnuch, A., Uter, W., Geier, J., et al., 2007a. Sensitization to 26 fragrances to be labelled according to current European regulation. Results of the IVDK and review of the literature. Contact Dermatitis 57, 1–10.

Schnuch, A., Brasch, J., Lessmann, H., et al., 2007b. A further characteristic of susceptibility to contact allergy: sensitization to a weak contact allergen is associated with polysensitization. Results of the IVDK. Contact Dermatitis 56, 331–337.

Schnuch, A., Brasch, J., Uter, W., 2008. Polysensitization and increased susceptibility in contact allergy: a review. Allergy 63, 156–167.

Schnuch, A., Westphal, G., Mössner, R., et al., 2010. Genetic factors in contact allergy – review and future goals. Contact Dermatitis 64, 2–23.

Schnuch, A., Oppel, E., Oppel, T., et al., 2011. Experimental inhalation of fragrance allergens in predisposed subjects: effects on skin and airways. Br. J. Dermatol. 162, 598–606.

Schoket, B., Horkay, I., Kosa, A., et al., 1990. Formation of DNA adducts in the skin of psoriasis patients, in human skin in organ culture, and in mouse skin and lung following topical application of coal-tar and juniper tar. J. Invest. Dermatol. 94, 241–246.

Schorr, W.F., 1975. Cinnamic aldehyde allergy. Contact Dermatitis 1, 108–111.

Schröder, V., Vollmer, H., 1932. The excretion of thymol, carvacrol, eugenol, and guaiacol and the distribution of these substances in the organism. Naunyn Schmiedebergs Arch. Exp. Pathol. Pharmakol. 168, 331–353.

Schuh, T.J., Hall, B.L., Kraft, J.C., et al., 1993. v-erbA and citral reduce the teratogenic effects of all-*trans* retinoic acid and retinol, respectively, in *Xenopus* embryogenesis. Development 119, 785–798.

Schuster, O., Haag, F., Priester, H., 1986. Transdermal absorption of terpenes from essential oils of Pinimenthol-S ointment. Med. Welt. 37, 100–102.

Sciarrone, D., Ragonese, C., Carnovale, C., et al., 2010. Evaluation of tea tree oil quality and ascaridole: a deep study by means of chiral and multi heart-cuts multidimensional gas chromatography system coupled to mass spectrometry detection. J. Chromatogr. A 1217, 6422–6427.

Scognamiglio, J., Jones, L., Vitale, D., et al., 2012. Fragrance material review on benzyl alcohol. Food Chem. Toxicol. 50, S140–S160.

Scolnik, M.D., Servadio, C., Abramovici, A., 1994a. Comparative study of experimentally induced benign and atypical hyperplasia in the ventral prostate of different rat strains. J. Androl. 15, 287–297.

Scolnik, M., Konichezky, M., Tykochinsky, G., et al., 1994b. Immediate vasoactive effect of citral on the adolescent rat ventral prostate. Prostate 25, 1–9.

Seawright, A., 1993. Comments on tea tree oil poisoning. Med. J. Aust. 159, 831.

Segal, R., Milo-Goldzweig, I., 1985. The hemolytic activity of citral – II. Glutathione depletion in citral treated erythrocytes. Biochem. Pharmacol 34, 4117–4119.

Seidenari, S., Di Nardo, A., Motolese, A., et al., 1990a. Erythema multiforme associated with contact sensitization: description of 6 clinical cases. G. Ital. Dermatol. Venereol. 125, 35–40.

Seidenari, S., Manzini, B.M., Danese, P., et al., 1990b. Patch and prick test study of 593 healthy subjects. Contact Dermatitis 23, 162–167.

Seidl, H., Kreimer-Erlacher, H., Back, B., et al., 2001. Ultraviolet exposure as the main initiator of p53 mutations in basal cell carcinomas from psoralen and ultraviolet A-treated patients with psoriasis. J. Invest. Dermatol. 117, 365–370.

Seife, M., Leon, J.L., 1954. Camphor poisoning following ingestion of nose drops. J. Am. Med. Assoc. 155, 1059–1060.

Seki, T., Tsuji, K., Hayato, Y., et al., 2000. Garlic and onion oils inhibit proliferation and induce differentiation of HL-60 cells. Cancer Lett. 160, 29–35.

Sekihashi, A., Yamamoto, A., Matsumura, Y., et al., 2002. Comparative investigation of multiple organs of mice and rats in the comet assay. Mutat. Res. 517, 53–74.

Sekizawa, J., Shibamoto, T., 1982. Genotoxicity of safrole-related chemicals in microbial test systems. Mutat. Res. 101, 127–140.

Select Committee on GRAS Substances, 1973. Evaluation of the health aspects of benzoic acid and sodium benzoate as food ingredients. U.S. Food & Drug Administration Report. NTIS Report No. PB-223 837.

Selvaag, E., Eriksen, B., Thune, P., 1994. Contact allergy due to tea tree oil and cross-sensitization to colophony. Contact Dermatitis 31, 124–125.

Selvaag, E., Holm, J.O., Thune, P., 1995. Allergic contact dermatitis in an aromatherapist with multiple sensitizations to essential oils. Contact Dermatitis 33, 354–355.

Selvi, R.T., Niranjali, S., 1998. Inhibition by eugenol of diethylnitrosamine-induced microsomal degranulation. Fitoterapia 69, 115–117.

Senatore, F., Della Porta, G., Reverchon, E., 1996. Constituents of *Vitex agnus-castus* L. essential oil. Flavour & Fragrance Journal 11, 179–182.

Sensch, O., Vierling, W., Brandt, W., et al., 2000. Effects of inhibition of calcium and potassium currents in guinea-pig cardiac contraction: comparison of β-caryophyllene oxide, eugenol, and nifedipine. Br. J. Pharmacol. 131, 1089–1096.

Seo, K.W., Kim, K.B., Kim, Y.J., et al., 2004. Comparison of oxidative stress and changes of xenobiotic metabolizing enzymes induced by phthalates in rats. Food Chem. Toxicol. 42, 107–114.

Seo, J.Y., Lim, S.S., Kim, J.R., et al., 2008. Nrf2-mediated induction of detoxifying enzymes by alantolactone present in Inula helenium. Phytother. Res. 22, 1500–1505.

Seo, K.A., Kim, H., Ku, H.Y., et al., 2008. The monoterpenoids citral and geraniol are moderate inhibitors of CYP2B6 hydroxylase activity. Chem. Biol. Interact. 174, 141–146.

Sepici, A., Gürbüz, I., Çevik, C., et al., 2004. Hypoglycaemic effects of myrtle oil in normal and alloxan-diabetic rabbits. J. Ethnopharmacol. 93, 311–318.

Serafino, A., Sinibaldi Vallebona, P., Andreola, F., et al., 2008. Stimulatory effect of Eucalyptus essential oil on innate cell-mediated immune response. BMC Immunol doi: 10.1186/1471-2172-9-17.

Serrano, G., Pujol, C., Cuadra, J., et al., 1989. Riehl's melanosis: pigmented contact dermatitis caused by fragrances. J. Am. Acad. Dermatol. 21, 1057–1060.

Sertel, S., Eichhorn, T., Plinkert, P.K., et al., 2011a. Cytotoxicity of Thymus vulgaris essential oil towards human oral cavity squamous cell carcinoma. Anticancer Res. 31, 81–87.

Sertel, S., Eichhorn, T., Plinkert, P.K., et al., 2011b. Chemical composition and antiproliferative activity of essential oil from the leaves of a medicinal herb, Levisticum officinale, against UMSCC1 head and neck squamous carcinoma cells. Anticancer Res. 31, 185–191.

Servadio, C., Abramovici, A., Sandbank, U., et al., 1986. Early stages of the pathogenesis of rat ventral prostate hyperplasia induced by citral. Eur. Urol. 12, 195–200.

Seth, G., Kokate, C.K., Varma, K.C., 1976. Effect of essential oil of Cymbopogon citrates Stapf. On central nervous system. Indian J. Exp. Biol. 14, 370–371.

Seto, T.A., Keup, W., 1969. Effects of alkylmethoxybenzene and alkylmethylenedioxybenzene essential oils on pentobarbital and ethanol sleeping time. Arch. Int. Pharmacodyn. Ther. 180, 232–241.

Sewell, J.S., 1925. Poisoning by eucalyptus oil. Br. Med. J. 1, 922.

Sezik, E., Tümen, G., Kirimer, N., et al., 1993. Essential oil composition of four Origanum vulgare subspecies of Anatolian origin. Journal of Essential Oil Research 5, 425–431.

Shaath, N.A., Azzo, N.R., 1993. Essential oils of Egypt. In: Charalambous, G. (Ed.), Food Flavors, Ingredients and Composition. Elsevier, Amsterdam, pp. 591–603.

Shafi, P.M., Saidutty, A., Clery, R.A., 2000. Volatile constituents of Zanthoxylum rhetsa leaves and seeds. Journal of Essential Oil Research 12, 179–182.

Shah, N.C., 1991. Chemical composition of the pericarp oil of Zanthxylum armatum DC. Journal of Essential Oil Research 3, 467–468.

Shahat, A., Ibrahim, A.Y., Hendawy, S.F., et al., 2011. Chemical composition, antimicrobial and antioxidant activities of essential oils from organically cultivated fennel cultivars. Molecules 16, 1366–1377.

Shahsavari, R., Ehsani-Zonouz, A., Houshmand, M., et al., 2009. Plasma glucose lowering effect of the wild Satureja khuzestanica Jamzad essential oil in diabetic rats: role of decreased gluconeogenesis. Pakistan Journal of Biological Sciences 12, 140–145.

Shalaby, A.S., El-Gamasy, A.M., Khattab, M.D., et al., 1988. Changes in the chemical composition of Mentha piperita and Mentha viridis oils during storage. Egyptian Journal of Horticulture 15, 225–240.

Shalaby, A.S., El-Gengaihi, S., Khattab, M., 1995. Oil of Melissa officinalis L., as affected by storage and herb drying. Journal of Essential Oil Research 7, 667–669.

Shankaran, V., Ikeda, H., Bruce, A.T., et al., 2001. IFNgamma and lymphocytes prevent primary tumour development and shape tumour immunogenicity. Nature 410, 1107–1111.

Shapiro, R., Frances, J., 2001. Cascarilla bark essential oil of El Salvador, new source and standard. Perfumer & Flavorist 26, 22–26.

Sharafi, S.M., Rasooli, I., Owlia, P., et al., 2010. Protective effects of bioactive phytochemicals from Mentha piperita with multiple health potentials. Pharmacognosy Magazine 6, 147–153.

Sharma, J.D., Dandiya, P.C., 1962. Studies in Acorus calamus Part VI. Pharmacological actions of asarone and beta-asarone on cardiovascular system and smooth muscles. Indian J. Med. Res 50, 61–65.

Sharma, R.A., Farmer, P.B., 2004. Biological relevance of adduct detection to the chemoprevention of cancer. Clin. Cancer Res. 10, 4901–4912.

Sharma, O.P., Sharma, S., Pattabhi, V., et al., 2007. A review of the hepatotoxic plant Lantana camara. Crit. Rev. Toxicol. 37, 313–352.

Sharma, P.R., Mondhe, D.M., Muthiah, S., et al., 2009. Anticancer activity of an essential oil from Cymbopogon flexuosus. Chem. Biol. Interact. 179, 160–168.

Sharma, M., Agrawal, S.K., Sharma, P.R., et al., 2010. Cytotoxic and apoptotic activity of essential oil from Ocimum viride towards COLO 205 cells. Food Chem. Toxicol. 48, 336–344.

Sharp, D.W., 1978. The sensitization potential of some perfume ingredients tested using a modified draize procedure. Toxicology 9, 261–271.

Shaughnessy, D.T., Setzer, R.W., DeMarini, D.M., 2001. The antimutagenic effect of vanillin and cinnamaldehyde on spontaneous mutation in Salmonella TA104 is due to a reduction in mutations at GC but not AT sites. Mutat. Res. 480–481, 55–69.

Shaughnessy, D.T., Schaaper, R.M., Umbach, D.M., et al., 2006. Inhibition of spontaneous mutagenesis by vanillin and cinnamaldehyde in Escherichia coli: dependence on recombinational repair. Mutat. Res. 602, 54–64.

Shea, K.M., 2003. Pediatric exposure and potential toxicity of phthalate plasticizers. Pediatrics 111, 1467–1474.

Sheen, L.Y., Sheu, S.F., Tsai, S.J., et al., 1999a. Effect of garlic active principle, diallyl disulphide, on cell viability, lipid peroxidation, glutathione concentration and its related enzyme activities in primary rat hepatocytes. Am. J. Chin. Med. 27, 95–105.

Sheen, L.Y., Wu, C.C., Lii, C.K., et al., 1999b. Metabolites of diallyl disulfide and diallyl sulfide in primary rat hepatocytes. Food Chem. Toxicol. 37, 1139–1146.

Sheen, L.Y., Wu, C.C., Lii, C.K., et al., 2001. Effect of diallyl sulfide and diallyl disulfide, the active principles of garlic, on the aflatoxin B(1)-induced DNA damage in primary rat hepatocytes. Toxicol. Lett. 122, 45–52.

Shehab, N., Lewis, C.L., Streetman, D.D., et al., 2009. Exposure to the pharmaceutical excipients benzyl alcohol and propylene glycol among critically ill neonates. Pediatr. Crit. Care Med. 10, 256–259.

Shelby, M.D., Erexson, G.L., Hook, G.J., et al., 1993. Evaluation of a three-exposure mouse bone marrow micronucleus protocol: results with 49 chemicals. Environ. Mol. Mutagen. 21, 160–179.

Shen, J., Niijima, A., Tanida, M., et al., 2005. Olfactory stimulation with scent of grapefruit oil affects autonomic nerves, lipolysis and appetite in rats. Neurosci. Lett. 380, 289–294.

Shenoi, S.D., Rao, R., 2007. Pigmented contact dermatitis. Indian J. Dermatol. Venereol. Leprol. 73, 285–287.

Sherry, C.J., Burnett, R.E., 1978. Enhancement of ethanol-induced sleep by whole oil of nutmeg. Experientia 34, 492–493.

Shieh, B., Lizuka, Y., Matsubara, Y., 1981. Monoterpenoid and sesquiterpenoid constituents of the essential oil of Hinoki (Chamaecyparis obtusa (Sieb. et Zucc.) Endl.). Journal of Agriculture Biology & Chemistry (Japan) 45, 1497–1499.

Shiina, Y., Funabashi, N., Lee, K., et al., 2008. Relaxation effects of lavender aromatherapy improve coronary flow velocity reserve in healthy men evaluated by transthoracic Doppler echocardiography. Int. J. Cardiol. 129, 193–197.

Shilling, W.H., Crampton, R.F., Longland, R.C., 1969. Metabolism of coumarin in man. Nature 221, 664–665.

Shim, C., Williams, M.H., 1986. Effect of odors in asthma. Am. J. Med. 80, 18–22.

Shimada, T., Shindo, M., Miyazawa, M., 2002. Species differences in the metabolism of (+)- and (-)-limonenes and their metabolites, carveols and carvones, by cytochrome P450 enzymes in liver microsomes of mice, rats, guinea pigs, rabbits, dogs, monkeys, and humans. Drug Metab. Pharmacokinet. 17, 507–515.

Shinde, U.A., Kulkarni, K.R., Phadke, A.S., et al., 1999a. Mast cell stabilizing and lipoxygenase inhibitory activity of Cedrus deodara (Roxb.) Loud. wood oil. Indian J. Exp. Biol. 37, 258–261.

Shinde, U.A., Phadke, A.S., Nair, A.M., et al., 1999b. Preliminary studies on the immunomodulatory activities of Cedrus deodara wood oil. Fitoterapia 70, 333–339.

Shipochliev, T., 1968. Pharmacological study of a group of essential oils. II. (in Bulgarian). Vet. Med. Nauki 5, 87–92.

Shoff, S.M., Grummer, M., Yatvin, M.B., et al., 1991. Concentration-dependent increase of murine P388 and B16 population doubling time by the acyclic monoterpene geraniol. Cancer Res. 51, 37–42.

Shtenberg, A.J., Ignatev, A.D., 1970. Toxicological evaluation of some combination of food preservatives. Food Cosmet. Toxicol. 8, 369–380.

Shulgin, A.T., 1966. Possible implication of myristicin as a psychotropic substance. Nature 210, 380–384.

Shusterman, D., Murphy, M.A., 2007. Nasal hyperreactivity in allergic and non-allergic rhinitis: a potential risk factor for non-specific building-related illness. Indoor Air 17, 328–333.

Shusterman, D., Murphy, M.A., Blames, J., 2003. Differences in nasal irritant sensitivity by age, gender, and allergic rhinitis status. Int. Arch. Occup. Environ. Health 76, 577–583.

Shwaireb, M.H., 1993. Caraway oil inhibits skin tumors in female BALB/c mice. Nutr. Cancer 19, 321–325.

Sibanda, S., Chigwada, G., Poole, M., et al., 2004. Composition and bioactivity of the leaf essential oil of *Heteropyxis dehniae* from Zimbabwe. J. Ethnopharmacol. 92, 107–111.

Sicé, J., Shubik, P., Feldman, R., 1957. Epithelial tumors induced by normal paraffins and derivatives. In: Twelfth International Congress on Occupational Health, vol. 3. Helsinki, p. 266.

Sidell, N., Verity, M.A., Nord, E.P., 1990. Menthol blocks dihydropyridine-insensitive Ca2+ channels and induces neurite outgrowth in human neuroblastoma cells. J. Cell. Physiol. 142, 410–419.

Sidibé, L., Chalchat, J.C., Garry, R.P., et al., 2001. Aromatic plants of Mali (IV): chemical composition of essential oils of *Cymbopogon citratus* (DC) Stapf and C. *giganteus* (Hochst.) Chiov. Journal of Essential Oil Research 13, 110–112.

Siegel, E., Wason, S., 1986. Camphor toxicity. Pediatr. Clin. North Am. 33, 375–379.

Sies, H., Stahl, W., 2004. Nutritional protection against skin damage from sunlight. Annu. Rev. Nutr. 24, 173–200.

Sigurdsson, S., Ogmundsdottir, H.M., Gudbjarnason, S., 2005. The cytotoxic effect of two chemotypes of essential oils from the fruits of *Angelica archangelica* L. Anticancer Res. 25, 1877–1880.

Silva, J., Abebe, W., Sousa, S.M., et al., 2003. Analgesic and anti-inflammatory effects of essential oils of *Eucalyptus*. J. Ethnopharmacol. 89, 277–283.

Silva Brum, L.F., Emanuelli, T., Souza, D.O., 2001a. Effects of linalool on glutamate release and uptake in mouse cortical synaptosomes. Neurochem. Res. 26, 191–194.

Silva Brum, L.F., Elisabetsky, E., Souza, D., 2001b. Effects of linalool on [(3)H]MK801 and [(3)H] muscimol binding in mouse cortical membranes. Phytother. Res. 15, 422–425.

Simmon, V.F., Kauhanen, K., Tardiff, R.G., 1977. Mutagenic activity of chemicals identified in drinking water. Dev. Toxicol. Environ. Sci. 2, 249–258.

Simons, C.T., Carstens, M.I., Carstens, E., 2003. Oral irritation by mustard oil: self-desensitization and cross-desensitization with capsaicin. Chem. Senses 28, 459–465.

Simpson, G.I., Jackson, Y.A., 2002. Comparison of the chemical composition of East Indian, Jamaican and other West Indian essential oils of *Myristica fragrans* Houtt. Journal of Essential Oil Research 14, 6–9.

Singh, A., Shukla, Y., 1998. Antitumour activity of diallyl sulfide on polycyclic aromatic hydrocarbon-induced mouse skin carcinogenesis. Cancer Lett. 131, 209–214.

Singh, A., Singh, S.P., Bamezai, R., 1999. Modulatory potential of clocimum oil on mouse skin papillomagenesis and the xenobiotic detoxication system. Food Chem. Toxicol. 37, 663–670.

Singh, A., Singh, S.P., Bamezai, R., 2000. Direct and translactational effect of arecoline alkaloid on the clocimum oil-modulated hepatic drug metabolizing enzymes in mice. Food Chem. Toxicol. 38, 627–635.

Singh, G., Kapoor, I.P., Singh, O.P., et al., 2000. Studies on essential oils, part 28: Chemical composition, antifungal and insecticidal activities of rhizome volatile oil of *Homalomena aromatica* Schott. Flavour & Fragrance Journal 15, 278–280.

Singh, B., Kumar, R., Bhandari, S., et al., 2007. Volatile constituents of natural *Boswellia serrata* oleo-gum-resin and commercial samples. Flavour & Fragrance Journal 22, 145–147.

Singh, G., Maurya, S., DeLampasona, M.P., et al., 2007. A comparison of chemical, antioxidant and antimicrobial studies of cinnamon leaf and bark volatile oils, oleoresins and their constituents. Food Chem. Toxicol. 45, 1650–1661.

Singh, G., Kapoor, I.P., Singh, P., et al., 2008. Chemistry, antioxidant and antimicrobial investigations on essential oil and oleoresins of *Zingiber officinale*. Food Chem. Toxicol. 46, 3295–3302.

Singhal, R.S., Kulkarni, P.R., Rege, D.V., 1997. Handbook of indices of food quality and authenticity. Woodhead Publishing, Abington.

Singhal, R.S., Kulkarni, P.R., Rege, D.V., 2001. In: Peter, K.V. (Ed.), Handbook of Herbs & Spices, vol. 1. CRC Press, Boca Raton.

Siveen, K.S., Kuttan, G., 2011. Augmentation of humoral and cell mediated immune responses by thujone. Int. Immunopharmacol. 11, 1967–1975.

Sivropoulou, A., Papanikolaou, E., Nikolaou, C., et al., 1996. Antimicrobial and cytotoxic activities of *Origanum* essential oils. J. Agric. Food Chem. 44, 1202–1205.

Sjöqvist, F., 1965. Psychotropic drugs (2). Interaction between monoamine oxidase (MAO) inhibitors and other substances. Proc. R. Soc. Med. 58, 967–978.

Skalli, S., Bencheikh, R.S., 2011. Epileptic seizures induced by fennel essential oil. Epileptic Discord. 13, 345–347.

Skoglund, R.R., Ware, L.L., Schanberger, J.E., 1977. Prolonged seizures due to contact and inhalation exposure to camphor: a case report. Clin. Pediatr. (Philadelphia) 16, 901–902.

Sköld, M., Börje, A., Matura, M., et al., 2002. Studies on the autoxidation and sensitizing capacity of the fragrance chemical linalool, identifying a linalool hydroperoxide. Contact Dermatitis 46, 267–272.

Sköld, M., Börje, A., Harambasic, E., et al., 2004. Contact allergens formed on air exposure of linalool. Identification and quantification of primary and secondary oxidation products and the effect on skin sensitization. Chem. Res. Toxicol. 17, 1697–1705.

Sköld, M., Karlberg, A.T., Matura, M., et al., 2005. The fragrance chemical beta-caryophyllene: air oxidation and skin sensitization. Food Chem. Toxicol. 44, 538–545.

Skovbjerg, S., Johansen, J.D., Rasmussen, A., et al., 2009. General practitioners' experiences with provision of healthcare to patients with self-reported multiple chemical sensitivity. Scand. J. Prim. Health Care 18, 1–5.

Skrebova, N., Brocks, K., Karlsmark, T., 1998. Allergic contact cheilitis from spearmint oil. Contact Dermatitis 39, 35.

Slamenová, D., Horváthová, E., Sramková, M., et al., 2007. DNA-protective effects of two components of essential plant oils carvacrol and thymol on mammalian cells cultured *in vitro*. Neoplasma 54, 108–112.

Slamenová, D., Horvathova, E., Marsalkova, L., et al., 2008. Carvacrol given to rats in drinking water reduces the level of DNA lesions induced in freshly isolated hepatocytes and testicular cells by H(2)O(2). Neoplasma 55, 394–399.

Slamenová, D., Horváthová, E., Wsólová, L., et al., 2009. Investigation of anti-oxidative, cytotoxic, DNA-damaging and DNA-protective effects of plant volatiles eugenol and borneol in human-derived HepG2, Caco-2 and VH10 cell lines. Mutat. Res. 677, 46–52.

Smith, W., 1844. Poisoning by oil of bitter almonds. Lancet 43 (1084), 335.

Smith, W., 1862. Royal Medical & Chirurgical Society: a case of poisoning by oil of wormwood (*Artemisia absinthium*). Lancet 80 (2049), 619.

Smith, A., Margolis, G., 1954. Camphor poisoning. Am. J. Pathol. 30, 857–869.

Smith, T.J., Guo, Z.Y., Thomas, P.E., et al., 1990. Metabolism of 4-(methylnitrosamino)-1-(3-pyridyl)-1-butanone in mouse lung microsomes and its inhibition by isothiocyanates. Cancer Res. 50, 6817–6822.

Smith, C.K., Moore, C.A., Elahi, E.N., et al., 2000. Human skin absorption and metabolism of the contact allergens, cinnamic aldehyde, and cinnamic alcohol. Toxicol. Appl. Pharmacol. 168, 189–199.

Smith, R.L., Adams, T.B., Doull, J., et al., 2002. Safety assessment of allylalcoxybenzene derivatives used as flavouring substances – methyl eugenol and estragole. Food Chem. Toxicol. 40, 851–870.

Smyth, H.F., Carpenter, C.P., Weil, C.S., 1951. Range-finding toxicity data: List IV. Arch. Ind. Hyg. Occup. Med. 4, 119–122.

Snyder, R.D., Drummond, P.D., 1997. Olfaction in migraine. Cephalalgia 17, 729–732.

Soares, M.C., Damiani, C.E., Moreira, C.M., et al., 2005. Eucalyptol, an essential oil, reduces contractile activity in rat cardiac muscle. Braz. J. Med. Biol. Res. 38, 453–461.

Soares, P.M., Assreuy, A.M., Souza, E.P., et al., 2005. Inhibitory effects of the essential oil of *Mentha pulegium* on the isolated rat myometrium. Planta Med. 71, 214–218.

Söderberg, T.A., Johansson, A., Gref, R., 1996. Toxic effects of some conifer resin acids and tea tree oil on human epithelial and fibroblast cells. Toxicology 107, 99–109.

Sœur, J., Marrot, L., Perez, P., et al., 2011. Selective cytotoxicity of *Aniba rosaeodora* essential oil towards epidermoid cancer cells through induction of apoptosis. Mutat. Res. 718, 24–32.

Sofuni, T., Hayashi, M., Matsuoka, A., et al., 1985. Mutagenicity tests on organic chemical contaminants in city water and related compounds. II. Chromosome aberration tests in cultured mammalian cells. Eisei Shikenjo Hokoku 103, 64–75.

Solheim, E., Scheline, R.R., 1973. Metabolism of alkenebenzene derivatives in the rat. I. p-methoxyallylbenzene (estragole) and p-methoxypropenylbenzene (anethole). Xenobiotica 3, 493–510.

Solheim, E., Scheline, R.R., 1980. Metabolism of alkenebenzene derivatives in the rat. III. Elemicin and isoelemicin. Xenobiotica 10, 371–380.

Soliman, F.M., El-Kashoury, E.A., Fathy, M.M., et al., 1994. Analysis and biological activity of the essential oil of Rosmarinus officinalis L. from Egypt. Flavour & Fragrance Journal 9, 29–33.

Solt, D.B., Chang, K., Helenowski, I., et al., 2003. Phenethyl isothiocyanate inhibits nitrosamine carcinogenesis in a model for study of oral cancer chemoprevention. Cancer Lett. 202, 147–152.

Someya, H., Higo, Y., Ohno, M., et al., 2008. Clastogenic activity of seven endodontic medications used in dental practice in human dental pulp cells. Mutat. Res. 650, 39–47.

Soni, B.P., Sherertz, E.F., 1997. Evaluation of previously patch-tested patients referred to a contact dermatitis clinic. Am. J. Contact Dermat. 8, 10–14.

Sonwa, M.M., 2000. Isolation and structure elucidation of essential oil constituents: comparative study of the oils of Cyperus alopecuroides, Cyperus papyrus and Cyperus rotundus. Dissertation, University of Hamburg, Faculty of Chemistry. www.sub.uni-hamburg.de/disse/372/diss.pdf.

Sørensen, J.M., Katsiotis, S.T., 2000. Parameters influencing the yield and composition of the essential oil from Cretan Vitex agnus-castus fuits. Planta Med. 66, 245–250.

Soukoulis, S., Hirsch, R., 2004. The effects of a tea tree oil-containing gel on plaque and chronic gingivitis. Aust. Dent. J. 49, 78–83.

Southwell, I., 1997. Tea tree oil composition, standards and monographs. Cosmetics, Aerosols & Toiletries in Australia. 10, 14–17.

Southwell, I.A., 2006. p-Cymene and organic peroxides as indicators of oxidation in tea tree oil. Rural Industries Research & Development Corporation Publication No: 06/112.

Southwell, I.A., Stiff, I.A., 1995. Chemical composition of an Australian geranium oil. Journal of Essential Oil Research 7, 545–547.

Southwell, I.A., Freeman, S., Rubel, D., 1997. Skin irritancy of tea tree oil. Journal of Essential Oil Research 9, 47–52.

Southwell, I.A., Russell, M., Smith, R.L., et al., 2000. Backhousia citriodora F. Muell. (Myrtaceae), a superior source of citral. Journal of Essential Oil Research 12, 735–741.

Southwell, I.A., Russell, M.F., Davies, N.W., 2011. Detecting traces of methyl eugenol in essential oils: tea tree oil, a case study. Flavour & Fragrance Journal doi: 10.1002/ffj.2067.

Sparks, T., 1985. Cinnamon oil burn. West. J. Med. 142, 835.

Sparnins, V.L., Barany, G., Wattenberg, L.W., 1988. Effects of organosulfur compounds from garlic and onions on benzo[a]pyrene-induced neoplasia and glutathione S-transferase activity in the mouse. Carcinogenesis 9, 131–134.

Spector, W.S. (Ed.), 1956. Handbook of toxicology vol. 1. Acute toxicities. WB Saunders, Philadelphia.

Sperber, E.F., Veliskova, J., Germano, I.M., et al., 1999. Age-dependent vulnerability to seizures. Adv. Neurol. 79, 161–169.

Spindler, P., Madsen, C., 1992. Subchronic toxicity study of peppermint oil in rats. Toxicol. Lett. 62, 215–220.

Spinner, J.R., 1920. The toxicology of eucalyptus and other essential oils, with special consideration for their abortifacient activity. Dtsch. Med. Wochenschr. 46, 389–391.

Spoerke, D.G., Vandenberg, S.A., Smolinske, S.C., et al., 1989. Eucalyptus oil: 14 cases of exposure. Vet. Hum. Toxicol. 31, 166–168.

Sporn, A., Dinu, I., Stanciu, V., 1965. Investigation of the toxicity of cinnamaldehyde. Igiena 14, 339–346.

Sreenan, C., Etches, P.C., Demianczuk, N., et al., 2001. Isolated mental developmental delay in very low birth weight infants: association with prolonged doxapram therapy for apnea. J. Pediatr. 139, 832–837.

Srinivas, S.R., 1986. Atlas of essential oils. Srinivas, New York.

Srivastava, A.K., Srivastava, S.K., Shah, N., 2001. Constituents of the rhizome essential oil of Curcuma amada Roxb. from India. Journal of Essential Oil Research 13, 63–64.

Stafstrom, C.E., 2007. Seizures in a 7-month-old child after exposure to the essential plant oil thuja. Pediatr. Neurol. 37, 446–448.

Stammati, A., Bonsi, P., Zucco, F., et al., 1999. Toxicity of selected plant volatiles in microbial and mammalian short-term assays. Food Chem. Toxicol. 37, 813–823.

Standen, M.D., Connellan, P.A., Leach, D.N., 2006. Natural killer cell activity and lymphocyte activation; investigating the effects of a selection of essential oils and components in vitro. Int. J. Aromather. 16, 133–139.

Stark, M.J., Burke, Y.D., McKinzie, J.H., et al., 1995. Chemotherapy of pancreatic cancer with the monoterpene perillyl alcohol. Cancer Lett. 96, 15–21.

Starke, J.C., 1967. Photoallergy to sandalwood oil. Arch. Dermatol. 96, 62–63.

Stashenko, E., et al., 1995. Catalytic transformation of copaiba (Copaifera officinalis) oil over zeolite. Journal of High Resolution Chromatography 18, 54–60.

Staudenmayer, H., 2001. Idiopathic environmental intolerances (IEI): myth and reality. Toxicol. Lett. 120, 333–342.

Staudenmayer, H., Selner, J.C., Buhr, M.P., 1993. Double-blind provocation chamber challenges in 20 patients presenting with "multiple chemical sensitivity" Regul. Toxicol. Pharmacol. 18, 44–53.

Steinberg, D., Avigan, J., Mize, C.E., 1966. Effects of dietary phytol and phytanic acid in animals. J. Lipid Res. 7, 684–691.

Steinemann, A.C., 2009. Fragranced consumer products and undisclosed ingredients. Environmental Impact Assessment Review 29, 32–38.

Steinhagen, W.H., Barrow, C.S., 1984. Sensory irritation structure-activity study of inhaled aldehydes in B6C3F1 and Swiss-Webster mice. Toxicol. Appl. Pharmacol. 72, 495–503.

Steinmann, A., Schatzle, M., Agathos, M., et al., 1997. Allergic contact dermatitis from black cumin (Nigella sativa) oil after topical use. Contact Dermatitis 36, 268–269.

Steinmetz, M.D., Joanny, P., Millet, Y., et al., 1985. Action d'huiles essentielles de sauge, thuya, hysope et de certains constituants, sur la respiration de coupes de cortex cérébral in vitro. Plantes Medicinales et Phytothérapie 19, 35–47.

Steinmetz, M.D., Vial, M., Millet, Y., 1987. Actions de l'huile essentielle de romarin et de certains de ses constituants (eucalyptol et camphre) sur le cortex cérébral de rat in vitro. J. Toxicol. Clin. Exp. 7 (4), 259–271.

Steltenkamp, R.J., Booman, K.A., Dorsky, J., et al., 1980a. Citral: a survey of consumer patch-test sensitization. Food Cosmet. Toxicol. 18, 413–417.

Steltenkamp, R.J., Booman, K.A., Dorsky, J., et al., 1980b. Cinnamic alcohol: A survey of consumer patch-test sensitization. Food Cosmet. Toxicol. 18, 419–424.

Stephen, W.H., Rishton, C.M., 1894. Case of pennyroyal poisoning. Provincial Medical Journal 1, 466.

Stern, R.S., 1998. Photocarcinogenicity of drugs. Toxicol. Lett. 102–103, 389–392.

Stern, R.S., Laird, N., 1994. The carcinogenic risk of treatments for severe psoriasis: photochemotherapy follow-up study. Cancer 73, 2759–2764.

Stern, R.S., Lange, R., 1988. Non-melanoma skin cancer occurring in patients treated with PUVA five to ten years after first treatment. J. Invest. Dermatol. 91, 120–124.

Stern, R.S., Lunder, E.J., 1998. Risk of squamous cell carcinoma and methoxsalen (psoralen) and UV-A radiation (PUVA). A meta-analysis. Arch. Dermatol 134, 1582–1585.

Stern, R.S., Laird, N., Melski, J., et al., 1984. Cutaneous squamous-cell carcinoma in patients treated with PUVA. N. Engl. J. Med. 310, 1156–1161.

Stern, R.S., Nichols, K.T., Väkevä, L.H., 1997. Malignant melanoma in patients treated for psoriasis with methoxsalen (psoralen) and ultraviolet A radiation (PUVA). The PUVA follow-up study. N. Engl. J. Med. 336, 1041–1045.

Stern, R.S., PUVA Follow-up Study, 2001. The risk of melanoma in association with long-term exposure to PUVA. J. Am. Acad. Dermatol. 44, 755–761.

Stevenson, C.S., 1937. Oil of wintergreen (methyl salicylate) poisoning. Report of three cases, one with autopsy, and a review of the literature. American Journal of Medical Science 193, 772–788.

Stich, H.F., Rosin, M.P., Brunnemann, K.D., 1986. Oral lesions, genotoxicity and nitrosamines in betel quid chewers with no obvious increase in oral cancer risk. Cancer Lett. 31, 15–25.

Stillwell, W.G., Carman, M.J., Bell, L., et al., 1974. The metabolism of safrole and 2',3'-epoxysafrole in the rat and guinea pig. Drug Metab. Dispos. 2, 489–498.

Stimpfl, T., Nasel, B., Nasel, C., et al., 1995. Concentration of 1,8-cineole in human blood during prolonged inhalation. Chem. Senses 20, 349–350.

Stingeni, L., Lapomarda, V., Lisi, P., 1995. Occupational hand dermatitis in hospital environments. Contact Dermatitis 33, 172–176.

Stoffelsma, J., De Roos, K.B., 1973. Identification of 2,4,6-trichloroanisole in several essential oils. J. Agric. Food Chem. 21, 738–739.

Stoner, G.D., Shimkin, M.B., Kniazeff, A.J., et al., 1973. Test for carcinogenicity of food additives and chemotherapeutic agents by the pulmonary tumor response in strain A mice. Cancer Res. 33, 3069–3085.

Storrs, F.J., 2007. Allergen of the year: fragrance. Dermatitis 18, 3–7.

Storrs, F.J., Rosenthal, L.E., Adams, R.M., et al., 1989. Prevalence and relevance of allergic reactions in patients patch tested in North America - 1984 to 1985. J. Am. Acad. Dermatol. 20, 1038–1045.

Stotz, S.C., Vriens, J., Martyn, D., et al., 2008. Citral sensing by TRANSient receptor potential channels in dorsal root ganglion neurons. PLoS ONE 3 (5), e2082.

Stratton, S.P., Dorr, R.T., Alberts, D.S., 2000. The state-of-the-art in chemoprevention of skin cancer. Eur. J. Cancer 36, 1292–1297.

Stratton, S.P., Saboda, K.L., Myrdal, P.B., et al., 2008. Phase 1 study of topical perillyl alcohol cream for chemoprevention of skin cancer. Nutr. Cancer 60, 325–330.

Strolin-Benedetti, M., Le Bourhis, B., 1972. Répartition dans l'organisme et élimination du trans-anéthole. Comptes Rendues des Séance de l'Académie des Sciences Paris 274 (D), 2378–2381.

Sudekum, M., Poppenga, R.H., Raju, N., et al., 1992. Pennyroyal oil toxicosis in a dog. J. Am. Vet. Med. Assoc. 200, 817–818.

Sugai, T., 1980. Standardization of fragrant allergens in patch tests. III. Studies on the suitable concentration of sandalwood series of fragrance materials. Skin Res. 22, 335–343.

Sugai, T., 1994. Group study IV – farnesol and lily aldehyde. Environ. Dermatol. 1, 213–214.

Sugiura, M., Hayakawa, R., Kato, Y., et al., 2000. Results of patch testing with lavender oil in Japan. Contact Dermatitis 43, 157–160.

Sugiura, S., Ogawa, K., Hirose, M., et al., 2003. Reversibility of proliferative lesions and induction of non-papillary tumors in rat urinary bladder treated with phenylethyl isothiocyanate. Carcinogenesis 24, 547–553.

Sukumaran, K., Kuttan, R., 1995. Inhibition of tobacco-induced mutagenesis by eugenol and plant extracts. Mutat. Res. 343, 25–30.

Sukumaran, K., Unnikrishnan, M.C., Kuttan, R., 1994. Inhibition of tumour promotion in mice by eugenol. Indian J. Physiol. Pharmacol. 38, 306–308.

Sullivan, J.B., Rumack, B.H., Thomas, H., et al., 1979. Pennyroyal oil poisoning and hepatotoxicity. J. Am. Med. Assoc. 242, 2873–2874.

Sultan, M.T., Butt, M.S., Anjum, F.M., 2009. Safety assessment of black cumin fixed and essential oil in normal Sprague Dawley rats: serological and hematological indices. Food Chem. Toxicol. 47, 2768–2775.

Summers, G.D., 1947. Case of camphor poisoning. Br. Med. J. 2, 1009.

Sun, C.M., Syu, W.J., Don, M.J., et al., 2003. Cytotoxic sesquiterpene lactones from the root of *Saussurea lappa*. Journal of Natural Products 66, 1175–1180.

Sun, W., Xu, Z., Wang, C., et al., 2005. Study on antioxidant activity of essential oils and its monomer from Pelargonium graveolens. Zhong Yao Cai 28, 87–89.

Sun, X.Y., Zheng, Y.P., Lin, D.H., et al., 2009. Potential anti-cancer activities of furanodiene, a sesquiterpene from *Curcuma wenyujin*. Am. J. Chin. Med. 37, 589–596.

Sundaram, S.G., Milner, J.A., 1993. Impact of organosulfur compounds in garlic on canine mammary tumor cells in culture. Cancer Lett. 74, 85–90.

Sundaram, S.G., Milner, J.A., 1996. Diallyl disulfide suppresses the growth of human colon tumor cell xenografts in athymic nude mice. J. Nutr. 126, 1355–1361.

Suneja, M., Belsito, D.V., 2001. Comparative study of Finn Chambers and T.R.U.E. test methodologies in detecting the relevant allergens inducing contact dermatitis. J. Am. Acad. Dermatol. 45, 836–839.

Sunil, V.R., Laumbach, R.J., Patel, K.J., et al., 2007. Pulmonary effects of inhaled limonene ozone reaction products in elderly rats. Toxicol. Appl. Pharmacol. 222, 211–220.

Surber, W., 1962. Étude de toxicité sous-chronique de la thujone sur rats: rapport final. Institut Battelle, Genève. Cited in: European Commission 2003 Opinion of the Scientific Committee on Food on Thujone. http://europa.eu.int/comm/food/fs/sc/scf/outcome_en.html

Sutton, J.D., Sangster, S.A., Caldwell, J., 1985. Dose-dependent variation in the disposition of eugenol in the rat. Biochem. Pharmacol. 34, 465–466.

Suzuki, T., Tomita, Y., 2008. Recent advances in genetic analyses of oculocutaneous albinism types 2 and 4. J. Dermatol. Sci. 51, 1–9.

Suzuki, Y., Sugiyama, K., Furuta, H., 1985. Eugenol-mediated superoxide generation and cytotoxicity in guinea pig neutrophils. Jpn. J. Pharmacol. 39, 381–386.

Svoboda, K.P., Ruzickova, G., Allan, R., et al., 2001. An investigation into drop sizes of essential oils using different dropper types. Int. J. Aromather. 10 (3/4), 99–103.

Swales, N.J., Caldwell, J., 1992. Cytotoxicity and depletion of glutathione (GSH) by cinnamaldehyde in rat hepatocytes. Hum. Exp. Toxicol. 10, 488–489.

Swanson, A.B., Chambliss, D.D., Blomquist, J.C., et al., 1979. The mutagenicities of safrole, estragole, eugenol, *trans*-anethole, and some of their known or possible metabolites for *Salmonella typhimurium* mutants. Mutat. Res. 60, 143–153.

Swanson, A.B., Miller, E.C., Miller, J.A., 1981. The side-chain epoxidation and hydroxylation of the hepatocarcinogens safrole and estragole and some related compounds by rat and mouse liver microsomes. Biochem. Biophys. Acta 673, 504.

Swenberg, J.A., Dietrich, D.R., McClain, R.M., et al., 1992. Species-specific mechanisms of carcinogenesis. IARC Sci. Publ. 116, 477–500.

Syed, T.A., Qureshi, Z.A., Ali, S.M., et al., 1999. Treatment of toenail onychomycosis with 2% butenafine and 5% *Melaleuca alternifolia* (tea tree) oil in cream. Trop. Med. Int. Health 4, 284–287.

Sylvestre, M., Legault, J., Dufour, D., et al., 2005. Chemical composition and anticancer activity of leaf essential oil of *Myrica gale* L. Phytomedicine 12, 299–304.

Sylvestre, M., Pichette, A., Lavoie, S., et al., 2007. Composition and cytotoxic activity of the leaf essential oil of *Comptonia peregrina* (L.) Coulter. Phytother. Res. 21, 536–540.

Szczot, M., Czyzewska, M.M., Appendino, G., et al., 2012. Modulation of GABAergic synaptic currents and current responses by α-thujone and dihydroumbellulone. J. Nat. Prod. 75, 622–629.

Tabacchi, R., Garnero, J., Bull, R., 1974. Contribution à l'étude de la composition de l'huile essentielle de fruits d'anise de Turque. Rivista Italiana EPPOS 56, 683–697.

Tabanca, N., Khan, S.I., Bedir, E., et al., 2004. Estrogenic activity of isolated compounds and essential oils of *Pimpinella* species from Turkey, evaluated using a recombinant yeast screen. Planta Med. 70, 728–735.

Tabatabaie, T., Floyd, R.A., 1996. Inactivation of glutathione peroxidase by benzaldehyde. Toxicol. Appl. Pharmacol. 141, 389–393.

Tada, H., Takeda, K., 1976. Sesquiterpenes of Lauraceae plants. IV. Germacranolides from *Laurus nobilis* L. Chem. Pharm. Bull. (Tokyo) 24, 667–671.

Taetle, R., Howell, S.B., 1983. Preclinical re-evaluation of benzaldehyde as a chemotherapeutic agent. Cancer Treat. Rep. 67, 561–566.

Tahti, H., Engelke, M., Vaalavirta, L., 1997. Mechanisms and models of neurotoxicity of n-hexane and related solvents. Arch. Toxicol. Suppl. 19, 337–345.

Takahashi, Y., Inaba, N., Kuwahara, S., et al., 2003. Antioxidative effect of citrus essential oil components on human low-density lipoprotein *in vitro*. Biosci. Biotechnol. Biochem. 67, 195–197.

Takanami, I., Utsunomiya, T., Onishi, H., et al., 1983. Costus root oil test in cancer patients: correlation with tumor stage. Gan No Rinsho 29, 1319–1322.

Takanami, I., Utsunomiya, T., Ohnishi, H., et al., 1984. Skin sensitization of costus root oil and peripheral lymphocyte count in gastric and colon cancers. Gan To Kagaku Ryoho 11, 81–86.

Takanami, I., Ishihara, T., Yanai, N., 1985. Cutaneous delayed hypersensitivity to costus root oil in lung cancer. Gan No Rinsho 31, 1362–1366.

Takanami, I., Ikeda, Y., Nakayama, H., 1987. Effect of costus root oil in murine tumors. Gan To Kagaku Ryoho 14, 2276–2279.

Takarada, K., Kimizuka, R., Takahashi, N., et al., 2004. A comparison of the antibacterial efficacies of essential oils against oral pathogens. Oral Microbiol. Immunol. 19, 61–64.

Takemoto, H., Ito, M., Shiraki, T., et al., 2008. Sedative effects of vapor inhalation of agarwood oil and spikenard extract and identification of their active components. Natural Medicines (Tokyo) 62, 41–46.

Takemura, M., Quarcoo, D., Niimi, A., et al., 2008. Is TRPV1 a useful target in respiratory diseases? Pulm. Pharmacol. Ther. 21, 833–839.

Takenaga, M., Hirai, A., Terano, T., et al., 1987. In vitro effect of cinnamic aldehyde, a main component of Cinnamomi Cortex, on human platelet aggregation and arachidonic acid metabolism. J. Pharmacobiodyn. 10, 201–208.

Takeuchi, H., Saoo, K., Yokohira, M., et al., 2003. Pretreatment with 8-methoxypsoralen, a potent human CYP2A6 inhibitor, strongly inhibits lung tumorigenesis induced by 4-(methylnitrosamino)-1-(3-pyridyl)-1-butanone in female A/J mice. Cancer Res. 63, 7581–7583.

Takeyoshi, M., Noda, S., Yamazaki, S., et al., 2004. Assessment of the skin sensitization potency of eugenol and its dimers using a non-radioisotopic modification of the local lymph node assay. J. Appl. Toxicol. 24, 77–81.

Takeyoshi, M., Iida, K., Suzuki, K., et al., 2008. Skin sensitization potency of isoeugenol and its dimers evaluated by a non-radioisotopic modification of the local lymph node assay and guinea pig maximization test. J. Appl. Toxicol. 28, 530–534.

Takizawa, Y., Noda, M., Kawamura, T., et al., 1985. Survey on mutagenicity of natural food additives II. Summary and conclusion. Mutat. Res. 147, 275.

Talalay, P., Fahey, J.W., 2001. Phytochemicals from cruciferous plants protect against cancer by modulating carcinogen metabolism. J. Nutr. 131 (Suppl. 11), 3027S–3033S.

Tam, C.C., Elston, D.M., 2006. Allergic contact dermatitis caused by white petrolatum on damaged skin. Dermatitis 17, 201–203.

Tamaoki, J., Chiyotani, A., Sakai, H., et al., 1995. Effect of menthol vapour on airway hyperresponsiveness in patients with mild asthma. Respir. Med. 89, 503–504.

Tamas, G., Weschler, C.J., Toftum, J., et al., 2006. Influence of ozone-limonene reactions on perceived air quality. Indoor Air 16, 168–178.

Tambe, Y., Tsujiuchi, H., Honda, G., et al., 1996. Gastric cytoprotection of the non-steroidal anti-inflammatory sesquiterpene, β-caryophyllene. Planta Med. 62, 469–470.

Tamir, I., Ambramovici, A., Milo-Goldzweig, I., et al., 1984. The haemolytic activity of citral: evidence for free radical participation. Biochem. Pharmacol. 33, 2945–2950.

Tamogami, S., Awano, K., Kitahara, T., 2001. Analysis of the enantiomeric ratios of chiral components in absolute jasmine. Flavor & Fragrance Journal 16, 161–163.

Tan, D.X., Pöeggeler, B., Reiter, R.J., et al., 1993. The pineal hormone melatonin inhibits DNA-adduct formation induced by the chemical carcinogen safreole in vivo. Cancer Lett. 70, 65–71.

Tan, P., Zhong, W., Cai, W., 2000. Clinical study on treatment of 40 cases of malignant brain tumor by elemene emulsion injection. Zhongguo Zhong Xi Yi Jie He Za Zhi 20, 645–648.

Tanaka, M., Tamura, K., Ide, H., 1996. Citral, an inhibitor of retinoic acid synthesis, modifies chick limb development. Dev. Biol. 175, 239–247.

Tanaka, S., Royds, C., Buckley, D., et al., 2004. Contact allergy to isoeugenol and its derivatives: problems with allergen substitution. Contact Dermatitis 51, 288–291.

Tandan, S.K., Singh, R., Gupta, S., et al., 1989. Subacute dermal toxicity study of Cedrus deodara wood essential oil. Indian Vet. J. 66, 1088.

Tanen, D.A., Danish, D.C., Reardon, J.M., et al., 2008. Comparison of oral aspirin versus topical applied methyl salicylate for platelet inhibition. Ann. Pharmacother. 42, 1396–1401.

Tanida, M., Niijima, A., Shen, J., et al., 2005. Olfactory stimulation with scent of essential oil of grapefruit affects autonomic neurotransmission and blood pressure. Brain Res. 1058, 44–55.

Tanida, M., Niijima, A., Shen, J., et al., 2006. Olfactory stimulation with scent of lavender oil affects autonomic neurotransmission and blood pressure in rats. Neurosci. Lett. 398, 155–160.

Tanojo, H., Boelsma, E., Junginger, H.E., et al., 1998. In vivo human skin barrier modulation by topical application of fatty acids. Skin Pharmacol. Appl. Skin Physiol. 11, 87–97.

Tao, G., Irie, Y., Li, D.J., et al., 2005. Eugenol and its structural analogs inhibit monoamine oxidase A and exhibit antidepressant-like activity. Bioorg. Med. Chem. 13, 4777–47788.

Tao, L., Zhou, L., Zheng, L., et al., 2006. Elemene displays anti-cancer ability on laryngeal cancer cells in vitro and in vivo. Cancer Chemother. Pharmacol. 58, 24–34.

Taraska, V., Pratt, M., 1997. Contact dermatitis in massage therapists. Am. J. Contact Dermat. 8, 63.

Tateo, F., Chizzini, F., 1989. The composition and quality of supercritical CO2 extracted cinnamon. Journal of Essential Oil Research 1, 165–168.

Tateo, F., Santamaria, L., Bianchi, L., et al., 1989. Basil oil and tarragon oil: composition and genotoxicity evaluation. In: Lawrence, B.M. (Ed.), 2005 The antimicrobial/biological activity of essential oils. Allured, Carol Stream, pp. 1–4.

Tatman, D., Huanbiao, M., 2002. Volatile isoprenoid constituents of fruits, vegetables and herbs cumulatively suppress the proliferation of murine B16 melanoma and human HL-60 leukemia cells. Cancer Lett. 175, 129–139.

Tava, A., 2001. Coumarin-containing grass: volatiles from sweet vernalgrass (Anthoxanthum odoratum L.). Journal of Essential Oil Research 13, 367–370.

Taveira, F.S., Andrade, E.H., Lima, W.N., et al., 2003. Seasonal variation in the essential oil of Pilocarpus microphyllus Stapf. Annals of the Brazilian Academy of Sciences 75, 27–31.

Tayama, S., 1996. Cytogenetic effects of piperonyl butoxide and safrole in CHO-K1 cells. Mutat. Res. 368, 249–260.

Taylor, H.S., 1905. A case of acute poisoning by eucalyptus oil. Lancet 166 (4283), 963–964.

Taylor, J.M., Jenner, P.M., Jones, W.I., 1964. A comparison of the toxicity of some allyl, propenyl, and propyl compounds in the rat. Toxicol. Appl. Pharmacol. 6, 378–387.

Taylor, J.M., Jones, W.I., Hagan, E.C., et al., 1967. Toxicity of oil of calamus (Jammu variety). Toxicol. Appl. Pharmacol. 10, 405.

Teissedre, P.L., Waterhouse, A.L., 2000. Inhibition of oxidation of human low-density lipoproteins by phenolic substances in different essential oils varieties. J. Agric. Food Chem. 48, 3801–3805.

Tekel, J., Holla, M., Vaverkova, S., 1997. Detemination of uracil herbicide residues and components in essential oil of Melissa officinalis L. in its main development phases. Journal of Essential Oil Research 9, 63–66.

Telci, I., Bayram, E., Yilmaz, G., et al., 2006. Variability in essential oil composition of Turkish Basils (Ocimum basilicum L.). Biochemical Systematics & Ecology 34, 489–497.

Temesvári, E., Németh, I., Baló-Banga, M.J., et al., 2002. Multicentre study of fragrance allergy in Hungary. Immediate and late type reactions. Contact Dermatitis 46, 325–330.

Temmink, J.H., Bruggeman, I.M., Bladeren, P.J., 1986. Cytomorphological changes in liver cells exposed to allyl and benzyl isothiocyanate and their cysteine and glutathione conjugates. Arch. Toxicol. 59, 103–110.

Temple, W.A., Smith, N.A., Beasley, M., 1991. Management of oil of citronella poisoning. Clin. Toxicol. 29, 257–262.

Tenenbein, M., 1990. Maternal-fetal toxicology: a clinician's guide. Dekker, New York.

Tennant, R.W., Margolin, B.H., Shelby, M.D., et al., 1987. Prediction of chemical carcinogenicity in rodents from in vitro genetic toxicity assays. Science 236, 933–941.

Terajima, Y., Ichikawa, H., Tokua, K., et al., 1988. Quantitative analysis of oakmoss. In: Lawrence, B.M., Mookherjee, B.D., Willis, B.J. (Eds.), Flavors & fragrances: a world perspective. Elsevier, Amsterdam, pp. 685–695.

Terblanché, F.C., Kornelius, G., 1996. Essential oil constituents of the genus Lippia (Verbenaceae) – a literature review. Journal of Essential Oil Research 8, 471–485.

Ternesten-Hasséus, E., Johansson, K., Löwhagen, O., et al., 2006. Inhalation method determines outcome of capsaicin inhalation in patients with chronic cough due to sensory hyperreactivity. Pulm. Pharmacol. Ther. 19, 172–178.

Ternesten-Hasséus, E., Löwhagen, O., Millqvist, E., 2007. Quality of life and capsaicin sensitivity in patients with airway symptoms induced by chemicals and scents: a longitudinal study. Environ. Health Perspect. 115, 425–429.

Teuscher, E., Melzig, M., Villmann, E., 1989. Components of essential oils as membrane active compounds. Planta Med. 55, 660–661.

Thappa, R.K., Agarwal, S.G., Kalia, N.K., et al., 1993. Changes in chemical composition of *Tagetes minuta* oil at various stages of flowering and fruiting. Journal of Essential Oil Research 5, 375–379.

Thappa, R.K., Kaul, P., Chisti, A.M., et al., 2005. Variability in the essential oil of *Angelica glauca* Edgew of different geographical regions. Journal of Essential Oil Research 17, 361–363.

Thejass, P., Kuttan, G., 2007a. Allyl isothiocyanate (AITC) and phenyl isothiocyanate (PITC) inhibit tumour-specific angiogenesis by downregulating nitric oxide (NO) and tumour necrosis factor- α (TNF-α) production. Nitric Oxide 16, 247–257.

Thejass, P., Kuttan, G., 2007b. Inhibition of endothelial cell differentiation and proinflammatory cytokine production during angiogenesis by allyl isothiocyanate and phenyl isothiocyanate. Integr. Cancer Ther. 6, 389–399.

Théron, E., Holeman, M., Potin-Gautier, M., et al., 1994. Authentication of *Ravensara aromatica* and *Ravensara anisata*. Planta Med. 60, 489–490.

Thomas, J.G., 1962. Peppermint fibrillation. (Letter). Lancet 279 (7222), 222.

Thomas, D.B., Pasternak, C.A., 1969. Vitamin A and the biosynthesis of sulphated mucopolysaccharides. Experiments with rats and cultured neoplastic mast cells. Biochem. J. 111, 407–412.

Thomassen, D., Slattery, J.T., Nelson, S.D., 1990. Menthofuran-dependent and independent aspects of pulegone hepatotoxicity: roles of glutathione. J. Pharmacol. Exp. Ther. 253, 567–572.

Thomassen, D., Pearson, P.G., Slattery, J.T., et al., 1991. Partial characterization of biliary metabolites of pulegone by tandem mass spectrometry. Detection of glucuronide, glutathione, and glutathionyl glucuronide conjugates. Drug Metab. Dispos. 19, 997–1003.

Thomassen, D., Knebel, N., Slattery, J.T., et al., 1992. Reactive intermediates in the oxidation of menthofuran by cytochromes P-450. Chem. Res. Toxicol. 5, 123–130.

Thompson, G.R., Booman, K.A., Dorsky, J., et al., 1983. Isoeugenol: a survey of consumer patch-test sensitization. Food Chem. Toxicol. 21, 735–7400.

Thompson, D., Constantin-Teodosiu, D., Egestad, B., et al., 1990. Formation of glutathione conjugates during oxidation of eugenol by microsomal; fractions of rat liver and lung. Biochem. Pharmacol. 39, 1587–1595.

Thompson, D.C., Constantin-Teodosiu, D., Moldéus, P., et al., 1991. Metabolism and cytotoxicity of eugenol in isolated rat hepatocytes. Chem. Biol. Interact. 77, 137–147.

Thompson, D.C., Perera, K., Fisher, R., Brendel, K., 1994. Cresol isomers: comparison of toxic potency in rat liver slices. Toxicol. Appl. Pharmacol. 125, 51–58.

Thompson, D.C., Perera, K., London, R., 1996. Studies on the mechanism of toxicity of 4-methylphenol (*p*-cresol): effects of deuterium labeling and ring substitution. Chem. Biol. Interact. 101, 1–11.

Thompson, D.C., Barhoumi, R., Burghardt, R.C., 1998. Comparative toxicity of eugenol and its quinone methide metabolite in cultured liver cells using kinetic fluorescence bioassays. Toxicol. Appl. Pharmacol. 149, 55–63.

Thorup, I., Würtzen, G., Carstensen, J., et al., 1983a. Short term toxicity study in rats dosed with peppermint oil. Toxicol. Lett. 19, 211–215.

Thorup, I., Würtzen, G., Carstensen, J., et al., 1983b. Short term toxicity study in rats dosed with pulegone and menthol. Toxicol. Lett. 19, 207–210.

Thrall, K.D., Poet, T.S., Corley, R.A., et al., 2000. A real-time *in-vivo* method for studying the percutaneous absorption of volatile chemicals. Int. J. Occup. Environ. Health 6, 96–103.

Thulin, M., Claeson, P., 1991. The botanical origin of scented myrrh (Bissabol or Habak Hadi). Econ. Bot. 45, 487–494.

Thune, P., Solberg, Y., McFadden, N., et al., 1982. Perfume allergy to oak moss and other lichens. Contact Dermatitis 8, 396–400.

Thyssen, J.P., 2007. Contact allergy epidemics and their controls. Contact Dermatitis 56, 185–195.

Tibballs, J., 1995. Clinical effects and management of eucalyptus oil ingestion in infants and young children. Med. J. Aust. 163, 177–180.

Timbrell, J.A., 2000. Principles of biochemical toxicology, third ed. Taylor & Francis, Padstow.

Tipton, D.A., Lyle, B., Babich, H., et al., 2003. In vitro cytotoxic and anti-inflammatory effects of myrrh oil on human gingival fibroblasts and epithelial cells. Toxicol. In Vitro. 17, 301–310.

Tisserand, R., 1977. The art of aromatherapy. CW Daniel, Saffron Walden.

To, L.P., Hunt, T.P., Andersen, M.E., 1982. Mutagenicity of *trans*-anethole, estragole, eugenol and safrole in the Ames *Salmonella typhimurium* assay. Bull. Environ. Contam. Toxicol. 28, 647–654.

Toaff, M.E., Abramovici, A., Sporn, J., et al., 1979. Selective oocyte degeneration and impaired fertility in rats treated with the aliphatic monoterpene, citral. J. Reprod. Fertil. 55, 347–352.

Todorov, S., Philianos, S., Petkov, V., et al., 1984. Experimental pharmacological study of three species from genus Salvia. Acta Physiol. Pharmacol. Bulg. 10 (2), 13–20.

Todorova, V.K., Harms, S.A., Luo, S., et al., 2003. Oral glutamine (AES-14) supplementation inhibits PI-3 k/Akt signaling in experimental breast cancer. JPEN J. Parenter. Enteral Nutr. 27, 404–410.

Tognolini, M., Barocelli, E., Ballabeni, V., et al., 2006. Comparative screening of plant essential oils: phenylpropanoid moiety as basic core for antiplatelet activity. Life Sci. 78, 1419–1432.

Tognolini, M., Ballabeni, V., Bertoni, S., et al., 2007. Protective effect of Foeniculum vulgare essential oil and anethole in an experimental model of thrombosis. Pharmacol. Res. 56, 254–260.

Tolnai, S., Morgan, J.F., 1962. Studies on the *in vitro* anti-tumor activity of fatty acids. VI. Derivatives of mono- and di-carboxylic and unsaturated fatty acids. Can. J. Biochem. 40, 1367.

Tomaino, A., Cimino, F., Zimbalatti, V., et al., 2005. Influence of heating on antioxidant activity and the chemical composition of some spice essential oils. Food Chem. 89, 549–554.

Tomatis, L., 1979. The predictive value of rodent carcinogenicity tests in the evaluation of human risks. Annu. Rev. Pharmacol. Toxicol. 19, 511–530.

Tominaga, H., Kobayashi, Y., Goto, T., et al., 2005. DPPH radical-scavenging effect of several phenylpropanoid compounds and their glycoside derivatives. Yakugaku Zasshi 125, 371–375.

Tong, M.M., Altman, P.M., Barnetson, R.S., 1992. Tea tree oil in the treatment of tinea pedis. Australas. J. Dermatol. 33, 145–149.

Topçu, G., Gören, A.C., 2007. Biological activity of diterpenoids isolated from Anatolian Lamiaceae plants. Rec. Nat. Prod. 1, 1–16.

Torrado, S., Torrado, S., Agis, A., et al., 1995. Effect of dissolution profile and (-)-α-bisabolol on the gastrotoxicity of acetylsalicylic acid. Pharmazie 50, 141–143.

Tosti, A., Guerra, L., Morelli, R., et al., 1990. Prevalence and sources ofens sensitization to emulsifiers: a clinical study. Contact Dermatitis 23, 68–72.

Toth, B., 2001. Species susceptibilities to chemical carcinogens: a critical appraisal of the roles of genetic and viral agents. In Vivo 15, 467–478.

Toulemonde, B., Beauverd, D., 1984. Contribution à l'étude d'une camomile sauvage du Maroc: l'huile essentielle d'*Ormenis mixta*. Parfums Cosmetiques Aromes 60, 65–67.

Toulemonde, B., Noleau, I., 1988. Volatile constituents of lovage (*Levisticum officinale* Koch). In: Lawrence, B.M., Mookherjee, B.D., Willis, B.J. (Eds.), Flavors & fragrances: a world perspective. Elsevier, Amsterdam, pp. 641–656.

Toussaint, 1982. Chemical composition of Curcuma longa L. and Curcuma xanthorriza Roxb. PhD Thesis, University of Hamburg.

Touvay, C., Vilain, B., Carre, C., et al., 1995. Effect of limonene and sobrerol on monocrotaline-induced lung alterations and pulmonary hypertension. Int. Arch. Allergy Immunol. 107, 272–274.

Towers, G.N., Arnason, T., Wat, C.K., 1979. Phototoxic polyacetylenes and their thiophene derivatives. Contact Dermatitis 5, 140–143.

Trabace, L., Avato, P., Mazzaccoli, M., et al., 1994. Choleretic activity of *Thapsia* chem. I, II, and III in rats: comparison with terpenoid constituents and peppermint oil. Phytother. Res. 8, 305–307.

Trattner, A., David, M., 2003. Patch testing with fine fragrances: comparison with fragrance mix, balsam of Peru and a fragrance series. Contact Dermatitis 49, 287–289.

Trattner, A., Hodak, E., David, M., 1999. Screening patch tests for pigmented contact dermatitis in Israel. Contact Dermatitis 40, 155–157.

Trattner, A., David, M., Lazarov, A., 2008. Occupational contact dermatitis due to essential oils. Contact Dermatitis 58, 282–284.

Traynor, N.J., Beattie, P.E., Ibbotson, S.H., et al., 2005. Photogenotoxicity of hypericin in HaCaT keratinocytes: Implications for St. John's Wort supplements and high dose UVA-1 therapy. Toxicol. Lett. 158, 220–224.

Treffel, P., Panisset, F., Humbert, P., 1993. Effect of pressure on in vitro percutaneous absorption of caffeine. Acta Derm. Venereol. 73, 200–202.

Tremblay, S., Avon, S.L., 2008. Contact allergy to cinnamon: case report. J. Can. Dent. Assoc. (Tor) 74, 445–461.

Treudler, R., Richter, G., Geier, J., et al., 2000. Increase in sensitisation to oil of turpentine: recent data from a multicenter study on 45,005 patients from the German-Austrian Information Network of Departments of Dermatology (IVDK). Contact Dermatitis 42, 68–73.

Tripathi, P., Tripathi, R., Patel, R.K., et al., 2013. Investigation of antimutagenic potential of *Foeniculum vulgare* essential oil on cyclophosphamide induced genotoxicity and oxidative stress in mice. Drug Chem. Toxicol. 36, 35–41.

Trivedi, A.H., Patel, R.K., Rawal, U.M., et al., 1994. Evaluation of chemopreventive effects of betel leaf on the genotoxicity of pan masala. Neoplasma 41, 177–181.

Troulakis, G., Tsatsakis, A.M., Tzatzarakis, M., et al., 1997. Acute intoxication and recovery following massive turpentine ingestion: clinical and toxicological data. Vet. Hum. Toxicol. 39, 155–157.

Truhaut, R., Le Bourhis, B., Attia, M., et al., 1989. Chronic toxicity/ carcinogenicity study of *trans*-anethole in rats. Food Chem. Toxicol. 27, 11–20.

Truitt, E.B., 1967. The pharmacology of myristicin and nutmeg. Public Health Service Publications Washington 1645, 215–222.

Truitt, E.B., Ebersberger, E.M., 1962. Evidence of monoamine oxidase inhibition by myristicin and nutmeg in vivo. Fed. Proc. 21, 418.

Truitt, E.B., Callaway, E., Braude, M.C., et al., 1961. The pharmacology of myristicin. J. Neuropsychiatr. 2, 205–210.

Truitt, E.B., Duritz, G., Ebersberger, E.M., 1963. Evidence of monoamine oxidase inhibition by myristicin and nutmeg. Proc. Soc. Exp. Biol. Med. 112, 647–650.

Tsai, R.S., Carrupt, P.A., Testa, B., et al., 1994. Structure-genotoxicity relationships of allylbenzenes and propenylbenzenes: a quantum chemical study. Chem. Res. Toxicol. 7, 73–76.

Tsai, J.F., Chuang, L.Y., Jeng, J.E., et al., 2001. Betel quid chewing as a risk factor for hepatocellular carcinoma: a case-control study. Br. J. Cancer 84, 709–713.

Tsai, J.F., Jeng, J.E., Chuang, L.Y., et al., 2004. Habitual betel quid chewing and risk for hepatocellular carcinoma complicating cirrhosis. Medicine (Baltimore) 83, 176–187.

Tsai, Y.C., Hsu, H.C., Yang, W.C., et al., 2007. α-Bulnesene, a PAF inhibitor isolated from the essential oil of *Pogostemon cablin*. Fitoterapia 78, 7–11.

Tsai, Y.S., Lee, K.W., Huang, J.L., et al., 2008. Arecoline, a major alkaloid of areca nut, inhibits p53, represses DNA repair, and triggers DNA damage response in human epithelial cells. Toxicology 249, 230–237.

Tsai, M.L., Lin, C.C., Lin, W.C., et al., 2011. Antimicrobial, antioxidant and anti-inflammatory activities of essential oils from five selected herbs. Biotechnol. Biochem. 75, 110377/1–110377/7.

Tsankova, E., Ognyanov, I., 1968. Öl von *Abies alba*. Reichstoffe, Aromen, Körperpflegemittel 18, 376.

Tsankova, E.T., Dyulgerov, A.S., Milenkov, B.K., 1993. Chemical composition of the Bulgarian sumac oil. J. Essential Oil Res. 5, 205–207.

Tsao, A.S., Kim, E.S., Hong, W.K., 2004. Chemoprevention of cancer. CA Cancer J. Clin. 54, 150–180.

Tsuchiya, T., Tanida, M., Uenoyama, S., et al., 1991. Effects of olfactory stimulation on the sleep time induced by pentobarbital administration in mice. Brain Res. Bull. 26, 397–401.

Tsuda, H., Uehara, N., Iwahori, Y., et al., 1994. Chemopreventive effects of beta-carotene, alpha-tocopherol and five naturally occurring antioxidants on initiation of hepatocarcinogenesis by 2-amino-3-methylimidazo[4,5-f] quinoline in the rat. Jpn. J. Cancer Res. 85, 1214–1219.

Tsuji, M., Fujisaki, Y., Yamachika, K., et al., 1974. Studies on d-limonene as a gallstone solubilizer (I) general pharmacological studies. Oyo yakuri 8, 1439–1459.

Tsuji, M., Fujisaki, Y., Arikawa, Y., 1975a. Studies on d-limonene, as gallstone solubilizer (II): Acute and subacute toxicities. Oyo Yakuri (Pharmacometrics) 9, 387–401.

Tsuji, M., Fujisaki, Y., Okubo, A., et al., 1975b. Studies on d-limonene as gallstone solubilizer (V). Effects on development of rat fetuses and offspring. Oyo Yakuri (Pharmacometrics) 10, 179–186.

Tsujimoto, Y., Hashizume, H., Yamazaki, M., 1993. Superoxide radical scavenging activity of phenolic compounds. Int. J. Biochem. 25, 491–494.

Tsuneki, H., Ma, E.L., Kobayashi, S., et al., 2005. Antiangiogenic activity of beta-eudesmol in vitro and in vivo. Eur. J. Pharmacol. 512, 105–115.

Tsutsulova, A.L., Antonova, R.A., 1984. Analysis of Bulgarian daisy oil. Maslo-Zhirovaya Promyshlennost 11, 23–24.

Tuberoso, C.I., Kowalczyk, A., Coroneo, V., et al., 2005. Chemical composition and antioxidant, antimicrobial, and antifungal activities of the essential oil of *Achillea ligustica* All. J. Agric. Food Chem. 53, 10148–10153.

Tucker, A.O., 1986. Frankincense and myrrh. Econ. Bot. 40, 425–433.

Tucker, A.O., Debaggio, T., 2000. The Big Book of Herbs. Interweave Press, Colorado.

Tucker, A.O., Maciarello, M.J., 1987. Plant identifications. In: Simon, J.E., Grant, L. (Eds.), Proceedings of the first national herb growing and marketing conference. Purdue University Press, West Lafayette, pp. 126–172.

Tucker, A.O., Maciarello, M.J., 1988. Nomenclature and chemistry of the Kazanlik damask rose. In: Lawrence, B.M., Mookherjee, B.D., Willis, B.J. (Eds.), Flavors & fragrances: a world perspective. Elsevier, Amsterdam, pp. 99–114.

Tucker, A.O., Maciarello, M.J., 1995. Two commercial oils of *Ravensara* from Madagascar: *R. anisata* Danguy and *R. aromatica* Sonn. (Lauraceae). J. Essential Oil Res. 7, 327–329.

Tucker, A.O., Maciarello, M.J., Adams, R.P., et al., 1991a. Volatile leaf oils of Caribbean Myrtaceae. I Three varieties of *Pimenta racemosa* (Miller) J. Moore of the Dominican Republic and the commercial bay oil. J. Essential Oil Res. 3, 323–329.

Tucker, A.O., Maciarello, M.J., Landrun, L.R., 1991b. Volatile leaf oils of Caribbean Myrtaceae. II *Pimenta dioica* (L.) Merr. of Jamaica. . J. Essential Oil Res. 3, 195–196.

Tucker, A.O., Maciarello, M.J., Sturtz, G., 1993. The essential oils of *Artemisia* 'Powis Castle' and its putative parents, *A. absinthium* and *A. arborescens*. J. Essential Oil Res. 5, 239–242.

Tucker, A.O., Maciarello, M.J., Charles, D.J., et al., 1997. Volatile leaf oil of the curry plant [*Helichrysum italicum* (Roth) G. Don subsp. *italicum*] and dwarf curry plant [subsp. *microphyllum* (Willd.) Nyman] in the North American herb trade. J. Essential Oil Res. 9, 583–585.

Tucker, A.O., Maciarello, M.J., Karchesy, J.J., 2000. Commercial "rose of cedar" oil, the wood oil of Port Orford cedar, *Chamaecyparis lawsoniana* (A. Murray) Parl. (Cupressaceae). J. Essential Oil Res. 12, 24–26.

Tuckler, V., Peck, C., Nesbitt, C., et al., 2002. Seizure in an infant from aniseed oil toxicity. Clin. Toxicol. 40, 689.

Tung, Y.T., Chua, M.T., Wang, S.Y., et al., 2008. Anti-inflammation activities of essential oil and its constituents from indigenous cinnamon (*Cinnamomum osmophloeum*) twigs. Bioresour. Technol. 99, 3908–3913.

Turgeon, D., Carrier, J.S., Chouinard, S., et al., 2003. Glucuronidation activity of the UGT2B17 enzyme toward xenobiotics. Drug Metab. Dispos. 31, 670–676.

Turkdogan, M.K., Ozbek, H., Yener, Z., et al., 2003. The role of *Urtica dioica* and *Nigella sativa* in the prevention of carbon tetrachloride-induced hepatotoxicity in rats. Phytother. Res. 17, 942–946.

Türkyilmaz, Z., Karabulut, R., Sönmez, K., et al., 2008. A striking and frequent cause of premature thelarche in children: *Foeniculum vulgare*. J. Pediatr. Surg. 43, 2109–2111.

Turner, S.D., Tinwell, H., Piegorsch, W., et al., 2001. The male rat carcinogens limonene and sodium saccharin are not mutagenic to male Big Blue rats. Mutagenesis 16, 329–332.

Turpeinen, M., 1988. Influence of age and severity of dermatitis on the percutaneous absorption of hydrocortisone in children. Br. J. Dermatol. 118, 517–522.

Tweats, D.J., Scott, A.D., Westmoreland, C., et al., 2007. Determination of genetic toxicity and potential carcinogenicity in vitro - challenges post the Seventh Amendment to the European Cosmetics Directive. Mutagenesis 22, 5–13.

Uc, A., Bishop, W.P., Sanders, K.D., 2000. Camphor hepatotoxicity. South Med. J. 93, 596–598.

Uedo, N., Tatsuta, M., Iishi, H., et al., 1999. Inhibition by *d*-limonene of gastric carcinogenesis induced by *N*-methyl-*N*´-nitro-*N*-nitrosoguanidine in Wistar rats. Cancer Lett. 137, 131–136.

Uehleke, H., Brinkschulte-Freitas, M., 1979. Oral toxicity of an essential oil from myrtle and adaptive liver stimulation. Toxicology 12, 335–342.

Ueng, Y.F., Hsieh, C.H., Don, M.J., 2005. Inhibition of human cytochrome P450 enzymes by the natural hepatotoxin safrole. Food Chem. Toxicol. 43, 707–712.

Uhl, M., Helma, C., Knasmüller, S., 2000. Evaluation of the single cell gel electrophoresis assay with human hepatoma (Hep G2) cells. Mutat. Res. 468, 213–225.

Ukelis, U., Kramer, P.J., Olejniczak, K., et al., 2008. Replacement of *in vivo* acute oral toxicity studies by *in vitro* cytotoxicity methods: opportunities, limits and regulatory status. Regul. Toxicol. Pharmacol. 51, 108–118.

Ündeger, U., Basaran, A., Degen, G.H., et al., 2009. Antioxidant activities of major thyme ingredients and lack of (oxidative) DNA damage in V79 Chinese hamster lung fibroblast cells at low levels of carvacrol and thymol. Food Chem. Toxicol. 47, 2037–2043.

Unger, P., Melzig, M.F., 2012. Comparative study of the cytotoxicity and genotoxicity of alpha- and beta-asarone. Sci. Pharm. 80, 663–668.

Usta, J., Kreydiyyeh, S., Knio, K., et al., 2009. Linalool decreases HepG2 viability by inhibiting mitochondrial complexes I and II, increasing reactive oxygen species and decreasing ATP and GSH levels. Chem. Biol. Interact. 180, 39–46.

Uter, W., Schnuch, A., Geier, J., et al., 2001. Association between occupation and contact allergy to the fragrance mix: a multifactorial analysis of national surveillance data. Occup. Environ. Med. 58, 392–398.

Uter, W., Ludwig, A., Balda, B.R., 2004. The prevalence of contact allergy differed between population-based and clinic-based data. J. Clin. Epidemiol. 57, 627–632.

Uter, W., Hegewald, J., Kränke, B., et al., 2008. The impact of meteorological conditions on patch test results with 12 standard series allergens (fragrances, biocides, topical ingredients). Br. J. Dermatol. 158, 734–739.

Uter, W., Schmidt, E., Geier, J., et al., 2010. Contact allergy to essential oils: current patch test results (2000–2008) from the Information Network of Departments of Dermatology (IVDK). Contact Dermatitis 63, 277–283.

Utsumi, M., Sugai, T., Shoji, A., et al., 1992. Incidence of positive reactions to sandalwood oil and its related fragrance materials in patch tests and a case of contact allergy to natural and synthetic sandalwood oil in a museum worker. Skin Res. 34, 209–213.

Uwaifo, A.O., 1984. The mutagenicities of seven coumarin derivatives and a furan derivative (nimbolide) isolated from three medicinal plants. J. Toxicol. Environ. Health 13, 521–530.

Uwaifo, A.O., Billings, P.C., Heidelberger, C., 1983. Mutation of Chinese hamster V79 cells and transformation and mutation of mouse fibroblast C3H/10 T1/2 clone 8 cells by aflatoxin B1 and four other furocoumarins isolated from two Nigerian medicinal plants. Cancer Res. 43, 1054–1058.

Valder, C., Neugebauer, M., Meier, M., et al., 2003. Western Australian sandalwood oil – new constituents of *Santalum spicatum* (R. Br.) A. DC. (Santalaceae). J. Essential Oil Res. 15, 178–186.

Valentini, G., Bellomaria, B., Arnold, N., 1998. L'Olio essenziale di *Vitex agnus-castus*. Riv. Ital. EPPOS 24, 13–18.

Valko, M., Izakovic, M., Mazur, M., et al., 2004. Role of oxygen radicals in DNA damage and cancer incidence. Mol. Cell. Biochem. 266, 37–56.

Vallance, W.B., 1955. Pennyroyal poisoning - a fatal case. Lancet 2, 850–851.

Valnet, J., 1964. Aromathérapie. Librairie Maloine, Paris (English translation: Valnet J 1990 The practice of aromatherapy. CW Daniel, Saffron Walden).

Van Beek, T.A., Kelis, R., Posthumus, M.A., et al., 1989. Essential oil of *Amyris balsamifera*. Phytochemistry 28, 1909–1911.

Van den Berg, V., Coeckelberghs, H., Vanhees, I., et al., 2002. HPLC-MS determination of the oxidation products of the reaction between alpha- and beta-pinene and OH radicals. Anal. Bioanal. Chem. 372, 630–638.

Van der Valk, P.G., de Groot, A.C., Bruynzeel, D.P., et al., 1994. Allergic contact eczema from tea tree oil. Ned. Tijdschr. Geneeskd. 138, 823–825.

Van Duuren, B.L., 1965. Carcinogenic epoxides, lactones and hydroperoxides. In: Mycotoxins Foodstuffs, Proc. Symp., Massachussets Institute of Technology 1964, pp. 275–285.

Van Duuren, B.L., Blazej, T., Goldschmidt, B.M., et al., 1971. Cocarcinogenesis studies on mouse skin and inhibition of tumor induction. J. Natl. Cancer Inst. 46, 1039–1044.

Van Duuren, B.L., Goldschmidt, B.M., 1976. Cocarcinogenic and tumor-promoting agents in tobacco carcinogenesis. J. Natl. Cancer Inst. 56, 1237–1242.

Van Iersel, M.L., Henderson, C.J., Walters, D.G., 1994. Metabolism of [3-^{14}C] coumarin in human liver microsomes. Xenobiotica 24, 795–803.

Van Iersel, M.L., Ploemen, J.P., Lo Bello, M., et al., 1997. Interactions of α, β-unsaturated aldehydes and ketones with human glutathione *S*-transferase P1-1. Chem. Biol. Interact. 108, 67–78.

Van Joost, T., Stolz, E., van der Hoek, J.C., 1985. Simultaneous allergy to perfume ingredients. Contact Dermatitis 12, 115–116.

Van Lookeren Campagne, J., 1939. Vergiftiging door oleum chenopodii. Ned. Tijdschr. Geneeskd. 83, 5472–5476.

Van Loveren, H., Cockshott, A., Gebel, T., et al., 2008. Skin sensitization in chemical risk assessment: report of a WHO/IPCS international workshop focusing on dose-response assessment. Regul. Toxicol. Pharmacol. 50, 155–161.

Van Miller, J.P., Weaver, E.P., 1987. Fourteen-day dietary minimum toxicity screen (MTS) in albino rats. Bushy Run Research Center, Export, PA Unpublished report to FEMA.

Van Zeeland, A.A., Vreeswijk, M.P., De Gruijl, F.R., et al., 2005. Transcription-coupled repair: impact on UV-induced mutagenesis in cultured rodent cells and mouse skin tumors. Mutat. Res. 577, 170–178.

Vance, S.H., Benghuzzi, H., Wilson-Simpson, F., et al., 2008. Thymoquinone supplementation and its effect on kidney tubule epithelial cells in vitro. Biomed. Sci. Instrum. 44, 477–482.

Vanithakumari, G., Sampathraj, R., Selvaraj, M., et al., 1998. Effect of short term treatment of eugenol on the seminal vesicles of adult albino rats. Indian J. Exp. Biol. 36, 1240–1244.

Vanscheidt, W., Rabe, E., Naser-Hijazi, B., et al., 2002. The efficacy and safety of a coumarin/troxerutin combination (SB-LOT) in patients with chronic venous insufficiency: a double blind placebo-controlled randomised study. Vasa. 31, 185–190.

Vardar-Unlu, G., Candan, F., Sokmen, A., et al., 2003. Antimicrobial and antioxidant activity of the essential oil and methanol extracts of *Thymus pectinatus* Fisch. et Mey. var. *pectinatus* (Lamiaceae). J. Agric. Food Chem. 51, 63–67.

Varma, S., Blackford, S., Statham, B.N., et al., 2000. Combined contact allergy to tea tree oil and lavender oil complicating chronic vulvovaginitis. Contact Dermatitis 42, 309–310.

Vasey, R.H., Karayannoppoulos, S.J., 1972. Camphorated oil. Br. Med. J. 1 (792), 112.

Vasil'ev, E.D., Il'nitskaia, S.I., Nikitenko, E.V., et al., 2005. Age- and sex-related differences in sensitivity to hepatotoxic action of estragole in mice. Ross. Fiziol. Zh. Im. I. M. Sechenova 91, 1066–1070.

Vassallo, J.D., Hicks, S.M., Daston, G.P., et al., 2004. Metabolic detoxification determines species differences in coumarin-induced hepatotoxicity. Toxicol. Sci. 80, 249–257.

Vaverkova, S., Holla, M., Tekel, J., 1995a. The effect of herbicides on the qualitative properties of healing plants. Pharmazie 50, 143–144.

Vaverkova, S., Tekel, J., Holla, M., 1995b. The effect of herbicides on the qualitative properties of medicinal plants. Pharmazie 50, 835–836.

Vaze, K., 2003. Lesser known essential oils of India, their composition and uses. FAFAI 5 (314), 47–58.

Vazquez, J.A., Zawawi, A.A., 2002. Efficacy of alcohol-based and alcohol-free melaleuca oral solution for the treatment of fluconazole-refractory oropharyngeal candidiasis in patients with AIDS. HIV Clin. Trials 3, 379–385.

Veien, N.K., Rosner, K., Skovgaard, G.L., 2004. Is tea tree oil an important contact allergen? Contact Dermatitis 50, 378–379.

Veiga, M.I., Asimus, S., Ferreira, P.E., et al., 2009. Pharmacogenomics of CYP2A6, CYP2B6, CYP2C19, CYP2D6, CYP3A4, CYP3A5 and MDR1 in Vietnam. Eur. J. Clin. Pharmacol. 65, 355–363.

Velasco-Neguerela, A., Perez-Alonso, M.J., 1990. Nuevos datos sobre la composición quimica de aceites essenciales procedentes de tomillos Ibericos. Botanica Complutensis 16, 91–97.

Veliskova, J., Velisek, L., Sperber, E.F., et al., 1994. The development of epilepsy in the paediatric brain. Seizure 3, 263–270.

Veliskova, J., Claudio, O.I., Galanopoulo, A.S., et al., 2004. Seizures in the developing brain. Epilepsia 45 (Suppl. 8), 6–12.

Vennekens, R., Owsianik, G., Nilius, B., 2008. Vanilloid transient receptor potential cation channels: an overview. Curr. Pharm. Des. 14, 18–31.

Verboom, P., Hakkaart-Van, L., Sturkenboom, M., et al., 2002. The cost of atopic dermatitis in the Netherlands: an international comparison. Br. J. Dermatol. 147, 716–724.

Verhulst, H.L., Page, L.A., Crotty, J.J., 1961. Communications from the national clearinghouse for poison control centers: camphor. Am. J. Dis. Child. 101, 536.

Vernin, G., 1991. Volatile constituents of the essential oil of *Santolina chamaecyparissus* L. J. Essential Oil Res. 3, 49–53.

Vernot, E.H., MacEwen, J.D., Haun, C.C., et al., 1977. Acute toxicity and skin corrosion data for some organic and inorganic compounds and aqueous solutions. Toxicol. Appl. Pharmacol. 42, 417–423.

Verrier, A.C., Schmitt, D., Staquet, M.J., 1999. Fragrance and contact allergens *in vitro* modulate the HLA-DR and E-cadherin expression on human epidermal Langerhans cells. Int. Arch. Allergy Immunol. 120, 56–62.

Verzera, A., Trozzi, A., Stagno D'Alcontres, I., et al., 1998. The composition of the volatile fraction of Calabrian bergamot essential oil. Riv. Ital. EPPOS 25, 17–38.

Vesselinovitch, S.D., Rao, K.V.N., Mihailovich, N., 1979. Transplacental and lactational carcinogenesis by safrole. Cancer Res. 39, 4378–4380.

Viana, G.S., do Vale, T.G., Silva, C.M., et al., 2000. Anticonvulsant activity of essential oils and active principles from chemotypes of *Lippia alba* (Mill.) N.E. Brown. Biol. Pharm. Bull. 23, 1314–1317.

Vidhya, N., Devaraj, S.N., 1999. Antioxidant effect of eugenol in rat intestine. Indian J. Exp. Biol. 37, 1192–1195.

Vidrich, V., Fusi, P., Michelozzi, M., et al., 1996. Analysis of essential oils from leaves and branches of different Italian provenances of *Pinus nigra* Arn. J. Essential Oil Res. 8, 377–381.

Vigushin, D.M., Poon, G.K., Boddy, A., et al., 1998. Phase I and pharmacokinetic study of *d*-limonene in patients with advanced cancer. Cancer Research Campaign Phase I/II Clinical Trials Committee. Cancer Chemother. Pharmacol 42, 111–117.

Vilaplana, J., Romaguera, C., 2000. Allergic contact dermatitis due to eucalyptol in an anti-inflammatory cream. Contact Dermatitis 43, 118–119.

Vilaplana, J., Romaguera, C., Grimalt, F., 1991. Contact dermatitis from geraniol in Bulgarian rose oil. Contact Dermatitis 24, 301–319.

Vilenchik, M.M., Knudson, A.G., 2000. Inverse radiation dose-rate effects on somatic and germ-line mutations and DNA damage rates. Proc. Natl. Acad. Sci. U. S. A. 97, 5381–5386.

Villar, D., Knight, M.J., Hansen, S.R., et al., 1994. Toxicity of Melaleuca oil and related essential oils applied topically on dogs and cats. Vet. Hum. Toxicol. 36, 139–142.

Viña, A., Murillo, E., 2003. Essential oil composition from twelve varieties of basil (*Ocimum* spp) grown in Colombia. J. Brazilian Chemical Society 14, 744–749.

Vishteh, A., Thomas, I., Imamura, T., 1986. Eugenol modulation of the immune response in mice. Immunopharmacology 12, 187–192.

Visscher, M.O., Chatterjee, R., Munson, K.A., 2000. Changes in diapered and nondiapered infant skin over the first month of life. Pediatr. Dermatol. 17, 45–51.

Vo, L.T., Chan, D., King, R.G., 2003. Investigation of the effects of peppermint oil and valerian on rat liver and cultured human liver cells. Clin. Exp. Pharmacol. Physiol. 30, 799–804.

Vocanson, M., Goujon, C., Chabeau, G., et al., 2006. The skin allergenic properties of chemicals may depend on contaminants - evidence from studies on coumarin. Int. Arch. Allergy Immunol. 140, 231–238.

Vocanson, M., Valeyrie, M., Rozières, A., et al., 2007. Lack of evidence for allergenic properties of coumarin in a fragrance allergy mouse model. Contact Dermatitis 57, 361–364.

Vogelstein, B., Kinzler, K.W., 1993. The multistep nature of cancer. Trends Genet. 9, 138–141.

Von der Hude, W., Seelbach, A., Basler, A., 1990. Epoxides: comparison of the induction of SOS repair in Escherichia coli PQ37 and the bacterial mutagenicity in the Ames test. Mutat. Res. 231, 205–218.

Von Rudloff, E., Lapp, M.S., Yeh, F.C., 1988. Chemosystematic study of *Thuja plicata*: multivariate analysis of leaf oil terpene composition. Biochem. Syst. Ecol. 16, 119–125.

Von Skramlik, E.V., 1959. Über die Giftigkeit und Verträglichkeit von ätherischen Ölen. Pharmazie 14, 435–445.

Vujosevic, M., Blagojevic, J., 2004. Antimutagenic effects of extracts from sage (*Salvia officinalis*) in mammalian system in vivo. Acta Vet. Hung. 52, 439–443.

Vuković-Gačić, B., Nikčević, S., Berić-Bjedov, T., et al., 2006. Antimutagenic effect of essential oil of sage (*Salvia officinalis* L.) and its monoterpenes against UV-induced mutations in *Escherichia coli* and *Saccharomyces cerevisiae*. Food Chem. Toxicol. 44, 1730–1738.

Wabner, D., 1993. Purity and pesticides. Int. J. Aromather. 5 (2), 27–29.

Wabner, D., Geier, K., Hauck, D., 2006. For a deeper understanding of tea tree oil: fresh is best – why we should only use fresh oil at any concentration. Int. J. Aromather. 16, 109–115.

Wacher, V.J., Wong, S., Wong, H.T., 2002. Peppermint oil enhances cyclosporine oral bioavailability in rats: comparison with D-alpha-tocopheryl poly(ethylene glycol 1000) succinate (TPGS) and ketoconazole. J. Pharm. Sci. 91, 77–90.

Waddell, W.J., 2003. Thresholds in Chemical Carcinogenesis: what are animal experiments telling us? Toxicol. Pathol. 31, 260–262.

Waddell, W.J., Crooks, N.H., Carmichael, P.L., 2004. Correlation of tumors with DNA adducts from methyl eugenol and tamoxifen in rats. Toxicol. Sci. 79, 38–40.

Wade, A.E., Holl, J.E., Hilliard, C.C., et al., 1968. Alteration of drug metabolism in rats and mice by an environment of cedarwood. Pharmacology 1, 317–328.

Wagner, H., Sprinkmeyer, L., 1973. Pharmacological effect of balm spirit. Dtsch. Apoth. Ztg. 113, 1159–1166.

Wagner, A.M., Wu, J.J., Hansen, R.C., et al., 2002a. Bullous phytophotodermatitis associated with high natural concentrations of furanocoumarins in limes. Am. J. Contact Dermat. 13, 10–14.

Wagner, J.E., Huff, J.L., Rust, W.L., et al., 2002b. Perillyl alcohol inhibits breast cell migration without affecting cell adhesion. J. Biomed. Biotech. 2, 136–140.

Wainman, T., Zhang, J., Weschler, C.J., Lioy, P.J., 2000. Ozone and limonene in indoor air: a source of submicron particle exposure. Environ. Health Perspect. 108, 1139–1145.

Wakazono, H., Gardner, I., Eliasson, E., et al., 1998. Immunochemical identification of hepatic protein adducts derived from estragole. Chem. Res. Toxicol. 11, 863–872.

Walde, A., Ve, B., Scheline, R.R., 1983. *p*-Cymene metabolism in rats and guinea-pigs. Xenobiotica 13, 503–512.

Waldman, N., 2011. Seizure caused by dermal application of over-the-counter eucalyptus oil head lice preparation. Clin. Toxicol. 49, 750–751.

Wallace, L.A., Nelson, W.C., Pellizzari, E., et al., 1991. Identification of polar volatile organic compounds in consumer products and common microenvironments. http://www.exposurescience.org/WNP91.

Wallengren, J., 2011. Tea tree oil attenuates experimental contact dermatitis. Arch. Dermatol. Res. 303, 333–338.

Waller, G.R., Price, G.H., Mitchell, E.D., 1969. Feline attractant, cis, trans-nepetalactone: metabolism in the domestic cat. Science 164, 1281–1282.

Waller, P., Shaw, M., Ho, D., et al., 2005. Hospital admissions for 'drug-induced' disorders in England: a study using the Hospital Episodes Statistics (HES) database. Br. J. Clin. Pharmacol. 59, 213–219.

Walter, B.M., Bilkei, G., 2004. Immunostimulatory effect of dietary oregano etheric oils on lymphocytes from growth-retarded, low-weight growing-finishing pigs and productivity. Tidjschrift Diergeneeskunde 129, 178–181.

Wan, S.H., Riegelman, S., 1972. Renal contribution to overall metabolism of drugs. I. Conversion of benzoic acid to hippuric acid. J. Pharm. Sci. 61, 1278–1284.

Wang, K., Su, C.Y., 2000. Pharmacokinetics and disposition of beta-elemene in rats. Yao Xue Xue Bao 35, 725–728.

Wang, L.H., Tso, M., 2002. Determination of 5-methoxypsoralen in human serum. J. Pharm. Biomed. Anal. 30, 593–600.

Wang, J., Zhang, H., Sun, Y., 1996. Phase III clinical trial of elemenum emulsion in the management of malignant pleural and peritoneal effusions. Zhonghua Zhong Liu Za Zhi 18, 464–467.

Wang, B.G., Hong, X., Li, L., et al., 2000. Chemical constituents of two Chinese Magnoliaceae plants, *Tsoongiodendron odorum* and *Manglietiastrum sinicum*, and their inhibition of platelet aggregation. Planta Med. 66, 511–515.

Wang, G., Li, X., Huang, F., et al., 2005. Antitumor effect of beta-elemene in non-small-cell lung cancer cells is mediated via induction of cell cycle arrest and apoptotic cell death. Cell. Mol. Life Sci. 62, 881–893.

Wang, S., Chen, Y., Gao, Z., et al., 2007. Gas chromatographic-mass spectrometric analysis of d-limonene in human plasma. J. Pharm. Biomed. Anal. 44, 1095–1099.

Wang, X.P., Ding, H.L., Geng, C.M., et al., 2008. Migraine as a sex-conditioned inherited disorder: evidences from China and the world. Neurosci. Bull. 24, 110–116.

Wang, Y.B., Qin, J., Zheng, X.Y., et al., 2010. Diallyl trisulfide induces Bcl-2 and caspase-3-dependent apoptosis via downregulation of Akt phosphorylation in human T24 bladder cancer cells. Phytomedicine 17, 363–368.

Wang, C.Y., Tsai, A.C., Peng, C.Y., et al., 2012. Dehydrocostuslactone suppresses angiogenesis in vitro and in vivo through inhibition of Akt/GSK-3β and mTOR signaling pathways. PLoS One 7, e31195.

Wangensteen, H., Molden, E., Christensen, H., et al., 2003. Identification of epoxybergamottin as a CYP3A4 inhibitor in grapefruit peel. Eur. J. Clin Pharmacol. 58, 663–668.

Wargovich, M.J., Woods, C., Eng, V.W., et al., 1988. Chemoprevention of N-nitrosomethylbenzylamine-induced esophageal cancer in rats by the naturally occurring thioether, diallyl sulfide. Cancer Res. 48, 6872–6875.

Warkany, J., Takacs, E., 1959. Experimental production of congenital malformations in rats by salicylate poisoning. Am. J. Pathol. 35, 315–331.

Warshaw, E.M., Zug, K.A., 1996. Sesquiterpene lactone allergy. Am. J. Contact Dermat. 7, 1–23.

Warshaw, E.M., Bucholz, H.J., Belsito, D.V., et al., 2009. Allergic patch test reactions associated with cosmetics: retrospective analysis of cross-sectional data from the North American Contact Dermatitis Group, 2001–2004. J. Am. Acad. Dermatol. 60, 23–38.

Watabe, T., Hiratsuka, A., Isobe, M., et al., 1980. Metabolism of d-limonene by hepatic microsomes to non-mutagenic epoxides toward *Salmonella typhimurium*. Biochem. Pharmacol. 29, 1068–1071.

Watabe, T., Hiratsuka, A., Ozawa, N., et al., 1981. A comparative study on the metabolism of d-limonene and 4-vinylcyclohex-1-ene by hepatic microsomes. Xenobiotica 11 (5), 333–344.

Watson, W.A., Litovitz, T.L., Rodgers, G.C., et al., 2003. 2002 Annual report of the American Association of Poison Control Centers Toxic Exposure Surveillance System. Am. J. Emerg. Med. 21, 353–421.

Watson, W.A., Litovitz, T.L., Klein-Schwartz, W., et al., 2004. 2003 Annual report of the American Association of Poison Control Centers Toxic Exposure Surveillance System. Am. J. Emerg. Med. 22, 335–404.

Watson, W.A., Litovitz, T.L., Rodgers, G.C., et al., 2005. 2004 Annual report of the American Association of Poison Control Centers Toxic Exposure Surveillance System. Am. J. Emerg. Med. 23, 589–666.

Wattenberg, L.W., 1983. Inhibition of neoplasia by minor dietary constituents. Cancer Res. 43 (5 Suppl.), 2448S–2453S.

Wattenberg, L.W., 1990. Inhibition of carcinogenesis by minor anutrient constituents of the diet. Proc. Nutr. Soc. 49, 173–183.

Wattenberg, L.W., 1991. Inhibition of azoxymethane-induced neoplasia of the large bowel by 3-hydroxy-3,7,11-trimethyl-1,6,10-dodecatriene (nerolidol). Carcinogenesis 12, 151–152.

Wattenberg, L.W., Coccia, J.B., 1991. Inhibition of 4-(methylnitrosamino)-1-(3-pyridyl)-1-butanone carcinogenesis in mice by d-limonene and citrus fruit oils. Carcinogenesis 12, 115–117.

Wattenberg, L.W., Lam, L.K., Fladmoe, A.V., 1979. Inhibition of chemical carcinogen-induced neoplasia by coumarins and α-angelicalactone. Cancer Res. 39, 1651–1654.

Wattenberg, L.W., Hanley, A.B., Barany, G., et al., 1985. Inhibition of carcinogenesis by some minor dietary constituents. Princess Takamatsu Symp. 16, 193–203.

Wattenberg, L.W., Sparnins, V.L., Barany, G., 1989. Inhibition of N-nitrosodiethylamine carcinogenesis in mice by naturally occurring organosulfur compounds and monoterpenes. Cancer Res. 49, 2689–2692.

Webb, W.K., Hansen, W.H., 1963. Chronic and subacute toxicology and pathology of methyl salicylate in dogs, rats and rabbits. Toxicol. Appl. Pharmacol. 5, 576–587.

Webb, N.J., Pitt, W.R., 1993. Eucalyptus oil poisoning in childhood: 41 cases in south-east Queensland. J. Paediatr. Child Health 29, 368–371.

Webb, D.R., Ridder, G.M., Alden, C.L., 1989. Acute and subchronic nephrotoxicity of d-limonene in Fischer 344 rats. Food Chem. Toxicol. 27, 639–650.

Webb, D.R., Kanerva, R.L., Hysell, D.K., et al., 1990. Assessment of the subchronic oral toxicity of d-limonene in dogs. Food Chem. Toxicol. 28, 669–676.

Wei, A., Shibamoto, T., 2007a. Antioxidant activities and volatile constituents of various essential oils. J. Agric. Food Chem. 55, 1737–1742.

Wei, A., Shibamoto, T., 2007b. Antioxidant activities of essential oil mixtures towards skin lipid squalene oxidized by UV irradiation. Cutan. Ocul. Toxicol. 26, 227–233.

Wei, Q., Harada, K., Ohmori, S., et al., 2006. Toxicity study of the volatile constituents og *Myoga* utilizing acute dermal irritation assays and the guinea-pig maximation test. J. Occup. Health 48, 480–486.

Wei, F.X., Liu, J.X., Wang, L., et al., 2008. Expression of bcl-2 and bax genes in the liver cancer cell line HepG2 after apoptosis induced by essential oils from *Rosmarinus officinalis*. Zhong Yao Cai 31, 877–879.

Weibel, H., Hansen, J., 1989a. Interaction of cinnamaldehyde (a sensitizer in fragrance) with protein. Contact Dermatitis 20, 161–166.

Weibel, H., Hansen, J., 1989b. Penetration of the fragrance compounds, cinnamaldehyde and cinnamyl alcohol, through human skin *in vitro*. Contact Dermatitis 20, 167–172.

Weil, A.T., 1965. Nutmeg as a narcotic. Econ. Bot. 19, 194–217.

Weil, A.T., 1966. The use of nutmeg as a psychotropic agent. Bull. Narc. 18, 15–23.

Weisbrod, S.D., Soule, J.B., Kimmel, P.L., 1997. Poison on line – acute renal failure caused by oil of wormwood purchased through the internet. N. Engl. J. Med. 337, 825–827.

Weisburger, J.H., Williams, G.M., 2000. The distinction between genotoxic and epigenetic carcinogens and implication for cancer risk. Toxicol. Sci. 57, 4–5.

Weiss, G., 1960. Hallucinogenic and narcotic-like effect of powdered myristica (nutmeg). Psychiatr. Q. 34, 346–356.

Weiss, J., Catalano, P., 1973. Camphorated oil intoxication during pregnancy. Pediatrics 52, 713–714.

Weiss, R.R., James, W.D., 1997. Allergic contact dermatitis from aromatherapy. Am. J. Contact Dermat. 8, 250–251.

Wen, Y.H., Sahi, J., Urda, E., et al., 2002. Effects of bergamottin on human and monkey drug-metabolizing enzymes in primary cultured hepatocytes. Drug Metab. Dispos. 30, 977–984.

Wenzel, D.G., Ross, C.R., 1957. Central stimulating properties of some terpenones. J. Am. Pharm. Assoc. 46, 77–82.

Wepierre, J., Cohen, Y., Valette, G., 1968. Percutaneous absorption and removal by the body fluids of 14C ethyl alcohol 3H perhydrosqualene and 14C-p-cymene. Eur. J. Pharmacol. 3, 47–51.

Weschler, C.J., Shields, H.C., 1999. Indoor ozone/terpene reactions as a source of indoor particles. Atmos. Environ. 33, 2301–2312.

Weschler, C.J., Shields, H.C., 2000. The influence of ventilation on reactions among indoor pollutants: modeling and experimental observations. Indoor Air 10, 92–100.

Wester, R.C., Maibach, H.I., 1983. Cutaneous pharmacokinetics: 10 stages to percutaneous absorption. Drug Metab. Rev. 14, 169–205.

Wester, R.C., Maibach, H.I., 2000. Understanding percutaneous absorption for occupational health and safety. Int. J. Occup. Environ. Health 6, 86–92.

Wester, R.C., Noonan, P.K., 1980. Relevance of international models for percutaneous absorption. Int. J. Pharm. 7, 99–110.

Westphal, G.A., Schnuch, A., Moessner, R., et al., 2003. Cytokine gene polymorphisms in allergic contact dermatitis. Contact Dermatitis 48, 93–98.

Weyerstahl, P., 1986. Isolation and synthesis of compounds from the essential oil of *Helichrysum italicum*. In: Brunke, E.J. (Ed.), Progress in essential oil research. De Gruyter, Berlin, pp. 177–195.

Weyerstahl, P., Marschall, H., Bork, W.R., et al., 1995. Constituents of the absolute of *Boronia megastigma* Nees. From Tasmania. Flavour Fragrance J. 10, 297–311.

Weyerstahl, P., Schneider, S., Marschall, H., 1996. Constituents of the Brazilian Cangerana oil. Flavour Fragrance J. 11, 81–94.

White, I.R., 1995. Phototoxic and photoallergic reactions. In: Rycroft, R.J., Menne, T., Frosch, P.J. et al., (Eds.), Textbook of contact dermatitis. Springer-Verlag, Berlin, p. 84.

White, T.J., Goodman, D., Shulgin, A.T., et al., 1977. Mutagenic activity of some centrally active aomatic amines in Salmonella typhimurium. Mutat. Res. 56, 199–202.

White, S.I., Friedmann, P.S., Moss, C., et al., 1986. The effect of altering area of application and dose per unit area on sensitization by DNCB. Br. J. Dermatol. 115, 663–668.

White, J.M., White, I.R., Glendinning, A., et al., 2007. Frequency of allergic contact dermatitis to isoeugenol is increasing: a review of 3636 patients tested from 2001 to 2005. Br. J. Dermatol. 157, 580–582.

Whitling, H.T., 1908. "Cures" for asthma: fatal case from an overdose of oil of sage. Lancet 171 (4415), 1074–1075.

Whyte, H.M., 1983. NHMRC workshop on non-pharmacological methods of lowering blood pressure: psychological methods of lowering blood pressure. Med. J. Aust. 2, S13–S16.

Wie, M.B., Won, M.H., Lee, K.H., et al., 1997. Eugenol protects neuronal cells from excitotoxic and oxidative injury in primary cortical cultures. Neurosci. Lett. 225, 93–96.

Wieslander, G., Norbäck, D., Björnsson, E., et al., 1997. Asthma and the indoor environment: the significance of emission of formaldehyde and volatile organic compounds from newly painted indoor surfaces. Int. Arch. Occup. Environ. Health 69, 115–124.

Wijesekera, R.O.B., 1973. The chemical composition and analysis of citronella oil. J. Natl. Sci. Council (Sri Lanka) 1, 67–81.

Wijesekera, R.O., 1978. The chemistry and technology of cinnamon. CRC Crit. Rev. Food Sci. Nutr. 10, 1–30.

Wild, C.P., Kleinjans, J., 2003. Children and increased susceptibility to environmental carcinogens: evidence or empathy? Cancer Epidemiol. Biomarkers Prev. 12, 1389–1394.

Wiley, H.M., Bigelow, W.D., 1908. Influence of benzoic acid and benzoates on digestion and health. Bulletin 84 pt. IV. Bureau of Chemistry, U.S. Department of Agriculture.

Wilhelm, K.P., Cua, A.B., Maibach, H.I., 1991. Skin aging. Effect on transepidermal water loss, stratum corneum hydration, skin surface pH, and casual sebum content. Arch. Dermatol. 127, 1806–1809.

Wilkins, C.K., Wolkoff, P., Clausen, P.A., et al., 2003. Upper airway irritation of terpene/ozone oxidation products (TOPS). Dependence on reaction time, relative humidity and initial ozone concentration. Toxicol. Lett. 143, 109–114.

Wilkinson, S.M., Beck, M.H., 1994. Allergic contact dermatitis from menthol in peppermint. Contact Dermatitis 30, 42–43.

Wilkinson, J.D., Andersen, K.E., Camarasa, J.G., et al., 1989. Preliminary results of the effectiveness of two forms of fragrance mix as screening agents for fragrance sensitivity. In: Frosch, P.J. et al., (Ed.), Current topics in contact dermatitis. Springer-Verlag, Heidelberg, pp. 127–131.

Willhite, C.C., 1986. Structure-activity relationships of retinoids in developmental toxicology. Toxicol. Appl. Pharmacol. 83, 563–575.

Williams, G.M., 2001. Mechanisms of chemical carcinogenesis and application to human cancer risk assessment. Toxicology 166, 3–10.

Williams, G.M., 2008. Application of mode-of-action considerations in human cancer risk assessment. Toxicol. Lett. 180, 75–80.

Williams, A.C., Barry, B.W., 1989. Essential oils as novel human skin penetration enhancers. Int. J. Pharm. 57, R7–R9.

Williams, A.C., Barry, B.W., 1991. Terpenes and the lipid-protein-partitioning theory of skin penetration enhancement. Pharm. Res. 8, 17–24.

Williams, P.L., Riviere, J.E., 1995. A biophysically based dermatopharmacokinetic compartment model for quantifying percutaneous penetration and absorption of topically applied agents. 1. Theory. J. Pharm. Sci. 84, 599–608.

Williams, L.R., Home, V., Asre, S., 1990. Oils of Melaleuca alternifolia: their antifungal activity against Candida albicans in perspective. Int. J. Aromather. 2, 12–13.

Williams, G.M., Iatropoulos, M.J., Jeffrey, A.M., et al., 2005a. Low dose non-linearities in experimental chemical hepatocarcinogenesis. (Abstract). Toxicol. Lett. 158S, S14.

Williams, G.M., Iatropoulos, M.J., Jeffrey, A.M., et al., 2005b. Thresholds for DNA-reactive (genotoxic) organic carcinogens. J. Toxicol. Pathol. 18, 69–77.

Williamson, E.M., 2000. Synergy – myth or reality? In: Ernst, E. (Ed.), Herbal Medicine. Butterworth-Heinemann, Oxford, pp. 43–58.

Williamson, E.A., 2010. Inhibition of cytochrome P450 2E1, cytochrome P450 3A6 and cytochrome P450 2A6 by citrus essential oils. MSc thesis, University of North Carolina, Greensboro.

Wilson, J.G., 1973. Present status of drugs as teratogens in man. Teratology 7, 3–15.

Wilson, B.J., 1979. Naturally occurring toxicants of foods. Nutr. Rev. 37, 305–312.

Wilson, J.D., 1980. The pathogenesis of benign prostatic hyperplasia. Am. J. Med. 68, 745–756.

Wilson, B.J., Garst, J.E., Linnabary, R.D., et al., 1977. Perilla ketone: a potent lung toxin from the mint plant, Perilla frutescens Britton. Science 197, 573–574.

Winder, C., 2002. Mechanisms of multiple chemical sensitivity. Toxicol. Lett. 128, 85–97.

Wingate, U.O., 1889. A case of poisoning by the oil of hedeoma (pennyroyal). Boston Medical & Surgical Journal 120, 536.

Winterbotham, L.P., 1914. Eucalyptus oil poisoning. Med. J. Aust. 2, 129–130.

Wiseman, R.W., Miller, E.C., Miller, J.A., et al., 1987. Structure-activity studies of the hepatocarcinogenicities of alkenylbenzene derivatives related to estragole and safrole on administration to preweanling male C57BL/6 J x C3H/HeJF1 mice. Cancer Res. 47, 2275–2283.

Wislocki, P.G., Borchert, P., Miller, J.A., et al., 1976. The metabolic activation of the carcinogen 1′-hydroxysafrole in vivo and in vitro and the electrophilic reactivities of possible ultimate carcinogens. Cancer Res. 36, 1686–1695.

Wislocki, P.G., Miller, E.C., Miller, J.A., et al., 1977. Carcinogenic and mutagenic activities of safrole, 1′-hydroxysafrole and some known or possible metabolites. Cancer Res. 37, 1883–1891.

Witthauer, W., 1922. Poisoning with eucalyptus oil. Klin. Wochenschr. 29, 1460–1461.

Woelk, H., Schläfke, S., 2010. A multi-center, double-blind, randomised study of the lavender oil preparation silexan in comparison to lorazepam for generalized anxiety disorder. Phytomedicine 17, 94–99.

Wöhrl, S., Hemmer, W., Focke, M., et al., 2001. The significance of fragrance mix, balsam of Peru, colophony and propolis as screening tools in the detection of fragrance allergy. Br. J. Dermatol. 145, 268–273.

Wolf, I.J., 1935. Fatal poisoning with oil of chenopodium in a Negro child with sickle cell anemia. Arch. Pediatr. 52, 126–130.

Wolf, R., Wolf, D., Tüzün, B., Tüzün, Y., 2001. Contact dermatitis to cosmetics. Clin. Dermatol. 19, 502–515.

Wolf, D.C., Allen, J.W., George, M.H., et al., 2006. Toxicity profiles in rats treated with tumorigenic and nontumorigenic triazole conazole fungicides: Propiconazole, triadimefon, and myclobutanil. Toxicol. Pathol. 34, 895–902.

Wolff, G.L., 1987a. Twenty-eight day gavage and encapsulated feed study on 1,8-cineole in Fischer 344 rats. NTP chemical no. 15 - NTP experiment nos: 5014-02 (encapsulated) and 5014-06 (gavage). Final report.

Wolff, G.L., 1987b. Twenty-eight day gavage and encapsulated feed study on 1,8-cineole in B6C3F1 hybrid mice. NTP chemical no. 15 - NTP experiment nos: 5014-03 (encapsulated) and 5014-07 (gavage). Final report.

Wolkoff, P., Clausen, P.A., Wilkins, C.K., et al., 1999. Formation of strong airway irritants in a model mixture of (+)-α-pinene/ozone. Atmos. Environ. 33, 693–698.

Wolkoff, P., Clausen, P.A., Wilkins, C.K., et al., 2000. Formation of strong airway irritants in terpene/ozone mixtures. Indoor Air 10, 82–91.

Wolkoff, P., Clausen, P.A., Larsen, K., et al., 2008. Acute airway effects of ozone-initiated d-limonene chemistry: importance of gaseous products. Toxicol. Lett. 181, 171–176.

Wondergem, R., Bartley, J.W., 2009. Menthol increase human glioblastoma intracellular Ca2+, BK channel activity and cell migration. J. Biomed. Sci doi: 10.1186/1423-0127-16-90.

Wondergem, R., Ecay, T.W., Mahieu, F., et al., 2008. HGF/SF and menthol increase human glioblastoma cell calcium and migration. Biochem. Biophys. Res. Commun. 372, 210–215.

Wondrak, G.T., Cabello, C.M., Villeneuve, N.F., et al., 2008. Cinnamoyl-based Nrf2-activators targeting human skin cell photo-oxidative stress. Free Radic. Biol. Med. 45, 385–395.

Wong, K.C., Tie, D.Y., 1993. The essential oil of the leaves of *Murraya koenigii* Spreng. J. Essential Oil Res. 5, 371–374.

Wong, K.C., Teng, Y.E., 1994. Volatile components of *Mimusops elengi* L. flowers. J. Essential Oil Res. 6, 453–458.

Wong, K.C., Ong, K.S., Lim, C.L., 1992. Composition of the essential oil of rhizomes of *Kaempferia galanga* L. Flavour Fragrance J. 7, 263–266.

Woo, D.C., Hoar, R.M., 1972. Apparent hydronephrosis as a normal aspect of renal development in late gestation of rats: the effect of methyl salicylate. Teratology 6, 191–196.

Woodruff, R.C., Mason, J.M., Valencia, R., et al., 1985. Chemical mutagenesis testing in *Drosophila*. V. Results of 53 coded compounds tested for the National Toxicology Program. Environ. Mutagen. 7, 677–702.

Woolf, A., 1999. Essential oil poisoning. Clin. Toxicol. 37, 721–727.

Woolverton, C.J., Fotos, P.G., Mokas, J., et al., 1986. Evaluation of eugenol for mutagenicity by the mouse micronucleus test. J. Oral Pathol. 15, 450–453.

Worm, M., Jeep, S., Sterry, W., et al., 1998. Perioral contact dermatitis caused by *L*-carvone in toothpaste. Contact Dermatitis 38, 338.

Worthen, D.R., Ghosheh, O.A., Crooks, P.A., 1998. The *in vitro* anti-tumor activity of some crude and purified components of blackseed, *Nigella sativa* L. Anticancer Res. 18, 1527–1532.

Wright, S.E., Baron, D.A., Heffner, J.E., 1995. Intravenous eugenol causes hemorrhagic lung edema in rats: proposed oxidant mechanisms. J. Lab. Clin. Med. 125, 257–264.

Wright, C.E., Laude, E.A., Grattan, T.J., et al., 1997. Capsaicin and neurokinin A-induced bronchoconstriction in the anaesthetised guinea-pig: evidence for a direct action of menthol on isolated bronchial smooth muscle. Br. J. Pharmacol. 121, 1645–1650.

Wu, H.B., Fang, Y.Q., 2004. Pharmacokinetics of *beta*-asarone in rats. Yao Xue Xue Bao 39, 836–838.

Wu, M.L., Tsai, W.J., Yang, C.C., et al., 1998a. Concentrated cresol intoxication. Vet. Hum. Toxicol. 40, 341–343.

Wu, W.Y., Luo, Y.J., Cheng, J.H., et al., 1998b. Therapeutic effect of *Curcuma aromatica* oil infused via hepatic artery against transplanted hepatoma in rats. Huaren Xiaohua Zazhi 6, 859–861.

Wu, W.Y., Xu, Q., Shi, L.C., et al., 2000. Inhibitory effects of *Curcuma aromatica* oil on proliferation of hepatoma in mice. World J. Gastroenterol. 6, 216–219.

Wu, C.C., Sheen, L.Y., Chen, H.W., et al., 2001. Effects of organosulfur compounds from garlic oil on the antioxidation system in rat liver and red blood cells. Food Chem. Toxicol. 39, 563–569.

Wu, C.C., Sheen, L.Y., Chen, H.W., et al., 2002. Differential effects of garlic oil and its three major organosulfur components on the hepatic detoxification system in rats. J. Agric. Food Chem. 50, 378–383.

Wu, C.C., Lii, C.K., Tsai, S.J., et al., 2004a. Diallyl trisulfide modulates cell viability and the antioxidation and detoxification systems of rat primary hepatocytes. J. Nutr. 134, 724–728.

Wu, C.C., Chung, J.G., Tsai, S.J., et al., 2004b. Differential effects of allyl sulfides from garlic essential oil on cell cycle regulation in human liver tumor cells. Food Chem. Toxicol. 42, 1937–1947.

Wu, M.T., Wu, D.C., Hsu, H.K., et al., 2004c. Constituents of areca chewing related to esophageal cancer risk in Taiwanese men. Dis. Esophagus 17, 257–259.

Wu, S.J., Ng, L.T., Lin, C.C., 2004d. Effects of vitamin E on the cinnamaldehyde-induced apoptotic mechanism in human PLC/PRF/5 cells. Clin. Exp. Pharmacol. Physiol. 31, 770–776.

Wyatt, R.M., Hodges, L.D., Kalafatis, N., et al., 2005. Phytochemical analysis and biological screening of leaf and twig extracts from *Kunzea ericoides*. Phytother. Res. 19, 963–970.

Wyllie, J.P., Alexander, F.W., 1994. Nasal instillation of 'Olbas Oil' in an infant. Arch. Dis. Child. 70, 357–358.

Wynder, E.L., Hoffman, D., 1967. Experimental contribution to tobacco smoke carcinogenesis. Dtsch. Med. Wochenschr. 88, 623.

Xiao, D., Singh, S.V., 2002. Phenethyl isothiocyanate-induced apoptosis in p53-deficient PC-3 human prostate cancer cell line is mediated by extracellular signal-regulated kinases. Cancer Res. 62, 3615–3619.

Xiao, D., Lew, K.L., Kim, Y.A., et al., 2006. Diallyl trisulfide suppresses growth of PC-3 human prostate cancer xenograft in vivo in association with Bax and Bak induction. Clin. Cancer Res. 12, 6836–6843.

Xiao, Y., Yang, F.Q., Li, S.P., et al., 2007. Furanodiene induces G(2)/M cell cycle arrest and apoptosis through MAPK signaling and mitochondria-caspase pathway in human hepatocellular carcinoma cells. Cancer Biol. Ther. 6, 1044–1050.

Xiao, D., Zeng, Y., Hahm, E.R., et al., 2009. Diallyl trisulfide selectively causes Bax- and Bak-mediated apoptosis in human lung cancer cells. Environ. Mol. Mutagen. 50, 201–212.

Xiufen, W., Hiramatsu, N., Matsubara, M., 2004. The antioxidative activity of traditional Japanese herbs. Biofactors 21, 281–284.

Xu, K., Thornalley, P.J., 2001. Signal transduction activated by the cancer chemopreventive isothiocyanates: cleavage of BID protein, tyrosine phosphorylation and activation of JNK. Br. J. Cancer 84, 670–673.

Xu, C., Rao, Y.S., Xu, B., et al., 2002. An in vivo pilot study characterizing the new CYP2A6*7, *8, and *10 alleles. Biochem. Biophys. Res. Commun. 290, 318–324.

Xu, M., Floyd, H.S., Greth, S.M., et al., 2004. Perillyl alcohol-mediated inhibition of lung cancer cell line proliferation: potential mechanisms for its chemotherapeutic effects. Toxicol. Appl. Pharmacol. 195, 232–246.

Yaacob, K.B., Abdullah, C.M., Joulain, D., 1989. Essential oil of Ruta graveolens L. J. Essential Oil Res. 1, 203–207.

Yadav, P., Dubey, N.K., Joshi, V.K., et al., 1999. Antidermatophytic activity of essential oil of *Cinnamomum* as a herbal ointment for cure of dermatomycosis. J. Med. Aromatic Plant Sci. 21, 347–351.

Yamada, K., Mimaki, Y., Sashida, Y., 1994. Anticonvulsive effects of inhaling lavender oil vapour. Biol. Pharm. Bull. 17, 359–360.

Yamaguchi, F., Tsutsui, T., 2003. Cell-transforming activity of fourteen chemical agents used in dental practice in Syrian hamster embryo cells. J. Pharmacol. Sci. 93, 497–500.

Yamamoto, H., 1995. Effect of atropine on cyanide-induced acute lethality in mice. Toxicol. Lett. 80, 29–33.

Yamamura, H., Ugawa, S., Ueda, T., et al., 2008. TRPM8 activation suppresses cellular viability in human melanoma. Am. J. Physiol. Cell Physiol. 295, C296–C301.

Yamano, S., Tatsuno, J., Gonzalez, F.J., 1990. The CYP2A3 gene product catalyzes coumarin 7-hydroxylation in human liver microsomes. Biochemistry 29, 1322–1329.

Yamasaki, M., Ebihara, S., Ebihara, T., et al., 2007. Cough reflex and oral chemesthesis induced by capsaicin and capsiate in healthy never-smokers. Cough 3, 9. http://dx.doi.org/10.1186/1745-9974-3-9.

Yan, B., Zhou, Y., Feng, S., et al., 2013. β-Elemene-Attenuated Tumor Angiogenesis by Targeting Notch-1 in Gastric Cancer Stem-Like Cells. Evid. Base. compl. Alternative Med. http://dx.doi.org/10.1155/2013/268468.

Yanaga, A., Goto, H., Nakagawa, T., et al., 2006. Cinnamaldehyde induces endothelium-dependent and –independent vasorelaxant action on isolated rat aorta. Biol. Pharm. Bull. 29, 2415–2418.

Yang, H., Wang, X., Yu, L., 1996. The antitumor activity of elemene is associated with apoptosis. Zhonghua Zhong Liu Za Zhi 18, 169–172.

Yang, Y.M., Conaway, C.C., Chiao, J.W., et al., 2002. Inhibition of benzo(a) pyrene-induced lung tumorigenesis in A/J mice by dietary N-acetylcysteine conjugates of benzyl and phenethyl isothiocyanates during the postinitiation phase is associated with activation of mitogen-activated protein kinases and p53 activity and induction of apoptosis. Cancer Res. 62, 2–7.

Yang, Q., Chen, Y., Shi, Y., et al., 2003. Association between ozone and respiratory admissions among children and the elderly in Vancouver, Canada. Inhal. Toxicol. 15, 1297–1308.

Yarosh, D.B., Boumakis, S., Brown, A.B., et al., 2002. Measurement of UVB-Induced DNA damage and its consequences in models of immunosuppression. Methods 28, 55–62.

Yashiki, M., Kojima, T., Miyazaki, T., et al., 1990. Gas chromatographic determination of cresols in the biological fluids of a non-fatal case of cresol intoxication. Forensic. Sci. Int. 47, 21–29.

Yatagai, M., Sato, T., Yakahashi, T., 1985. Terpenes of leaf oils from Cupressaceae. Biochem. Syt. Ecol. 13, 377–385.

Yayi, E., Moudachirou, M., Chalchat, J.C., 2001. Chemotyping of three *Ocimum* species from Benin: O. *basilicum*, O. *canum* and O. *gratissimum*. J. Essential Oil Res. 13, 13–17.

Yea, S.S., Jeong, H.S., Choi, C.Y., et al., 2006. Inhibitory effect of anethole on T-lymphocyte proliferation and interleukin-2 production through down-regulation of the NF-AT and AP-1. Toxicol. In Vitro 20, 1098–1105.

Yeruva, L., Pierre, K.J., Carper, S.W., et al., 2006. Jasmonates induce apoptosis and cell cycle arrest in non-small cell lung cancer lines. Exp. Lung Res. 32, 499–516.

Yi, T., Cho, S.G., Yi, Z., et al., 2008. Thymoquinone inhibits tumor angiogenesis and tumor growth through suppressing AKT and extracellular signal-regulated kinase signalling pathways. Mol. Cancer Ther. 7, 1789–1796.

Yip, A.S., Chow, W.H., Tai, Y.T., et al., 1990. Adverse effect of topical methyl salicylate ointment on warfarin anticoagulation: an unrecognized potential hazard. Postgrad. Med. J. 66, 367–369.

Yokley, K.A., Tran, H., Schlosser, P.M., 2008. Sensory irritation response in rats: modeling, analysis and validation. Bull. Math. Biol. 70, 555–588.

Yokota, H., Yuasa, A., 1990. Induction of liver microsomal UDP-glucuronyltransferase in the rat administered with a plant phenol, eugenol. Nihon Juigaku Zasshi 52, 105–111.

Yokota, H., Hoshino, J., Yuasa, A., 1986. Suppressed mutagenicity of benzo[a]pyrene by the liver S9 fraction and microsomes from eugenol-treated rats. Mutat. Res. 172, 231–236.

Yokota, H., Hashimoto, H., Motoya, M., et al., 1988. Enhancement of UDP-glucuronyltransferase, UDP-glucose dehydrogenase, and glutathione S-transferase activities in rat liver by dietary administration of eugenol. Biochem. Pharmacol. 37, 799–802.

Yoo, Y.S., 1986. Mutagenic and antimutagenic activities of flavoring agents used in foodstuffs. J. Osaka Shiritso Daigaku Igaku Zasshi 34, 267–288.

Yoo, C.B., Han, K.T., Cho, K.S., et al., 2005. Eugenol isolated from the essential oil of Eugenia caryophyllata induces a reactive oxygen species-mediated apoptosis in HL-60 human promyelocytic leukemia cells. Cancer Lett. 225, 41–52.

Yoshioka, M., Tamada, T.T., 2005. Aromatic factors of anti-platelet aggregation in fennel oil. Biogenic Amines 19, 89–96.

Yoshida, N., Takagi, A., Kitazawa, H., et al., 2005. Inhibition of P-glycoprotein-mediated transport by extracts of and monoterpenoids contained in Zanthoxyli fructus. Toxicol. Appl. Pharmacol. 209, 167–173.

Yoshida, N., Koizumi, M., Adachi, I., et al., 2006. Inhibition of P-glycoprotein-mediated transport by terpenoids contained in herbal medicines and natural products. Food Chem. Toxicol. 44, 2033–2039.

Yosipovitch, G., Xiong, G.L., Haus, E., et al., 1998. Time-dependent variations of the skin barrier function in humans: transepidermal water loss, stratum corneum hydration, skin surface pH, and skin temperature. J. Invest. Dermatol. 110, 20–23.

You, W.C., Chang, Y.S., Heinrich, J., 2001. An intervention trial to inhibit the progression of precancerous gastric lesions: compliance, serum micronutrients and S-allyl cysteine levels, and toxicity. Eur. J. Cancer Prev. 10, 257–263.

Youdim, K.A., Deans, S.G., 1999. Dietary supplementation of thyme (Thymus vulgaris L.) essential oil during the lifetime of the rat: its effects on the antioxidant status in liver, kidney and heart tissues. Mech. Ageing Dev. 109, 163–175.

Young, A.R., Magnus, I.A., Davies, A.C., et al., 1983. A comparison of the phototumorigenic potential of 8-MOP and 5-MOP in hairless albino mice exposed to solar stimulated radiation. Br. J. Dermatol. 108, 507–518.

Young, A.R., Potten, C.S., Chadwick, C.A., et al., 1988. Inhibition of UV radiation-induced DNA damage by a 5-methoxypsoralen tan in human skin. Pigment Cell Res. 1, 350–354.

Young, A.R., Walker, S.L., Kinley, J.S., et al., 1990. Phototumorigenesis studies of 5-methoxypsoralen in bergamot oil: evaluation and modification of risk of human use in an albino mouse skin model. J. Photochem. Photobiol. 7, 231–250.

Young, A.R., Potten, C.S., Chadwick, C.A., et al., 1991. Photoprotection and 5-MOP photochemoprotection from UVR-induced DNA damage in humans: the role of skin type. J. Invest. Dermatol. 97, 942–948.

Young, D.G., Chao, S., Casabianca, H., et al., 2007. Essential oil of Bursera graveolens (Kunth) Triana et Planch from Ecuador. J. Essential Oil Res. 19, 525–526.

Yourick, J.J., Bronaugh, R.L., 1997. Percutaneous absorption and metabolism of coumarin in human and rat skin. J. Appl. Toxicol. 17, 153–158.

Youssefi, A.A., Arutyunyan, R., Emerit, I., 1994. Chromosome damage in PUVA-treated human lymphocytes is related to active oxygen species and clastogenic factors. Muat. Res. 309, 185–191.

Yu, T.H., Wu, C.M., Liou, Y.C., 1989. Volatile compounds from garlic. J. Agric. Food Chem. 37, 725–730.

Yu, S.G., Hildebrandt, L.A., Elson, C.E., 1995a. Geraniol, an inhibitor of mevalonate biosynthesis, suppresses the growth of hepatomas and melanomas transplanted to rats and mice. J. Nutr. 125, 2763–2767.

Yu, S.G., Anderson, P.J., Elson, C.E., 1995b. Efficacy of β-ionone in the chemoprevention of rat mammary carcinogenesis. J. Agric. Food Chem. 43, 2144–2147.

Yu, J.C., Jiang, Z.T., Li, R., et al., 2003. Chemical composition of the essential oils of Brassica juncea (L.) Coss. grown in different regions, Hebei, Shaanxi and Shandong, of China. J. Food Drug Analysis 11, 22–26.

Yu, S.S., Pai, S., Neuhaus, I.M., et al., 2007. Diagnosis and treatment of pigmentary disorders in Asian skin. Facial Plast. Surg. Clin. North Am. 15, 367–380.

Yu, F.S., Yang, J.S., Yu, C.S., et al., 2011. Safrole induces apoptosis in human oral cancer HSC-3 cells. J. Dent Res. 90, 168–174.

Yu, F.S., Huang, A.C., Yang, J.S., et al., 2012. Safrole induces cell death in human tongue squamous cancer SCC-4 cells through mitochondria-dependent caspase activation cascade apoptotic signaling pathways. Environ. Toxicol. 27, 433–444.

Yuan, J.H., Dieter, M.P., Bucher, J.R., et al., 1992. Toxicokinetics of cinnamaldehyde in F344 rats. Food Chem. Toxicol. 30, 997–1004.

Yuan, J.H., Goehl, T.J., Abdo, K., et al., 1995. Effects of gavage versus dosed feed administration on the toxicokinetics of benzyl acetate in rats and mice. Food Chem. Toxicol. 33, 151–158.

Yuan, J., Gu, Z.L., Chou, W.H., et al., 1999. Elemene induces apoptosis and regulates expression of bcl-2 protein in human leukemia K562 cells. Chung Kuo Yao Li Hsueh Pao 20, 103–106.

Yun, C.H., Lee, H.S., Lee, H.Y., et al., 2003. Roles of human liver cytochrome P450 3A4 and 1A2 enzymes in the oxidation of myristicin. Toxicol. Lett. 137, 143–150.

Yuri, T., Danbara, N., Tsujita-Kyutoku, M., et al., 2004. Perillyl alcohol inhibits human breast cancer cell growth in vitro and in vivo. Breast Cancer Res. Treat. 84, 251–260.

Yusof, W., Gan, S.H., 2009. High prevalence of CYP2A6*4 and CYP2A6*9 alleles detected among a Malaysian population. Clin. Chim. Acta 403, 105–109.

Zaitsev, A.N., Maganova, N.B., 1975. Embryotoxic effects of some aromatizers for food products. Vopr. Pitan. 3, 64–68.

Zaitsev, A.N., Rakhmanina, N.L., 1974. Some data on the toxic properties of derivatives of phenylethanol and cinnamic alcohol. Vopr. Pitan. 5, 48–53.

Zajdela, F., Bisagni, E., 1981. 5-methoxypsoralen, the melanogenic additive in sun-tan preparations, is tumorigenic in mice exposed to 365 nm u.v. radiation. Carcinogenesis 2, 121–127.

Zamith, H.P., Vidal, M.N., Speit, G., et al., 1993. Absence of genotoxic activity of β-myrcene in the in vivo cytogenetic bone marrow assay. Braz. J. Med. Biol. Res. 26, 93–98.

Zanchin, G., Dainese, F., Trucco, M., et al., 2007. Osmophobia in migraine and tension-type headache and its clinical features in patients with migraine. Cephalalgia 27, 1061–1068.

Zangerl, A.R., Green, E.S., Lampmon, R.L., et al., 1997. Phenological chamges in primary and secondary chemistry of reproductive parts of wild parsnip. Phytochemistry 44, 825–831.

Zangouras, A., Caldwell, J., Hutt, J., et al., 1981. Dose-dependent conversion of estragole in the rat and mouse to the carcinogenic metabolite 1′-hydroxyestragole. Biochem. Pharmacol. 30, 1383–1386.

Zani, F., Massimo, G., Benvenuti, S., et al., 1991. Studies on the genotoxic properties of essential oils with Bacillus subtilis rec-assay and Salmonella/microsome reversion assay. Planta Med. 57, 237–241.

Zarghami, N.S., Heinz, D.E., 1971. Volatile constituents of saffron: monoterpene aldehyde and isophorone related compounds of saffron. Phytochemistry 10, 2755–2761.

Zarzuelo, A., Crespo, E., 2002. The medicinal and non-medicinal uses of thyme. In: Stahl-Biskup, E., Sáez, F. (Eds.), Thyme, the genus Thymus. Medicinal & Aromatic Plants - Industrial Profiles. Taylor & Francis, London, pp. 263–292.

Zaynoun, S.T., Johnson, B.E., Frain-Bell, W., 1977a. A study of bergamot and its importance as a phototoxic agent. II. Factors which affect the phototoxic reaction induced by bergamot oil and psoralen derivatives. Contact Dermatitis 3, 225–239.

Zaynoun, S.T., Johnson, B.E., Frain-Bell, W., 1977b. A study of oil of bergamot and its importance as a phototoxic agent. I. Characterisation and quantification of the photoactive component. Br. J. Dermatol 96, 475–482.

Zedlitz, S., Kaufmann, R., Boehncke, W.H., 2002. Allergic contact dermatitis from black cumin (Nigella sativa) oil-containing ointment. Contact Dermatitis 46, 188.

Zeiger, E., Anderson, B., Haworth, S., et al., 1987. Salmonella mutagenicity tests: III. Results from the testing of 255 chemicals. Environ. Mutagen. 9 (Suppl. 9), 1–109.

Zeiger, E., Anderson, B., Haworth, S., et al., 1988. Salmonella mutagenicity tests: IV. Results from the testing of 300 chemicals. Environ. Mol. Mutagen. 12, 1–157.

Zeiger, E., Haseman, J.K., Shelby, M.D., et al., 1990. Evaluation of four in vitro genetic toxicity tests for predicting rodent carcinogenicity: confirmation of earlier results with 41 additional chemicals. Environ. Mol. Mutagen. 16 (Suppl. 18), 1–14.

Zeiger, E., Anderson, B., Haworth, S., et al., 1992. Salmonella mutagenicity tests: V. Results from the testing of 311 chemicals. Environ. Mol. Mutagen. 19 (Suppl. 21), 2–141.

Zelikoff, J.T., Belman, S., 1985. Effect of onion and garlic oil on 3T3 cell transformation. In Vitro 21, 41A.

Zeller, A., Horst, K., Rychlik, M., 2009. Study of the metabolism of etragole in humans consuming fennel tea. Chem. Res. Toxicol. 22, 1929–1937.

Zeng, T., Zhang, C.L., Zhu, Z.P., 2008. Diallyl trisulfide (DATS) effectively attenuated oxidative stress-mediated liver injury and hepatic mitochondrial dysfunction in acute ethanol-exposed mice. Toxicology 252, 86–91.

Zeytinoglu, M., Aydin, S., Öztürk, Y., et al., 1998. Inhibitory effects of carvacrol on DMBA induced pulmonary tumorigenesis in rats. Acta Pharm. Turcica 40, 93–98.

Zeytinoglu, H., Incesu, Z., Baser, K.H., 2003. Inhibition of DNA synthesis by carvacrol in mouse myoblast cells bearing a human N-RAS oncogene. Phytomedicine 10, 292–299.

Zhang, L., Barritt, G.J., 2006. TRPM8 in prostate cancer cells: a potential diagnostic and prognostic marker with a secretory function? Endocr. Relat. Cancer 13, 27–38.

Zhang, S.Y., Robertson, D., 2000. A study of tea tree oil ototoxicity. Audiol. Neurootol. 5, 64–68.

Zhang, Z., Chen, H., Chan, K.K., et al., 1999. Gas chromatographic-mass spectrometric analysis of perillyl alcohol and metabolites in plasma. J. Chromatogr. B 728, 85–95.

Zhang, X.H., Lowe, D., Giles, P., 2001. A randomized trial of the effects of garlic oil upon coronary heart disease risk factors in trained male runners. Blood Coagul. Fibrinolysis 12, 67–74.

Zhang, Y., Jiang, X., Chen, B., 2004. Reproductive and developmental toxicity in F(1) Sprague-Dawley male rats exposed to di-n-butyl phthalate in utero and during lactation and determination of its NOAEL. Reprod. Toxicol. 18, 669–676.

Zhang, Z.M., Yang, X.Y., Deng, S.H., et al., 2007. Anti-tumor effects of polybutylcyanoacrylate nanoparticles of diallyl trisulfide on orthotopic transplantation tumor model of hepatocellular carcinoma in BALB/c nude mice. Chin. Med. J. 120, 1336–1342.

Zhang, Y.K., Zhang, X.H., Li, J.M., et al., 2009. A proteomic study on a human osteosarcoma cell line Saos-2 treated with diallyl trisulfide. Anticancer Drugs 20, 702–712.

Zhao, Q., Bowles, E.J., Zhang, H.Y., 2008. Antioxidant activities of eleven Australian essential oils. Nat. Prod. Commun. 3, 837–842.

Zhao, J., Zhang, J.S., Yang, B., et al., 2010. Free radical scavenging activity and characterization of sesquiterpenoids in four species of Curcuma using a TLC bioautography assay and GC-MS analysis. Molecules 15, 7547–7557.

Zheljazkov, V., Zhalnov, I., 1995. Effect of herbicides on yield and quality of Coriandrum sativum L. J. Essential Oil Res. 7, 633–639.

Zheng, G., Kenney, P.M., Zhang, J., et al., 1992a. Inhibition of benzo[a] pyrene-induced tumorigenesis by myristicin, a volatile aroma constituent of parsley leaf oil. Carcinogenesis 13, 1921–1923.

Zheng, G., Kenney, P.M., Lam, L.K., 1992b. Myristicin: a potential cancer chemoprotective agent from parsley leaf oil. J. Agric. Food Chem. 40, 107–110.

Zheng, G., Kenney, P.M., Lam, L.K., 1992c. Sesquiterpenes from clove (Eugenia caryophyllata) as potential anticarcinogenic agents. J. Nat. Prod. 55, 999–1003.

Zheng, G., Kenney, P.M., Lam, L.K., 1992d. Anethofuran, carvone and limonene: potential cancer chemopreventive agents from dill weed oil and caraway oil. Planta Med. 58, 338–341.

Zheng, G., Kenney, P.M., Lam, L.K., 1993a. Potential anticarcinogenic natural products isolated from lemongrass oil and galanga root oil. J. Agric. Food Chem. 41, 153–156.

Zheng, G., Kenney, P.M., Lam, L.K., 1993b. Chemoprevention of benzo[a] pyrene-induced forestomach cancer in mice by natural phthalides from celery seed oil. Nutr. Cancer 19, 77–86.

Zheng, S., Yang, H., Zhang, S., et al., 1997. Initial study on naturally occurring products from traditional Chinese herbs and vegetables for chemoprevention. J. Cell Biochem. Suppl. 27, 106–112.

Zheng-kui, L., Ying-fang, H., 1986. A study on the volatile flavor constituents of Sichuan preserved vegetable (Brassica juncea Czern. et Coss.) (content % sample B). Acta Botanica Sinica 28, 199–306.

Zhong, Z., Chen, X., Tan, W., et al., 2011. Germacrone inhibits the proliferation of breast cancer cell lines by inducing cell cycle arrest and promoting apoptosis. Eur. J. Pharmacol. 667, 50–55.

Zhong, Z.F., Hoi, P.P., Wu, G.S., et al., 2012. Anti-angiogenic effect of furanodiene on HUVECs in vitro and on zebrafish in vivo. J. Ethnopharmacol. 141, 721–727.

Zhou, J.Y., Tang, F.D., Mao, G.G., et al., 2003. Effect of Eucalyptus globulus oil on activation of nuclear factor-kappaB in THP-1 cells. Zhejiang Da Xue Xue Bao Yi Xue Ban 32, 315–318.

Zhou, H.L., Deng, Y.M., Xie, Q.M., 2006. The modulatory effects of the volatile oil of ginger on the cellular immune response in vitro and in vivo in mice. J. Ethnopharmacol. 105, 301–305.

Zhou, G.D., Moorthy, B., Bi, J., et al., 2007. DNA adducts from alloxyallylbenzene herb and spice constituents in cultured human (HepG2) cells. Environ. Mol. Mutagen. 48, 715–721.

Zhou, L., Zhang, K., Li, J., et al., 2013. Inhibition of vascular endothelial growth factor-mediated angiogenesis involved in reproductive toxicity induced by sesquiterpenoids of Curcuma zedoaria in rats. Reprod. Toxicol. 37, 62–69.

Zhu, L., Li, Y., Li, B., et al., 1993. Aromatic plants and essential constituents. South China Institute of Botany, Hong Kong.

Zhu, L., Ding, D., Lawrence, B.M., 1994. The Cinnamomum species in China: resources for the present and future. Perfumer Flavorist 19, 17–22.

Zhu, L., Li, Y., Li, B., et al., 1995. Aromatic plants and essential constituents (supplement 1). South China Institute of Botany, Hong Kong.

Zhu, H., Rockhold, R.W., Baker, R.C., et al., 2001. Effects of single or repeated dermal exposure to methyl parathion on behavior and blood cholinesterase activity in rats. J. Biomed. Sci. 8, 467–474.

Zibrowski, E.M., Hoh, T.E., Vanderwolf, C.H., 1998. Fast wave activity in the rat rhinencephalon: elicitation by the odors of phytochemicals, organic solvents, and a rodent predator. Brain Res. 800, 207–215.

Ziegler, M., Brandauer, H., Ziegler, E., et al., 1991. A different aging model for orange oil: deterioration products. J. Essential Oil Res. 3, 209–220.

Zimmermann, F.K., Scheel, I., Resnick, M.A., 1989. Induction of chromosome loss by mixtures of organic solvents including neurotoxins. Mutat. Res. 224, 287–303.

Zimmermann, T., Seiberling, M., Thomann, P., et al., 1995. The relative bioavailability and pharmacokinetics of standardized myrtol. Arzneimittelforschung 45, 1198–1201.

Zoghbi M das, G., Andrade, E.H., Oliveira, J., et al., 2006. Yield and chemical composition of the essential oil of the stems and rhizomes of Cyperus articulatus L. cultivated in the State of Pará, Brazil. J. Essential Oil Res. 18, 10–12.

Zolotovich, G., Nachev, C., Siljanovska, K., et al., 1967. Cytotoxic effect of carbonyl compounds isolated from essential oils. C. R. Acad. Bulgare Sci. 20, 1213–1216.

Zolotovich, G., Silyanovska, K., Stoichev, S., et al., 1969. Cytotoxic effect of essential oils and their individual components. II. Oxygen-containing compounds excluding alcohols. Parfümerie und Kosmetik 50, 257.

Zondek, B., Bergmann, E., 1938. Phenol methyl esters as estrogenic agents. Biochem. J. 32, 641–645.

Zou, L., Liu, W., Yu, L., 2001. *Beta*-Elemene induces apoptosis of K562 leukemia cells. Zhonghua Zhong Liu Za Zhi 23, 196–198.

Zou, X., Liu, S.L., Zhou, J.Y., et al., 2012. Beta-asarone induces LoVo colon cancer cell apoptosis by up-regulation of caspases through a mitochondrial pathway in vitro and in vivo. Asian Pac. J. Cancer Prev. 13, 5291–5298.

Zrira, S.S., Benjilali, B.B., 1996. Seasonal changes in the volatile oil and cineole contents of five *Eucalyptus* species growing in Morocco. J. Essential Oil Res. 8, 19–24.

Zrira, S.S., Benjilali, B.B., Fechtal, M.M., et al., 1992. Essential oils of twenty-seven *Eucalyptus* species grown in Morocco. J. Essential Oil Res. 4, 259–264.

Zu, Y., Yu, H., Liang, L., et al., 2010. Activities of ten essential oils towards *Propionibacterium acnes* and PC-3, A-549 and MCF-7 cancer cells. Molecules 15, 3200–3210.

Zwaving, J.H., Bos, R., 1992. Analysis of the essential oils of five Curcuma spp. Flavour Fragrance J. 7, 19–22.

Zwaving, J.H., Bos, R., 1996. Composition of the essential oil from the root of *Sassafras albidum* (Nutt.) Nees. J. Essential Oil Res. 8, 193–195.

Index

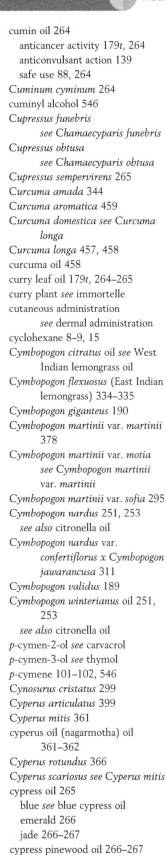